Surgical Critical Care Therapy

Ali Salim • Carlos Brown • Kenji Inaba
Matthew J. Martin
Editors

Surgical Critical Care Therapy

A Clinically Oriented Practical Approach

Springer

Editors
Ali Salim
Brigham and Womens's Hospital
Harvard Medical School
Boston, MA, USA

Carlos Brown
Dell Medical School
University of Texas at Austin
Austin, TX, USA

Kenji Inaba
Division of Trauma Surgery, Rm C5L100
University of Southern California
Los Angeles, CA, USA

Matthew J. Martin
Trauma and Emergency Surgery Service
Legacy Emanuel Medical Center
Portland, OR, USA

ISBN 978-3-030-10099-5 ISBN 978-3-319-71712-8 (eBook)
https://doi.org/10.1007/978-3-319-71712-8

Softcover re-print of the Hardcover 1st edition 2018

Printed on acid-free paper

This Springer imprint is published by the registered company Springer International Publishing AG part of Springer Nature.
The registered company address is: Gewerbestrasse 11, 6330 Cham, Switzerland

Preface

The field of surgical critical care is constantly expanding, evolving, and undergoing rapid change. Providers are experiencing increasing volumes of complex surgical cases and clinically challenging postoperative patients from a wide variety of surgical subspecialties. With the introduction of new technologies, less invasive surgery, balanced resuscitation strategies, and an aging population, updating and communicating improved care techniques for the critically ill surgical patient are crucial. As critical care providers, our goal is to deliver optimal, evidence-based care supported by relevant policies and data; however, there is no comprehensive source that provides concise and practical guidance to surgical intensivists and multidisciplinary ICU team members.

The *Surgical Critical Care Therapy* textbook will provide a comprehensive, state-of-the-art review of the field and will serve as a valuable resource for clinicians, surgeons, and researchers with an interest in surgical critical care. The chapters focus on the management of common problems and critical decision-making scenarios that arise in the Surgical Intensive Care Unit. For example, several well-designed randomized prospective trials have recently altered the way we care for surgical patients presenting with traumatic brain injury, hemorrhagic shock, acute respiratory distress syndrome, and sepsis. The protocols, care bundles, guidelines, and checklists that show improved process measures and patient outcomes will be discussed in detail throughout the book.

We hope that this textbook will help guide patient management and stimulate future investigative efforts. Each chapter is written by widely recognized and established experts in the field who share numerous tips and wisdom gained over the course of their careers. We also believe that this textbook will become an invaluable resource for residents preparing for their in-service exams or the critical care portions of their general surgery board exams and for all fellowship-trained intensivists who are taking the surgical critical care board examinations.

We wish to thank the professional editorial efforts of Springer and to acknowledge our peers and family members for their support throughout this project. Without the help of so many, this project could not have been brought to fruition.

Austin, TX, USA — Carlos Brown
Los Angeles, CA, USA — Kenji Inaba
Tacoma, WA, USA — Matthew J. Martin
Boston, MA, USA — Ali Salim

Contents

Contributors

Craig R. Ainsworth Burn Intensive Care Unit, Burn Center, US Army Institute of Surgical Research, Brooke Army Medical Center, JBSA Fort Sam Houston, TX, USA

Uniformed Services University of the Health Sciences, Bethesda, MD, USA

Hasan B. Alam Department of General Surgery, University of Michigan, Ann Arbor, MI, USA

Deidra Allison Dell Seton Medical Center at University of Texas, Surgical Intensive Care Unit, Austin, TX, USA

Jared L. Antevil Division of Cardiothoracic Surgery, Department of Surgery, Walter Reed National Military Medical Center, Bethesda, MD, USA

Reza Askari Department of Surgery, Brigham and Women's Hospital, Harvard Medical School, Boston, MA, USA

Trauma, Burn, and Surgical Critical Care, Brigham and Women's Hospital, Boston, MA, USA

Jayson Aydelotte Department of Surgery and Perioperative Care, Dell Medical School at the University of Texas-Austin, Austin, TX, USA

Asad Azim Department of Surgery, University of Arizona, Tucson, AZ, USA

Chad G. Ball Department of Surgery, University of Calgary, Foothills Medical Center, Calgary, AB, Canada

Jessica Ballou Oregon Health and Science University, Portland, OR, USA

Brittany K. Bankhead-Kendall Dell Medical School, University of Texas at Austin, Austin, TX, USA

James M. Bardes Division of Trauma, Emergency Surgery and Surgical Critical Care, Los Angeles County and Univeristy of Southern California Medical Center, Los Angeles, CA, USA

Galinos Barmparas Department of Surgery, Division of Acute Care Surgery and Surgical Critical Care, Cedars-Sinai Medical Center, Los Angeles, CA, USA

Brian C. Beldowicz Department of Surgery, Division of Trauma, UC Davis Health, Acute Care Surgery and Surgical Critical Care, Sacramento, CA, USA

Elizabeth Benjamin Division of Trauma, Emergency Surgery and Surgical Critical Care, Los Angeles County and Univeristy of Southern California Medical Center, Los Angeles, CA, USA

Andrew C. Bernard Department of Surgery, University of Kentucky, Lexington, KY, USA

Robel Beyene Division of Trauma and Surgical Critical Care, Vanderbilt University Medical Center, Nashville, TN, USA

Bishwajit Bhattacharya Section of General Surgery, Trauma and Surgical Critical Care, Department of Surgery, Yale School of Medicine, New Haven, CT, USA

Walter L. Biffl Scripps Memorial Hosptial La Jolla, San Diego, CA, USA

David W. Bliss Department of Surgery, Keck School of Medicine of the University of Southern California, Division of Pediatric Surgery, Children's Hospital Los Angeles, Los Angeles, CA, USA

Karen J. Brasel Department of Surgery, Division of Trauma, Critical Care, and Acute Care Surgery, Oregon Health and Science University, Portland, OR, USA

Stacy Brethauer Digestive Disease and Surgery Institute, Cleveland Clinic, Cleveland, OH, USA

Eric Bui Department of Surgery, UCSF East Bay – Highland Hospital, Oakland, CA, USA

Marko Bukur Department of Surgery, Bellevue Hospital Center, New York, NY, USA

Division of Trauma and Surgical Critical Care, New York University School of Medicine, New York, NY, USA

Samuel Cemaj Department of Surgery, University of Nebraska Medical Center, Omaha, NE, USA

Julietta Chang Massachusetts General Hospital, Department of General Surgery, Boston, MA, USA

Aaron M. Cheng University of Washington, Department of Surgery, Division of Cardiothoracic Surgery Co-Director, Cardiothoracic ICU, University of Washington Medical Center Director, Thoracic Surgery, Harborview Medical Center, Seattle, WA, USA

Kevin K. Chung Department of Medicine, Brooke Army Medical Center, JBSA-Fort Sam Houston, TX, USA

Uniformed Services University of the Health Sciences, Bethesda, MD, USA

David J. Ciesla Department of Surgery, University of South Florida College of Medicine, Tampa, FL, USA

Mark Cipolle Department of Surgery – Surgical Critical Care, Christiana Care Health System, Newark, DE, USA

Damon Clark University of Southern California Keck School of Medicine, Keck Hospital, Norris Cancer Hospital and LAC-USC, Department of Surgery, Acute Care Surgery and Surgical Critical Care, Los Angeles, CA, USA

Christine S. Cocanour Department of Surgery, Division of Trauma, UC Davis Health, Sacramento, CA, USA

Ellie Cohen Hennepin County Medical Center in Minneapolis, Minneapolis, MI, USA

Christos Colovos Department of Surgery, Cedars-Sinai Medical Center, Los Angeles, CA, USA

Charles H. Cook Division of Acute Care Surgery, Trauma, Surgical Critical Care, Harvard Medical School, Boston, MA, USA

Zara Cooper Department of Trauma, Burn, and Surgical Critical Care, Brigham and Women's Hospital, Boston, MA, USA

Ben Coopwood Department of Surgery, Dell Medical School, University of Texas at Austin, Austin, TX, USA

Martin A. Croce University of Tennessee Health Science Center, Memphis, TN, USA

Bruce A. Crookes Department of Surgery, General Surgery Division, Medical University of South Carolina, Charleston, SC, USA

Daniel G. Cuadrado General and Thoracic Surgery, Department of Surgery, Madigan Army Medical Center, Tacoma, WA, USA

Mitchell J. Daley Department of Pharmacy, Dell Seton Medical Center at the University of Texas, Austin, TX, USA

Benjamin L. Davis Division of Acute Care Surgery, University of Arkansas for Medical Sciences, Little Rock, AR, USA

Kimberly Davis Section of General Surgery, Trauma and Surgical Critical Care, Department of Surgery, Yale School of Medicine, New Haven, CT, USA

Marc de Moya Division of Trauma, Acute Care Surgery, Medical College of Wisconsin, Froedtert Hospital, Milaukee, WI, USA

Joseph J. DuBose Division of Vascular Surgery, David Grant Medical Center, Travis AFB, CA, USA

Jeremiah J. Duby Department of Pharmacy Services, UC Davis Health, Sacramento, CA, USA

Touro University, College of Pharmacy, Vallejo, CA, USA

UCSF School of Pharmacy, San Francisco, CA, USA

Alexander L. Eastman Department of Surgery, Division of Burns, Trauma, and Critical Care, University of Texas Southwestern, Dallas, TX, USA

Matthew J. Eckert Department of Surgery, Madigan Army Medical Center, Joint Base Lewis-McChord, Tacoma, WA, USA

Alexandra Edwards Department of Surgery, University of Kentucky, Lexington, KY, USA

Margaret K. M. Ellis Department of Anesthesiology and Perioperative Medicine, Oregon Health and Science University, Portland, OR, USA

Charity H. Evans Department of Surgery, University of Nebraska Medical Center, Omaha, NE, USA

Paul M. Evans Division of Acute Care Surgery, Department of Surgery, Grady Memorial Hospital, Atlanta, GA, USA

Peter Fagenholz Division of Trauma/Acute Care Surgery, Massachusetts General Hospital, Harvard Medical School, Boston, MA, USA

Stephen A. Fann Department of Surgery, General Surgery Division, Medical University of South Carolina, Charleston, SC, USA

Dina M. Filiberto University of Tennessee Health Science Center, Memphis, TN, USA

Damon Forbes Pulmonary & Critical Care Service, Womack Army Medical Center, Ft. Bragg, NC, USA

Jamie Golden Department of Surgery, Keck School of Medicine of the University of Southern California, Division of Pediatric Surgery, Children's Hospital Los Angeles, Los Angeles, CA, USA

Eduardo Gonzalez Department of Surgery, University of Colorado, Denver, CO, USA

Daniel Grabo Department of Trauma, Acute Care Surgery and Surgical Critical Care, West Virginia University, Morgantown, WV, USA

Daniel L. Gramins Division of Cardiovascular & Thoracic Surgery, Sulpizio Cardiovascular Center, UC San Diego Health System, La Jolla, CA, USA

Amar Gupta Department of General Surgery, Foothills Medical Center, Calgary, AB, Canada

Adil H. Haider Center for Surgery and Public Health (CSPH), Brigham and Women's Hospital, Boston, MA, USA

David A. Hampton R Adams Cowley Shock Trauma Center, University of Maryland Medical Center, Baltimore, MD, USA

Wendy F. Hansen Department of Obstetrics and Gynecology, University of Kentucky College of Medicine, Lexington, KY, USA

Alyssa Fitzpatrick Harlow Center for Surgery and Public Health (CSPH), Brigham and Women's Hospital, Boston, MA, USA

Elliott R. Haut Department of Surgery, Anesthesiology/Critical Care Medicine (ACCM), and Emergency Medicine, Johns Hopkins University School of Medicine, Baltimore, MD, USA

Johns Hopkins University Bloomberg School of Public Health, Baltimore, MD, USA

Thomas J. Herron Department of Surgery, University of South Florida College of Medicine, Tampa, FL, USA

Michael Hernon Department of Surgery, Boston University School of Medicine, Boston Medical Center, Boston, MA, USA

Sameer A. Hirji Department of Surgery, Brigham and Women's Hospital, Harvard Medical School, Boston, MA, USA

Athena Hobbs Department of Clinical Pharmacy, Baptist Memorial Health Care & The University of Tennessee Health Science Center – Memphis, Memphis, TN, USA

Emily K. Hodge Department of Pharmacy, Dell Seton Medical Center at the University of Texas, Austin, TX, USA

John B. Holcomb Department of Surgery, McGovern Medical School, University of Texas Health Science Center at Houston (UTHealth), Houston, TX, USA

Cindy H. Hsu Department of Emergency Medicine and Surgery, University of Michigan, Ann Arbor, MI, USA

Aaron R. Jensen Department of Surgery, Keck School of Medicine of the University of Southern California, Division of Pediatric Surgery, Children's Hospital Los Angeles, Los Angeles, CA, USA

Christian Jones Department of Surgery, Johns Hopkins University School of Medicine, Baltimore, MD, USA

Bellal Joseph Department of Surgery, University of Arizona, Tucson, AZ, USA

Gregory J. Jurkovich Department of Surgery, Division of Trauma, UC Davis Health, Acute Care Surgery and Surgical Critical Care, Sacramento, CA, USA

Kyle J. Kalkwarf Department of Surgery, McGovern Medical School, University of Texas Health Science Center at Houston (UTHealth), Houston, TX, USA

George Kasotakis Department of Surgery, Boston University School of Medicine, Boston Medical Center, Boston, MA, USA

Andrew S. Kaufman General Surgery Resident, Department of Surgery, Walter Reed National Military Medical Center, Bethesda, MD, USA

Edward Kelly Harvard Medical School, Division of Trauma, Burns, and Surgical Critical Care, Department of Surgery, Brigham and Women's Hospital, Boston, MA, USA

Uzer Khan Department of Surgery, Division of Trauma, Acute Care and Critical Care, Ruby Memorial Hospital, WVU Medicine, Morgantown, WV, USA

Andrew W. Kirkpatrick Regional Trauma Services, Departments of Surgery, Critical Care Medicine, University of Calgary, Calgary, AB, Canada

Lisa M. Kodadek Department of Surgery, Johns Hopkins University School of Medicine, Baltimore, MD, USA

John Kuckelman Department of Surgery, Madigan Army Medical Center, Joint Base Lewis-McChord, Tacoma, WA, USA

Eric J. Ley Department of Surgery, Cedars-Sinai Medical Center, Los Angeles, CA, USA

George Paul Liao Department of Surgery, Division of Acute Care Surgery and Surgical Critical Care, Cedars-Sinai Medical Center, Los Angeles, CA, USA

Tarek Madni Department of Surgery, Division of Burns, Trauma, and Critical care, University of Texas Southwestern, Dallas, TX, USA

Darren J. Malinoski Department of Surgery, Oregon Health & Science University, Portland, OR, USA

Daniel Margulies Section of Trauma, Emergency Surgery & Surgical Intensive Care and Professor of Surgery, Cedars-Sinai Medical Center, Los Angeles, CA, USA

University of California at Los Angeles David Geffen School of Medicine, Los Angeles, CA, USA

Matthew J. Martin Trauma and Emergency Surgery Service, Legacy Emanuel Medical Center, Portland, OR, USA

Robert G. Martindale Department of Surgery, Oregon Health & Science University, Portland, OR, USA

Maher M. Matar Department of Surgery, Division of General Surgery, The Ottawa Hospital, Ottawa, Ontario, Canada

Paul B. McBeth Departments of Surgery and Critical Care Medicine, Foothills Medical Centre, Calgary, AB, Canada

Nicolas Melo Department of Surgery, Division of Acute Care Surgery, Cedars-Sinai Medical Center, Los Angeles, CA, USA

Maureen Mercante Department of Surgery – Surgical Critical Care, Christiana Care Health System, Newark, DE, USA

Ernest E. Moore Department of Surgery, University of Colorado Denver, Denver, CO, USA

Department of Surgery, Denver Health, Denver, CO, USA

Hunter B. Moore Department of Surgery, University of Colorado, Denver, CO, USA

Filip Moshkovsky Department of Surgery – Surgical Critical Care, Christiana Care Health System, Newark, DE, USA

Philip S. Mullenix Division of Cardiothoracic Surgery, Department of Surgery, Walter Reed National Military Medical Center, Bethesda, MD, USA

Stephanie Nitzschke Department of Trauma, Burn, Surgical Critical Care & Emergency General Surgery, Brigham and Women's Hospital, Boston, MA, USA

Kathleen O'Connell Department of Surgery, University of Washington, Seattle, WA, USA

E. Charles Osterberg University of Texas – Dell Medical School, Austin, TX, USA

Douglas R. Oyler Department of Pharmacy, University of Kentucky Chandler Medical Center, Lexington, KY, USA

Erin Palm Los Angeles County, University of Southern California Medical Center, Los Angeles, CA, USA

Caroline Park Department of Acute Care Surgery, LAC-USC Medical Center, Los Angeles, CA, USA

Charles S. Parsons Department of Surgery, Beth Israel Deaconess Medical Center, Harvard Medical School, Boston, MA, USA

Dave D. Paskar Divisions of General Surgery Trauma & Critical Care Medicine, University of Toronto, Toronto, ON, Canada

Danielle Pigneri Department of Surgery, Division of Trauma, UC Davis Health, Sacramento, CA, USA

Priya S. Prakash Department of Surgery, Division of Trauma and Acute Care Surgery, Pritzker School of Medicine, University of Chicago, Chicago, IL, USA

R. Lawrence Reed II Revenue Cycle Services, IU Health, Department of Surgery, IU Health Methodist Hospital, Indianapolis, IN, USA

Trista D. Reid Division of General and Acute Care Surgery, UNC Department of Surgery, University of North Carolina at Chapel Hill, Chapel Hill, NC, USA

Patrick M. Reilly Department of Surgery, Division of Trauma, Surgical Critical Care, and Emergency Surgery, Perelman School of Medicine, University of Pennsylvania, Philadelphia, PA, USA

Peter Rhee Division of Acute Care Surgery, Department of Surgery, Grady Memorial Hospital, Atlanta, GA, USA

Sandro B. Rizoli Department of Trauma & Acute Care Surgery, St. Michael's Hospital, University of Toronto, Toronto, ON, Canada

Dusten T. Rose Department of Pharmacy, Dell Seton Medical Center at the University of Texas, Austin, TX, USA

Evan Ross Department of Surgery, The University of Texas Medical Branch, Galveston, TX, USA

Javid Sadjadi Department of Surgery, University of California San Francisco East Bay, Oakland, CA, USA

Joseph V. Sakran Division of Acute Care Surgery, Emergency General Surgery, The Johns Hopkins University, Baltimore, MD, USA

Ali Salim Division of Trauma, Burn, Surgical Critical Care and Emergency General Surgery, Brigham and Women's Hospital, Harvard Medical School, Boston, MA, USA

Mitchell B. Sally Department of Surgery, Oregon Health & Science University, Portland, OR, USA

Pablo G. Sanchez University of Pittsburgh, Department of Cardiothoracic Surgery, Division of Lung Transplant and Lung Failure, University of Pittsburgh Medical Center, Associate Director of Lung Transplant and ECLS, Pittsburgh, PA, USA

Jack Sava Department of Trauma, MedStar Washington Hospital Center, Washington, DC, USA

Martin A. Schreiber Division of Trauma, Surgical Critical Care, and Acute Care Surgery, Oregon Health and Science University, Portland, OR, USA

Anupamaa Seshadri Department of Surgery, Brigham and Women's Hospital, Boston, MA, USA

David A. Spain Department of Surgery, Stanford University, Stanford, CA, USA

Nicole A. Stassen Department of Surgery, Acute Care Surgery Division, University of Rochester Medical Center, Rochester, NY, USA

Deborah M. Stein R Adams Cowley Shock Trauma Center, University of Maryland Medical Center, Baltimore, MD, USA

Ian J. Stewart Combat Casualty Care Research, Clinical Investigation Facility, David Grant USAF Medical Center, Travis AFB, CA, USA

Aaron Strumwasser Los Angeles County, University of Southern California Medical Center, Los Angeles, CA, USA

Sharven Taghavi Department of Surgery, Brigham and Women's Hospital, Harvard Medical School, Boston, MA, USA

James M. Tatum Department of Surgery, Cedars-Sinai Medical Center, Los Angeles, CA, USA

Pedro G. R. Teixeira Department of Surgery and Perioperative Care, University of Texas at Austin, Dell Medical School, Austin, TX, USA

Marc D. Trust Department of Surgery and Perioperative Care, University of Texas at Austin, Dell Medical School, Austin, TX, USA

Jeffrey S. Upperman Department of Surgery, Keck School of Medicine of the University of Southern California, Division of Pediatric Surgery, Children's Hospital Los Angeles, Los Angeles, CA, USA

Tarsicio Uribe-Leitz Center for Surgery and Public Health (CSPH), Brigham and Women's Hospital, Boston, MA, USA

Gary Vercruysse Director of Emergency General Surgery, University of Michigan, Ann Arbor, MI, USA

Gregory P. Victorino Department of Surgery, University of California San Francisco East Bay, Oakland, CA, USA

Elizabeth Warnack Department of Surgery, Bellevue Hospital Center, New York, NY, USA

Division of Trauma and Surgical Critical Care, New York University School of Medicine, New York, NY, USA

Alison Wilson WVU Critical Care and Trauma Institute, Department of Surgery, Ruby Memorial Hospital, WVU Medicine, Morgantown, WV, USA

Franz S. Yanagawa Department of Surgery, Johns Hopkins University School of Medicine, Baltimore, MD, USA

Daniel Dante Yeh Department of Surgery, Ryder Trauma Center, Miami, FL, USA

Traumatic Brain Injury

1

Asad Azim and Bellal Joseph

Introduction

Traumatic brain injury (TBI) is a non-degenerative, non-congenital disruption of brain function from an external force that leads to a permanent or a temporary impairment of cognitive and/or physical functions—it may or may not be associated with a diminished or altered state of consciousness. The external forces that create the injury may be the result of a variety of insults, including acceleration or deceleration, compression, penetrating objects, and complex mechanisms like blast injuries. TBI is the leading cause of death and disability among trauma patients. According to an estimate, about 2.5 million TBIs occur every year. Of those, about 50,000 people die, and approximately 80,000–90,000 survivors suffer severe lifelong neurological disabilities [1]. The external cause of injury ("mechanism of injury") associated with TBI varies with age and demographics. Males aged 0–4 have the highest rates of TBI-related visits, whereas adults aged 75 years and older have the highest rate of TBI-related hospitalizations and deaths (1). Falls are the leading mechanism of injury of TBI, accounting for 40% of all TBI-related emergency department (ED) visits (2). They cause more than half (55%) of all TBIs among children aged 0–14 years and 81% of all TBIs among adults aged 65 years and older. The second leading mechanism of injury is unintentional blunt trauma, accounting for 15% of all TBI-related ED visits (1). Motor vehicle collisions and assaults are the third and fourth leading mechanisms of injury, accounting for 14% and 10% of TBI-related ED visits, respectively [2].

A. Azim (✉) · B. Joseph
Department of Surgery, University of Arizona, Tucson, AZ, USA
e-mail: asadazim@surgery.arizona.edu

Types of Primary Injuries

Various types of primary TBI are summarized below.

- *Subdural Hematoma (SDH)*: SDH is the most common type of traumatic brain lesion and occurs in about 20–40% of severely head-injured patients. SDH originates in the space between the dura and the arachnoid matter of the meninges [3]. It results from damage and tearing of cortical bridging veins, which drain the cerebral cortical surface into the dural venous sinuses. The presentation can be acute, subacute, or chronic. Patients have variable loss of consciousness (LOC). On CT imaging, SDH appears to be crescent-shaped. It tends to be associated with underlying cerebral injury and thus usually has a poor prognosis [4].
- *Epidural Hematoma (EDH)*: EDH is a form of intracranial bleed between the dura mater and the inner table of the skull. It results from tearing of arterial dural vessels, i.e., middle meningeal artery. The most common site is temporal, where the bone is very thin and susceptible to fracture. On CT imaging, EDH appears to be lenticular-shaped. EDH is usually due to skull injury rather than brain injury, although brain injury certainly can occur with them. Morbidity and mortality associated with EDH is primarily due to the mass effect from the hematoma, which, if left unchecked, can lead to brain herniation [5].
- *Subarachnoid Hemorrhage (SAH)*: SAH results from disruption of small pial vessels between the subarachnoid and the pia mater of the meninges. Trauma is the most common cause of SAH. Patients with traumatic SAH have 70% higher risk of developing cerebral contusion and 40% higher risk of developing subdural hematoma [6]. SAH is a marker of the severity of TBI. The positive predictive value of SAH (>1 cm) for poor outcome is 72–80%. On CT imaging, SAH appears as hyper-attenuating material filling the subarachnoid space [7].
- *Intraparenchymal Hemorrhage (IPH)*: This is a form of intracerebral bleed in which there is bleeding within the brain parenchyma. IPH, along with cerebral edema, may

A. Salim et al. (eds.), *Surgical Critical Care Therapy*, https://doi.org/10.1007/978-3-319-71712-8_1

disrupt and compress adjacent brain tissue, constituting an immediate medical emergency. On CT imaging, IPH appears as the accumulation of blood within different intracranial spaces, most commonly as a lobar hemorrhage [8].

- *Intraventricular Hemorrhage (IVH)*: IVH refers to bleeding into the ventricular system of the brain, where cerebrospinal fluid is produced and circulates toward the subarachnoid space. It commonly results from an intracerebral hemorrhage with ventricular reflex. On CT imaging, blood appears as hyper-dense material in the ventricles that is best seen in the occipital horns. Blood in ventricular system also predisposes these patients to post-traumatic hydrocephalus. IVH is also a marker of severity of injury and is associated with adverse outcomes [9].
- *Cerebral Contusion*: Contusion is bruising of brain tissue often caused by a blow to the head. When this happens, the blood-brain barrier loses its integrity, thereby creating a heterogeneous region. This type of lesion usually occurs in coup or contrecoup injuries. It manifests in cortical tissue and can be associated with multiple microhemorrhages and small vessels that leak into brain tissue. The most common regions of the brain affected are the frontal and anterior temporal lobes. Cerebral contusions often take 12–24 h to evolve and may be absent on an initial head CT scan [10].
- *Cerebral Concussion*: This is the most common type of TBI. It occurs with a head injury caused by acceleration/deceleration forces or contact forces. It can result in rapid-onset, short-lived impairment of neurological function that resolves spontaneously. Concussions are a clinical diagnosis as there are no CT scan findings associated with it. The key signs and symptoms of a concussion are confusion and amnesia [11].
- *Diffuse Axonal Injury (DAI)*: A DAI is the most common and devastating type of TBI, resulting from extensive damage to white matter tracts over a widespread area. This injury develops from traumatic shearing forces that occur when the head is rapidly accelerated or decelerated. DAI is commonly seen in motor vehicle collisions and shaken baby syndrome. The sites frequently involved in DAI are the frontal and the temporal lobes. CT imaging usually appears normal. Newer imaging modalities, such as diffusion tensor imaging, are more sensitive than a standard MRI for detecting a white matter tract injury [12].

Secondary Brain Injury

Secondary brain injury is a consequence of pathological processes set in motion at the time of primary insult. Mechanism behind secondary brain injury is complex. It is purposed that it is due to the liberation of proinflammatory cytokines and chemicals as result of primary injury that leads to cerebral edema neuronal death and disruption of the blood-brain barrier [13]. The common pathways that contribute to this damage are the liberation of excitatory amino acids, platelet-activating factors, and oxygen free radicals and ubiquitous nitric oxide radicals [14]. While little can be done to limit primary injury, the main goals of current TBI management strategies are targeted at limiting secondary brain injury. With recent advances and better understanding of cellular and biochemical functions, it has become more clear that inadequate blood flow and substrate delivery result in exacerbation of secondary injury [15]. Hence, ensuring adequate nutritional supply and avoiding hypoxia and hypotension can help limit secondary brain injury and enhance neuronal recovery [16].

Emergency Management

History and Physical Examination

A history and physical examination should be obtained, including the events preceding a trauma, a description of the actual event, and complete description of the patient's neurological status. History of medications as well as medications given in the prehospital setting should be determined. Special attention should be paid to medications with the ability to alter the neurological examination, including sedatives or psychopharmacologics, paralytics, atropine (for cardiac resuscitation), and other mydriatics (for evaluation of ocular trauma). Primary and secondary surveys should be performed thoroughly evaluating for systemic injuries. Open lacerations and a vigorous scalp hemorrhage may lead to hypovolemia.

Neurological Assessment

An accurate neurological examination is necessary in order to make a correct diagnosis as well as to plan appropriate treatment strategies. The exam may be limited or altered by age, language, sedative or paralytic medication, alcohol intoxication, or illicit drug abuse. It is crucial to monitor trends that appear in neurological examinations overtime because they fluctuate based on the patient's improving or declining condition. The accuracy and completeness of a neurological exam is based on the alertness and cooperativeness of the patient. The extent of the examination must be tailored to each patient's neurological ability.

- *Pupillary Response*: Documenting pupillary abnormality is important, and it has a high diagnostic and prognostic utility [17]. Pupillary asymmetry is defined as a difference of >1 mm between the pupils. A dilated pupil is defined as a diameter of a pupil >4 mm. A fixed pupil shows no response to bright light. Orbital trauma, hypotension, and hypoxia are common causes of pupillary dilation. Hypoxia and hypotension should be corrected before herniation can be excluded as a cause of pupillary dilation. Orbital trauma can be ruled out by using direct and consensual response for each pupil.

- *Glasgow Coma Scale (GCS)*: An important component of a primary survey is to obtain an accurate GCS. It has become the standard for the objective measurement of the severity of a TBI. A GCS assesses a patient's neurological status based on three components: motor function, verbalization, and eye opening (Table 1.1). A patient who is neurologically intact can receive a maximum score of 15, and the most severely injured patient can get a minimum score of 3. If the patient is intubated, the verbal component is given a score of "q," and the overall score is annotated with a "T." A GCS 13–15 defines a mild TBI—such patients are usually awake and have no focal deficits. A GCS 9–12 is considered a moderate TBI, in which patients have altered sensorium and focal neurological deficits. Patients with a GCS 3–8 have a severe TBI. Usually, they will not follow commands, and they fit the criteria of comatose state [17].

Airway, Breathing, and Circulation

Clinicians should adhere to the basic principles of trauma resuscitation, including rapid assessment and maintenance of an airway, breathing, and circulation [18]. The maintenance of an unobstructed and clear airway is of the utmost importance as hypoxia is the most critical factor leading to adverse outcomes in TBI patients. A multicenter trial has shown that mortality rises by 17% in patients that experience hypoxic episodes following a TBI [19]. Regarding patients with a GCS <9, guidelines recommend that skilled personnel should intubate them by rapid sequence induction. During intubation, the cervical spine should be considered injured until proven otherwise, and it must be protected.

Once the airway is secured, the patient must be ventilated appropriately to maintain normocarbia ($PaCO_2$ 35–40 mmHg). Monitoring of oxygen saturation and capnography is recommended in severely injured patients to avoid unrecognized hypoxemia or changes in ventilation. A study of 11,000 TBI patients showed that both hypo- and hypercarbia were associated with increased mortality in TBI patients [20]. In patients with signs of brain herniation, transient hyperventilation may be an option.

Hypotension is a major secondary brain insult. Studies have shown that even a single episode of hypotension is associated with a dramatic increase in mortality in TBI patients [21]. It should be treated with appropriate fluid resuscitation and blood products to achieve euvolemia. Recent studies have shown that maintaining systolic blood pressure above 100 mmHg is associated with decreased mortality and better neurological outcomes in TBI patients [22].

Table 1.1 Glasgow Coma Scale

Score	Motor	Verbal	Eye opening
6	Obeys command	–	–
5	Localizes to pain	Oriented	–
4	Withdraws to pain	Confused	Spontaneously
3	Flexes arm	Words/phrases	To voice
2	Extends arm	Makes sounds	To pain
1	No response	No response	Remain closed

Radiological Assessment

Computed Axial Tomography (CT) Scan CT scan remains the investigation of choice for patients presenting with head trauma. In a single, rapid pass, without patient repositioning, scans of the head, neck, chest, abdomen, and pelvis can be performed. Additionally, administration of contrast also allows for a CT angiogram reconstruction in order to evaluate vasculature of the head and neck. CT scan findings after trauma include SDH, EDH, SAH, IPH, IVH, contusions, hydrocephalus, cerebral edema or anoxia, skull fractures, ischemic/infarction (if >12 h old), and mass effect resulting in midline shift. Indications for an initial post-traumatic head CT scan include GCS ≤14, unresponsiveness, focal deficit, amnesia for the injury, altered mental status, and signs of basilar skull fracture [23].

Magnetic Resonance Imaging (MRI) MRI scans have better parenchymal resolution and can evaluate infarction, ischemia, edema, and DAI. An MRI is also helpful to determine a ligamentous injury of the spine or a traumatic cord injury. It is generally performed after the initial trauma evaluation and resuscitation have been completed. MRIs have limited availability, slower image acquisition time, image interference by monitoring devices, and a greater cost. Although their use in the initial assessment of trauma is not routinely recommended because intracranial surgical lesions seen on an MRI can also be identified on a CT scan [24], their use in the ICU setting can play a crucial role in evaluating DAI.

Intensive Care Unit Management

Monitoring

Blood Pressure Systolic blood pressure (SBP) plays a critical role in a secondary brain injury cascade after a severe TBI. TBI patients admitted with a systolic blood pressure of less than 85 mmHg have mortality rates as high as 35%, compared to only 6% in patients with a higher SBP [19]. Autoregulatory vasodilation plays a critical role in maintaining cerebral perfusion. After disruption of cerebral autoregulation, which is a common event following severe TBI, cerebral perfusion relies on SBP. Hence, a low SBP leads to cerebral ischemia, which is recognized as the single most important secondary insult. In order to decrease mortality and improve clinical outcomes following a TBI, SBP should be maintained at ≥100 mmHg for patients 50–69 years old or at ≥110 mmHg for patients 15–49 years old or over 70 years old (5).

Intracranial Pressure (ICP) The concept of intracranial pressure is based on the Monro-Kellie hypothesis. Assuming that the skull is a closed space, the hypothesis states that there is a balance between brain, blood volume, and CSF. Increase in the volume of one constituent (e.g., cerebral edema) or an addition of a constituent (i.e., hemorrhage or tumor) mandates a compensatory decrease in other constituents in order to maintain ICP. The management of raised ICP varies greatly in clinical practice, and there are inconsistent reports about the utility of ICP monitoring on clinical outcomes and survival of TBI patients. According to the recently updated Brain Trauma Foundation (BTF 4th Edition 2016) guidelines, ICP monitoring should be performed in all salvageable patients with severe TBI (GCS 3–8) and an abnormal head CT, a normal head CT scan with a SBP of ≤90 mmHg, posturing, or age ≥40 years [25]. Studies have shown that treating ICP above 22 mmHg is recommended to reduce overall mortality [26]. Moreover, management of severe TBI using information from ICP monitoring is associated with reduced in-hospital and 2-week post-injury mortality. A vast majority of patients with severe TBI meet the criteria for ICP monitoring based on these guidelines. However, only a small subset of these patients receives ICP monitoring based on institutional guidelines. A prospective multicenter controlled trial performed in Ecuador demonstrated that there is no difference in clinical outcomes in patients who underwent ICP monitoring compared to those who were managed with an established protocol of neuroimaging and clinical examination [27]. Medical management remains the standard of care for elevated ICP, with a possible role for ICP monitoring and operative intervention in a subset of patients. However, further studies are required to better define subset of patients requiring ICP monitoring.

Cerebral Perfusion Pressure Monitoring (CPP) A traumatically injured brain is at a high risk of a local cerebral ischemia around the area of primary insult as well as global ischemia due to loss of cerebral circulation. In such a situation, maintaining adequate cerebral perfusion is of prime importance. CPP is defined as the pressure gradient across the cerebral vascular bed between blood inflow and outflow. It is calculated as the difference between mean arterial pressure (MAP) and ICP. Studies have shown that a CPP of less than 50 mmHg is associated with a high risk of cerebral ischemia and secondary brain injury. The BTF guidelines recommend a target CPP value between 60 and 70 mmHg for improved survival and favorable outcomes [25]. TBI management includes CPP monitoring in the "bundle" of care; however, the impact of CPP-based management of TBI patients remains unclear. There is some evidence which suggests that the management of TBI patients' using information from CPP monitoring is associated with 2-week post-injury mortality.

Treatment

Hyperosmolar Therapy

An injured brain is highly susceptible to secondary ischemia from either systemic hypotension or diminished cerebral perfusion (attributable to intracranial hypertension, cerebral edema, and inflammation). The objective of hemodynamic therapy in TBI is to ensure adequate brain perfusion and to keep intracranial pressure within normal limits. There are various methods for controlling ICP; however, one of the key pharmacological interventions is hyperosmolar therapy [24–29]. Such therapies reduce ICP by two distinct methods. One commonly accepted mechanism is via establishment of an osmolar gradient across the blood-brain barrier, with the gradient favoring the flow into the circulation. Another mechanism, which explains the rather more rapid action of osmolar agents, is improvement in the rheology of the blood due to plasma expansion as well as decreased hematocrit, which leads to decreased viscosity and more efficient cerebral blood flow (CBF). It is believed that the two most commonly utilized hyperosmolar agents, that is, hypertonic saline and mannitol, utilize both mechanisms [29].

- *Mannitol*: Mannitol is a naturally occurring sugar alcohol used clinically for its osmotic diuretic properties. It has been accepted as an effective tool for reducing intracranial pressure. Although there has never been a randomized comparison of mannitol with a placebo, both the BTF and the European Brain Injury Consortium identify level II and III evidence to support its use for the treatment of intracranial hypertension after a TBI. Mannitol can be administered as a bolus in response to raised ICP or as a continuous drip in a prophylactic fashion [29]. Studies have shown that bolus infusion is superior to continuous therapy; however, a difference of opinion still exists concerning the two modes of administration. Although mannitol plays a vital role in controlling ICP in severe TBI patients, its eventual diuretic effect is undesirable in hypotensive patients, and appropriate monitoring and aggressive fluid resuscitation are required to replenish fluid loss and to maintain SBP within target limits. Clinicians should be cautious, however, because mannitol therapy can accumulate in extracellular space if the infusion rates are higher than the excretion of the drug. This leads to a phenomenon known as the "rebound effect" movement of water back into the brain.

- *Hypertonic Saline*: While hyperosmolar therapy has been utilized to reduce elevated intracranial pressure and edema in TBIs for nearly five decades, the use of hypertonic saline (HTS) as a hyperosmolar agent has only recently become a popular choice for both resuscitation and maintenance therapy in TBI patients. Physiologically, the sodium content is what determines the amount of volume increased intravascularly during initial resuscitation. HTS was initially used as a volume expander in the resuscitation of patients with hemorrhagic shock on the battlefield as a low-volume resuscitation fluid. It was observed that in patients with hemorrhagic shock and TBI, resuscitation with HTS was associated with better survival [30]. In patients with severe TBI and increased ICP or brain edema, a serum sodium level Na + up to 150–155 mEq/L may be acceptable [31]. At our institution, the serum Na + should be maintained below 158 mEq/L. Further studies on animal and humans revealed that this decrease in mortality is attributed to a reduction in ICP and cerebral edema, which was due to hyperosmolar effects of HTS. There is no consensus about the exact makeup of HTS. Concentrations of 3%, 5%, 7.2%, 10%, and 23.4% have all been referred to in the literature. The most commonly used concentration of HTS is 3%, though, recently, 5% saline has become more prevalent. In comparison with 3% HTS, studies have demonstrated that 5% HTS has a sustained higher serum osmolarity and serum sodium concentration within the first 72 h, without any increase in adverse effects [32]. Over time, HTS evolved as an alternative to mannitol in treating cerebral edema and raised ICP following a TBI. HTS has been shown to have more profound and sustained effects on ICP, immune modulation, neurological recovery, and survival. Moreover, known adverse effects of mannitol, like renal injury, worsening of heart failure, and osmotic diuresis, make HTS a better contender for hyperosmolar therapy for the management of TBI. Although there is not enough evidence to support its definitive superiority over mannitol, HTS has clear logistical advantages over mannitol in the treatment of TBI.

Decompressive Craniectomy (DC) Cerebral edema can result from a combination of several pathophysiological mechanisms associated with primary and secondary injury following a TBI. As the skull is a closed cavity, increase in intracranial contents (i.e., cerebral edema) results in brain tissue displacement causing cerebral herniation ultimately leading to severe disability or death. DC is defined as the surgical removal of a portion of the skull and the opening of the underlying dura for the purpose of relieving elevated ICP. A lot of controversy exists regarding the role of DC in the management of severe TBI due to variation in surgical techniques, timing, and the patient population in the recent literature published in the last decade. According to current BTF guidelines, bifrontal DC is not recommended to improve outcomes as measured by the Glasgow Coma Outcome Scale-Extended (GOS-E) score at 6 months post-injury. However, a large frontotemporoparietal DC (not less than 12 × 15 or 15 cm diameter) is recommended to reduce mortality and improve neurological outcomes in patients with a severe TBI with a diffuse injury and ICP values >20 mmHg refractory to medical treatment [25]. A recent randomized controlled trial of DC for refractory traumatic intracranial hypertension (RESCUEicp Trial) [33] has shown that it is associated with lower mortality but higher rates of a vegetative state at 6 months. In contrast to a DC as a last-tier therapy, an early DC as a primary treatment has the advantage of rapid ICP control of elevated ICP; there is, however, increased risk of a number of potential complications that include infections, subdural hygromas, hydrocephalus, syndrome of trephined, and cerebral infarction [34].

Prophylactic Hypothermia Suspended animation, the ability to put a person's biological processes on hold, has long been a staple of science fiction. Interest in the field blossomed in the 1950s as a direct consequence of the space race. However, most of the studies to date have utilized whole-body cooling, and this technique is associated with an increased risk of adverse effects, including coagulopathy, hypotension, and infections in patients [35]. In order to minimize such effects and gain maximum benefits of therapeutic hypothermia, a novel method of selective brain cooling (SBC) has been devised. It uses bilateral common carotid artery (CCA) cooling cuffs that can achieve rapid reductions in core brain temperature without significant changes in normal body temperature [36]. Potential neuroprotective effects of SBC are mediated by reducing the hemoglobin accumulation, inhibition of injury-mediated upregulation of HO-1, which, in turn, ameliorates brain edema. Compared to standard therapy, a recent international, multi-institutional, randomized controlled trial (Eurotherm 3235) that examined the effects of titrated therapeutic hypothermia (32–35°C) as a treatment for raised ICP demonstrated worse outcomes with lower Glasgow Outcome Scale-Extended (GOS-E) scores among patients with therapeutic brain cooling. These findings in the interim analysis were considered harmful, and the trial was stopped in 2014 [37]. Another multi-institutional trial to access the utility of therapeutic hypothermia for 48–72 h with slow rewarming after severe TBI in children was conducted. It was also terminated early due to ineffectiveness of the therapy as compared to a standard treatment [38]. Therefore, in keeping with the results of these randomized trials, the previously ascertained therapeutic benefit of hypothermia on mortality and neurological outcome in TBI patients is minimal, and recommendations for its use cannot be made.

Ventilation Therapy Severe TBI patients require airway protection because they are at increased risk of aspiration or compromised respiratory drive. In addition to normal ventilation, which is currently the goal for severe TBI patients, sometimes these patients may require transient hyperventilation to treat intracranial hypertension and cerebral herniation. Under normal circumstances, $PaCO_2$ is a strong determinant of CBF, and a range between 20 and 80 mmHg CBF is linearly responsive to $PaCO_2$. Low $PaCO_2$ therefore causes a decrease in CBF by cerebrovascular constriction, while a high $PaCO_2$ increases CBF via cerebrovascular dilation. Older studies suggested that cerebral hyperemia is more common than cerebral ischemia; hence they recommended hyperventilation as a management therapy for TBI patients. However, this has been falsified by recent studies demonstrating cerebral ischemia as a major culprit, thereby changing the long-standing recommendations concerning ventilation therapy. Current guidelines state that prolonged prophylactic hyperventilation with partial pressure of carbon dioxide in arterial blood ($PaCO_2$) of 25 mmHg or less is not recommended. Hyperventilation can be used as a temporizing measure to reduce elevated ICP; however, it should be avoided during first 24 h post-injury when CBF is typically reduced. The optimal timing for tracheostomy has been controversial. A common perception is that early tracheostomy may reduce the necessity for mechanical ventilation. In a prospective randomized clinical trial of trauma patient, early tracheostomy (within 7 days) was associated with reduction in duration of mechanical ventilation. In addition, reduction in hospital and ICU length of stay was also observed in the early tracheostomy group [39]. According to Eastern Association for the Surgery of Trauma (EAST), early tracheostomy (within 3–7 days of TBI) should be performed as it decreases the total days of mechanical ventilation and ICU length of stay [40]. However, none of the randomized clinical trials have demonstrated survival benefit of early tracheostomy [41].

Anesthetic Analgesics and Sedatives Anesthetics, analgesics, and sedatives are widely used therapies in acute TBI as either prophylaxis or to control ICP and seizures. Barbiturates have historically been used to control ICP, presumably by preventing unnecessary movements, metabolic suppression, and alteration of cerebral vascular tone [42]. Anesthetic, analgesic, and sedative therapy also carries with it high morbidity. Side effects include hypotension, decreased cardiac output, as well as increased intrapulmonary shunting, which leads to hypoxia and decreased cerebral perfusion. For these reasons, high-dose barbiturates (barbiturate coma) should not be initiated unless hemodynamic stability is insured in victims of refractory intracranial hypertension following TBI [43].

Steroids Steroids were introduced in the early 1960s as a treatment for brain edema [44]. Experimental evidence accumulated indicates that steroids were useful in the restoration of altered vascular permeability in brain edema, reduction of cerebrospinal fluid production, and attenuation of free radical production. Several randomized controlled trials demonstrated benefits with the use of methylprednisolone for 24 h; however, meta-analysis of these randomized trials failed to demonstrate any conclusive benefit of steroids in TBI. The most conclusive evidence was brought forward after the CRASH (Corticosteroid Randomization After Significant Head Injury) trial in over 10,000 TBI patients that demonstrated an 18% higher risk of death 2 weeks post-injury in patients who were randomized to receive corticosteroids for 48 h [45].

Nutrition Following TBI there is a cascade of inflammatory cytokines released into the blood stream that initiates rapid catabolism and increased energy expenditure. Therefore, TBI patients require appropriate nutritional support at the right time for optimal recovery. Nutritional support after TBI provides patients with appropriate substrates, essential nutrients, and enough calories to inhibit catabolism and promote rapid neurological recovery [46]. Based on this evidence, current BTF guidelines and the American Association of Neurological Surgeons' (AANS) guidelines recommend initiation of enteral nutrition within 72 h and full nutritional replacement by the seventh day [25]. Recent studies have shown that initiation of tube feeds as early as within the first 24 h of injury can interfere with post-injury acute phase response, which is an immediate protective response of the body to protect primary host functions. This can lead to slower recovery and higher incidence of pneumonia in these TBI patients [47]. For optimal clinical results and rapid recovery in TBI, nutrition can be safely started after the first 24 h post-injury and should advance toward optimal nutritional goals over the next 48–72 h.

Seizure Prophylaxis Acute symptomatic seizures occur as a result of severe TBI. Post-traumatic seizures (PTS) are classified as "early" when they occur within 7 days of injury and "late" when they occur after 7 days of injury. Rate of PTS in patients with severe TBI is as high as 12%, whereas rate of subclinical seizures detected by electroencephalography is as high as 20–25% [48]. Risk factors for early PTS include the following: GCS of $\leq$10; immediate seizures; post-traumatic amnesia lasting longer than 30 min; a linear or depressed skull fracture; a penetrating head injury; subdural, epidural, or intracerebral hematoma; cortical contusion; age $\leq$65 years; and chronic alcoholism. The BTF recommends use of phenytoin to decrease the incidence of early PTS; however, neither phenytoin nor valproic acid has shown any benefit in limiting late PTS. Levetiracetam (Keppra), a relatively newer drug, has recently gained popularity for seizure prophylaxis for various pathologies, including TBI [49]. However, current evidence is insufficient to recommend for or against its use over other available agents.

Beta Blocker

Animal model studies of TBI have shown an increase in sympathoadrenal activity after TBI. This increase in sympathetic activity by surge in catecholamine has shown to be directly associated with increased mortality, lower neurological recover, and increase in hospital stay [50].Based on these findings, beta blockers have been studied as a potential therapeutic option after brain injury. In a murine model of TBI, propranolol was administrated after induction of TBI. Propranolol-treated mice demonstrated improved survival and histological recovery [51]. Several retrospective studies have shown an independent association of beta blockers with survival [52, 53]. Despite optimistic results, early beta-blockade use is not indicated routinely. Propranolol may be the ideal agent because of its nonselective inhibition and its lipophilic properties allowing it to penetrate the blood-brain barrier. In a randomized placebo controlled clinical trial, early administration of propranolol after TBI was associated with improved survival after controlling for confounding factors, demonstrating its potential role in TBI [54]. Another randomized placebo controlled trial is currently ongoing to evaluate the role of beta blockers in traumatic brain injury by decreasing adrenergic or sympathetic hyperactivity [55].

Most of the modern ICUs utilize guidelines for the management of TBI and ICP. Figure 1.1 shows the intracranial pressure monitoring guidelines which is implemented at our level I trauma center.

Complications

Coagulopathy TBI is often associated with disturbances in the coagulation profile. Coagulopathy affects up to one-third of TBI patients [56]. Mechanisms by which TBI induces coagulopathy include local and systemic inflammation, which lead to the release of tissue factor, activation of the protein C pathways, platelet dysfunction, and disseminated intravascular coagulation. Coagulopathy after TBI is a dynamic process that goes through stages of hypercoagulability and hypocoagulability ultimately leading to a state of bleeding diathesis [56]. TBI coagulopathy is diagnosed with traditional measures of coagulation, such as prothrombin time, activated partial thromboplastin time, and international normalized ratio. It has also been shown that development of coagulopathy after TBI is associated with higher mortality. In recent years, viscoelastic tests such as thromboelastography (TEG) and rotational thromboelastometry (ROTEM) have been frequently used to assess TBI coagulopathy. These coagulation tests are both more sensitive and specific than conventional assays. They are also more efficient in predicting therapy for TBI-induced coagulopathy [57].

The reversal of TBI coagulopathy requires the replacement of coagulation factors. Classically, fresh frozen plasma (FFP) has been used to reverse both acquired and induced TBI coagulopathy. Studies have demonstrated that prothrombin complex concentrate (PCC), when used in conjunction with FFP, is associated with complete and more rapid reversal of coagulopathy, without any increase in complications compared to FFP alone [58, 59]. PCC, in conjunction with FFP, also leads to a faster time to craniotomy in all patients with TBI-induced coagulopathy. While recombinant factor VIIa has been shown as an effective therapy in reversing coagulopathy, there is no difference in its effectiveness when compared with PCC [58, 60].

Thromboembolic Events

TBI patients are at increased risk of developing deep venous thrombosis (DVT) with rates as high as 20–30% even with appropriate mechanical prophylaxis. Pharmacological prophylaxis with low molecular weight heparin is the first-line therapy to limit thromboembolic events. Due to high risk of bleeding in TBI patients, thromboprophylaxis in head-injured patients must weigh the dangers of pulmonary embolism with risk of bleeding. The challenge in deciding when to initiate pharmacologic prophylaxis lies in determining when the risk of progression of intracranial hemorrhage has become sufficiently low. American College of Surgeons Trauma Quality Improvement Program (ACS-TQIP) best practice guidelines recommend that in patient with minimal risk of progression, pharmacological prophylaxis can be started if the repeat head CT scan is stable at 24 h. For patients with moderate risk defined as subdural/epidural hematoma >8 mm or intraventricular hemorrhage >2 cm or if the progression is seen on repeat head CT at 24 hours, DVT prophylaxis should be delayed up to 72 h until the repeat head CT scan is stable. In patients with ICP monitor placement, craniotomy, or evidence of progression at 72 h, IVC filter placement should be considered [61].

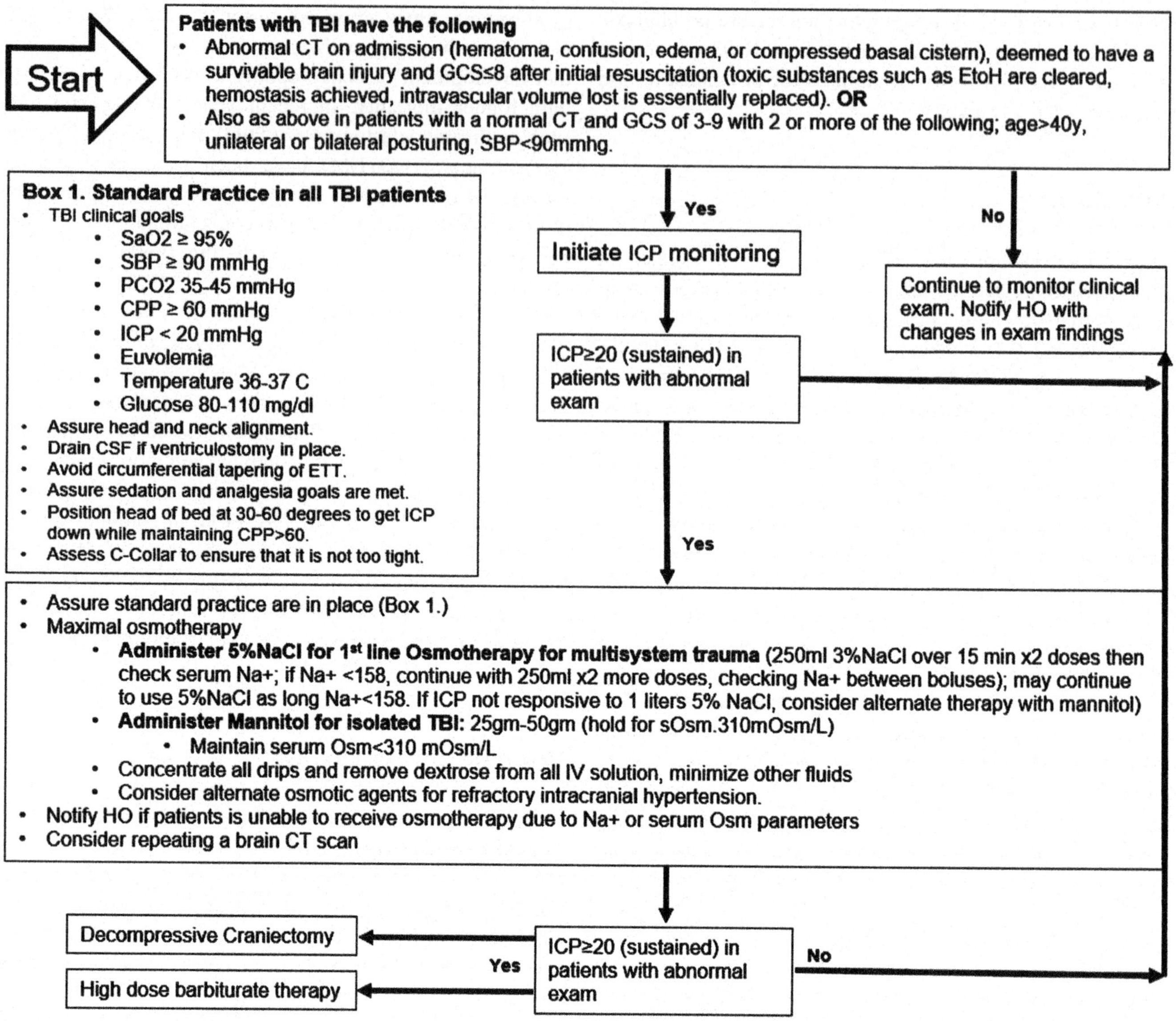

Fig. 1.1 Intracranial pressure monitoring guidelines SaO_2, oxygen saturation; SBP, systolic blood pressure; PCO_2, partial pressure of carbon dioxide; GCS, Glasgow Coma Scale; HO, house officer; CPP, cerebral perfusion pressure; ICP, intracranial pressure; ETT, endotracheal tube

Role of Acute Care Surgeon in Acute Management of TBI

Traditionally, patients with a suspected TBI are first seen by trauma surgeons for initial evaluation and receive an initial head CT scan, followed by neurosurgical consultation, regardless of the severity of injury, clinical presentation, or associated risk factors. Recently, this approach has been challenged for two fundamental reasons. First, the vast majority of these patients never undergo any form of neurosurgical intervention and are managed nonoperatively by the critical care surgeons in the ICU [62]. Indiscriminate use of repeat imaging in these patients results in unwarranted expenditure of valuable human and financial resources. Second, because TBI is a clinical diagnosis, the decision about neurosurgical intervention or a repeat head CT scan can be unfailingly predicted by considering the size of initial head bleed, close clinical examination, and the presence of risk factors for bleed progression, such as antiplatelet and anticoagulation medication [63]. For the abovementioned reasons, several studies have suggested that patients with TBI undergoing nonoperative management can be reliably followed for any sign of neurological decline without a routine repeat head imaging [64, 65]. Some institutes have developed their own guidelines to manage TBI patients based on well-known risk factors for neurosurgical consultation, such as the use of antiplatelet/anticoagulant medications, intoxication, and clinical examination. The Brain Injury Guidelines (BIG) (Table 1.2.) formulated at the University of Arizona demonstrated safe and effective management of TBI patients. Based on BIG, a subset of TBI patients with mini-

Table 1.2 Brain injury guidelines

Variables	BIG 1	BIG 2	BIG 3
LOC	Yes/No	Yes/No	Yes/No
Neurologic examination	Normal	Normal	Abnormal
Intoxication	No	No/Yes	No/Yes
CAMP	No	No	Yes
Skull Fracture	No	Non-displaced	Displaced
SDH	≤4 mm	5–7 mm	≥8 mm
EDH	≤4 mm	5–7 mm	≥8 mm
IPH	≤4 mm, 1 location	3–7 mm, 2 locations	≥8 mm, multiple locations
SAH	Trace	Localized	Scattered
IVH	No	No	Yes
	Therapeutic plan		
Hospitalization	No Observation (6h)	Yes	Yes
RHCT	No	No	Yes
NSC	No	No	Yes

BIG brain injury guidelines, *CAMP* Coumadin, Aspirin, Plavix, *EDH* epidural hemorrhage, *IVH* intraventricular hemorrhage, *IPH* intraparenchymal hemorrhage, *LOC* loss of consciousness, *NSC* neurosurgical consultation, *RHCT* repeat head computed tomography, *SAH* subarachnoid hemorrhage, *SDH* subdural hemorrhage

mal injury can be managed reliably via neuro-examination without the need for neurosurgical consultation or repeat head CT scans [66]. This practice has resulted in a significant reduction in the use of valuable resources (such as neurosurgical consultation, repeat CT scans, and hospital costs) without affecting patient care.

Brain Death and Organ Donation

"Brain death" denotes the absence of any neurological activity in a patient whose core temperature is >32.8 C, whose mental status is not impacted by sedating or paralyzing medications, who is completely resuscitated with a SBP >90 mmHg, and whose oxygen saturations are above 90%. In brain-dead patients, pupils are fixed and dilated; there are no observable corneal oculocephalic, oculovestibular, gag, or cough reflexes [67]. No movement to deep central or peripheral pain and no spontaneous breathing is seen on disconnection from the ventilator with $PaCO_2 > 60$ mmHg (i.e., apnea test). If the brain death protocol is equivocal, one can perform secondary tests, such as a cerebral angiography to show absence of CBF or a cerebral ribonucleotide angiogram to show absent uptake.

In 1999, TBI was the cause of brain death for more than 40% of the individuals from whom organs were procured. Many efforts have been made to date to improve organ donation rates following brain death. Administration of levothyroxine (T4) after brain death has emerged as one of the most effective therapies. It has led to an increase in both the quantity and quality of organs available for transplantation. More recent studies have shown that initiation of levothyroxine therapy before declaration of brain death further increases the yield of organ donation in such individuals. Currently, administration of T4 alone, or in combination with corticosteroids, is the prime therapy available to enhance organ donation rates following brain death.

References

1. Prevention I. Control: traumatic brain injury,"Centers for Disease Control and Prevention,". National Center for Injury Prevention and Control, Division of Unintentional Injury Prevention, http://www.cdc.gov/traumaticbraininjury. 2014.
2. CDC. https://www.cdc.gov/traumaticbraininjury/pdf/blue_book.pdf. CDC. 2016.
3. Wilberger JE Jr, Harris M, Diamond DL. Acute subdural hematoma: morbidity, mortality, and operative timing. J Neurosurg. 1991;74(2):212–8.
4. MAEDA M. Surgical treatment of chronic subdural hematoma in 500 consecutive cases: clinical characteristics, surgical outcome, complications, and recurrence rate. Neurol Med Chir. 2001;41(8):371–81.
5. Teasdale GM, et al. Risks of acute traumatic intracranial haematoma in children and adults: implications for managing head injuries. BMJ. 1990;300(6721):363–7.
6. Armin SS, Colohan AR, Zhang JH. Traumatic subarachnoid hemorrhage: our current understanding and its evolution over the past half century. Neurol Res. 2006;28(4):445–52.
7. Servadei F, et al. Traumatic subarachnoid hemorrhage: demographic and clinical study of 750 patients from the European brain injury consortium survey of head injuries. Neurosurgery. 2002;50(2):261–9.
8. Chang EF, Meeker M, Holland MC. Acute traumatic intraparenchymal hemorrhage: risk factors for progression in the early post-injury period. Neurosurgery. 2006;58(4):647–56.
9. Atzema C, et al. Prevalence and prognosis of traumatic intraventricular hemorrhage in patients with blunt head trauma. J Trauma Acute Care Surg. 2006;60(5):1010–7.
10. Werner C, Engelhard K. Pathophysiology of traumatic brain injury. Br J Anaesth. 2007;99(1):4–9.
11. Gennarelli TA. Mechanisms and pathophysiology of cerebral concussion. J Head Trauma Rehabil. 1986;1(2):23–9.
12. Smith DH, Meaney DF, Shull WH. Diffuse axonal injury in head trauma. J Head Trauma Rehabil. 2003;18(4):307–16.
13. Klatzo I. Pathophysiological aspects of brain edema. Acta Neuropathol. 1987;72(3):236–9.
14. Karibe H, et al. Mild intraischemic hypothermia suppresses consumption of endogenous antioxidants after temporary focal ischemia in rats. Brain Res. 1994;649(1):12–8.
15. Chesnut RM, et al. The role of secondary brain injury in determining outcome from severe head injury. J Trauma. 1993;34(2):216–22.
16. Robertson CS, et al. Prevention of secondary ischemic insults after severe head injury. Crit Care Med. 1999;27(10):2086–95.
17. Marmarou A, et al. Prognostic value of the Glasgow coma scale and pupil reactivity in traumatic brain injury assessed pre-hospital and on enrollment: an IMPACT analysis. J Neurotrauma. 2007;24(2):270–80.
18. Gentleman D, et al. Guidelines for resuscitation and transfer of patients with serious head injury. BMJ. 1993;307(6903):547–52.
19. Haddad SH, Arabi YM. Critical care management of severe traumatic brain injury in adults. Scand J Trauma Resusc Emerg Med. 2012;20(1):12.
20. Davis DP, et al. Prehospital airway and ventilation management: a trauma score and injury severity score-based analysis. J Trauma Acute Care Surg. 2010;69(2):294–301.

21. Manley G, et al. Hypotension, hypoxia, and head injury: frequency, duration, and consequences. Arch Surg. 2001;136(10):1118–23.
22. Vos P, et al. EFNS guideline on mild traumatic brain injury: report of an EFNS task force. Eur J Neurol. 2002;9(3):207–19.
23. Maas AI, et al. Prediction of outcome in traumatic brain injury with computed tomographic characteristics: a comparison between the computed tomographic classification and combinations of computed tomographic predictors. Neurosurgery. 2005;57(6):1173–82.
24. Wilberger JE Jr, Deeb Z, Rothfus W. Magnetic resonance imaging in cases of severe head injury. Neurosurgery. 1987;20(4):571–6.
25. Carney N, et al. Guidelines for the management of severe traumatic brain injury, fourth edition. Neurosurgery. 2016;80(1):6–15.
26. Talving P, et al. Intracranial pressure monitoring in severe head injury: compliance with Brain Trauma Foundation guidelines and effect on outcomes: a prospective study: clinical article. J Neurosurg. 2013;119(5):1248–54.
27. Chesnut RM, et al. A trial of intracranial-pressure monitoring in traumatic brain injury. N Engl J Med. 2012;367(26):2471–81.
28. Burgess S, et al. A systematic review of randomized controlled trials comparing hypertonic sodium solutions and mannitol for traumatic brain injury: implications for emergency department management. Ann Pharmacother. 2016;50(4):291–300.
29. Hinson HE, Stein D, Sheth KN. Hypertonic saline and mannitol therapy in critical care neurology. J Intensive Care Med. 2013;28(1):3–11.
30. Wade CE, et al. Individual patient cohort analysis of the efficacy of hypertonic saline/dextran in patients with traumatic brain injury and hypotension. J Trauma Acute Care Surg. 1997;42(5S):61S–5S.
31. Froelich M, et al. Continuous hypertonic saline therapy and the occurrence of complications in neurocritically ill patients. Crit Care Med. 2009;37(4):1433–41.
32. Joseph B, et al. The physiological effects of hyperosmolar resuscitation: 5% vs 3% hypertonic saline. Am J Surg. 2014;208(5):697–702.
33. Hutchinson P, et al. Decompressive craniectomy in traumatic brain injury: the randomized multicenter RESCUEicp study (www.RESCUEicp.com). In: Brain edema XIII. New York: Springer; 2006. p. 17–20.
34. Cooper DJ, et al. Decompressive craniectomy in diffuse traumatic brain injury. N Engl J Med. 2011;364(16):1493–502.
35. Shiozaki T, et al. A multicenter prospective randomized controlled trial of the efficacy of mild hypothermia for severely head injured patients with low intracranial pressure. Mild Hypothermia Study Group in Japan. J Neurosurg. 2001;94(1):50–4.
36. Yao C, et al. Selective brain cooling in rats ameliorates intracerebral hemorrhage and edema caused by penetrating brain injury: possible involvement of heme oxygenase-1 expression. J Neurotrauma. 2011;28(7):1237–45.
37. Andrews PJ, et al. European society of intensive care medicine study of therapeutic hypothermia (32-35 degrees C) for intracranial pressure reduction after traumatic brain injury (the Eurotherm3235Trial). Trials. 2011;12:8.
38. Adelson PD, et al. Comparison of hypothermia and normothermia after severe traumatic brain injury in children (cool kids): a phase 3, randomised controlled trial. Lancet Neurol. 2013;12(6):546–53.
39. Rodriguez JL, et al. Early tracheostomy for primary airway management in the surgical critical care setting. Br J Surg. 1990;77(12):1406–10.
40. Holevar M, et al. Practice management guidelines for timing of tracheostomy: the EAST Practice Management Guidelines Work Group. J Trauma Acute Care Surg. 2009;67(4):870–4.
41. Sugerman HJ, et al. Multicenter, randomized, prospective trial of early tracheostomy. J Trauma Acute Care Surg. 1997;43(5):741–7.
42. Roberts I, Sydenham E. Barbiturates for acute traumatic brain injury. Cochrane Libr. 2012;(12):CD000033.
43. Roberts DJ, et al. Sedation for critically ill adults with severe traumatic brain injury: a systematic review of randomized controlled trials. Crit Care Med. 2011;39(12):2743–51.
44. Ransohoff J. The effects of steroids on brain edema in man. In: Steroids and brain edema. Berlin: Springer; 1972. p. 211–7.
45. Roberts I, et al. Effect of intravenous corticosteroids on death within 14 days in 10008 adults with clinically significant head injury (MRC CRASH trial): randomised placebo-controlled trial. Lancet. 2004;364(9442):1321–8.
46. Chiang YH, et al. Early enteral nutrition and clinical outcomes of severe traumatic brain injury patients in acute stage: a multi-center cohort study. J Neurotrauma. 2012;29(1):75–80.
47. Azim A, et al. Early feeds not force feeds: enteral nutrition in traumatic brain injury. J Trauma Acute Care Surg. 2016;81(3):520–4.
48. Annegers JF, et al. A population-based study of seizures after traumatic brain injuries. N Engl J Med. 1998;338(1):20–4.
49. Jones KE, et al. Levetiracetam versus phenytoin for seizure prophylaxis in severe traumatic brain injury. Neurosurg Focus. 2008;25(4):E3.
50. Haider W, et al. Urinary catecholamine excretion and thyroid hormone blood level in the course of severe acute brain damage. Eur J Intensive Care Med. 1975;1(3):115–23.
51. Liu M. Protective effects of propranolol on experimentally head-injured mouse brains. J Formos Med Assoc = Taiwan yi zhi. 1995;94(7):386–90.
52. Arbabi S, et al. Beta-blocker use is associated with improved outcomes in adult trauma patients. J Trauma Acute Care Surg. 2007;62(1):56–62.
53. Cotton BA, et al. Beta-blocker exposure is associated with improved survival after severe traumatic brain injury. J Trauma Acute Care Surg. 2007;62(1):26–35.
54. Ko A, et al. Early propranolol after traumatic brain injury is associated with lower mortality. J Trauma Acute Care Surg. 2016;80(4):637–42.
55. Patel MB, et al. Decreasing adrenergic or sympathetic hyperactivity after severe traumatic brain injury using propranolol and clonidine (DASH after TBI study): study protocol for a randomized controlled trial. Trials. 2012;13(1):177.
56. Harhangi B, et al. Coagulation disorders after traumatic brain injury. Acta Neurochir. 2008;150(2):165–75.
57. Lancé MD. A general review of major global coagulation assays: thrombelastography, thrombin generation test and clot waveform analysis. Thromb J. 2015;13(1):1.
58. Joseph B, et al. Prothrombin complex concentrate versus fresh-frozen plasma for reversal of coagulopathy of trauma: is there a difference? World J Surg. 2014;38(8):1875–81.
59. Joseph B, et al. Prothrombin complex concentrate: an effective therapy in reversing the coagulopathy of traumatic brain injury. J Trauma Acute Care Surg. 2013;74(1):248–53.
60. Stein DM, et al. Recombinant factor VIIa: decreasing time to intervention in coagulopathic patients with severe traumatic brain injury. J Trauma Acute Care Surg. 2008;64(3):620–8.
61. ACS TQIP Best Practice Guidelines. 2017. Available from https://www.facs.org/quality-programs/trauma/tqip/best-practice.
62. Patel NY, et al. Traumatic brain injury: patterns of failure of nonoperative management. J Trauma Acute Care Surg. 2000;48(3):367–75.
63. Joseph B, et al. Repeat head computed tomography in anticoagulated traumatic brain injury patients: still warranted. Am Surg. 2014;80(1):43–7.
64. Brown CV, et al. Does routine serial computed tomography of the head influence management of traumatic brain injury? A prospective evaluation. J Trauma Acute Care Surg. 2004;57(5):939–43.
65. Joseph B, et al. A three-year prospective study of repeat head computed tomography in patients with traumatic brain injury. J Am Coll Surg. 2014;219(1):45–51.
66. Joseph B, et al. The BIG (brain injury guidelines) project: defining the management of traumatic brain injury by acute care surgeons. J Trauma Acute Care Surg. 2014;76(4):965–9.
67. Rowland LP. Guidelines for the determination of death report of the medical consultants on the diagnosis of death to the President's Commission for the Study of Ethical Problems in Medicine and Biomedical and Behavioral Research. Neurology. 1982;32(4):395.

Intracranial Pressure

2

David A. Hampton and Deborah M. Stein

Background

Cranial injuries related to enemy combatants, hunting, or natural disasters have influenced human evolution. The ability to adequately address these injuries determined which early humans survived. Throughout Africa, Asia, and South America, archeologist have excavated skulls which have holes of various sizes across the cranium [1]. Many of these skulls had more than one hole, and many were found in various stages of healing. Trepanation, derived from the Greek trypanon meaning a borer or auger, was a procedure used to create holes in the skull to relieve pressure after injury or to release evil spirits in the mentally ill [2, 3].

The Edwin Papyrus, an Egyptian medical treatise drafted in 1600 BC by a physician working with pyramid construction teams, describes numerous injuries sustained by the workforce [1, 4]. The document details 48 cases of which 27 were related to head trauma. The Papyrus was the first descriptive medical documentation of cranial structures, the meninges, the brain's surface, cerebral spinal fluid, and cranial injury and their associated physiologic deficit. Given its detail and utility, it was believed the Papyrus was later utilized as a textbook for military trauma [1].

Traumatic Brain Injury

In modern times, cranial injuries commonly occur after a motor vehicle accident, assault, athletic collision, or ground level fall [5, 6]. The sudden acceleration and deceleration resulting in translational and rotational forces moving the brain within the cranial vault causes it to impact against the immobile cranium resulting in a focal injury [7–9]. Diffuse injury can occur secondary to shock waves from the initial strike or cavitation injury from a foreign body translating through the brain parenchyma [10, 11]. This injury pattern is commonly known as a traumatic brain injury (TBI). TBI is the signature injury of the recent Middle East conflicts. As of 2016, there were 357,000 United States service members diagnosed with a TBI [12]. In 2000 there were 1.7 million individuals in the United States who sustained a TBI. Fifty two thousand died, 275,000 were hospitalized, and 1.3 million were released from the emergency department. In total, this resulted in an estimated $60 billion economic burden [13].

TBIs are gradated into three tiers – mild, moderate, and severe – based upon the presenting Glasgow Coma Scale (GCS) (Table 2.1). The GCS is a reliable objective measure of a patients' consciousness based upon three physical examination criteria – eye, motor, and verbal responses [14, 15]. The summation of the individual component scales ranges from 3 to 15. The TBI's severity is based upon this composite number.

A mild TBI is defined as a GCS greater than or equal to 13. These patients will usually have a history of a brief loss of consciousness, amnesia to the event, confusion, and may perseverate when asked questions. Patients afflicted with a mild TBI usually do not require an inpatient admission and are managed on an outpatient basis. A moderate TBI is classified as a GCS less than 13 but greater than or equal to 9. This injury is associated with a prolonged loss of consciousness, neurologic deficits, and radiographic findings, i.e., subdural, epidural, or subarachnoid hemorrhage [16]. Unlike the mild TBI, these patients require further observation as an inpatient.

A severe TBI is classified as a GCS less than or equal to 8. These patients will usually have radiographic evidence of an intracranial hemorrhage. Additionally, depending on their level of consciousness, the patient may have an abnormal neurologic examination with respect to motor function and pupillary or other cranial nerve responsiveness. These patients are at a high risk for respiratory failure and a

D. A. Hampton · D. M. Stein (✉)
R Adams Cowley Shock Trauma Center, University of Maryland Medical Center, Baltimore, MD, USA
e-mail: dstein@umm.edu

A. Salim et al. (eds.), *Surgical Critical Care Therapy*, https://doi.org/10.1007/978-3-319-71712-8_2

Table 2.1 Glasgow Coma Scale [14]

Eyes		Motor		Verbal	
Scale	Response	Scale	Response	Scale	Response
4	Open spontaneously	6	Follows commands	5	Oriented (appropriate responses)
3	Open to voice	5	Localizes to pain	4	Confused
2	Open to painful stimulus	4	Withdrawals from pain	3	Inappropriate words
1	No response	3	Decorticate (flexion) posture	2	Inappropriate sounds
		2	Decerebrate (extensor) posture	1	No response
		1	No response		

potentially elevated intracranial pressure (ICP) secondary to the physical insult sustained. A TBI can result in an elevated ICP secondary to cerebral edema, hyperemia, hematoma formation, presence of a foreign body, or depressed skull fracture.

Physiology

The adult cranium volume is approximately 1400–1700 mls. The intracranial contents by volume are: brain parenchyma (80%), CSF (10%), and blood (10%) [17]. The ICP generated is the force exerted by the three tissue volumes against the intracranial surface area. ICP varies by age. An adult ICP is <10–15 mmHg, while a child's is <3–7 mmHg. The Monro-Kellie hypothesis states the volume of tissue within the cranium is conserved; therefore when one tissue volume expands, for example, secondary to brain edema, vascular injury, or outflow obstruction, an equal decrease must occur in one or both of the other two (Fig. 2.1). Compensatory mechanisms, such as the removal of CSF or blood, to relieve pressure, are the body's immediate response. The cranium is a non-expansile vault, and the force is considered to be distributed evenly; therefore the pressure-related effects are experienced throughout the cranial vault. In the event the compensatory mechanisms fail or are inadequate, the rising pressure can result in intracranial hypertension (IC-HTN), ICP ≥20 mmHg. Aside from the aforementioned physical changes, IC-HTN can occur or be exacerbated by seizure activity, Valsalva maneuvers, venous sinus thrombosis, systemic hypertension, or obstruction of CSF circulation.

An elevation in ICP can adversely affect cerebral blood flow (CBF). Brain function and survival are dependent upon adequate CBF and oxygen delivery [18]. Cerebral perfusion is dependent upon the driving pressure and resistance encountered. Analogous to Ohm's law, the current through a conductor is directly proportional to the change in voltage across it; the CBF is equal to the change in pressure across the brain [19]:

$$\mathrm{CBF} = \frac{\mathrm{CAP} - \mathrm{JVP}}{\mathrm{CVR}} \tag{2.1}$$

where CAP is carotid artery pressure, JVP is jugular venous pressure, and CVR is the cerebrovascular resistance. The CBF is not typically directly measured; therefore the cerebral perfusion pressure (CPP) is often used as an indirect surrogate. CPP is defined as:

$$\mathrm{CPP} = \mathrm{MAP} - \mathrm{ICP} \tag{2.2}$$

the difference between the MAP, the forward driving pressure, and the ICP, the pressure retarding it.

Autoregulation

Cerebrovascular autoregulation maintains a constant CBF over a wide range of perfusion pressures (Fig. 2.2). This cerebral autoregulation allows for shifts in pressure without adversely affecting CBF [20, 21]. This mechanism allows for adequate oxygen and nutrients to be delivered while removing carbon dioxide and other metabolic waste products. The majority of this regulation occurs within the immense arteriolar network where the greatest changes in resistance can occur.

After an intracranial insult, autoregulation may become dysfunctional. Conditions which result in an elevated ICP will decrease the CPP and cause cerebral ischemia. Conversely, an elevated MAP can increase the CPP leading to hyperemia or worsening of cerebral edema [21–23]. Under these conditions, knowledge of the signs associated with and elevated ICP will directly affect patient outcomes.

Clinical Signs and Symptoms

In the setting of an evolving intracranial injury, clinical manifestations of the cerebral insult may develop. Commonly an elevated ICP is associated with headache, depressed consciousness, and emesis. Additionally, the compression of the brain stem will result in respiratory lability. As the CBF decreases secondary to the elevated ICP, the sympathetic nervous system will stimulate vascular alpha-1 adrenergic receptors causing an increase in systemic vascular resistance and systolic blood pressure. This response is an innate mechanism to maintain adequate CBF. However, the aortic baroreceptors will sense the new onset hypertension and stimulate the parasympathetic response, the vagus nerve, resulting in bradycardia. The constellation of bradycardia,

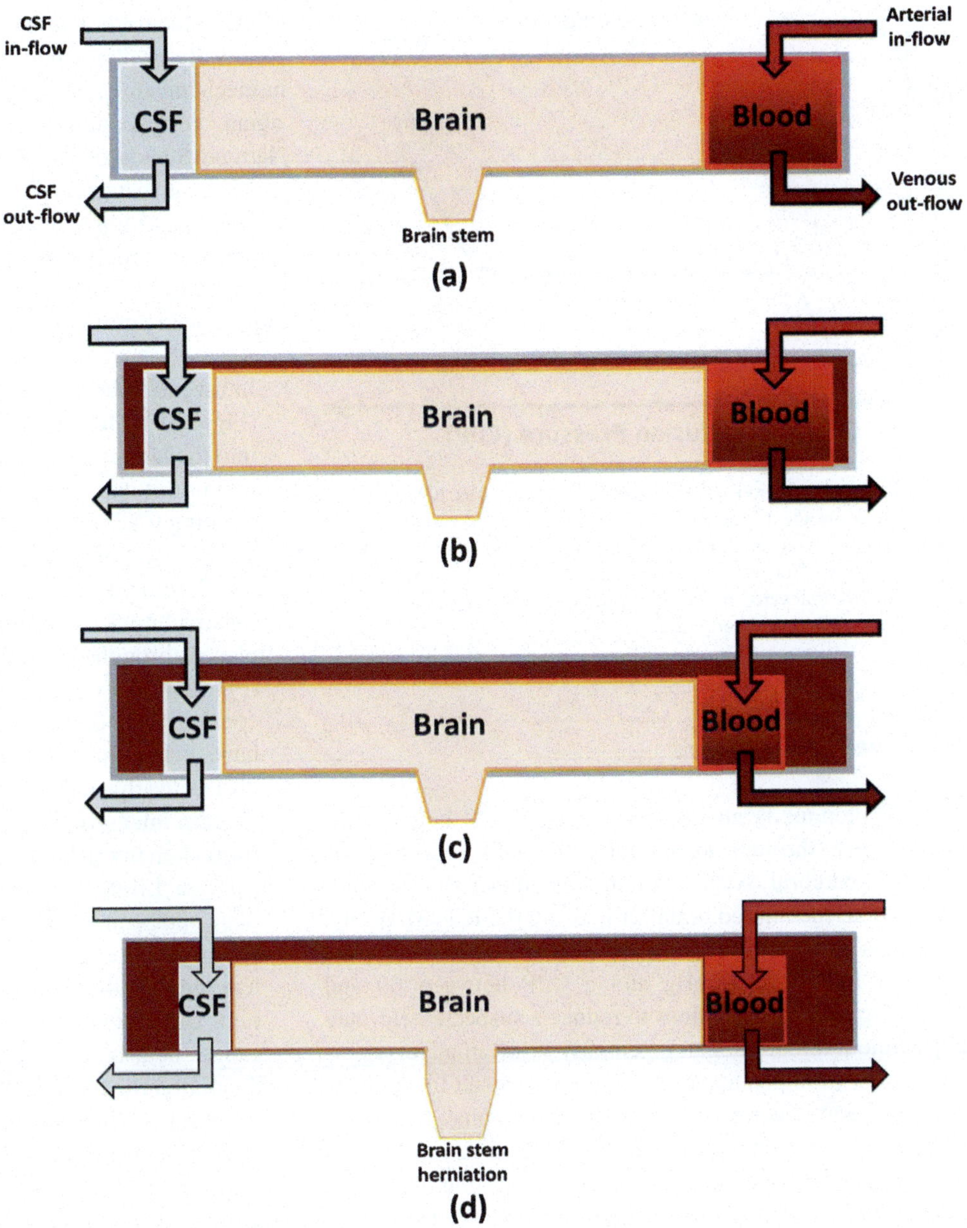

Fig. 2.1 Monro-Kellie Doctrine – (**a**) Intracranial contents – CSF, brain parenchyma, and blood; (**b**, **c**) an increasing intracranial mass/insult results in compensatory removal of blood and CSF, reducing overall compression of the brain parenchyma in order to maintain constant intracranial volume; (**d**) when compensatory mechanisms are exhausted, continued increasing ICP results in brain herniation

hypertension, and respiratory lability is known as Cushing's reflex [17, 18]. This reflex can be an early sign that the compensatory mechanisms are exhausted, and brain herniation will occur to further relieve the developing IC-HTN.

Brain herniation is classified by the structure herniating or the anatomic landmark traversed.

- Subfalcine herniation is the most common form. It occurs when the frontal lobe is displaced beneath the falx cerebri resulting in contralateral hydrocephalus secondary to obstruction of the foramen of Monro and compression of the anterior cerebral artery manifesting as contralateral lower extremity weakness [24].
- Central herniation occurs secondary to downward pressure resulting in bilateral uncal herniation and a lateral gaze deficit secondary to a cranial nerve VI palsy [25].
- Uncal herniation, a variant of transtentorial herniation, results in the uncus and medial temporal lobe exiting through the tentorial incisura and compressing against the brain stem and tentorial edge. This can result in ipsilateral hemiparesis also known as Kernohan-Woltman notch phenomenon [24].
- Tonsillar herniation occurs when the cerebellar tonsils transit below the foramen magnum. This is often caused by a posterior fossa hematoma or fourth ventricle obstruction and can result in respiratory depression, blood pressure instability, and sudden death [25].

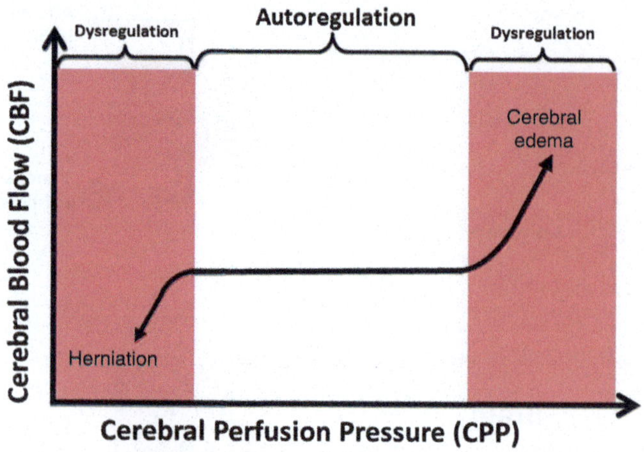

Fig. 2.2 Autoregulation – The cerebral blood flow is held constant over a wide range of perfusion pressures. Elevated pressures and exhaustion of or dysfunctional compensatory mechanisms can result in cerebral edema. Conversely, a decreased cerebral perfusion pressure can result from elevated intracranial pressures and present as reduced cerebral blood flow and herniation

Invasive ICP Monitors

An ICP monitor is an invasive device which helps direct patient care through maximizing the CPP, resulting in improved cerebral oxygenation and avoidance of a secondary insult to the injured brain [26]. Using the ICP, MAP, and Eq. 2.2, a clinician will be able to achieve their therapeutic goals: a ICP < 20 mmHg and a CPP between 60 and 70 mmHg [27]. Interventions to reduce a suspected elevated ICP without a monitor can potentially result in adverse outcomes. For example, hyperventilation will result in vasoconstriction and decreased intracranial volume; however prolonged hyperventilation is complicated by decreased oxygen delivery and the potential for cerebral ischemia. Given these potential complications, ancillary monitoring such as venous oxygen content ($CvjO_2$) or brain tissue oxygenation ($PbrO_2$) is often beneficial.

Currently an ICP monitor is recommended for patients with a post-resuscitation GCS ≤ 8 and radiographic evidence of intracranial pathology such as herniation, contusion, basal cistern compression, cerebral edema, or intracranial hemorrhage [18, 27]. Additionally, ICP monitors can be indicated for patients after a traumatic head injury with normal CT scans. In this patient population, it has been shown that individuals who meet two or more of these criteria: (1) SBP < 90 mmHg, (2) posturing on physical examination, and (3) age > 40 years old, have been found to have an intracranial hemorrhage 60% of the time [27–29].

The first ICP monitors were passive devices, U-shaped tubes directly communicating with the CSF and the atmosphere [30]. The CSF back pressure was an indirect measure of ICP. Modern ICP monitors have been engineered to utilize solid-state or fiber-optic transducers which convert changes in mechanical resistance or light reflection into an electrical signal corresponding to pressure [31]. The American National Standards Institute/Association for the Advancement of Medical Instrumentation standards require these devices to function within a range of 0–100 mmHg with a ± 2 mmHg error from 0 to 20 mmHg and a ± 10% error from 21 to 100 mmHg [32]. The invasive monitors have been designed to be placed within one of four intracranial sites:

- Intraventricular – This is the gold standard location (Fig. 2.3b). The monitor's pressure sensing arm is inserted into the lateral ventricle. Aside from being used as an ICP monitor, it can also provide a therapeutic intervention by draining CSF to relieve pressure as needed. These devices can be complicated by infection [33, 34] and potentially misplacement due to collapsed ventricles.
- Subarachnoid – The Richmond bolt is a hollow screw placed through the skull and terminates against the dura (Fig. 2.3c). A dural puncture allows CSF and the ICP to communicate directly with the transducer. These devices have a low infection risk; however, they can become obstructed by debris. They are infrequently utilized in modern intensive care units.
- Intraparenchymal – These monitors, such as the Camino® (Integra LifeSciences Corporation), are a cable with a fiber-optic transducer tip placed within the brain's parenchyma (Fig. 2.3d). The device is technically less challenging than the EVD to deploy and has a lower infection rate. Unlike the EVD, it is only a measurement tool and cannot be used to remove CSF. Additionally, it is dependent upon the tissue in which it is embedded.
- Epidural – This device does not enter the brain parenchyma or penetrate the dura (Fig. 2.3e). It is an optical transducer which is placed against the dura. Its accuracy is limited by the dura damping the true ICP. It is infrequently utilized, but due to low hemorrhagic complications, it may be useful in coagulopathic patients.

These monitors transduce the ICP as a continuous waveform. The waveform amplitude is usually shallow with small perturbations secondary to B- and C-waves which correspond to respiratory variation and the cardiac cycle, respectively [18, 19]. A persistent waveform elevation, an A-wave, lasting minutes to hours, is associated with loss of autoregulation and the need for an urgent intervention.

The utility of ICP monitoring has been repeatedly questioned. The American College of Surgeons (ACS) Trauma Quality Improvement Program (TQIP) database was interrogated to determine the relationship between ICP monitoring and mortality [35]. The TQIP database is a repository of trauma patient data compiled from participating ACS

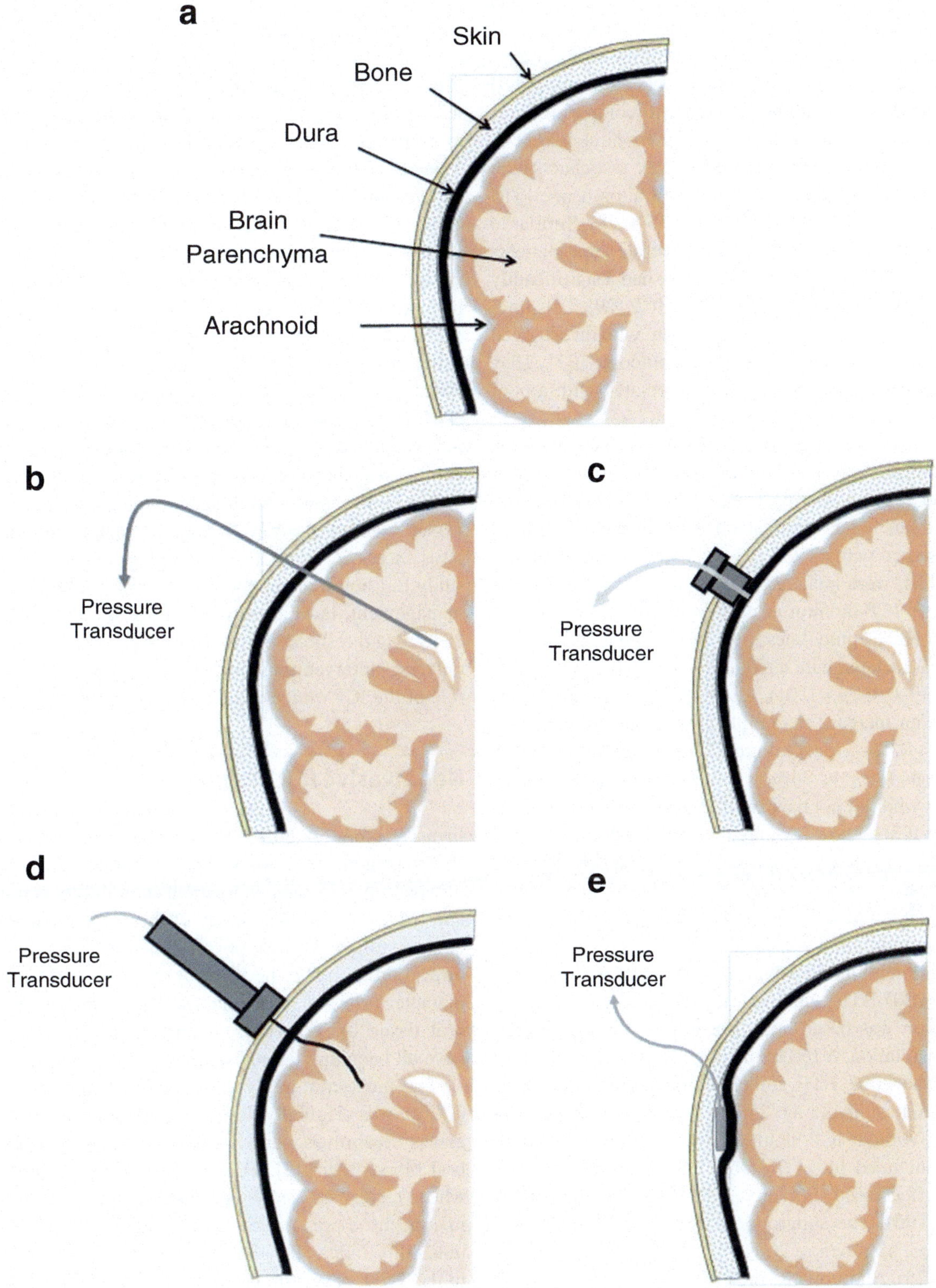

Fig. 2.3 Sagittal cross sections of the skull, brain parenchyma, and intracranial pressure monitors – (**a**) identification of the tissue layers from the skin to brain parenchyma, (**b**) intraventricular pressure transducer/extraventricular drain with sensor/drain within the lateral ventricle, (**c**) subdural pressure transducer with open communication between the subdural space and sensor, (**d**) intraparenchymal sensor also known as Camino sensor with sensor implanted within the brain parenchyma, and (**e**) epidural intracranial pressure sensor within the epidural space

level-I and level-II trauma centers from the United States and Canada. This database was designed as a platform to compare interventions and risk-adjusted outcomes between participating centers [36]. Over 10,500 patients with severe TBI were investigated. The adjusted odds ratio comparing mortality in those with and without an ICP monitor was 0.44 (95% CI, 0.31–0.63). Lower mortality was associated with institutions with higher rates of ICP monitor usage. The adjusted odds ratio was 0.52 (95% CI, 0.35–0.78). Similar to the TQIP study, Narayan's group demonstrated that patients with a severe TBI and an ICP > 20 mmHg had a significantly poorer prognosis than those with a lower ICP [29]. This finding was corroborated by Marmarou's group who investigated the relationship between ICP, SBP, and outcome [37]. They also found an ICP > 20 mmHg was associated with a poor outcome.

Converse to these findings, a 7-year retrospective review of 1646 patients registered in the National Trauma Data Bank found ICP monitoring worsened survival [38]. Adult trauma patients who experienced a blunt mechanism of injury, presented with a GCS ≤ 8 and had a CT scan demonstrating a TBI, were included. Less than half of the patients underwent an ICP monitor as directed by the Brain Trauma Foundation (BTF) guidelines [39]. In this study, ICP monitoring was associated with a reduction in survival (OR, 0.54; 95% CI, 0.39–0.76; $p < 0.01$). Additionally, it was also associated with an increase in complications: pneumonia (37% vs 23%, $p < 0.001$), renal failure (2.7% vs 1.1%, $p = 0.02$), and infections (39% vs 24%, $p < 0.001$), as compared with the patients who did not have an ICP monitor. These finding did propose ICP monitoring may not be helpful, the pressure lowering interventions employed were misappropriated potentially causing patient harm, or the appropriate interventions were undertaken however were not performed at the appropriate time.

The aforementioned study was performed with patients prior to the 2007 BTF guidelines. Prior to 2007 ICP monitoring utilization was based upon practitioner clinical experience or consultation. A recent meta-analysis investigated the impact of the 2007 BTF guidelines on patient outcomes. Eighteen studies involving 25,229 patients (ICP monitor ($n = 7637$), without ICP monitor ($n = 17{,}862$)) with severe TBI were included [40]. The pool data demonstrated ICP monitoring decreased mortality (RR, 0.85; 95% CI, 0.73–0.98; $p < 0.05$). The subgroup analysis demonstrated this effect was not seen before 2007 (RR, 1.18, 95% CI = 0.89–1.56, $p = 0.25$). Additionally, mortality decreased after 2007 (R, 0.72, 95% CI = 0.63–0.83, $p < 0.01$). This finding was also noted as a 31% reduction in in-hospital mortality in patients treated after 2007 (RR, 0.69, 95% CI = 0.56–0.85, $p < 0.01$). There was no difference seen in in-hospital mortality prior to 2007 (RR, 1.30, 95% CI = 0.91–1.85, $p = 0.16$).

After the introduction of the 2007 BTF guidelines demonstrated the utility of an ICP monitor, the Benchmark Evidence from South American Trials: Treatment of Intracranial Pressure (BEST:TRIP) trial was developed to determine if ICP monitoring versus radiographic imaging and clinical examination improved patient outcomes [41]. This was a 3-year, multicenter, controlled trial which enrolled 324 patients with a TBI who presented with a GCS of 3–8 or demonstrated a decline in their GCS during the initial 48 hours of admission. Patients were randomized to either receiving an intraparenchymal pressure monitor with maintenance of their ICP below 20 mmHg ($n = 157$) or to an imaging-clinical examination group which received care based upon the participating hospital's pretrial protocol ($n = 167$). There was no difference in the 14-day mortality (30% versus 21%, $p = 0.18$), 6-month mortality (41% versus 39%, $p = 0.60$), or ICU length of stay (12 days versus 9 days, $p = 0.25$). The number of days receiving brain-specific treatments was higher in the imaging-clinical examination group, 4.8 days versus 3.4 days ($p = 0.002$). There were, however, more decubitus ulcers in the ICP-monitored group. The BEST:TRIP study did not demonstrate a superiority in either method of management, but did raise concerns regarding the use of a 20 mmHg threshold, injury pattern-specific treatments versus universal interventions, and the potential need to revise the role of the ICP monitor in TBI management [42].

Noninvasive ICP Monitors

Invasive monitors continue to be the accepted standard for ICP management; however they are limited by their duration of use, infection risk, and patient immobility. A noninvasive approach can eliminate many of these complications. These devices utilize known physical parameters which have a direct correlation to the ICP. For example, optic nerve sheath diameter (ONSD), tympanic membrane displacement, cerebral tissue oxygenation, or cerebral blood flow velocities have all been utilized to estimate ICP.

The most commonly used method, transcranial doppler (TCD), was originally described as a noninvasive method to assess cerebrovascular dynamics through changes in cerebral blood flow [43]. TCD is a low-cost, portable monitor whose results are easily reproducible. Increases in ICP result in concentric pressure on the vasculature and changes in the pulsatility index (PI) – qualitative and quantitative changes in the TCD waveform morphology. The device is limited by its signal attenuation through tissue, a patient's presence of absence of an acoustic window, and changes in ICP which did not affected the vasculature. Additionally, it can be technically challenging to perform and typically requires significant training to attain proficiency. Previously validated

Table 2.2 Brain Trauma Foundation guidelines [27]

Threshold	Recommendations	
Systolic blood pressure	Patients 15–49-year-old:≥ 110 mmHg Patients 50–69-year-old: ≥ 100 mmHg Patients > 70-year-old: ≥ 110 mmHg	Decreases mortality and improves outcomes
Intracranial pressure	ICP > 22 mmHg is associated with increased mortality	
Cerebral perfusion pressure	CPP ≥ 60 and ≤ 70 mmHg. The minimum optimal threshold is currently unclear and is dependent upon the patient autoregulatory status	

mathematical models which estimated the ICP based upon arterial blood pressure and TCD-obtained blood flow velocity were used to assess the potential clinical applications for TCD measurements [44]. These tests demonstrated a significant correlation ($r = 0.98$, $p < 0.01$) between measured and estimated ICP and a significant correlation ($r = 0.9$, $p < 0.01$) between autoregulation indices when using the measured versus estimated ICPs.

Other discussed noninvasive ICP measures are changes in the ONSD and quantitative pupillometry. The optic nerve sheath is an extension of the subarachnoid space. Intracranial pressures are transmitted through the sheath into the retrobulbar space, changing the sheath's diameter. These changes can be noted on transpupillary ultrasound. Quantitative pupillometry is a measure of pupillary size and light reflexes. The dynamic changes noted, size, dilation, and constriction velocity, comprise the neurological pupil index, NPi. The NPi scale is 1–5; an NPi < 3 is considered abnormal. Our institution recently investigated noninvasive measures, TCD, ONSD, and NPi, correlation with early CT findings in brain trauma [45]. One hundred intubated adult trauma patients with CT evidence of a TBI or GCS < 12 were included in the study. The number of patients with a TCD PI >1.3 (71.4% vs 51%, $p = 0.04$) and NPi < 3 (38.8% vs 17.7%, $p = 0.02$) was significantly higher in the group with radiographic TBI findings. When these variables were combined with age > 40 and lactate levels, a logistic regression model demonstrated an ROC of 0.72, which is comparable with other prediction models. Even with these promising results, noninvasive ICP measures are not commonly used.

Clinical Thresholds

During the initial evaluation of a head-injured patient, avoidance of hypoxia and hypotension has been shown to improve outcomes [46]. Adherence to this guidance is started in the prehospital setting and continues throughout a patient's hospitalization. Additionally established clinical practice guidelines dictate endotracheal intubation for a GCS less than 8, maintaining an oxygen saturation, S_pO_2, > 90%, or partial pressure of oxygen, PO_2, > 60 mmHg, and avoidance of hypotension [47, 48].

The Brain Trauma Foundation (BTF) was established to support TBI research. Their first TBI management guidelines were developed in 1995. Most recently, they reviewed 189 publications to support their current treatment goals [27]. Maintenance of a minimum SBP based upon age and an ICP < 22 mmHg has resulted in improved patient outcomes (Table 2.2). A CPP between 60 and 70 mmHg is also associated with improved patient outcomes. The optimal CPP threshold has not been established and may also be associated with an intact autoregulation status.

Radiography

During the initial patient evaluation, the mechanism of injury and physical examination findings may lead the clinician to believe a patient has a TBI. A computerized tomography (CT) scan may provide radiographic evidence of potential causes for a presenting neurologic deficit. Indications for a CT scan include (1) GCS < 15, (2) loss of consciousness >5 min, (3) antegrade amnesia, (4) basilar or depressed skull fracture, (5) penetrating injury, (6) pupillary or neurologic deficit, (7) known bleeding diathesis, or (8) anticoagulant therapy [18]. A non-contrast CT scan is the standard of care.

Clinical Interventions

The ABCs of the primary survey apply to all trauma patients [10]. In the head-injured population, priority is given to maintenance of oxygenation, end-organ perfusion, and avoidance of hypotension. A hypotensive episode in concert with hypoxemia can result in vasoconstriction, ICP elevation, and ischemia. The algorithms to manage elevated ICP are often institution dependent. The ACS Committee on Trauma (COT) has developed a three-tiered approach (Tables 2.3, 2.4, and 2.5) [49]. They created a systematic, escalating management intervention approach based upon the most current literature. Similarly, our institution has developed a

Table 2.3 Three-tiered management of intracranial pressure – Tier 1 [49]

Tier 1
Head of bed elevated at 30 degrees (reverse Trendelenburg) to improve cerebral venous outflow
Sedation and analgesia using recommended short-acting agents (e.g., propofol, fentanyl, midazolam) in intubated patients
Ventricular drainage performed intermittently. Continuous drainage is not recommended unless an additional ICP monitor is placed; as when the drain is open, it does not accurately reflect the true ICP
Repeat CT imagine and neurological examination should be considered to rule out the development of a surgical mass lesion and guide treatment
If ICP remains > 20–25 mmHg, proceed to tier 2

Table 2.4 Three-tiered management of intracranial pressure – Tier 2 [49]

Tier 2
In patients with a parenchymal ICP monitor an EVD should be considered to allow for intermittent CSF drainage
Hyperosmolar therapy should be given intermittently as needed for ICP elevation and not on a routine schedule Mannitol should be administered in intermittent boluses (0.25 – 1.0 gm/kg body weight). Caution should be taken in the hypovolemic patient when osmotic diuresis is instituted with mannitol. The serum sodium and osmolality must be assessed frequently (every 6 h) and additional doses should be held if serum osmolality exceeds 320 mOsm/L. Mannitol may also be held if there is evidence of hypovolemia. Hypertonic saline may be administered in intermittent boluses of 3% sodium chloride solution (250 ml over ½ h) or other concentrations (e.g. 30cc of 23.4%). Serum sodium and osmolality must be assessed frequently (every 6 h) and additional doses should be held if serum sodium exceeds 160 mEq/L
Cerebral autoregulation should be assessed. If the patient is not autoregulating, the CPP goal should be lowered to reduce ICP (to no less than 50 mmHg). Additional neuromonitoring (e.g. $PbtO_2$, $SjvO_2$, CBF) may help determine optimal CPP
$PaCO_2$ goal of 30 – 35 mmHg should be maintained, as long as brain hypoxia is not encountered. Additional neuromonitoring neuromonitoring (e.g. $PbtO_2$, $SjvO_2$, CBF) may help determine optimal $PaCO_2$
Repeat CT imaging and neurological examination should be considered to rule out development of a surgical mass lesion and guide treatment
Neuromuscular paralysis achieved with a bolus "test dose" of a neuromuscular blocking agent should be considered if the above measures fail to adequately lower ICP and restore CPP. If there is a positive response, continuous infusion of a neuromuscular blocking agent should be employed
If ICP remains ≥ 20 – 25 mmHg proceed to Tier 3

tiered approach to ICP management which is based upon guidelines established by the Brain Trauma Foundation [28, 50]. Analogous to the ACS guidelines, it also starts with non-invasive interventions (Fig. 2.4a) and escalates thereafter (Fig. 2.4b).

Table 2.5 Three-tiered management of intracranial pressure – Tier 3 [49]

Tier 3
Decompressive hemi-craniectomy or bilateral craniectomy should only be performed if treatments in tiers 1 and 2 are not sufficient or are limited by development of side effects of medical treatment
Neuromuscular paralysis via continuous infusion of neuromuscular blocking agent can be employed if there is a positive response to a bolus dose. The infusion should be titrated to maintain at least two twitches (out of a train of four) using a peripheral nerve stimulator. Adequate sedation must be utilized
Barbiturate or propofol (anesthesia dosage) coma may be induced for those patients who have failed to respond to aggressive measures to control malignant intracranial hypertension; however it should only be instituted if a test dose of barbiturate or propofol results in a decrease in ICP, thereby identifying the patient as a "responder." hypotension is a frequent side effect of high-dose therapy with these agents. Meticulous volume resuscitation should be ensured, and infusion of vasopressor/inotropes may be required. Prolonged use of high dose of propofol can lead to propofol infusion syndrome. Continuous EEG may be used to ensure targeting of the infusion to burst suppression
Hypothermia (<36 °C) is not currently recommended as an initial TBI treatment. Hypothermia should be reversed for "rescue" or salvage therapy after reasonable attempts at ICP control via the previous tier 3 treatments have failed

Management of IC-HTN

Systemic Interventions

Mannitol

If the routine measures have failed to achieve the ICP goals, manipulation of the blood-brain osmotic gradient is a secondary option. Mannitol ($C_6H_8(OH)_6$) is a polyol, sugar alcohol, found in marine algae, mushrooms, and tree sap [51]. Mannitol has two mechanisms of action: (1) a rheologic agent which reduces blood viscosity, thus improving microvascular flow and oxygen delivery, and (2) an osmotic diuretic which initially increases intravascular volume and subsequently cardiac output. It is initially given as a 1 g/kg bolus with repeat dosing at 0.25–0.5 g/kg as needed every 6–8 h. The effects are usually immediate, are maximal after 1 h, and can last for 4–24 h [52]. Repeated uses have been associated with a reversal of the osmotic gradient secondary to blood-brain barrier damage. Additionally, care must be taken to avoid hypovolemia from diuresis which can lower systemic pressure and cerebral perfusion pressure. When mannitol is administered, attention should be given to serum sodium, serum osmolality, and renal function surveillance. The treatment endpoints are a serum sodium of 150 mEq, serum osmolality of 320 mOsm/L [53], or any signs of a decreasing renal function.

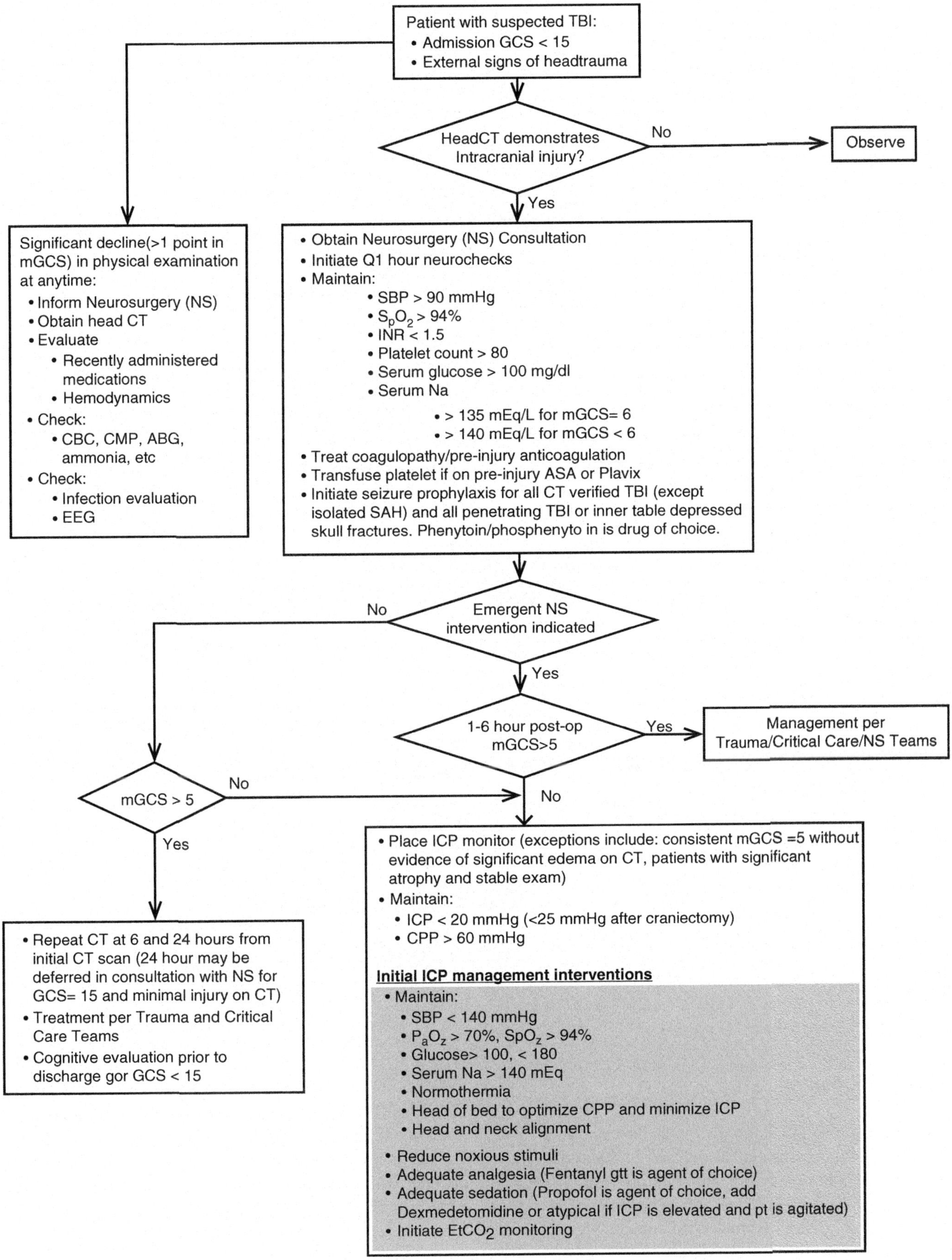

Fig. 2.4 (**a**, **b**) R Adams Cowley Shock Trauma Center Elevated Intracranial Pressure Management Algorithm

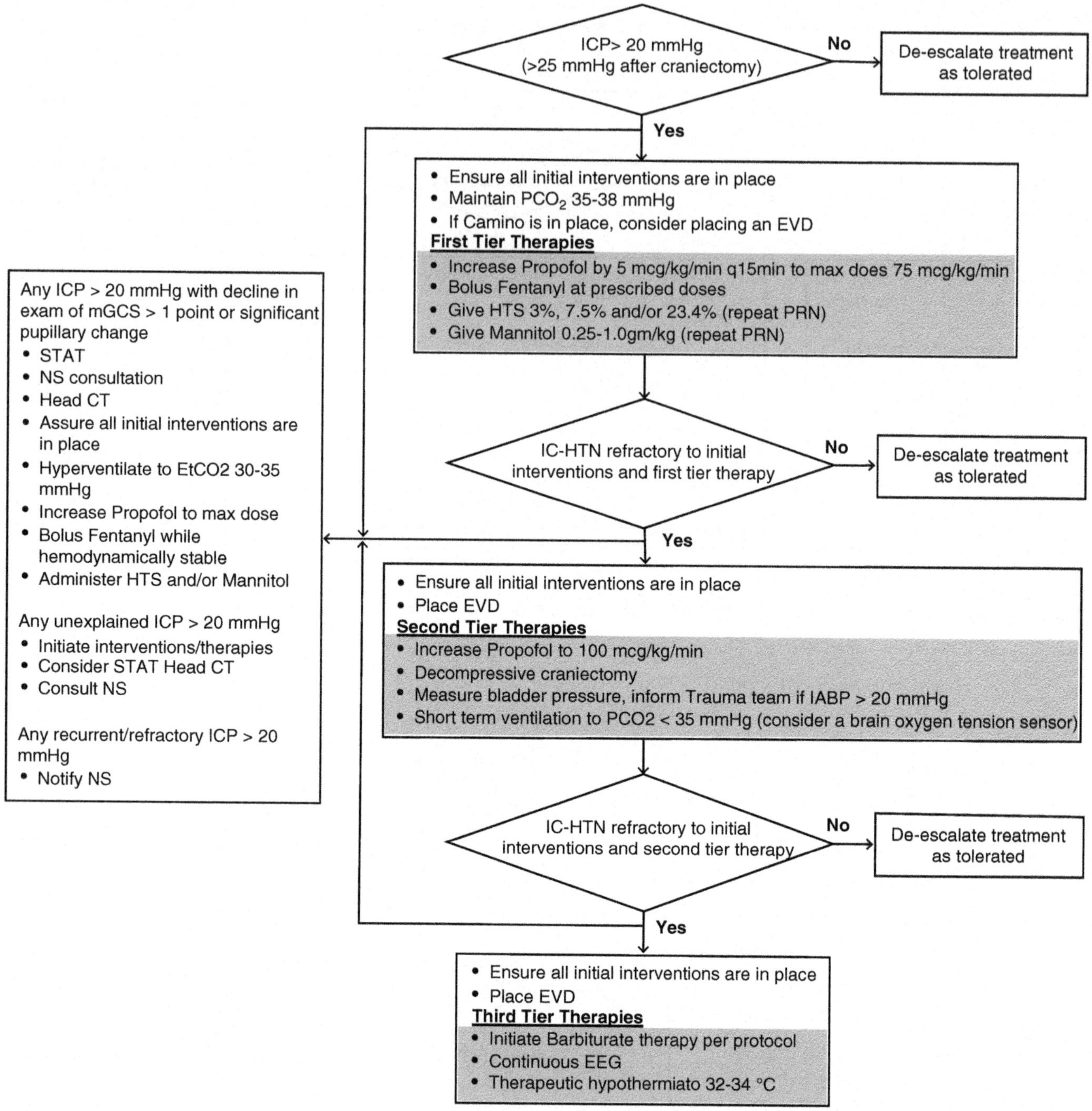

Fig. 2.4 (continued)

Hypertonic Saline

Hypertonic saline (HTS) also increases the osmotic gradient resulting in fluid being pulled into the intravascular space [18, 54]. HTS is dosed as a bolus of 2%, 3%, 7.5%, and 23.4%. Two percent HTS can be administered through a peripheral line, though secondary to concerns for phlebitis, higher concentrations should be given through a central line. The benefits of hypertonic solutions may include an increase in circulating blood volume and maintenance of euvolemia. Central pontine myelinolysis is a known complication in patients with chronic hyponatremia; this is rarely seen in patients with normonatremia.

CSF Removal

The intraventricular ICP monitor's outlet valve, also known as an extraventricular drain (EVD), can be utilized to remove CSF. By placing the valve at a specific height in relation to the auricle, the device will act as a release valve if the ICPs are higher than the desired target pressure threshold [18]. The EVD can be manually used to remove CSF when a threshold is exceeded or a patient's clinical presentation warrants further removal of fluid. By following the patient's clinical examination and tolerance of the desired ICP, an assessment of the EVD's utility and potential removal can be made.

Hyperventilation

Hyperventilation (HPV) is a two-phase process: (1) inspiration, the movement of air into the lungs, and (2) expiration, the removal of CO_2 and other gases from the alveoli. The exchanged CO_2 is in equilibrium with the arterial blood; therefore an increased minute ventilation, respiratory rate times tidal volume, will evacuate a larger volume of CO_2 and decrease the $PaCO_2$. The reduced $PaCO_2$ will cause cerebral vasoconstriction and lower the ICP. Hyperventilation is indicated for: (1) clinical signs of IC-HTN, (2) IC-HTN unresponsive to other interventions, or (3) known hyperemia [18].

A $PaCO_2$ of 30–35 mmHg is the intervention's goal [18]. A $PaCO_2$ reduction from 35 to 29 mmHg will lower the ICP by 25–30%. Hyperventilation below a $PaCO_2$ of 30 mmHg has not been shown to consistently lower the ICP and may further exacerbate the CBF deficit and autoregulation dysfunction [55]. This effect has a rapid onset, < 30 sec, the maximal benefit is seen within 8 min, and the resultant decreased ICP is usually seen for approximately 1 hour. Secondary to concerns for cerebral ischemia and dysfunctional autoregulation, HPV is not recommended within the first 5 days after an injury.

Analgesia

Pain control after trauma is an essential element in patient care; however hypotension is a common side effect of some opioid medications. Administration can result in vasodilation, inhibition of the baroreflexes, and histamine release, all of which lower systolic blood pressure. Patients with an acute TBI are dependent upon their MAP to maintain CBF.

Three commonly used opioids, fentanyl, sufentanil, and morphine, were investigated to determine their effect on ICP [56]. A study population was divided into three groups. Each was given a loading dose followed by a titrated infusion of one drug. A difference in ICP between the three groups was not seen, nor was there a difference in CPP. Additionally, the CPP was not significantly different from individual baseline pressures. The investigators concluded that a slow titration of opioids could be given without encountering adverse hemodynamic effects.

Analogous to these findings, morphine's and fentanyl's effects on cerebral hemodynamics were studied in adult trauma patients with severe TBI [57]. The patients were randomized to receive equivalent doses of either drug. Approximately half of the study population was found to have dysfunctional autoregulation. Even though both opioids caused an increased in ICP and decrease in MAP and CPP, the CBF was unaffected. These findings were seen in patients with and without intact autoregulation. Even though opioid-induced vasodilation was seen, CBF remained intact secondary to other compensatory mechanisms. The opioids are safe to use in patients afflicted with a TBI. The dose and frequency should be selected on clinical judgment and patient tolerance.

Barbiturates

When IC-HTN does not resolve or is poorly controlled, a chemically induced coma may be a fail-safe noninvasive option. Barbiturate usage has been demonstrated to lower the brain's metabolic rate, decrease its oxygen demand, and reduce CBF [58, 59]. Pentobarbital (Nembutal), a short-acting barbiturate, is given in a 5–20 mg/kg loading bolus, followed by a 1–3 mg/kg/h infusion. The therapy can be titrated based upon ICP or burst suppression seen on electroencephalography [60]. Once a therapeutic level has been achieved, the ability to easily perform serial neurologic examinations will be lost. Barbiturate usage has been complicated by hypotension which is correctable by fluid administration or additional vasopressor support. Its routine usage has largely fallen out of favor due to the significant side effect profile and is typically reserved for refractory malignant hypertension as a third-line agent.

Temperature Management

Hypothermia

Therapeutic hypothermia (TH) is the induction of 32–35 °C degree cooling to attenuate secondary injuries. This intervention has been shown to decrease ICP, reduce cerebral edema, and, in some early studies, improve patient outcomes. Study results though have not been consistent. Qiu's group investigated adult patients with a severe TBI randomized to 33–35 °C for 3–5 days versus normothermia [61]. The hypothermia group demonstrated a lower mortality rate (25.6% vs

Table 2.6 Glasgow Outcome Scale

Scale	Outcome
1	Death
2	Vegetative state
3	Severe disability
4	Moderate disability
5	Good recovery

51.2%, $p < 0.05$) and a faster 2-year recovery rate (65.1% vs 37.2%, $p < 0.05$). Additionally the hypothermic group presented a decreased extradural pressure at 24 h (27.3 mmHg ±4.8 mmHg vs 32.6 mmHg ±3.0 mmHg, $p < 0.05$), at 48 h (29.4 mmHg ±4.5 mmHg vs 34.8 mmHg ±6.0 mmHg, $p < 0.05$), and at 72 h (26.4 mmHg ±4.1 mmHg vs 31.8 mmHg ±4.5 mmHg, $p < 0.05$). These encouraging results did not address the duration of cooling necessary to achieve a mortality reduction or favorable outcome.

Jiang's group randomized trauma patients with a severe TBI to long-term, 5 ± 1.3 days, versus short-term, 2 ± 0.6 days, mild hypothermia, 33–35 °C [62]. A favorable Glasgow Outcome Scale (GOS) was seen more often in the long-term group (43.5% vs 29.0%, $p < 0.05$), while an unfavorable outcome was seen more often in the short-term group (56.5% vs 71.0%, $p < 0.05$). The GOS (see Table 2.6) is a metric rating patients by physical disability in performing defined tasks rather than cognitive impairment [63, 64]. Upon rewarming the patients, the short-term group experienced a significant rebound in ICP as compared with the long-term group at the same time point. This was thought to be secondary to dysfunctional autoregulation.

Analogous to these studies, a multicenter randomized clinical trial was performed to determine the effect of early TH on patient outcomes [65]. Adult trauma patients with severe brain injury were randomized to early cooling to 33 °C for 48 h or normothermia. There was no difference in the number of patients who experienced a poor outcome in either group (60% (hypothermia group) vs 56% (normothermia group), RR, 1.08; 95% CI, 0.76–1.53; $p = 0.67$). Additionally, patient mortality was equivalent (23% (hypothermia group) vs 18% (normothermia group), RR, 1.3; 95% CI, 0.58–2.89; $p = 0.52$). Secondary to these early findings, the trial was terminated due to futility.

The European Study of Therapeutic Hypothermia for Intracranial Pressure Reduction after Traumatic Brain Injury (the Eurotherm3235 Trial) was a 5-year multinational randomized controlled trial which also encountered similar results [66]. This study investigated therapeutic hypothermia usage as commonly performed in routine ICU protocols. Three hundred and eighty-seven adult trauma patients with a closed TBI and ICP > 20 mmHg for at least 5 min after initial ICP-lowering interventions were eligible. Patients were randomized to the standard of care group versus the intervention group – therapeutic hypothermia plus standard of care.

Table 2.7 Extended Glasgow Outcome Scale

Scale	Outcome
1	Death
2	Vegetative state
3	Lower severe disability
4	Upper severe disability
5	Lower moderate disability
6	Upper moderate disability
7	Lower good recovery
8	Upper good recovery

The primary outcome, mortality, favored the control group (HR, 1.45; 95% CI, 1.01–2.10; $p = 0.047$). A favorable extended GOS (eGOS), a score of 5–8, was more common in the control group (25.7% vs 36.5%, $p = 0.03$). The eGOS (see Table 2.7) subdivided three of the GOS categories into lower and upper tiers, increasing the measure's sensitivity [67]. The adjusted eGOS odds ratio (OR, 1.53; 95% CI, 1.02–2.30; $p = 0.04$) demonstrated a worse outcome for the hypothermia group. This study was also stopped secondary to safety concerns and the inability to demonstrate that the standard of care supplemented with TH resulted in better outcomes than the standard of care alone.

When the pediatric population was considered, a similar outcome was encountered. A multicenter, multinational, randomized controlled trial investigated children afflicted with severe TBI [68]. Seventy-seven patients were recruited over a 4-year period. They were randomized to the hypothermia group – rapidly cooled with 4 °C saline to 34–35 °C followed by surface cooling to 32–33 °C for 48 h – versus the normothermia group, maintenance of 36.5–37.5 °C. A difference in mortality, complications, or adverse events was not demonstrated. Similar to the aforementioned studies, this trial was also terminated early secondary to futility.

Given all injury patterns, current TH studies have not consistently demonstrated an all-cause mortality reduction [28]. Despite early enthusiasm based on a number of small single center trials, the most recent high quality large studies have failed to demonstrate a benefit and have questionably been associated with harm. Based on current available evidence, TH cannot be recommended as a standard of care intervention but may have a role in malignant IC-HTN untreatable by other means.

Other Considerations

Antiepileptics

Seizure activity is a well-known complication in patients presenting with a GCS < 10, depressed skull fracture, contusion, or intracranial hemorrhage [10]. Increased metabolic activity can lead to elevated ICPs. Phenytoin (Dilantin) and fosphenytoin (Cerebyx) are anticonvulsant which stabilizes sodium efflux from neurons reducing their excitability. Phenytoin has been shown to decrease the seizure risk during the 7-day period immediately following an injury [69]. It is administered as an 18 mg/kg loading dose followed by 100 mg given three times per day. Routine serum levels are followed to ensure the patient is within a therapeutic range. An additional phenytoin bolus can be given, or the routine dose can be held in order to maintain a patient within the therapeutic window. Phenytoin use has been complicated by cardiovascular collapse, pancytopenia, and Stevens-Johnson syndrome.

Although there is no data to support its use, levetiracetam, Keppra, an antiepileptic which acts as a neuromodulator by binding to synaptic vesicle glycoproteins and inhibiting presynaptic calcium channels, is being used by some institutions. It has a decreased side effect profile as compared to phenytoin and does not require surveillance of serum concentration levels. This makes the medication an attractive choice, but large studies demonstrating efficacy are lacking.

Paroxysmal Sympathetic Hyperactivity

The constellation of fever, posturing, tachycardia, hypertension, and diaphoresis is commonly known as "sympathetic storming," paroxysmal sympathetic hyperactivity (PSH), or paroxysmal autonomic dysfunction. Normally a balance between the sympathetic and parasympathetic nervous systems exists. An increase in the sympathetic nervous system discharge is theorized to occur secondary to a disassociation or uncoupling from the parasympathetic system. The clinical presentation can occur hours to weeks after a TBI. A discrete radiographic lesion has not been identified; however diffuse axonal injury has been a common finding.

These hyperactive episodes have been noted to occur after rapid increases in ICP [70], spontaneously, or in association with a noxious trigger such as deep pulmonary suctioning, repositioning, or ambient noise [71]. All events result in a catecholamine surge. Untreated storming can lead to a secondary injury. For example, hyperventilation results in vasoconstriction and decreased CBF and tissue oxygenation. Conversely, hypertensive episodes can cause increased blood flow leading to cerebral edema and potential exacerbation of intracranial hemorrhage. Patients with PSH have experienced longer ICU stays, increased healthcare costs, and worse eGOS scores [70]. Given the numerous organ systems involved, a singular intervention will not comprehensively address autonomic dysfunction, rather a multimodal approach is employed (Table 2.8).

Invasive Interventions

Hematoma Evacuation

After a traumatic event, increased ICPs can occur secondary to hematoma formation, cerebral edema, or CSF obstruction. An acute subdural hematoma (ASDH) results from torn bridging veins and subsequent formation of a crescentic mass against the inner table. ASDHs are associated with a high level of mortality, 50–90%, secondary to the associated brain injury [18]. In the adult population, an ASDH whose thickest point is greater than 1 cm should undergo surgical evacuation. This is usually performed through a craniotomy flap large enough to evacuate the gelatinous hematoma but also adequate enough to identify and address the source of bleeding. A greater than 4-hour delay in evacuation is associated with increased mortality [72]. Patients who underwent an ASDH evacuation within 4 h of injury had a significantly lower mortality than those who did not (30% vs 90%, $p < 0.0001$). This 4-hour intervention threshold was not supported by a similar study which did not find an association with time to intervention and mortality [73].

Epidural hematomas (EDH) occur secondary to temporoparietal skull fractures compromising the middle meningeal artery. They are seen less frequently than ASDHs. The resulting extravascular arterial pressure dissects the dura off the

Table 2.8 Paroxysmal sympathetic hyperactivity treatment options

Indication	Medication	Mechanism of action	Physical effect
Fever	Acetaminophen	Inhibition of cyclooxygenase	Antipyretic
	Bromocriptine	Dopamine receptor agonist	Lowers the hypothalamic temperature threshold, reducing the fever potential
	Chlorpromazine	Dopamine antagonist	Antipyretic
Dystonia	Benzodiazepine	γ-aminobutyric acid receptor type-A receptor agonist	Muscle relaxant, anticonvulsant
	Dantrolene	Inhibits release of intracellular calcium	Decrease muscle tonicity
Tachycardia, Hypertension	Clonidine	α_2-receptor agonist	Adrenergic blockade
	Dexmedetomidine	α_2-adrenergic receptor agonist	Adrenergic blockade
	Propranolol	Nonselective β-blocker	Decrease serum catecholamine levels and metabolic demand
Pain	Morphine	μ-, δ-, κ-receptor agonist	Analgesia

inner table creating a lenticular-shaped mass. These injuries are associated with a 20–55% mortality [18]. Mortality is usually secondary to uncal herniation causing respiratory arrest. Similar to the ASDH, surgical evacuation is required for a symptomatic EDH or radiographic evidence of the thickest measurement greater than 1 cm. Aside from hematoma evacuation and obtaining hemostasis, the surgical objective is to obliterate the potential epidural space by re-approximating the dura against the inner table.

Currently, the Randomized Evaluation of Surgery with Craniectomy for patients Undergoing Evacuation of Acute Subdural Haematoma (RESCUE-ASDH) is a multicenter randomized trial comparing the clinical and cost-effectiveness of a decompressive craniectomy versus craniotomy [74]. This 5-year study will be conducted over 20 international sites with a 1000 patient recruiting goal. The primary endpoint will be the eGOS at a 1-year interval post-injury. The secondary endpoints will be the eGOS at 6 months, hospitalization data, radiographic findings at 1 year, and healthcare utilization data. In a finance capitation healthcare model, this study may help dictate the intervention with greatest outcome per dollar spent.

Decompressive Craniectomy

A decompressive craniectomy (DC) is a well-known and frequently utilized intervention. Decompressive craniectomy involves removing a portion of the skull and allowing the swollen or compromised brain to expand into the extracranial environment. Bone removal alone can result in a 15% ICP reduction. When combined with opening the dura, a 70% reduction can be achieved [75]. This invasive maneuver has been shown to improve cerebral tissue oxygenation [76], cerebral perfusion pressure, and blood flow [77, 78]. While this can be a lifesaving intervention, DC can be complicated by meningitis or empyema requiring a potential second invasive procedure, i.e., cranioplasty.

Decompressive craniectomy is a highly invasive and potentially morbid procedure, and its utility and timing have been extensively studied. Decompressive craniectomies can be performed during the initial surgical decompression (primary or prophylactic) or for refractory IC-HTN (secondary or therapeutic). The indications for each and respective outcomes were recently investigated [79]. Seventy patients with a moderate to severe TBI were divided into primary or secondary DC groups based upon the care given. While a significant difference in GCS and ISS was not seen, the primary DC group had one or both pupils dilated (37.2% vs 4.0%, p = 0.002) and were older (46.3 + 18.5 years old vs 29.7 + 11.3 years old, $p < 0.001$) as compared to the secondary DC group. Additionally, the primary DC group was predominantly a Marshall grade V (79.1%) vs the secondary DC group which was predominantly a Marshall grade III (84.6%), $p < 0.001$. The Marshall grade, which is divided into six tiers, I–VI, is a head injury severity classification (Table 2.9). As expected, each DC group demonstrated a significant decrease in pre- and postoperative ICP – primary DC group (33.5 ± 12.3 mmHg vs 9.1 ± 4.6 mmHg, $p < 0.001$) and secondary DC group (31.1 + 6.0 mmHg vs 14.5 + 11.6 mmHg, $p = 0.046$). When outcomes were examined, the primary group had a lower GOS (2.89 vs 3.69, $p = 0.02$) and a higher mortality rate (40.9% vs 15.4%, $p = 0.026$). Finally, when the determinants for outcome were scrutinized, the odds of death and poor outcome in the primary DC group were significantly higher for patients with a Marshall grade ≥ 4 (OR, 9.72, $p = 0.04$ and OR, 7.50, $p = 0.025$), SDH (OR, 10.62, $p = 0.03$ and OR, 14.06, $p = 0.003$), and age ≥ 40 (OR, 5.83, $p = 0.018$ and OR, 10.56, $p = 0.001$), respectively. These outcome determinants were nonsignificant in the secondary DC group. This study demonstrated that DC timing should be based upon the pathology addressed: surgical lesion (primary) vs intractable IC-HTN (secondary). Additionally this group found differences in population characteristics and physical examination findings which may also serve as indicators for DC timing and outcome.

Table 2.9 Marshall CT classification for head injury

Category	Definition
Diffuse injury I	No visible intracranial pathology seen on CT
Diffuse injury II	Cisterns are present with midline shift (0-5 mm) and/or lesion densities present no high- or mixed-density lesion >25 ml; may include bone fragments and foreign bodies
Diffuse injury III	Cisterns compressed or absent with midline shift (0-5 mm), no high- or mixed-density lesion >25 ml
Diffuse injury IV	Midline shift >5 mm, no high- or mixed-density lesion >25 ml
Diffuse injury V(Evacuated mass lesion)	Any lesion surgically evacuated
Diffuse injury VI(Nonevacuated mass lesion)	High- or mixed-density lesion >25 ml, not surgically evacuated

The timing for a DC was also investigated in the *Decompressive Craniectomy in Diffuse Traumatic Brain Injury (DECRA)* study which was a multicenter, randomized controlled trial designed to determine the efficacy of bifrontotemporoparietal decompressive craniectomy in patients poorly controlled by first-tier interventions [80]. This 8-year study enrolled 155 adult patients. As compared with patients receiving the standard of care, the surgical intervention arm demonstrated a decreased ICP (14.4 ± 6.8 mmHg vs 19.1 ± 8.9 mmHg, $p < 0.001$), fewer mechanical ventilation days (11 days IQR(8,15) vs 15 days IQR (12, 20), $p < 0.001$), and shorter ICU stay (13 days IQR(10–18) vs 18 days IQR (13–24), $p < 0.001$). These patients also had a lower median eGOS (3, IQR(2,5) vs 4, IQR (3–5), $p = 0.03$) and a higher risk for an unfavorable outcome (51% vs 42%, $p = 0.02$). The poor surgical outcomes in this study were thought to be secondary to extracranial cerebral expansion causing axonal stretch [81, 82] and neuronal injury [83, 84] or known surgical complications, i.e., wound infection or hematoma [85]. There have been a number of criticisms of this study including problems with randomization, the fact that the ICP threshold of >20 mmHg for >15 min does not reflect most clinical practice, and a high crossover rate from the standard care arm to the surgical arm.

Contrary to the DECRA study, the Randomized Evaluation of Surgery with Craniectomy for Uncontrollable Elevation of Intracranial Pressure (RESCUEicp) trial evaluated the efficacy of a craniectomy as a third-tier intervention to refractory IC-HTN. This was a 10-year international, multicenter, randomized trial which enrolled 389 patients [86]. The study demonstrated a decreased 6-month mortality in the surgical group (26.9% vs 48.9%). Regarding the eGOS scores, the surgical group also demonstrated higher rates of vegetative states (8.5% vs 2.1%); lower severe disability, dependent on others for care (21.9% vs 14.4%); and lower upper severe disability, independent at home (15.4% vs 8.0%). In contrast to the DECRA trial, this study utilized craniectomy as a third-tier intervention rather than a second-tier. Additionally, they also included patients with an intracranial hematoma and utilized both unilateral and bilateral decompressive craniectomies. This may have led to the improved patient outcomes.

Multiple Compartment Management

Abdominal compartment syndrome is a well-known constellation of intraperitoneal complications, abdominal distension and decreased urine output; intrathoracic complications, decreased pulmonary compliance and poor cardiac output; and vascular complications, decreased venous return. The pliable diaphragm allows for transmission of intraperitoneal pressure to the thorax leading to the aforementioned presentation. Additionally, the open vascular communication will also act as a conduit to transmit pressure. Elevated intra-abdominal pressure (IAP) can escalate to organ compromise resulting in a surgical emergency requiring a pressure-relieving decompressive laparotomy (DL). In patients with a TBI, elevated IAP and intrathoracic pressures (ITP) can manifest as an increase in ICP. This is known as multiple compartment syndrome (MCS). Currently accepted ICP management interventions target the cranial vault and do not directly address IAP and ITP.

MCS and its relationship with ICP and poor outcomes have been well documented. One study reported on 17 cases of intractable ICP elevation requiring a decompressive laparotomy [87]. All patients had maximized current ICP management interventions. Fourteen had undergone a decompressive craniectomy. The ICP decreased from 30.0 ± 4.0 mmHg pre-laparotomy to 17.5 ± 3.2 mmHg after the intervention. All survivors were noted to have a significant decrease in pre- and post-DL, 22 ± 5.8 mmHg versus 16 ± 5.1 mmHg, $p < 0.02$. This decrease was sustained after the procedure. Mortality was associated with a transient decrease in ICP and a nonsignificant change in pre- and post-DL, 20.2 ± 6.7 mmHg versus 23 ± 7.8 mmHg, $p = 0.2$.

Scalea's group investigated current ICP management therapies and the serial application of DC and DL to treat MCS [88]. One hundred and two patients with refractory IC-HTN were studied. Seventy-eight underwent DC. They demonstrated a significant difference in pre- and post-DC ICP, 24 ± 11 mmHg versus 14 ± 8 mmHg, $p < 0.05$. The remaining 24 patients were treated for MCS and underwent a dual DC and DL for MCS. The DC was performed first in 15 patients (DC/DL), and the DL was performed first in the remaining 9 patients (DL/DC). The DC/DL group experienced a decrease in ICP 34 ± 13 mmHg versus 20 ± 12 mmHg, $p < 0.05$, while the DL/DC group experienced a decrease in ICP 25 ± 10 mmHg versus 13 ± 10 mmHg, $p < 0.05$. There was no difference in mortality between the DC and MCS groups, 31% versus 42%, p = NS. It was noted that MCS patients had a significantly higher ISS, pre-DC ICP, and first 7 day of hospitalization fluid requirement as compared with the DC-alone group. It is still difficult to identify the sentinel element for MCS and is most likely multifactorial. Fluid resuscitation related to maintenance of CPP, hypotension, and ICP management goals is one potential adverse factor resulting in MCS. The mean airway pressure was also noted to be higher in the group treated for MCS. This also could be a product of fluid administration leading to interstitial edema resulting in increased ventilator driving pressures. Additionally, the elevated ventilator settings can limit venous return, causing hepatic congestion and edema leading to elevated IAP and poor superior vena caval return resulting in an elevated ICP.

Conclusion

As demonstrated by the multiple well-healed holes found in excavated skulls, early man's ICP management intervention, trepanation, was most likely based upon anecdotal evidence, continued survival. In the modern day, a more advanced form of trepanation, decompressive craniotomy or craniectomy, is utilized within our management armamentarium. We do, however, have multiple other less invasive options available prior to entertaining that ancient intervention. Through evidence-based medicine, numerous guidelines have been developed and incorporated into our daily clinical practices. The Brain Trauma Foundation and other professional organizations continue to refine ICP management recommendations in an effort to improve patient survival. Unlike early man, we will continue to manage and refine our clinical approach to ICP management and improve upon our patient outcomes.

References

1. Hajar R. The air of history: early medicine to galen (part I). Heart Views. 2012;13(3):120–8. https://doi.org/10.4103/1995-705X.102164.
2. Ghannaee Arani M, Fakharian E, Sarbandi F. Ancient legacy of cranial surgery. Arch Trauma Res. 2012;1(2):72–4. https://doi.org/10.5812/atr.6556.
3. Woods M. Ancient medical technology: from herbs to scalpels. Mineapolis: Twenty-first Century Books; 2011.
4. Feldman RP, Goodrich JT. The edwin smith surgical papyrus. Childs Nerv Syst. 1999;15(6–7):281–4.
5. Centers for Disease Control and Prevention. Injury prevention and control: Traumatic brain injury and concussion. https://www.cdc.gov/traumaticbraininjury/index.html. Updated 2016. Accessed 31 Dec 2016.
6. Kushner D. Mild traumatic brain injury: toward understanding manifestations and treatment. Arch Intern Med. 1998;158(15):1617–24.
7. Hardman JM, Manoukian A. Pathology of head trauma. Neuroimaging Clin N Am. 2002;12(2):175–87. vii.
8. Morrison AL, King TM, Korell MA, Smialek JE, Troncoso JC. Acceleration-deceleration injuries to the brain in blunt force trauma. Am J Forensic Med Pathol. 1998;19(2):109–12.
9. Shaw NA. The neurophysiology of concussion. Prog Neurobiol 2002;67(4):281–344. S0301008202000187 [pii].
10. Trauma. 7. New York: McGraw Hill; 2013.
11. Saatman KE, Duhaime AC, Bullock R, et al. Classification of traumatic brain injury for targeted therapies. J Neurotrauma. 2008;25(7):719–38. https://doi.org/10.1089/neu.2008.0586.
12. Defense and Veterans Brain Injury Center. DOD worldwide numbers for TBI. http://dvbic.dcoe.mil/dod-worldwide-numbers-tbi. Updated 2016. Accessed 28 Dec 2016.
13. Centers for Disease Control and Prevention, National Center for Injury Prevention and Control, Division of Unintentional Injury Prevention. Get the stats on traumatic brain injury in the United States. https://www.cdc.gov/traumaticbraininjury/pdf/BlueBook_factsheet-a.pdf. Updated 2016. Accessed 03 Jan 2017.
14. Jennett B, Teasdale G. Aspects of coma after severe head injury. Lancet. 1977;1(8017):878–81. S0140-6736(77)91201-6 [pii].
15. Middleton PM. Practical use of the glasgow coma scale; a comprehensive narrative review of GCS methodology. Australas Emerg Nurs J. 2012;15(3):170–83. https://doi.org/10.1016/j.aenj.2012.06.002.
16. Geocadin R, Bhardwaj A, Mirski M, et al. Traumatic brain injury. Totowa: Humana Press; 2004.
17. Kaye A. Brain tumors: an encyclopedic approach. 2nd ed. New York: Churchill Livingstone; 2001.
18. Greenberg M. Handbook of neurosurgery. 6th ed. New York: Thieme Medical Publishers; 2006.
19. Wilkins R, editor. Neurosurgery. 2nd ed. New York: McGraw-Hill; 1996.
20. Strandgaard S, Andersen GS, Ahlgreen P, Nielsen PE. Visual disturbances and occipital brain infarct following acute, transient hypotension in hypertensive patients. Acta Med Scand. 1984;216(4):417–22.
21. Strandgaard S, Paulson OB. Cerebral blood flow and its pathophysiology in hypertension. Am J Hypertens. 1989;2(6 Pt 1):486–92.
22. Lassen NA, Agnoli A. The upper limit of autoregulation of cerebral blood flow--on the pathogenesis of hypertensive encepholopathy. Scand J Clin Lab Invest. 1972;30(2):113–6.
23. Kaplan NM. Management of hypertensive emergencies. Lancet. 1994;344(8933):1335–38. S0140-6736(94)90696-3 [pii].
24. Brazis P, Masdeu J, Biller J. Localization in clinical neurology. Baltimore: Lippincott Williams & Wilkins; 2007.
25. Blumenfeld H. Neuroanatomy through clinical cases. Sunderland: Sinauer Associates; 2002.
26. Brain Trauma Foundation, American Association of Neurological Surgeons, Congress of Neurological Surgeons, et al. Guidelines for the management of severe traumatic brain injury. VI. Indications for intracranial pressure monitoring. J Neurotrauma. 2007;24(Suppl 1):S37–44. https://doi.org/10.1089/neu.2007.9990.
27. Carney N, Totten AM, O'Reilly C, et al. Guidelines for the management of severe traumatic brain injury, fourth edition. Neurosurgery. 2016. https://doi.org/10.1227/NEU.0000000000001432.
28. Bullock MR, Povlishock JT. Guidelines for the management of severe traumatic brain injury. Editor's commentary. J Neurotrauma. 2007;24 Suppl 1:2 p preceding S1. https://doi.org/10.1089/neu.2007.9998.
29. Narayan RK, Kishore PR, Becker DP, et al. Intracranial pressure (ICP): to monitor or not to monitor? A review of our experience with severe head injury. J Neurosurg. 1982;56(5):650–9. https://doi.org/10.3171/jns.1982.56.5.0650.
30. Guillaume J, Janny P. Continuous intracranial manometry; importance of the method and first results. Rev Neurol (Paris). 1951;84(2):131–42.
31. Kawoos U, McCarron RM, Auker CR, Chavko M. Advances in intracranial pressure monitoring and its significance in managing traumatic brain injury. Int J Mol Sci. 2015;16(12):28979–97. https://doi.org/10.3390/ijms161226146.
32. Association for the Advancement of Medical Instrumentation Imperial County Planning & Development Services, American National Standards Institute. Intracranial pressure monitoring devices; 1993.
33. Mayhall CG, Archer NH, Lamb VA, et al. Ventriculostomy-related infections. A prospective epidemiologic study. N Engl J Med. 1984;310(9):553–9. https://doi.org/10.1056/NEJM198403013100903.
34. Holloway KL, Barnes T, Choi S, et al. Ventriculostomy infections: the effect of monitoring duration and catheter exchange in 584 patients. J Neurosurg. 1996;85(3):419–24. https://doi.org/10.3171/jns.1996.85.3.0419.
35. Alali AS, Fowler RA, Mainprize TG, et al. Intracranial pressure monitoring in severe traumatic brain injury: results from the American College of Surgeons Trauma Quality Improvement Program. J Neurotrauma. 2013;30(20):1737–46. https://doi.org/10.1089/neu.2012.2802.
36. Hemmila MR, Nathens AB, Shafi S, et al. The trauma quality improvement program: pilot study and initial demonstration of feasibility. J Trauma. 2010;68(2):253–62. https://doi.org/10.1097/TA.0b013e3181cfc8e6.
37. Marmarou A, Anderson R, Ward JD. Impact of ICP instability and hypotension on outcome in patients with severe head trauma. J Neurosurg. 1991;75(Supplement):s59–66.
38. Shafi S, Diaz-Arrastia R, Madden C, Gentilello L. Intracranial pressure monitoring in brain-injured patients is associated with worsening of survival. J Trauma. 2008;64(2):335–40. https://doi.org/10.1097/TA.0b013e31815dd017.
39. The Brain Trauma Foundation. The American Association of Neurological Surgeons. The Joint Section on Neurotrauma and

Critical Care. Indications for intracranial pressure monitoring. J Neurotrauma. 2000;17(6–7):479–91. https://doi.org/10.1089/neu.2000.17.479.
40. Shen L, Wang Z, Su Z, et al. Effects of intracranial pressure monitoring on mortality in patients with severe traumatic brain injury: a meta-analysis. PLoS One. 2016;11(12):e0168901. https://doi.org/10.1371/journal.pone.0168901.
41. Chesnut RM, Temkin N, Carney N, et al. A trial of intracranial-pressure monitoring in traumatic brain injury. N Engl J Med. 2012;367(26):2471–81. https://doi.org/10.1056/NEJMoa1207363.
42. Chesnut RM. Intracranial pressure monitoring: headstone or a new head start. The BEST TRIP trial in perspective. Intensive Care Med. 2013;39(4):771–4. https://doi.org/10.1007/s00134-013-2852-9.
43. Cardim D, Robba C, Bohdanowicz M, et al. Non-invasive monitoring of intracranial pressure using transcranial doppler ultrasonography: is it possible? Neurocrit Care. 2016;25(3):473–91. https://doi.org/10.1007/s12028-016-0258-6.
44. Schmidt B, Czosnyka M, Klingelhofer J. Clinical applications of a non-invasive ICP monitoring method. Eur J Ultrasound. 2002;16(1–2):37–45. S0929826602000447 [pii].
45. Glaser J, Vasquez M, Cardarelli C, et al. Through the looking glass: early non-invasive imaging in TBI predicts the need for interventions. Trauma Sur Acute Care Open. 2016;1(1):1–6.
46. Morrison CA, Carrick MM, Norman MA, et al. Hypotensive resuscitation strategy reduces transfusion requirements and severe postoperative coagulopathy in trauma patients with hemorrhagic shock: preliminary results of a randomized controlled trial. J Trauma. 2011;70(3):652–63. https://doi.org/10.1097/TA.0b013e31820e77ea.
47. McHugh GS, Engel DC, Butcher I, et al. Prognostic value of secondary insults in traumatic brain injury: results from the IMPACT study. J Neurotrauma. 2007;24(2):287–93. https://doi.org/10.1089/neu.2006.0031.
48. Kunth T, Letarte P, Ling G, et al. Guidelines for the field management of combat-related head trauma. 1st ed. New York: Brain Trauma Foundation; 2005.
49. American College of Surgeons Trauma Quality Improvement Program. ACS TQIP best practices in the management of traumatic brain injury. https://www.facs.org/~/media/files/quality%20programs/trauma/tqip/traumatic%20brain%20injury%20guidelines.ashx. Updated 2016. Accessed 07 Jan 2017.
50. Bullock R, Chesnut R, Clifton G, et al. Part 1: guidelines for the management of severe head trauma. In: Brain Trauma Foundation, editor. Management and prognosis of severe traumatic brain injury. 2nd ed. New York: Brain Trauma Foundation; 2000.
51. Shawkat H, Westwood M, Mortimer A. Mannitol: a review of its clinical uses; 2012.
52. Jafar JJ, Johns LM, Mullan SF. The effect of mannitol on cerebral blood flow. J Neurosurg. 1986;64(5):754–9. https://doi.org/10.3171/jns.1986.64.5.0754.
53. Diringer MN, Zazulia AR. Osmotic therapy: fact and fiction. Neurocrit Care. 2004;1(2):219–33. NCC:1:2:219 [pii].
54. Mortazavi MM, Romeo AK, Deep A, et al. Hypertonic saline for treating raised intracranial pressure (ICP): literature review with meta-analysis. J Neurosurg. 2012;116(1):210–21. https://doi.org/10.3171/2011.7.JNS102142.
55. Obrist WD, Langfitt TW, Jaggi JL, Cruz J, Gennarelli TA. Cerebral blood flow and metabolism in comatose patients with acute head injury. Relationship to intracranial hypertension. J Neurosurg. 1984;61(2):241–53. https://doi.org/10.3171/jns.1984.61.2.0241.
56. Lauer KK, Connolly LA, Schmeling WT. Opioid sedation does not alter intracranial pressure in head injured patients. Can J Anaesth. 1997;44(9):929–33. https://doi.org/10.1007/BF03011963.
57. de Nadal M, Munar F, Poca MA, Sahuquillo J, Garnacho A, Rossello J. Cerebral hemodynamic effects of morphine and fentanyl in patients with severe head injury: absence of correlation to cerebral autoregulation. Anesthesiology. 2000;92(1):11–9.
58. Marshall LF, Shapiro HM, Rauscher A, Kaufman NM. Pentobarbital therapy for intracranial hypertension in metabolic coma. Reye's syndrome. Crit Care Med. 1978;6(1):1–5.
59. Nordstrom CH, Messeter K, Sundbarg G, Schalen W, Werner M, Ryding E. Cerebral blood flow, vasoreactivity, and oxygen consumption during barbiturate therapy in severe traumatic brain lesions. J Neurosurg. 1988;68(3):424–31. https://doi.org/10.3171/jns.1988.68.3.0424.
60. Clifton GL, Miller ER, Choi SC, Levin HS. Fluid thresholds and outcome from severe brain injury. Crit Care Med. 2002;30(4):739–45.
61. Qiu WS, Liu WG, Shen H, et al. Therapeutic effect of mild hypothermia on severe traumatic head injury. Chin J Traumatol. 2005;8(1):27–32.
62. Jiang JY, Xu W, Li WP, et al. Effect of long-term mild hypothermia or short-term mild hypothermia on outcome of patients with severe traumatic brain injury. J Cereb Blood Flow Metab. 2006;26(6):771–76. 9600253 [pii].
63. Wilson JT, Pettigrew LE, Teasdale GM. Structured interviews for the glasgow outcome scale and the extended glasgow outcome scale: guidelines for their use. J Neurotrauma. 1998;15(8):573–85. https://doi.org/10.1089/neu.1998.15.573.
64. Jennett B, Bond M. Assessment of outcome after severe brain damage. Lancet. 1975;1(7905):480–4.
65. Clifton GL, Valadka A, Zygun D, et al. Very early hypothermia induction in patients with severe brain injury (the national acute brain injury study: hypothermia II): a randomised trial. Lancet Neurol. 2011;10(2):131–9. https://doi.org/10.1016/S1474-4422(10)70300-8.
66. Andrews PJ, Sinclair HL, Rodriguez A, et al. Hypothermia for intracranial hypertension after traumatic brain injury. N Engl J Med. 2015;373(25):2403–12. https://doi.org/10.1056/NEJMoa1507581.
67. Teasdale GM, Pettigrew LE, Wilson JT, Murray G, Jennett B. Analyzing outcome of treatment of severe head injury: a review and update on advancing the use of the glasgow outcome scale. J Neurotrauma. 1998;15(8):587–97. https://doi.org/10.1089/neu.1998.15.587.
68. Adelson PD, Wisniewski SR, Beca J, et al. Comparison of hypothermia and normothermia after severe traumatic brain injury in children (cool kids): a phase 3, randomised controlled trial. Lancet Neurol. 2013;12(6):546–53. https://doi.org/10.1016/S1474-4422(13)70077-2.
69. Temkin NR, Dikmen SS, Wilensky AJ, Keihm J, Chabal S, Winn HR. A randomized, double-blind study of phenytoin for the prevention of post-traumatic seizures. N Engl J Med. 1990;323(8):497–502. https://doi.org/10.1056/NEJM199008233230801.
70. Hinson HE, Sheth KN. Manifestations of the hyperadrenergic state after acute brain injury. Curr Opin Crit Care. 2012;18(2):139–45. https://doi.org/10.1097/MCC.0b013e3283513290.
71. Lemke DM. Riding out the storm: sympathetic storming after traumatic brain injury. J Neurosci Nurs. 2004;36(1):4–9.
72. Seelig JM, Becker DP, Miller JD, Greenberg RP, Ward JD, Choi SC. Traumatic acute subdural hematoma: major mortality reduction in comatose patients treated within four hours. N Engl J Med. 1981;304(25):1511–8. https://doi.org/10.1056/NEJM198106183042503.
73. Wilberger JE Jr, Harris M, Diamond DL. Acute subdural hematoma: morbidity, mortality, and operative timing. J Neurosurg. 1991;74(2):212–8. https://doi.org/10.3171/jns.1991.74.2.0212.
74. University of Cambridge Department of Clinical Neurosciences. The official RESCUE-ASDH trial web site. http://www.rescueasdh.org/home. Updated 2016. Accessed 02 Jan 2017.
75. Jourdan C, Convert J, Mottolese C, Bachour E, Gharbi S, Artru F. Evaluation of the clinical benefit of decompression

hemicraniectomy in intracranial hypertension not controlled by medical treatment. Neurochirurgie. 1993;39(5):304–10.
76. Jaeger M, Soehle M, Meixensberger J. Effects of decompressive craniectomy on brain tissue oxygen in patients with intracranial hypertension. J Neurol Neurosurg Psychiatry. 2003;74(4):513–5.
77. Kunze E, Meixensberger J, Janka M, Sorensen N, Roosen K. Decompressive craniectomy in patients with uncontrollable intracranial hypertension. Acta Neurochir Suppl. 1998;71:16–8.
78. Schneider GH, Bardt T, Lanksch WR, Unterberg A. Decompressive craniectomy following traumatic brain injury: ICP, CPP and neurological outcome. Acta Neurochir Suppl. 2002;81:77–9.
79. Al-Jishi A, Saluja RS, Al-Jehani H, Lamoureux J, Maleki M, Marcoux J. Primary or secondary decompressive craniectomy: different indication and outcome. Can J Neurol Sci. 2011;38(4):612–20. M0Q2UM4871541226 [pii].
80. Cooper DJ, Rosenfeld JV, Murray L, et al. Decompressive craniectomy in diffuse traumatic brain injury. N Engl J Med. 2011;364(16):1493–502. https://doi.org/10.1056/NEJMoa1102077.
81. Cooper PR, Hagler H, Clark WK, Barnett P. Enhancement of experimental cerebral edema after decompressive craniectomy: implications for the management of severe head injuries. Neurosurgery. 1979;4(4):296–300.
82. Stiver SI. Complications of decompressive craniectomy for traumatic brain injury. Neurosurg Focus. 2009;26(6):E7. https://doi.org/10.3171/2009.4.FOCUS0965.
83. Chung RS, Staal JA, McCormack GH, et al. Mild axonal stretch injury in vitro induces a progressive series of neurofilament alterations ultimately leading to delayed axotomy. J Neurotrauma. 2005;22(10):1081–91. https://doi.org/10.1089/neu.2005.22.1081.
84. Staal JA, Dickson TC, Gasperini R, Liu Y, Foa L, Vickers JC. Initial calcium release from intracellular stores followed by calcium dysregulation is linked to secondary axotomy following transient axonal stretch injury. J Neurochem. 2010;112(5):1147–55. https://doi.org/10.1111/j.1471-4159.2009.06531.x.
85. Gooch MR, Gin GE, Kenning TJ, German JW. Complications of cranioplasty following decompressive craniectomy: analysis of 62 cases. Neurosurg Focus. 2009;26(6):E9. https://doi.org/10.3171/2009.3.FOCUS0962.
86. Hutchinson PJ, Kolias AG, Timofeev IS, et al. Trial of decompressive craniectomy for traumatic intracranial hypertension. N Engl J Med. 2016;375(12):1119–30. https://doi.org/10.1056/NEJMoa1605215.
87. Joseph DK, Dutton RP, Aarabi B, Scalea TM. Decompressive laparotomy to treat intractable intracranial hypertension after traumatic brain injury. J Trauma. 2004;57(4):687–93; discussion 693–5. 00005373-200410000-00001 [pii].
88. Scalea TM, Bochicchio GV, Habashi N, et al. Increased intra-abdominal, intrathoracic, and intracranial pressure after severe brain injury: multiple compartment syndrome. J Trauma. 2007;62(3):647–56. discussion 656. https://doi.org/10.1097/TA.0b013e31802ee542.

Spinal Cord Injury

3

Michael Hernon and George Kasotakis

Introduction

Spinal cord injury, the devastating sequela of spinal trauma, results in a wide spectrum of neurologic disability – depending on level and severity – with major emotional and financial ramifications for both patients and caretakers. Despite advances in imaging technology, critical and surgical care, specialized in-hospital management, and skilled rehabilitation, morbidity and mortality from spinal cord injury remain very high.

Approximately 17,000 new spinal cord injuries occurred in 2016 in the United States alone, according to the National Spinal Cord Injury Statistical Center [1]. There has been a steady rise in the incidence of spinal cord injuries over the past decade, with approximately 6000 more cases recorded annually now compared to 2009. This rise is most likely secondary to heightened awareness and improved diagnostic modalities and documentation. The prevalence of spinal cord injuries has also been on the rise, likely due to better acute and long-term management, with an estimated 282,000 people living with it in the United States alone.

The overwhelming majority of patients diagnosed with spinal cord injury are males with an average age of 42 years. The most common mechanism of injury is motor vehicle collisions, followed by falls, acts of violence, and sporting accidents. The latter account for less than 9% of all spinal cord injuries; however, they appear to receive a disproportionate amount of media attention.

The healthcare expenditure associated with spinal cord injuries is extraordinary, with an estimated annual cost of over five billion dollars in the United States alone [2]. Unsurprisingly, the costs incurred per patient correlate closely with the degree of neurologic impairment. Life expectancy is also significantly reduced in spinal cord injury victims. Mortality is the highest during the first year after diagnosis, compared to each subsequent year, and the two most common causes of death are pneumonia and sepsis.

M. Hernon · G. Kasotakis (✉)
Department of Surgery, Boston University School of Medicine, Boston Medical Center, Boston, MA, USA
e-mail: gkasot@bu.edu

Acute Management

Any suspicion for vertebral column injury (high-energy impact or high-intensity deceleration force, asymmetry in or loss of sensorimotor function) requires immediate in-line spinal immobilization, including rigid cervical collar, lateral support, and full spinal immobilization on a hard backboard. The spine must remain in a neutral position, and any patient movement should be conducted using the logrolling technique. Maintaining appropriate oxygenation and ventilation is crucial, in order to minimize secondary insult to the highly oxygen-sensitive neurons, and securing the airway – typically with an endotracheal tube – may be necessary, especially in high spinal cord injuries, in which partial or complete denervation of the diaphragm and accessory respiratory muscles may have occurred. Intubation in patients with suspected spinal cord injury may prove technically challenging in the setting of spinal immobilization, due to inability to hyperextend the neck and directly visualize the vocal cords.

The second mainstay toward preventing secondary insult is to promote hemodynamic stability, as even minor blood pressure fluctuations may further injure the spinal cord neural cells and adversely affect long-term outcomes. Appropriate resuscitation should be considered in all patients with suspected or confirmed spinal cord injury, in addition to quickly addressing any other potential source of hemodynamic instability. Patients with high spinal cord injuries may present with neurogenic shock, typically manifesting as hypotension and bradycardia in a warm and flushed patient, due to a decrease in the sympathetic tone enervating the heart

A. Salim et al. (eds.), *Surgical Critical Care Therapy*, https://doi.org/10.1007/978-3-319-71712-8_3

and peripheral vascular system. Vasopressors are commonly used in such patients, in an attempt to restore part of the vascular tone and maintain a perfusing pressure. Norepinephrine (an alpha and beta-1 adrenergic agonist) is one of the most commonly used pressors to support the low peripheral vascular resistance while increasing heart rate and cardiac output with its positive chronotropic and inotropic effects. Phenylephrine (pure alpha adrenergic agonist) is avoided in general, as its unopposed alpha adrenergic activity may worsen bradycardia. Phenylephrine may be considered in low spinal cord injuries, in which tachycardia may be present as a compensatory mechanism. Atropine can also be considered acutely for bradycardia, until positive chronotropy can be achieved medically or transcutaneous pacing is available.

Classification of Injury and Clinical Diagnosis of Spinal Cord Injury

The American Spinal Injury Association (ASIA) impairment scale is used by many centers to quantify the degree of neurological impairment (Fig. 3.1). The neurological level of injury is considered the most caudal level at which sensory and motor functions are intact. The motor level is considered the most caudal level at which a muscle group has full range of motion against gravity but no resistance, while the sensory level is the most caudal dermatome to have normal sensation to pinprick and crude touch (Fig. 3.2). The skeletal level on injury correlates with radiological findings.

There are multiple spinal cord syndromes that are classic in appearance, due to the neurologic pathways they affect:

Complete cord transection is the most common of all spinal cord syndromes and typically follows a severely displaced vertebral body fracture or olisthesis that significantly compromises the spinal canal (Fig. 3.3). It typically manifests with loss of sensorimotor and autonomic function below the level of the injury.

Central cord syndrome occurs typically in the elderly with degenerative disease resulting from hyperextension. The syndrome is seen with motor dysfunction of the upper extremities, particularly the distal muscle groups. Sensory dysfunction is usually variable, but most commonly seen is loss of pain and temperature sensation in the upper extremities with sacral sparing and usual preservation of bladder and bowel function (Fig. 3.4).

Anterior cord syndrome is usually secondary to a vascular insult of the anterior spinal artery, commonly presenting as complete motor dysfunction below the level of injury, in addition to pain and temperature sensory dysfunction with intact vibration. Bladder and bowel function are also usually impaired with anterior cord syndrome (Fig. 3.4).

Brown-Sequard syndrome is most commonly caused by penetrating trauma to the cord and results in complete loss of half of the spinal cord. It clinically manifests as ipsilateral motor and proprioception loss with contralateral loss of pain and temperature sensation (Fig. 3.4).

Cauda equina syndrome is a syndrome with compression of the lumbar plexus resulting in lower extremity paralysis with bowel and bladder dysfunction in addition to perineal sensory deficits.

Spinal shock, not to be confused with neurogenic shock (described below), manifests as a syndrome of flaccid paralysis with areflexia that over time becomes tonic paralysis with hyperreflexia.

Diagnostic Workup

After initial stabilization, diagnosing vertebral body fractures is essential to treatment. For this purpose, the gold standard diagnostic modality currently is a fine-cut multi-view helical computed tomography (CT) scan. This has supplanted plain radiographs in most trauma centers around the world. Clinical examination with direct palpation of the spine is of course the main stay of initial evaluation to assess for pain, deformity, or any step-offs. Any abnormalities identified during clinical examination, typically mandate diagnostic imaging.

Patients with suspected spinal cord injury who are unable to have a proper clinical examination due to altered mental status (sedated, mechanically ventilated patients, or those with clinically significant brain injury) will commonly require diagnostic imaging to clear cervical spinal precautions. CT imaging has been found to be the most sensitive imaging modality in detecting fractures and usually the first to be obtained; however, magnetic resonance imaging (MRI) is superior in diagnosing ligamentous injuries and spinal cord hematomas that may be missed otherwise in as many as 23.6% of all patients with a negative c-spine CT [3] and should be considered in subjects with unexplained neurologic findings.

Treatment

The primary injury is classified as the mechanical injury to the cord itself which can be classified as compression, laceration, contusion, impaction, and shear injury [4]. The role of surgery is to stabilize the column and aid in preventing further spinal cord trauma. Secondary injuries occur after the initial injury and relate to the pathological changes that arise following a spinal cord injury including a neuroinflammatory cascade and immune dysregulation. Clinical investigation is ongoing in an effort to identify therapeutic agents that may improve neurological function and minimize this secondary injury.

Spinal Immobilization

Spinal immobilization for 6–8 weeks remains the mainstay of treatment for all stable fractures, to allow for fracture union to occur spontaneously. This immobilization can be achieved with collars for the cervical spine or braces (that limit the mobility of the torso) for the thoracic and lumbar spine. The majority of compression fractures can be managed nonoperatively with the exception of injuries showing significant kyphosis >30° or anterior height loss >40% [5].

Surgical Fixation

Surgical fixation is recommended in cases where the structural integrity and stability of the vertebral column is compromised. Historical teaching recommended surgical fixation to take place after patients were stabilized systemically; however, newer data suggest that early operative intervention may improve neurological outcomes [6] and afford lower pneumonia rates and shorter duration of mechanical ventilation and hospital stays [7]. Class II evidence is now available from multiple prospective and retrospective reviews demonstrating the superiority of early decompression and stabilization with in the first 72 h of presentation, compared to delayed (>7 days) surgical management.

Corticosteroids

Corticosteroids have been studied as an adjunct toward minimizing secondary injury and improving neurologic function. The basis for steroid use in spinal cord injury has been twofold: their anti-inflammatory effects may decrease local edema and hence cord compression; they may minimize lipid peroxidation on neuron cell membranes, enhancing their survival and function [8].

Fig. 3.1 The American Spinal Injury Association (ASIA) impairment scale (Adapted from http://asia-spinalinjury.org/wp-content/uploads/2016/02/International_Stds_Diagram_Worksheet.pdf)

A	**Complete**	No sensory or motor function of Sacral Dermatome S4-5
B	**Incomplete**	Only sensory function including Sacral Dermatome S4-5 below level of injury intact
C	**Incomplete**	Motor Function intact below level of injury with ½ muscle groups motor score < 3 (ROM against gravity)
D	**Incomplete**	Motor function intact below level of injury with ½ muscle groups motor score > 3 (ROM against gravity)
E	**Normal**	Motor and sensory function intact

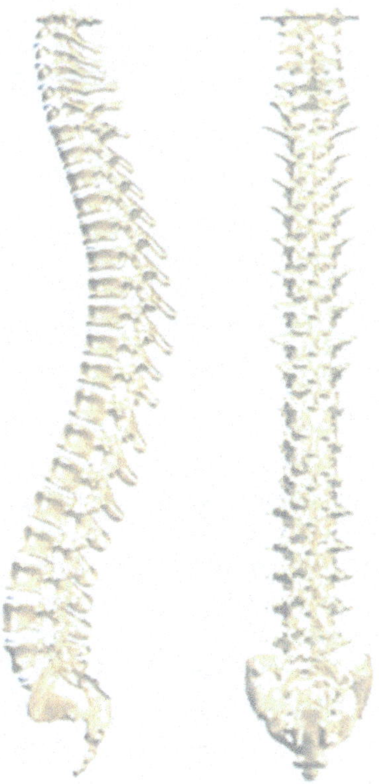

Spinal Cord Level	Function
C_3-C_5	Diaphragrm Function
C_5-C_6	Elbow Flexion (Bicep Function)
C_6-C_7	Elbow Extension (Tricep function)
C_7-C_8	Wrist Flexion
T_1-T_6	Intercostal/abdominal muscle function
L_1-L_4	Thigh flexion
L_2-L_4	Thigh adduction
L_4-S_1	Thigh abduction, knee flexion, foot dorsiflexion
L_5-S_2	Leg extension, plantar flexion

Fig. 3.2 (**a**) Neurologic findings at various levels of spinal cord injury. (**b**) Spinal cord dermatome map

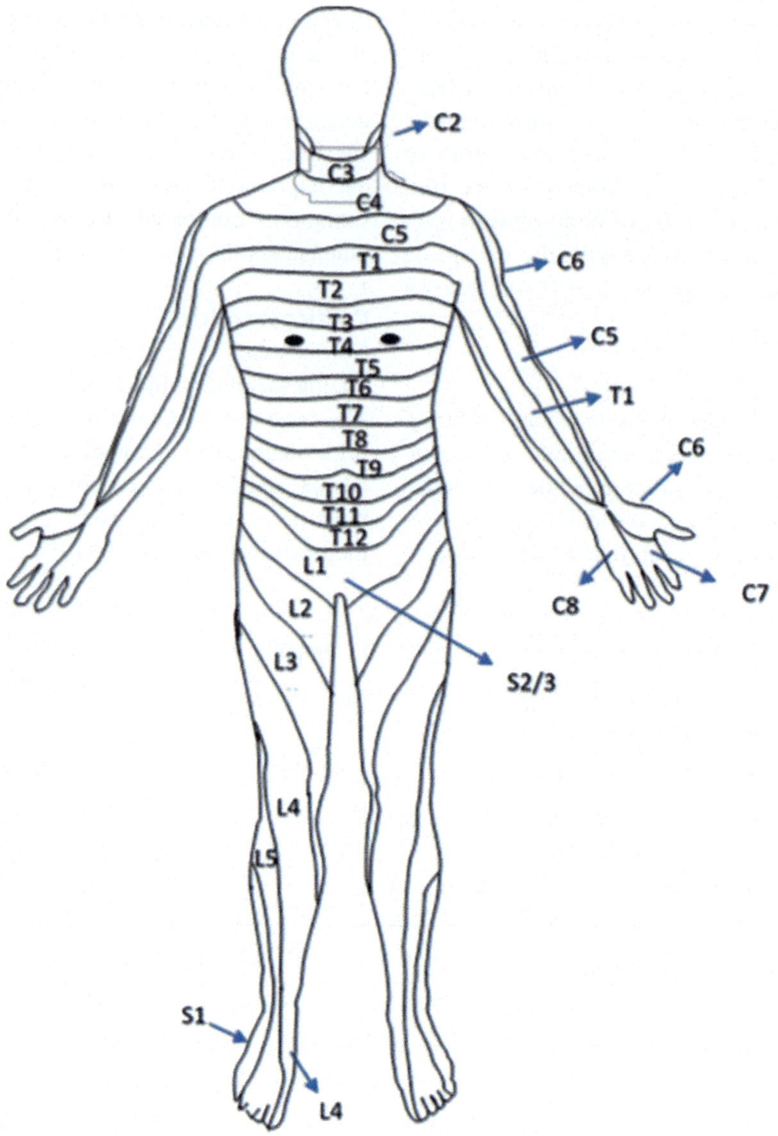

Fig. 3.2 (continued)

The role of corticosteroids in the treatment of blunt spinal cord injuries has been a topic of controversy. The NASCIS I (methylprednisolone ×10 days post-injury [9]) and II (methylprednisolone vs. naloxone and placebo [10]) trials failed to demonstrate improvement in the long-term neurologic outcome, with a higher incidence of steroid-related adverse events (wound infections, gastrointestinal hemorrhage, and thromboembolic events). A subgroup that received methylprednisolone within 8 h post-injury demonstrated improved neurologic recovery, a finding that led to the NASCIS III (methylprednisolone vs. tirilazad mesylate within 8 h after injury) trial. The 1-year neurologic recovery was slightly improved in the steroid group, again at the expense of a high incidence of infectious complications. With these findings, recent guidelines advocate against the use of corticosteroids in spinal cord injuries due to their limited efficacy and high rates of infectious complications [11].

Gangliosides

Gangliosides are glycosphingolipids that are abundant in neural membranes and appear to play a key role in cell-cell signal transduction. Results from an early phase III clinical trial were encouraging in reducing mortality and improving neurologic function [12]; however, those did not materialize in subsequent studies and meta-analyses [13, 14] and are thus not currently recommended.

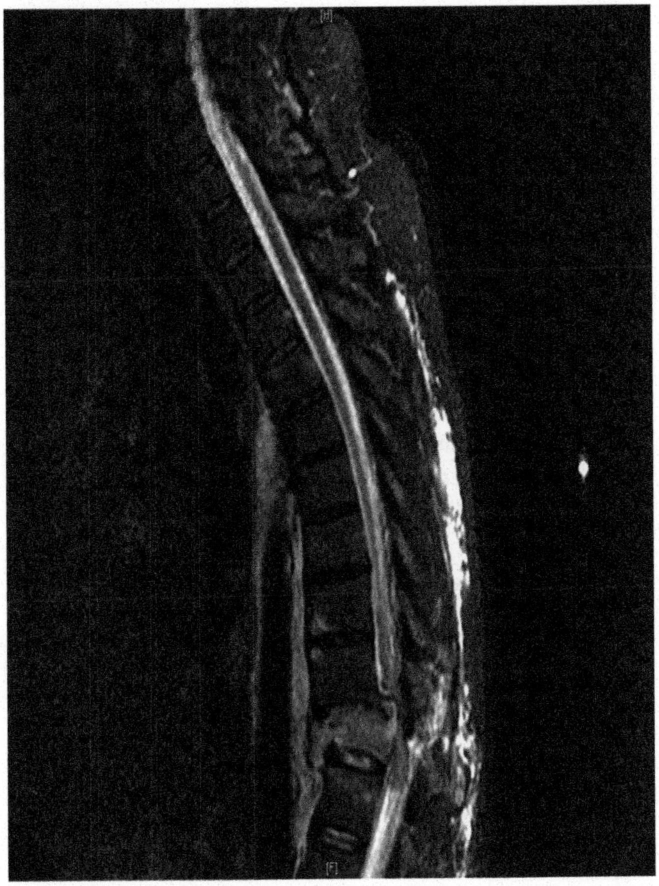

Fig. 3.3 Traumatic burst fracture of T11 resulting in significant retropulsion with near complete spinal cord disruption

Riluzole

Riluzole, a known anticonvulsant, is used in the treatment of amyotrophic lateral sclerosis. Its neuroprotective effect is mediated by calcium influx inhibition and prevention of neuronal excitotoxicity [15]. It has been surmised that Riluzole may have a role in aiding functional recovery following spinal cord injury, and a recent phase 1 trial demonstrated enhanced motor recovery at 3 months when compared to a controlled registry [16]. Currently, a phase III trial is being undertaken by the AOSpine North America Research Network.

Systemic Hypertension

Systemic hypertension, defined as a mean arterial pressure of 85 mm Hg, commonly achieved with the use of pressors – typically norepinephrine – has been found to have a beneficial effect on neurological outcome in spinal cord injuries. The "MAP push," as it is commonly called, is undertaken for 5–7 days post-injury. Multiple studies have demonstrated this MAP push to improve recovery with better long-term ASIA scores, especially when used in the acute period [17, 18].

Hypothermia

Research is ongoing on the role of hypothermia toward improving functional outcomes after spinal cord injury. The premise is that lower core temperatures may decelerate the neuron metabolic processes and lessen the destructive secondary injury cascade. However, most studies are preliminary at this point [19], and larger prospective multicenter randomized trials are pending.

Systemic Sequelae of Spinal Cord Injury

Spinal cord injury has been found to impact most systemic functions. The highest impact is seen in patients with high cervical injuries and low ASIA scores. Patients with clinically significant spinal cord injuries are found to have the lowest morbidity and mortality rates when cared for in an ICU setting, although both early and late systemic complications are common.

Pulmonary

Respiratory complications are the most common following spinal cord injury, likely due to weakened respiratory muscles and inability to handle secretions leading to aspiration, pneumonia, atelectasis, and even acute respiratory distress syndrome. Mortality may be as high as 18–30% in quadriplegics secondary to pulmonary complications [20]. It is of the utmost importance to be mindful of potential high vertebral column instability, should the need for intubation arise and maintain spinal cord alignment at all times. To this end, fiberoptic endoscopy and video laryngoscopy may prove invaluable in accessing the airway safely.

In intubated spinal cord injury victims, aggressive pulmonary therapy is crucial in minimizing pulmonary morbidity and associated mortality. Bronchodilators, chest physiotherapy, frequent pulmonary toilet, and rotational bed therapy have all been shown to improve respiratory complications. Tracheostomy may also be required in the setting of a high spinal cord injury that affects the respiratory muscles. Early versus late tracheostomy has been debated for many years. In patients having undergone spinal surgery via anterior neck incisions, this usually precludes early tracheostomy secondary to surgical healing and risk of hardware infection. A recent meta-analysis demonstrated no difference in the duration of mechanical ventilation, ventilator-associated pneumonia risk, and mortality, while the only benefit achieved was less sedation required [21]. In cases of complete phrenic denervation of the diaphragm (injuries above the C3 level), percutaneous stimulation of the diaphragm may be consid-

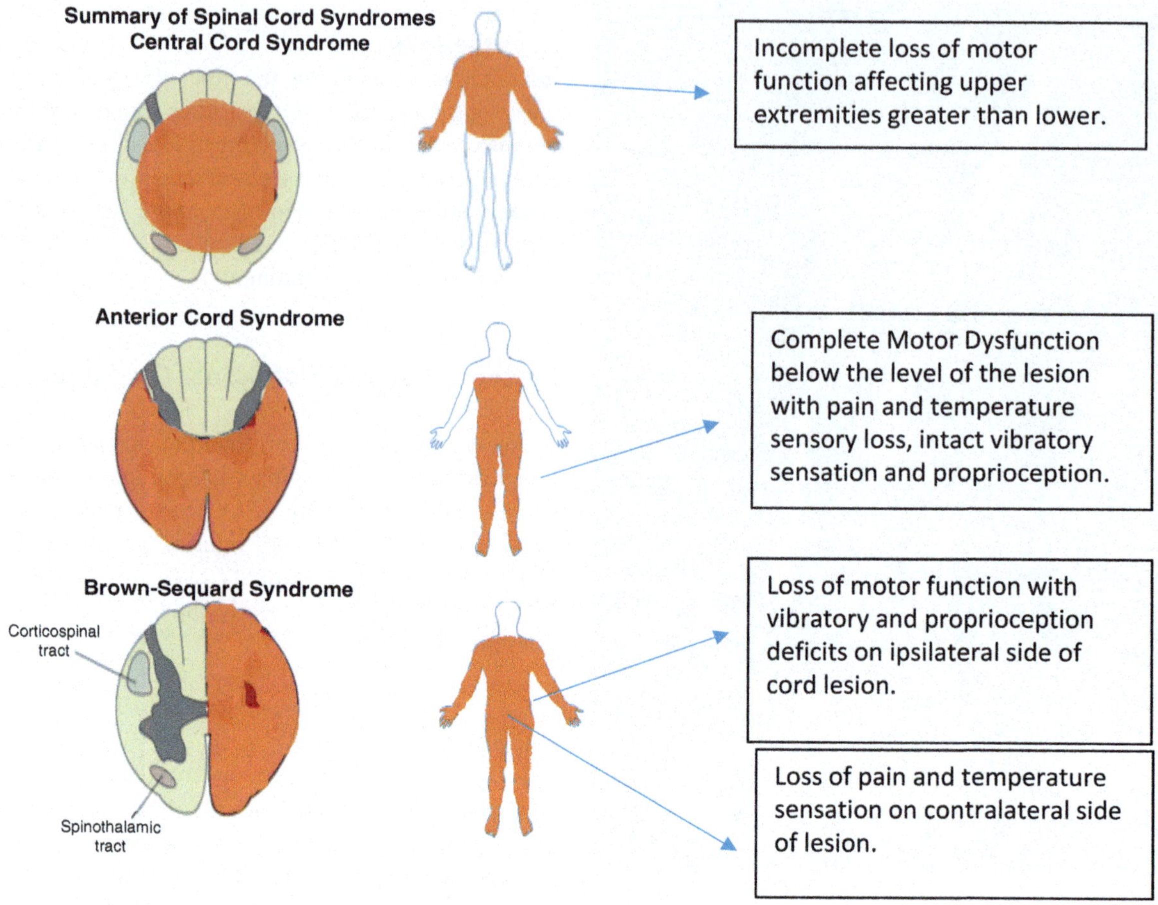

Fig. 3.4 Spinal cord syndromes

ered, via exogenous electrical stimulation. Electrodes are attached to the diaphragmatic muscle typically with laparoscopy, while a pacemaker is implanted in the abdominal subcutaneous tissue. Compared to long-term mechanical ventilation, fewer pulmonary complications, improved venous return, physiologic breathing, phonation and swallowing, and enhanced patient mobility can be achieved with significant cost savings [22].

Cardiovascular

Hemodynamic instability is seen in spinal cord injury especially in patients with injuries above T6. This results in sympathetic disruption and an unopposed vagal tone which results in bradycardia and profound hypotension secondary to vasodilation. This is termed *neurogenic shock*. The treatment of neurogenic shock is supportive with fluid resuscitation and vasopressor administration, typically norepinephrine. Vasodilation may also occur with lower spinal cord injuries, although in this setting, reflex tachycardia may be present, as the sympathetic enervation to the heart is maintained. Phenylephrine may be utilized in such instances. Although compensatory mechanisms typically develop in the chronic phase in the majority of cases, an oral alpha 1 adrenergic agonist, such as midodrine, may be considered, to minimize dependence on intravenous vasoactive drips [23].

Gastrointestinal

High rates of ileus and gastrointestinal immobility have been described in spinal cord injury patients. Gastric and small bowel dilatation should be avoided with nasogastric decompression as needed. Enteral nutritional support may be initiated once the ileus has improved.

Gastric and duodenal stress ulcers are also common following spinal cord injury. Many studies have demonstrated a 3–5% risk of developing these ulcers, and H_2RA blockade is commonly indicated in the acute setting.

Genitourinary

Bladder dysfunction is common after cervical and thoracic spinal cord injuries. After the initial decompression with Foley catheterization for the first 3–5 days following injury, bladder training and decannulation may be entertained. This is described as intermittent bladder catheterization to maintain urinary volumes less than 500 cc. This aids in regaining at least partial urinary bladder function over time.

Urinary tract infections are also common following spinal cord injury secondary to high rates of bladder dysfunction, urinary retention, and need for repeat catheterization. It is important to obtain cultures (to address the high rates of multidrug-resistant organisms) and manage as a complicated urinary tract infection.

Thromboembolic Disease

Thromboembolic events in spinal cord injury patients are also common and typically occur in the first 3 months after trauma, while patients are immobile and procoagulant [24]. The risk eventually normalizes with enhanced mobility with physical therapy and rehabilitation and as the host antithrombogenic pathways are upregulated to counteract the blood stasis. Low-molecular-weight heparin with pneumatic compression stockings is recommended for prevention of thromboembolic events in spinal cord injury victims, as it has been demonstrated to be superior to unfractionated heparin [25]. The timing of initiation of thromboprophylaxis remains a topic of debate. Inferior vena caval interruption with removable filters can be entertained in the acute setting in patients with contraindication to chemical thromboprophylaxis.

Prognosis

The degree of neurologic disability varies greatly from patient to patient depending on type and severity of injury, as well as spinal cord level involved. Providing a reasonable expectation for long-term neurologic function and disability is crucial in aiding patients and families understand the long-term consequences of their injury and resources that will likely be required. The type and level of spinal cord injury, degree of motor and sensory function loss, age, comorbidities, and concurrent injuries are important in predicting long-term recovery [26]. MRI may also aid in determining prognosis, by providing detailed information of the extent of the spinal cord injury and integrity of the surrounding supporting structures.

Conclusion

Spinal cord injuries can inflict devastating long-term neurologic and functional limitations to patients, with significant emotional and financial ramifications. Spinal cord injury victims experience very high morbidity and mortality. Short- and long-term rehabilitation with aggressive physical and occupational therapy is crucial in aiding in improving long-term neurological function. Surgical stabilization of the encompassing vertebral column as indicated and minimizing secondary injury in a closely monitored setting are current mainstays of management.

References

1. National Spinal Cord Injury Statistical Center. Facts and figures at a glance. Birmingham, AL: University of Alabama at Birmingham; 2016.
2. Ma VY, Chan L, Carruthers KJ. Incidence, prevalence, costs, and impact on disability of common conditions requiring rehabilitation in the United States: stroke, spinal cord injury, traumatic brain injury, multiple sclerosis, osteoarthritis, rheumatoid arthritis, limb loss, and back pain. Arch Phys Med Rehabil. 2014;95:986–95. e1.
3. Maung AA, Johnson DC, Barre K, et al. Cervical spine MRI in patients with negative CT: a prospective, multicenter study of the Research Consortium of New England Centers for Trauma (ReCONECT). J Trauma Acute Care Surg. 2017;82:263–9.
4. Bracken MB, Webb SB Jr, Wagner FC. Classification of the severity of acute spinal cord injury: implications for management. Paraplegia. 1978;15:319–26.
5. Tezer M, Erturer RE, Ozturk C, Ozturk I, Kuzgun U. Conservative treatment of fractures of the thoracolumbar spine. Int Orthop. 2005;29:78–82.
6. McLain RF, Benson DR. Urgent surgical stabilization of spinal fractures in polytrauma patients. Spine (Phila Pa 1976). 1999;24:1646–54.
7. McKinley W, Meade MA, Kirshblum S, Barnard B. Outcomes of early surgical management versus late or no surgical intervention after acute spinal cord injury. Arch Phys Med Rehabil. 2004;85:1818–25.
8. Hall ED, Yonkers PA, Andrus PK, Cox JW, Anderson DK. Biochemistry and pharmacology of lipid antioxidants in acute brain and spinal cord injury. J Neurotrauma. 1992;9(Suppl 2):S425–42.
9. Bracken MB, Shepard MJ, Hellenbrand KG, et al. Methylprednisolone and neurological function 1 year after spinal cord injury. Results of the National Acute Spinal Cord Injury Study. J Neurosurg. 1985;63:704–13.
10. Bracken MB, Shepard MJ, Collins WF, et al. A randomized, controlled trial of methylprednisolone or naloxone in the treatment of acute spinal-cord injury. Results of the Second National Acute Spinal Cord Injury Study. N Engl J Med. 1990;322:1405–11.
11. Hurlbert RJ, Hadley MN, Walters BC, et al. Pharmacological therapy for acute spinal cord injury. Neurosurgery. 2013;72(Suppl 2):93–105.
12. Mocchetti I. Exogenous gangliosides, neuronal plasticity and repair, and the neurotrophins. Cell Mol Life Sci. 2005;62:2283–94.
13. Chinnock P, Roberts I. Gangliosides for acute spinal cord injury. Cochrane Database Syst Rev. 2005;(2):CD004444.
14. Zhai HW, Gong ZK, Sun J, et al. Ganglioside with nerve growth factor for the recovery of extremity function following spinal cord injury and somatosensory evoked potential. Eur Rev Med Pharmacol Sci. 2015;19:2282–6.
15. Schwartz G, Fehlings MG. Evaluation of the neuroprotective effects of sodium channel blockers after spinal cord injury: improved behavioral and neuroanatomical recovery with riluzole. J Neurosurg. 2001;94:245–56.
16. Grossman RG, Fehlings MG, Frankowski RF, et al. A prospective, multicenter, phase I matched-comparison group trial of safety,

pharmacokinetics, and preliminary efficacy of riluzole in patients with traumatic spinal cord injury. J Neurotrauma. 2014;31:239–55.
17. Hawryluk G, Whetstone W, Saigal R, et al. Mean arterial blood pressure correlates with neurological recovery after human spinal cord injury: analysis of high frequency physiologic data. J Neurotrauma. 2015;32:1958–67.
18. Martin ND, Kepler C, Zubair M, Sayadipour A, Cohen M, Weinstein M. Increased mean arterial pressure goals after spinal cord injury and functional outcome. J Emerg Trauma Shock. 2015;8:94–8.
19. Dietrich WD, Levi AD, Wang M, Green BA. Hypothermic treatment for acute spinal cord injury. Neurotherapeutics. 2011;8:229–39.
20. Thietje R, Pouw MH, Schulz AP, Kienast B, Hirschfeld S. Mortality in patients with traumatic spinal cord injury: descriptive analysis of 62 deceased subjects. J Spinal Cord Med. 2011;34:482–7.
21. Meng L, Wang C, Li J, Zhang J. Early vs late tracheostomy in critically ill patients: a systematic review and meta-analysis. Clin Respir J. 2016;10:684–92.
22. Dalal K, DiMarco AF. Diaphragmatic pacing in spinal cord injury. Phys Med Rehabil Clin N Am. 2014;25:619–29. viii.
23. Kim T, Jwa CS. Effect of alpha-1-adrenergic agonist, midodrine for the management of long-standing neurogenic shock in patient with cervical spinal cord injury: a case report. Korean J Neurotrauma. 2015;11:147–50.
24. Giorgi Pierfranceschi M, Donadini MP, Dentali F, et al. The short- and long-term risk of venous thromboembolism in patients with acute spinal cord injury: a prospective cohort study. Thromb Haemost. 2013;109:34–8.
25. Maung AA, Schuster KM, Kaplan LJ, Maerz LL, Davis KA. Risk of venous thromboembolism after spinal cord injury: not all levels are the same. J Trauma. 2011;71:1241–5.
26. Hsieh CH, DeJong G, Groah S, Ballard PH, Horn SD, Tian W. Comparing rehabilitation services and outcomes between older and younger people with spinal cord injury. Arch Phys Med Rehabil. 2013;94:S175–86.

Analgesia, Sedation, and Delirium in the ICU

4

Douglas R. Oyler and Andrew C. Bernard

Pain and Analgesia

The incidence of moderate-to-severe pain in the ICU is over 50% and is similar between medical and surgical patients [1]. A comprehensive list of risk factors for pain has not been developed, but pain in the ICU may be associated with the disease process or injury, invasive procedures (including mechanical ventilation), medication administration, and mobilization [2]. Untreated pain can lead to hyperglycemia, tachycardia, myocardial oxygen supply/demand mismatch, coagulopathy, immunosuppression, as well as development of hyperalgesia, chronic pain, and post-traumatic stress disorder (PTSD) [2–5].

Pain Assessment

Adequate treatment of pain must first begin with appropriate assessment. Pain is a subjective phenomenon that is best assessed using the patient's self-report, typically using a 0–10 rating scale [6]. Unfortunately, many patients may be unable to self-report pain, and the clinician must rely on other reproducible ways to assess pain. In this instance, the most valid tools to assess pain in the ICU are the Behavioral Pain Scale (BPS) and Critical Care Pain Observation Tool (CPOT) (Tables 4.1 and 4.2) [6]. These scales have been validated in patients with brain injury, with delirium, and in French and English [7, 8]. Vital signs may be a cue to begin further assessment of pain but should not be used alone for pain assessment.

D. R. Oyler
Department of Pharmacy, University of Kentucky Chandler Medical Center, Lexington, KY, USA

A. C. Bernard (✉)
Department of Surgery, University of Kentucky, Lexington, KY, USA
e-mail: andrew.bernard@uky.edu

Treatment of Pain with Opioids

Opioids have long been considered the mainstay of analgesia in the ICU and are the most frequently used class of medications for treatment of pain [9]. Opioids are available in a variety of dosage forms, and each regimen must be individually tailored for a patient's needs based on pharmacokinetic and pharmacodynamic properties of the drugs used. A review of these basic properties of opioids can be found in Table 4.3. Morphine and fentanyl are the most commonly used opioids in the ICU.

In general, opioids used in the ICU are intravenous; however, enteral formulations should be considered for patients with adequate gastrointestinal function. Although relative potencies between opioids may differ, when opioids are titrated to similar analgesic endpoints, there are no differences in efficacy [6]. Continuous versus intermittent dosing of medications should be based on patient characteristics (e.g., severity and duration of pain) as well as pharmacokinetics of the drug being used [11].

Although opioids are considered the most effective class of medications for provision of analgesia, their use is not without adverse effects. Of particular concern is the risk for dependence and abuse, as drug overdose is currently the leading cause of injury-related death in most US states (outpacing both deaths from motor vehicle collisions and gun-related deaths) [12], and the majority of first-time drug abusers obtain medications directly from a prescriber. Additionally, opioids cause dose-dependent respiratory and central nervous system depression, slow gastrointestinal time and may lead to development of ileus, and may be immunosuppressive [13].

Treatment of Pain with Non-opioid Analgesics

Because of the limitations of opioid analgesics, particularly respiratory depression, constipation, and the development of tolerance to analgesic effects, several non-opioid analgesics

A. Salim et al. (eds.), *Surgical Critical Care Therapy*, https://doi.org/10.1007/978-3-319-71712-8_4

Table 4.1 Behavioral Pain Scale

Item	Description	Score
Facial expression	Relaxed	1
	Partially tightened (e.g., brow lowering)	2
	Fully tightened (e.g., eyelid closing)	3
	Grimacing	4
Upper limb movements	No movement	1
	Partially bent	2
	Fully bent with finger flexion	3
	Permanently retracted	4
Compliance with mechanical ventilation	Tolerating movement	1
	Coughing but tolerating ventilation for most of the time	2
	Fighting ventilator	3
	Unable to control ventilation	4

A score of 5 or higher warrants treatment of pain

have been recommended to reduce opioid requirements or obviate the need for opioids altogether [6]. These may include nonsteroidal anti-inflammatory drugs (NSAIDs), N-methyl D-aspartate (NMDA) antagonists, skeletal muscle relaxants, α_2-receptor agonists, and antiepileptics. There is presently no evidence regarding comparative efficacy of opioids and non-opioids in the ICU. General pharmacologic characteristics of select non-opioid analgesics can be found in Table 4.4.

NSAIDs may be the most efficacious adjuvant therapy to opioids for treatment of acute pain, and the wide variety of available dosage forms is also appealing. NSAIDs have been shown to reduce opioid requirements and nausea and vomiting, constipation, sedation, and heterotopic ossification when compared with opioids alone in critically ill trauma patients [14]. However, the use of NSAIDs in the critically ill is complicated by risk of gastrointestinal bleeding and renal failure. Inconsistent data suggests NSAIDs may also increase the risk of fracture nonunion/malunion or infection [15, 16] and should be used cautiously in patients with fractures. NSAIDs should not be used for perioperative pain in patients undergoing coronary artery bypass graft surgery, and emerging low-quality data suggests postoperative NSAID use may be linked with anastomotic leak [17].

Acetaminophen may be classified as an NSAID; however the drug has no anti-inflammatory properties. Acetaminophen may reduce opioid requirements by up to 20% [18] and is safe when used in doses lower than 4000 mg per day. In doses >4000 mg per day or in high-risk populations (e.g., elderly, malnourished, pre-existing hepatic or renal dysfunction), acetaminophen may increase risk of hepatocellular damage; in these populations acetaminophen should be used cautiously with the total daily dose not exceeding 2000 mg per day.

Table 4.2 Critical Care Pain Observation Tool

Indicator	Description	Score	
Facial expression	No muscular tension observed	Relaxed, neutral	0
	Presence of frowning, brow lowering, orbit tightening, and levator contraction	Tense	1
	All of the above facial movements plus eyelid tightly closed	Grimacing	2
Body movements	Does not move at all (does not necessarily mean absence of pain)	Absence of movements	0
	Slow, cautious movements, touching or rubbing the pain site, seeking attention through movements	Protection	1
	Pulling tube, attempting to sit up, moving limbs/thrashing, not following commands, striking at staff, trying to climb out of bed	Restlessness	2
Muscle tensionevaluation by passive flexion and extension of upper extremities	No resistance to passive movements	Relaxed	0
	Resistance to passive movements	Tense, rigid	1
	Strong resistance to passive movements, inability to complete them	Very tense or rigid	2
Compliance with the ventilator (intubated patients) ORvocalization (extubated patients)	Alarms not activated, easy ventilation	Tolerating ventilator or movement	0
	Alarms stop spontaneously	Coughing but tolerating	1
	Asynchrony: Blocking ventilation, alarms frequently activated	Fighting ventilator	2
	Talking in normal tone or no sound	Talking in normal tone or no sound	0
	Sighing, moaning	Sighing, moaning	1
	Crying out, sobbing	Crying out, sobbing	2
Total, range			0–8

A score of 3 or higher warrants treatment of pain

Table 4.3 Pharmacology of intravenous opioids used in the ICU [6, 10]

Opioid	Equianalgesic dose (mg)	Onset (min)	Duration	Half-life	Metabolic pathway	Active metabolites	Intermittent dosing	Continuous infusion	Notes
Morphine	10	5–10	3–6 h	1.5–4.5 h	Glucuronidation	Yes	2–4 mg q1–2 h	2–30 mg/h	Histamine release may cause hypotension
Hydromorphone	1.5	5–15	4–5 h	2–3 h	Glucuronidation	No	0.2–0.6 mg q1–2 h	0.5–3 mg/h	Generally used in patients tolerant to morphine/fentanyl
Fentanyl	0.1	1–2	0.5–2 h	2–4 h	N-dealkylation, CYP 3A4/5 substrate	No	0.35–0.5 mcg/kg q30–60 min	0.7–10 mcg/kg/h	May cause less hypotension than morphine
Remifentanil	0.1	1–3	3–10 min	3–10 min	Plasma esterase hydrolysis	No	N/A	1.5 mcg/kg once, then 0.5–1.5 mcg/kg/h	No accumulation in organ dysfunction Dose based on IBW if weight > 130% IBW
Methadone	N/A[a]	15	8 h	8–59 h	N-demethylation, CYP 3A4/5, 2D6, 2B6, 1A2 substrate	Yes	2.5–10 mg q8–12 h	N/A	Unpredictable pharmacokinetics May slow opioid tolerance Monitor QTc

[a]Estimation of equianalgesic dose using conventional dosing tables may underestimate methadone potency as the potency of the drug relative to other opioids rises with increasing dose

Table 4.4 Pharmacology of non-opioid analgesics used in the ICU

Non-opioid (route)	Onset (min)	Duration (h)	Half-life (h)	Metabolic pathway	Active metabolites	Dosing	Notes
Ibuprofen (PO)	25	4–6	1.8–2.4	Oxidation	No	400 mg q4–6h	See text for precautions
Ketorolac (IM/IV)	10	4–6	2.4–8.6	Hydroxylation, conjugation, renal excretion	No	15–30 mg q6 h	See text for precautions Max dose 120 mg per day for 5 days
Acetaminophen (IV)	5–10	4–6	2–3	Glucuronidation, sulfonation	No	1000 mg q6 h	Expensive, use PO when able See text for precautions Max dose ≤4 g per day
Acetaminophen (PO/PR)	30–60	4–6	2–3	Glucuronidation, sulfonation	No	325–1000 mg q4–6 h	See text for precautions Max dose ≤4 g per day
Cyclobenzaprine (PO)	<60	12–24	18	N-demethylation	No	5 mg two to three times daily	ADRs include somnolence, arrhythmia, xerostomia, bone marrow suppression Similar structure to TCA; caution with serotonergic drugs Not recommended in the elderly
Clonidine (PO)	30–60	6–12	12.7–13.7	Hydroxylation, renal excretion	No	0.1 mg q6 h	Dose requires renal adjustment ADRs include sedation, bradycardia, hypotension Abrupt withdrawal can cause severe hypertension Max dose 2 mg per day
Gabapentin (PO)	60–180	4–8	5–7	Renal excretion	No	100–1200 mg three times daily	Dose requires renal adjustment ADRs include sedation, confusion, dizziness, ataxia Abrupt withdrawal can cause seizures
Carbamazepine (PO)	240–300	6–12	25–65[a]	Oxidation	No	50–100 mg twice daily	Multiple drug interactions ADRs include nystagmus, dizziness, lethargy, aplastic anemia, agranulocytosis May cause SJS-TEN in patients with HLA-B1502 gene Max dose 1200 mg per day
Ketamine (IV)	30–40 sec	5–10 min	2–3	N-demethylation	Yes	0.1–0.5 mg/kg, then 0.05–0.4 mg/kg/h	May attenuate opioid tolerance May cause hallucinations or psychiatric disturbances

PO orally, *PR* rectally, *IV* intravenously, *max* maximum, *ADR* adverse drug reaction, *TCA* tricyclic antidepressant, *SJS-TEN* Stevens-Johnson syndrome/toxic epidermal necrolysis

[a]Due to auto-induction of metabolism, half-life of carbamazepine decreases to 12–17 h over days to weeks and may require q6h dosing

NMDA antagonists such as ketamine and methadone have shown broad applicability in reducing opioid requirements in the surgical and trauma populations [19]. Opioid receptor activation (by exogenous opioids like morphine) induces protein kinase C gamma-mediated phosphorylation of NMDA receptors on the same cell, causing a cascade of events ultimately leading to downregulation of opioid receptors and so-termed opioid-induced hyperalgesia; NMDA antagonism may blunt this response [20]. Ketamine has been most commonly used for management of procedural sedation/analgesia. It has been postulated to raise intracranial pressure (ICP); however a recent meta-analysis showed ketamine caused similar changes in ICP when compared with opioids for analgesia and concluded traumatic brain injury is not a contraindication to its use [21]. Limited available evidence suggests methadone may expedite opioid weaning and reduce length of mechanical ventilation [22]. However methadone has unique and complicated pharmacokinetics, and use by inexperienced practitioners may increase the risk of overdose and death [23].

Skeletal muscle relaxants, including benzodiazepines, generally have limited utility as analgesics in the ICU. Some drugs, such as tizanidine and baclofen, may improve spasticity after spinal cord injury [24], but the sedative effects of these medications, which may be synergistic with opioids, likely limit broad utilization. Benzodiazepines may reduce anticipatory pain and spasticity, but use in the ICU has been associated with delirium and excess sedation (discussed under "Sect. 2.2").

Clonidine and dexmedetomidine act via inhibition of neurotransmitter release through α_2-receptor activation. This action results in synergistic effects with opioids as well as light sedation and anxiolysis. Dexmedetomidine has consistently shown an ability to reduce opioid requirements in sedation trials in a variety of ICUs; clonidine is less lipophilic than dexmedetomidine and may therefore cause more pronounced hypotension and bradycardia at equianalgesic doses. α_2-receptor agonists are discussed in more depth in Sect. 2.4.

Anticonvulsants (e.g., gabapentin and carbamazepine) are primarily used in patients with neuropathic pain and have been shown to provide superior pain relief for this indication when compared to opioids alone [25]. Multiple studies of gabapentin in the perioperative setting support a potential role for this medication as an adjunct to opioids for non-neuropathic as well [26, 27]. However, the validity of many gabapentin studies has been questioned [28], and recent data suggests the sedative risk of gabapentinoids in concert with opioids may outweigh the benefit if used in a broad population of patients [29].

Epidural Analgesia

For select patient populations in the ICU, epidural analgesia may be preferred over intravenous administration of opioids. In patients undergoing abdominal aortic surgery, thoracic epidural analgesia is superior to parenteral opioids alone for reduction of myocardial infarction, pain, time to extubation, postoperative respiratory failure, and ICU length of stay [30, 31]. The Eastern Association for the Surgery of Trauma also recommends epidural analgesia for patients older than 65 with four or more rib fractures, younger patients with more traumatic rib fractures, or older patients with fewer based on an association with mortality reduction in this population [32]. Epidurals may cause postoperative heart failure, infections, or respiratory failure and should not be placed in patients receiving full anticoagulation. In patients with traumatic rib fractures that cannot receive an epidural placement, transdermal lidocaine or paravertebral blocks should be considered [33, 34]. Transversus abdominis plane (TAP) blocks may be considered in select cases where thoracic epidural analgesia is not possible after abdominal surgery [35, 36].

Nonpharmacologic Therapies

In general, nonpharmacologic therapies (e.g., acupuncture, relaxation) have not been well-studied in the critically ill and are not recommended as the sole means of analgesia. Relaxation, in addition to pharmacologic therapy, is recommended for procedural analgesia, particularly chest tube removal [6].

Summary/Thoughts on Analgesia in the ICU

Pain is commonplace in the ICU regardless of visible injury, and patients usually require pharmacologic analgesia. In unstable patients, particularly those without intact gastrointestinal function, intravenous fentanyl (generally via continuous infusion with intermittent boluses for procedural/acute pain) is preferred. Although evidence is limited, some components of non-opioid analgesia can be utilized in most patients and should generally be attempted. Patients should be maintained on the lowest effective dose of opioids that provides analgesia, and daily attempts at weaning pain medications should be considered. Procedural pain should be anticipated, and prophylactic utilization of analgesics to prevent procedural pain is strongly encouraged.

Agitation and Sedation

Anxiety and agitation occur in up to 70% of ICU patients and may lead to unintended patient harm [37]. Anxiety—a feeling of fear or dread regarding a proposed or real threat to homeostasis—in the ICU is generally poorly assessed and poorly managed. Agitation, which may be the manifestation of behavior related to anxiety (or delirium, pain, hypoxia, hypoglycemia, or drug/alcohol withdrawal), has traditionally received more attention because it may pose a significant threat to patient well-being. Efforts to reduce agitation through other means such as provision of analgesia, reorientation, and optimization of sleep patterns should be attempted before administration of sedatives [6]. Indeed, utilization of so-called analgosedation—utilization of analgesics without sedatives—has shown to reduce mechanical ventilation time in a randomized trial [38]. Pharmacology of commonly used sedatives is reviewed in Table 4.5.

Depth of Sedation

Numerous well-conducted trials have now shown that sedation minimization, either through daily interruption of sedatives or utilization of a sedation protocol, shortens duration of mechanical ventilation and ICU length of stay [39–42].

Table 4.5 Pharmacology of sedatives used in the ICU

Sedative	Onset (min)	Duration (after bolus)	Half-life (h)	Metabolic pathway	Active metabolites	Dosing	Notes
Benzodiazepines							
Diazepam	2–5	2–4 h	20–120	CYP 450 metabolism	Yes	0.03–0.1 mg/kg q0.5–6 h prn	Avoid continuous infusion
Midazolam	1–5	1–2 h	3–11	CYP 450 metabolism	Yes	0.02–0.1 mg/kg, then 0.04–0.2 mg/kg/h	Infusion associated with prolonged emergence from sedation
Lorazepam	15–20	2–6 h	8–15	Conjugation	No	0.02–0.04 mg/kg, then 0.01–0.1 mg/kg/h[a]	Propylene glycol toxicity associated with infusion
Non-benzodiazepines							
Propofol	1–2	3–10 min	Short term 3–12, Long term 50 ± 18.6	Glucuronidation	No	25 mcg/kg over 5 min, then 5–50 mcg/kg/min	Contains 1.1 kcal/mL Concern for PRIS at high doses for prolonged periods
Dexmedetomidine	5–10	60–120 min	1.8–3.1	N-methylation, N-glucuronidation, CYP 450 metabolism	No	1 mcg/kg over 10 min, then 0.2–0.7 mcg/kg/h[b]	Does not produce deep sedation
Ketamine	30–40 sec	5–10 min	2–3	N-demethylation	Yes	0.1–0.5 mg/kg, then 0.05–0.4 mg/kg/h	May attenuate opioid tolerance May cause hallucinations or psychiatric disturbances

PRIS propofol-related infusion syndrome
[a]Maximum lorazepam bolus = 2 mg, maximum infusion rate = 10 mg/h
[b]Dexmedetomidine bolus is associated with hypotension and bradycardia and should be used with caution. Continuous infusion rates up to 1.5 mcg/kg/h have been studied

Daily interruption of sedation (discontinuation of intravenous sedation for as long as the patient tolerates, followed by resumption of sedation at 50% of the pre-interruption dose if needed) can usually be attempted during a spontaneous breathing trial. Patients on neuromuscular blocking agents (NMBAs) or those receiving sedation for treatment of intracranial hypertension or refractory status epilepticus are not appropriate for sedation interruption.

In most patients, light sedation is preferable to deep sedation [6] regardless of the medication used. Depth of sedation is best assessed using subjective scales such as the Richmond Agitation-Sedation Scale (RASS) or Sedation-Agitation Scale (SAS). Elements of the RASS and SAS can be found in Tables 4.6 and 4.7. Other subjective sedation scales are less valid and reliable and are therefore not recommended for general ICU use [6]. Utilization of objective markers of sedation (e.g., bispectral index, Narcotrend Index, auditory evoked potentials, Patient State Index, and state entropy) should only be considered for patients in whom subjective scales are unreliable, such as those receiving NMBAs.

Table 4.6 Richmond Agitation-Sedation Scale (RASS)

Scale	Label	Description
+4	Combative	Combative, violent, immediate danger to staff
+3	Very agitated	Pulls to remove tubes or catheters; aggressive
+2	Agitated	Frequent nonpurposeful movement, fights ventilator
+1	Restless	Anxious, apprehensive, movements not aggressive
0	Alert and calm	Spontaneously pays attention to caregiver
−1	Drowsy	Not fully alert, but has sustained awakening to voice (eyes open and contact >10 seconds)
−2	Light sedation	Briefly awakens to voice (eyes open and contact <10 seconds)
−3	Moderate sedation	Movement or eye opening to voice (no eye contact)
−4	Deep sedation	No response to voice, but movement or eye opening to physical stimulation
−5	Unarousable	No response to voice or physical stimulation

Table 4.7 Riker Sedation-Agitation Scale (SAS)

Scale	Label	Description
7	Dangerous agitation	Pulling at ETT, trying to remove catheters, climbing over bedrail, striking at staff, thrashing side-to-side
6	Very agitated	Requiring restraint and frequent verbal reminding of limits, biting ETT
5	Agitated	Anxious or physically agitated, calms to verbal instructions
4	Calm and cooperative	Calm, easily arousable, follows commands
3	Sedated	Difficult to arouse but awakens to verbal stimuli or gentle shaking, follows simple commands but drifts off again
2	Very sedated	Arouses to painful stimuli but does not communicate or follow commands, may move spontaneously
1	Unarousable	Minimal or no response to noxious stimuli, does not communicate or follow commands

ETT endotracheal tube

Sedation with Benzodiazepines

Benzodiazepines were traditionally the most commonly used sedatives in the ICU owing to their amnestic properties and generally accepted safety profile. However, more recent data suggests these medications may be associated with an increased incidence of delirium and delayed emergence from sedation, particularly when used as prolonged/continuous infusions or in susceptible populations (e.g., those with renal or hepatic dysfunction, obese patients, and the elderly) [6]. Furthermore, benzodiazepines may cause respiratory and hemodynamic compromise, particularly when used in combination with opioids. Finally, with prolonged use, tolerance to the sedative effects of benzodiazepines does develop. In any patient receiving benzodiazepines, drug interactions (particularly with select proton-pump inhibitors, macrolides, and azole antifungals) should be considered.

The benzodiazepines used in the ICU include lorazepam, midazolam, and diazepam, of which lorazepam is the most potent. Furthermore, lorazepam is cleared through hepatic conjugation, which may reduce accumulation in select patient populations, particularly those with alcoholic cirrhosis. However, lorazepam is uncommonly used as a continuous infusion sedative because the parenteral formulations of the drug contain propylene glycol which may cause metabolic acidosis and acute kidney injury. In patients receiving continuous infusion lorazepam, frequent monitoring of the osmolar gap is recommended [43].

Diazepam is the least potent of the intravenously available benzodiazepines and should not be used as a continuous infusion because of its long half-life and active metabolites. Diazepam is most commonly used for substance abuse/withdrawal disorders since the pharmacokinetics of the drug produce a stable taper with intermittent dosing.

Midazolam is the most commonly used continuous infusion benzodiazepine because of the drug's quick uptake into fatty tissues and relatively short duration of action. However, because of its active metabolites and redistribution from fatty tissues with prolonged use, extended infusions of midazolam should generally be avoided. The most common indications for continuous infusion benzodiazepines are treatment of refractory status epilepticus and deep sedation in patients with the acute respiratory distress syndrome requiring NMBA administration.

Sedation with Propofol

Propofol is a short-acting sedative/amnestic that primarily acts as a $GABA_A$ receptor antagonist, although it also has effects on sodium channels and the endocannabinoid system [44, 45]. Likely owing to its shorter half-life and rapid cessation of sedation when the drug is discontinued, propofol has been shown to reduce duration of mechanical ventilation when compared to benzodiazepines [46–50].

Because of its high lipid solubility, propofol is commercially available as a 10% lipid emulsion containing 1.1 kcal/mL. Depending on the infusion rate, the caloric contribution of a propofol infusion may be significant and should be factored into nutrient intake. Additionally, hypertriglyceridemia may occur in as many as 18% of patients requiring propofol for over 24 h, and serum triglycerides should be routinely monitored in these patients [51]. There is clinical evidence that 20% lipid emulsions may be associated with fat deposition in extracorporeal membrane oxygenation (ECMO) circuits [52]; therefore, propofol should be used with caution in this population. Fospropofol is a water-soluble prodrug that may circumvent most of the common complications associated with propofol; however experience in the ICU setting is extremely limited.

Propofol-related infusion syndrome (PRIS), characterized by bradycardia, cardiovascular collapse, high anion gap metabolic acidosis, rhabdomyolysis, hepatomegaly, and lipemia, is a rare but serious complication of propofol use. The pathophysiology of PRIS is complex, but the syndrome is most common in patients with multiple risk factors such as the use of high-dose infusions (e.g., >4 mg/kg/h) for >48–72 h, presence of shock, use of catecholamines or corticosteroids, and carbohydrate depletion [53]. In adults, the mortality associated with PRIS may be over 80%; therefore the best treatment is prevention, but ECMO, renal replacement therapy, and blood exchange have been occasionally used to successfully treat PRIS [54, 55].

Sedation with α_2-Receptor Agonists

Dexmedetomidine is a centrally acting α_2-receptor agonist with sedative, analgesic, and sympatholytic properties that produces a pattern of sedation that is lighter than other available sedatives with less respiratory depression. Compared with benzodiazepines, sedation with dexmedetomidine has been shown to reduce duration of mechanical ventilation and improve patient interaction [49] as well as reduce ICU length of stay [56] and incidence of delirium/coma at comparable sedation levels in one study [57]. Because dexmedetomidine does not reliably produce deep sedation, alternative agents are strongly encouraged in patients requiring deep sedation (e.g., patients receiving NMBAs). Dexmedetomidine does produce dose-dependent hypotension and bradycardia—especially with bolus doses—and should be used with caution in hemodynamically unstable patients.

To date, only two small studies have evaluated clonidine use for sedation in the ICU [58, 59]. These studies suggest enteral clonidine may be an appropriate, cost-effective alternative to dexmedetomidine for sedation. Because clonidine is less lipophilic than dexmedetomidine, higher than normal doses of the drug have been reported to be required for full sedative effects (e.g., 0.3–0.5 mg every 6 h) [59]. Tolerability appears to be similar to dexmedetomidine.

Sedation with Ketamine

Ketamine is a lipophilic cyclohexamine anesthetic [60]. Compared to older derivatives (e.g., phencyclidine), ketamine exhibits less psychiatric adverse effects, lower potency, and shorter duration of action. The drug has a high volume of distribution, low protein binding, and active metabolites that are by-products of hepatic, renal, pulmonary, and gastrointestinal metabolism. Norketamine, the principle active metabolite of ketamine, is an analgesic with a potency approximately 20–30% that of ketamine. Because of norketamine kinetics, ketamine requirements decrease with time when used as a continuous infusion for analgesia/sedation.

Ketamine primarily acts through antagonism at glutamate-binding sites—mainly NMDA receptors—to provide analgesic, psychosensory, amnestic, and neuroprotective effects. Ketamine also interacts with opioid (mu, delta, and kappa), monoaminergic, cholinergic, nicotinic, and muscarinic receptors. At high concentrations, ketamine agonizes GABA receptors as well. Opioid receptor binding is not antagonized by naloxone.

Continuous infusion ketamine is gaining popularity as a benzodiazepine-sparing sedative for continuous infusion in the ICU. At present, limited data exists regarding the safety and efficacy of long-term sedation (>24 h) with ketamine. Case reports and small retrospective studies suggest ketamine has similar tolerability to other sedatives including propofol and benzodiazepines [61, 62]. The most commonly reported adverse reactions are tachydysrhythmias and worsened agitation.

Summary/Thoughts on Sedation in the ICU

Agitation is commonplace in the ICU; however universal utilization of sedative agents has not been shown to improve patient outcomes. Oftentimes, anxiolysis or sedation can be achieved through nonpharmacologic means or through provision of adequate analgesia. When sedation is required, the lowest effective level of sedation should be sought using validated scales such as the RASS or SAS. The use of nonbenzodiazepines (e.g., propofol, dexmedetomidine) is associated with improvements in duration of mechanical ventilation and ICU length of stay when compared with benzodiazepines, but the impact on other clinically meaningful parameters such as mortality and delirium remains unclear. The use of ketamine and clonidine, while appealing based on the drugs' pharmacologies, requires further investigation.

Delirium

Delirium is an acute brain dysfunction characterized by altered wakefulness and cognition and is associated with adverse outcomes including mortality [63]. Numerous risk factors exist for delirium. Prophylactic or therapeutic pharmacologic strategies are unproven, making nonpharmacologic prevention the most important approach to delirium. There are three types of delirium: hypoactive (quiet), hyperactive (agitated), and mixed, with hypoactive being most common [64].

Outcomes Associated with Delirium in the ICU

Delirium affects 35–80% of adult ICU patients [65] and as many as 25% of critically ill children [66]. Delirium duration may be a more potent predictor of mortality, period of ventilation, and ICU length of stay than age or even APACHE II score [67].

Delirium may prolong ICU length of stay by up to 10 days, and each day of delirium increases length of hospitalization by 20% and mortality by 10% [68]. Delirium in the ICU has lasting effects, impairing post-discharge cognition; however it does not appear to significantly affect post-discharge mortality [69]. A report from the American Association of Retired Persons considered delirium a leading cause of preventable injury [70].

Delirium increases cost by as much as $9000 per case and is expected to increase total US healthcare cost by $6–20 billion annually [71]. By increasing patient acuity, delirium increases care intensity and stresses the nursing workforce. Thus decreasing delirium may decrease nursing workload [72].

Detecting and Monitoring Delirium

Monitoring organ function and dysfunction is standard in the ICU, and this practice should apply to the central nervous system. Though delirium represents brain organ dysfunction, it is notoriously under-screened and under-documented, remaining undiagnosed in two thirds of those affected [63]. Since the incidence of delirium is expected to increase as the population ages, effective screening is imperative [73]. Techniques for delirium screening originally developed for the ICU have now been translated into 20 languages and modified for non-ICU areas [74]. All methods are based upon the fundamental symptom of inattention. Five delirium assessment tools have been assessed against the American Psychiatric Association's Diagnostic and Statistical Manual (DSM), but we will discuss the two most common and well-validated tools: the Confusion Assessment Method for the ICU (CAM-ICU) and the Intensive Care Delirium Screening Checklist (ICDSC).

The Confusion Assessment Method was modified for the ICU by Wes Ely. In 2001, CAM-ICU was validated to be highly sensitive compared to a delirium expert using DSM criteria and have high inter-rater reliability among nurses and intensivists [75]. The CAM-ICU is initiated if the patient has an acute change in mental status and has documented inattention; the evaluation is deemed to be positive if it confirms altered mental status and also disordered thinking (Fig. 4.1). The ICDSC was described by Bergeron in 2001 (Fig. 4.2). While CAM-ICU is performed at one moment of time, the ICDSC is performed over at least 8 h, allowing a summative and therefore theoretically more complete assessment. Both methods are of adequate sensitivity and specificity according to an analysis pooling nine studies of CAM-ICU (80.0% sensitive and 95.9% specific) and four studies of ICDSC (74% sensitive and 81.9% specific) [76]. Both CAM-ICU and ICDSC are more prone to indicate the presence of delirium at deeper levels of sedation [77]; therefore ICU delirium assessment or clinical investigation should be wary of the effects of short-term sedation biasing assessment or results rapidly reversible, sedation-related delirium does not carry the untoward effects of true delirium [78].

Risk Factors for Development of Delirium

Prevention of delirium is the best treatment; therefore risk factor recognition and reduction are critical. Delirium is multifactorial in most cases [79]. Risk factors fall into three categories: patient-related, environmental, and iatrogenic [80]. Patient-related risk factors include critical illness (RR 1.13 per 1 point increase in APACHE II score), age over 65, hypertension, alcohol use, and smoking [73, 79]. In older patients, dementia, prior delirium events, and prior falls each double the risk of delirium [81]. Recent data also suggests constipation lasting >5 days is independently associated with development of delirium in ventilated ICU patients [82].

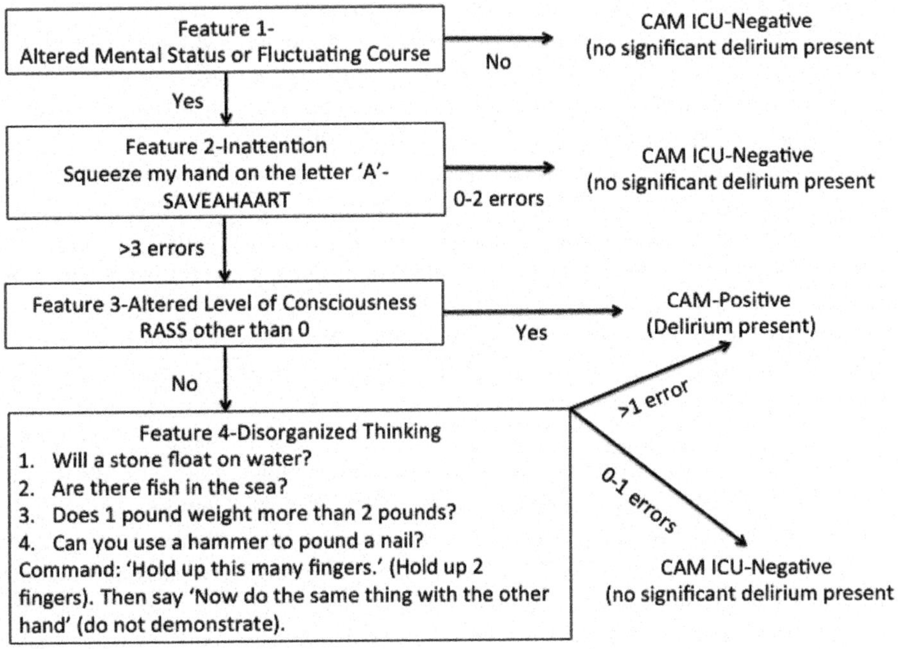

Fig. 4.1 Confusion Assessment Method for the ICU (CAM-ICU)

Fig. 4.2 Intensive Care Delirium Screening Checklist (ICDSC)

Item	Point Value
1. Altered level of consciousness Agitation (RASS 1 to 4, SAS 5 to 7) at any point, or Light sedation (RASS -1 to -3, SAS 2 or 3) with no recent sedative	1
2. Inattention Difficulty following instructions or conversation Easily distracted by external stimuli	1
3. Disorientation Any error in identifying name, place, or date	1
4. Hallucinations, delusion, or psychosis	1
5. Psychomotor agitation or slowing Hyperactivity requiring the use of sedative drugs or restraints, or Clinically relevant psychomotor slowing	1
6. Inappropriate speech or mood Inappropriate emotion, or Disorganize or incoherent speech, or Sexual or inappropriate interactions, or Apathy or overly demanding	1
7. Sleep-wake cycle disturbances Frequent awakening or <4 hours sleep at night (not caused by caregivers), or Sleeping during much of the day	1
8. Fluctuation of any of the above symptoms over a 24 hour period	1
TOTAL	8 points

Scoring: 0=normal, 1-3=subsyndromal delirium, 4-8=delirium
Items 1-4 require a focused bedside assessment, which cannot be completed if the patient is deeply sedated or comatose (i.e., SAS=1 or RASS=-4 or -5).
Items 5-8 are based on observations throughout the entire shift. Information from the prior 24 hours should be obtained for items 7 and 8.
RASS = Richmond Agitation Sedation Scale; SAS = Riker Sedation Agitation Scale

Environmental factors are those that primarily worsen sleep deprivation (e.g., alterations in circadian rhythms, interruptions in sleep for lab monitoring, persistent noise in the ICU, etc.) [83]. Surgical procedures are associated with more delirium, and mechanical ventilation triples the risk [73, 79]. In older, more vulnerable patients, even transfers between care areas nearly triple the risk [81]. Acute kidney injury (AKI) increases risk of delirium in a dose-dependent fashion with severity of AKI, and renal replacement therapy may abrogate some of these effects, suggesting an interplay between the brain and renal organ systems [84]. Noxious stimuli including catheters (vascular, bladder, gastric), lack of visitors, and lack of daylight also contribute to delirium [85].

Medications may contribute to delirium. Benzodiazepines were strongly implicated in original descriptions of ICU delirium [86], but subsequent investigations suggest this relationship is more complex than previously perceived. Intermittent benzodiazepine use has not been associated with the same risk of delirium as continuous infusion, and many studies do not differentiate between rapidly reversible, sedation-related delirium from benzodiazepines and true delirium [87]. However, benzodiazepines have been shown to reduce slow wave sleep and REM sleep, which may influence delirium [88]. In general, less sedation is better when the outcome desired is less brain dysfunction. The Awakening and Breathing Controlled trial showed that patients managed with a strategy of regular awakening had fewer ventilator days, shorter ICU and hospital durations, and lower mortality [89]. The number of opioid doses has been associated with ICU delirium in trauma patients, but the correlation is far weaker than with benzodiazepines [90]. The use of proton-pump inhibitors is associated with a 1.7-fold relative risk increase [81]. Various high-quality studies have reported disparate results regarding the impact of systemic corticosteroid administration in delirium, and further research is needed in this area before definitive conclusions can be made [91, 92]. Cessation of home statin therapy has been shown to increase incidence of delirium in a mixed medical/surgical cohort of patients with sepsis [93].

Delirium Prevention

The most important strategy in the prevention of delirium is minimization of sedation. While intermittent benzodiazepines may not increase risk as much as previously believed, continuous infusion of benzodiazepines should generally be avoided due to complex pharmacokinetic interactions in obese patients or those with underlying organ dysfunction [87]. Studies comparing dexmedetomidine to benzodiazepines with respect to delirium vary in design and do not all measure delirium in the same manner, making them difficult to interpret collectively [94]. Dexmedetomidine does permit faster awakening, lighter sedation, and less sleep disturbance than benzodiazepines, all effects which reduce delirium [83]. In general, when sedation is required, nonbenzodiazepines such as dexmedetomidine or propofol are preferred.

Knowing the multitude of nonpharmacologic risk factors associated with delirium development, reduction strategies require a systematic approach to apply multiple interventions. A delirium prevention bundle including sleep promotion, sedation and pain management, sensory stimulation, and mobility reduces incidence of delirium by up to 78% [72]. A nonpharmacologic prevention intervention including reorientation, opening and closing of blinds, music, and eye and ear care, bundled together, reduced total time in delirium [95]. Early mobilization is an important delirium prevention strategy and bundle component. Compliance with ABCDEF bundle (awakening and breathing coordination, choice of drugs, delirium monitoring and management, early mobility, and family engagement) increases survival and reduces coma and delirium [96].

Sleep hygiene is a common theme in delirium prevention bundles. Many ICU patients get less than 2 h of sleep and fewer than 6% get any REM sleep [97]. Earplugs reduce delirium risk by almost half, and compliance with this simple therapy is good (86%) [98]. Eye masks and bright light therapy have been used to enhance sleep quality and restore circadian rhythm [83]. Additional prospective clinical trials are underway to evaluate the efficacy of prevention interventions including mobility, sleep quality, and sedation management [99]. An advantage of these trials is that, unlike interventional studies including drug studies, unlikely harmful side effects and risk make enrollment easier.

Pharmacologic Prophylaxis of Delirium

Multicomponent interventions reduce the incidence of delirium compared to usual care, and the effect is the same in medical and surgical patients. Unfortunately, the severity or duration of delirium is not affected, and no single agent has proven efficacy. Pre-existing dementia reduces likelihood that any combination of interventions will be effective [100]. There is some evidence that BIS-guided anesthesia reduces the incidence of delirium postoperatively compared to BIS-blinded anesthesia or clinical judgment [100].

Evidence from small studies provides support for but cannot prove efficacy of any particular agent in the ICU. Incidence of delirium was lower with use of an atypical antipsychotic (olanzapine) compared to placebo in a postoperative ward population, but lower scores on Mini-mental Status Exam suggest that this therapy also impairs cognition [101]. Paucity of supporting evidence leaves olanzapine therapy unproven. Single-dose risperidone has been suggested for use in the postoperative cardiac surgery population, but again evidence is limited [102]. Empiric low-dose dexmedetomidine reduces CAM-measured delirium in the first 7 days after non-cardiac surgery [103], but most other studies fail to prove that dexmedetomidine administration is itself the mechanism reducing delirium [94].

Melatonin has been used as a sleep aid and may reduce delirium occurrence in hospitalized patients but remains unproven in the ICU [100]. Theoretical benefit of melatonin in ICU delirium is based upon enhanced quality and amount of sleep and evidence showing decreased melatonin metabolites in mechanically ventilated patients, which coincided with delirium [104]. Melatonin could be as efficacious as some nonpharmacologic measures based on data from healthy volunteers in an ICU environment [105]. Ramelteon, a melatonin receptor agonist, has also been reported to decrease delirium incidence [106]. Benefits of melatonin and melatonin receptor agonists remain unproven with respect to delirium reduction, but numerous multicenter trials are underway [107]. The standard dosage in these trials is 0.5–5 mg melatonin nightly for up to 2 weeks during the ICU stay.

Delirium Treatment

Pharmacologic treatment of delirium is marginally effective at best (Table 4.8). Options include typical antipsychotics, for which the mechanism of action is unknown, atypical antipsychotics, antiepileptics, and cholinesterase inhibitors. Haloperidol has traditionally been a mainstay of delirium treatment, but recent randomized trials suggest a lack of efficacy with regard to reduction in both delirium incidence and duration [108, 109]. Additionally, use of haloperidol is associated with an increased incidence of adverse effects, particularly extrapyramidal symptoms, when compared to newer antipsychotics, and use is generally not recommended [6, 110].

Atypical antipsychotics lack a strong evidence base in ICU delirium compared to the non-ICU population [111]. Randomized prospective data for quetiapine in escalating doses (plus as-needed haloperidol) showed reduced delirium

Table 4.8 Antidelirium therapies used in the ICU

Medication	Recommended for prevention	Recommended for treatment	Typical dose	Metabolic pathway	Active metabolites	Notes
Haloperidol (IM/IV)	No	No	2.5–5 mg TID	Oxidation	Yes	High risk of EPS, QT prolongation
Quetiapine (PO)	No	Yes, with nonpharmacologic therapy	25–100 mg BID	CYP 450 metabolism	Yes	Lower risk of EPShigh risk of QT prolongation, sedationstop when delirium resolved
Risperidone (PO)	No	No	1 mg 1–3×/day	CYP 450 metabolism	Yes	Lower risk of EPS, high risk of QT prolongation, sedation, tremor, and fever limited evidence
Olanzapine (PO)	No	No	5–10 mg BID	Glucuronidation, CYP 450 metabolism	Yes	Lower risk of EPS, QT prolongationhigh risk of sedation, weakness, hypotension, liver dysfunction Limited evidence
Valproate (PO)	No	No	250–500 mg TID-QID	Glucuronidation, oxidation	Yes	High risk of sedation, thrombocytopenia, tremorassociated with increased mortality in acute phase of TBI Limited evidence
Melatonin (PO)	Yes, with nonpharmacologic therapy	Yes, with nonpharmacologic therapy	3–10 mg HS	Hydroxylation	No	Limited evidence
Ramelteon (PO)	Yes, with nonpharmacologic therapy	No	8 mg HS	Oxidation	Yes	Limited evidence

EPS extrapyramidal symptoms, *TBI* traumatic brain injury

duration, but this study was limited by sample size [112]. A later study of patients who had received quetiapine showed reduced delirium duration compared to patients who did not, but this study was retrospective [113]. Additionally, these medications carry the risks of serious adverse reactions including arrhythmias, sedation (which is additive to other medications including opioids), and extrapyramidal symptoms. Furthermore, without an active diagnosis of delirium, antipsychotic use has been associated with increased length of stay and hospital mortality [114]. Additionally, multiple studies have shown the antipsychotics initiated in the ICU are frequently continued on hospital discharge without a valid indication, increasing the risks associated with polypharmacy and risk of metabolic consequences associated with long-term use of second-generation antipsychotics [115, 116]. Given the paucity of therapeutic evidence and clear risks associated with this class of medications, broad use of atypical antipsychotics in the ICU as prophylaxis or therapy for delirium cannot be recommended.

Valproate has shown some early promise in decreasing not only agitation but also delirium and opioid requirement, but this drug too needs much further study [117]. Additionally, use of cholinesterase inhibitors such as rivastigmine, approved for dementia, is not recommended [6].

Delirium Summary

Delirium is perhaps the most common organ dysfunction in ICU patients. Screening and documentation are the first step. Prevention is the best cure and avoidance of deep sedation is the best prevention. Nonpharmacologic therapies work and are best bundled into a plan of care for delirium reduction in the ICU culture. Once delirium occurs, the pharmacologic options are few and have numerous side effects.

Final Thoughts

Pain, agitation, and delirium are common occurrences in the ICU and can carry significant consequences if left unaddressed. That said, overutilization of medications is associated with longer ventilation times, increased complications, and higher mortality. Appropriate stewardship of sedatives, targeting the lightest level of sedation possible, should be pursued. For delirium, prevention is the most effective treatment; normalizing the patient's environment through commonsense measures that often get overlooked (e.g., providing hearing aids or eyeglasses, promoting healthy sleep, and encouraging early mobility) is the mainstay of reducing its occurrence (Fig. 4.3). Perhaps most importantly, the surgeon must ensure appropriate provision of analgesia using both

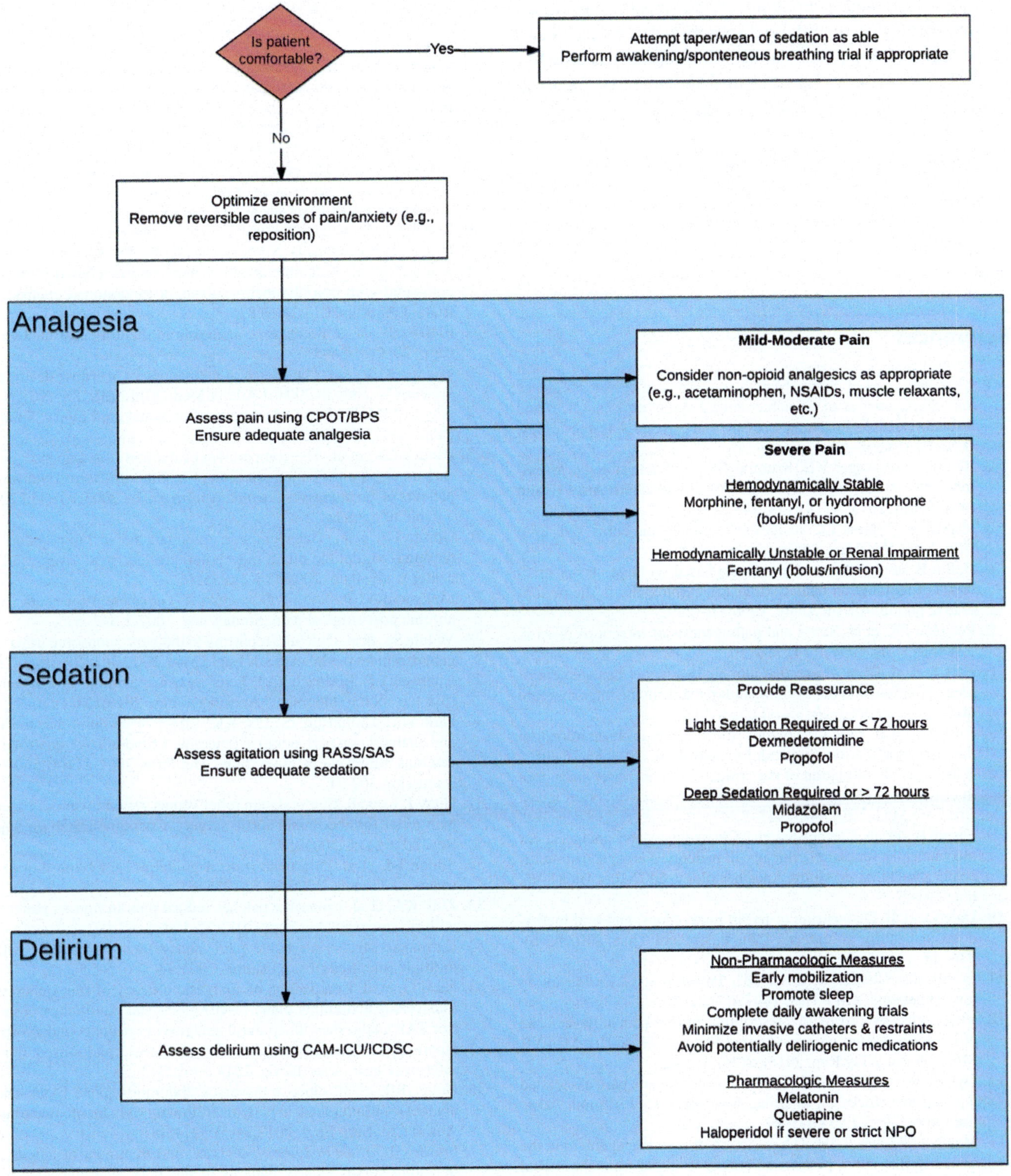

Fig. 4.3 Treatment approach for pain, agitation, and delirium

pharmacologic and nonpharmacologic means. Given the recent explosion in opioid use disorders and overdose deaths in the United States, the clear benefit of opioids as effective analgesics must be weighed against the potential for long-term consequences associated with their use.

Acknowledgment All authors report no conflicts of interest, including pharmaceutical or industry support, regarding any of the information contained in this report. No relevant funding from any organization was provided to any of the authors regarding this manuscript or the ideas contained herein.

References

1. Chanques G, et al. A prospective study of pain at rest: incidence and characteristics of an unrecognized symptom in surgical and trauma versus medical intensive care unit patients. Anesthesiology. 2007;107(5):858–60.
2. Reardon DP, Anger KE, Szumita PM. Pathophysiology, assessment, and management of pain in critically ill adults. Am J Health Syst Pharm. 2015;72(18):1531–43.
3. Hedderich R, Ness TJ. Analgesia for trauma and burns. Crit Care Clin. 1999;15(1):167–84.
4. Beilin B, et al. Effects of anesthesia based on large versus small doses of fentanyl on natural killer cell cytotoxicity in the perioperative period. Anesth Analg. 1996;82(3):492–7.
5. Peterson PK, et al. Stress and pathogenesis of infectious disease. Rev Infect Dis. 1991;13(4):710–20.
6. Barr J, et al. Clinical practice guidelines for the management of pain, agitation, and delirium in adult patients in the intensive care unit. Crit Care Med. 2013;41(1):263–306.
7. Joffe AM, et al. Validation of the critical-care pain observation tool in brain-injured critically ill adults. J Crit Care. 2016;36:76–80.
8. Kanji S, et al. Validation of the critical care pain observation tool in critically ill patients with delirium: a prospective cohort study. Crit Care Med. 2016;44(5):943–7.
9. Payen JF, et al. Current practices in sedation and analgesia for mechanically ventilated critically ill patients: a prospective multicenter patient-based study. Anesthesiology. 2007;106(4):687–95. quiz 891-2
10. Dale O, et al. Disposition of nasal, intravenous, and oral methadone in healthy volunteers. Clin Pharmacol Ther. 2002;72(5): 536–45.
11. Erstad BL, Chopda S, Esser MJ. Prescribing of analgesics in trauma patients. Am J Ther. 1997;4(1):27–30.
12. Vital signs: overdoses of prescription opioid pain relievers and other drugs among women--United States, 1999–2010. MMWR Morb Mortal Wkly Rep. 2013;62(26):537–42.
13. Oyler DR, et al. Nonopioid management of acute pain associated with trauma: focus on pharmacologic options. J Trauma Acute Care Surg. 2015;79(3):475–83.
14. Malchow RJ, Black IH. The evolution of pain management in the critically ill trauma patient: emerging concepts from the global war on terrorism. Crit Care Med. 2008;36(7 Suppl):S346–57.
15. Marquez-Lara A, et al. Nonsteroidal anti-inflammatory drugs and bone-healing: a systematic review of research quality. JBJS Rev. 2016;4(3):1–14
16. Pountos I, et al. Do nonsteroidal anti-inflammatory drugs affect bone healing? a critical analysis. ScientificWorldJournal. 2012;2012:606404.
17. Bhangu A, et al. Postoperative nonsteroidal anti-inflammatory drugs and risk of anastomotic leak: meta-analysis of clinical and experimental studies. World J Surg. 2014;38(9):2247–57.
18. Elia N, Lysakowski C, Tramer MR. Does multimodal analgesia with acetaminophen, nonsteroidal antiinflammatory drugs, or selective cyclooxygenase-2 inhibitors and patient-controlled analgesia morphine offer advantages over morphine alone? meta-analyses of randomized trials. Anesthesiology. 2005;103(6):1296–304.
19. Guillou N, et al. The effects of small-dose ketamine on morphine consumption in surgical intensive care unit patients after major abdominal surgery. Anesth Analg. 2003;97(3):843–7.
20. Roeckel LA, et al. Opioid-induced hyperalgesia: cellular and molecular mechanisms. Neuroscience. 2016;338:160–82.
21. Wang X, et al. Ketamine does not increase intracranial pressure compared with opioids: meta-analysis of randomized controlled trials. J Anesth. 2014;28(6):821–7.
22. Elefritz JL, et al. Methadone analgesia in the critically ill. J Crit Care. 2016;34:84–8.
23. Weimer MB, et al. The source of methadone in overdose deaths in Western Virginia in 2004. J Addict Med. 2011;5(3):188–202.
24. Adams MM, Hicks AL. Spasticity after spinal cord injury. Spinal Cord. 2005;43(10):577–86.
25. Pandey CK, et al. The comparative evaluation of gabapentin and carbamazepine for pain management in Guillain-Barre syndrome patients in the intensive care unit. Anesth Analg. 2005;101(1):220–5. table of contents
26. Gordh TE, et al. Gabapentin in traumatic nerve injury pain: a randomized, double-blind, placebo-controlled, cross-over, multicenter study. Pain. 2008;138(2):255–66.
27. Melemeni A, Staikou C, Fassoulaki A. Gabapentin for acute and chronic post-surgical pain. Signa Vitae. 2007;2:S42–51.
28. Vedula SS, et al. Outcome reporting in industry-sponsored trials of gabapentin for off-label use. N Engl J Med. 2009;361(20):1963–71.
29. Kharasch ED, Eisenach JC. Wherefore Gabapentinoids?: was there rush too soon to judgment? Anesthesiology. 2016;124(1):10–2.
30. Park WY, Thompson JS, Lee KK. Effect of epidural anesthesia and analgesia on perioperative outcome: a randomized, controlled veterans affairs cooperative study. Ann Surg. 2001;234(4):560–9. discussion 569-71
31. Guay J, Kopp S. Epidural pain relief versus systemic opioid-based pain relief for abdominal aortic surgery. Cochrane Database Syst Rev. 2016;(1):CD005059.
32. Simon BJ, et al. Pain management guidelines for blunt thoracic trauma. J Trauma. 2005;59(5):1256–67.
33. Zink KA, et al. Lidocaine patches reduce pain in trauma patients with rib fractures. Am Surg. 2011;77(4):438–42.
34. Karmakar MK, et al. Acute pain management of patients with multiple fractured ribs. J Trauma. 2003;54(3):615–25.
35. Niraj G, et al. Comparison of analgesic efficacy of four-quadrant transversus abdominis plane (TAP) block and continuous posterior TAP analgesia with epidural analgesia in patients undergoing laparoscopic colorectal surgery: an open-label, randomised, non-inferiority trial. Anaesthesia. 2014;69(4):348–55.
36. Brady RR, et al. Open transversus abdominis plane block and analgesic requirements in patients following right hemicolectomy. Ann R Coll Surg Engl. 2012;94(5):327–30.
37. Fraser GL, et al. Frequency, severity, and treatment of agitation in young versus elderly patients in the ICU. Pharmacotherapy. 2000;20(1):75–82.
38. Strom T, Martinussen T, Toft P. A protocol of no sedation for critically ill patients receiving mechanical ventilation: a randomised trial. Lancet. 2010;375(9713):475–80.
39. Kress JP, et al. Daily interruption of sedative infusions in critically ill patients undergoing mechanical ventilation. N Engl J Med. 2000;342(20):1471–7.

40. Mehta S, et al. Daily sedation interruption in mechanically ventilated critically ill patients cared for with a sedation protocol: a randomized controlled trial. JAMA. 2012;308(19):1985–92.
41. Kollef MH, et al. The use of continuous i.v. sedation is associated with prolongation of mechanical ventilation. Chest. 1998;114(2):541–8.
42. Treggiari MM, et al. Randomized trial of light versus deep sedation on mental health after critical illness. Crit Care Med. 2009;37(9):2527–34.
43. Barnes BJ, et al. Osmol gap as a surrogate marker for serum propylene glycol concentrations in patients receiving lorazepam for sedation. Pharmacotherapy. 2006;26(1):23–33.
44. Haeseler G, et al. High-affinity blockade of voltage-operated skeletal muscle and neuronal sodium channels by halogenated propofol analogues. Br J Pharmacol. 2008;155(2):265–75.
45. Fowler CJ. Possible involvement of the endocannabinoid system in the actions of three clinically used drugs. Trends Pharmacol Sci. 2004;25(2):59–61.
46. Aitkenhead AR, et al. Comparison of propofol and midazolam for sedation in critically ill patients. Lancet. 1989;2(8665):704–9.
47. Hall RI, et al. Propofol vs midazolam for ICU sedation : a Canadian multicenter randomized trial. Chest. 2001;119(4):1151–9.
48. Carson SS, et al. A randomized trial of intermittent lorazepam versus propofol with daily interruption in mechanically ventilated patients. Crit Care Med. 2006;34(5):1326–32.
49. Jakob SM, et al. Dexmedetomidine vs midazolam or propofol for sedation during prolonged mechanical ventilation: two randomized controlled trials. JAMA. 2012;307(11):1151–60.
50. Muellejans B, et al. Sedation in the intensive care unit with remifentanil/propofol versus midazolam/fentanyl: a randomised, open-label, pharmacoeconomic trial. Crit Care. 2006;10(3):R91.
51. Devlin JW, Lau AK, Tanios MA. Propofol-associated hypertriglyceridemia and pancreatitis in the intensive care unit: an analysis of frequency and risk factors. Pharmacotherapy. 2005;25(10):1348–52.
52. Lee HM, et al. What are the adverse effects associated with the combined use of intravenous lipid emulsion and extracorporeal membrane oxygenation in the poisoned patient? Clin Toxicol (Phila). 2015;53(3):145–50.
53. Mirrakhimov AE, et al. Propofol infusion syndrome in adults: a clinical update. Crit Care Res Pract. 2015;2015:260385.
54. Mayette M, et al. Propofol infusion syndrome resuscitation with extracorporeal life support: a case report and review of the literature. Ann Intensive Care. 2013;3(1):32.
55. Walli A, et al. Propofol infusion syndrome in refractory status epilepticus: a case report and topical review. Case Rep Emerg Med. 2016;2016:3265929.
56. Chen K, et al. Alpha-2 agonists for long-term sedation during mechanical ventilation in critically ill patients. Cochrane Database Syst Rev. 2015;(1):Cd010269.
57. Riker RR, et al. Dexmedetomidine vs midazolam for sedation of critically ill patients: a randomized trial. JAMA. 2009;301(5):489–99.
58. Farasatinasab M, et al. A randomized placebo-controlled trial of clonidine impact on sedation of mechanically ventilated ICU patients. Iran J Pharm Res. 2015;14(1):167–75.
59. Gagnon DJ, et al. Transition from dexmedetomidine to enteral clonidine for ICU sedation: an observational pilot study. Pharmacotherapy. 2015;35(3):251–9.
60. Mion G, Villevieille T. Ketamine pharmacology: an update (pharmacodynamics and molecular aspects, recent findings). CNS Neurosci Ther. 2013;19(6):370–80.
61. Benken ST, Goncharenko A. The future of intensive care unit sedation: a report of continuous infusion ketamine as an alternative sedative agent. J Pharm Pract. 2017;30(5):576–581. doi: 10.1177/0897190016646293. Epub 2016 May 2.
62. Umunna BP, et al. Ketamine for continuous sedation of mechanically ventilated patients. J Emerg Trauma Shock. 2015;8(1):11–5.
63. Pisani MA, et al. A research algorithm to improve detection of delirium in the intensive care unit. Crit Care. 2006;10(4):R121.
64. Pandharipande P, et al. Motoric subtypes of delirium in mechanically ventilated surgical and trauma intensive care unit patients. Intensive Care Med. 2007;33(10):1726–31.
65. Skrobik Y. Delirium prevention and treatment. Crit Care Clin. 2009;25(3):585–91.
66. Joyce C, et al. Evaluation of the safety of quetiapine in treating delirium in critically ill children: a retrospective review. J Child Adolesc Psychopharmacol. 2015;25(9):666–70.
67. Shehabi Y, et al. Delirium duration and mortality in lightly sedated, mechanically ventilated intensive care patients. Crit Care Med. 2010;38(12):2311–8.
68. Ely EW, et al. Delirium as a predictor of mortality in mechanically ventilated patients in the intensive care unit. JAMA. 2004;291(14):1753–62.
69. Salluh JI, et al. Outcome of delirium in critically ill patients: systematic review and meta-analysis. BMJ. 2015;350:h2538.
70. LL RJL. The nature and extent of medical injury in older patients. In: The public policy institute. Washington, DC: AARP; 2000.
71. Milbrandt EB, et al. Costs associated with delirium in mechanically ventilated patients. Crit Care Med. 2004;32(4):955–62.
72. Smith CD, Grami P. Feasibility and effectiveness of a delirium prevention bundle in critically ill patients. Am J Crit Care. 2016;26(1):19–27.
73. Huai J, Ye X. A meta-analysis of critically ill patients reveals several potential risk factors for delirium. Gen Hosp Psychiatry. 2014;36(5):488–96.
74. Brummel NE, et al. Implementing delirium screening in the ICU: secrets to success. Crit Care Med. 2013;41(9):2196–208.
75. Ely EW, et al. Evaluation of delirium in critically ill patients: validation of the Confusion Assessment Method for the Intensive Care Unit (CAM-ICU). Crit Care Med. 2001;29(7):1370–9.
76. Gusmao-Flores D, et al. The Confusion Assessment Method for the Intensive Care Unit (CAM-ICU) and Intensive Care Delirium Screening Checklist (ICDSC) for the diagnosis of delirium: a systematic review and meta-analysis of clinical studies. Crit Care. 2012;16(4):R115.
77. Haenggi M, et al. Effect of sedation level on the prevalence of delirium when assessed with CAM-ICU and ICDSC. Intensive Care Med. 2013;39(12):2171–9.
78. Patel SB, et al. Rapidly reversible, sedation-related delirium versus persistent delirium in the intensive care unit. Am J Respir Crit Care Med. 2014;189(6):658–65.
79. Inouye SK, Westendorp RG, Saczynski JS. Delirium in elderly people. Lancet. 2014;383(9920):911–22.
80. Truman B, Ely EW. Monitoring delirium in critically ill patients. Using the confusion assessment method for the intensive care unit. Crit Care Nurse. 2003;23(2):25–36. quiz 37-8
81. Otremba I, Wilczynski K, Szewieczek J. Delirium in the geriatric unit: proton-pump inhibitors and other risk factors. Clin Interv Aging. 2016;11:397–405.
82. Smonig R, et al. Constipation is independently associated with delirium in critically ill ventilated patients. Intensive Care Med. 2016;42(1):126–7.
83. Flannery AH, Oyler DR, Weinhouse GL. The impact of interventions to improve sleep on delirium in the ICU: a systematic review and research framework. Crit Care Med. 2016;44(12):2231–40.
84. Siew ED, et al.. Acute kidney injury as a risk factor for delirium and coma during critical illness. Am J Respir Crit Care Med. 2017;195(12):1597–1607.
85. Brummel NE, Girard TD. Preventing delirium in the intensive care unit. Crit Care Clin. 2013;29(1):51–65.

86. Pandharipande P, et al. Lorazepam is an independent risk factor for transitioning to delirium in intensive care unit patients. Anesthesiology. 2006;104(1):21–6.
87. Zaal IJ, et al. Benzodiazepine-associated delirium in critically ill adults. Intensive Care Med. 2015;41(12):2130–7.
88. Weinhouse GL, Schwab RJ. Sleep in the critically ill patient. Sleep. 2006;29(5):707–16.
89. Girard TD, et al. Efficacy and safety of a paired sedation and ventilator weaning protocol for mechanically ventilated patients in intensive care (awakening and breathing controlled trial): a randomised controlled trial. Lancet. 2008;371(9607):126–34.
90. Mehta S, et al. Prevalence, risk factors, and outcomes of delirium in mechanically ventilated adults. Crit Care Med. 2015;43(3):557–66.
91. Wolters AE, et al. Systemic corticosteroids and transition to delirium in critically ill patients. Crit Care Med. 2015; 43(12):e585–8.
92. Schreiber MP, et al. Corticosteroids and transition to delirium in patients with acute lung injury. Crit Care Med. 2014;42(6):1480–6.
93. Morandi A, et al. Statins and delirium during critical illness: a multicenter, prospective cohort study. Crit Care Med. 2014;42(8):1899–909.
94. Nelson S, et al. Defining the role of Dexmedetomidine in the prevention of delirium in the intensive care unit. Biomed Res Int. 2015;2015:635737.
95. Rivosecchi RM, et al. Nonpharmacological interventions to prevent delirium: an evidence-based systematic review. Crit Care Nurse. 2015;35(1):39–50. quiz 51
96. Barnes-Daly MA, Phillips G, Ely EW. Improving hospital survival and reducing brain dysfunction at seven California community hospitals: implementing PAD guidelines via the ABCDEF bundle in 6,064 patients. Crit Care Med. 2017;45(2):171–8.
97. Maldonado JR. Delirium in the acute care setting: characteristics, diagnosis and treatment. Crit Care Clin. 2008;24(4):657–722. vii
98. Litton E, et al. The efficacy of earplugs as a sleep hygiene strategy for reducing delirium in the ICU: a systematic review and meta-analysis. Crit Care Med. 2016;44(5):992–9.
99. Wassenaar A, et al. The impact of nUrsiNg DEliRium preventive INnterventions in the intensive care unit (UNDERPIN-ICU): a study protocol for a multi-centre, stepped wedge randomized controlled trial. Int J Nurs Stud. 2016;68:1–8.
100. Siddiqi N, et al. Interventions for preventing delirium in hospitalised non-ICU patients. Cochrane Database Syst Rev. 2016;(3):Cd005563.
101. Larsen KA, et al. Administration of olanzapine to prevent postoperative delirium in elderly joint-replacement patients: a randomized, controlled trial. Psychosomatics. 2010;51(5):409–18.
102. Prakanrattana U, Prapaitrakool S. Efficacy of risperidone for prevention of postoperative delirium in cardiac surgery. Anaesth Intensive Care. 2007;35(5):714–9.
103. Su X, et al. Dexmedetomidine for prevention of delirium in elderly patients after non-cardiac surgery: a randomised, double-blind, placebo-controlled trial. Lancet. 2016;388(10054):1893–902.
104. Mekontso Dessap A, et al. Delirium and circadian rhythm of melatonin during weaning from mechanical ventilation: an ancillary study of a weaning trial. Chest. 2015;148(5):1231–41.
105. Huang HW, et al. Effect of oral melatonin and wearing earplugs and eye masks on nocturnal sleep in healthy subjects in a simulated intensive care unit environment: which might be a more promising strategy for ICU sleep deprivation? Crit Care. 2015;19:124.
106. Hatta K, et al. Preventive effects of ramelteon on delirium: a randomized placebo-controlled trial. JAMA Psychiat. 2014;71(4):397–403.
107. Walker CK, Gales MA. Melatonin receptor agonists for delirium prevention. Ann Pharmacother. 2017;51(1):72–78. doi: 10.1177/1060028016665863. Epub 2016 Aug 20.
108. Girard TD, et al. Feasibility, efficacy, and safety of antipsychotics for intensive care unit delirium: the MIND randomized, placebo-controlled trial. Crit Care Med. 2010;38(2):428–37.
109. Page VJ, et al. Effect of intravenous haloperidol on the duration of delirium and coma in critically ill patients (hope-ICU): a randomised, double-blind, placebo-controlled trial. Lancet Respir Med. 2013;1(7):515–23.
110. Skrobik YK, et al. Olanzapine vs haloperidol: treating delirium in a critical care setting. Intensive Care Med. 2004;30(3):444–9.
111. Devlin JW, et al. Quetiapine for intensive care unit delirium: the evidence remains weak. Pharmacotherapy. 2016;36(2):e12-3. discussion e13-4
112. Devlin JW, et al. Efficacy and safety of quetiapine in critically ill patients with delirium: a prospective, multicenter, randomized, double-blind, placebo-controlled pilot study. Crit Care Med. 2010;38(2):419–27.
113. Michaud CJ, et al. Impact of quetiapine treatment on duration of hypoactive delirium in critically ill adults: a retrospective analysis. Pharmacotherapy. 2015;35(8):731–9.
114. Swan JT, et al. Antipsychotic use and diagnosis of delirium in the intensive care unit. Crit Care. 2012;16(3):R84.
115. Flurie RW, et al. Hospital delirium treatment: continuation of antipsychotic therapy from the intensive care unit to discharge. Am J Health Syst Pharm. 2015;72(23 Suppl 3):S133–9.
116. Tomichek JE, et al. Antipsychotic prescribing patterns during and after critical illness: a prospective cohort study. Crit Care. 2016;20(1):378.
117. Gagnon DJ, et al. Valproate for agitation in critically ill patients: a retrospective study. J Crit Care. 2017;37:119–25.

Alcohol Withdrawal

5

Uzer Khan and Alison Wilson

Introduction

Definition

Alcohol withdrawal syndrome (AWS) is considered to be a conglomeration of symptoms that develops when an individual, with chronic and heavy intake of alcohol, ceases or decreases the intake. These symptoms have been listed in the DSM-5 (Diagnostic and Statistical Manual of Mental Disorders) criteria used to diagnose the disorder [1]:

A. Cessation of (or reduction in) alcohol use that has been heavy and prolonged
B. Two (or more) of the following developing within several hours to a few days after criterion A:
   (a) Autonomic hyperactivity
   (b) Increasing tremor
   (c) Insomnia
   (d) Nausea or vomiting
   (e) Transient visual, tactile, or auditory hallucinations or illusions
   (f) Psychomotor agitation
   (g) Anxiety
   (h) Generalized tonic-clonic seizures

Although the criteria are an attempt to standardize some elements of alcohol withdrawal, individuals presenting with the disorder are invariably positioned on a spectrum. The majority of individuals will have symptoms that are mild and that can be managed as an outpatient. Three to five percent of those presenting in withdrawal, however, will present with symptoms that would be classified as severe, including seizure activity and/or delirium tremens [2].

Epidemiology

According to a 2013 survey, alcohol users amount to over 136 million in the United States. Of these, about eight million are affected by alcohol *dependence* annually, with about 50% of this suffering alcohol withdrawal if alcohol intake is reduced [3, 4]. Such disorders not only affect adequate social functioning but are also associated with the development of significant medical comorbidities and, ultimately, a lifespan shortened by up to a decade [2].

Pathophysiology

Alcohol intake produces its sedative and inhibitory effects through action on two receptors in the central nervous system. It *stimulates* γ-aminobutyric acid (GABA) receptors and *inhibits* *N*-methyl-D-aspartate (NMDA) receptors. With repeated exposure to alcohol, GABA (and specifically $GABA_A$) receptors are down regulated, and NMDA receptors are upregulated. The result is *tolerance* and the need for increasing doses of alcohol to achieve similar effects.

Furthermore, if ingestion of alcohol decreases in a state of alcohol tolerance, *withdrawal symptoms* begin to appear. These symptoms are, in general, the opposite of the inhibitory effects alcohol primarily engenders and revolve around the development of generalized autonomic and sympathetic stimulation as well as psychomotor agitation. These findings include anxiety, tremors, hyperthermia, tachycardia, hypertension, tachypnea, and insomnia [2, 4].

U. Khan
Department of Surgery, Division of Trauma, Acute Care and Critical Care, Ruby Memorial Hospital, WVU Medicine, Morgantown, WV, USA

A. Wilson (✉)
WVU Critical Care and Trauma Institute, Department of Surgery, Ruby Memorial Hospital, WVU Medicine, Morgantown, WV, USA
e-mail: awilson@hsc.wvu.edu

A. Salim et al. (eds.), *Surgical Critical Care Therapy*, https://doi.org/10.1007/978-3-319-71712-8_5

Withdrawal

Mild to Moderate Alcohol Withdrawal

Cessation of alcohol ingestion can produce a withdrawal state. These symptoms can develop as early as 8 h after the normalization of blood alcohol levels. Typically, symptoms peak at the 72-h mark and subside by approximately 7 days [2]. During this period of withdrawal, scoring systems help to evaluate the severity of the syndrome. The Clinical Institute Withdrawal Assessment of Alcohol Scale, revised (CIWA-Ar) [5], is a scoring system designed to help the clinician assess and manage the alcohol withdrawal state. A score can range from 0 to 67 with higher levels indicating more severe symptoms (Table 5.1):

- Scores <8 indicate mild alcohol withdrawal and will often not require the use of medication for treatment.
- Scores ranging from 8 to 15 indicate moderate alcohol withdrawal and will often be treated with low-moderate dose benzodiazepine therapy.
- Scores >15 indicate severe alcohol withdrawal and will likely require close monitoring to prevent progression to seizures and delirium tremens.

Severe Alcohol Withdrawal

More severe symptoms, as mentioned, are consistent with the development of severe alcohol withdrawal syndrome. Untreated, this can progress to the development of seizures and withdrawal delirium with a published mortality rate of 1–4% [2, 6, 7]. The DSM-5 criteria for the diagnosis of delirium are summarized as follows:

A. Decreased attention and awareness
B. Disturbance in attention, awareness, memory, orientation, language, visuospatial ability, perception, or all of these abilities that is a change from the normal level and fluctuates in severity during the day
C. Disturbances in memory, orientation, language, visuospatial ability, or perception
D. No evidence of coma or other evolving neurocognitive disorders

Death is usually secondary to complications from seizures, arrhythmias, hyperthermia, or concomitant medical disorders [2, 8].

CIWA-Ar scores are helpful not only to assist in diagnosing alcohol withdrawal but can help direct therapy. There is a linear relationship, for example, between CIWA-Ar scores and benzodiazepine requirements. Although practiced nurses can conduct the evaluation in 2 min and it has high inter-rater reliability, it is limited by requiring a degree of patient interaction. Hence, the CIWA-Ar can be confounded if patients are, for example, intubated. For such situations, studies have reported the successful use of scales such as the Richmond Agitation-Sedation Scale (RASS), Riker Sedation Analgesia Scale, and the Minnesota Detoxification Scale [9, 10].

Management

Patients undergoing severe alcohol withdrawal and those with marked tremulousness, diaphoresis, hallucinations, and generally severe psychomotor and sympathetic stimulation should be managed in an ICU setting. Other indications for ICU care include withdrawal despite elevated blood alcohol levels, hemodynamic instability, associated organ system failure, previous history of withdrawal complications, and persistent hyperthermia (>39 °C). With initiation of therapy, any persistent increase or high doses of medications to control symptoms should also result in a transfer to the ICU [11].

Once inpatient management is implemented, basic delirium prophylaxis should be instituted. Specifically, patients will often demonstrate confusion and agitation – it will be up to the healthcare providers to provide patient and constant reorientation. Rooms should be quiet and unstimulating during the nighttime. Interruptions should occur only when absolutely necessary, in order to promote sleep hygiene.

Wernicke's Encephalopathy

Many patients undergoing alcohol withdrawal are malnourished and, therefore, at risk for Wernicke's encephalopathy (WE). WE is a syndrome of encephalopathy, oculomotor dysfunction, and ataxia – untreated it can progress to coma and death. This syndrome develops from thiamine deficiency; hence, thiamine supplementation is warranted in the treatment of alcoholics who are at risk due to malnutrition, poor GI absorption of nutrients, and diminished liver storage capability as well as utilization (see below).

Of note, it is classically taught that thiamine requirements are dependent on metabolic demand and glucose intake [12]. Hence, glucose administration prior to thiamine supplementation would precipitate WE and should be withheld until thiamine is administered. This is corroborated by animal studies but has *not* been unequivocally shown in humans where case reports are ambiguous. Hence, the clinician should give due consideration to the substantial harms associated with hypoglycemia, the treatment of which should not be delayed while awaiting thiamine. Acute glucose delivery and repletion, as opposed to a prolonged glucose infusion, is likely to be safe [13].

Table 5.1 CIWA-Ar (Clinical Institute Withdrawal Assessment of Alcohol Scale, Revised) scoring system

Nausea and vomiting: Ask, "Do you feel sick to your stomach? Have you vomited?" Observation 0, no nausea or vomiting 1, mild nausea with no vomiting 2 3 4, intermittent nausea with dry heaves 5 6 7, constant nausea, frequent dry heaves, and vomiting	*Tactile disturbances*: Ask, "Have you any itching, pins and needles sensations, any burning, any numbness, or do you feel bugs crawling on or under your skin?" Observation 0, none 1, very mild itching, pins and needles, burning, or numbness 2, mild itching, pins and needles, burning, or numbness 3, moderate itching, pins and needles, burning, or numbness 4, moderately severe hallucinations 5, severe hallucinations 6, extremely severe hallucinations 7, continuous hallucinations
Tremor: Arms extended and fingers spread apart. Observation 0, no tremor 1, not visible but can be felt fingertip to fingertip 2 3 4, moderate, with patient's arm extended 5 6 7, severe, even with arms not extended	*Auditory disturbances*: Ask, "Are you more aware of sounds around you? Are they harsh? Do they frighten you? Are you hearing anything that is disturbing to you? Are you hearing things you know are not there?" Observation 0, not present 1, very mild harshness or ability to frighten 2, mild harshness or ability to frighten 3, moderate harshness or ability to frighten 4, moderately severe hallucinations 5, severe hallucinations 6, extremely severe hallucinations 7, continuous hallucinations
Paroxysmal sweats: Observation 0, no sweat visible 1, barely perceptible sweating, palms moist 2 3 4, beads of sweat obvious on forehead 5 6 7, drenching sweats	*Visual disturbances*: Ask, "Does the light appear to be too bright? Is its color different? Does it hurt your eyes? Are you seeing anything that is disturbing to you? Are you seeing things you know are not there?" Observation 0, not present 1, very mild sensitivity 2, mild sensitivity 3, moderate sensitivity 4, moderately severe hallucinations 5, severe hallucinations 6, extremely severe hallucinations 7, continuous hallucinations
Anxiety: Ask, "Do you feel nervous?" Observation 0, no anxiety, at ease 1, mildly anxious 2 3 4, moderately anxious, or guarded, so anxiety is inferred 5 6 7, equivalent to acute panic states as seen in severe delirium or acute schizophrenic reactions	*Headache*, fullness in head: Ask, "Does your head feel different? Does it feel like there is a band around your head?" Do not rate for dizziness or lightheadedness. Otherwise, rate severity 0, not present 1, very mild 2, mild 3, moderate 4, moderately severe 5, severe 6, very severe 7, extremely severe
Agitation: Observation 0, normal activity 1, somewhat more than normal activity 2 3 4, moderately fidgety and restless 5 6 7, paces back and forth during most of the interview or constantly thrashes about	*Orientation and clouding of sensorium*: Ask, "What day is this? Where are you? Who am I?" 0, oriented and can do serial additions 1, cannot do serial additions or is uncertain about date 2, disoriented for date by no more than 2 calendar days 3, disoriented for date by more than 2 calendar days 4, disoriented for place or person

Total CIWA-Ar score (maximum = 67):____________

Rater's initials: ____________

"Banana Bags" or Multivitamin Bags

Due to the mentioned macro- and micronutrient deficiencies alcohol withdrawal patients are susceptible to, many institutions will nutritionally supplement patients presenting with alcoholism. Due to the poor bioavailability of orally administered medications in patients with alcoholism, IV supplementation is often utilized.

To this end, most institutions compound an intravenous combination of a variety of nutritional supplements. This "banana bag" generally consists of 100 mg of thiamine, 1 mg of folic acid, 1–2 g of magnesium, and a multivitamin combined in 0.9% normal saline or D5W. It is the multivitamin which imparts the characteristic yellow color of this concoction.

The 100 mg dose of thiamine is generally considered insufficient and ineffective in the prevention of WE. This dose appears to have been arbitrarily chosen by two authors in the 1950s based on what seemed, subjectively, to be a high dose [14]. Furthermore, it appears that thiamine's pharmacokinetics favor intermittent dosing rather than a continuous infusion for optimal absorption into the CNS. In addition, there is insufficient evidence regarding the dosage and desirability of supplementing magnesium and folate.

Therefore, there is concern that the standard "banana bag" is insufficient to prevent Wernicke's encephalopathy in at-risk groups. Flannery et al. in their review, instead, recommend the following [13]:

- 200–500 mg IV thiamine every 8 h for at least 72 h or until WE is ruled out.
- 64 mg/kg magnesium sulfate (approximately 4–5 g for most adults) on day 1, followed by 32 mg/kg on days 2–4 (approximately 2–3 g).
- 400–1000 mcg IV folate.
- IV multivitamin is unlikely to be harmful in this setting; however, it is also unlikely to show benefit in alcoholics with deficiencies. Identification of individual nutrient deficiencies with implemented focused, definitive repletion makes the most sense.
- Isotonic IV fluids are ideal for intravascular volume repletion; however, many patients with alcoholism present in a starved state. These patients may suffer alcoholic ketoacidosis which is often not identified. This is likely to resolve more rapidly by the administration of dextrose-containing solutions.

Pharmacologic Therapy

Along with addressing any underlying comorbid conditions and preventing the development of complications such as WE and malnutrition, the provider caring for a patient in alcohol withdrawal will need to prevent the development of grand mal seizures. This is generally accomplished through the administration of benzodiazepines [15, 16]. Benzodiazepines bind directly to a specific site on the $GABA_A$ receptors to induce sedation and hypnosis and to exert their anticonvulsant effects. The most common agents employed are lorazepam (Ativan), diazepam (Valium), and chlordiazepoxide (Librium). Diazepam and chlordiazepoxide may be preferred in general due to their long action and metabolism to active metabolites – these metabolites may prevent recurrent withdrawal events. Conversely, lorazepam may be superior in patients with liver failure where drugs that generate active metabolites may not be cleared in a predictable fashion.

Benzodiazepines remain the first-line agents in the treatment of alcohol withdrawal, due to their sedating and anticonvulsant effects, and are identified as such in the most recent iteration of the American Psychiatric Association guidelines [17] as well as those of the World Health Organization [18].

There are two general strategies to accomplish the goal of seizure prevention and agitation control.

Fixed-Schedule Therapy

This involves the administration of a set dose of benzodiazepine tapered at a predetermined rate. Medication administration is independent of symptomatology and, therefore, can result in overdosing. This in turn may result in untoward respiratory complications and unnecessarily prolonged inpatient stays relative to symptom-triggered protocols. The only advantage of this regimen is that it involves relatively infrequent assessments, and therefore interventions, by healthcare providers. An example of a fixed-schedule therapy is as follows [19]:

- First 48 h: Lorazepam 2 mg PO every 4 h for a total of 12 doses
- After first 48 h taper as follows:
  - 1 mg every 4 h for six doses (24 h)
  - 0.5 mg every 4 h for six doses (24 h)
- An "as needed" dose of lorazepam may be administered for any worsening withdrawal symptoms (CIWA-Ar >30) until the score was less than 30 for two consecutive assessments.

Symptom-Triggered Therapy

A variety of retrospective and prospective trials have demonstrated the superiority of the symptom-triggered approach to the management of alcohol withdrawal instead of a fixed-schedule therapy [19–22]. These trials have shown equal therapeutic efficacy in preventing seizures while using less overall dose of medications and over a less total time period. Moreover, symptom-triggered therapy allows the subset of patients that require *no medications* for their alcohol withdrawal to avoid being empirically sedated [21]. To determine the amount of benzodiazepine to use, a CIWA-Ar score (see above) is calculated. Although not specifically validated, initially the assessment intervals will likely be as frequent as every 10–15 min with de-escalation proceeding as CIWA scores decrease to hourly and even every 4–6 h.

An example of a symptom-triggered protocol is as follows [19]. In this protocol assessments are done every 4 h:

- For CIWA-Ar score <5, administer 0 mg of lorazepam.
- For CIWA-Ar score 6–9, administer 0.5 mg of lorazepam.
- For CIWA-Ar score 10–19, administer 1 mg of lorazepam.
- For CIWA-Ar score 20–29, administer 2 mg of lorazepam.
- For CIWA-Ar score 30–39, administer 3 mg of lorazepam.
- For CIWA-Ar score >40, administer 4 mg of lorazepam.
- If the score is >30, the patient is assessed hourly and given 3–4 mg of lorazepam until the score is <30 for two consecutive checks.

Adjuncts to Benzodiazepine Therapy

Phenobarbital

The use of phenobarbital in the treatment of AWS is inherently attractive due to pharmacologic synergy; it theoretically exhibits with benzodiazepines (the former increases the duration of GABA inhibition; the latter increases the frequency of chloride channel opening). Nevertheless, the evidence supporting its use as monotherapy or as an adjunct is limited. One study comparing a single emergency room dose of phenobarbital 10 mg/kg plus symptom-triggered therapy versus symptom-triggered therapy alone resulted in fewer ICU admissions for alcohol withdrawal [23]. Other studies have limited its use to refractory alcohol withdrawal [9, 10]. These retrospective trials demonstrated a reduced need for mechanical ventilation and reduced ICU length of stay. In these trials escalating doses of benzodiazepine were used until a trigger dose was hit at which point phenobarbital, also in an escalating fashion, was initiated. An example of this protocol follows:

- Diazepam dose escalation until 100–150 mg/dose.
- If agitation persists despite maximal diazepam dose, add escalating doses of IV phenobarbital (65, 130, and 260) to IV diazepam.
- If agitation persists, intubate and initiate continuous sedation.

Propofol

Propofol is a $GABA_A$ agonist and NMDA antagonist. Due to its heavy respiratory depressant effects, its use is limited to severe, refractory alcohol withdrawal in patients who are already receiving high-dose benzodiazepines and who have required intubation. Several case series, cohort studies, and retrospective reviews have demonstrated its use to be safe [4]. Propofol may be initiated at 0.3–1.25 mg/kg body weight up to 4 mg/kg/h for up to 48 h [2].

Dexmedetomidine

Dexmedetomidine (DEX) is an α_2 receptor agonist that blunts sympathetic autonomic activity (by decreasing norepinephrine synthesis) and promotes parasympathetic activity by activating receptors in the medullary vasomotor center. Its mechanism of action is similar to clonidine although it has a much higher specificity for α_2 than α_1 receptors (1600:1 for DEX vs 200:1 for clonidine). Hence, its clinical effects revolve around anxiolysis, sedation, analgesia, and sympatholysis [4]. As a sedative-analgesic, the lack of respiratory depression is touted as a major advantage. Randomized trials have also demonstrated a protective effect against delirium [25–27], although that assertion has recently been challenged [28]. The major adverse effect of DEX is bradycardia. When using DEX, it should be borne in mind that DEX does not have anticonvulsant or GABA receptor activity and, therefore, is insufficient as monotherapy for alcohol withdrawal – its use is strictly adjunctive.

The recommended dose of DEX includes a loading dose of 1 mcg/kg over *10 min* followed by a maintenance infusion of 0.2–0.7 mcg/kg/h. The loading dose may be omitted if the patient is already adequately sedated on another sedative regimen (and DEX is being used to switch over) or if there is concern for hemodynamic compromise. Limiting titration of the maintenance dose to no more frequently than every 30 min may also improve hemodynamic tolerance. Although the FDA's maximum dose is recommended at 0.7 mcg/kg/h, large trials have confirmed the safety of the drug at doses of up to 1.5 mcg/kg/h [24, 25]. Additional doses beyond this level appear to have limited therapeutic efficacy.

The available literature is insufficient to help generate a formal recommendation about the use of DEX in alcohol withdrawal [27–29]; the two randomized trials addressing this issue are relatively small and underpowered [30, 31]. The summary of the literature suggests that adding DEX to patients already receiving benzodiazepines can reduce the doses required of the latter. Effects on ICU length of stay, hospital length of stay, and intubation rates are variable.

Miscellaneous Adjuncts

Baclofen is a $GABA_B$ receptor agonist. Studies, detailing its use in the inpatient ICU environment, are limited. A recent Cochrane review [32] identified only two randomized controlled trials with a total of 81 patients. Its use may have potential in decreasing total benzodiazepine dose in a patient with AWS.

Ketamine works as an NMDA antagonist. Only a single, small (23 patients), unmatched retrospective review [33] has evaluated its use in AWS. This study demonstrated a trend toward decrease in total benzodiazepine use in the first 12 h after initiation, but this trend was nonsignificant. Hence, ketamine does not appear to have any impact on the management of AWS, and therefore its use should be limited until further studies can more emphatically support its use.

The uses of anticonvulsants such as valproic acid or carbamazepine as adjuncts to benzodiazepines have also been evaluated. The literature is sparse [34]. A 2014 Cochrane review [35] has, thus, concluded that the use of anticonvulsants should be guided by individual clinical risk/benefit as the available evidence is of limited quantity and low quality.

Atypical and typical antipsychotics have been shown to decrease the seizure threshold and should be used with care and only as adjuncts in AWS. Moreover, they may prolong the QT interval and predispose to cardiac complications. A diagnostic imperative to consider is whether a patient is suffering from AWS or ICU delirium as therapies will differ accordingly. The timing of onset of symptoms may be relevant. Validated screening tools such as the Confusion Assessment Method for the ICU (CAM-ICU) or the Intensive Care Delirium Screening Checklist (ICDSC) may also be of benefit.

Enteral and Intravenous Ethanol

Bypassing the preceding pharmacologic discussion provided in this text and leapfrogging to the obvious notion of providing withdrawing patients with ethanol (enteral or intravenous) to suppress their symptoms is an ostensibly sensible notion. Ethanol's use may seem to be specifically reasonable in situations where the sedative effects of benzodiazepines are particularly troublesome such as in the frequent neurologic assessment required for patients suffering traumatic brain injury or strokes. Indeed, avoiding the respiratory depressant and sedative effects of benzodiazepines is the primary argument for the use of ethanol in AWS.

Nevertheless, the few studies that have evaluated the use of ethanol deem it to be, at best, non-inferior to benzodiazepines, and with no demonstrable advantage with regard to sedation and respiratory depression.

The use of *enteral* ethanol has recently been evaluated in a cardiac critical care unit as a supplement to a standard lorazepam protocol [36]. This pilot study concluded that supplemental use of ethanol was safe but demonstrated no improvement in ICU or hospital length of stay and no difference in cardiac complications. Another study conducted among neurocritical care patients similarly found no difference in CIWA score change during the first 24 h, as well as no improvement in relative sedation [37].

Studies evaluating the use of *intravenous* ethanol demonstrate essentially similar findings with a similar degree of uncertainty. It is unclear what blood alcohol levels (BAL) are necessary to maintain AWS prophylaxis or treatment. Gower and Kersten suggest that a detectable BAL is not necessary to maintain therapeutic efficacy [38], whereas Hansbrough et al. recommend maintaining levels between 0.2 and 0.8 mg/ml [39]. The latter may require volume administration of over 200–400 ml/h of 5% ethanol in healthy adults which can, in turn, generate the significant problems associated with fluid overload and hyponatremia. Part of the reason behind this uncertainty is that it is unknown *how* BALs contribute to successful alcohol withdrawal prophylaxis. Eggers et al. studied alcohol withdrawal in their ICU population and noted that IV Ethanol was associated with a 41% failure rate. Moreover, the total ethanol dose and actual blood alcohol levels did not differ between groups that were successful in their AWS prophylaxis and those that were not [40]. Moreover, benzodiazepines appear to be better tolerated than anticipated. Weinberg et al. evaluated 50 trauma patients admitted to the ICU in whom they compared a fixed-schedule diazepam protocol to their institutional IV ethanol protocol [41]. They noted superior symptom control in the benzodiazepine group with no episodes of oversedation.

In addition to the questionable efficacy of ethanol described in the preceding discussion, there are ethical imperatives worth discussing. Enteral ethanol is established to be a strong relapse trigger in addiction medicine. The provision of enteral ethanol may be construed as a valid therapeutic modality, exposes the patient to taste and behavioral cues, and may be misinterpreted as reinforcement for the patient's continued drinking [42]. Evaluating and treating the intoxicated trauma patient is an enormous responsibility and opportunity for the healthcare provider. A recent systematic review collated information from 12 separate studies and noted that, in over 3000 trauma recidivists, 41% of trauma recidivism was related to the use of alcohol [43]. Moreover, after intervention, abstinence rates of 60% have been documented [44], as well as a 47% reduction in injuries requiring either emergency department or trauma center admission [44]. This underscores not only the need for early alcohol intervention but also for a consistent message delivered by all healthcare disciplines caring for the patient.

In light of the evidence cited above, ethanol's pharmacokinetic inconsistency, narrow and unclear therapeutic window, high failure rates, and ethical considerations, published guidelines have recommended against the routine use of ethanol, enteral or intravenous, in the treatment or prophylaxis of AWS [7, 11, 15].

Summary

The current evidence maintains that benzodiazepines are effective as first-line agents in the treatment of AWS. Symptom-triggered protocols have been shown to decrease the total amount of benzodiazepine use as well as the total duration of therapy. Patients refractory to, or who are predicted to be refractory to, high-dose benzodiazepine therapy may benefit from a dose of phenobarbital. This dose has been shown to be effective whether given upfront prior to the initiation of benzodiazepines or when a patient is noted to be refractory after multiple doses have been administered. At this time, the safety and efficacy profile of longer-term barbiturate infusions is unclear. In addition, dexmedetomidine may also promote a benzodiazepine-sparing effect. Its use is particularly beneficial due to the lack of a respiratory depressant effect but should not be used as monotherapy due to the absence of an anticonvulsant effect. Propofol may also be considered as an adjunct. There is no suggestion that its benzodiazepine-sparing effect is superior to DEX, and it may increase duration of ventilation and ICU length of stay. Nevertheless, it may be considered in patients who are already ventilated and have adverse hemodynamic reactions to DEX. Based on the current state of the literature, the use of baclofen, ketamine, anticonvulsants, antipsychotics, and ethanol should all be considered very carefully particularly in the ICU setting.

References

1. American Psychiatric Association. Diagnostic and statistical manual of mental disorders. 5th ed. Washington, DC: American Psychiatric Association; 2013.
2. Schuckit MA. Recognition and management of withdrawal delirium (delirium tremens). N Engl J Med. 2014;371(22):2109–13.
3. Kosten TR, O'Connor PG. Management of drug and alcohol withdrawal. N Engl J Med. 2003;18(348):1786–95.
4. Schmidt KJ, Doshi MR, Holzhausen JM, Natavio A, Cadiz M, Winegardner JE. Treatment of severe alcohol withdrawal. Ann Pharmacother. 2016;50(5):389–401.
5. Sullivan JT, Sykora K, Schneiderman J, Naranjo CA, Sellers EM. Assessment of alcohol withdrawal: the revised clinical institute withdrawal assessment for alcohol scale (CIWA-Ar). Br J Addict. 1989;84(11):1353–7.
6. Mainerova B, Prasko J, Latalova K, et al. Alcohol withdrawal delirium - diagnosis, course and treatment. Biomed Pap Med Fac Univ Palacky Olomouc Czech Repub. 2015;159(1):44–52.
7. Mayo-Smith MF, Beecher LH, Fischer TL, et al. Management of alcohol withdrawal delirium. An evidence-based practice guideline. Arch Intern Med. 2004;164(13):1405–12.
8. Khan A, Levy P, DeHorn S, et al. Predictors of mortality in patients with delirium tremens. Acad Emerg Med. 2008;15(8):788–90.
9. Gold JA, Rimal B, Nolan A, Nelson LS. A strategy of escalating doses of benzodiazepines and phenobarbital administration reduces the need for mechanical ventilation in delirium tremens. Crit Care Med. 2007;35(3):724–30.
10. Duby JJ, Berry AJ, Ghayyem P, et al. Alcohol withdrawal syndrome in critically ill patients: protocolized versus nonprotocolized management. J Trauma Acute Care Surg. 2014;77(6):938–43.
11. Carlson RW, Kumar NN, Wong-Mckinstry E, et al. Alcohol withdrawal syndrome. Crit Care Clin. 2012;28(4):549–85.
12. Schabelman E, Kuo D. Glucose before thiamine for Wernicke encephalopathy: a literature review. J Emerg Med. 2012;42(4):488–94.
13. Flannery AH, Adkins DA, Cook AM. Unpeeling the evidence for the banana bag: evidence-based recommendations for the management of alcohol-associated vitamin and electrolyte deficiencies in the ICU. Crit Care Med. 2016;44(8):1545–52.
14. Donnino MW, Vega J, Miller J, Walsh M. Myths and misconceptions of Wernicke's encephalopathy: what every emergency physician should know. Ann Emerg Med. 2007;50(6):715–21.
15. Mayo-Smith MF. Pharmacological management of alcohol withdrawal. A meta-analysis and evidence-based practice guideline. American Society of Addiction Medicine Working Group on Pharmacological Management of Alcohol Withdrawal. JAMA. 1997;9(2):144–51.
16. Lejoyeux M, Solomon J, Adès J. Benzodiazepine treatment for alcohol-dependent patients. Alcohol Alcohol. 1998;33(6):563–75.
17. Kleber HD, Weiss RD, Anton Jr. RF, et al. American Psychiatric Association. [Online]; 2006 [cited 2017 Jan. Available from https://www.psychiatry.org/psychiatrists/practice/clinical-practice-guidelines.
18. World Health Organization. [Online]; 2012 [cited 2017 Jan. Available from http://www.who.int/mental_health/mhgap/evidence/alcohol/q2/en/.
19. Weaver MF, Hoffman HJ, Johnson RE, Mauck K. Alcohol withdrawal pharmacotherapy for inpatients with medical comorbidity. J Addict Dis. 2006;25(2):17–24.
20. Saitz R, Mayo-Smith MF, Roberts MS, et al. Individualized treatment for alcohol withdrawal. A randomized double-blind controlled trial. JAMA. 1994;272(7):519–23.
21. Daeppen JB, Gache P, Landry U, et al. Symptom-triggered vs fixed-schedule doses of benzodiazepine for alcohol withdrawal: a randomized treatment trial. Arch Intern Med. 2002;162(10):1117–21.
22. Jaeger TM, Lohr RH, Pankratz VS. Symptom-triggered therapy for alcohol withdrawal syndrome in medical inpatients. Mayo Clin Proc. 2001;76(7):695–701.
23. Rosenson J, Clements C, Simon B, et al. Phenobarbital for acute alcohol withdrawal: a prospective randomized double-blind placebo-controlled study. J Emerg Med. 2013;44(3):592–8.
24. Pandharipande PP, Pun BT, Herr DL, et al. Effect of sedation with dexmedetomidine vs lorazepam on acute brain dysfunction in mechanically ventilated patients: the MENDS randomized controlled trial. JAMA. 2007;298(22):2644–53.

25. Riker R, Shehabi Y, Bokesch P, et al. Dexmedetomidine vs midazolam for sedation of critically ill patients: a randomized trial. JAMA. 2009;301(5):489–99. Skrupky LP, Drewry AM, Wessman B, et al. Clinical effectiveness of a sedation protocol minimizing benzodiazepine infusions and favoring early dexmedetomidine: a before-after study. Crit Care. 2016;19(136).
26. Crispo AL, Daley MJ, Pepin JL, et al. Comparison of clinical outcomes in nonintubated patients with severe alcohol withdrawal syndrome treated with continuous-infusion sedatives: dexmedetomidine versus benzodiazepines. Pharmacotherapy. 2014;34(9):910–7.
27. Lizotte RJ, Kappes JA, Bartel BJ, et al. Evaluating the effects of dexmedetomidine compared to propofol as adjunctive therapy in patients with alcohol withdrawal. Clin Pharmacol. 2014;31(6):171–7.
28. Frazee EN, Personett HA, Leung JG, et al. Influence of dexmedetomidine therapy on the management of severe alcohol withdrawal syndrome in critically ill patients. J Crit Care. 2014;29(2):298–302.
29. Mueller SW, Preslaski CR, Kiser TH, et al. A randomized, double-blind, placebo-controlled dose range study of dexmedetomidine as adjunctive therapy for alcohol withdrawal. Crit Care Med. 2014;42(5):1131–9.
30. Bielka K, Kuchyn I, Glumcher F. Addition of dexmedetomidine to benzodiazepines for patients with alcohol withdrawal syndrome in the intensive care unit: a randomized controlled study. Ann Intensive Care. 2015;5(33)
31. Liu J, Wang LN. Baclofen for alcohol withdrawal. Cochrane Database Syst Rev. 2013;28(2):1–33, CD008502.
32. Wong A, Benedict NJ, Armahizer MJ, Kane-Gill SL. Evaluation of adjunctive ketamine to benzodiazepines for management of alcohol withdrawal syndrome. Ann Pharmacother. 2015;49(1):14–9.
33. Eyer F, Schreckenberg M, Hecht D, et al. Carbamazepine and valproate as adjuncts in the treatment of alcohol withdrawal syndrome: a retrospective cohort study. Alcohol Alcohol. 2011;46(2):177–84.
34. Pani PP, Trogu E, Pacini M, Maremmani I. Anticonvulsants for alcohol dependence. Cochrane Database Syst Rev. 2014;(2): CD008544.
35. Fullwood JE, Mostaghimi Z, Granger CB, et al. Alcohol withdrawal prevention: a randomized evaluation of lorazepam and ethanol--a pilot study. Am J Crit Care. 2013;22(5):398–406.
36. Gipson G, Tran K, Hoang C, Treggiari M. Comparison of enteral ethanol and benzodiazepines for alcohol withdrawal in neurocritical care patients. J Clin Neurosci. 2016;31:88–91.
37. Gower WE, Kersten H. Prevention of alcohol withdrawal symptoms in surgical patients. Surg Gynecol Obstet. 1980;151(3): 382–4.
38. Hansbrough JF, Zapata-Sirvent RL, Carroll WJ, et al. Administration of intravenous alcohol for prevention of withdrawal in alcoholic burn patients. Am J Surg. 1984;148(2):266–9.
39. Eggers V, Tio J, Neumann T, et al. Blood alcohol concentration for monitoring ethanol treatment to prevent alcohol withdrawal in the intensive care unit. Intensive Care Med. 2002;28(10):1475–82.
40. Weinberg JA, Magnotti LJ, Fischer PE, et al. Comparison of intravenous ethanol versus diazepam for alcohol withdrawal prophylaxis in the trauma ICU: results of a randomized trial. J Trauma. 2008;64(1):99–104.
41. DiPaula B, Tommasello A, Solounias B, McDuff D. An evaluation of intravenous ethanol in hospitalized patients. J Subst Abus Treat. 1998;15(5):437–42.
42. Nunn J, Erdogan M, Green RS. The prevalence of alcohol-related trauma recidivism: a systematic review. Injury. 2016;47(3): 551–8.
43. Gentilello LM, Duggan P, Drummond D, et al. Major injury as a unique opportunity to initiate treatment in the alcoholic. Am J Surg. 1988;156(6):558–61.
44. Gentilello LM, Rivara FP, Donovan DM, et al. Alcohol interventions in a trauma center as a means of reducing the risk of injury recurrence. Ann Surg. 1999;230(4):473.

6 Brain Death Evaluation and Determination

Anupamaa Seshadri and Ali Salim

Introduction

Brain death is an important concept for the surgical intensivist to be aware of. As "brain death" has been a controversial subject since the inception of term, the development of a clear definition and standard diagnostic requirements of brain death have been critically important. The first important step in establishing brain death as a clear medical entity was the passage of the Uniform Determination of Death Act (UDDA) in 1981, which provided a legal definition of death. This reads, "An individual who has sustained either (1) irreversible cessation of circulatory and respiratory functions, or (2) irreversible cessation of all functions of the entire brain, including the brain stem, is dead. A determination of death must be made with accepted medical standards" [1]. The dilemma posed by this legislation, however, is that it does not specify the "accepted medical standards" that are required for the determination of neurological death. Therefore, medical societies including the American Academy of Neurology (AAN) have since published guidelines in order to assist physicians in standardizing the determination of brain death [2, 3].

This chapter delineates the basic diagnosis of brain death as described by the AAN guidelines, including the cardinal findings of brain death required for diagnosis as well as confirmatory tests that can be used as ancillary evidence of brain death. These criteria are important for every surgical intensivist to know, particularly because surgical critical care physicians are often involved in the care of patients with severe brain injury. Furthermore, this knowledge assists the surgical intensivist in giving prognosis to a patient's family, allowing them to prepare for end-of-life care as well as for potential organ donation.

A. Seshadri
Department of Surgery, Brigham and Women's Hospital, Boston, MA, USA

A. Salim (✉)
Division of Trauma, Burn, Surgical Critical Care and Emergency General Surgery, Brigham and Women's Hospital, Harvard Medical School, Boston, MA, USA
e-mail: asalim1@bwh.harvard.edu

Cardinal Findings of Brain Death

The American Academy of Neurology (AAN) published practice parameters in 1995 to define the medical standards required for the determination of brain death, with an update in 2010 to help improve uniformity in diagnosis [2, 3]. The recommendations were based upon peer-reviewed literature, textbooks across multiple disciplines, as well as expert opinion.

These practice parameters described the three cardinal findings in brain death: coma or unresponsiveness, absence of brainstem reflexes, and apnea. Prior to being able to determine the presence or absence of these cardinal findings, multiple physiological prerequisites must be met. These are demonstrated in our institutional guidelines for determination of brain death (Table 6.1). First, it is required that there be clinical or neuroimaging evidence of an acute central nervous system (CNS) catastrophe which would lead to potential brain death. Second, there must be no complicating medical condition that could potentially lead to a misdiagnosis or altered clinical assessment of neurological function. In similar fashion, there must be no drug intoxication or poisoning that could affect the physician's ability to test neurologic function, including drugs normally used for sedation, like benzodiazepines, in the critically ill. One suggested guideline is to conduct the neurological examination after five to seven times of the elimination half-life of any such drug that the patient has been exposed to has elapsed [4]. Finally, the patient must not be hypothermic, which is defined as a core temperature ≥32 °C. With these parameters, there has been no report to date of recovery of neurologic function in adults after the clinical diagnosis of brain death.

There is geographic variation in the number and timing of neurologic examinations required for the determination of brain death. Most states in the United States state that one neurologic exam with the cardinal findings is sufficient to pronounce brain death. However, some states require two clinical evaluations, which the guidelines suggest can be spaced 6 h apart, with the caveat that this spacing is arbitrary

A. Salim et al. (eds.), *Surgical Critical Care Therapy*, https://doi.org/10.1007/978-3-319-71712-8_6

Table 6.1 Brigham and Women's Hospital institutional guidelines on the determination of brain death

Institutional guidelines for declaration of death by neurologic criteria	
Preconditions (all must be present)	Coma, irreversible and cause known
	Absence of severe acid-base, electrolyte, or endocrine abnormality
	Normothermia (core temperature > 36.5 °C)
	Systolic blood pressure ≥ 90 mmHg with or without pressors
	No spontaneous respirations
Examination (all must be present)	Pupils nonreactive to bright light
	Corneal reflex absent
	Oculocephalic reflex absent (if cervical spine integrity ensured)
	No facial movement to noxious stimuli at supraorbital nerve
	Gag reflex absent
	Cough reflex absent to tracheal suctioning
	Absence of motor response to noxious stimuli in all four limbs (spinally mediated reflexes permissible)
Apnea test (must be performed at least once; if indeterminate, proceed to ancillary testing)	Apnea with $PaCO_2 \geq 60$ mmHg or increase in $PaCO_2$ of ≥20 mmHg over baseline normal $PaCO_2$ after 8 min
Ancillary tests (not required)	Cerebral angiogram
	HMPAO SPECT nuclear medicine brain scan
	Electroencephalogram
	Transcranial Doppler

and not evidence-based. All physicians in most US states are legally allowed to perform these examinations, but some states or individual hospitals have more strict requirements of expertise for a physician to declare brain death. Because of the profound implications of the diagnosis of brain death, it is reasonable that any physician performing this evaluation be not only intimately familiar with the criteria but also has demonstrated competence in the brain death examination.

First, a comprehensive neurological exam is required to establish the unresponsiveness of the patient as well as the absence of brainstem reflexes. The AAN defines coma or unresponsiveness as a lack of cerebral motor response to pain in all extremities; the guidelines define pain stimuli as nail-bed pressure and supraorbital pressure. There are numerous brainstem reflexes that are required to be tested by the AAN practice parameters. Pupillary reflex is defined as pupillary light response with pupil size 4–9 mm. Ocular movement is determined by evaluating the oculocephalic reflex and oculovestibular reflex. For determining the presence or absence of the oculocephalic reflex, the head is turned quickly to each side. If the reflex is present, the eyes will move to focus on the side the head was originally facing, and if the reflex is absent, there will be no ocular movement, and the eyes will continue to look straight ahead. The oculovestibular reflex can be determined by elevating the head 30 degrees and infusing 50 cc of ice water into an external auditory canal. If the reflex is present, there will be a nystagmus toward the ear that was infused, and if the reflex is absent, there will be no eye movement. Facial sensation or motor function is determined by the corneal reflex, jaw reflex, or grimacing to deep pressure. Pharyngeal or tracheal reflexes are determined by the presence or absence of cough or gag. In this way, a thorough neurological exam can determine both unresponsiveness as well as the absence of brainstem reflexes.

The third cardinal finding in brain death is apnea. Prior to conducting the apnea test, strict physiologic factors must be measured to determine that there is no other reason for the patient to become apneic. First, the patient must be normothermic with a more strict definition of core temperature ≥ 36.5 °C. Second, the patient must either be euvolemic or hypovolemic (defined as positive fluid balance in the 6 h prior to testing) and must be normotensive with a systolic blood pressure ≥ 90 mmHg. Third, the patient should have a normal PCO_2, which is not clearly defined in the literature but is suggested in the guidelines to be an arterial $PCO_2 \geq 40$ mmHg. Furthermore, the patient should have a normal PO_2, which again is not clearly defined in the literature, but for which the guidelines suggest to preoxygenate the patient prior to testing to obtain an arterial $PO_2 \geq 200$ mmHg.

After it is determined that the patient meets these physiologic criteria, the patient should be connected to a pulse oximeter and disconnected from the mechanical ventilator. Delivery of 100% O_2 at 6 L/min should be given through a catheter at the carina without positive pressure. During the test, the patient should be monitored closely for any evidence of respiratory movements. The patient's arterial PO_2, PCO_2, and pH should be measured after 8 min of being disconnected from the ventilator. Once these tests are drawn, the patient can then be reconnected to the ventilator. If there was no evidence of respiratory movement during the observed 8-min period and the measured arterial PCO_2 is either ≥60 mmHg or if there is a 20 mmHg increase of PCO_2 over a baseline normal PCO_2, the apnea test is deemed positive and indicative of brain death because of a lack of ventilation. If these parameters are not met, the diagnosis of brain death is not supported. In this case, if the patient remained hemodynamically stable through the procedure, the test can be repeated for a longer period of time (approximately 10–15 min) after repeat preoxygenation to better determine whether the patient is able to ventilate without assistance.

Should the patient's systolic blood pressure drop below 90 mmHg or should hypoxia to O_2 saturation of <85% for more than 30 s during the test, the patient can be reconnected to the ventilator before the 8-min test period is completed. Arterial blood should be drawn and analyzed at that time. If the arterial PCO2 is ≥60 mmHg or there is an increase in arterial PCO_2 of ≥20 mmHg over a baseline normal PCO_2, the apnea test indicates brain death. If these parameters are not met, the result is indeterminate, and additional confirmatory tests are required. In the case of desaturation, the procedure can be retried with the use of a T-piece, CPAP to 10 cm H_2O, and 100% O_2 at 12 L/min, to try to prevent hypoxia from ending the test before determination can be made.

Difficulties and Strategies in Clinical Diagnosis of Brain Death

In some conditions where there may be interference with the clinical diagnosis of brain death, confirmatory tests may be required. For example, patients with severe facial trauma or preexisting pupillary abnormalities cannot be adequately ruled out through testing brainstem reflexes because of their underlying conditions. Furthermore, the presence of toxic levels of several drugs including sedatives, anticholinergics, antiepileptics, and neuromuscular blocking agents can affect the patient's neurological exam and prevent diagnosis, and these agents may not always be able to be weaned prior to testing. The apnea test may not be able to be performed in patients with sleep apnea or severe pulmonary disease resulting in chronic retention of CO_2 as well as in patients with high cervical spinal cord injuries. For these patients, confirmatory imaging is recommended.

There are some clinical manifestations that may be seen by the practitioner that may appear to be evidence of brainstem function but are actually compatible with brain death. These include occasional spontaneous nondirected movement of limbs, respiratory-like movements that do not result in significant tidal volumes, sweating or blushing, normal blood pressure without pressor support, deep tendon reflexes, and the Babinski reflex. Despite the presence of these signs, if the patient has unresponsiveness, lack of brainstem reflexes, and apnea, the patient meets the criteria for brain death.

Confirmatory Tests for Brain Death

Adjunctive tests are sometimes required to provide corroborative evidence of brain death. These may also be used as confirmation in order to make the diagnosis of brain death earlier, which is considered useful for facilitating possible transplantation. The updated AAN guidelines specify three preferred tests: conventional cerebral angiography, nuclear brain scan, and electroencephalography (EEG) [3]. CT angiography, MR angiography, and transcranial Doppler studies are also used in practice for ancillary testing [3].

The most sensitive imaging test for determining brain death is cerebral angiography. In a patient with brain death, intracranial pressure rises, resulting in diminished cerebral perfusion pressure. Because of this, there will be no intracerebral filling at the level of the carotid bifurcation or the circle of Willis evident on cerebral angiograph. The external carotid circulation is usually patent, and the filling of the superior sagittal sinus may be delayed. While this is still considered the gold standard ancillary test for neurologic death, the test is invasive and requires that the patient be stable for transfer to the angiography suite. Of note, patients with open skull defects, such as decompressive craniectomies, have been shown to have false-negative results with a small amount of residual flow in patients that are clinically brain dead because intracranial pressure may not exceed cerebral perfusion pressure [5].

A nuclear medicine brain scan can be performed to determine brain death and may be preferred as it is a less invasive option. The AAN guidelines specifically recommend Technetium-99 m hexamethylpropyleneamineoxime (Tc-99 m HMPAO) scanning, which uses a lipophilic agent that can cross the blood brain barrier [6, 7]. In the brain dead patient, there is no uptake of isotope in the brain parenchyma, demonstrating lack of cerebral perfusion (Fig. 6.1). This may be referred to as the "hollow skull phenomenon" [2]. Munari et al. compared Tc-99m HMPAO SPECT brain scans to four-vessel angiography in 20 patients, demonstrating 100% congruency of findings between the two studies [8]. The specificity of radionuclide brain scans for the absence of cerebral perfusion has been shown to be virtually 100% [9].

EEG is a convenient adjunct for diagnosing brain death, as it can be performed bedside for critically ill patients. Brain death is diagnosed by the absence of electrical activity for at least 30 min, which constitutes electrocerebral silence (ECS). This requires that the recording adheres to the minimal technical criteria as adopted by the American Electroencephalographic Society [2]. Somatosensory evoked potentials can also be performed with bilateral absence of response to median nerve stimulation being indicative of brain death [2].

Computed tomography angiography (CTA) has not yet been included in the AAN guidelines but is beginning to be widely used because it is a noninvasive test that is widely available. Furthermore, many patients that are being potentially evaluated for brain death may also be receiving head CT scans for medical management purposes, making CT angiography cost-effective as well. The purpose of a CT angiography is to determine lack of brain perfusion via non-opacification of intracerebral vessels, similar to a conventional cerebral angiography. A three-phase scan of the head and neck can be performed with a noncontrast phase, an arterial phase, and a venous phase, in order to fully evaluate perfusion of the brain [10, 11]. One meta-analysis from 2015

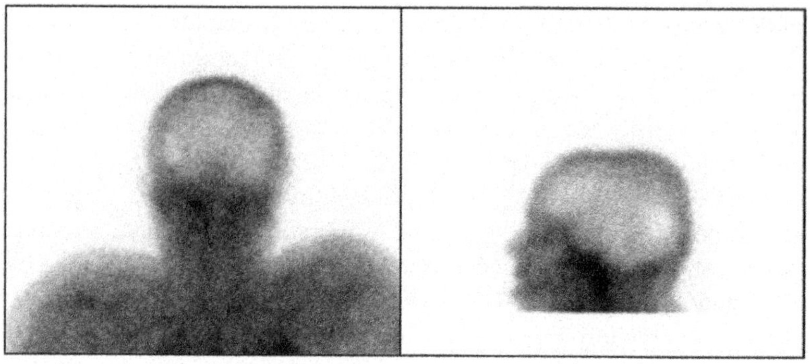

Fig. 6.1 Tc-99m nuclear medicine brain scan of patient demonstrating "hollow skull" sign, indicative of lack of cerebral perfusion and brain death

evaluating the sensitivity of CTA for brain death showed a wide range between 52.4% and 100%, but this reflects heterogeneity in the number of opacified vessels required to diagnose brain death by each individual study within the analysis [12]. The first CTA score for brain death, developed by Dupas et al., required lack of opacification of seven intracerebral vessels including the pericallosal arteries, cortical segments of the middle cerebral arteries (MCAs), internal cerebral veins (ICVs), and one great cerebral vein per patient [13]. With this seven-point system, Combes et al. found CTA to be 69.7% sensitive compared to conventional angiography [8]. Frampas et al. then developed a simpler four-point score, requiring lack of opacification of the cortical segments of the MCAs and the ICVs [14]. This group then reevaluated the patients studied in Combes et al.'s study and, using the four-point scale, found improved sensitivity of 81.4%. A subsequent case series compared the two scoring systems and found them both to have the same sensitivity of 72.7% [15]. There is not yet a consensus on which and how many vessels are required to lack opacification on CTA for confirmation of brain death. Therefore, further large-scale studies are likely required before CTA will be included in the AAN guidelines.

Magnetic resonance angiography (MRA) has also been used to evaluate cerebral perfusion for the assessment of brain death. Similar to CTA, MRA evaluates several intracranial vessels for the absence of opacification and can show intraparenchymal lesions such as infarcted tissue, microhemorrhages, or cerebral edema [16]. MRA is a significantly longer study than a CTA to perform, however, and therefore its use may be limited in unstable patients. Similar to CTA, there is again no consensus on which or how many vessels are required to be examined for determination of brain death. Therefore, MRA also requires more study prior to being included in the AAN guidelines.

Transcranial Doppler (TCD) ultrasonography is a newer imaging modality that can be used to evaluate cerebral perfusion and is appealing in that it is a noninvasive test that can be performed at the bedside. Indications of cerebral circulatory arrest on TCD include oscillating or reverberating flow and systolic spikes, which develop from intracranial pressure being higher than diastolic blood pressure in the brain dead patient [17, 18]. The specific intracranial vessels evaluated are typically the internal carotid artery and the middle cerebral artery. Confirmation is further determined by evaluation of the extracranial common carotid artery, internal carotid artery, and vertebral artery [17]. This can be challenging in up to 10–15% of patients due to difficulty in penetrating the temporal bone barrier, which can lead to a false finding of no flow [19]. A meta-analysis performed by Monteiro et al. showed an 89–95% sensitivity for TCD in diagnosis of cerebral circulatory arrest, including patients whose vessels were unable to be localized with TCD as a negative result, with a 99% specificity [18]. As in all ultrasound modality tests, TCD is operator-dependent and requires the performance of the test to be done by a skilled and practiced ultrasonographer if the test is to be considered reliable. There are also several reports in the literature of skull defects leading to false-negative results, and this should be taken into account when using TCD [20–23].

Documentation

At the time of diagnosis of brain death, proper documentation is critically important. The documented time of death is defined by the AAN as the time the arterial PCO_2 reaches the target value of either ≥60 mmHg or >20 mmHg above a normal baseline arterial PCO_2 during an apnea test. Should a confirmatory test be required, the time of death is documented as the time that the confirmatory test was officially interpreted. Once brain death is determined, federal and state law requires the physician to contact the appropriate local organ procurement organization.

References

1. Uniform Determination of Death Act, 12 uniform laws annotated 589 (West 1993 and West suppl 1997).
2. The quality standards subcommittee of the American Academy of Neurology. Practice parameters for determining brain death in adults (summary statement). Neurology. 1995;45:1012–4.
3. The quality standards subcommittee of the American Academy of Neurology. Evidence-based guideline update: determining brain death in adults. Neurology. 2010;74:1911–8.
4. Wijdicks EFM. Brain death. Handb Clin Neurol. 2013;118:191–203.
5. Escudero D, et al. Diagnosing brain death by CT perfusion and multislice CT angiography. Neurocrit Care. 2009;11:261–71.
6. Conrad GR, et al. Scintigraphy as a confirmatory test of brain death. Semin Nuc Med. 2003;33(4):312–23.
7. Zuckier LS, et al. Radionuclide studies in the determination of brain death: criteria, concepts, and controversies. Semin Nucl Med. 2008;38:262–73.
8. Munari M, et al. Confirmatory tests in the diagnosis of brain death: comparison between SPECT and contrast angiography. Crit Care Med. 2005;33(9):2068–73.
9. Sinha P, et al. Scintigraphic confirmation of brain death. Semin Nucl Med. 2012;42:27–32.
10. Berenguer CM, et al. Brain death confirmation: comparison of computed tomographic angiography with nuclear medicine perfusion scan. J Trauma. 2010;68:553–9.
11. Combes J-C, et al. Reliability of computed tomographic angiography in the diagnosis of brain death. Transplant Proc. 2007;39:16–20.
12. Brasil S, et al. Role of computed tomography angiography and perfusion tomography in diagnosing brain death: a systematic review. J Neuroradiol. 2015. https://doi.org/10.1016/j.neurad.2015.07.006.
13. Dupas B, et al. Diagnosis of brain death using two-phase spiral CT. Am J Neuroradiol. 1998;19:641–7.
14. Frampas E, et al. CT angiography for brain death diagnosis. Am J Neuroradiol. 2009;30:1566–70.
15. Shankar JJS, et al. CT perfusion for confirmation of brain death. Am J Neuroradiol. 2013;34:1175–9.
16. Matsumura A, et al. Magnetic resonance imaging of brain death. Neurol Med Chir (Tokyo). 1996;36(3):166–71.
17. Ducrocq X, et al. Consensus opinion on diagnosis of cerebral circulatory arrest using Doppler-sonography. J Neurol Sci. 1998;159:145–50.
18. Monteiro LM, et al. Transcranial Doppler ultrasonography to confirm brain death: a meta-analysis. Intensive Care Med. 2006;32:1937–44.
19. Lampl Y, et al. Diagnosing brain death using the transcranial Doppler with a transorbital approach. Arch Neurol. 2002;39:58–60.
20. Azevedo E, et al. Transcranial Doppler and brain death. Transplant Proc. 2000;32:2579–81.
21. Cabrer C, et al. Persistence of intracranial diastolic flow in transcranial Doppler sonography exploration of patients in brain death. Transplant Proc. 2003;35:1642–3.
22. Dosemeci L, et al. Utility of transcranial Doppler ultrasonography for confirmatory diagnosis of brain death: two sides of the coin. Transplantation. 2004;77(1):71–5.
23. Ducrocq X, et al. Brain death and transcranial Doppler: experience in 130 cases of brain dead patients. J Neurol Sci. 1998;160:41–6.

Management of the Potential Organ Donor

7

Margaret K. M. Ellis, Mitchell B. Sally, and Darren J. Malinoski

Systems and Processes of Organ Donation

Introduction

There is a well-established shortage of organs available for transplantation, with approximately 124,000 Americans on the Organ Procurement and Transplantation Network (OPTN) waiting list [1]. This culminates in 22 Americans dying each day while waiting for an organ transplant. Contributing to this shortage is the fact that, on average, only three out of a possible eight organs are transplanted from each organ donor [1].

There are two general categories of organ donors, living and deceased, with the latter being divided into those that are declared dead by either neurologic or circulatory criteria. In 2013 OPTN reported that 58% of all transplanted organs came from donors after neurologic determination of death, also referred to as brain death (BD). This is important, for multiple studies have demonstrated that deceased donor grafts result in inferior outcomes when compared to living donors in terms of initial function, long-term survival, and rejection. When these inferior outcomes result in the need for repeat transplantation, the organ shortage is exacerbated [1]. Efforts to improve the management of donors after brain death (DBDs) prior to recovery of organs are needed to increase the quality and quantity of organs available for transplantation.

After BD, despite cessation of all brain function, the rest of the body's organs can continue to function, albeit under considerable physiologic stress. Critical care management of potential organ donors is aimed at stabilizing the hemodynamic, endocrine, respiratory, inflammatory, and metabolic derangements concomitant with brainstem herniation. This chapter will highlight current best practices and the available evidence supporting the management of potential brain-dead organ donors. When assessing the effectiveness of different strategies, multiple outcomes are examined, including conversion rates (% of potential organ donors that go on to donate transplantable organs), organs transplanted per donor (OTPD), individual organ transplantation rates, and both initial and long-term graft function and survival.

M. K. M. Ellis
Department of Anesthesiology and Perioperative Medicine, Oregon Health and Science University, Portland, OR, USA

M. B. Sally · D. J. Malinoski (✉)
Department of Surgery, Oregon Health & Science University, Portland, OR, USA
e-mail: darren.malinoski@va.gov

Brain Death and Catastrophic Brain Injury Guidelines

When a patient has a severe neurologic injury that is deemed "non-survivable" by either neurology or neurosurgery, it is termed a catastrophic brain injury (CBI). In such cases, standard neurocritical care practices are implemented, with the exception of efforts to manage intracranial pressure (ICP). Many institutions have adopted catastrophic brain injury guidelines (CBIGs), which include clinical pathways and checklists designed to aid in the medical management of the multi-system pathophysiology of severe brain injury and brainstem herniation. Some patients will have an improvement of neurologic status with these measures and will become candidates for neurologic intervention and ICP management. For patients who do not improve and regress to BD or whose families decide to withdraw life-sustaining measures, these efforts preserve the option of organ donation for those who choose it. Of note, >50% of adults in the USA are registered organ donors [2] and, for those patients who have not made a first-person declaration on a state registry, >75% of families say "yes" when appropriately approached regarding the option of donation [3]. Needless to say, the desire and intent to donate organs is prevalent among patients and their families.

The American Academy of Neurology has published evidence-based guidelines on determining BD, which is a complex process involving a comprehensive clinical exami-

A. Salim et al. (eds.), *Surgical Critical Care Therapy*, https://doi.org/10.1007/978-3-319-71712-8_7

nation, excluding confounding factors, and performing an apnea test [4]. Many care centers have adopted checklists to protocolize this determination, as it can involve upward of 25 individual assessments. These protocols ensure confidence in the determination prior to initiation of the authorization process for donation. Recent recommendations from the Neurocritical Care Society have indicated a 72-h care period after brain injury to determine prognosis prior to discussions regarding prognosis and withdrawal of life-sustaining treatments [5]. If, however, all brainstem reflexes are lost and BD is suspected, formal testing can and should occur at any time. Determination of BD is addressed in detail in another chapter of this text.

Coordination of Care/Organ Procurement Organization Involvement

Most organ procurement organizations (OPOs), in collaboration with the donor hospitals they serve, have protocols for referring patients with a severe neurologic injury and "imminent death." In patients with a neurologic injury that requires mechanical ventilation, specific clinical triggers for notification of an OPO include (1) a Glasgow coma scale score (GCS) of five or less, (2) loss of a brainstem reflex, or (3) if a family discussion is being planned that may result in withdrawal of life-sustaining therapy. It is important to note that referral to the OPO does not change the patient's course of management; rather, it simply alerts the OPO to the presence of a patient with a catastrophic brain injury, allowing them to review the patient's history and to be prepared to approach the family, if appropriate. After referral (often done by nursing or administration) and initial evaluation by the OPO, if the patient regresses to BD or the patient's family decides to withdraw life-sustaining measures, the OPO meets with the family and makes a request of authorization for donation. It has been shown that trained requesters from OPOs have better success with obtaining authorization for donation from families compared to requests made by the treating physician [6, 7]. This success may be attributable to avoidance of a perceived conflict of interest, a more thorough explanation of the process, or more time spent with the family.

After authorization for donation, the OPO assumes direction of the care of the potential organ donor, much of which is directed at the bedside by OPO-specific protocols. These protocols usually target critical care parameters to best optimize the function of all organ systems.

Donor Management Goals

Inconsistent donor management practices may account for part of the shortage of organs available for transplantation. Donor management goals (DMGs) represent a checklist of critical care endpoints that reflect the normal physiologic goals of any critically ill patient. The values assessed during donor management were originally based on a series of Canadian task force recommendations [8] and were designed to represent normal hemodynamic, respiratory, endocrine, acid-base, and renal values, typically targeted in standard ICU management. They were initially seen as a way to standardize care for all potential donors in an area in which practice patterns varied, there were conflicting goals between different organ systems (e.g., hydrating the kidneys versus drying out the lungs), and there was a paucity of evidence-based guidelines. The DMG Bundle utilized by many OPOs consists of a checklist of nine critical care endpoints that are examined at four standardized time points during the process of donor management, which typically lasts between 24 and 48 h. The current set of DMGs utilized by several OPOs is displayed in Fig. 7.1.

The timeline of the clinical course of a potential organ donor is displayed in Fig. 7.2. The process begins with neurologic injury. At this point in the process, the patient is being managed with current critical care standard practices by the referring hospital as described above. If the patient triggers local standards for referral, a referral is made to the OPO for evaluation of a potential organ donor. This process of referral is the first time point in donor management, labeled "Referral." If the patient declines neurologically, and proceeds to BD, the trained practitioners from the OPO request authorization for donation. If authorization is granted or the patient is already on a state registry, the OPO takes over donor management from the critical care providers in the hospital. This time point for recording donor critical care targets is labeled "Authorization." The next major time point in donor management is labeled "Allocation," which represents the time when organ offers are being made to potential recipients, about 12–18 h after authorization and after OPOs have gathered enough data to inform an organ offer. The final time point is that of "Prior to OR," which is just prior to organ recovery in the operating room, marking the conclusion of donor management.

Achieving any seven of the nine DMGs results in the "DMG Bundle being met" at any given time point. Previous studies have found that meeting the DMG Bundle during donor management is associated with more OTPD. In addition, the status of the DMG Bundle at the time of authorization, which reflects the care provided by donor hospital staff prior to the OPO assuming care of the potential organ donor, has been associated with both increased organ utilization and

Fig. 7.1 Current donor management goal (DMG) components and values

UNITED NETWORK FOR ORGAN SHARING DONOR MANAGEMENT GOALS

Donor management goal	***parameter***
Mean arterial pressure (mmHg)	60-110
Central venous pressure (mmHg)	4-12
Left ventricular ejection fraction (%)	≥50%
Low-dose vasopressors*, number of agents	≤1
Arterial blood gas pH	7.3-7.5
PaO2:FiO2 ratio	≥300
Serum sodium (mEq/L)	≤155
Urine output (mL/kg/h over 4h)	≥0.5
Glucose (mg/dL)	≤180

mmHg = millimeter of mercury; PaO2 = arterial partial pressure of oxygen; FiO2 = fraction of inspired oxygen
*less than or equal one vasopressor used and at a low dose (dopamine ≤ 10 mcg/kg/min; phenylephrine ≤ 1 mcg/kg/min; norepinephrine ≤ 0.2 mcg/kg/min), with any dose of epinephrine resulting in the element not being met

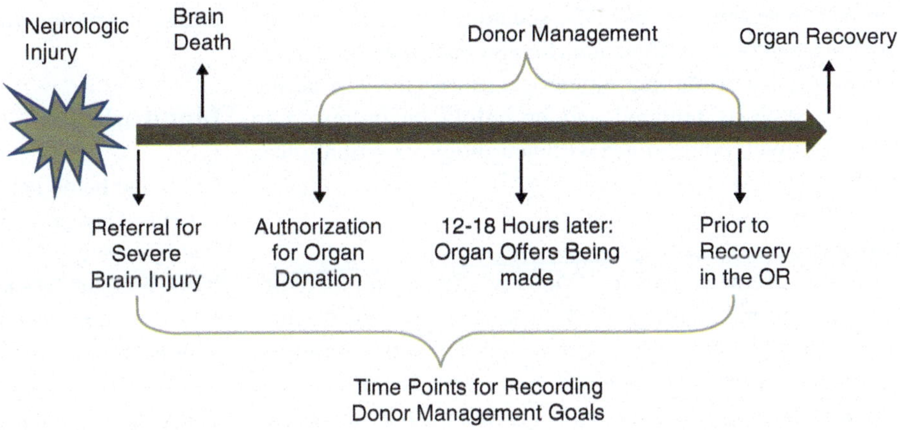

Fig. 7.2 Potential organ donor timeline

improved graft function in the recipient [9–14]. This highlights the importance of continuing aggressive critical care measures until the OPO is able to determine suitability for donation, even in the face of a poor prognosis.

Strategies for Critical Care Management of Potential Organ Donors

The following sections will address the pathophysiology, monitoring, and treatment of each organ system that is affected by CBIs, brainstem herniation, and BD. DMGs are *bolded* when they are specifically addressed in the context of the management of individual organ systems. Of note, many of the recommendations included below are based on an expert consensus guidelines document created by a joint task force of the Society of Critical Care Medicine (SCCM), the American College of Chest Physicians (ACCP), and Association of Organ Procurement Organizations (AOPO) [15].

Neurologic

Physiologic Consequences of Severe Neurologic Injury and Herniation Syndrome

The central nervous system is responsible for regulation of the processes of the entire body; when it is irreversibly damaged and eventually ceases to function, this regulation is lost and widespread dysfunction takes place. As a testament to the broad impact of BD on the physiology of the rest of the body, the most common non-neurologic issues encountered when brainstem herniation occurs are hypotension, diabetes insipidus, disseminated intravascular coagulation, cardiac arrhythmias, pulmonary edema, and metabolic acidosis [16, 17].

Monitoring

Due to the loss of temperature regulation by the hypothalamus, all patients should have their temperature monitored continuously. Serial neurologic examination is crucial to assess the progression of the patient's neurologic injury and to prompt definitive testing if BD is suspected.

Critical Care Management

Sedation and Analgesia Sedation and analgesia should be provided as deemed necessary by the patient's team, based upon bedside assessment. However, as patients progress to brainstem herniation and BD, sedation and analgesia are no longer necessary. Providers should base these decisions upon serial bedside neurologic assessments. Short-acting agents, such as fentanyl and propofol, are preferred to avoid as much interference with neurologic examination as possible.

Temperature Management Wide swings in temperature often occur in the setting of BD as the hypothalamic regulation of body temperature is lost, and active rewarming is frequently necessary to maintain normothermia in potential organ donors. Current guidelines recommend avoidance of hypothermia and hyperthermia, with a goal temperature between 36 and 37 °Celsius. However, mounting evidence for an association between mild hypothermia and renal protection in models of cardiac arrest prompted further investigation for the role of temperature management in potential organ donors after catastrophic neurologic injury. A recent multicenter trial of targeted temperature management in DBDs compared rates of delayed graft function (DGF) in recipients of kidneys from donors randomized to either mild hypothermia (34–35 °C) or normothermia (36.5–37.5 °C). The reduction in DGF rates in the hypothermia group was so compelling that the study was stopped early for efficacy [18]. While this is not yet the standard practice, targeted temperature management is a promising therapy for improving transplantation outcomes.

Cardiovascular

Cardiovascular Derangements in Severe Neurologic Injury

Catastrophic neurologic injury and brainstem herniation syndrome are associated with hemodynamic instability, which is often severe. Catecholamine surges due to neurologic injury may lead to myocardial stunning, manifested by acutely decreased ejection fraction and myocardial wall motion abnormalities in a nonvascular distribution. Arrhythmias are also common as a consequence of autonomic instability, excessive circulating catecholamine levels, and acute myocardial dysfunction. Traumatic blood loss, aggressive initial resuscitation, and loss of hormonal regulation of sodium and water homeostasis from disruption of the hypothalamic-pituitary axis all contribute to dynamic changes in volume status. When intracranial pressure has increased such that the pons is compressed, many patients will display the Cushing reflex (profound hypertension and bradycardia). When medullary function (including vagal cardiac innervation) ceases, sympathetic tone becomes unopposed, and sympathetic storm may occur. Finally, as all spinal reflexes are lost, sympathetic tone is abolished, leading to unopposed sympathoplegia and peripheral vasodilation [17].

Monitoring

Given the hemodynamic instability expected in this group of patients, invasive hemodynamic monitoring is necessary. Patients should have an arterial line placed for beat-to-beat blood pressure monitoring, and central venous access is necessary to monitor central venous pressure (CVP) as well as for administration of vasoactive medications. Furthermore, assessments of right and left intracardiac filling pressures, cardiac output and index, mixed venous oxygen saturation, stroke volume, and fluid responsiveness are recommended, either with invasive monitoring (pulmonary artery catheterization) or noninvasive (pulse-contour analysis) technologies [15].

Echocardiography is an important tool in cardiovascular monitoring and diagnosis. Transthoracic echocardiography (TTE) can be used to acquire real-time data regarding cardiac function. Transesophageal echocardiography (TEE) is useful when TTE data is inconclusive or TTE cannot be performed [15].

Critical Care Management

Optimizing Perfusion Maintaining optimal perfusion to all organs is paramount in the aggressive management of patients with catastrophic neurologic injury, and remains crucial even after declaration of BD in an organ donor, when the focus of management shifts to organ preservation. The target *mean arterial pressure* (MAP) for organ perfusion in this population is 60–110 mmHg. Achieving this MAP frequently requires a combination of vasoactive medication administration and volume resuscitation.

Vasoactive Medications The use of *low-dose vasopressors* and inotropes to support hemodynamics is supported by limited evidence [15]. Any catecholamine use in the donor has been associated with improved renal graft survival in recipients [19]; however, epinephrine use in the donor has also been associated with higher levels of serum creatinine prior to organ recovery [20]. In addition, an RCT in DBDs found that low-dose dopamine (≤5 mcg/kg/min) infusion in donors led to a significant reduction in DGF in the recipient [21]. Finally, arginine vasopressin, which is frequently administered as part of hormonal replacement therapy, has been associated with increased OTPD [22].

Intravascular volume status Hypovolemia is commonly found in patients with catastrophic neurologic injury upon initial presentation. This should be corrected through aggressive fluid resuscitation. Despite the long-held concern that optimal lung and kidney preservation required conflicting resuscitation goals, more recent evidence has suggested that targeting euvolemia (defined in the *UNOS Region 5 DMGs as CVP 4–12*) improves utilization of lungs, hearts, kidneys, and pancreata [23]. Specific targets of volume resuscitation included in the SCCM/ACCP/AOPO guidelines, in addition to CVP, include mean arterial pressure of at least 60 mmHg, urine output at least 1 mL/kg/h, and the reduction of vasopressor requirements [15].

Choice of Resuscitation Fluid Crystalloid solutions are considered first line during initial volume resuscitation; however, concern for volume overload when large quantities of crystalloid are administered for resuscitation has prompted the study of colloid solutions for resuscitation, including synthetic colloids such as hydroxyethyl starch (HES). While initially promising as a means to reduce the amount of crystalloid required for resuscitation [24], subsequent studies have suggested either no difference or an increased risk in delayed graft function in patients who received kidneys from DNDDs treated with low-molecular-weight HES [25]. Given the lack of demonstrable benefit and the compelling evidence for harm associated with HES use in living patients, it cannot be recommended as a safe strategy for volume resuscitation in potential organ donors. Colloids other than HES, such as albumin, may provide a safer alternative, but evidence is currently inconclusive, and ongoing study in this area is needed [26–28]. At this time, isotonic crystalloid solutions remain the recommended fluid for resuscitation in potential organ donors.

Echocardiography Echocardiography is an important tool for assessment of the potential organ donor. It can be used to guide resuscitation and identify cardiac dysfunction. As myocardial function is extremely important in preserving systemic perfusion, achieving a *left ventricular ejection fraction (LVEF) of ≥50%* is one of the goals of donor management. Given that there is often significant but transient myocardial dysfunction associated with the acute phase of catastrophic neurologic injury, serial echocardiographic assessments over 12–24 h are often necessary, particularly in patients in whom procurement of the heart for donation is being considered [15].

Respiratory

Respiratory Derangements in Severe Neurologic Injury

Patients with catastrophic neurologic injuries and brainstem herniation syndrome will universally require endotracheal intubation and mechanical ventilation for airway protection, oxygenation, and ventilation. These patients are also at risk for neurogenic pulmonary edema, volume overload and cardiogenic pulmonary edema, transfusion-associated lung injury (TRALI), and acute respiratory distress syndrome (ARDS). Trauma patients may also have chest wall injuries, pulmonary contusions, or pleural processes (pneumothorax, hemothorax) requiring chest tube drainage.

Monitoring and Diagnostics

All patients should have an arterial blood gas (ABG) performed on admission and serially throughout their management in the ICU to inform ventilator adjustments in order to provide optimal levels of ventilation and oxygenation. Bronchoscopy may be necessary for bronchoalveolar lavage (BAL) to obtain cultures in patients with suspected infections and for pulmonary hygiene and airway clearance in potential lung donors. Chest X-rays should be obtained following procedures such as intubation and central line placement and as needed to evaluate changes in pulmonary status.

Critical Care Management

Lung-Protective Ventilation Strategy Support for lung-protective ventilation strategies (low tidal volume, high PEEP, low FiO_2) is strong in the critically ill. These strategies have been shown to reduce both pulmonary and extrapulmonary complications in various populations, including ARDS, trauma, sepsis, and high-risk surgery patients [29–32]. A European RCT also demonstrated improved lung graft recovery when lung-protective ventilation strategies were used during the time period between clinical exams for BD testing [33]. Research into the protective effect of low tidal volumes upon transplantation outcomes for organs other than lungs is ongoing.

Lung-protective ventilation strategies consist most importantly of high PEEP and low tidal volume, which is defined as between 4 and 8 ml/kg of predicted body weight (PBW), a calculated value based upon the patient's sex and height. Each institution may have its own procedures to guide titration of PEEP and FiO_2, but in general, increased PEEP is preferred over increased FiO_2 as a strategy for improving oxygenation due to the protective effect of PEEP against atelectasis and the detrimental effects of oxygen toxicity.

Oxygenation and Ventilation Goals The targets for ventilator adjustment are slightly different in the prospective organ donor than in other patient populations. While hypercarbia is permissible in most lung-protective ventilation strategies and is likely safe in the prospective donor population as well, apnea testing to diagnose BD should not be performed unless the $PaCO_2$ is within the range of normocarbia (35–45 mmHg) [15]. Furthermore, while the goal FiO_2 and PEEP titration in many lung-protective ventilation strategies is a PaO_2 of >60 mmHg, the oxygenation goal in prospective organ donors is *a P:F ratio of ≥300.*

Renal/Electrolytes

Renal and Electrolyte Derangements in Severe Neurologic Injury

Most derangements of renal function and electrolyte and acid-base homeostasis in severe neurologic injury are consequences of hemodynamic or endocrine instability. For example, hemodynamic instability places patients at risk of renal hypoperfusion, tissue hypoperfusion, and metabolic acidosis, while endocrine dyscrasias alter sodium and water homeostasis, leading to hypernatremia and hyperosmolality. Preservation of renal function is a critical goal in the management of the potential organ donor. Not only is a lower terminal creatinine (the last creatinine measured before organ procurement) associated with a lower incidence of delayed graft function in kidney transplant recipients [34, 35], but it has also been identified as an independent predictor of an increased number of organs transplanted per donor [11]. Acid-base derangements are also common in patients with catastrophic neurologic injuries and may be multifactorial. Elevated lactate levels can represent tissue hypoperfusion and may be useful as a marker for adequacy of resuscitation; investigation for inclusion of serum lactate as a donor management goal is ongoing.

Monitoring

All patients with catastrophic brain injury should have a Foley catheter placed during their initial resuscitation in order to be able to monitor strict intake and output measurements. A serum metabolic panel, including electrolytes (sodium, potassium, magnesium, calcium, phosphate, chloride, and bicarbonate) and serum blood urea nitrogen (BUN) and creatinine, should be obtained upon admission and serially throughout the patient's ICU stay in order to monitor effectiveness of therapy and identify new derangements. Arterial blood gases should also be obtained upon admission to assess acid-base status and tissue perfusion and then serially to monitor the effectiveness of resuscitation. Serial lactate measurements may also be considered to guide resuscitation.

Critical Care Management

Renal Perfusion/Urine Output Goal Urine output is monitored as a surrogate of renal perfusion in potential organ donors. Fluid resuscitation and vasopressors should be administered to maintain euvolemia (per the cardiovascular section above) and achieve a *goal urine output of ≥0.5–1 ml/kg/h*. In patients who develop polyuria, diabetes insipidus should be considered as a possible cause, and evaluation should proceed as described in the endocrine section below.

Acid/Base and Electrolyte Management Physiologically *normal pH (7.3–7.5)* is a goal in the management of patients with catastrophic neurologic injury, as derangements in pH can have adverse effects on coagulation and cardiovascular stability. If metabolic acidosis persists despite adequate resuscitation, euvolemia, and MAP within goal range, administration of bicarbonate-containing solutions may be considered. One recommended regimen consists of an addition of 50–150 mmol/L sodium bicarbonate to the patient's IV fluids [15]. Close attention should be paid to the patient's sodium levels when administering additional sodium in the form of sodium bicarbonate, and the makeup of the IV fluid may need to be altered to prevent hypernatremia. In general, *a sodium goal of ≤155* is targeted, as higher levels in the donor are associated with worse liver graft outcomes [36, 37].

Hematologic/Infectious Disease

Hematologic and Immunologic Derangements in Severe Neurologic Injury

Patients who present with severe neurologic injury are prone to derangements in the hematologic and immunologic systems. Anemia is common; patients may have experienced hemorrhage from non-neurologic sites of trauma or have nonhemorrhagic anemia as a consequence of prolonged illness. Coagulopathy, a common problem in this patient population, can be dilutional, consumptive, or due to trauma or medical illness and is exacerbated by hypothermia and acidosis [38]. Disseminated intravascular coagulation (DIC) is particularly common in traumatic brain injury patients and is thought to be a consequence of the release of tissue factor from areas of injured brain [39]. Finally, numerous factors, including indwelling catheters, mechanical ventilation, the immunomodulatory effects of medications (opioids, corticosteroids, catecholamines, etc.), and hospitalization itself, place patients with catastrophic brain injury at increased risk of infection and sepsis. The risk of bacteremia or other infections increases with the length of ICU admission [15].

Monitoring

Complete blood count (CBC) and coagulation studies, including fibrinogen, should be assessed on admission and then as needed based on clinical evidence of anemia or coagulopathy. In patients with difficult-to-diagnose coagulopathies, thromboelastography (TEG) may be a useful assessment, although little to no data currently exists to guide its use in organ donors. Given the potential for poor outcomes of untreated infections for both the donor and recipient, intensivists should continually assess patients for evidence of infection or sepsis, with a low threshold to culture blood, BAL fluid, and urine if infection is suspected.

Management

Management of Anemia Current OPO guidelines vary regarding target serum hematocrit (ranging from 21 to 30%); further prospective randomized studies are needed to inform evidence-based practices in this area. Interestingly, in a recent propensity analysis, blood transfusion in the donor was associated with a lower risk of delayed kidney graft function in the recipient. This effect was seen most strongly in donors who received large-volume blood transfusions [40]. A potential explanation for this protective effect is downregulation of the dysfunctional inflammatory processes associated with brainstem herniation syndrome due to the immunosuppressive effects of transfusion. Still, at this time, the optimal hemoglobin level in organ donors is unknown, and decisions regarding blood transfusion should be guided by clinical status and accepted critical care guidelines.

Management of Coagulopathy Particularly in cases of massive blood loss or trauma as the etiology of brain injury, patients with catastrophic brain injuries may also present with coagulopathy. Management of coagulopathy should be based upon clinical status and laboratory assessment. Given the high risk for DIC, fibrinogen should be included in the workup of coagulopathy, and consideration should be given to cryoprecipitate administration if fibrinogen levels are low.

Management of Infections Intensivists should have a low threshold to send cultures in patients in whom infection is suspected. All potential sites of infection should be assessed with cultures and imaging as appropriate in any critically ill patients, and broad-spectrum antibiotics should be initiated. Culture data may guide management of antibiotic choice and duration in both the donor and the recipient. Sepsis, if present, should be managed according to established critical care guidelines. OPO practices regarding the use of prophylactic antibiotics vary.

Endocrine

Endocrine Derangements in Severe Neurologic Injury

Diabetes Insipidus (DI) Due to the irreversible loss of hypothalamic function and subsequent cessation of antidiuretic hormone (ADH) production, DNDDs are at risk for severe central DI. Without ADH to stimulate reabsorption of water in the kidney, large volumes of dilute urine are produced (specific gravity <1.005 and/or urine osmolality <200 mOsm/kg H_2O), leading to hypovolemia, hyperosmolality, and hypernatremia [17].

Hyperglycemia The combination of catecholamine and steroid administration, the administration of dextrose-containing solutions, and the hormonal derangements leading to insulin resistance and increased gluconeogenesis may all lead to hyperglycemia in potential organ donors.

Corticosteroid Deficiency While dysfunction of the hypothalamic-pituitary axis occurs in brainstem herniation syndrome, it is not clear that patients with catastrophic neurologic injuries have clinically significant adrenal insufficiency; corticosteroid administration for the treatment of hypocortisolism is not currently recommended. However, as a consequence of brainstem herniation, inflammatory and immunologic mediators are upregulated. The activation of these mediators has been shown to adversely affect graft function in transplant recipients, and corticosteroid administration in donors has been recommended as a strategy to mitigate the negative effects of inflammatory cascade activation.

Acute Hypothyroidism While loss of pituitary function in BD should theoretically lead to reduced levels of thyroid-stimulating hormone (TSH), blood levels are not consistently low when tested in patients with brainstem herniation syndrome. However, levels of T3 and T4 are often low, and peripheral conversion of T4 to T3 is impaired as a result of the inflammatory response to CBI and BD [41]. Given the association between clinical hypothyroidism and decreased myocardial function, significant acute hypothyroidism in patients with brainstem herniation often manifests as hemodynamic instability or reduced left ventricular ejection fraction (LVEF).

Monitoring and Diagnostics

Patients should be monitored for hemodynamic instability with invasive and noninvasive monitors as described in the cardiovascular section above. Frequent laboratory assessment of serum electrolytes, particularly blood glucose and serum sodium, is important in monitoring for hyperglycemia and diabetes insipidus. In patients with suspected or confirmed diabetes insipidus, serial urinalysis (specifically looking at urine specific gravity and/or osmolality) and serum osmolality should be performed to assess the adequacy of therapy. Routine laboratory testing for thyroid and adrenal function is not recommended; however, echocardiographic findings may inform treatment with thyroid hormone replacement as described below.

Management

Diabetes Insipidus DI should be managed with a combination of volume resuscitation with hypotonic saline (0.25% or 0.5%) and hormonal replacement with desmopressin and/or vasopressin [15]. Desmopressin may be particularly useful in patients who are also coagulopathic due to its stimulation of von Willebrand factor release. Vasopressin serves a dual role as a vasopressor and has been shown to improve transplant outcomes as described above [22]. The goals of DI management are euvolemia, a decrease of urine output to no greater than 4 mL/kg/h, and sodium levels ≤155 mEq/L [15].

Hyperglycemia Current recommendations from the Society of Critical Care Medicine advocate for the *avoidance of hyperglycemia above 180 mg/dL* [42]. Poor glucose control in DNDDs has been associated with elevated terminal serum creatinine in kidney donors prior to organ recovery [43], which has been independently associated with higher rates of DGF [34, 35]. Recently, a study of prospectively collected characteristics of over 1600 DNDDs was performed using multivariate analysis to determine the effect of hyperglycemia on OTPD and renal graft function; better function was associated with better glucose control, with the best outcomes occurring in the group in whom hyperglycemia >180 mg/dL was avoided [44]. This evidence suggests that the generally accepted critical care guideline for glucose control of ≤180 md/dL is also appropriate for DNDDs. Hyperglycemia should be managed with insulin, either via intermittent dosing or infusion per each institution's protocol.

Corticosteroids High-dose corticosteroids should be administered for their anti-inflammatory effects. Current dosing regimens include intravenous methylprednisolone 1000 mg bolus, 15 mg/kg bolus, or 250 mg bolus followed by 100 mg/h infusion. If possible, due to its potential to suppress human leukocyte antigen (HLA) expression, methylprednisolone administration should be started after blood has been collected for tissue typing [15].

Acute Hypothyroidism Currently, evidence suggests that hemodynamically unstable donors or prospective cardiac donors with EF <45% may benefit from thyroid hormone replacement [15]. Dosing regimens vary; no difference in efficacy between T3 and T4 has been demonstrated. Common regimens include (1) 4 μg intravenous bolus of T3 followed by infusion at 3 μg/h or (2) 20 μg intravenous bolus of T4 followed by infusion at 10 μg/h.

Conclusion

There is a persistent shortage of organs available for transplantation, and thousands of people die each year waiting for a lifesaving transplant. Caring for potential deceased organ donors is a complex process due to the severe, widespread physiologic derangements that occur in the setting of catastrophic brain injury, brainstem herniation, and brain death. Standardized goals and guidelines for patient care, a focus on multidisciplinary collaboration and coordination of donation processes, and a growing field of research in the field of organ donor management have begun to narrow the gap between the supply and demand of transplantable organs. The critical care provider's role is crucial in ensuring that patients with catastrophic brain injuries maximize both their chances for clinical improvement and the potential to preserve the option of organ donation for their families.

References

1. Organ Procurement and Transplantation Network Data. December 29, 2016]; Available from https://optn.transplant.hrsa.gov/data/.
2. Donate Life America 2015 Annual Update. December 29, 2016]; Available from https://www.donatelife.net/wp-content/

uploads/2016/06/2015-DLA_Annual-Report_FINAL-for-onscreen-viewing.pdf.
3. OPTN, Organ Procurement and Transplantation Network Data, January 2008–June 2010. 2010.
4. Machado C, et al. Evidence-based guideline update: determining brain death in adults: report of the quality standards Subcommittee of the American Academy of Neurology. Neurology. 2011;76(3):307. author reply 308-9.
5. Souter MJ, et al. Recommendations for the Critical Care Management of devastating brain injury: prognostication, psychosocial, and ethical management : a position statement for healthcare professionals from the Neurocritical Care Society. Neurocrit Care. 2015;23(1):4–13.
6. Siminoff LA, et al. Factors influencing families' consent for donation of solid organs for transplantation. JAMA. 2001;286(1):71–7.
7. Rodrigue JR, Cornell DL, Howard RJ. Organ donation decision: comparison of donor and nondonor families. Am J Transplant. 2006;6(1):190–8.
8. Shemie SD, et al. Organ donor management in Canada: recommendations of the forum on Medical Management to optimize donor organ potential. CMAJ. 2006;174(6):S13–32.
9. Malinoski DJ, et al. Achieving donor management goals before deceased donor procurement is associated with more organs transplanted per donor. J Trauma. 2011;71(4):990–5. discussion 996.
10. Malinoski DJ, et al. The impact of meeting donor management goals on the development of delayed graft function in kidney transplant recipients. Am J Transplant. 2013;13(4):993–1000.
11. Malinoski DJ, et al. The impact of meeting donor management goals on the number of organs transplanted per donor: results from the United Network for Organ Sharing Region 5 prospective donor management goals study. Crit Care Med. 2012;40(10):2773–80.
12. Franklin GA, et al. Optimization of donor management goals yields increased organ use. Am Surg. 2010;76(6):587–94.
13. Hagan ME, et al. Attaining specific donor management goals increases number of organs transplanted per donor: a quality improvement project. Prog Transplant. 2009;19(3):227–31.
14. Patel MS, et al. The impact of meeting donor management goals on the number of organs transplanted per donor: a prospective study from the UNOS Region 45 Donor Management Goals Workgroup. JAMA Surg. 2014;149(9):969–75.
15. Kotloff RM, et al. Management of the potential organ donor in the ICU: Society of Critical Care Medicine/American College of Chest Physicians/Association of Organ Procurement Organizations Consensus Statement. Crit Care Med. 2015;43(6):1291–325.
16. Salim A, et al. Complications of brain death: frequency and impact on organ retrieval. Am Surg. 2006;72(5):377–81.
17. Smith M. Physiologic changes during brain stem death--lessons for management of the organ donor. J Heart Lung Transplant. 2004;23(9 Suppl):S217–22.
18. Niemann CU, et al. Therapeutic hypothermia in deceased organ donors and kidney-graft function. N Engl J Med. 2015;373(5):405–14.
19. Schnuelle P, et al. Effects of catecholamine application to brain-dead donors on graft survival in solid organ transplantation. Transplantation. 2001;72(3):455–63.
20. Blasco V, et al. Impact of intensive care on renal function before graft harvest: results of a monocentric study. Crit Care. 2007;11(5):R103.
21. Schnuelle P, et al. Effects of donor pretreatment with dopamine on graft function after kidney transplantation: a randomized controlled trial. JAMA. 2009;302(10):1067–75.
22. Plurad DS, et al. Arginine vasopressin significantly increases the rate of successful organ procurement in potential donors. Am J Surg. 2012;204(6):856–60.
23. Abdelnour T, Rieke S. Relationship of hormonal resuscitation therapy and central venous pressure on increasing organs for transplant. J Heart Lung Transplant. 2009;28(5):480–5.
24. Randell T, Orko R, Höckerstedt K. Perioperative fluid management of the brain-dead multiorgan donor. Acta Anaesthesiol Scand. 1990;34(7):592–5.
25. Patel MS, et al. The impact of hydroxyethyl starch use in deceased organ donors on the development of delayed graft function in kidney transplant recipients: a propensity-adjusted analysis. Am J Transplant. 2015;15(8):2152–8.
26. Blasco V, et al. Comparison of the novel hydroxyethylstarch 130/0.4 and hydroxyethylstarch 200/0.6 in brain-dead donor resuscitation on renal function after transplantation. Br J Anaesth. 2008;100(4):504–8.
27. Giral M, et al. Effect of brain-dead donor resuscitation on delayed graft function: results of a monocentric analysis. Transplantation. 2007;83(9):1174–81.
28. Darby JM, et al. Approach to management of the heartbeating 'brain dead' organ donor. JAMA. 1989;261(15):2222–8.
29. Serpa Neto A, et al. Association between use of lung-protective ventilation with lower tidal volumes and clinical outcomes among patients without acute respiratory distress syndrome: a meta-analysis. JAMA. 2012;308(16):1651–9.
30. The Acute Respiratory Distress Syndrome Network, et al. Ventilation with lower tidal volumes as compared with traditional tidal volumes for acute lung injury and the acute respiratory distress syndrome. N Engl J Med. 2000;342(18):1301–8.
31. Lipes J, Bojmehrani A, Lellouche F. Low tidal volume ventilation in patients without acute respiratory distress syndrome: a paradigm shift in mechanical ventilation. Crit Care Res Prac. 2012;2012:416862.
32. Futier E, et al. A trial of intraoperative low-tidal-volume ventilation in abdominal surgery. N Engl J Med. 2013;369(5):428–37.
33. Mascia L, et al. Effect of a lung protective strategy for organ donors on eligibility and availability of lungs for transplantation: a randomized controlled trial. JAMA. 2010;304(23):2620–7.
34. Heilman RL, et al. Transplanting kidneys from deceased donors with severe acute kidney injury. Am J Transplant. 2015;15(8):2143–51.
35. Farney AC, et al. Evolving experience using kidneys from deceased donors with terminal acute kidney injury. J Am Coll Surg. 2013;216(4):655–6.
36. Figueras J, et al. The deleterious effect of donor high plasma sodium and extended preservation in liver transplantation. A multivariate analysis. Transplantation. 1996;61(3):410–3.
37. Cywinski JB, et al. Association between donor-recipient serum sodium differences and orthotopic liver transplant graft function. Liver Transpl. 2008;14(1):59–65.
38. Hefty TR, et al. Disseminated intravascular coagulation in cadaveric organ donors. Incidence and effect on renal transplantation. Transplantation. 1993;55(2):442–3.
39. Stein SC, Smith DH. Coagulopathy in traumatic brain injury. Neurocrit Care. 2004;1(4):479–88.
40. De La Cruz JS, et al. The impact of blood transfusions in deceased organ donors on the outcomes of 1,884 renal grafts from United Network for Organ Sharing Region 5. J Trauma Acute Care Surg. 2015;79(4 Suppl 2):S164–70.
41. Novitzky D, et al. Hormonal therapy of the brain-dead organ donor: experimental and clinical studies. Transplantation. 2006;82(11):1396–401.
42. Jacobi J, et al. Guidelines for the use of an insulin infusion for the management of hyperglycemia in critically ill patients. Crit Care Med. 2012;40(12):3251–76.
43. Blasi-Ibanez A, et al. Predictors associated with terminal renal function in deceased organ donors in the intensive care unit. Anesthesiology. 2009;110(2):333–41.
44. Sally MB, et al. Determining optimal threshold for glucose control in organ donors after neurologic determination of death: a United Network for Organ Sharing Region 5 Donor Management Goals Workgroup prospective analysis. J Trauma Acute Care Surg. 2014;76(1):62–8.

Care of the Postop Craniectomy/ Craniotomy Patient

8

Filip Moshkovsky, Maureen Mercante, and Mark Cipolle

History of Craniotomy for Evacuation of Traumatic Hematoma of the Brain

The craniotomy is a procedure with ancient Greek roots with the most descriptive explanation found in a translation of Hippocrates' *On Injuries of the Head*, where he described the use of a trepan, a type of saw, to repair skull fractures [1]. The craniotomy has been refined since Hippocrates' explanation and is widely performed today as a means to remove a large hematoma from the surface of the brain, thereby, lowering the intracranial pressure and reducing the resulting mass effect and/or midline shift. Not all acute or traumatic hematomas need to be evacuated and may be treated medically. Deciding when to surgically evacuate a traumatic hematoma is often up to the discretion of each individual neurosurgeon. Treatment guidelines have been developed by the American Academy of Neurological Surgery to help determine which patients would benefit from surgical evacuation of an intracranial hemorrhage.

Indications for Surgical Treatment of Traumatic Hematoma of the Brain

Bullock et al. established guidelines for the AANS and Brain Trauma Foundation for surgical treatment and timing of evacuation of traumatic subdural hematomas [2]. While these guidelines are from 2006, due to the new format of the Brain Trauma Foundation's Living Guidelines (2016), only *updates* are included in the most recent guidelines. The indications for surgical evacuation of traumatic mass lesions have not been updated in the Brain Trauma Foundation Guidelines. They remain as they were written in 2006 [3].

- An acute SDH with a thickness greater than 10 mm or a midline shift greater than 5 mm on computed tomographic (CT) scan should be surgically evacuated, regardless of the patient's Glasgow Coma Scale (GCS) score.
- All patients with acute SDH in coma (GCS score less than 9) should undergo intracranial pressure (ICP) monitoring.
- A comatose patient (GCS score less than 9) with a SDH less than 10 mm thick and a midline shift less than 5 mm should undergo surgical evacuation of the lesion if the GCS score decreased between the time of injury and hospital admission by 2 or more points and/or the patient presents with asymmetric or fixed and dilated pupils and/or the ICP exceeds 20 mm Hg.

It is important that all clinicians who care for post-craniotomy/craniectomy patients in the ICU setting are familiar with these guidelines. Additionally, Pascual and Prieto have further categorized the guidelines for surgical treatment of all types of acute traumatic hemorrhages based primarily upon class III scientific evidence [4]. These recommendations are found in Table 8.1.

Once it has been determined that surgery is indicated, plans should be made to transport the patient to the operating room for evacuation of the hematoma as soon as possible.

Explanation of Craniotomy for Evacuation of Traumatic Acute Epidural Hematoma

Pascual and Prieto describe the craniotomy procedure for a traumatic subdural hematoma in a broad outline form as follows [4]:

1. The patient is placed in supine position with a roll placed under the shoulder, and the head turned almost 90 degrees away from the surgeon, supported on a donut or with the Mayfield three-pin head holder.

F. Moshkovsky · M. Mercante · M. Cipolle (✉)
Department of Surgery – Surgical Critical Care, Christiana Care Health System, Newark, DE, USA
e-mail: mcipolle@christianacare.org

A. Salim et al. (eds.), *Surgical Critical Care Therapy*, https://doi.org/10.1007/978-3-319-71712-8_8

Table 8.1 Indications for evacuation of intracrianal hemorrhages adapted from Pascual and Prieto [4]

Location of hematoma	Indication for surgical treatment
Epidural hematoma	Volume >30 cm^3
Subdural hematoma	Thickness >10 mm or midline shift >5 mm regardless of GCS
	Thickness <10 mm or midline shift <5 mm, and GCS < 9 points and decreased ≥2 points between injury and hospital admission
	Asymmetrical or fixed and dilated pupils
	ICP > 20 mmHg
Parenchymal lesions	Progressive neurologic deterioration referable to the lesion
	Medically refractory high ICP, mass effect signs on CT, or volume >50 cm^3
	GCS score = 6–8 points, frontal or temporal contusions ≥20 cm^3 and midline shift ≥5 mm and/or cisternal compression on CT
Posterior fossa lesions	Mass effect on CT scan (distortion, dislocation/obliteration of the fourth ventricle, compression/loss of visualization of basal cisterns, hydrocephalus)
	Neurologic dysfunction or deterioration
Depressed cranial fractures	Open (compound) cranial fractures depressed greater than the thickness of the cranium (to prevent infection)

2. The scalp is marked in a question mark shape over the site of the hematoma.
3. The skin incision is started about 1 cm in front of the tragus at the zygomatic arch, and curved backward and upward above the auricle, reaching the midline in a question mark shape, ending in the hairline if possible.
4. In the event of a rapidly deteriorating patient, the temporal portion of the incision is quickly opened and a burr hole is placed.
5. The surgeon should always be aware of the middle meningeal artery during turning of the bone flap and be ready to quickly address bleeding should any occur.
6. Once the bone flap is removed, the hematoma can carefully be removed with suction, irrigation, and cup forceps. Bleeding can be addressed with bipolar electrocautery.
7. After the hematoma has been removed, the surgeon can place a small opening in the dura to rule out an underlying subdural hematoma.
8. The dura is the repaired using silk sutures.
9. The bone flap is then reapplied to the edges, with placement of a subgaleal drain.
10. The superficial fascia and then the galea are approximated, and skin staples are used to close the skin margins.

The patient should then be returned to the intensive care unit in stable condition for ongoing management by the trauma and/or neurocritical care team. The neurosurgeon should remain available to assist in guiding care and to make additional treatment recommendations.

Decompressive Craniectomy for Treatment of Refractory Intracranial Hypertension

The use of decompressive craniectomy (DC) for treatment of intracranial hypertension has been debated for decades. The Brain Trauma Foundation, in their most recent Guidelines for the Management of Severe Traumatic Brain Injury, 4th Edition (2016), offers no level I evidence for or against craniectomy but stated the following:

Level II A

- Based on the results of the DECRA trial, bifrontal DC is not recommended to improve outcomes as measured by the Glasgow Outcome Scale-Extended (GOS-E) at 6 months post-injury in severe TBI patients with diffuse injury (without mass lesions) and with ICP elevation to values >20 mm Hg for more than 15 min within a 1-hour period that are refractory to first-tier therapies. However, this procedure has been demonstrated to reduce ICP and to minimize days in the intensive care unit (ICU) [5].
- A large frontotemporoparietal DC (not less than 12 × 15 cm or 15 cm diameter) is recommended over a small frontotemporoparietal DC for reduced mortality and improved neurologic outcomes in patients with severe TBI.

Since publication of these recommendations, a new, larger study investigating the efficacy of bifrontal craniectomy has been published, primarily in Europe. The Randomized Evaluation of Surgery with Craniectomy for Uncontrollable Elevation of Intracranial Pressure (RESCUEicp) concluded the following:

"At 6 months, decompressive craniectomy for severe and refractory intracranial hypertension after TBI resulted in a mortality that was 22% points lower than that with medical management. Surgery also was associated with higher rates of a vegetative state, lower severe disability, and upper severe disability compared to medical management. The rates of moderate disability and good recovery with surgery were similar to those with medical management." So it seems, while decompressive craniectomy reduces mortality in patients with severe TBI and intracranial hypertension, "favorable" long-term neurologic functional outcomes are worse compared to patients who underwent medical management only [6].

Hemicraniectomy is also performed for cerebral edema caused by malignant middle cerebral artery (MCA) stroke. A recent meta-analysis indicated that there was an odds ratio of 5.56 for reduction in mortality and an odds ratio of 2.04 (both statistically significant) for obtaining a "favorable" long-term outcome in patients who underwent a decompressive hemicraniectomy for a malignant MCA stroke when compared to patients who did not undergo the procedure [7]. However, these beneficial effects seem to be diminished and lose statistical significance in patients older than 60 years of age [7].

Immediate Postoperative Care

Patients that require an emergent decompressive craniectomy or craniotomy will need to be cared for in an intensive care unit postoperatively. Generally, these patients will go to either a neurocritical care or surgical critical care/trauma intensive care unit. It is important for the nursing staff and providers to be aware of the required monitoring that will be needed and treatment plans that will be employed and have a heightened awareness of important neurologic changes that may have a subtle presentation.

Since all patients requiring decompressive craniectomies or craniotomies will require ICU level of care, a system-based approach to these patients will ensure that every patient receives the same complete and optimal care. Immediate postoperative care of the patient will require obtaining laboratory data as well as establishing monitoring that will guide treatment. Common types of monitoring for post-craniectomy/craniotomy patients are cardiac and respiratory monitoring, invasive blood pressure monitoring, intracranial pressure monitoring, as well as EEG monitoring for those at high risk of seizures. The postsurgical care that is most specific to patients after craniectomy/craniotomy is closely related to the etiology requiring the neurosurgical intervention. Common postsurgical care is described below, and general guidelines are provided. It is important to remember that the following content must be used in the context of the underlying process necessitating the craniectomy/craniotomy.

Postoperative Drains

Knowing the area of the brain that was injured requiring surgical intervention is important. For traumatic brain injury patients, a frontotemporoparietal (FTP) hemicraniectomy is common and often is concomitant with evacuation of a space-occupying lesion, often a hematoma, on that side [3]. Some patient's may have bifrontal decompressive craniotomies for a more diffuse process causing generalized cerebral edema despite little evidence supporting improved outcomes [3]. This approach is most commonly performed in patients that have failed medical management of ongoing cerebral edema and is part of the tier approach to traumatic brain injury. Drains are often placed at the time of the craniectomy/craniotomy for monitoring, draining, or both. The most commonly placed drains are in the subgaleal or subdural space. An external ventricular drain (EVD) may be used for monitoring as well as treatment of elevated intracranial pressure (ICP). The Brain Trauma Foundation guidelines recommend the consideration of continuous drainage over intermittent drainage of the CSF [3]. These drains need to be frequently evaluated to ensure that they are functioning properly, and drain care consists of keeping the area clean, dry, and covered. Drain management, removal, and monitoring will be determined by the neurosurgeon. The removal of drains is generally attempted as early as possible, and it has been demonstrated that removal of subdural drains as early as 48 hours results in no increase in reoperation rate compared to removing these drains later [8]. It's imperative that the nursing staff caring for these neurologically ill and injured patients have a thorough understanding of, and skills to manage, an EVD. A major advantage of an EVD over other devices is that it can be used not only to monitor the ICP but can also be used to treat an elevated ICP via drainage of CSF.

Postoperative Exam

Post-craniectomy patients require immediate detailed neurological exam to establish a baseline, and this should be clearly documented and easily accessed by all providers. The Glasgow Coma Scale (GCS) is a well-recognized and internationally accepted neurological assessment tool allowing providers from different disciplines to use common language in the exam of the patient. The GCS scale does have significant limitations, and a more detailed neurological exam including pupillary exam, tone, strength, and sensory exam as well as a degree of wakefulness may help in determining changes in the neurological exam sooner and more precisely potentially advancing to a higher tier of ICP management sooner which is described below.

Postoperative Elevated ICP

Elevated ICP may have detrimental effects on the perfusion of the brain; therefore, monitoring and treating elevated ICP is the cornerstone in the care of patients with severe traumatic brain injury defined as a GCS 3–8 with an abnormal head CT [3]. Studies have shown that patients with an ICP

Table 8.2 Tiered approach to elevated ICP

Tier 1	Head of bed elevated at 30 degrees (reverse Trendelenburg) to improve cerebral venous outflow
	Sedation and analgesia using recommended short-acting agents (e.g., propofol, fentanyl, midazolam) in intubated patients
	Ventricular drainage performed intermittently. Continuous drainage is not recommended unless an additional ICP monitor is placed, as when the drain is open, it does not accurately reflect the true ICP
	Repeat CT imaging and neurological examination should be considered to rule out the development of a surgical mass lesion and guide treatment
	If ICP remains 20–25 mmHg, proceed to tier 2
Tier 2	In patients with a parenchymal ICP monitor, an EVD should be considered to allow for intermittent CSF drainage
	Hyperosmolar therapy should be given intermittently as needed for ICP elevation and not on a routine schedule
	Mannitol should be administered in intermittent boluses (0.25–1 gm/kg body weight). Caution should be taken in the hypovolemic patient when osmotic diuresis is instituted with mannitol. The serum sodium and osmolality must be assessed frequently (every 6 h), and additional doses should be held if serum osmolality exceeds 320 mosm/l. mannitol may also be held if there is evidence of hypovolemia
	Hypertonic saline may be administered in intermittent boluses of 3% sodium chloride solution (250 ml over ½ h) or other concentrations (e.g., 30 cc of 23.4%). Serum sodium and osmolality must be assessed frequently (every 6 h), and additional doses should be held if serum sodium exceeds 160 meq/l. generally, targeting a serum sodium of 145–155 meq/L is a reasonable goal in patients with an elevated ICP
	Cerebral autoregulation should be assessed. If the patient is not autoregulating, the CPP goal should be lowered to reduce ICP (to no less than 50 mmHg). Additional neuromonitoring (e.g., PbtO2, SjvO2, CBF) may help determine optimal CPP
	PaCO2 goal of 30–35 mmHg should be maintained, as long as brain hypoxia is not encountered. Additional neuromonitoring (e.g., PbtO2, SjvO2, CBF) may help determine optimal PaCO2
	Repeat CT imaging and neurological examination should be considered to rule out development of a surgical mass lesion and guide treatment
	Neuromuscular paralysis achieved with a bolus test dose of a neuromuscular blocking agent should be considered if the above measures fail to adequately lower ICP and restore CPP. If there is a positive response, continuous infusion of a neuromuscular blocking agent should be employed (tier 3)
	If ICP remains greater than 20 mmHg, proceed to tier 3
Tier 3	Decompressive hemicraniectomy or bilateral craniectomy should only be performed if treatments in tiers 1 and 2 are not sufficient or are limited by development of side effects of medical treatment
	Neuromuscular paralysis via continuous infusion of a neuromuscular blocking agent can be employed if there is a positive response to a bolus dose. The infusion should be titrated to maintain at least two twitches (out of a train of four) using a peripheral nerve stimulator. Adequate sedation must be utilized
	Barbiturate or propofol (anesthesia dosage) coma may be induced for those patients who have failed to respond to aggressive measures to control malignant intracranial hypertension; however it should only be instituted if a test dose of barbiturate or propofol results in a decrease in ICP, thereby identifying the patient as a responder. Hypotension is a frequent side effect of high-dose therapy with these agents. Meticulous volume resuscitation should be ensured and infusion of vasopressor/inotropes may be required. Prolonged use or high dose of propofol can lead to propofol infusion syndrome. Continuous EEG may be used to ensure targeting of the infusion to burst suppression

above 22 mmHg have worse outcomes compared to patients without an elevated ICP and aggressive treatment to decrease the ICP will decrease morbidity and mortality [3]. ICP monitoring is paramount in directing the treatments in a tier step approach to manage an elevated ICP. Details of when to consider ICP monitoring and management of an elevated ICP are further covered in another chapter. In addition to the Brain Trauma Foundation Guidelines, the American College of Surgeons Trauma Quality Improvement Program (ACS TQIP) Best Practices in the Management of Traumatic Brain Injury describes and established the three-tiered management of intracranial pressure as a "best practice" [9]. This TQIP best practice is consistent with the recommendations in the latest version of the Brain Trauma Foundation Guidelines [3]. Decompressive craniectomy is in the third tier of management of increased intracranial pressure. Once decompressive craniotomy has been accomplished, it is important to remember to continue with the guidelines and the recommendations found in the tier approach; below is the three-tiered approach as found in the ACS TQIP for the management of elevated ICP (>20–25 mmHg) or low cerebral perfusion pressure (CPP) (<60 mmHg) and discussed by the Brain Trauma Foundation (Table 8.2).

Postoperative Pain and Sedation

It is important to remember that post-craniectomy patients have undergone major surgery and pain control is very important as this will decrease the catecholamine surge which may potentially have undesirable consequences [10]. If the patient is intubated postoperatively, it is important to remember that pain should be treated before initiating sedation. Withholding pain medication or sedation for prolonged periods of time may increase ICP to an undesirable level with detrimental effects. Of course, frequent "sedation holidays" should occur for accurate neurologic examinations which are the cornerstone of ICU management of the neurologically injured patients.

Postoperative Nutrition

Some of the other important aspects to consider in the postoperative patient is the timing of initiating nutrition. The BTF recommends starting nutrition within the first 5 days. Intubated patients may have tube feeds started via an oral or nasal enteric tube provided there is no significant ileus or gastroparesis. In patients that are not intubated, it's advisable to have a bedside or formal swallowing evaluation prior to initiating feeding since many of these patients will have dysphagia secondary to their neurologic insult.

Postoperative VTE Prophylaxis

While there has been some controversy and concern over the use of venous thromboembolism chemoprophylaxis while a drain or EVD is in place, the Neurocritical Care Society (NCS) recommends the use of prophylactic doses of either low molecular weight heparin or unfractionated heparin even while the EVD is in place [11]. The NCS guideline recommends starting VTE chemoprophylaxis within the first 3 days after injury and within 1 day after EVD insertion [11]. Full anticoagulation is not recommended in the immediate postoperative period in these patients [11]. Mechanical VTE prophylaxis is recommended during and immediately following craniotomy/craniectomy. VTE chemoprophylaxis should be started within 24 h after the procedure and should not be held for monitoring devices or drains in place [12]. Treatment doses of anticoagulants should only be initiated after discussion with the neurosurgery team.

Postoperative Antibiotic Prophylaxis

Antibiotic prophylaxis for drain placement has also been addressed by the NCS consensus statement for EVD management. Their recommendation is to give one dose of antibiotics before a drain is placed. They do not recommend prophylactic antimicrobial treatment for the entire duration of EVD drain use. Also, in order to reduce the infection rates associated with drains, the earliest removal as possible is a best practice standard [11]. There is no evidence to suggest that giving antibiotics post-craniectomy/craniotomy beyond the perioperative dose reduces surgical site or CSF infection [13, 14].

Postoperative Seizure Treatment and Prophylaxis

Seizure treatment and/or prophylaxis must be evaluated in postsurgical patient. Craniectomy or craniotomy itself may not increase the risk of seizures, but the reason leading to the surgery such as traumatic brain injury may be an indication for seizure prophylaxis. If the patient was treated for seizures prior to surgery, then it would be prudent to continue with the seizure treatment postsurgery. Regarding seizure prophylaxis, the BTF recommends 1 week of seizure prophylaxis in patients with severe TBI. If there has been no evidence of seizure activity in 1 week, this prophylaxis may be discontinued [3].

Complications of Craniotomy and Craniectomy

Craniotomy and craniectomy surgery is not without risk of secondary injury. Multiple complications can arise from surgically opening the once tightly closed and protective layers covering the brain, such as hygroma, hydrocephalus, and infection of the cranial incision, syndrome of the trephined, normal perfusion pressure breakthrough, and cerebral infarction. Associated symptoms, expected timing of onset, and treatment recommendations will be discussed so providers will be able to anticipate the needs of the postsurgical craniotomy patient.

Hygroma

The most common complication associated with decompressive brain surgery is a hygroma [15]. Patients with a hygroma may display a decline in their neurologic exams which may precipitate an urgent CT scan for evaluation. The incidence is as high as 92% and most hygromas occur on the same side as the initial injury and many will occur within the first postoperative week [15]. Postoperative hygromas may enlarge for up to 4 weeks, and they often resolve spontaneously in months. Only 10% of patients required drainage of their hygromas. However, should they become so large that drainage is necessary, this is done by one of four methods: twist drill, burr hole, percutaneous drainage system, or craniotomy [16].

Hydrocephalus

The incidence of developing hydrocephalus as a direct result of decompressive craniectomy has been debated and studied extensively with widely varying results due to a variety of study inclusions [17]. It is a well-recognized complication that can occur within 4 weeks after surgery with the incidence being widely variable (0–88%). However, the risk factors are also controversial, and it has been suggested that the surgery itself may not be a cause of hydrocephalus. Rather, the risk of hydrocephalus increases with "age, intraventricular hemorrhage, blood thickness greater than or equal to 5 millimeters, and a diffuse distribution of blood rather than a focal hemorrhage" [18]. A decline in neurologic function or an arrest in rehabilitation milestones should elicit an additional CT scan of the brain to rule out hydrocephalus. In these patients, a shunting device, such as a ventriculostomy, can be inserted until a cranioplasty can be performed. If hydrocephalus persists after cranioplasty, a more permanent ventricular peritoneal shunt can be placed [16, 18].

Infection of Craniotomy Incision

Even the most minor surgical procedure carries a risk of infection because the protective layer of skin is opened, allowing for the entry of bacteria. Most common after neurosurgery, infections present as meningitis, epidural abscess, subdural empyema, and brain abscess. Two independent risk factors are leakage of cerebrospinal fluid and male sex. The most common pathogens are *Staphylococcus aureus* and *Propionibacterium acnes*[19]. Even with prophylactic antibiotic treatment prior to surgery, infections still occur. Symptoms of post-neurosurgical infections are fever, elevated white blood cell count, edema, erythema, and purulence in the area or around the incision, decline in Glasgow Coma Scale score, agitation, and/or seizure. The diagnosis can be made with CT scanning and CSF cultures, a complete blood count, erythrocyte sedimentation rate, and C-reactive protein level. Broad-spectrum antibiotics should be started early and tapered as CSF and/or wound culture data return [15]. Infectious disease specialists may be a vital resource when there is a concern for a CSF infection. Surgical evacuation and debridement may be needed for more severe infections associated with the operative site [19].

Syndrome of the Trephined

Syndrome of the trephined is also referred to as "sunken flap syndrome." A systemic review by Ashayeri et al. in *Neurosurgery* define it as a poorly understood complication of craniectomy, characterized most commonly by unexplained neurological dysfunction in patients with acquired skull defects and subsequent improvement after secondary cranial reconstruction (i.e., cranioplasty) [20]. Symptoms are described as long-term neurological deficits beginning weeks to months after craniectomy, with clinical improvement after cranioplasty has been done. Symptoms can range dramatically among patients but usually include motor weakness, cognitive and language difficulty, headache, seizures, and cranial nerve changes. As stated in the definition, the definitive treatment is cranioplasty, and most patients do have a good recovery after cranioplasty, though with varying timeframes [20].

Normal Perfusion Pressure Breakthrough

Normal perfusion pressure breakthrough (NPPB), which sometimes occurs after surgical resection of an arteriovenous malformation (AVM), remains a misunderstood phenomenon ever since 1978 when it was originally proposed by Spetzler et al. Several studies have attempted to explain its occurrence, but none have definitively proven the mechanism behind the theory. AVMs are high-flow vascular shunts between arteries and veins without capillary beds in between. When an AVM is resected, the previously hypotensive cerebral perfusion pressure becomes normalized [21]. This new influx of blood can cause edema and hemorrhage, which in turn can lead to neurologic changes such as hemiplegia and neglect. Several studies have confirmed that keeping the systolic blood pressure on the lower end of normal (90–100 mm Hg), and gradually allowing blood pressure to normalize, will prevent or resolve neurologic side effects [21].

Cerebral Infarction

Cerebral infarction can occur after traumatic brain injury as a secondary injury. Similar secondary injury can occur after a neurosurgical procedure involving craniectomy and craniotomy. This is secondary to edema that causes the brain to be in a hyperemic state due to its high demand for oxygen and quick refilling of the vessels after compression is relieved [15]. In addition, brain strangulation and herniation can be caused by brain compression, venous compression, and diminished blood flow against this sharp edge of remaining skull leading to infarct [15]. It is recommended that the bone flap should be larger to allow for brain swelling without compression of the vessels or brain tissue against the cranial defect [3, 15].

References

1. Hippocrates. (400 B.C.). On injuries of the head, Part 21. Translated by Francis Adams. Retrieved from http://classics.mit.edu/Hippocrates/headinjur.21.21.html
2. Bullock M, Chestnut R, Ghajar J, Gordon D, Hartl R, Newell D, et al. Surgical management of acute subdural hematomas. Neurosurgery. 2006;58(3):16–24. https://doi.org/10.1227/01.NEU.0000210364.29290.C9.

3. Brain Trauma Foundation. (2016). Guidelines for the management of severe traumatic brain injury, 4th ed. Retrieved from https://braintrauma.org/uploads/03/12/Guidelines_for_Management_of_Severe_TBI_4th_Edition.pdf
4. Pascual JM, Prieto R. Surgical management of severe closed head injury in adults. In: Quiñones-Hinjosa A, editor. Schmidek & Sweet operative neurosurgical techniques. Philadelphia: Elsevier Saunders; 2012. p. 1527–30.
5. Cooper DJ, Rosenfeld JV, Arabi YM, et al. Decompressive craniectomy in diffuse traumatic brain injury. N Engl J Med. 2011;364:1493–502. https://doi.org/10.1056/NEJMoa1102077.
6. Hutchinson PJ, Kolias AG, Timofeev IS, Corteen EA, Czonsnyka M, Timothy J, Kirkpatrick PJ. Trial of decompressive craniectomy for traumatic intracranial hypertension. N Engl J Med. 2016;375(12):1128. https://doi.org/10.1056/NEJMoa1605215.
7. Quereshi AL, Ishfaq MF, Rahman HA, Thomas AP. Hemicraniectomy versus conservative treatment in large hemispheric ischemic stroke patients: a meta-analysis of randomized controlled trials. J Stroke Cerebrovasc Dis. 2016;25(9):2209–14.
8. David Panczykowski, Benjamin Zusman, David Okonkwo, Joshua Bauer, Ava Puccio. Early discontinuation of subdural drain following evacuation of acute subdural hematoma does not increase risk of reoperation. Presented in Neurotrauma 2016. National Neurotrauma Society. June 26th, 2016. Accessed PubMed 14 Feb 2017.
9. ACS TQIP. https://www.facs.org/~/media/files/quality%20programs/trauma/tqip/traumatic %20brain%20injury%20guidelines.ashx. 2015. Accessed 13 Feb 2017.
10. Lewis KS, Whipple JK, Michael KA, Quebbeman EJ. Effect of analgesic treatment on the physiological consequences of acute pain. Am J Hosp Pharm. 1994;51(12):1539–54.
11. Fried HI, Nathan BR, Shaun Rowe A, et al. The insertion and Management of external ventricular drains: an evidence- based consensus statement - a statement for healthcare professionals from the Neurocritical Care Society. Neurocrit Care. 2016;24(1):61–81.
12. Nyquist P, Bautista C, Jichici D, et al. Prophylaxis of venous thrombosis in Neurocritical care patients: an evidence-based guideline: a statement for healthcare professionals from the Neurocritical Care Society. Neurocrit Care. 2016;24(1):47–60.
13. Cao Y, Pu K, Li Q, et al. The role of antibiotic prophylaxis in the clean neurosurgery. World Neurosurg. 2017;pii: S1878-8750(16)31423-1. doi:https://doi.org/10.1016/j.wneu.2016.12.108.
14. Korinek AM, Baugnon T, Golmard JL, et al. Risk factors for adult nosocomial meningitis after craniotomy: role of antibiotic prophylaxis. Neurosurgery. 2008;62(Suppl 2):532–9. https://doi.org/10.1227/01.neu.0000316256.44349.b1.
15. Webb S, Timmons SD. Surgical management of traumatic brain injury. In: Winn B, Dacey, editors. Youman's neurological surgery. Philadelphia: Elsevier Saunders; 2011. p. 3475–548.
16. Arabi B, Chesler D, Maulucci C, Blacklock T, Alexander M. Dynamics of subdural hygroma following decompressive craniectomy: a comparative study. Neurosurg Focus. 2009;26(6):E8. Retrieved from http://thejns.org/doi/10.3171/2009.3.FOCUS0947.
17. Ding J, Guo Y, Tian H. The influence of decompressive craniectomy on the development of hydrocephalus: a review. Arq Neuropsiquiatr. 2014;72(9):715–20. Retrieved from https://doi.org/10.1590/0004-282X20140106.
18. Greenberg MS. Posttraumatic hydrocephalus. In: Handbook of neurosurgery. New York: Theime Publishers; 2010. p. 906.
19. McClelland S, Hall WA. Postoperative central nervous system infection: incidence and associated factors in 2111 neurosurgical procedures. Clin Infect Dis. 2007;45(1):55–9. https://doi.org/10.1086/518580.
20. Ashayeri K, Jackson E, Huang J, Brem H, Gordon CH. Syndrome of the trephined: a systematic review. Neurosurgery. 2016;79(4):525–34. https://doi.org/10.1227/NEU.0000000000001366.
21. O'Connor TE, Fargen KM, Mocco J. Normal perfusion pressure breakthrough following AVM resection: a case report and review of the literature. Open J Mod Neurosurg. 2013;3:66–71. Retrieved from http://file.scirp.org/pdf/OJMN_2013101516172598.pdf

9 Arrhythmia Evaluation and Management in the Surgical ICU

Edward Kelly

Introduction

Critically ill surgical patients may experience cardiac dysrhythmias for a wide variety of reasons, including preexisting cardiac disease; myocardial irritation from acid-base disturbances, electrolyte abnormalities, or sepsis; myocardial ischemia; or toxic effects of medications. While nonsustained, benign rhythms such as premature ventricular contractions (PVCs) can be observed in almost all patients, the prevalence of sustained dysrhythmias in mixed medical/surgical (non-cardiothoracic) ICU populations has been reported as 12%, with high correlation with mortality, especially with ventricular dysrhythmias. Thus, it is vital for the surgical intensivist to have expertise in recognition and treatment of cardiac dysrhythmias.

Effective management of cardiac dysrhythmias depends on rapid diagnosis and prompt intervention, often requiring a multimodality approach, which may include simultaneous correction of electrolytes and pH, pharmacological measures for rate control, pressors, specific antiarrhythmic medications, electrical pacing, or cardioversion. Intervention should be carefully tailored to the patient's specific dysrhythmia, its underlying cause, and the patient's own coexisting medical and surgical condition. To facilitate prompt diagnosis, this chapter is organized by categories of the major classes of cardiac dysrhythmia. In discussion of treatment, emphasis will be placed on both rapid intervention for arrhythmia and treatment of underlying causes.

E. Kelly (✉)
Harvard Medical School, Division of Trauma, Burns, and Surgical Critical Care, Department of Surgery, Brigham and Women's Hospital, 75 Francis Street, Boston, 02116 MA, USA
e-mail: Ekelly1@partners.org

Anatomy of the Conducting System

Electrical impulses are generated and conducted through the heart via anatomically distinct tracts called the conducting system. Normally, specialized pacemaking cells in the sinoatrial (SA) node originate the impulse or action potential (AP). The impulse propagates through the cardiomyocytes of the atrium, triggering atrial muscular contraction. Once the impulse arrives at the atrioventricular junction, the atrioventricular (AV) node is triggered. The AV node functions both to delay the entry of the impulse into the ventricle (thereby enabling the completion of atrial contraction before initiation of ventricular contraction) and to facilitate organized conduction of the impulse to the larger mass of the ventricle. The AV node transmits the impulse into a specialized conducting tract, the AV bundle, or bundle of His, which allows more rapid conduction. The AV bundle divides into separate branches to the left and right ventricles, which then further divide into a network of conducting fibers, the Purkinje fibers. On the left, where the ventricle is thicker, the bundle further divides into anterior and posterior bundle branches. Much like a parallel network of electrical wiring, this arrangement enables rapid organized contraction of the thick muscular ventricles.

Electrophysiology Review

Normal cardiac function relies on regulated generation and conduction of electrical impulses in the myocardium and conducting system to enable organized contraction. A comprehensive review of cardiac electrophysiology is beyond the scope of this chapter, but a brief summary is provided in order to better comprehend diagnosis and management. Action potentials originate in the heart due to the function of ion channels in the cellular membrane, leading to controlled changes in the electrical polarization of the membrane. These occur in discrete phases, as indicated in Fig. 9.1.

A. Salim et al. (eds.), *Surgical Critical Care Therapy*, https://doi.org/10.1007/978-3-319-71712-8_9

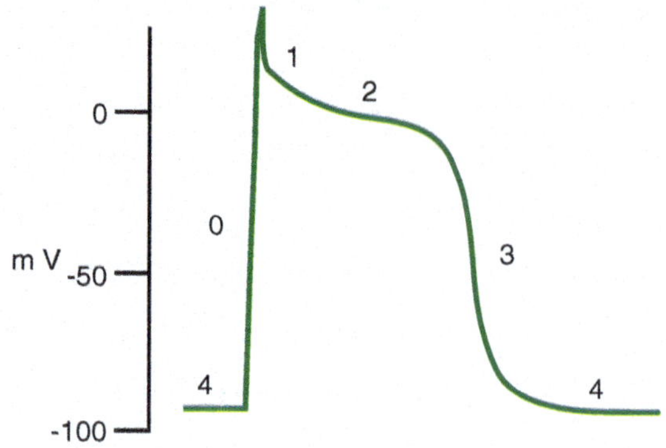

Fig. 9.1 Cardiomyocyte phases of depolarization

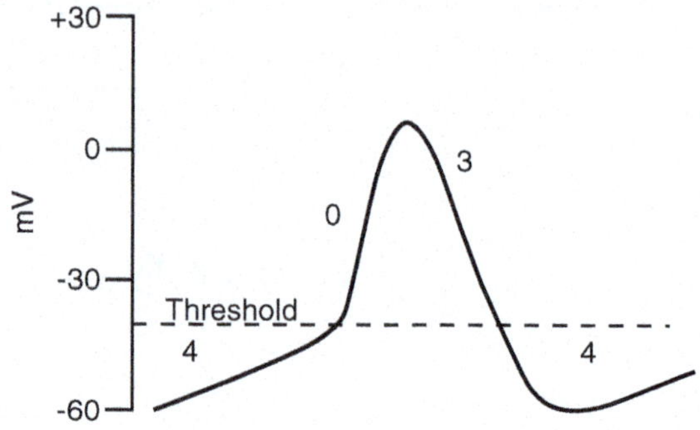

Fig. 9.2 Pacemaking cell phases of depolarization

In a cardiac myocyte at rest (phase 4), the cell membrane is polarized at about −90 mV potential energy (external vs. cell interior). The negative electrical potential, or resting transmembrane potential (TMP), of the cell interior is maintained by the inward rectifier potassium channels that facilitate movement of K^+ ion out of the cell. These channels are not voltage dependent. Depolarization (phase 0) occurs when the resting membrane potential is raised to the threshold voltage of −70 mV, either by an action potential arising from a pacemaker cell or any other source (e.g., external electrical pacer). In response to the threshold voltage being reached, fast sodium channels are opened, which enable entry of Na^+ ion in the cell. This results in the membrane potential becoming net positive or depolarizing. Fast Na+ channels are time dependent and close while the membrane is still depolarized. While the TMP is greater than −40 mV, the voltage-dependent long calcium channels open and prolong depolarization by facilitating movement of Ca^{++} into the cell and promoting Ca++ release from the sarcoplasmic reticulum.

When the time-dependent Na channels close, phase 1 begins, and the TMP rapidly deflects toward the negative (repolarization), facilitated by K^+ exiting the cells via K channels. These K channels are voltage dependent and open transiently, only while the membrane is depolarized. This results in a sharp, limited decrease in TMP. Throughout repolarization, the cell is refractory to initiation of a second action potential.

Phase 2 is characterized as the plateau phase, where TMP decreases very gradually through the sustained activity of the long (L-type) Ca^{++} channels. Increased sarcoplasmic Ca^{++} triggers the muscular contraction of the heart during this phase.

In late repolarization, or phase 3, the TMP decreases sharply again as the Ca^{++} channels close, and the inward rectifier K^+ channels restore the resting TMP. During phase 3, the cell membrane is only relatively refractory to new action potentials and can be depolarized by an aberrant or externally applied action potential (e.g., an external electrical pacer) stimulating the voltage-dependent channels. In clinical terms, this is seen as the R-on-T phenomenon, when an aberrant depolarization disrupts the organized conduction of electrical impulses within the ventricle, leading to chaotic propagation of aberrant signals, resulting in ventricular dysrhythmias. Once late repolarization is complete, the cell reenters phase 4, the TMP returns to −90 mV, and the membrane is no longer refractory.

In specialized pacemaking cells primarily in the SA and AV nodes, but also found in other locations, phase 4 does not have a stable resting TMP, as shown in Fig. 9.2. Pacemaking cells exhibit a property known as automaticity or a regularly pulsating TMP. Rapid depolarization is absent, as there are no fast Na^+ channels in these cells. Instead, the TMP rises gradually during phase 4 due to the action of slow Na^+ channels conducting Na^+ ion inward. As the TMP rises to −50 mV, transient (T-type) Ca^{++} channels open, conducting Ca^{++} inward. This Ca^{++} flux is brief in comparison with the L-type Ca^{++} channels but carries the TMP into the positive, depolarizing the cell. L-type Ca^{++} channels are also present in pacer cells and contribute to prolonging depolarization, as is in other cardiomyocytes. Phase 0 depolarization in pacer cells is thus dependent on both T- and L-type Ca^{++} channels. Pacer cells do not exhibit a phase 1 or phase 2; instead phase 3 begins as the Ca^{++} channels close, and the inward rectifier K^+ channel repolarizes the cell membrane. Phase 4 resumes as the slow Na^+ channels open again and the TMP gradually rises again.

Automaticity can be displayed by cardiac myocytes and in the conducting system, and automaticity is subject to both adrenergic stimulation and parasympathetic inhibition. In terms of generation of arrhythmias, this means that completing pacing sites can lead to aberrant contractions, such as atrial premature beats (APCs) and ventricular premature beats (VPCs). In terms of therapy, adrenergic beta stimulation (e.g., with isoproterenol) or muscarinic inhibition (e.g., with atropine) can be used to treat bradycardia, and beta blockade can be used to treat supraventricular tachycardia.

Reentry is the formation of an abnormal circuit that allows a sustained, unregulated depolarization impulse to travel through the myocardium. This circuit may involve only the atria, only the ventricles, or the entire heart. In normal conduction, there exist branch points, where an impulse travels down several pathways at the same time (e.g., the division of the AV bundle), and the refractory period prevents conduction in the retrograde direction. When the refractory period is shorter in one branch than the other (e.g., in ischemic conditions or due to medications or electrolyte abnormalities), the impulse can be conducted retrograde through the non-refractory channel back to the branch point, until it reaches another non-refractory section of the common channel, and depolarizes that pathway in the anterograde direction again. This leads to an unregulated circular pattern of impulses (circus movement) that can depolarize the downstream branches of the circuit.

Classification of Antiarrhythmic Drugs

Based on their primary effects on the ion channels that govern depolarization and repolarization, antiarrhythmic medications are commonly classified according to the scheme of Singh and Williams, shown in Table 9.1. While it is helpful to understand the pharmacological action of these medications and understanding pharmacology will enable better management of adverse effects, many commonly used antiarrhythmics have several mechanisms of action, and the primary mechanism of action does not always predict the clinical effects with precision.

Although not classified among the typical antiarrhythmic medications, adenosine can be used in diagnosis of tachyarrhythmia when there is uncertainty regarding supraventricular or ventricular origin. Adenosine is an endogenous nucleoside-signaling molecule with diverse physiological effects, which depend on the type and location of its four receptors. In the microcirculation of the myocardium, the A_{2A} receptor predominates in the coronary smooth muscle, which results in coronary vasodilation and can be used for pharmacological stress testing. In the SA and AV node, the A1 receptor predominates and functions to inhibit the slow Na and long Ca channels, producing hyperpolarization and slowing electrical conduction, which is its main clinical use in the ICU. Ventricular rate will briefly decrease in response to a single intravenous dose of adenosine in cases of supraventricular tachycardia, but ventricular tachyarrhythmia will be unaffected by adenosine. In addition, slowing conduction through the AV node with adenosine will convert reentrant tachyarrhythmias that involve the AV node, such as Wolff-Parkinson-White syndrome or AV nodal reentrant tachycardia. Of note, adenosine should be used with caution in patients with history of first- or second-degree heart block or abnormal infranodal conduction. Complete heart block can ensue, and external pacing should be available with use of adenosine for this reason. Alternatively, in a stable, cooperative patient, a vagal maneuver such as a Valsalva can be employed. Vagal maneuvers lead to reflex parasympathetic stimulation, thus decreasing AV nodal conduction.

Cardioversion

Direct current cardioversion (DCCV) is an often useful maneuver for certain dysrhythmias in hemodynamically unstable patients. DCCV involves application of electrical leads on the chest, or directly onto the heart if the chest is open, and delivery of an electrical countershock to depolarize the myocardium all at once, which stops all electrical conduction, both normal and aberrant. Standard equipment enables the delivery of the shock as a biphasic electrical discharge, which delivers the energy through the chest wall in opposite vectors sequentially. This approach is useful in overcoming the electrical impedance of the thorax. Using a

Table 9.1 Singh-Vaughan Williams classification

Class	Primary mechanism	Pharmacological effect	Example drug	Adverse cardiovascular effects
I	Fast Na^+ channel inhibition	Reduced phase 0 slope and maximum depolarization		Decreased contractility Tachycardia due to vagal inhibition
Ia		Moderate reduction in phase 0 slope; increased AP duration; increased refractory period	Quinidine	Qt interval prolongation
Ib		Minor reduction in phase 0 slope; reduced AP duration; shortened refractory period	Lidocaine	Vasodilation
Ic		Major reduction in phase 0 slope; no effect on AP duration or refractory period	Flecainide	PR interval prolongation
II	Cardiac beta adrenergic receptor blockade	Block sympathetic response; reduced slope of phase 4 (automaticity)	Metoprolol	Decreased contractility, arterial vasodilation
III	K^+ channel inhibition	Prolonged phase 3 repolarization, increased AP duration and refractory period	Ibutilide	Qt interval prolongation, ventricular tachycardia
IV	L-type Ca^{++} channel inhibition in nodes	Prolonged refractory period, decreased pacer rate	Diltiazem	High-degree AV block, vasodilation

biphasic defibrillator, the typical energy delivered in a single countershock is 50 Joules (J); with monophasic defibrillation, 350 J is usually required. In dysrhythmias with discernible R waves (e.g., atrial fibrillation), the countershock should be delivered using the synchronized setting of the defibrillator. This enables the device to deliver the shock after the late depolarization period has occurred, in order to prevent the R-on-T phenomenon and avoid precipitating ventricular fibrillation. In patients with no discernible R waves (e.g., ventricular fibrillation), the asynchronous setting is appropriate. After defibrillation, there is a refractory period, then normal electrical conduction resumes, and the SA node will resume normal generation of pacer potentials and sinus rhythm will be restored. If a competing abnormal pacing center or centers resume function before the SA node, the arrhythmia will continue. For this reason, it is almost always necessary to use DCCV in combination with some other therapy to treat the underlying cause of the arrhythmia. This approach is discussed in detail in the next sections.

Tachycardias

Sinus Tachycardia

Sinus tachycardia (ST) is defined as sinus rhythm with rate greater than 100 beats per minute (Fig. 9.3) and is the most common dysrhythmia observed in critically ill patients. It may be considered primarily as a physiological response to a wide variety of stressors: pain, fever, sepsis, anemia, hemorrhage, alcohol withdrawal, and delirium, to name just a few. In these clinical situations, there is excessive sympathetic stimulation to the conducting system, resulting in increased automaticity in the SA node and decreased conduction time in the AV node and infranodal conducting system. Unexplained ST should prompt the clinician to investigate and treat the underlying cause, rather than applying a remedy (such as beta blockers) prematurely. When ST is a compensatory physiological response, for example, in the case of hemorrhagic shock, slowing the heart rate with beta blockers, without treating the cause of hemorrhage and resuscitating with blood, will worsen hypotension and decrease oxygen delivery, resulting in a more severe state of shock.

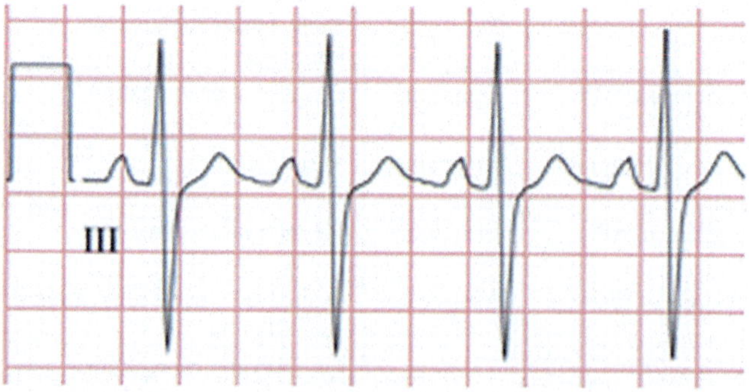

Fig. 9.3 Sinus tachycardia: There is a P wave preceding every R wave, the PR interval is constant, and the rate is greater than 100

However, there are indications for rate control in some cases of ST. In patients with thyroid storm, delirium tremens, pheochromocytoma, and blunt myocardial injury, when ST is a manifestation of a non-compensatory response to a pathological state, rate control of ST is required. Uncontrolled ST can lead to life-threatening myocardial demand ischemia, a condition which results from increased myocardial oxygen demand arising from tachycardia in conjunction with diminished myocardial perfusion due to higher wall tension and ventricular stiffness, again arising from tachycardia. Demand ischemia can be recognized on electrocardiography (ECG) with ST change in the distribution of the ischemic territory, often accompanied by new conduction abnormalities. Troponin may be elevated in this context, especially if the ischemia is not treated promptly, and uncontrolled demand ischemia may progress to a type 2 myocardial infarction (MI).

Class II (beta blockers) or class IV (calcium channel blockers) antiarrhythmics are appropriate for rate control in ST, when used in combination with correction of the underlying diagnosis. Both of these classes can cause hypotension and should be used with caution, especially if demand ischemia is suspected, as hypotension will further compromise oxygen delivery to the myocardium. Sinus tachycardia does not respond to cardioversion, and adenosine is contraindicated due to hypotension.

Atrial Fibrillation

Atrial fibrillation (AF), the most common sustained dysrhythmia overall, is characterized by rapid, unorganized generation or propagation of electrical impulses in the atrial chambers, leading to unpredictable triggering of the AV node. Recent evidence indicates that the majority of the abnormal impulses arise from the pulmonary vein orifices in the posterior atria, which can be targeted for surgical or catheter-based interventions. On ECG, AF appears as a chaotic baseline without discernible organized P waves and irregularly spaced R waves (Fig. 9.4). Measuring the R-R interval may be helpful to exclude rhythms that appear to be irregular, such as second-degree heart block. The ventricular response is often rapid, greater than 120 beats per minute, corresponding to a rapid peripheral pulse described as "irregularly irregular."

If the atrial impulses are rapid and regular, but the ventricular response is irregular, the condition is termed atrial flutter. Common clinical factors associated with AF in critically ill patients include electrolyte disturbances, especially

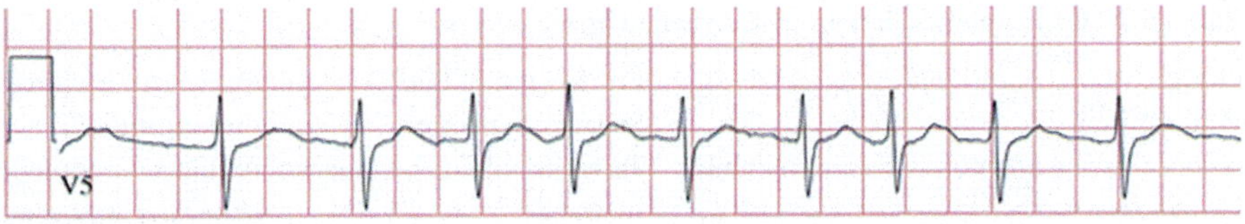

Fig. 9.4 Atrial fibrillation: There are no discernable P waves, and the R waves appear at irregular intervals

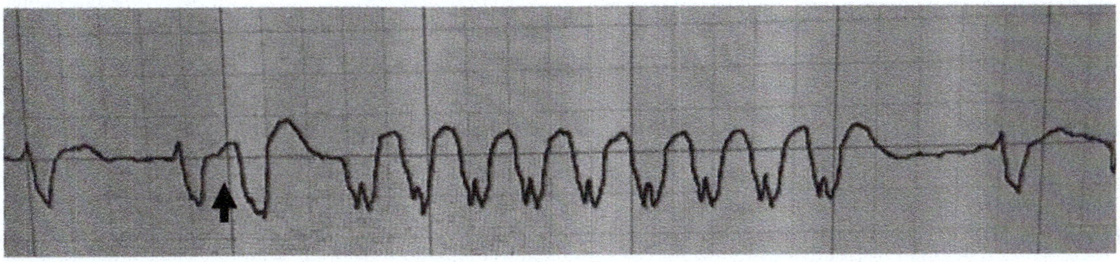

Fig. 9.5 Ventricular tachycardia: There is an R wave during the T wave (R on T, arrow) that has triggered a wide complex rapid rhythm without P waves, lasting for 9 beats

hypokalemia and hypomagnesemia, acidosis, fever, sepsis, and fluid volume overload. Thyrotoxicosis and withdrawal states are also highly associated with elevated AF risk. Control of AF requires correction of any of these factors but often also requires specific antiarrhythmic medication. In patients with a stable blood pressure and no signs of compromised cardiac function, rate control of ventricular response can be achieved with class II or class IV antiarrhythmics. If AF persists for longer than 24 h, risk of atrial thrombosis and cardioembolism becomes significant, and anticoagulation should be considered in appropriate patients. AF may trigger a rapid ventricular response, decreased cardiac function, and cardiogenic shock. In this urgent clinical setting, electrical cardioversion should be considered. In less severe cases where conversion to sinus rhythm is indicated, class III medications are effective.

Ventricular Tachycardia

Ventricular tachycardia (VT) is almost always a life-threatening rhythm in critically ill patients, as it is usually associated with significant myocardial ischemia and severely compromised cardiac function. On ECG (Fig. 9.5), VT characteristically appears as a tachycardia of 100–280 beats per minute of wide ventricular complexes (>0.14 milliseconds). Atrial complexes are not seen, but atrial tachycardias with aberrant ventricular conduction can easily be confused for VT. If necessary, a single dose of intravenous adenosine can be administered to produce temporary AV nodal block to differentiate these rhythms.

VT may arise from increased automaticity in ventricular foci or from the development of reentrant circuits within the ventricle. Metabolic derangements such as hypokalemia, acidosis, catecholamine surge, thyrotoxicosis, and ischemia are important factors in the generation of VT in critically ill patients and should be corrected promptly. Additional factors include pro-arrhythmic effects of many medications used in the ICU (Table 9.2) and myocardial ischemia. Patients with myocardial scarring after STEMI are at elevated risk for VT, especially if there is depressed ventricular function and when one of the metabolic risk factors appears. VT in these cases is almost always monomorphic (all of the ventricular complexes have the same shape), reflecting a focal region of the myocardium that is generating uncontrolled impulses.

Polymorphic VT refers to wide ventricular complex tachycardia where the shapes of the complexes are not uniform. With one notable exclusion, the origin of this arrhythmia is nearly always myocardial ischemia and carries a high mortality on that basis. The notable exclusion is torsade de pointes (TdP), which is characterized as a tachycardia with a "pulsating baseline" or "rotating axis." In critically ill patients, this arrhythmia is most often the result of adverse drug effects that cause prolongation of the Qt interval, leading to reentry circuits in the myocardium.

VT is usually associated with hemodynamic instability or frank cardiac arrest (pulseless VT). In these urgent cases, the recommended treatment is urgent electrical cardioversion, cardiopulmonary resuscitation, correction of any underlying metabolic disturbances, and treatment of myocardial ischemia. In the more unusual case of VT with a stable pulse, class I or class III antiarrhythmic medications are indicated. When the VT is ischemia-related, or associated with myocardial scarring, recurrence is common, and consideration should be given to advanced therapies such as ablation or implantation of an automated cardioverter-defibrillator (AICD).

Table 9.2 Common medications with arrhythmogenic effects

Drug	Primary use in ICU	Pharmacological effect	Associated dysrhythmia
Haloperidol	Sedative hypnotic	Prolongation of repolarization	Ventricular tachycardia
Lidocaine and other class I antiarrhythmics	Tachyarrhythmia treatment	Prolongation of repolarization	Ventricular tachycardia
Dobutamine	Inotrope	Increased intracellular cAMP	Atrial and ventricular tachycardia
Fluoroquinolones	Antibiotic	Prolonged phase 3	Torsade de pointes
Micafungin	Antifungal	Prolonged phase 3	Atrial and ventricular tachycardia
Ondansetron	Antiemetic	Prolonged phase 3	Torsade de pointes

Ventricular Fibrillation

Ventricular fibrillation (VF) is never considered a stable rhythm and is the leading cause of sudden cardiac arrest. It is characterized by multiple reentrant impulses arising in the ventricle and propagating at random. As such, VF should be treated promptly with cardiopulmonary resuscitation (CPR) and electrical defibrillation. It is characterized on ECG as disorganized electrical impulses without pulses or cardiac contraction. On echocardiography it is easily identified as a quivering (fibrillating) ventricle. In some cases the electrical activity on ECG may be very low in amplitude, so-called fine VT, and may resemble asystole. If the clinical context suggests VF, it is advisable to attempt electrical cardioversion in these cases.

The primary underlying cause of VF is myocardial ischemia, but in hospitalized, critically ill patients, other risk factors are prominent. These include cardiomyopathy, drug toxicity, and sepsis. These severe underlying conditions require rapid effective intervention, but once a VF or VT arrest has occurred, survival depends on undelayed defibrillation. As with VT, an episode of ventricular fibrillation arrest should prompt consideration for advanced therapies such as AICD.

Bradycardias

Sinus Bradycardia

Sinus bradycardia (SB) refers to sinus rhythm with a rate less than 60 beats per minute (BPM). There is a wide array of risk factors and causes, and in some patients, especially trained athletes, it may be a normal adaptation. The more prominent associated factors include medications (especially beta blockers, calcium channel blockers, sedatives, and opioids), hypothyroidism, and seizure. In urgent cases, atropine may be used as first-line therapy, but for sustained symptomatic SB, temporary or permanent pacing may be required.

Atrioventricular Block

First Degree

First-degree atrioventricular block (1AVB) is characterized by prolongation of the PR interval, which is normally 120–200 ms. Common risk factors include electrolyte abnormalities especially hypokalemia, myocardial ischemia, myocarditis, and side effects of medications, especially class II and class IV antiarrhythmics. While 1AVB is not directly life-threatening, some of the underlying causes may be and should be urgently investigated and corrected. In addition, 1AVB is a marker of AV node dysfunction, and caution should be exercised when using medications which delay AV conduction in patients with 1AVB. Treatment of 1AVB is targeted at the underlying cause, but the PR interval should be closely monitored until the block resolves.

Second Degree

Second-degree AV block (2AVB) is characterized by intermittent nonconduction of atrial impulses to the ventricle and is divided into two types: Mobitz type 1, where the PR interval becomes longer with every atrial impulse until there is a nonconducted impulse or "dropped beat," and Mobitz type 2, where the PR interval does not change, and may be of normal duration, but there is a nonconducted impulse at regular intervals (e.g., after every two conducted impulses, there is a nonconducted impulse).

Mobitz type I is usually due to drug effects or ischemia of the AV node and is not usually life-threatening or associated with progression to a more severe condition. This rhythm may initially appear to be irregular until the PR interval is measured and the successive prolongation is recognized.

Mobitz type II is usually due to structural damage to the infranodal conducting system (e.g., due to myocardial infarction, myocarditis, sarcoidosis, or cardiac injury), leading to widening of the ventricular complexes. Mobitz II is associated with a high risk of progression to complete heart block and sudden cardiac death. For this reason, urgent diagnosis of the underlying cause is mandatory, as is rapidly establishing pacing access.

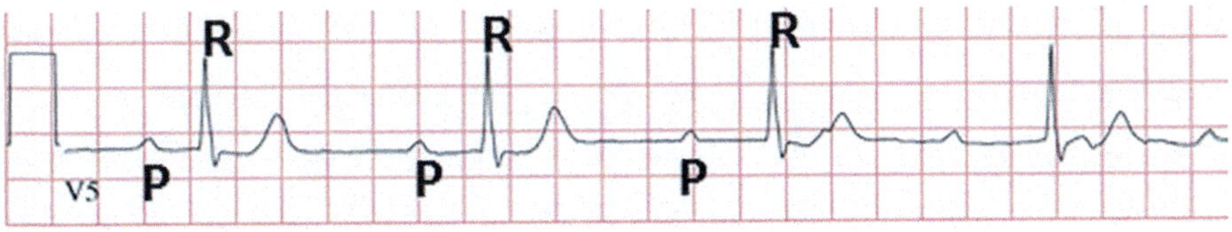

Fig. 9.6 Third-degree heart block: There are regular P waves and regular R waves, but the PR interval is not constant; ventricular conduction is completely independent from atrial impulses

Third Degree

Third-degree, or complete, heart block (CHB) refers to complete lack of conduction through the AV node. In this condition, the ventricular complexes are generated distal to the AV node by junctional or ventricular myocytes that have automaticity (junctional or ventricular escape rhythm). These impulses are not conducted through the ventricle as rapidly and efficiently and appear as abnormally wide complexes on ECG (Fig. 9.6). Junctional and ventricular escape rhythms are not as fast as sinus rhythm and are often associated with diminished cardiac output and cardiogenic shock.

CHB can occur as a result of ischemia or infarction (inferior wall STEMI) of the AV node, drug effects especially with class II or class IV antiarrhythmics, and inflammatory conditions involving the conducting system. Urgent diagnosis of the underlying cause is essential, as is rapid establishment of pacing.

Pacing Access

In many cases of AVB, treatment requires urgent temporary pacing or even establishment of long-term internal pacing. Every intensive care unit should have an external defibrillator/pacer unit available and ready for emergency use. These devices use transcutaneous contact paddles placed at the cardiac apex and on the mid-back to detect cardiac activity and deliver electrical pacing impulses. The unit can be set for synchronous or asynchronous pacing, the desired rate, and the desired current to deliver. Transcutaneous pacing is appropriate for the emergency setting, but it is uncomfortable in awake patients, can lead to skin burns with prolonged use, and is subject to loss of capture if the patient moves.

If pacing is required for a prolonged period, temporary transvenous access is preferred. In this approach, a temporary pacing wire is placed into the cardiac chambers using a central venous access sheath. The placement of the wire can be guided using fluoroscopy, or it can be done at the bedside using ECG sensing via the wire as a guide. Once the wire is in place, the external pacer is activated, and electrical pacer potentials (pacer spikes) will be observed on the ECG monitor. As the electrical output is increased to produce capture (mechanical contraction of the heart resulting from pacer impulses), the threshold current (the minimal setting that produces capture) should be recorded. If feasible, the output should be set for double the threshold current.

Conclusion

Critically ill surgical patients with cardiac dysrhythmias present a challenge to the intensivist for rapid diagnosis, careful evaluation, and prompt decision-making from among a wide array of therapeutic choices. Most often, the dysrhythmia will appear as a consequence of a noncardiac condition; thus there will be more than one objective for treatment, and antiarrhythmic options may be limited by the underlying condition. To provide the best care and ensure the best outcome, it is imperative to approach the patient as a whole and not to treat the conduction abnormality in isolation.

Suggested Readings

1. Annane D, Sebille V, Duboc D, Le Heuzey J, Sadoul N, Bouvier E, Bellissant E. Incidence and prognosis of sustained arrhythmias in critically ill patients. AJRCCM. 2008;178:20–5.
2. Barnes BJ, Hollands JM. Drug-induced arrhythmias. Crit Care Med. 2010;38(6 Suppl):S188–97.
3. Layland J, Carrick D, Lee M, Oldroyd K, Berry C. Adenosine physiology, pharmacology, and clinical applications. J Am Coll Cardiol Intv. 2014;7:581–91.
4. Zipes DP, Camm AJ, et al. AHA/ESC 2006 Guidelines for management of patients with ventricular arrhythmias and the prevention of sudden cardiac death. Circulation. 2006;114:e385–484.
5. January CT, Wann LS, et al. A report of the American College of Cardiology/American Heart Association Task Force on Practice Guidelines and the Heart Rhythm Society. Circulation. 2014;129:000.

Acute Coronary Syndrome

10

Daniel L. Gramins

As noted by the American College of Cardiology/American Heart Association Task Force on Practice Guidelines, "Acute Coronary Syndrome (ACS) has evolved as a useful operational term that refers to a spectrum of conditions compatible with acute myocardial ischemia and/or infarction due to an abrupt reduction in coronary blood flow" [1]. The critical tools for the clinician to place patients on this spectrum and prioritize their care are the electrocardiogram (ECG) and troponin assays, the specific cardiac biomarkers of necrosis (Box 10.1). A key branch point is the presence of ST-segment elevation (ST elevation) or new left bundle branch block on a patient's ECG, which is pathognomonic of an ST elevation myocardial infarction (STEMI). STEMI is an indication for immediate coronary angiography to determine if there is an opportunity for reperfusion therapy to open a likely completely occluded coronary artery [1]. The absence of persistent ST elevation on the ECG is suggestive of non-ST elevation acute coronary syndrome (NSTE-ACS) which can be further subdivided on the basis of cardiac biomarkers of necrosis. If cardiac biomarkers are elevated and the clinical context is appropriate, the patient is considered to have a non-ST elevation myocardial infarction (NSTEMI). Otherwise, the patient is deemed to have unstable angina (UA) [1].

The role of the critical care surgeon in acute coronary syndrome is to recognize the presence of this clinical syndrome in the perioperative or trauma patient. Recognition is the crucial first step in rescuing these patients. Once a patient is found to have ACS, proper assignment to STEMI or NSTE-ACS pathways will guide the urgency of consultations and interventions by cardiologists and cardiac surgeons. The critical care surgeon will need to remain engaged as the subject matter expert with regard to the patient's ability to tolerate various anticoagulation, intervention, and cardiac surgical therapies in relation to their current condition and potential need for further surgical intervention.

D. L. Gramins (✉)
Division of Cardiovascular & Thoracic Surgery, Sulpizio Cardiovascular Center, UC San Diego Health System, La Jolla, CA, USA
e-mail: drgramins@ucsd.edu

Epidemiology and Pathogenesis

In the United States, the most current estimate is that each year over 780,000 persons will experience an acute coronary syndrome, with a median age at presentation of 68 years and a male-to-female ratio of 3:2. Approximately 30% will have STEMI and 70% NSTE-ACS [1].

Postoperative ischemia occurs most frequently on days 1 and 2 [2]. In a recent prospective perioperative ACS study conducted in Finland in which investigators monitored troponin levels before and after surgery on inpatients, 7% of noncardiac surgical patients sustained a perioperative myocardial infarction (MI), with vascular surgery patients having a rate of 11%. The perioperative MI patients' 90-day mortality was 30%, compared to just over 5% of postoperative patients who did not have a perioperative MI [3]. In another study from Canada, patients experiencing an MI after noncardiac surgery had an in-hospital mortality rate of 15–25%, and patients who had a cardiac arrest had a hospital mortality rate of 65% [4].

In 2012 the European Society of Cardiology, American College of Cardiology Foundation, American Heart Association, and the World Heart Federation Task Force for the Universal Definition of Myocardial Infarction convened to update an expert consensus document, titled "Third Universal Definition of Myocardial Infarction" [5].

Box 10.1 Definition of myocardial infarction

Criteria for acute myocardial infarction

The term acute myocardial infarction (MI) should be used when there is evidence of myocardial necrosis in a clinical setting consistent with acute myocardial ischaemia. Under these conditions any one of the following criteria meets the diagnosis for MI:

(continued)

A. Salim et al. (eds.), *Surgical Critical Care Therapy*, https://doi.org/10.1007/978-3-319-71712-8_10

- Detection of a rise and/or fall of cardiac biomarker values [preferably cardiac troponin (cTn)] with at least one value above the 99th percentile upper reference limit (URL) and with at least one of the following:
  - Symptoms of ischaemia.
  - New or presumed new significant ST-segment–T wave (ST–T) changes or new left bundle branch block (LBBB).
  - Development of pathological Q waves in the ECG.
  - Imaging evidence of new loss of viable myocardium or new regional wall motion abnormality.
  - Identification of an intracoronary thrombus by angiography or autopsy.
- Cardiac death with symptoms suggestive of myocardial ischaemia and presumed new ischaemic ECG changes or new LBBB, but death occurred before cardiac biomarkers were obtained, or before cardiac biomarker values would be increased.
- Percutaneous coronary intervention (PCI) related MI is arbitrarily defined by elevation of cTn values (>5 × 99th percentile URL) in patients with normal baseline values (≤99th percentile URL) or a rise of cTn values >20% if the baseline values are elevated and are stable or falling. In addition, either (i) symptoms suggestive of myocardial ischaemia or (ii) new ischaemic ECG changes or (iii) angiographic findings consistent with a procedural complication or (iv) imaging demonstration of new loss of viable myocardium or new regional wall motion abnormality are required.
- Stent thrombosis associated with MI when detected by coronary angiography or autopsy in the setting of myocardial ischaemia and with a rise and/or fall of cardiac biomarker values with at least one value above the 99th percentile URL.
- Coronary artery bypass grafting (CABG) related MI is arbitrarily defined by elevation of cardiac biomarker values (>10 × 99th percentile URL) in patients with normal baseline cTn values (≤99th percentile URL). In addition, either (i) new pathological Q waves or new LBBB, or (ii) angiographic documented new graft or new native coronary artery occlusion, or (iii) imaging evidence of new loss of viable myocardium or new regional wall motion abnormality.

Criteria for prior myocardial infarction

Any one of the following criteria meets the diagnosis for prior MI:

- Pathological Q waves with or without symptoms in the absence of non-ischaemic causes.
- Imaging evidence of a region of loss of viable myocardium that is thinned and fails to contract, in the absence of a non-ischaemic cause.
- Pathological findings of a prior MI.

The diagnostic criteria presented above were updated as troponin assays have become more sensitive. The requirement for a rising and falling pattern is necessary to distinguish acute processes in patients who have chronic troponin elevations, such as patients with structural heart disease or renal failure [5].

The Third Universal Definition of Myocardial Infarction recognizes five types of MI based upon their pathogenesis [5] (Table 10.1):

Type 1: Spontaneous MI (related to atherosclerotic plaque rupture, ulceration, fissuring, erosion, or dissection with resulting intraluminal thrombus in one or more of the coronary arteries leading to decreased myocardial blood flow or distal platelet emboli with ensuing myocyte necrosis.

Type 2: MI secondary to ischemic imbalance (myocardial injury with necrosis where a condition other than coronary artery disease contributes to an imbalance between MVO2, e.g., coronary endothelial dysfunction, coronary artery spasm, coronary embolism, tachy–/bradyarrhythmias, anemia, respiratory failure, hypotension, and hypertension with or without LVH).

Type 3: MI resulting in death when biomarker values are unavailable (cardiac death with symptoms suggestive of myocardial ischemia, new ECG changes, but death prior to blood samples or before cardiac biomarkers could rise).

Type 4a: MI related to percutaneous coronary intervention.

Type 4b: MI related to stent thrombosis (stent thrombosis detected by coronary angiography or autopsy with myocardial ischemia and a cardiac biomarker elevation.

Type 5: MI related to coronary artery bypass grafting.

Based upon the epidemiology of ACS, the critical care surgeon will most frequently encounter the Type 2 MI, followed by Type 1. However, as increasing numbers of patients present for surgery after previous percutaneous coronary interventions with drug-eluting stents, the incidence of Type 4b MI will increase.

Acute coronary syndrome is caused by the sudden imbalance between myocardial oxygen consumption, or

Table 10.1 Universal classification of myocardial infarction

Type 1: Spontaneous myocardial infarction
Spontaneous myocardial infarction related to atherosclerotic plaque rupture, ulceration, fissuring, erosion, or dissection with resulting intraluminal thrombus in one or more of the coronary arteries leading to decreased myocardial blood flow or distal platelet emboli with ensuing myocyte necrosis. The patient may have underlying severe CAD but on occasion non-obstructive or no CAD.
Type 2: Myocardial infarction secondary to an ischaemic imbalance
In instances of myocardial injury with necrosis where a condition other than CAD contributes to an imbalance between myocardial oxygen supply and/or demand, e.g. coronary endothelial dysfunction, coronary artery spasm, coronary embolism, tachy–/brady-arrhythmias, anaemia, respiratory failure, hypotension, and hypertension with or without LVH.
Type 3: Myocardial infarction resulting in death when biomarker values are unavailable
Cardiac death with symptoms suggestive of myocardial ischaemia and presumed new ischaemic ECG changes or new LBBB, but death occurring before blood samples could be obtained, before cardiac biomarker could rise, or in rare cases cardiac biomarkers were not collected.
Type 4a: Myocardial infarction related to percutaneous coronary intervention (PCI)
Myocardial infarction associated with PCI is arbitrarily defined by elevation of cTn values >5 × 99th percentile URL in patients with normal baseline values (≤99th percentile URL) or a rise of cTn values >20% if the baseline values are elevated and are stable or falling. In addition, either (i) symptoms suggestive of myocardial ischaemia, or (ii) new ischaemic ECG changes or new LBBB, or (iii) angiographic loss of patency of a major coronary artery or a side branch or persistent slow-or no-flow or embolization, or (iv) imaging demonstration of new loss of viable myocardium or new regional wall motion abnormality are required.
Type 4b: Myocardial infarction related to stent thrombosis
Myocardial infarction associated with stent thrombosis is detected by coronary angiography or autopsy in the setting of myocardial ischaemia and with a rise and/or fall of cardiac biomarkers values with at least one value above the 99th percentile URL.
Type 5: Myocardial infarction related to coronary artery bypass grafting (CABG)
Myocardial infarction associated with CABG is arbitrarily defined by elevation of cardiac biomarker values >10 × 99th percentile URL in patients with normal baseline cTn values (≤99th percentile URL). In addition, either (i) new pathological Q waves or new LBBB, or (ii) angiographic documented new graft or new native coronary artery occlusion, or (iii) imaging evidence of new loss of viable myocardium or new regional wall motion abnormality.

Thygesen et al. [5] Or:
Kristian Thygesen et al. *Circulation*. 2012;126:2020–2035

demand, and myocardial oxygen supply. In a STEMI, this imbalance is the result of coronary artery obstruction, usually due to acute plaque rupture. Other mechanisms can lead to ACS, including acute coronary insufficiency from vasospasm, embolism, and arteritis; noncoronary causes of myocardial oxygen supply and demand mismatch from surgical stress or critical illness, hypertrophic cardiomyopathy, and aortic stenosis; and myocardial injury from infection, trauma, and drugs (Table 10.2).

Table 10.2 Elevations of cardiac troponin values because of myocardial injury [5]

Injury related to primary myocardial ischaemia
Plaque rupture
Intraluminal coronary artery thrombus formation
Injury related to supply/demand imbalance of myocardial ischaemia
Tachy-/brady-arrhythmias
Aortic dissection or severe aortic valve disease
Hypertrophic cardiomyopathy
Cardiogenic, hypovolaemic, or septic shock
Severe respiratory failure
Severe anaemia
Hypertension with or without LVH
Coronary spasm
Coronary embolism or vasculitis
Coronary endothelial dysfunction without significant CAD
Injury not related to myocardial ischaemia
Cardiac contusion, surgery, ablation, pacing, or defibrillator shocks
Rhabdomyolysis with cardiac involvement
Myocarditis
Cardiotoxic agents, e.g. anthracyclines, herceptin
Multifactorial or indeterminate myocardial injury
Heart failure
Stress (Takotsubo) cardiomyopathy
Severe pulmonary embolism or pulmonary hypertension
Sepsis and critically ill patients
Renal failure
Severe acute neurological diseases, e.g. stroke, subarachnoid haemorrhage
Infiltrative diseases, e.g. amyloidosis, sarcoidosis
Strenuous exercise

Kristian Thygesen et al. *Circulation*. 2012;126:2020–2035

Evaluation and Diagnosis

The single greatest challenge for the critical care surgeon is diagnosing ACS in the perioperative or the polytrauma patient. Some patients will have silent ischemia, which will only be detected with cardiac troponins. Symptoms of ACS can be masked by similar postsurgical symptoms. NSTE-ACS usually presents as retrosternal pressure-type chest pain which radiates to the arms, neck, or jaw. It may be accompanied by diaphoresis, dyspnea, nausea, abdominal pain, and syncope, all findings which can occur in normal postoperative patients. Exertional dyspnea is the most common angina equivalent, but nausea and vomiting, diaphoresis, fatigue, and syncope may manifest. Atypical symptoms such as epigastric pain, indigestion, and pleuritic pain can confound the diagnosis.

The physical examination is often more useful for finding an alternative diagnosis to NSTE-ACS. However, signs of heart failure should help make the diagnosis. The differential diagnosis of NSTE-ACS includes nonischemic cardiovascular causes of chest pain such as acute aortic syndrome, aortic dissection, pulmonary embolism, and pericarditis and non-cardiovascular causes of chest, back, or upper abdominal discomfort including pulmonary causes, gastrointestinal causes, musculoskeletal causes, and even psychiatric disorders.

An ECG is the first critical diagnostic test after obtaining the patient's vital signs. Comparison to a pre-event ECG is extremely helpful. Persistent ST elevation in two contiguous leads, new left bundle branch block, or anterior ST depression indicative of a posterior MI should trigger an emergent cardiology consultation and an institutional STEMI response with immediate activation of the cardiac catheterization lab.

If the initial ECG is normal, or unchanged, then it should be repeated at 15- to 30-min intervals during the first hour of symptoms, and if the symptoms remit but recur. New ST depression, horizontal or down-sloping, is suggestive of NSTE-ACS. Transient ST changes (>0.5 mm) or a new T wave inversion (>2 mm) suggests acute ischemia but can also be seen in pulmonary embolism. A normal or unchanged ECG does not exclude an NSTE-ACS. At this point, an urgent cardiology consultation to assist with ECG interpretation and diagnosis is appropriate.

A chest X-ray is important to quickly identify potential pulmonary causes of chest pain. A widened mediastinum may suggest an aortic dissection. A computed tomography scan of the chest with appropriately timed intravenous contrast can demonstrate pulmonary embolism and aortic dissection. A transthoracic echocardiogram is useful for identifying a pericardial effusion and tamponade physiology, as well as cardiac wall motion abnormalities suggestive of NSTE-ACS.

Cardiac troponins are the most sensitive and specific biomarkers for NSTE-ACS and will rise within a few hours of symptom onset in the event of an NSTEMI. A level should be obtained at symptom onset and then at 3–6 h. A troponin value above the 99th percentile of the upper reference level is required. In addition, a serial increase or decrease of >20% is needed if the initial value is elevated due to an underlying medical condition (tachyarrhythmia, hypotension, hypertension, cardiac trauma, acute heart failure, myocarditis, pericarditis, acute pulmonary embolism, and noncardiac conditions including sepsis, burns, respiratory failure, renal failure, acute neurological diseases, and drug toxicity). Chronic troponin elevations can be due to left ventricular hypertrophy and ventricular dilatation.

Additional troponin levels can be obtained after 6 h if symptoms return or ECG changes become suspicious for ACS. Also, B-type natriuretic peptide levels can be measured to detect new or worsening heart failure. Creatinine kinase myocardial isoenzyme and myoglobin do not add to making the diagnosis of ACS and do not need to be ordered.

Relief of chest pain with sublingual nitroglycerin or "gastrointestinal cocktails" neither predicts nor excludes ACS.

Treatment of STEMI

The critical care surgeon plays an important role in the treatment of STEMI in the perioperative or polytrauma patient, having the most insight into the patient's ability to be safely anticoagulated for coronary catheterization in light of their recent surgery or trauma, as well as the patient's ability to comply with a 12-month course of dual antiplatelet therapy (DAPT) given their medical and surgical comorbid conditions, and their social situation as it relates to their ability to comply with a post-percutaneous coronary intervention (PCI) medication regimen.

The conventional treatment of STEMI involves immediate transfer of the patient to the cardiac catheterization laboratory for diagnostic coronary angiography and percutaneous coronary intervention (PCI) to restore flow in the culprit obstructed coronary artery. The goal of first medical contact to balloon time of 90 min also applies to inpatients with STEMI. However, patients sustaining a STEMI in a surgical facility without coronary intervention capabilities, such as an outpatient surgical center or smaller community hospital, still benefit from PCI outside of the 90-min interval, up to 12 h after the onset of the event. Therefore, having a transfer plan to the nearest STEMI receiving facility is a must for surgeons and anesthesiologists who practice in these facilities. Systemic fibrinolytic treatment guidelines exist for patients without immediate access to facilities with the necessary interventional cardiology capabilities, but systemic fibrinolytics are contraindicated in almost all trauma and surgical patients [6].

Current guidelines recommend pretreatment with non-enteric coated aspirin, either 162 mg or 325 mg, and the initiation of either unfractionated heparin or bivalirudin. The goal activated clotting time (ACT) is at least 200 s and over 250 s if heparin will be used as monotherapy. In the catheterization laboratory, when imaging demonstrates that the patient is an anatomic candidate for percutaneous coronary intervention (PCI), the patient is loaded with a P2Y12 inhibitor, either clopidogrel or ticagrelor, and flow is restored in the stenosed or occluded coronary artery with a combination of balloon angioplasty and manual thrombus aspiration as needed, followed by stenting with either a drug-eluting stent (DES) or a bare metal stent (BMS). In the infrequent case of a patient whose anatomy is not amenable to PCI, emergent coronary artery bypass grafting (CABG) is recommended. For this reason, enoxaparin and P2Y12 inhibitors, while options under current STEMI treatment protocols, should be avoided until the patient's anatomy is clear, to reduce the risk of excessive operative hemorrhage if CABG must be performed without delay [6].

In fact, under current STEMI guidelines, PCI with a DES has a Class III (harm) recommendation for patients who are unable to tolerate or comply with a prolonged course of DAPT because of the increased risk of stent thrombosis with premature discontinuation of one or both agents. Also, prasugrel, another P2Y12 inhibitor, is contraindicated in patients with a history of prior CVA or TIA [6].

In patients who are not considered candidates for immediate PCI due to comorbid conditions, a delayed invasive management strategy is chosen for their STEMI. Class I indications for later cardiac catheterization include the development of cardiogenic shock or severe heart failure, intermediate- or high-risk findings on pre-discharge noninvasive ischemia testing, or myocardial ischemia that is spontaneous or provoked by minimal exertion during hospitalization [6]. Intra-aortic balloon pump (IABP) counterpulsation has a Class IIa indication for mechanical support in these patients, and percutaneous ventricular assist devices remain under evaluation as well, with a Class IIb indication [6].

One could readily envision the above scenario playing out in a neurosurgical patient, who sustains a STEMI in the first 1–3 days after a craniotomy or spine surgery and who would not be eligible for anticoagulation and DAPT, but several days later it would be safe to proceed.

Treatment of NSTE-ACS

The goals of treatment for the NSTE-ACS patient are the relief of ischemia and the prevention of MI and death. Stable patients with an NSTE-ACS diagnosis should be moved to a telemetry-capable unit for continuous cardiac monitoring and treated with antianginal, antiplatelet, and anticoagulant therapy (17). Further invasive treatment may follow an early invasive strategy (coronary angiography and revascularization within 24 h) or an ischemia-guided strategy. NSTE-ACS patients with continuing angina, hemodynamic instability, uncontrolled arrhythmias, or a large MI should be moved to an ICU if they are not already there [1].

Patients suspected of having an NSTE-ACS should receive oral antiplatelet therapy as soon as possible. For patients without an aspirin allergy or gastrointestinal contraindications, non-enteric coated, chewable aspirin, either 162 mg or 325 mg, should be given, and a maintenance dose of aspirin (81 mg to 325 mg daily) should be continued indefinitely. Due to the contribution of higher aspirin doses to bleeding with multimodality therapy, selecting 162 mg followed by 81 mg would be prudent. In patients unable to take aspirin, a loading dose of clopidogrel followed by a daily maintenance dose should be administered. In the absence of knowledge about the patient's coronary anatomy, the smaller clopidogrel loading dose (300 mg) is suggested. A P2Y12 inhibitor (clopidogrel or ticagrelor) in addition to aspirin should be administered for up to 12 months in all patients with NSTE-ACS without contraindications [1]. In patients with NSTE-ACS treated with an early invasive strategy and dual antiplatelet therapy with intermediate–/high-risk features, a glycoprotein IIb/IIIa inhibitor may be considered as part of initial antiplatelet therapy. These agents have some benefit in medical patients, at a cost of increased periprocedural bleeding, and their use should probably be discouraged in postoperative patients.

In addition to antiplatelet therapy, patients with NSTE-ACS should be anticoagulated. Options include enoxaparin, bivalirudin, fondaparinux, or unfractionated heparin [1]. For perioperative patients, heparin is the easiest agent to reverse in the event of bleeding or if the patient is found to require CABG for revascularization instead of PCI.

Supplemental oxygen should be administered to patients with NSTE-ACS with arterial oxygen saturation less than 90%, respiratory distress, or other high-risk features of hypoxemia [1]. These patients should also receive sublingual nitroglycerin up to three doses, at which point intravenous nitroglycerin is indicated for the treatment of persistent ischemia, heart failure, or hypertension. Nitrates should not be given to patients with NSTE-ACS who recently received a phosphodiesterase inhibitor, within 24 h of sildenafil or vardenafil and within 48 h of tadalafil [1]. Most patients requiring continuous nitroglycerin to relieve their angina move to an early invasive strategy. Another adjunct for patients with persistent ischemia is intra-aortic balloon pump (IABP) counterpulsation. While the physiology of IABP use is well understood, its current application is driven by clinical experience and observational studies. When rigorously studied, IABP use fails to deliver a statistically significant benefit for patients with cardiogenic shock [1].

Oral beta-blocker therapy should be initiated in the first 24 h in NSTE-ACS patients who do not have heart failure, evidence of a low cardiac output state, increased risk for cardiogenic shock (>70 years of age, heart rate >110 beats per minute, systolic BP <120 mm Hg), or contraindications to beta-blockade including a ECG PR interval of >0.24 s, second- or third-degree heart block without a cardiac pacemaker, or active asthma or reactive airway disease (Class I) [1]. While the beta-blockers metoprolol succinate, carvedilol, and bisoprolol are recommended for continuing therapy, common sense guides many practitioners to start with small doses of shorter-acting beta-1 selective oral metoprolol tartrate or intravenous esmolol and then titrate the dose while monitoring the patient's hemodynamics for hypotension and their respiratory status for signs of bronchospasm. In patients with a respiratory contraindication to beta-blockers, a nondihydropyridine calcium channel blocker (CCB) (verapamil or diltiazem) can be given as initial therapy, with the same caveats regarding heart failure, shock, and conduction abnormalities [1]. These CCBs are also recommended when beta-blockers are not successful or their side effect profile is not tolerated and for patients with coronary artery spasm.

Other recommended medications for the NSTE-ACS patient include high-intensity statin therapy (atorvastatin 80 mg daily), as well as ACE inhibitors in all patients with a left ventricular ejection fraction of less than 40%, and in those with hypertension, diabetes mellitus, or stable chronic kidney disease. Angiotensin receptor blockers (ARBs) are recommended for those patients who are ACE inhibitor intolerant [1]. As a practical matter, it is best to start these medications when one is sure that the patient will not require CABG surgery and that their renal function is indeed stable.

Anemic patients require special consideration. Gastrointestinal, surgical, or traumatic hemorrhage often contributes to the myocardial oxygen supply and demand mismatch that leads to an ACS. However, there is no proven benefit with transfusion in hemodynamically stable patients with a hemoglobin in the 7–8 grams per deciliter range and definitely no benefit above 8 grams per deciliter [1]. The critical care surgeon is best positioned to decide if the patient is hemodynamically stable and to guide decision-making on blood component therapy.

Cocaine and methamphetamine users on a trauma or surgical service also require special handling. Specifically, in these patients, when acutely intoxicated, the use of beta-blockers can precipitate coronary spasm from unopposed alpha stimulation. Instead, benzodiazepines and nitroglycerin should be used until the patient is no longer acutely intoxicated, at which time conventional medical therapy can be implemented [1].

In summary, the critical care surgeon plays an important role in recognizing the presence of acute coronary syndrome in the perioperative and trauma patients under their care. Understanding the protocols and pharmacologic treatment of ACS, in the context of the specific patient and their appropriateness for these therapies, will lead to better care for surgical patients and the prevention of avoidable morbidity and death.

References

1. Amsterdam E, et al. 2014 AHA/ACC guideline for the Management of Patients with non-ST-elevation acute coronary syndromes. Circulation. 2014;130:e344–426. e359.
2. Jassal D. Perioperative cardiac management. Medscape online 11/16/2015.
3. Ollila A, et al. Perioperative myocardial infarction in non-cardiac surgery patients: a prospective observational study. Scand J Surg. 2016;106:180–6.
4. Devereaux P, et al. Perioperative cardiac events in patients undergoing non-cardiac surgery: a review of the magnitude of the problem, the pathophysiology of the events and methods to estimate and communicate risk. Can Med Assoc J. 2005;173(6):627–39.
5. Thygesen K, et al. Third universal definition of myocardial infarction. Circulation. 2012;126(16):2020–35.
6. O'Gara P, et al. 2013 ACCF/AHA guideline for the management of ST-elevation myocardial infarction: a report of the American College of Cardiology Foundation/American Heart Association task force on practice guidelines. Circulation. 2013;128:e481.

11 Hemodynamic Monitoring

Nicole A. Stassen

Introduction

Webster defines monitoring as "to watch, keep track of, or check usually for a special purpose." [1] The primary goal in the management of critically ill patients includes the assessment and manipulation of the circulatory system to ensure adequate tissue delivery of oxygen and essential metabolic substrates. The hemodynamic status of critically ill patients is complex; it may include varying degrees of hypovolemia, left and right ventricular dysfunction, abnormalities of vascular tone, and microvascular dysfunction. These acute impairments are often further complicated by chronic comorbidities. Physical examination and conventional hemodynamic monitoring cannot adequately assess the nature and extent of such hemodynamic dysfunction [2–4]. Appropriate hemodynamic monitoring can assist with both identifying the presence and causes of hemodynamic instability and therefore may allow for targeting therapeutic approaches. Hemodynamic monitoring can therefore be viewed as a means to minimize the uncertainty that often surrounds the patient's hemodynamic status [5–7].

Medical history, clinical manifestations (such as skin turgor, blood pressure, pulse rate, and urine output), and routine laboratory tests are important but of limited sensitivity and specificity in critically ill patients [8]. As the understanding of hemodynamics and critical illness has evolved, more sophisticated circulatory monitoring technologies have been developed. The ideal hemodynamic monitor is reliable, noninvasive, cost-effective, and easy to use. At the current time, the surgical intensivist's toolbox when approaching a critically ill patient who requires advanced hemodynamic monitoring can be divided into the following categories:

N. A. Stassen (✉)
Department of Surgery, Acute Care Surgery Division, University of Rochester Medical Center, Rochester, NY, USA
e-mail: nicole_stassen@urmc.rochester.edu

- Noninvasive hemodynamic monitors
  - Ultrasound
  - Thoracic bioelectric impedance
- Invasive hemodynamic monitors
  - Pulmonary artery catheter
  - Arterial catheter – pulse contour wave analysis
  - Central venous pressure monitor
  - Esophageal Doppler monitor

Hemodynamic monitoring devices should be selected on a patient-specific basis, either alone or in combination with other hemodynamic monitors. Detailed physical examination along with other clinical data provides a framework for assessment of the underlying pathophysiology of the patient against which all information obtained from hemodynamic monitors can be interpreted. The correct application of hemodynamic data necessitates the integration of various variables that may complement each other in order to provide the whole clinical picture. The purpose of this section is to explore the selection of currently available hemodynamic monitoring methods which can be used to optimize a patient's status in the intensive care unit.

Noninvasive Monitoring

Ultrasound

The role of point-of-care echocardiography performed by intensivists who are not trained in cardiology is constantly growing due to its immediate availability and diagnostic value. The literature continues to confirm that brief, goal-directed transthoracic echocardiography performed by intensivists is feasible and reliable in assessing some causes of shock [9–12]. It can assist in the rapid, accurate, and noninvasive diagnosis of a broad range of acute cardiovascular diseases. The availability of echocardiography has appropriately decreased the need for invasive procedures needed to diagnose life-threatening conditions. To define the scope of point-

A. Salim et al. (eds.), *Surgical Critical Care Therapy*, https://doi.org/10.1007/978-3-319-71712-8_11

of-care cardiac ultrasound in the intensive care unit, *Critical Care Medicine* has published two comprehensive supplements describing the technique and applications [13, 14]. Critical care societies worldwide have developed expert statements on training standards in critical care ultrasonography [10–12, 15, 16]. These publications define the differences between binary point-of-care examinations at the bedside and formal cardiology-driven echocardiogram. Intensivist-performed, brief echocardiographic examinations should not be used to replace formal echocardiograms but, instead, as an adjunct to physical examination.

Point-of-care cardiac ultrasound is noninvasive and can be performed immediately at the bedside as an extension of the physical examination [17–19]. It does not require advanced technology. It can be performed with a simple two-dimensional ultrasound machine. It is performed at the bedside by the intensivist, who can tailor the scope of the test depending on the clinical condition of the patient [20–23]. There are numerous publications regarding goal-directed point-of-care echocardiography to guide resuscitation, with different acronyms for a variety of focused bedside cardiac ultrasound protocols [9, 19, 22, 24–30]. The common denominator in all of these protocols is that they evaluate a combination of cardiac function, volume status, and fluid responsiveness. In essence point-of-care cardiac ultrasound is problem oriented and centered on guiding immediate therapy dictated by the patient's symptoms. The diagnostic targets of this simplified examination are gross cardiac contractility and anatomy (left and right ventricle size and function) as well as volume status and presence of a pericardial effusion with and without tamponade physiology.

All cardiac imaging should be performed with a phased array, low-frequency probe (typically 2–5 MHz). The basic study requires two-dimensional imaging, although more advanced semiqualitative examinations require the use of M mode and color Doppler. The ideal windows for this test are subcostal long axis, subcostal inferior vena cava, parasternal long axis, parasternal short axis, and apical four chamber. On occasion, not all windows are required to obtain target information necessary to change therapy, especially since the test can be repeated to address the effectiveness of the therapy change [9, 19, 22, 24–30]. Visualization of the inferior vena cava can be obtained in several places: the subcostal echocardiographic view, the right midclavicular line, and the posterior right mid-axillary line [31].

Patient volume status can be assessed with point-of-care ultrasound by evaluation of the inferior vena cava and the overall myocardium. An empty heart and/or a flat IVC, collapsing >50% during the respiratory cycle, can be diagnostic of hypovolemia in a hypotensive patient [32–34]. During positive-pressure inspiration, the increased intrathoracic pressure transmits to the right atrium reducing venous return causing inferior vena cava dilation, whereas during expiration, the decreased intrathoracic pressure increases venous return and decreases inferior vena cava diameter. The dynamic changes in inferior vena cava diameter will be greater the more volume responsive a subject is. Studies in septic patients demonstrated that changes in inferior vena cava diameter > 12% or inferior vena cava collapsibility index ≥18% differentiated volume responders from non-responders. The overall size of the inferior vena cava is not as important as the variability [35, 36]. In hypovolemia, the ventricular walls will also come together or "kiss."

It is well established in the literature that visual estimations of global cardiac function are equivalent to more detailed measurements [37–40]. While making an assessment of global cardiac function, the intensivist needs to address the inward motion of the endocardium, the presence of thickening of the myocardium, the longitudinal motion of the mitral annulus, and the overall geometry of the ventricle. The current recommendation of the American Society of Echocardiography is to assess left ventricular function on the short-axis view at the level of the mitral valve [16]. This interpretation takes into consideration only the radial function of the ventricle. It is also important to use the apical views to look at the longitudinal function of the heart as well as how the left and right ventricles are interacting. The intensivist only needs to be able to detect if there is a decrease in global cardiac activity [41]. Identification of the lack of cardiac activity is of great utility during medical and surgical resuscitation. A "standstill heart" is highly predictive of mortality and can help triage efforts effectively [42–44]. Evaluation of the function and the size of the right ventricle can be very useful for the clinician in guiding immediate treatment with anticoagulation for pulmonary embolus. Right ventricular enlargement in the presence of a massive pulmonary embolus is predictive of poor outcome. In acute cases of pulmonary hypertension, the right ventricle becomes large, but the ventricular wall is thin. In cases of chronic pulmonary hypertension, the right ventricle is large, but the muscle is thicker, since time allows for compensation. These factors will help the operator differentiate the acuity of the process accordingly [45–47].

Point-of-care cardiac ultrasound in any window has a high diagnostic application when it comes to fluid in the pericardium and visualization of cardiac tamponade physiology (right heart compression) [48, 49]. Pitfalls that may preclude detection of pericardial effusion include the presence of a hemothorax, pneumothorax, or having a defect in the pericardium decompressing the blood into the thoracic cavity [50].

Point-of-care cardiac ultrasound needs to be performed by the clinician at the bedside, helping to increase the utility of the information obtained and thereby assisting in optimizing patient management. One of its current limitations compared with the other commonly used hemodynamic monitoring devices is that it does not provide continuous data.

Also, information gained by point-of-care cardiac ultrasound is user dependent. Intensivists need to be competent in both the performance and the interpretation of the exam. Appropriate use and knowledge on the ultrasound machine, ability to obtain the standard echocardiogram windows, critical interpretation of the images acquired, and clinical integration of the findings and the use of the information obtained to guide patient therapy are essential to competency in point-of-care cardiac ultrasound [13, 51, 52].

Thoracic Bioelectric Impedance

Impedance cardiography in the measurement of cardiovascular performance was introduced in the late 1960s [53]. It is a grossly noninvasive method to continuously monitor stroke volume and cardiac output. It is based on the measurement of changes in the thoracic impedance to an electrical current that is produced by the fluctuations in thoracic blood volume with each cardiac cycle. Depending on the equation used, the theory behind impedance cardiography models the thorax as a cylinder or a truncated cone that is homogenously perfused with blood of a specific resistivity based on the hematocrit [54, 55]. The thorax has a steady state mean base impedance. Spot or band electrodes placed on the patient's thorax are used to emit and sense a low-voltage (2.5–4.0 mA), high-frequency (70–100 kHz), alternating electrical current through the thorax [53]. The electrical impedance is inversely proportional to the volume of thoracic fluids, implying that the pulsatile decrease in total thoracic impedance can be used in several mathematical models to estimate the beat-to-beat stroke volume as well as cardiac output.

There are many limitations and pitfalls with impedance cardiography. The models used for estimating hemodynamic parameters from impedance cardiography are based on nomograms based on age, height, weight, and gender to estimate the volume of electrically participating tissue that introduces a margin of inaccuracy. Alteration in electrode position can drastically change cardiac output measurements. It vases the measurement of ventricular ejection time on distance between QRS complexes on EKG precluding its use in patients with arrhythmias. It is also subject to interference from mechanical ventilation. Newer generation methods have overcome some of these limitations by having faster signal processing, better signal filters, improved EKG triggering, and respiratory filtering [56].

Results have been highly inconsistent in the critically ill population with problems including underestimation of high cardiac output and overestimation of low cardiac output, particularly in the setting of positive-pressure ventilation, arrhythmias, and pulmonary disorders (due to changes in thoracic cavity configuration and surface area). It is also highly unreliable in the presence of valvular disease and intracardiac shunts. Currently it is still not used as frequently in the United States as other methods of hemodynamic monitoring.

Invasive Monitoring

Pulmonary Artery Catheter

The introduction of pulmonary artery catheter in the 1970s was accompanied with great optimism. Unfortunately, clinical studies, including the PAC-Man and ESCAPE trials, have failed to show a consistent benefit with routine use of pulmonary artery catheter in the intensive care unit [57–63]. Pulmonary arterial catheterization is an invasive procedure. It requires the insertion of a central venous port and passage of a catheter across two heart valves. Inflation of the catheter once in a pulmonary artery may cause rupture of that vessel with disastrous consequences. Furthermore, the continual presence of a pulmonary artery catheter increases the likelihood of arrhythmias, catheter-related bloodstream infections, and endocarditis [57, 58]. Despite the criticism regarding its use, this invasive hemodynamic tool continues to find a role in the management of a subset of critically ill patients [64–66]. It remains very useful when used for the appropriate indication and interpreted by clinicians with adequate expertise in the analysis and application of data obtained from pulmonary artery catheter. The indications for placement of a pulmonary artery catheter in critically ill patients include acute myocardial infarction complicated by shock; severe heart failure; differentiation between various causes of shock; severe left ventricular failure to guide therapy, including inotropes, vasodilators, and diuretics; cardiac tamponade (when clinical and echocardiographic findings are inconclusive); assessment of level and magnitude of intracardiac shunt; and severe pulmonary hypertension to guide therapy.

The pulmonary artery catheter can directly measure right atrial pressure, right ventricular pressure, pulmonary artery pressure, pulmonary capillary wedge pressure, and cardiac output. Cardiac output is measured by either thermodilution or Fick principle-derived equations. The thermodilution method assumes three major conditions: complete mixing of the indicator and blood, constant blood flow, and lack of loss of indicator between the site of injection and place of detection. These assumptions introduce the possibility for inaccurate cardiac output assessment via thermodilution methods. Tricuspid regurgitation, arrhythmias, intracardiac shunts, extremes of cardiac output, slow injection, incorrect volume or temperature of injectate, and improper positioning of the catheter can all cause inaccuracy of cardiac output when thermodilution is used. Cardiac output calculation using the Fick principle is based on the conservation of mass so that the total uptake or release of a substance by an organ is the product of blood flow to that organ multiplied by the arteriovenous concentration difference. The inaccuracy of the Fick method is mostly related to the oxygen consumption parameter that is often estimated. Cardiac index, systemic vascular resistance, pulmonary vascular resistance, stroke volume index, left ventricular stroke work index, and right ventricular work index can all be derived from pulmonary artery catheter data. The data above can be used to help differentiate the etiology of shock as well as guide therapeutic interventions.

The major reservations and concerns regarding the use of the pulmonary artery catheter given its level of invasiveness and the lack of evidence supporting improved outcomes, as well as the decreased familiarity and training in PAC, have triggered the search for less-invasive hemodynamic monitoring methods. However, no study has used pulmonary artery catheter-derived variables to drive treatment protocols of proven benefit to determine whether pulmonary artery-specific data result in better outcomes than do data derived from less-invasive devices, such as the central venous catheter and echocardiography.

Arterial Catheter: Pulse Contour Wave Analysis

Given the unreliability of sphygmomanometers at blood pressure extremes, invasive arterial blood pressure monitoring is often needed in hemodynamically unstable patients. Stroke volume can be estimated by analyzing arterial pressure waveforms. There are several commercially available devices that use the pulse contour wave analysis for continuous stroke volume and cardiac output measurement. These systems can be broadly divided into two groups, those requiring calibration (PiCCO and lithium dilution cardiac output [LiDCO]) and the uncalibrated systems (FloTrac). The PiCCO system (Pulsion Medical Systems, Germany) requires a thermistor-tipped arterial line to measure downstream temperature changes after the injection of a cold indicator via a central venous catheter. It uses pulse contour wave analysis according to a modified Wesseling algorithm with periodic thermal dilution calibration to continuously measure SV and calculate the cardiac output, stroke volume variation, pulse pressure variation, and systemic vascular resistance. The LiDCO system (LiDCO Ltd., UK) uses pulse contour wave analysis along with dye dilution (lithium) calibration to measure cardiac output. For calibration, a small dose of lithium is injected into a vein, where an ion-selective electrode sensor mounted on a peripheral arterial line plots the concentration of lithium over time to calculate the cardiac output. For pulse contour wave analysis, this system uses an algorithm based on the law of conservation of power for continuous cardiac output calculations. It assumes that the net power change in the arterial tree is equal to the amount of blood entering (stroke volume) minus that of blood leaving. Once calibrated for compliance, the linear relationship between power and flow can be obtained and converted to nominal stroke volume that is then converted to an actual stroke volume. The FloTrac or Vigileo system (Edwards Lifesciences, California, USA) is designed around the application of advanced statistical principles to the arterial pressure tracing, resulting in the creation of a proprietary algorithm that recalibrates itself constantly, rending external calibration unnecessary. It is based on a principle of the linear relation between pulse pressure and stroke volume. The arterial pressure waveform is sampled every 20 seconds at 100 Hz, allowing the arterial pulsatility to be derived from the standard deviation of the pressure wave over 20 seconds, which is then multiplied by the patient-specific aortic compliance to obtain stroke volume. It can be unreliable with arterial waveform artifact, aortic regurgitation, intense peripheral vasoconstriction, severe cardiac dysfunction, and irregular heart rate or tachycardia.

Besides cardiac output monitoring, pulse contour wave analysis methods can be used for evaluating volume status and fluid responsiveness.

Stroke volume variation and pulse pressure variation calculated during the inspiratory and expiratory phases of mechanical ventilation are continuously monitored dynamic variables to optimize fluid therapy. They are based on beat-to-beat changes in left ventricular output during positive-pressure ventilation. During inspiration, the reduction in left ventricular stroke volume causes a decrease in systemic blood pressure and pulse pressure at end-inspiration. Appreciating how the venous return changes with the various pathologic states, in addition to its alterations in the setting of positive-pressure ventilation, helps in the diagnosis and management of the common hemodynamic profiles encountered in shock [67, 68]. Two meta-analyses suggested that both stroke volume variation and pulse pressure variation are accurate predictors of fluid responsiveness in hemodynamically unstable patients under controlled mechanical ventilation [69, 70]. Several clinical trials have documented that a stroke volume variation SVV >10% or a pulse pressure variation >13–15% in a mechanically ventilated patient on a tidal volume of ≥8 ml/kg or greater is highly predictive of volume responsiveness [71–73]. Although better than conventional static parameters, stroke volume variation and pulse pressure variation have limited value in predicting fluid responsiveness in these patients who were ventilated using low tidal volumes (<8 cc/kg), which is the commonly accepted ventilation strategy in patients with acute respiratory distress syndrome [74, 75]. With low tidal volume ventilation, the cyclic changes in intrathoracic pressures were not significant enough to induce preload variations [76]. A major problem of using pulse pressure variation or stroke volume variation is the need for a constant heart rate so that diastolic filling time is not contributing to the preload effect of the positive-pressure breath. Thus, in patients with frequent premature ventricular contractions or atrial fibrillation, the accuracy of these parameters degrades markedly.

Central Venous Monitor

Central venous pressure, a measure of right atrium pressure, can be estimated by transducing a central venous catheter with its tip placed in the superior vena cava or right atrium [77]. Positive-pressure breathing cyclically increases in intrathoracic pressure by forcing the expanding lungs to passively expand the chest wall. This causes central venous pressure to increase proportionally. Since central venous pressure is the back pressure to systemic venous return to the heart, these cyclic increases in central venous pressure cause reciprocal cyclic decreases in venous return. End-expiratory central venous pressure is often taken as an estimate of the intravascular state. A low central venous pressure (<8 mmHg) is presumed to reflect a low circulating blood volume and a high central venous pressure an expanded blood volume [78, 79]. Central venous pressure has been suggested as a measure for preload; however, its validity in predicting fluid responsiveness is nonexistent across numerous studies. Except for extremely low values, static levels of central venous pressure are often unreliable in predicting volume expansion responders [80, 81]. Dynamic changes of central venous pressure in response to fluids or in relation to the respiratory cycle have been investigated in evaluating preload responsiveness with some conflicting evidence [82, 83]. Caution should be used when using central venous pressure variation because it can be altered by a host of factors independent of volume status, including changes in tidal volumes, abdominal pressure, and vascular tone [84, 85]. Using the dynamic changes in central venous pressure during spontaneous ventilation, Magder et al. predicted that those patients breathing spontaneously who displayed a decrease in CVP of >1 mmHg would be volume responsive, whereas those who did not would not be volume responsive [86]. Regrettably, central venous pressure variation does not reliably predict a patient's response to fluid challenges [87–89].

Esophageal Doppler Monitor

Esophageal Doppler monitoring was initially introduced in 1971 by Side and Gosling and subsequently modified by Singer in 1998. An esophageal Doppler monitor is a minimally invasive hemodynamic device that evaluates the CO and fluid status based on the assessment of descending aortic blood flow [90–93]. Using a Doppler probe inserted into the esophagus, the velocity of the descending aortic blood flow can be determined by the frequency shift as the waves get reflected of the moving red blood cells. The spectral analysis of the Doppler shift provides the velocity waveforms. This waveform is used to estimate stroke volume and cardiac output. The probe is about 6–7 mm in diameter and is inserted orally or nasally in intubated patients. The probe is usually inserted to the distal esophagus where it is closest and most parallel to the aorta. Contraindications to EDM placement include pharyngeal and esophageal disease (pharyngeal pouch, esophageal stent, cancer, stricture, surgery) or significant systemic coagulopathy.

Two major assumptions are the basis of CO measurements using EDM. Because the probe measures blood flow in the descending aorta, it presumes a fixed percentage of CO to supply the coronary, cerebral, and brachiocephalic circulation and adjusts for it with a correction factor. This percentage is reliable in young healthy patients but can be highly variable depending on the metabolic activity of different organs or the pathologic state. The second assumption is the cross-sectional area of the descending aorta because using the nomogram might not be applicable to all patients. The M-mode option does not completely resolve this problem because the diameter of the aorta is dynamic and changes with alterations in vascular tone, volume status, and pulse pressure [94, 95]. Other limitations in the use of EDM include operator dependence, accurate probe position, and issues with dislodgement. It is inaccurate in aortic regurgitation, aneurysm, or coarctation. Also most studies were done in subjects with hypovolemic shock, and it is less extensively studied in cardiogenic and distributive shocks.

There has been a sizable body of evidence to evaluate the validity of EDM-derived measures and to support their clinical value in critically ill patients. Most of the studies were performed in hemodynamically stable patients. More recent data have provided evidence for its use in hemodynamically unstable cohorts [92, 96, 97]. Esophageal Doppler monitoring is a minimally invasive, safe, and easy means to continuous, real-time circulatory monitoring that requires minimal training and can safely be used for a prolonged period of time without significant complications. In clinical practice, EDM has been best studied and shown to be most useful in goal-directed optimization of preload in intravascularly volume-depleted patients. This is especially true when emphasis is placed on the trend of change in stroke volume and cardiac output as opposed to absolute values. Further studies are needed to confirm the same level of reliability in its usefulness in guiding vasoactive and inotropic agents' use [98–100].

Conclusion

The one-size-fits-all, noninvasive, easy-to-use, cost-effective, and reliable hemodynamic monitor remains elusive. In the meantime, current monitoring devices should continue to be selected on a patient-specific basis, either alone or in combination with other hemodynamic monitors, until the gold standard hemodynamic monitoring tool is developed. The monitoring of physiological variables in the intensive care unit per se cannot improve outcome unless it is followed by correct therapeutic interventions. Making the "correct" decision is not always straightforward even when hemodynamic monitoring is utilized, due to the potential for misinterpretation of the monitored parameters, the failure to identify their relative importance, and the remaining uncertainty regarding the exact nature of the physiological impairment.

Disclosure I have no commercial or financial conflicts of interest related to this manuscript.

References

1. Merriam-Webster dictionary. [Internet]. Available from http://www.merriam-webster.com.
2. Saugel B, Ringmaier S, Holzapfel K, Schuster T, Phillip V, Schmid RM, Huber W. Physical examination, central venous pressure, and chest radiography for the prediction of transpulmonary thermodilution-derived hemodynamic parameters in critically ill patients: a prospective trial. J Crit Care. 2011;26:402–10.
3. Saugel B, Kirsche SV, Hapfelmeier A, Phillip V, Schultheiss C, Schmid RM, Huber W. Prediction of fluid responsiveness in patients admitted to the medical intensive care unit. J Crit Care. 2013;28:537. e1-9
4. Perel A, Saugel B, Teboul JL, Malbrain ML, Belda FJ, Fernandez-Mondejar E, Kirov M, Wendon J, Lussmann R, Maggiorini M. The effects of advanced monitoring on hemodynamic management in critically ill patients: a pre and post questionnaire study. J Clin Monit Comput. 2016;30:511–8.
5. Vincent JL, Rhodes A, Perel A, Martin GS, Della Rocca G, Vallet B, Pinsky MR, Hofer CK, Teboul JL, de Boode WP, Scolletta S, Vieillard-Baron A, De Backer D, Walley KR, Maggiorini M, Singer M. Clinical review: update on hemodynamic monitoring—a consensus of 16. Crit Care. 2011;15:229.
6. Cecconi M, De Backer D, Antonelli M, Beale R, Bakker J, Hofer C, Jaeschke R, Mebazaa A, Pinsky MR, Teboul JL, Vincent JL, Rhodes A. Consensus on circulatory shock and hemodynamic monitoring. Task force of the European Society of Intensive Care Medicine. Intensive Care Med. 2014;40:1795–815.
7. Teboul JL, Saugel B, Cecconi M, De Backer D, Hofer CK, Monnet X, Perel A, Pinsky MR, Reuter DA, Rhodes A, Squara P, Vincent JL, Scheeren TW. Less invasive hemodynamic monitoring in critically ill patients. Intensive Care Med. 2016;42:1350–9.
8. Michard F, Teboul JL. Predicting fluid responsiveness in ICU patients: a critical analysis of the evidence. Chest 2002, 121:2000–2008. Vincent JL, Weil MH: fluid challenge revisited. Crit Care Med. 2006;34:1333–7.
9. Beaulieu Y. Bedside echocardiography in the assessment of the critically ill. Crit Care Med. 2007;35(5 Suppl):S235–49.
10. Beaulieu Y. Specific skill set and goals of focused echocardiography for critical care clinicians. Crit Care Med. 2007;35 (5 Suppl):S144–9.
11. Sloth E. Echocardiography in the ICU. Intensive Care Med. 2006;32(8):1283.
12. Sloth E, Larsen KM, Schmidt MB, Jensen MB. Focused application of ultrasound in critical care medicine. Crit Care Med. 2008;36(2):653–4.
13. Neri L, Storti E, Lichtenstein D. Toward an ultrasound curriculum for critical care medicine. Crit Care Med. 2007;35 (5 Suppl):S290–304.
14. Kendall JL, Hoffenberg SR, Smith RS. History of emergency and critical care ultrasound: the evolution of a new imaging paradigm. Crit Care Med. 2007;35(5 Suppl):S126–30.
15. Mayo PH, Beaulieu Y, Doelken P, Feller-Kopman D, Harrod C, Kaplan A, Oropello J, Vieillard-Baron A, Axler O, Lichtenstein D, et al. American College of Chest Physicians/la Societe de reanimation de langue Francaise statement on competence in critical care ultrasonography. Chest. 2009;135(4):1050–60.
16. Cahalan MK, Abel M, Goldman M, Pearlman A, Sears-Rogan P, Russell I, Shanewise J, Stewart W, Troianos C. American Society of Echocardiography and Society of Cardiovascular Anesthesiologists task force guidelines for training in perioperative echocardiography. Anesth Analg. 2002;94(6):1384–8.
17. Pershad J, Myers S, Plouman C, Rosson C, Elam K, Wan J, Chin T. Bedside limited echocardiography by the emergency physician is accurate during evaluation of the critically ill patient. Pediatrics. 2004;114(6):e667–71.
18. Via G, Hussain A, Wells M, Reardon R, ElBarbary M, Noble VE, Tsung JW, Neskovic AN, Price S, Oren-Grinberg A, et al. International evidencebased recommendations for focused cardiac ultrasound. J Am Soc Echocardiogr. 2014;27(7):683.
19. Vignon P, Dugard A, Abraham J, Belcour D, Gondran G, Pepino F, Marin B, Francois B, Gastinne H. Focused training for goal-oriented hand-held echocardiography performed by noncardiologist residents in the intensive care unit. Intensive Care Med. 2007;33(10):1795–9.
20. Alherbish A, Priestap F, Arntfield R. The introduction of basic critical care echocardiography reduces the use of diagnostic echocardiography in the intensive care unit. J Crit Care. 2015;30(6):1419. e7–1419.e11. Cowie B. Focused cardiovascular ultrasound performed by anesthesiologists in the perioperative period: feasible and alters patient management. J Cardiothorac Vasc Anesth. 2009;23(4):450–456.
21. Fedson S, Neithardt G, Thomas P, Lickerman A, Radzienda M, DeCara JM, Lang RM, Spencer KT. Unsuspected clinically important findings detected with a small portable ultrasound device in patients admitted to a general medicine service. J Am Soc Echocardiogr. 2003;16(9):901–5.
22. Ferrada P, Anand RJ, Whelan J, Aboutanos MA, Duane T, Malhotra A, Ivatury R. Limited transthoracic echocardiogram: so easy any trauma attending can do it. J Trauma. 2011;71(5):1327–31.
23. Ferrada P, Wolfe L, Anand RJ, Whelan J, Vanguri P, Malhotra A, Goldberg S, Duane T, Aboutanos M. Use of limited transthoracic echocardiography in patients with traumatic cardiac arrest decreases the rate of nontherapeutic thoracotomy and hospital costs. J Ultrasound Med. 2014;33(10):1829–32.
24. Carr BG, Dean AJ, Everett WW, BS K, Mark DG, Okusanya O, Horan AD, Gracias VH. Intensivist bedside ultrasound (INBU) for volume assessment in the intensive care unit: a pilot study. J Trauma. 2007;63(3):495–500.
25. Atkinson PR, McAuley DJ, Kendall RJ, Abeyakoon O, Reid CG, Connolly J, Lewis D. Abdominal and cardiac evaluation with sonography in shock (ACES): an approach by emergency physi-

cians for the use of ultrasound in patients with undifferentiated hypotension. Emerg Med J. 2009;26(2):87–91.
26. Breitkreutz R, Price S, Steiger HV, Seeger FH, Ilper H, Ackermann H, Rudolph M, Uddin S, Weigand MA, Muller E, et al. Focused echocardiographic evaluation in life support and peri-resuscitation of emergency patients: a prospective trial. Resuscitation. 2010;81(11):1527–33.
27. Ferrada P, Murthi S, Anand RJ, Bochicchio GV, Scalea T. Transthoracic focused rapid echocardiographic examination: real-time evaluation of fluid status in critically ill trauma patients. J Trauma. 2011;70(1):56–62. Jensen MB, Sloth E, Larsen KM, Schmidt MB. Transthoracic echocardiography for cardiopulmonary monitoring in intensive care. Eur J Anaesthesiol. 2004;21(9):700Y707.
28. Manasia AR, Nagaraj HM, Kodali RB, Croft LB, Oropello JM, Kohli-Seth R, Leibowitz AB, DelGiudice R, Hufanda JF, Benjamin E, et al. Feasibility and potential clinical utility of goal-directed transthoracic echocardiography performed by noncardiologist intensivists using a small hand-carried device (SonoHeart) in critically ill patients. J Cardiothorac Vasc Anesth. 2005;19(2):155–9.
29. Perera P, Mailhot T, Riley D, Mandavia D. The RUSH exam: rapid ultrasound in shock in the evaluation of the critically lll. Emerg Med Clin North Am. 2010;28(1):29–56. vii
30. Rose JS, Bair AE, Mandavia D, Kinser DJ. The UHP ultrasound protocol: a novel ultrasound approach to the empiric evaluation of the undifferentiated hypotensive patient. Am J EmergMed. 2001;19(4):299–302. Fletcher SN, Grounds RM. Critical care echocardiography: cleared for take up. Br J Anaesth. 2012;109(4):490–492.
31. Ferrada P. Image-based resuscitation of the hypotensive patient with cardiac ultrasound: an evidence-based review. J Trauma Acute Care Surg. 2016;80(3):511–8.
32. Leung JM, Levine EH. Left ventricular end-systolic cavity obliteration as an estimate of intraoperative hypovolemia. Anesthesiology. 1994;81(5):1102–9.
33. Maizel J, Airapetian N, Lorne E, Tribouilloy C, Massy Z, Slama M. Diagnosis of central hypovolemia by using passive leg raising. Intensive Care Med. 2007;33(7):1133–8.
34. Zengin S, Al B, Genc S, Yildirim C, Ercan S, Dogan M, Altunbas G. Role of inferior vena cava and right ventricular diameter in assessment of volume status: a comparative study: ultrasound and hypovolemia. Am J Emerg Med. 2013;31(5):763–7.
35. Barbier C, Loubieres Y, Schmit C, et al. Respiratory changes in inferior vena cava diameter are helpful in predicting fluid responsiveness in ventilated septic patients. Intensive Care Med. 2004;30:1740–6.
36. Feissel M, Michard F, Faller JP, et al. The respiratory variation in inferior vena cava diameter as a guide to fluid therapy. Intensive Care Med. 2004;30:1834–7.
37. Gudmundsson P, Rydberg E, Winter R, Willenheimer R. Visually estimated left ventricular ejection fraction by echocardiography is closely correlated with formal quantitative methods. Int J Cardiol. 2005;101(2):209–12.
38. Kaul S, Stratienko AA, Pollock SG, Marieb MA, Keller MW, Sabia PJ. Value of two-dimensional echocardiography for determining the basis of hemodynamic compromise in critically ill patients: a prospective study. J Am Soc Echocardiogr. 1994;7(6):598–606.
39. Moore CL, Rose GA, Tayal VS, Sullivan DM, Arrowood JA, Kline JA. Determination of left ventricular function by emergency physician echocardiography of hypotensive patients. Acad Emerg Med. 2002;9(3):186–93.
40. Sabia P, Abbott RD, Afrookteh A, Keller MW, Touchstone DA, Kaul S. Importance of two-dimensional echocardiographic assessment of left ventricular systolic function in patients presenting to the emergency room with cardiac-related symptoms. Circulation. 1991;84(4):1615–24.
41. Expert Round Table on Echocardiography in ICU. International consensus statement on training standards for advanced critical care echocardiography. Intensive Care Med. 2014;40(5):654–66.
42. Cureton EL, Yeung LY, Kwan RO, Miraflor EJ, Sadjadi J, Price DD, Victorino GP. The heart of the matter: utility of ultrasound of cardiac activity during traumatic arrest. J Trauma Acute Care Surg. 2012;73(1):102–10.
43. Blaivas M, Fox JC. Outcome in cardiac arrest patients found to have cardiac standstill on the bedside emergency department echocardiogram. Acad Emerg Med. 2001;8(6):616–21.
44. Hernandez C, Shuler K, Hannan H, Sonyika C, Likourezos A, Marshall JCAUSE. Cardiac arrest ultra-sound ExamVa better approach to managing patients in primary non-arrhythmogenic cardiac arrest. Resuscitation. 2008;76(2):198–206.
45. Ribeiro A, Lindmarker P, Juhlin-Dannfelt A, Johnsson H, Jorfeldt L. Echocardiography Doppler in pulmonary embolism: right ventricular dysfunction as a predictor of mortality rate. Am Heart J. 1997;134(3):479–87.
46. Bova C, Greco F, Misuraca G, Serafini O, Crocco F, Greco A, Noto A. Diagnostic utility of echocardiography in patients with suspected pulmonary embolism. Am J Emerg Med. 2003;21(3):180–3.
47. Labovitz AJ, Noble VE, Bierig M, Goldstein SA, Jones R, Kort S, Porter TR, Spencer KT, Tayal VS, Wei K. Focused cardiac ultrasound in the emergent setting: a consensus statement of the American Society of Echocardiography and American College of Emergency Physicians. J Am Soc Echocardiogr. 2010;23(12):1225–30.
48. Levitt MA, Jan BA. The effect of real time 2-D-echocardiography on medical decision-making in the emergency department. J Emerg Med. 2002;22(3):229–33.
49. Plummer D. Principles of emergency ultrasound and echocardiography. Ann Emerg Med. 1989;18(12):1291–7.
50. Ball CG, Williams BH, Wyrzykowski AD, Nicholas JM, Rozycki GS, Feliciano DVA. Caveat to the performance of pericardial ultrasound in patients with penetrating cardiac wounds. J Trauma. 2009;67(5):1123–4.
51. Wright J, Jarman R, Connolly J, Dissmann P. Echocardiography in the emergency department. Emerg Med J. 2009;26(2):82–6.
52. Cerqueira MD, Arrighi JA, Geiser EA. Physician certification in cardiovascular imaging: rationale, process, and benefits. JACC Cardiovasc Imaging. 2008;1(6):801–8.
53. Jensen L, Yakimets J, Teo KA. Review of impedance cardiography. Heart Lung. 1995;24:183–93.
54. Kubicek WG, Karnegis JN, Patterson RP, et al. Development and evaluation of an impedance cardiac output system. Aerosp Med. 1966;37:1208–12.
55. Sramek BB, Rose DM, Miyamoto A. Stroke volume equation with a linear base impedance model and its accuracy, as compared to thermodilution and magnetic flow meter techniques in humans and animals. Proceedings of Sixth International Conference on electrical Bioimpedance. Zadar (Yugoslavia), 1983. p. 38–41.
56. Nagel JG, Shyu LY, Reddy SP, et al. New signal processing techniques for improved precision of noninvasive impedance cardiography. Ann Biomed Eng. 1989;17:517–34.
57. Harvey S, Harrison D, Singer M, et al. Assessment of the clinical effectiveness of pulmonary artery catheters in management of patients in intensive care (PACMan): a randomized controlled trial. Lancet. 2005;366:472–7.
58. Binanay C, Califf RM, Hasselblad V, et al. Evaluation study of congestive heart failure and pulmonary artery catheterization effectiveness. JAMA. 2005;294(13):1625–33.
59. Morris AM, Bender JS, Smith-Meek MA, Jones CE. Routine pulmonary artery catheterization does not reduce morbidity and

mortality of elective vascular surgery: results of a prospective randomized trial. Ann Surg. 1997;226(3):229–37.
60. Connors AF, Speroff T, Dawson NV, et al. The effectiveness of right heart catheterization in the initial care of critically ill patients. JAMA. 1996;276:889–97.
61. Rhodes A, Cusack RJ, Newman PJ, et al. A randomized controlled trial of the pulmonary artery catheter in critically ill patients. Intensive Care Med. 2002;28:256–64.
62. Isaacson IJ, Lowdon JD, Berry AJ, et al. The value of pulmonary artery catheter and central venous monitoring in patients undergoing abdominal aortic reconstruction surgery: a comparative study of two selected, randomized, groups. J Vasc Surg. 1990;12:754–60.
63. Soni N. Swan song for the swan-Ganz catheter? The use of pulmonary artery catheters probably needs re-evaluation-but they should not be banned. BMJ. 1996;3313:763–4.
64. Morris AM, Chapman RH, Gardner RM. Frequency of wedge pressure errors in the ICU. Crit Care Med. 1985;13:705–8.
65. Iberti TJ, Fischer EP, Leibowitz AB, et al. A multicenter study of physicians' knowledge of the pulmonary artery catheter. JAMA. 1990;264:2928–32.
66. Gnaegi A, Feihl F, Perret C. Intensive care physicians' insufficient knowledge of right heart catheterization at the bedside: time to act? Crit Care Med. 1997;25:213–20.
67. Michard F, Boussat S, Chemla D, et al. Relation between respiratory changes in arterial pulse pressure and fluid responsiveness in septic patients with acute circulatory failure. Am J Respir Crit Care Med. 2000;162:134–8.
68. Funk DJ, Jacobsohn E, Kumar A. The role of venous return in critical illness and shock: part II-shock and mechanical ventilation. Crit Care Med. 2013;41:573–9.
69. Marik PE, Cavallazzi R, Vasu T, Hirani A. Dynamic changes in arterial waveform derived variables and fluid responsiveness in mechanically ventilated patients: a systematic review of the literature. Crit Care Med. 2009;37:2642–7.
70. Hong JQ, He HF, Chen ZY, ZS D, Liu WF, Weng PQ, Huang HB. Comparison of stroke volume variation with pulse pressure variation as a diagnostic indicator of fluid responsiveness in mechanically ventilated critically ill patients. Saudi Med J. 2014;35:261–8.
71. Berkenstadt H, Margalit N, Hadani M, et al. Stroke volume variation as a predictor of fluid responsiveness in patients undergoing brain surgery. Anesth Analg. 2001;92:984–9.
72. Montenij LJ, de Waal EE, Buhre WF. Arterial waveform analysis in anesthesia and critical care. Curr Opin Anaesthesiol. 2011;24:651–6.
73. Michard F. Changes in arterial pressure during mechanical ventilation. Anesthesiology. 2005;103:419–28.
74. Vallee F, Richard JCM, Mari A, Gallas T, Arsac E, Verlaan PS, Chousterman B, Samii K, Genestal M, Fourcade O. Pulse pressure variations adjusted by alveolar driving pressure to assess fluid responsiveness. Intensive Care Med. 2009;35:1004–10.
75. Lakhal K, Ehrmann S, Benzekri-Lefevre D, Runge I, Legras A, Dequin P, Mercier E, Wolff M, Regnier B, Boulain T. Respiratory pulse pressure variation fails to predict fluid responsiveness in acute respiratory distress syndrome. Crit Care. 2011;15:R85.
76. Oliveira-Costa CD, Friedman G, Vieira SR, Fialkow L. Pulse pressure variation and prediction of fluid responsiveness in patients ventilated with low tidal volumes. Clinics (Sao Paulo). 2012;67:773–8.
77. Cook DJ, Simel DL. Does this patient have abnormal central venous pressure? JAMA. 1996;275(8):630–4.
78. Pinsky MR. The hemodynamic consequences of mechanical ventilation: an evolving story. Intensive Care Med. 1997; 23:493–503.
79. Bendjelid K, Romand JA. Fluid responsiveness in mechanically ventilated patients: a review of indices used in intensive care. Intensive Care Med. 2003;29:352–60.
80. Marik PE, Baram M, Vahid B. Does central venous pressure predict fluid responsiveness? A systematic review of the literature and the tale of seven mares. Chest. 2008;134:172–8.
81. Marik PE, Cavallazzi R. Does the central venous pressure predict fluid responsiveness. An updated meta-analysis and a plea for some common sense. Crit Care Med. 2013;41:1774–81.
82. Teboul JL, Monnet X. Prediction of volume responsiveness in critically ill patients with spontaneous breathing activity. Curr Opin Crit Care. 2008;14:334–9.
83. Magder S, Lagonidis D, Erice F. The use of respiratory variations in right atrial pressure to predict the cardiac output response to PEEP. J Crit Care. 2001;16:108–14.
84. Magder S. How to use central venous pressure measurements. Curr Opin Crit Care. 2005;11:264–70.
85. Barnes GE, Laine GA, Giam PY, et al. Cardiovascular response to elevation of intra-abdominal hydrostatic pressure. Am J Phys. 1985;248:R208–13.
86. Magder S, Georgiadis G, Cheong T. Respiratory variations in right atrial pressure predict the response to fluid challenge. J Crit Care. 1992;7:76–85.
87. Kumar A, Anel R, Bunnell E, et al. Pulmonary artery occlusion pressure and central venous pressure fail to predict ventricular filling volume, cardiac performance, or the response to volume infusion in normal subjects. Critical Care Med. 2004;32:691–9.
88. Malbrain MLI. It wise not to think about intraabdominal hypertension in the ICU? Curr Opin Crit Care. 2004;10:132–45.
89. Pinsky MR. Clinical significance of pulmonary artery occlusion pressure. Intensive Care Med. 2003;29:175–8.
90. Vieillard-Baron A, Slama M, Charron C, et al. A pilot study on safety and clinical utility of a single-use 72-hour indwelling transesophageal echocardiography probe. Intensive Care Med. 2013;39:629–35.
91. Singer M. Oesophageal doppler. Curr Opin Crit Care. 2009;15(3):244–8.
92. Dark PM, Singer M. The validity of trans-esophageal Doppler ultrasonography as a measure of cardiac output in critically ill adults. Intensive Care Med. 2004;30:2060–6.
93. Schober P, Loer SA, Schwarte LA. Perioperative hemodynamic monitoring with trans-esophageal Doppler technology. Anesth Analg. 2009;109(2):340–53.
94. Kamal GD, Symreng T, Starr J. Inconsistent esophageal Doppler cardiac output during acute blood loss. Anesthesiology. 1990;72:95–9.
95. List W, Gravenstein N, Banner T, et al. Interaction in sheep between mean arterial pressure and cross sectional area of the descending aorta: implications for esophageal Doppler monitoring. Anesthesiology. 1987;67:178.
96. Seoudi HM, Perkal MF, Hanrahan A, et al. The esophageal Doppler monitor in mechanically ventilated surgical patients: does it work? J Trauma. 2003;55(4):720–5.
97. Valtier B, Cholley BP, Belot JP, et al. Noninvasive monitoring of cardiac output in critically ill patients using transesophageal Doppler. Am J Respir Crit Care Med. 1998;158:77–83. 90
98. Lefrant J, Bruelle P, Aya A, et al. Training is required to improve the reliability of esophageal Doppler to measure cardiac output in critically ill patients. Intensive Care Med. 1998;24:347–52.
99. Madan AK, UyBarreta VV, Aliabadi-Wahle S, et al. Esophageal Doppler ultrasound monitor versus pulmonary artery catheter in the hemodynamic management of critically ill surgical patients. J Trauma. 1999;46(4):607–11.
100. Singer M, Bennett ED. Noninvasive optimization of left ventricular filling using esophageal Doppler. Crit Care Med. 1991;19(9):1132–7.

Endpoints of Resuscitation

12

Benjamin L. Davis and Martin A. Schreiber

Introduction

There are many methods for measuring the adequacy of resuscitation in a patient in shock, but none is universally applicable and few appear to be without significant limitations. As in so many areas of medicine, the constellation of findings from multiple modalities and the patient's trajectory must be interpreted and acted upon, occasionally with imperfect data. Further, given the disparate settings and situations in which resuscitations are performed, the methods of guiding resuscitation must be tailored to local capabilities.

While under-resuscitation often has grave consequences, over-resuscitation also leads to worse outcomes [1, 2]. In this chapter, we attempt to present a concise review of available endpoints of resuscitation and caveats to their use, as well as the limitations to available modalities.

Hemodynamic Endpoints

Mean Arterial Pressure

Mean arterial pressure (MAP) can be obtained quickly and provides nearly instantaneous and continuous results making it one of the most widely used resuscitation parameters. Despite its widespread use – including as a critical parameter in the Advanced Trauma Life Support and Surviving Sepsis Campaign Guidelines – blood pressure monitoring is not without limitations [3, 4]. There is no universal goal for blood pressure for all patients, and MAP goals must be individualized according to patients' comorbidities, pathophysiology, and the patient response to interventions [5]. Additionally, in the setting of hemorrhage, convincing data has shown that permissive hypotension (until bleeding is definitively controlled) is safe and may even lead to better outcomes. This is likely related to disruption of clot at higher pressure, hypothermia, and the dilutional coagulopathy that is a well described consequence of large doses of crystalloid [6, 7]. Based on the Committee on Tactical Combat Casualty Care, the current battlefield protocol is to give no fluid to patients that have a normal pulse and mentation [8]. In civilian practice, controlled resuscitation to hypotensive goals has been shown to be safe [9].

A traditional cuff pressure is sufficient in most clinical settings, though patients in shock – usually from hemorrhage or sepsis in our trauma/surgical ICU – usually get an arterial catheter to provide "beat-to-beat" monitoring of the response to ongoing fluid and blood product resuscitation. It would be rare to have a massive transfusion or pressor-dependent patient without an arterial line. Other common indications for invasive blood pressure monitoring in our TSICU are the brain-injured patient requiring intracranial pressure monitoring and patients with traumatic aortic injury, both groups in which blood pressure derangements may have immediate and devastating consequences [10, 11].

Central Venous Pressure

Central venous pressure (CVP) monitoring is theoretically a reflection of cardiac preload and overall volume status, and that is the basis of its use to help guide resuscitation. Like MAP, it is one of the fundamental parameters of the Surviving Sepsis Campaign Guidelines, the target being 8–12 mmHg. However, recent criticisms of the Surviving Sepsis Guidelines include studies showing lack of survival benefit with goal-directed therapy [12–14]. Absolute CVP values may be unreliable due to the non-volume-related variables that affect CVP, namely, positive pressure ventilation and pulmonary hypertension, especially if no measurement of cardiac output is obtained [15]. However, trends in CVP as a resuscitation

B. L. Davis
Division of Acute Care Surgery, University of Arkansas for Medical Sciences, Little Rock, AR, USA

M. A. Schreiber (✉)
Division of Trauma, Surgical Critical Care, and Acute Care Surgery, Oregon Health and Science University, Portland, OR, USA
e-mail: schreibm@ohsu.edu

A. Salim et al. (eds.), *Surgical Critical Care Therapy*, https://doi.org/10.1007/978-3-319-71712-8_12

proceeds may be more helpful for gauging volume status, assuming other variables are not changing [16]. Additionally, there may be significant variability in the manner in which CVP is actually measured at the bedside [17]. Because of this, we seldom place central venous catheters (CVC) for the sole purpose of monitoring CVP, though if a CVC is in place, we will use a trended CVP as a supplemental data point along with other clinical data.

Cardiac Output Monitoring: Pulmonary Artery Catheter and Pulse Contour Wave Analysis

Due to studies showing lack of survival benefit from the use of pulmonary artery catheters (PAC), their use has waned and is often discouraged [18–22]. The PAC is no longer routinely a part of resuscitations in our TSICU; the possible exception being in the rare patient who is unstable but the source of instability is not clear and other modalities are unhelpful for whatever reason. This most frequently occurs in patients with acute kidney injury and complex cardiac disorders in which standard physiologic parameters are not reliable.

Pulse contour wave analysis is a less invasive method of determining cardiac output. The pulse wave is analyzed via an arterial line to determine a stroke volume, from which cardiac output may be calculated. Concerns about this method's reliability in critically ill patients have dampened our enthusiasm, and it is not a routine part of our practice [23] (See Fig. 12.1).

Mixed/Central Venous Oxygen Saturation

A PAC is required to obtain a true mixed venous oxygen saturation (SvO_2), as the sample is taken from the pulmonary artery itself. A central venous oxygen saturation ($ScvO_2$) is not a true mixed venous oxygen saturation, and the absolute value of $ScvO_2$ is usually higher than the SvO_2, though the difference is constant enough to make $ScvO_2$ – which only requires a specialized central line to obtain – a useful value [24]. The Surviving Sepsis Guidelines suggest a goal of 65 mmHg for SvO_2 and 70 mmHg for $ScvO_2$, and others have shown that correction of $ScvO_2$ correlates with survival [25].

Echocardiography

Several studies have shown that echocardiography performed at the bedside – by surgeons with commonly available ultrasound machines – correlates well with more invasive means of assessing cardiac output [26]. In a series of studies, Ferrada et al. showed that an initial inferior vena cava diameter <2 cm correlates with worse outcomes in trauma patients, that fluid resuscitation has an identifiable and consistent impact on caval diameter, and that echocardiography is a viable option for directing trauma resuscitations [27–29].

On a practical level, a relatively straightforward, repeatable, and reproducible method of assessing cardiac function and volume shows great promise. The fact that it can be done

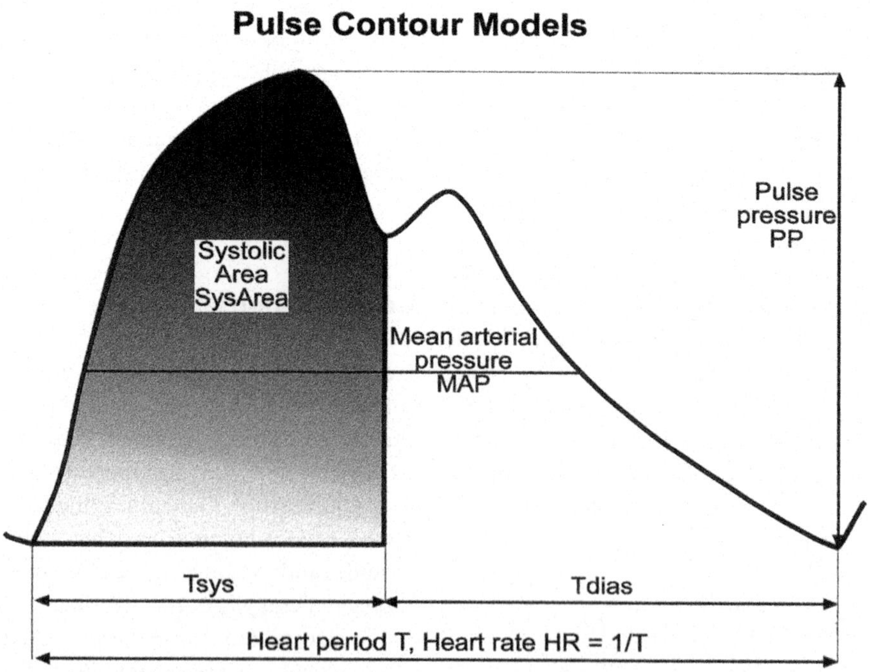

Fig. 12.1 Caption for pulse contour models. A typical tracing of a pulse wave and representation of systolic area measurements used to derive cardiac output measurements (Source: http://www.physiology.org/doi/abs/10.1152/ajpheart.2001.281.3.h1148)

with equipment that is already available in most ICUs contributes to its value. Additionally, an extended FAST exam with thoracic and abdominal views may be performed in tandem with the echocardiogram. Several of our attending trauma surgeons use bedside ultrasound to evaluate at least the IVC, and our trauma/surgical critical care fellows have a dedicated rotation for hands-on experience in the performance and interpretation of echocardiograms.

One major limitation of transthoracic echocardiography is that trauma patients may have a large amount of subcutaneous emphysema which limits the exam. We will occasionally request a transesophageal echo in this case, but given the more invasive nature of this approach, we usually reserve it for patients with known or suspected cardiac disease which is thought to be confounding our resuscitation.

Metabolic Endpoints

Lactate and Base Deficit

Lactate – the final product of anaerobic metabolism – accumulates in the setting of tissue dysoxia. It has been established that a lactate level of 3.4 mmol/L on presentation is a predictor of in-hospital death [30] and that failure to clear lactate over time – specifically within 48 h – is associated with increased mortality [31–33]. Further, lactate-guided resuscitations may lead to better results than those guided by other markers [34, 35]. In practice, a lactate is obtained and followed for our most seriously injured trauma patients as well as in septic patients. This is usually done with traditional lab testing, though in emergencies a lactate obtained from an arterial blood gas sample is often much faster, especially when analyzed as a point of care test as with the iSTAT system. As long as a patient remains stable, lactate levels are not followed if normal or once significant correction is observed.

Base deficit is defined as the amount of base required to raise the pH of 1 l of whole blood to the normal range based on the pCO_2. Higher values of base deficit reflect more severe metabolic acidosis, and unlike a simple pH measurement, respiratory compensation does not affect this value [36]. Several studies have shown that higher base deficits predict trauma mortality, transfusion requirements, and organ failure [37–39]. Like lactate levels, base deficit is obtained early in a resuscitation, and if abnormal, repeated base deficits are followed to help ensure adequate resuscitation. Unlike lactate, base deficit can be affected by high chloride-containing resuscitation fluids which produce hyperchloremic acidosis. Elevated base deficit secondary to hyperchloremic acidosis does not correlate with increased mortality as in the case of lactic acidosis [40].

Novel Metabolic Markers

When compared to traditional, clinical markers of shock such as SBP, base deficit, pulse, shock index, and tissue oxygen saturation, novel markers (ADAMTS14, heat shock protein 27, and sP-selectin) were found to be better predictors of multi-organ dysfunction and death in hemorrhaging patients [41]. However, this study was small ($N = 17$) and these tests are not widely available. Such markers show promise but are not yet a part of our practice.

Regional Endpoints

Mental Status and Urine Output

If shock is defined as evidence of diminished end-organ perfusion, then monitoring the function of end organs seems to be a reasonable goal with regard to guidance of resuscitation. We still use mental status and urine output (0.5 mg/kg/h in adults) as evidence that the brain and kidneys are adequately perfused, keeping in mind that certain conditions may result in normal or even elevated urine output in an under-resuscitated individual (diabetes insipidus, for example). While we do not base a resuscitation solely on those findings, they can offer fairly good insight into the patient's overall status and can quickly alert us to a decompensating patient.

Gastric Tonometry/Sublingual Capnography/Near-Infrared Spectrometry

Measurement of CO_2 concentration in the gastric mucosa (gastric tonometry) and in the sublingual mucosa theoretically provides an estimate of systemic perfusion, but these modalities have not yet been shown to be reproducible and result in improved resuscitation. One meta-analysis reported reduced mortality with gastric tonometry-guided therapy, but the authors point out that the benefit was mostly seen in patients with a normal intramucosal pH on admission [42]. This calls into question whether the results are generalizable to the most critically ill patients. Further, gastric tonometry does not appear to correlate well with traditional metabolic markers [43, 44]. Adequate studies regarding sublingual capnography are lacking.

Near-infrared spectrometry uses a probe on the thenar eminence to measure peripheral tissue oxygen saturation (StO_2) of the muscle tissue. Studies have shown worse outcomes with low initial StO_2 [45, 46]. It appears that StO_2 correlates with base deficit but not with MAP, $ScvO_2$, or heart rate [47]. Very little clinical data exists to guide the use of this modality in critical care. Similar to CVP, absolute values obtained appear to be less useful than trends.

Correction of Coagulopathy and the Thrombelastogram as a Resuscitation Endpoint

In approximately 10% of trauma patients, coagulopathy is present on admission [48]. Large volumes of cold crystalloid exacerbate this coagulopathy through acidosis and hypothermia, as does ongoing hemorrhage (Tieu). In trauma patients who present with normal coagulation, coagulopathy may be acquired through the same mechanisms. The feared consequence of this coagulopathy is exsanguinating hemorrhage despite surgical control of bleeding injuries, and so hemostasis and correction of coagulopathy would seem to be reasonable endpoints of resuscitation.

Traditional measures of coagulation can be used for identification of coagulopathy, though, if available, we increasingly recommend thrombelastograms (TEG) to determine coagulopathy in the injured patient. This practice is based on data that show the international normalized ratio overestimates coagulopathy [49] and data that indicates that hyperfibrinolysis is the cause of coagulopathy in a significant portion of coagulopathic trauma patients [50, 51]. Some authors have gone so far as to say that traditional coagulation studies are inappropriate for guidance of monitoring and treatment of coagulopathy in trauma [52].

The anti-fibrinolytic tranexamic acid (TXA) has gained acceptance as an adjunct to balanced resuscitation in recent years following the CRASH-2 trial [53]. However, it has been shown that not all massively bleeding patients will be hyperfibrinolytic and suggested that TEG can be used to help identify which patients are at risk of fibrinolysis shutdown, increased mortality, and thrombotic complications from TXA administration [54]. Other work suggests that balanced resuscitation strategies such as that described in the Prospective Observational Multicenter Massive Transfusion Trial (PROMMTT) may prevent the development of hyperfibrinolysis [55, 56].

It appears then that TEG shows great promise as a guide to transfusion and will be an important endpoint in the resuscitation of the hemorrhaging patient, though as yet there are no head-to-head trials comparing it to traditional endpoints (Figs. 12.2, 12.3, and 12.4).

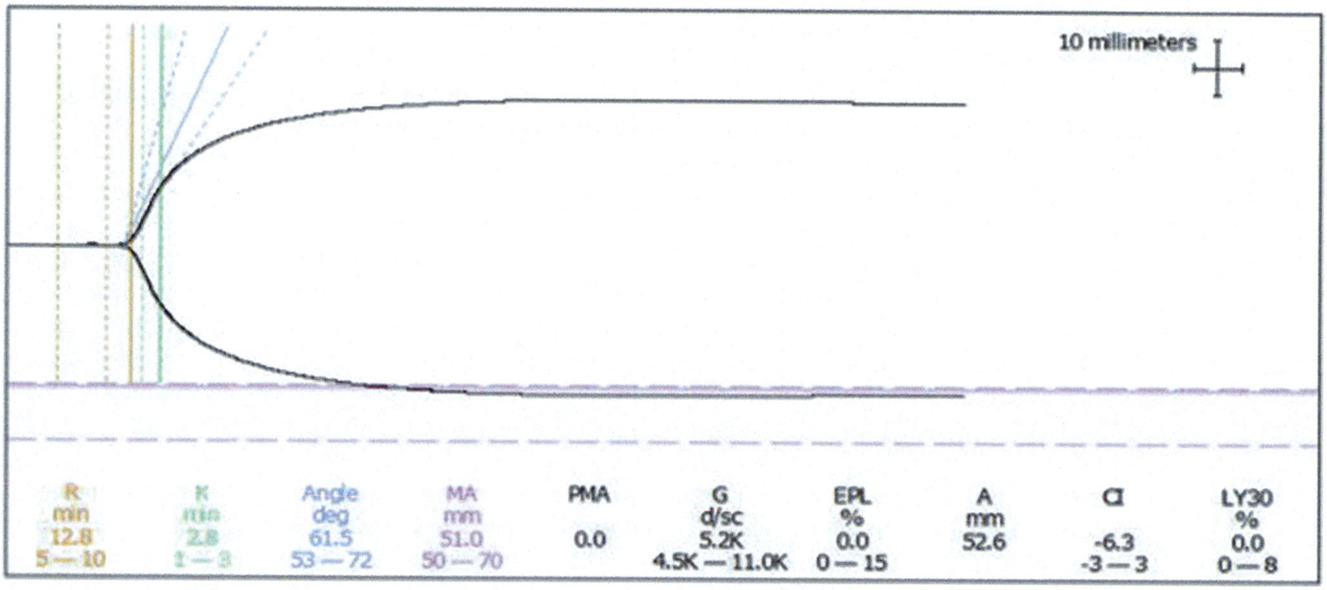

Fig. 12.2 TEG 1 – elevated *R* time in a patient status post-complex resection of a large pancreatic mass who received a 14 l of crystalloid in addition to 6 units PRBC, 6 units of FFP, and one apheresis of platelets during the course of a 16-h operation. The patient arrived in our TSICU with ongoing coagulopathic hemorrhage (Source: Sean McCully, MD, OHSU)

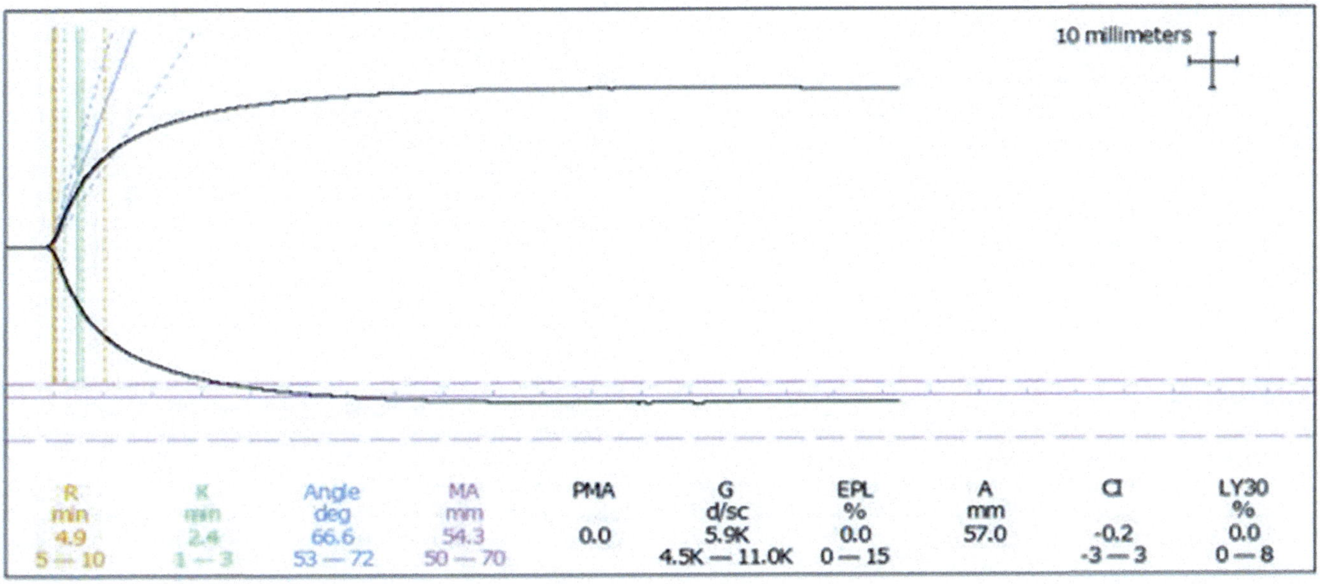

Fig. 12.3 TEG 2 – same patient as TEG 1, note corrected R time after balanced blood product resuscitation with minimized crystalloid (Source: Sean McCully, MD, OHSU)

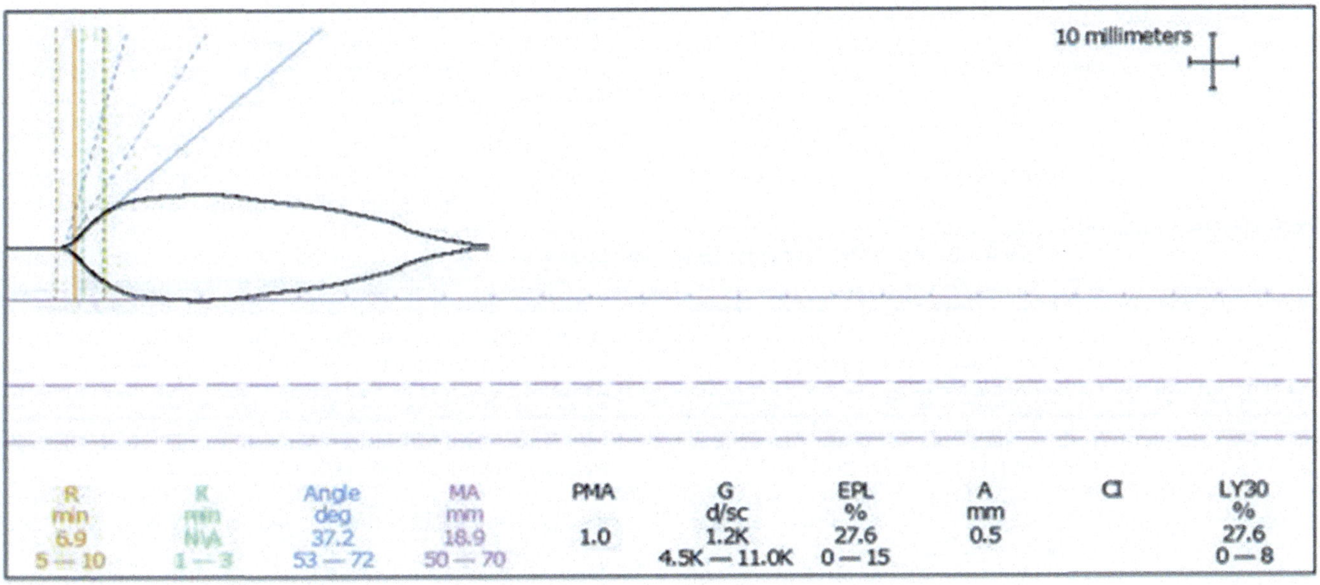

Fig. 12.4 TEG 3 – TEG showing fibrinolysis after severe head injury (Source: Sean McCully, MD, OHSU)

Conclusion

There is no universal endpoint to resuscitation. Patient factors, such as comorbidities, along with the underlying pathophysiology and type of shock will determine which endpoints are most appropriate. Given the disparate settings in which medical care is provided, local conditions and resources will by necessity have an impact on the choice of endpoint.

References

1. Murphy CV, Schramm GE, Doherty JA, Reichley RM, Gajic O, Afessa B, Micek ST, Kollef MH. The importance of fluid management in acute lung injury secondary to septic shock. Chest. 2009;136:102–9.
2. Boyd JH, Forbes J, Nakada TA, Walley KR, Russell JA. Fluid resuscitation in septic shock: a positive fluid balance and elevated central venous pressure are associated with increased mortality. Crit Care Med. 2011;39(2):259–65.
3. American College of Surgeons. Advanced trauma life support (ATLS): advanced trauma life support for doctors (student course manual). 9th ed. Chicago: American College of Surgeons; 2012.
4. Dellinger RP, Levy MM, Rhodes A, et al. Surviving sepsis campaign: international guidelines for management of severe sepsis and septic shock: 2012. Crit Care Med. 2013;41:580–637.
5. Kato R, Pinsky MR. Personalizing blood pressure management in septic shock. Ann of Intensive Care. 2015;5(1):41.
6. Tieu BH, Holcomb JB, Schreiber MA. Coagulopathy: its pathophysiology and treatment in the injured patient. World J Surg. 2007;31:1055–64.
7. Schreiber MA. Coagulopathy in the trauma patient. Curr Opin Crit Care. 2005;11:590–7.
8. Butler FK Jr, Blackbourne LH. Battlefield trauma care then and now: a decade of tactical combat casualty care. J Trauma Acute Care Surg. 2012;73(6 Suppl 5):S395–402.
9. Schreiber MA, Meier EN, Tisherman SA, et al. A controlled resuscitation strategy is feasible and safe in hypotensive trauma patients: results of a prospective randomized pilot trial. J Trauma Acute Care Surg. 2015;78:687–95. discussion 695–697
10. Manley G, Knudson MM, Morabito D, Damron S, Erickson V, Pitts L. Hypotension, hypoxia, and head injury: frequency, duration, and consequences. Arch Surg. 2001;136(10):1118–23.
11. Fabian TC, Davis KA, Gavant ML, et al. Prospective study of blunt aortic injury: helical CT is diagnostic and antihypertensive therapy reduces rupture. Ann Surg. 1998;227:666.
12. Mouncey PR, Osborn TM, Power GS, et al. Trial of early, goal-directed resuscitation for septic shock. N Engl J Med. 2015;372:1301–11.
13. ARISE Investigators; ANZICS Clinical Trials Group, Peake SL, et al. Goal directed resuscitation for patients with early septic shock. N Engl J Med. 2014;371:1496–506.
14. ProCESS Investigators, Yealy DM, Kellum JA, et al. A randomized trial of protocol-based care for early septic shock. N Engl J Med. 2014;370:1683–93.
15. Magder S. Central venous pressure: A useful but not so simple measurement. Crit Care Med. 2006;34(8):2224–7.
16. Magder S. Understanding central venous pressure: not a preload index? Curr Opin Crit Care. 2015;21(5):369–75.
17. Figg KK, Nemergut EC. Error in Central Venous Pressure Measurement. Anesthesia and Analgesia. 2009;08:1209–11.
18. Connors AF Jr, Speroff T, Dawson NV, et al. The effectiveness of right heart catheterization in the initial care of critically ill patients. JAMA. 1996;276:889–97.
19. Shah MR, Hasselblad V, Stevenson LW, et al. Impact of the pulmonary artery catheter in critically ill patients: meta-analysis of randomized clinical trials. JAMA. 2005;294:1664–70.
20. National Heart, Lung, and Blood Institute Acute Respiratory Distress Syndrome (ARDS) Clinical Trials Network, Wheeler AP, Bernard GR, Thompson BT, et al. Pulmonary-artery versus central venous catheter to guide treatment of acute lung injury. N Engl J Med. 2006;354:2213–24.
21. Rajaram SS, Desai NK, Kalra A, et al. Pulmonary artery catheters for adult patients in intensive care. Cochrane Database Syst Rev. 2013;2:CD003408.
22. Gidwani UK, Mohanty B, Chatterjee K. The pulmonary artery catheter: a critical reappraisal. Cardiol Clin. 2013;31:545–65.
23. Argueta E, Berdine G, Pena C, Nugent KM. FloTrac monitoring system: what are its uses in critically ill medical patients? Am J Med Sci. 2015;349:352–6.
24. Reinhart K, Kuhn HJ, Hartog C, Bredle DL. Continuous central venous and pulmonary artery oxygen saturation monitoring in the critically ill. Intensive Care Med. 2004;30:1572–8.
25. Hernandez G, Luengo C, Bruhn A, et al. When to stop septic shock resuscitation: clues from a dynamic perfusion monitoring. Ann Intensive Care. 2014;4:30. 30-014-0030-z. eCollection 2014
26. Gunst M, Matsushima K, Sperry J, et al. Focused bedside echocardiography in the surgical intensive care unit: comparison of 3 methods to estimate cardiac index. J Intensive Care Med. 2011;26:255–60.
27. Ferrada P, Vanguri P, Anand RJ, et al. Flat inferior vena cava: indicator of poor prognosis in trauma and acute care surgery patients. Am Surg. 2012;78:1396–8.
28. Ferrada P, Vanguri P, Anand RJ, et al. A, B, C, D, echo: limited transthoracic echocardiogram is a useful tool to guide therapy for hypotension in the trauma bay: a pilot study. J Trauma Acute Care Surg. 2013;74:220–3.
29. Ferrada P, Evans D, Wolfe L, et al. Findings of a randomized controlled trial using limited transthoracic echocardiogram (LTTE) as a hemodynamic monitoring tool in the trauma bay. J Trauma Acute Care Surg. 2014;76:31–7. discussion 37–38
30. Strnad, M, et al. Predictors of mortality and prehospital monitoring limitations of blunt trauma patints. Biomed Res Int. 2015;Epub 2015 Feb 1. https://www.hindawi.com/journals/bmri/2015/983409/
31. Abramson D, Scalea TM, Hitchcock R, et al. Lactate clearance and survival following injury. J Trauma. 1993;35:584–8. discussion 588–589
32. McNelis J, Marini CP, Jurkiewicz A, et al. Prolonged lactate clearance is associated with increased mortality in the surgical intensive care unit. Am J Surg. 2001;182:481–5.
33. Husain FA, Martin MJ, Mullenix PS, et al. Serum lactate and base deficit as predictors of mortality and morbidity. Am J Surg. 2003;185:485–91.
34. Jones AE, Shapiro NI, Trzeciak S, et al. Lactate clearance vs central venous oxygen saturation as goals of early sepsis therapy: a randomized clinical trial. JAMA. 2010;303:739–46.
35. Jansen TC, van Bommel J, Schoonderbeek FJ, et al. Early lactate-guided therapy in intensive care unit patients: a multicenter, open-label, randomized controlled trial. Am J Respir Crit Care Med. 2010;182:752–61.
36. Davis JW, Parks SN, Kaups KL, et al. Admission base deficit predicts transfusion requirements and risk of complications. J Trauma. 1996;41:769–74.
37. Mutschler M, Nienaber U, Brockamp T, et al. Renaissance of base deficit for the initial assessment of trauma patients: a base deficit-based classification for hypovolemic shock developed on data from 16 305 patients derived from the trauma register DGU. Crit Care. 2013;17:R42.

38. Rutherford EJ, Morris JA, Reed GW, Hall KS. Base deficit stratifies mortality and determines therapy. J Trauma. 1992;33:417–23.
39. Eberhard LW, Morabito DJ, Matthay MA, et al. Initial severity of metabolic acidosis predicts the development of acute lung injury in severely traumatized patients. Crit Care Med. 2000;28:125–31.
40. Brill SA, Stewart TR, Brundage SI, Schreiber MA. Base deficit does not predict mortality when secondary to hyperchloremic acidosis. Shock. 2002;17(6):459–62.
41. Furmaga W, et al. Novel markers predict death and organ failure following hemorrhagic shock. Clin Chim Acta. 2015;440:87–92.
42. Zhang X, Xuan W, Yin P, Wang L, Wu X, Wu Q. Gastric tonometry guided therapy in critical care patients: a systematic review and meta-analysis. Crit Care. 2015;19:22. https://doi.org/10.1186/s13054-015-0739-6.
43. Miami Trauma Clinical Trials Group. Splanchnic hypoperfusion-directed therapies in trauma: a prospective, randomized trial. Am Surg. 2005;71:252–60.
44. Hameed SM, Cohn SM. Gastric tonometry: the role of mucosal pH measurement in the management of trauma. Chest. 2003;123(5 Suppl):475S–81S.
45. Cohn SM, Nathens AB, Moore FA, et al. Tissue oxygen saturation predicts the development of organ dysfunction during traumatic shock resuscitation. J Trauma. 2007;62:44–54. discussion 54–55
46. Lima A, van Bommel J, Jansen TC, et al. Low tissue oxygen saturation at the end of early goal-directed therapy is associated with worse outcome in critically ill patients. Crit Care. 2009;5(13 Suppl):S13.
47. Payen D, Luengo C, Heyer L, et al. Is thenar tissue hemoglobin oxygen saturation in septic shock related to macrohemodynamic variables and outcome? Crit Care. 2009;5(13 Suppl):S6.
48. Holcomb JB. Damage control resuscitation. J Trauma. 2007;62(6 Suppl):S36–7.
49. McCully SP, Fabricant LJ, Kunio NR, Groat TL, Watson KM, Differding JA, Deloughery TG, Schreiber MA. The International Normalized Ratio overestimates coagulopathy in stable trauma and surgical patients. Journal of Trauma and Acute Care Surgery Issue. 2013;75(6):947–53.
50. Ives C, Inaba K, Branco BC, et al. Hyperfibrinolysis elicited via thromboelastography predicts mortality in trauma. J Am Coll Surg. 2012;215:496–502.
51. Schochl H, Voelckel W, Maegele M, Solomon C. Trauma-associated hyperfibrinolysis. Hamostaseologie. 2012;32:22–7.
52. Johansson PI. Coagulation monitoring of the bleeding traumatized patient. Curr Opin Anaesthesiol. 2012;25:235–41.
53. CRASH-2 trial collaborator. Effects of tranexamic acid on death, vascular occlusive events, and blood transfusion in trauma patients with significant haemorrhage (CRASH-2): a randomised, placebo-controlled trial. Lancet. 2010;376:23–32.
54. Moore HB, Moore EE, Gonzalez E, et al. Hyperfibrinolysis, physiologic fibrinolysis, and fibrinolysis shutdown: the spectrum of postinjury fibrinolysis and relevance to antifibrinolytic therapy. J Trauma Acute Care Surg. 2014;77:811–7.
55. Holcomb JB, Wade CE, Michalek JE, Chisholm GB, Zarzabal LA, Schreiber MA, Gonzalez EA, Pomper GJ, Perkins JG, Spinella PC, Williams KL, Park MS. Increased plasma and platelet to red blood cell ratios improves outcome in 466 massively transfused civilian trauma patients. Ann Surg. 2008;248(3):447–58.
56. Moore HB, Moore EE, Gonzalez E, et al. Plasma is the physiologic buffer of tissue plasminogen activator-mediated fibrinolysis: rationale for plasma-first resuscitation after life-threatening hemorrhage. J Am Coll Surg. 2015;220:872–9.

Care for the Postoperative Cardiac Surgery Patient

13

Andrew S. Kaufman, Philip S. Mullenix, and Jared L. Antevil

The views and opinions expressed in this chapter are those of the authors and do not necessarily reflect the official policy or position of any agency of the US government.

Introduction

Standardized pathways are one of the key foundations for the postoperative care of cardiac surgical patients – structured care criteria rooted in the best available evidence contribute to greater efficiency in care delivery and enhance patient safety [1]. Such pathways are only a starting place, however. Contrary to some popular lore, every cardiac surgical patient, procedure, and postoperative course is unique. A pathway dictating the baseline plan of care allows the critical care patient team to dedicate time and effort toward dynamic or unexpected events when they occur.

In this chapter, a review of general management principles and techniques relevant to the care of cardiac surgical patients will be followed by guidance for the management of more specific clinical scenarios. Finally, this chapter will present some considerations unique to particular cardiac surgical procedures.

General Management: Receiving the Patient

When a patient is transferred from the cardiac surgery operating room (OR) to the intensive care unit (ICU), a "team huddle" is critical, to convey key information about the patient, the operative procedure, and early plans for care. Ideally, this patient care transition should involve the cardiac surgeon, anesthesiologist, receiving intensivist, and primary receiving nurse. At a minimum, the transferring team should convey patient information (baseline cardiac function, significant comorbidities), pertinent details from the operative procedure (conduct of the procedure, difficulty of intubation, any transfusions, any unexpected findings/events), and current state (cardiac function on post-procedure transesophageal echocardiogram [TEE], most recent cardiac output/index, current vasoactive drips, current pacing regimen, and most recent underlying rhythm). In addition, the team should discuss initial plans for care – including the goals for blood pressure, expected goals concerning timing for extubation, and any significant deviations from the normal postoperative pathway plan.

Upon a cardiac surgical patient's transition to ICU care, initial cardiac assessment should include determination of a patient's heart rate and rhythm, cardiac output, pulmonary artery (PA) pressures, and systemic blood pressure. Assessment of clinical perfusion should include an arterial blood gas (ABG) and mixed venous oxygen saturation assessment, examination of extremity pulses and perfusion, and a determination of initial urine output. Baseline chest tube output should be noted, as should the character of ongoing drainage. The ICU nurses should attempt to maintain chest tube patency by hooking all drains to immediate suction (20 cm H2O) and by gentling "milking" any visible clot within the tubes (aggressive "stripping" of mediastinal drains is not advised). A portable chest radiograph (CXR) should be performed to assess position of the endotracheal tube, central line and PA catheter. Lung fields should be evaluated on CXR for pneumothorax and/or pleural effusion. ABG results and arterial oxygen saturation levels should be assessed to determine appropriate initial ventilator settings. Warming measures (warm blankets, Bair Hugger, and warming of all IV infusions) should be instituted for any patient arriving in the ICU with a temperature below 36–36.5 °C. If an orogastric tube is not already in place, one should be placed to low suction in order to prevent gastric distention after extubation.

A. S. Kaufman
General Surgery Resident, Department of Surgery, Walter Reed National Military Medical Center, Bethesda, MD, USA

P. S. Mullenix · J. L. Antevil (✉)
Division of Cardiothoracic Surgery, Department of Surgery, Walter Reed National Military Medical Center, Bethesda, MD, USA
e-mail: Jared.L.Antevil.mil@mail.mil

A. Salim et al. (eds.), *Surgical Critical Care Therapy*, https://doi.org/10.1007/978-3-319-71712-8_13

General Management: Hemodynamic Monitoring

Traditionally, a PA catheter is placed after anesthetic induction for all patients undergoing cardiac surgery. PA catheter use is no longer universal for these procedures; specifically, PA catheters are omitted in some centers for isolated coronary artery bypass grafting (CABG), particularly for patients with preserved left ventricular (LV) function. Just as in most other ICU populations, there is no hard evidence that PA catheter use has a measurable clinical benefit for cardiac surgery patients [2]. When utilized, the PA catheter provides a useful tool to monitor intravascular volume (through interpretation of the pulmonary capillary wedge pressure and/or pulmonary arterial diastolic pressure), monitor for the development of new or worsening pulmonary hypertension, and to assess cardiac output. Many institutions utilize an advanced fiber optic PA catheter, which allows for continual assessment of cardiac output and mixed venous oxygen saturation.

Even with a PA catheter in appropriate position, the absolute values of PA pressure, cardiac output, and mixed venous oxygen saturation can often be deceptive in the early postoperative period. Given a new post-op heart patient with low cardiac output but with normal urine output, warm extremities with brisk pulses, and a normal serum lactate level, there is likely no cause for immediate concern (and certainly no reason to implement major changes in treatment). In other words, clinical markers indicating adequate end-organ perfusion trump PA catheter data every time. While absolute values do not necessarily correlate with a patient's true physiological state, changes in cardiac output and PA pressures (particularly a sudden or persistent decline in cardiac output or increase in PA pressure) should always be investigated. These findings may precede evidence of end-organ dysfunction by a significant interval [3].

There is a relative decrease in cardiac output for many patients after initial separation from cardiopulmonary bypass, which is typically followed by steady recovery over the first 24 h after surgery [4]. However, one must always be cognizant of alternative explanations for an early decline in cardiac output, most notably bleeding, tamponade, or ischemia (all of which are covered in detail later in this chapter).

Mixed venous oxygen saturation values from a PA catheter (assessed with a manual blood gas from the distal PA catheter port or using an oximetric PA catheter) can be a highly valuable tool. In general, a mixed venous oxygen saturation above 60% suggests adequate tissue-level perfusion [5]. Once again, its absolute value should be interpreted with caution and in the context of other clinical indicators of organ perfusion.

If a PA catheter is not in place, central venous pressure (CVP) measurement can provide some information about a patient's intravascular volume status. Because of the inherent compliance in the venous system, CVP measurements do not correlate well with volume status, other than at the extremes [6]. However, CVP interpretation over time for a given patient (particularly after therapeutic intervention) can certainly be of value. The absence of a significant increase in CVP after volume administration can be either suggestive of ongoing bleeding or more generally suggestive of the need for continued volume resuscitation. Although PA catheter and CVP measurements are described in the medical literature for the diagnosis of tamponade, these measurements do not correlate well with the presence or absence of tamponade after cardiac surgery [7].

Radial artery pressure monitoring is standard for all cardiac surgical cases. However, radial arterial pressures are often inaccurate in the early period after separation from cardiopulmonary bypass [8, 9]. Most often, radial pressure readings are artificially low, presumably due to peripheral vasoconstriction. An artificially low radial arterial pressure reading can be associated with unrecognized hypertension (HTN) or can prompt the administration of inappropriate vasopressor medications. Either of these scenarios can have disastrous consequences with regard to fresh cannulation sites and suture lines. Because accurate arterial pressure assessment is critical during this early postoperative period, many centers have adopted routine femoral arterial pressure monitoring (in addition to radial) for cardiac surgical patients [10]. At a minimum, radial pressures should be correlated with noninvasive pressure measurements and with clinical examination. If there is any doubt as to the accuracy of radial pressures, femoral arterial monitoring should be instituted immediately.

General Management: Sedation/Analgesia

Most institutions utilize propofol or dexmedetomidine infusion for sedation in the early postoperative period after cardiac surgery. The latter agent is being used with increasing frequency due to its less pronounced vasodilatory affects [11]. Most patients are sedated on initial admission to the ICU. Prior to awakening a patient and considering extubation, sedation allows for assessment of hemodynamic stability, adequate rewarming, the absence of surgical bleeding, and acceptable acid-base status (all of which are requisites for safe extubation after cardiac surgery).

Because propofol has no analgesic properties, it is typically supplemented with intravenous (IV) narcotics based on nursing assessment. For patients with normal renal function, IV ketorolac can be an extremely effective analgesic adjunct after cardiac surgery. Ketorolac may be particularly helpful after extubation and for younger patients (who often experience a higher degree of pain after median sternotomy). Some centers avoid ketorolac use after CABG, as there is a black box warning against the use of nonsteroidal anti-inflammatory medications in this setting [12]. However, the evidentiary basis for this Food and Drug Association (FDA) warning is scant, and many centers have reported excellent results utilizing ketorolac for CABG patients [13].

"Fast-track pathways" designed to minimize ventilator time and ICU stay are utilized in some cardiac surgery centers, particularly for lower risk patients/procedures. Such pathways have demonstrated some success in achieving these goals [14], although they have not been widely adopted overall.

After extubation, adequate pain control can be achieved in most patients with intermittent IV morphine for the first 24–48 h, after which patients may be transitioned to oral narcotics. Patient-controlled analgesia with IV hydromorphone or morphine can be helpful if a patient is requiring frequent narcotic dosing. There is some evidence that oral gabapentin may reduce narcotic requirements after sternotomy [15, 16].

General Management: Ventilator Management

In the absence of significant preexisting pulmonary disease, ventilator management for cardiac surgical patients is generally straightforward. However, cardiac surgery patients often require higher tidal volumes than those typically utilized for medical patients or other surgical patients. The period of apnea during cardiopulmonary bypass predisposes them to postoperative atelectasis [17]. Appropriate tidal volumes for most patients are in the range of 6–8 ml/kg for ideal body weight [18]. Almost all patients undergoing cardiac surgery will have some degree of transient pulmonary edema due to a systemic inflammatory response and/or a state of relative fluid overload. As such, it is not uncommon for patients to require higher oxygen concentrations in the early period after cardiac surgery.

General Management: Inotropes

Depending on a patient's preoperative left or right ventricular function and the conduct of a particular operation, some patients undergoing cardiac surgery will arrive in the ICU on a continuous inotropic infusion. In other patients, the addition of a new inotrope may be indicated during their ICU course. The selection of a particular agent to augment ventricular function is a complex decision, driven in no small part by a particular surgeon's, anesthesiologist's, or intensivist's personal experience (and training). The most commonly utilized inotropic agents after cardiac surgery are epinephrine, dopamine, milrinone, and norepinephrine.

Epinephrine exerts a strong inotropic effect and a moderate vasopressor effect, the combination of which is often very effective at improving cardiac output, blood pressure and clinical perfusion at lower-dose infusion rates. Its use is associated with tachycardia, increased myocardial oxygen demand, and an increased risk for ectopy and arrhythmias (particularly at higher doses). In addition, the use of epinephrine can contribute to a persistent lactic acidosis after cardiac surgery in some patients [19]. Low-dose epinephrine infusion (rates of 0.01–0.05 mcg/kg/min) is generally well tolerated by most patients and represents the first-line inotrope in most scenarios after cardiac surgery.

Dopamine is classically described to have dose-dependent response effects, with low doses exerting vasodilatation in the renal vascular bed, moderate doses associated with a primary inotropic effect, and higher doses exerting a primary vasoconstrictor effect [20]. In reality, the various physiologic effects of dopamine are not compartmentalized by infusion dosing level nor are they entirely predictable for a given patient. Regardless, a low-dose dopamine infusion is utilized postoperatively on a routine basis for many cardiac surgery patients. The use of dopamine does promote tachycardia and both atrial and ventricular arrhythmias.

Milrinone, a phosphodiesterase inhibitor, augments both right and left ventricular function and promotes vasodilatation. Both of these effects occur via increased production of cyclic AMP. In addition, milrinone is a relatively potent pulmonary arterial vasodilator. Because of this physiologic profile, milrinone is often used for patients undergoing mitral valve surgery, those with significant right ventricular dysfunction, and for patients with pulmonary hypertension. Because of its vasodilatory properties, it should be used with caution in any patient with marginal systemic pressures. In situations where milrinone is clearly the preferred inotropic medication (such as in a patient with right ventricular dysfunction and pulmonary hypertension), its use may necessitate concomitant vasopressor support utilizing norepinephrine or phenylephrine.

Norepinephrine exerts some inotropic effect, but because of its potent vasopressor effect, it is not optimal for use to augment cardiac output, as the increase in afterload may offset augmentation of cardiac contractility [20]. In general, the use of both norepinephrine and epinephrine simultaneously in the same patient should be discouraged – because they are both adrenergic agents competing for the many of the same receptors; their use in tandem may lead to unpredictable effects.

All inotropic medications have complex physiological profiles and are associated with some risk of arrhythmias and other side effects. The one possible exception is IV calcium bolus therapy. Although its effect is transient, calcium (generally administered in 1 or 2 g doses of calcium chloride) will often markedly augment cardiac function (and blood pressure) with no appreciable side effects. At a minimum, calcium replacement is indicated for cardiac surgical patients (to keep ionized calcium >5 mg/dL), and calcium should be considered a "go to" medication in any non-bleeding patient with new hypotension. The use of IV calcium in this setting will often buy the clinician a little time to determine the next most appropriate therapy.

General Management: Vasopressors

Transient peripheral vasodilatation, or "vasoplegia," is very common following cardiac surgery with cardiopulmonary bypass (CPB), likely because of the pro-inflammatory effects of bypass. In the setting of preserved cardiac output and end-organ perfusion, low- to moderate-dose continuous vasopressor support is perfectly appropriate for this normally transient condition (which generally resolves in the first 12–24 h after cardiac surgery). However, when hypotension coincides with decreased cardiac output, vasopressor support is not indicated and may be deleterious. In this scenario, volume resuscitation and/or inotropic support represent more appropriate therapy.

In most cases, the treatment of peripheral vasodilatation with preserved cardiac function and perfusion involves the administration of either phenylephrine or norepinephrine infusion (with the former providing for more selective alpha-adrenergic peripheral vasoconstriction). One must resist the temptation to bolus these medications or to make multiple hemodynamic interventions simultaneously, which may lead to a "seesaw" in blood pressure. Patients are often quite hemodynamically labile in the early postoperative period, particularly those with low intravascular volume or decreased left ventricular compliance (from left ventricular hypertrophy). It is much better to tolerate a systolic pressure in the 60s or 70s mmHg for a few minutes while awaiting the effects of a new vasopressor agent or dose than to overshoot (and subject fresh cannulation sites and suture lines to supraphysiologic pressures). The mantra in managing hypotension after cardiac surgery should be fine-tuning and patience.

"Adequate" blood pressure in the early postoperative period is best defined as the lowest blood pressure that supports satisfactory end-organ perfusion, which may vary for a given patient. For most cardiac surgical cases, a systolic blood pressure goal of 90–120 mmHg or a mean arterial pressure in the 60s–70s mmHg is appropriate. For elderly patients, patients with known peripheral vascular disease/carotid stenosis, or those with severe long-standing HTN, a higher blood pressure goal may be appropriate. In the setting of postoperative bleeding, most surgeons would advocate a systolic blood pressure goal in the low 90s mmHg.

Rarely, patients may manifest severe and refractory vasoplegia, unresponsive to higher doses of alpha-adrenergic agonists. Just as in other ICU patients, the addition of "background" treatment with a non-titrated vasopressin infusion at a rate of 0.04 units/min may be beneficial in such cases. There is some evidence that vasopressin may be particularly effective in counteracting the vasoplegia that can be associated with oral angiotensin-converting enzyme (ACE) inhibitor or angiotensin receptor blocker (ARB) use in the preoperative period [21]. For refractory vasoplegia after cardiac surgery, the use of methylene blue (typically dosed at 1.5–2 mg/kg over 20 min) may be very beneficial [22], with minimal risk of significant deleterious effects.

When a patient manifests significant persistent vasoplegia and vasopressor requirements outside of the immediate postoperative period, one must consider the possibility of an alternate explanation to the normal "post-pump" physiological state. In particular, the patient should be assessed for abdominal complications such as pancreatitis (due to cardiopulmonary bypass) or mesenteric ischemia (due to emboli or a low-flow state). Adrenal insufficiency should be considered in every patient with persistent vasoplegia, as transient adrenal suppression has been described after a single induction dose of etomidate [23]. Although rare in the first 24–48 h after cardiac surgery, one must also consider the possibility of sepsis/bacteremia.

General Management: Hypertension

The maximum acceptable systemic pressure for a cardiac surgical patient will vary depending on a surgeon's preference, institutional practices, and the characteristics of a given patient/surgical procedure. Generally speaking, in the absence of high chest tube output, the maximal systolic pressure should be maintained at less than 120–130 mmHg during the early postoperative period. For patients with ongoing bleeding (whether medical or surgical), the surgical team may direct a more aggressive pressure management strategy (such as a systolic goal of less than 100–110 mmHg) to avoid the exacerbation of bleeding. For patients with known carotid artery stenosis and for elderly patients with long-standing/severe HTN, the surgical team may direct a higher initial blood pressure goal. In general, for patients following a normal postoperative course, maximal pressure goals are relaxed to 130–140 mmHg after the morning of the first postoperative day, although again blood pressure goals will be individualized for a given patient, scenario, and surgeon's preference.

Early blood pressure control is most often achieved using the following agents (alone or in combination) via IV continuous infusion: nitroglycerin, sodium nitroprusside, or nicardipine. Less commonly, esmolol or labetalol infusion may be appropriate. As with vasopressors, the agent of choice to reduce systemic arterial pressure may vary based on surgeon/institutional preference and practice. Also as with vasopressor use in the early postoperative period, the titration for vasodilator agents should be judicious and deliberate (to avoid wild swings in pressure). In addition to the pharmacologic treatment of hypertension in the early period after cardiac surgery, the appropriate treatment of pain and/or anxiety must not be overlooked in the sedated patient and may significantly improve blood pressure control.

There are several important characteristics and factors relevant to the use of each of these common antihypertensive drip medications. Nitroglycerin has some favorable properties for CABG patients in particular, as it potentially may induce the vasodilatation of both native coronary arteries and the left internal mammary artery (LIMA) pedicle (the standard CABG graft to the anterior wall). Nitroglycerin is inexpensive and has rapid effect and a short half-life, approximately 4 min [24]. It is therefore one of the mainstays for early blood pressure control after cardiac surgery. Sodium nitroprusside is a more potent vasodilator than nitroglycerin, and because it exerts less relative venous dilation compared with nitroglycerin, it may allow for blood pressure control without the need to administer additional IV fluid. It is more expensive than nitroglycerin and can cause cyanide toxicity with prolonged infusion and/or higher infusion rates but is also a cornerstone of blood pressure management at many institutions. Nicardipine is being used with increasing frequency for postoperative HTN, as it is highly effective and has a favorable side effect profile (unusual tachycardia or gastrointestinal effects). Although nicardipine has a short half-life of 2 min, its hemodynamic effects are more persistent than either nitroglycerin or sodium nitroprusside [24].

Once patients are beyond the first postoperative day, the need for IV infusion to control systemic pressure is very unusual. Most patients by this time can be started on oral agents, and goals for blood pressure control need not be quite as stringent. Nearly all CABG patients who are not on vasopressors should be started on an oral beta-blocker beginning the first postoperative day – generally metoprolol with a starting dose of 12.5–25 mg twice daily or carvedilol for patients with heart failure/reduced LV function. Valve surgery patients may also benefit from a beta-blocker to reduce the risk of atrial arrhythmias, although all medications with potential effects on conduction must be used with caution in valve surgery patients, who often have some degree of atrioventricular (AV) nodal or sinoatrial (SA) nodal dysfunction after surgery. Other blood pressure medications (calcium channel blockers, ACE inhibitors/ARBs, oral nitrates, etc.) can also be started in the ICU if needed for blood pressure control. However, most centers avoid the use of ACE inhibitors/ARB medications for at least the first several days after surgery. In addition to the titration of oral agents, persistent HTN later in the postoperative period may be managed with doses of IV metoprolol or labetalol (when associated with an elevated heart rate) or IV hydralazine (when associated with a normal or low heart rate).

General Management: Antiplatelet and Anticoagulant Medications

With very few exceptions, every cardiac surgical patient should be on aspirin through surgery, generally 325 mg daily for CABG patients (including on the night of surgery, given per rectum or via an orogastric tube if needed) and at least 81 mg daily for valve procedures. Many CABG patients are eventually started on dual antiplatelet therapy postoperatively (aspirin and clopridigrel), but this is rarely relevant for their ICU course.

Although previous literature suggested that venous thromboembolism (VTE) is rare in cardiac surgical patients, these patients are in fact all in a high-risk category for VTE [25]. Therefore, the combination of sequential compression devices (typically omitted on the vein harvest leg for a CABG patient) and pharmacologic prophylaxis (unfractionated subcutaneous heparin, typically 5000 mg Q8hrs, or prophylactic-dose low-molecular-weight heparin [LMWH]) is appropriate for most patients. Some surgeons will hold any heparin in patients with bleeding issues, and others will hold aspirin in patients with significant thrombocytopenia, so the use of these medications should be verified with the surgical team.

Warfarin is a mandatory medication for all mechanical heart valve patients. Warfarin is also prescribed for several months by many surgeons for patients undergoing a tissue mitral valve replacement or mitral repair and is prescribed for several months after tissue aortic valve replacement by some surgeons [26]. In the absence of an ongoing bleeding diathesis and/or coagulopathy, most patients can be started on warfarin on the first postoperative day (or once extubated). Bridging IV heparin is never needed for tissue valves or mitral repair but is used by some surgical groups after mechanical heart valve replacement. Studies show that bridging may slightly reduce the thromboembolism rate but may be associated with higher risk of bleeding [27, 28]. Patients anticoagulated preoperatively with warfarin or a novel oral anticoagulant (e.g., dabigatran, rivaroxaban) can generally be started back on their home dose prior to discharge, but there should rarely be a need to restart this medication during a patient's ICU course.

General Management: Other Medications

Because all patients are markedly fluid positive after cardiopulmonary bypass, most cardiac surgical patients should be started on diuretic therapy beginning on the first postoperative day. The timing, specific medication, route, and dose for diuretics will vary a great deal based on institutional and surgeon preference. For most patients with preserved renal function, an initial regimen of furosemide 20 mg IV twice daily is an appropriate starting place. Diuretics should be initiated with caution in patients with severe left ventricular hypertrophy (who may require higher intravascular volume to maintain adequate left ventricular filling due to reduced LV compliance). Diuretics should also be initiated with caution in patients with persistent vasopressor requirements and those with evidence of reduced end-organ perfusion (particularly renal).

All CABG patients without a contraindication (and many valve patients) are generally continued on statin therapy through surgery. In addition to the favorable longer-term effects of this medication class on lipid profile, there is some evidence that perioperative statin use may reduce the incidence of atrial fibrillation, and statins have been shown to have anti-inflammatory properties [29–31]. However, in a recent study comparing perioperative rosuvastatin to placebo for cardiac surgery patients, patients receiving perioperative statin therapy were at an increased risk for acute kidney injury [32]. Therefore, the use of statins in the immediate perioperative period is not without controversy.

The use of antifibrinolytic medications after cardiac surgery is standard practice at most institutions, as there is strong evidence that they reduce bleeding and transfusion requirements in this setting [33]. Antifibrinolytic medications include aprotinin (serine protease inhibitor, no longer in use in the USA due to safety concerns) and the lysine analogs: ε-aminocaproic acid (EACA) and tranexamic acid (TXA). Both EACA and TXA are renally excreted with similar half-lives (2–3 h) and conflicting data regarding relative efficacy. Therefore, the choice between the two lysine analogs is often based on institutional availability and cost. Dosing regimens for lysine analogs are variable, but both medications are typically administered as an IV bolus after skin incision and are sometimes re-dosed in the CPB circuit. In many institutions, EACA or TXA is given via a continuous infusion for 6–8 h thereafter. Therefore, depending on institutional protocols and practice, some cardiac surgical patients will arrive to the ICU with a lysine analog infusion.

Perioperative antibiotics should be continued through 48 h after cardiac surgery, with the last dose of IV antibiotics typically administered on the morning of the second postoperative day.

General Management: Temporary Pacing

Most patients undergoing cardiac surgery will have temporary epicardial pacing leads placed at the time of surgery. Most surgeons will place both atrial and ventricular pacing leads at the time of any cardiac valvular procedure, as valvular procedures place the AV node complex at risk for transient or permanent injury. The exception is patients with "permanent" atrial fibrillation, in whom atrial pacing is not possible (and in whom no atrial wires should be placed). The use of epicardial pacing leads after isolated CABG is variable between surgeons and institutions, with some surgeons placing atrial leads only, some placing only ventricular leads, some utilizing both, and others not placing any. For patients with an existing permanent pacemaker (and/or internal cardiac defibrillator [ICD]), the device will have been inactivated prior to surgery (either by placement of a magnet or more commonly by formal programming). For these patients, most surgeons will place epicardial temporary leads, which can be removed at the time of reactivation of a patient's permanent device settings.

Pacing leads allow for the treatment of postoperative bradycardia/heart block and for augmentation of cardiac output in the early postoperative period. In addition, there is some evidence that supraphysiologic atrial pacing may suppress the development of atrial arrhythmias in the early postoperative period [34, 35].

By convention, atrial wires are generally brought out through the skin to the right of midline and ventricular leads to the left. Some surgeons will utilize two wires on both an atrium and a ventricle, and others will place only a single wire on one or both chambers, relying on a "ground" lead placed through the skin for the other pacer cable connection.

The convention for pacing mode description (and nursing orders for pacing) indicates that the first letter of the mode description refers to the chamber(s) paced – "A" for atrium, "V" for ventricle, or "D" for dual pacing (both chambers). The second letter refers to the chamber(s) sensed. The third letter reflects the pacer's response to sensing a native electrical signal – "I" if the pacer is inhibited by a sensed native electrical signal; in "D" response mode, the pacer generator's response to a sensed native signal will vary to optimize AV synchrony. For example, when a pacemaker is placed in an AAI mode, the atrium is paced and sensed, and the pacer does not fire (or is "inhibited") when a native atrial signal is detected in the prescribed time interval. In the absence of a native atrial signal, the pacer in this mode will trigger an atrial beat (after which the AAI mode would rely on normal AV nodal and ventricular conduction). There are two additional mode categories for pacing, but for cardiac surgical patients, a three-letter mode designation is adequate.

Most patients will arrive to the ICU after cardiac surgery in an "asynchronous" pacing mode (DOO if both atrial and ventricular leads are in place, otherwise either AOO or VOO). Intraoperative pacer use is generally limited to these asynchronous modes, as otherwise interference from electrocautery use impedes reliable pacing. Upon arrival to the ICU, pacing should be changed to a "synchronous" mode (typically DDD, AAI, or VVI), whereby pacing is coordinated with native conduction. Otherwise there is a risk that the device will deliver an inappropriately timed ventricular signal that can trigger a malignant arrhythmia (e.g., the "R on T" phenomenon, where an ectopic beat takes place on the T-wave of the preceding beat). Patients with A and V wires should usually be placed in DDD pacing mode, with AAI pacing for those with only A wires and VVI if only V wires are in place. For most pacemaker generator devices, the pacing generator can simply be placed in DDD mode, which allows for dual pacing, atrial pacing (by plugging in only A wires or turning V output to zero), or ventricular pacing (by plugging in only V wires or turning A output to zero). In general, isolated ventricular pacing should be avoided except as a "bailout" method to pace patients with complete heart block and no functional atrial wires. The loss of coordinated atrial function with ventricular pacing will compromise cardiac output. The loss of an "atrial kick" will reduce cardiac output by 20% for most patients but can be associated with a greater than 30% detriment in those with underlying heart disease [36].

Nurses should be instructed to check pacing lead "thresholds" daily in any patient with a need for ongoing pacing. This is done by turning each output (A and V) to maximal level (generally 20 mA for V output and 10 mA for A output) and then reducing output until reliable pacing capture is lost. The pacer generator output should generally be set 1–2 mA above this threshold. A high pacing threshold may indicate impending failure of temporary epicardial wires. Typical wire life span has been reported at 4–5 days [37].

Unless otherwise directed by the cardiac surgeon, most patients will arrive to the ICU paced at a rate of 80 or 90 bpm (with some obviously having a native rate in excess of the set pacer rate). In general, the ICU nurses should pause the patient's pacer for an initial 12-lead electrocardiogram (ECG); although if there is any report that a patient may be "pacer-dependent," the surgeon or anesthesiologist should confirm that it is safe to briefly hold pacing. In most cases if the patient is in sinus rhythm with an adequate rate on the morning of the first postoperative day, pacing can be discontinued and the pacer wires capped or placed to a pacer generator with a typical "backup "rate of 40 bpm.

AV node dysfunction is exceedingly rare after CABG, whereas up to 20% of patients will have transient AV block after valve surgery, particularly after re-operative or tricuspid valvular procedures [38]. Sinus node dysfunction may also occur after cardiac surgery, particularly after the maze procedure for atrial fibrillation. In most cases, SA node dysfunction and AV block are transient phenomena (likely related to myocardial edema and the effects of cardioplegia), with less than 5% of valve surgery patients and less than 2% of CABG patients requiring permanent pacemaker implantation [39]. Therefore, it is rare that a "permanent" pacemaker is indicated prior to the fifth postoperative day [39].

"Pacer-dependent patients," defined as those with an absent or non-perfusing native rhythm, demand certain precautions in the ICU until an adequate rhythm ensues (or until an intravascular/endocardial pacing system is in place). Specifically, temporary pacing means (transcutaneous pacer pads and either a pacing PA catheter kit or temporary transvenous pacer wire kit) should be immediately available.

If previously functional temporary epicardial leads cease to function (in spite of maximal output from the pacer generator), there are several bedside maneuvers that may restore epicardial pacing. The simplest maneuver is to reverse polarity on the pacing leads by simply swapping the connections of the two atrial or the two ventricular wires on the pacing cable connector. If this does not work, placement of an additional "ground" wire (Fig. 13.1) through the skin will allow for the trial of different pacing combinations (e.g., one A lead with ground, other A lead with ground), as there need only be a single functional A or V lead for adequate pacing. Finally, one should always consider switching to a new set of pacing cables, as these are an occasional source of pacing failure.

In addition to the use of temporary pacing for patients with bradycardia and/or heart block, temporary pacing can be a simple and very effective means to augment cardiac output. Because pacing at a higher rate decreases relative available time for diastolic filling (thereby reducing stroke volume), the relationship between heart rate and cardiac output is not directly linear. However, for most patients with a low cardiac output and lower heart rate, an increase in pacing rate up to 90 or 100 bpm will significantly augment cardiac output. There are certain patient groups (most notably those with surgery for aortic stenosis and those with severe, longstanding HTN) whose decreased LV compliance demands a longer period for adequate diastolic filling. In such patients, an increase in heart rate may actually reduce cardiac output.

The timing for removal of temporary epicardial pacing leads is highly variable. They are never removed in a pacer-dependent patient until a more reliable means for pacing is in place. For non-pacer-dependent patients, some surgeons will remove the wires as early as the first or second postoperative day, whereas others will leave them in place until the patient is nearing hospital discharge. The argument for later removal is that some patients, particularly those who underwent valve surgery, will develop rhythm disturbances after the second or third postoperative day. The argument for early removal is that a patient is more likely to be in a monitored setting, facilitating the early recognition of bleeding or tamponade after epicardial pacer wire removal. Some cardiac surgeons will leave epicardial wires in place permanently by cutting them just below the level of the skin at the time of discharge. Avoiding pacer wire removal may be particularly indicated for older patients, anticoagulated patients, and/or those with friable tissues.

Based on your institutional protocols, when wire removal is indicated, this is accomplished by cutting the skin suture holding the wire(s) in place and then pulling with steady, firm force at a 45-degree angle. If any significant resistance is encountered, removal should be deferred to the surgical team, or the wire(s) should simply be cut at the skin. After pacer wire removal, most institutions place patients on bed

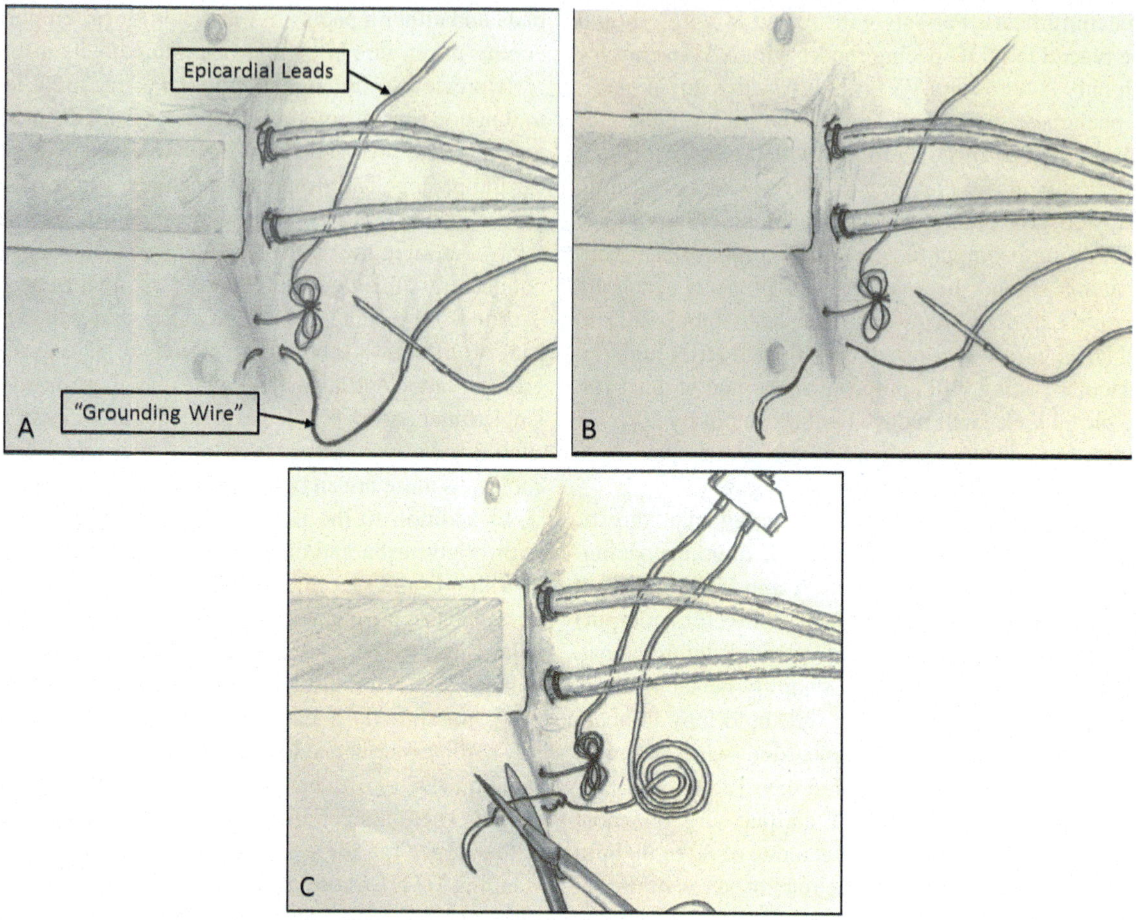

Fig. 13.1 Placement of a cutaneous "ground wire" for temporary epicardial pacing; (**a**) and (**b**) temporary pacemaker wire sewn to the skin; (**c**) exposed portion of the wire is twisted around itself, needle is cut, and the lead is hooked up to a pacing cable (paired with an existing epicardial atrial or ventricular pacing wire)

rest for 1–2 h and ensure that close monitoring is in place. The risk of clinically significant bleeding following pacer wire removal is very low but may necessitate emergent surgical intervention [40].

General Management: Glycemic Control

Strong evidence supporting a mortality benefit (and significant reduction in morbidity) with the use of strict glycemic control for critically ill patients was derived from a study of mostly cardiac surgical patients, which was reported in 2001 [41]. The proposed glucose goal of 80–110 mg/dL from this landmark study can be associated with a significant risk for hypoglycemia [41]. As a result, most institutions presently target a less aggressive glucose goal (< 180–200 mg/dL). A glucose control protocol (employing continuous insulin infusion as needed and sliding scale insulin) should be utilized for at least the first 24 h after cardiac surgery (and ideally for at least 48 h). Beyond the initial period, glycemic control for cardiac surgical patients may be managed in a typical fashion.

General Management: Criteria for Transfusion

There are no evidence-based transfusion criteria specific to the postoperative cardiac surgical population. However, there is compelling evidence linking blood transfusion in postoperative cardiac surgical patients with increases in perioperative and long-term mortality, morbidity, and resource utilization [42, 43]. Red blood cell transfusions should be administered with the intent of improving oxygen delivery, for a patient in whom there are clinical indicators of inadequate tissue perfusion coupled with anemia. In the absence of evidence of end-organ dysfunction, ischemia, or symptoms related to anemia, most institutions utilize a hemoglobin transfusion trigger of 7.0–7.5 mg/dL for stable patients [44]. For patients with ongoing/severe bleeding after cardiac surgery, a more aggressive approach to red blood cell transfusion is critical to maintain adequate tissue-level oxygenation. A typical hemoglobin transfusion trigger for a bleeding patient may be 8.0–9.0 mg/dL (depending on the degree of bleeding, a patient's stability, and a patient's comorbid conditions).

The transfusion of fresh frozen plasma (FFP), cryoprecipitate, or platelets is not typically indicated based on any particular coagulation parameters, fibrinogen level, or platelet count. Rather, these additional blood products are reserved for use in the face of clinical coagulopathy and bleeding. More recently, there is evidence that directed blood component therapy utilizing point of care thromboelastography (TEG) or ROTEM (TEM Systems, Inc. Durham, NC, USA) testing may be the optimal means to direct postoperative transfusion in the setting of bleeding or clinical coagulopathy [45]. The mechanical effects of cardiopulmonary bypass impair platelet function. Therefore, a normal platelet count in a bleeding postoperative patient should not preclude platelet transfusion in the appropriate clinical setting.

Specific Management: Intra-aortic Balloon Pump Management

For the appropriate patient, intra-aortic balloon pump (IABP) counterpulsation therapy can provide a highly effective means to improve cardiac output, by reducing systemic afterload and augmenting coronary perfusion, and can favorably influence the myocardial blood flow supply/demand ratio. An IABP may be in place preoperatively for some cardiac surgical patients – most often those with an acute coronary syndrome and ongoing ischemia/shock or those with acute heart failure/shock due to valvular disease. In this setting, the IABP is left in place through the cardiac surgical procedure and can generally be removed at an interval between 12 h and 2 days after surgery. In some patients with severely impaired LV function, an IABP will be placed electively just prior to (or during) cardiac surgery to facilitate weaning from cardiopulmonary bypass and to support hemodynamic stability during the early postoperative period. An IABP may be placed on bypass for a patient in whom separation from cardiopulmonary bypass has been unsuccessful in spite of high-dose vasoactive pharmacologic support. Finally, there are rare circumstances where an IABP may be placed postoperatively for a cardiac surgical patient in the ICU, typically for a patient with reduced LV function and a persistent low cardiac output state with ongoing poor perfusion.

Absolute contraindications to IABP placement are significant aortic valve insufficiency and aortic dissection, whereas relative contraindications include abdominal aortic aneurysm (increased risk for embolic complications) and advanced peripheral vascular disease (increased risk of limb ischemia) [46].

IABP placement involves either placing the device using TEE or fluoroscopic guidance directly via the femoral artery or more commonly placing the balloon device via a femoral arterial sheath (which is included in the IABP kit). Rarely, IABP placement intraoperatively may occur via the axillary/subclavian artery or by direct aortic insertion, which is generally used in a salvage setting for a patient with planned temporary closure and anticipated return to the OR.

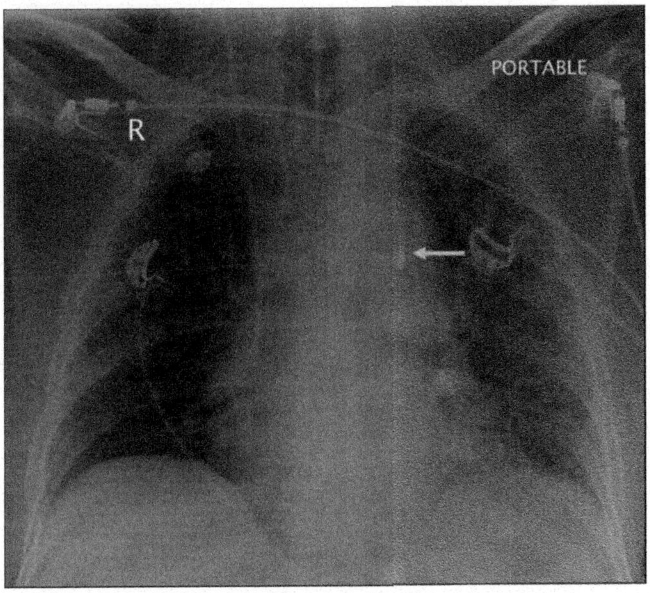

Fig. 13.2 Chest radiograph demonstrating appropriate intra-aortic balloon pump position, as indicated by visualization of the radio-opaque tip marker (arrow) in the proximal descending thoracic aorta, distal to level of left subclavian artery takeoff

After placement, the balloon pump is generally started at 1:1 support (meaning that the balloon inflates/deflates with every cardiac cycle). IABP support may be reduced to 1:2 if tolerated. The 1:3 setting is generally utilized only for a brief interval (20–30 min) during consideration of IABP removal to assess whether a patient's hemodynamics and perfusion will support IABP removal. There are three available triggers for balloon inflation (during early diastole) and deflation (just prior to systole) – the device can be triggered based on rhythm/ECG (most often used), arterial blood pressure, or pacemaker input. The use of a rhythm trigger requires that IABP leads be in place on the patient. Most modern IABP devices have sophisticated software that will determine and automatically implement the optimal trigger and timing for balloon function, so unless you have extensive IABP experience, the "auto" setting is recommended.

A chest x-ray is needed to confirm IABP placement. The IABP has a radio-opaque marker near the device tip, which should be visualized in the proximal descending aorta (Fig. 13.2). Placement of the device too far proximally can occlude the left subclavian artery and affect left upper extremity blood flow, whereas overly distal placement can affect perfusion to the renal arteries. When a patient arrives in the ICU with an IABP in place, the ICU team must always verify that the device is adequately secured to the patient's groin/thigh, as patient movement may otherwise displace the position of the IABP. Additional sutures may need to be placed.

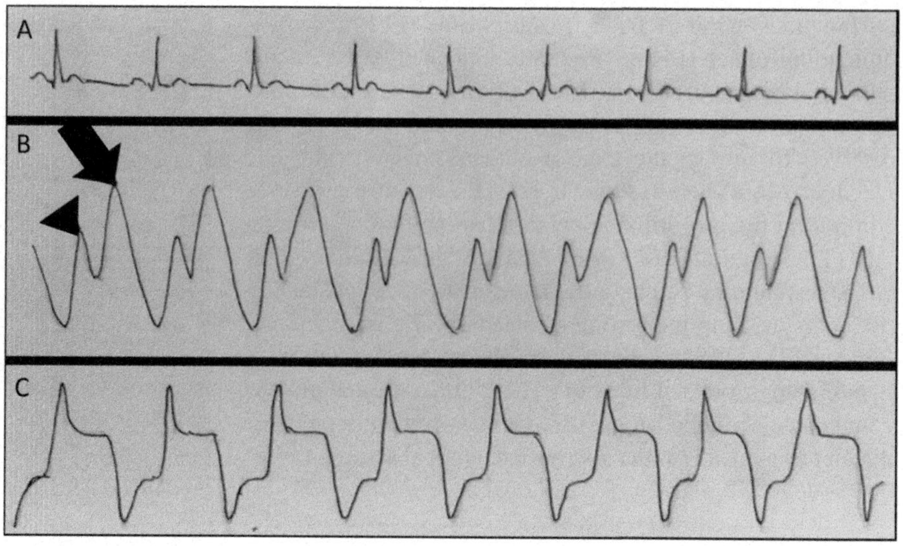

Fig. 13.3 Typical intra-aortic balloon pump console display; (**a**), trace and number reflect rhythm and heart rate, respectively; (**b**), trace reflects arterial blood pressure from site of balloon pump transducer, with numbers reflecting systolic, diastolic, and mean pressures; (**c**), trace reflects balloon pressure waveform and displays the numeric "augmented diastolic" blood pressure; note that on arterial pressure trace, the augmented diastolic pressure (arrow) is well above systolic blood pressure (arrowhead)

If the IABP is functioning correctly, the augmented diastolic arterial pressure, as displayed on the console, will be the highest reading, followed by systolic pressure, and finally the un-augmented diastolic pressure (Fig. 13.3). Vasoactive drip titration should generally target an augmented diastolic pressure in the 90s and a mean arterial pressure of 60–70 mmHg on the IABP console. The central monitor readings, such as a radial arterial line pressure tracings, such not be used. Although data is limited, anticoagulation is generally not indicated/necessary for IABP placement after cardiac surgery [47].

The chief complication associated with IABP use is limb malperfusion/ischemia, due to either embolism or due to compromise of flow from the device/sheath itself. Both of these complications are much more common in patients with advanced peripvheral vascular disease, for whom an IABP should be placed/used with extreme caution. While an IABP is in place, pedal pulses must be monitored closely. The loss of detectable pedal signals demands immediate IABP removal. For a patient who is truly dependent on IABP support, this scenario may require contralateral placement of a new device.

When femoral IABP removal is directed by the surgical team (generally after ensuring that the underlying indication has been corrected or resolved and that there is not a significant ongoing coagulopathy), this can usually be accomplished at the bedside. After ensuring that the IABP is not critical for a patient's continued stability (by assessing blood pressure, cardiac output, and perfusion during an interval of 1:3 support), the sutures holding the device/sheath are cut, the IABP is placed on "standby," and the device is removed. If the IABP is placed via a femoral arterial sheath, the IABP device cannot be removed through the sheath due to sizing. Instead, the IABP is backed up to the sheath until there is resistance, after which the sheath and balloon are removed as a unit. After the device and sheath are out, the distal femoral artery is firmly occluded for a single heartbeat, and then the proximal femoral artery (well above the insertion site) is transiently occluded – both these measures are intended to reduce the risk of the embolization of thrombus/debris. Next, firm pressure is applied over the insertion site in the femoral artery (which is generally 1–2 cm *cephalad to* the site of skin insertion) for a minimum of 30 min. Pedal pulses should be assessed periodically during this time, as overly aggressive pressure can occlude arterial flow to the limb and lead to thrombotic occlusion. After 30 min of direct pressure, a pressure dressing, sandbag, or a compression assist device is placed, and the ICU nursing team continues pulse monitoring. The patient should remain on bed rest (with hips not flexed beyond 30°) for several hours after removal, and the IABP site should be monitored regularly for bleeding or hematoma. In a patient with new hypotension or progressive anemia after IABP removal, one must always be cognizant of the possibility of retroperitoneal bleeding. In some circumstances (ongoing coagulopathy, severe vascular disease, surgeon preferences), the cardiac surgical team may opt to remove the IABP device/sheath surgically via direct cutdown and repair. This procedure may be accomplished either at the bedside or during a return to the OR.

Specific Management: Postoperative Bleeding

Unlike most other surgical procedures, a certain amount of bleeding is not only tolerated but is expected after cardiac surgery. All cardiac patients will have some combination of pleural and mediastinal chest tubes/drains. Acceptable output from chest drains will vary a great deal based on the type and conduct of a cardiac surgical procedure and the modus operandi of the surgeon. For example, while 250 ml total tube output may not be cause for concern in the first hour after a redo double valve with CABG x 3, a similar drain output in a patient who underwent a "routine" two-vessel CABG certainly demands attention.

Generally speaking, total chest tube output of less than 100 ml/hour in the presence of clinically patent drains predicts a very low likelihood that there is surgical bleeding. In contrast, drain output over 150–200 ml/hour should always be of concern, particularly after the first hour in the ICU, during which initial tube output may reflect the evacuation of retained irrigation fluid vice ongoing bleeding. One must be cognizant that a reduction in chest tube output in a previously bleeding patient is not always a positive development. In particular, if sudden cessation of drain output coincides with deteriorating hemodynamics, this is a scenario highly suggestive of tamponade. Just as important as (if not more important than) the hourly drain output is the trend over time. Chest tube output of 150 ml in the third hour after ICU arrival in a patient with previous hourly outputs of 300 ml and 200 ml is certainly of less concern than the same output in a patient with hourly drainage of less than 50 ml/hour for the first two hours.

The fundamental decision in a postoperative cardiac surgical patient with excessive mediastinal/pleural drain output is whether operative management is indicated. There are three general categories of postoperative bleeding: (1) massive exsanguination with arrest or imminent arrest; (2) bleeding that is less dramatic, but which will clearly require emergency re-exploration; or (3) bleeding felt to be medically manageable. The cardiac surgical literature supports an aggressive surgical approach in the face of persistent significant bleeding [48]. Early return to the OR is often preferred over expectant management and continued blood product transfusions, particularly if bleeding persists after the correction of coagulopathy and hypothermia.

For the clinical scenario of massive bleeding with arrest or imminent arrest, immediate surgical management is paramount and may need to be performed in the ICU. From the standpoint of sterility, lighting, and resource availability, it is always preferable to manage bleeding in the OR. However, in rare instances, a patient's condition may not allow sufficient time to mobilize the patient and necessary resources. Concomitant with bedside re-exploration, blood products should be obtained immediately, including activation of a massive transfusion protocol. The cardiac surgical team should be immediately mobilized, as all patients surviving bedside ICU re-exploration will need to be taken to the OR for more definitive management, washout, and temporary or permanent closure.

There are relatively new, evidence-based guidelines for bedside re-exploration in postoperative cardiac surgical patients [49], which should be reviewed and customized for each institution. Some of the key elements of these recommendations include the immediate availability of a streamlined set of necessary instruments/supplies and ensuring appropriate training of all ICU team members who might assist in this scenario. The initial steps in emergent bedside sternal re-exploration can be summarized as follows: place a large drape (do not attempt a sterile surgical skin prep); cut through the skin incision (cut around skin staples if used in skin closure) and cut through the sutures closing the soft tissues/fascia; cut and remove all sternal wires; and carefully place a retractor and gradually open the retractor blades. In the setting of bleeding with tamponade, the action of opening the sternum is often all that is needed to allow for the temporary restoration of perfusion (allowing for transport to the OR for more definitive management). If there is massive, ongoing bleeding immediately apparent after sternal retractor placement (such as from an aortic or venous cannulation site, a cardiac or great vessel suture line, or an avulsed coronary graft), unless you have extensive cardiac surgical experience, attempt digital control to temporize the bleeding while blood products are administered and resources are mobilized for definitive control of the bleeding source in the OR by a cardiac surgeon.

In the setting of significant ongoing bleeding clearly indicating re-exploration, but absent arrest or impending arrest, once again blood products should be obtained and the cardiac surgical OR team should be mobilized. The bedside chest re-entry cart should be placed in close proximity to the patient's room in case bedside re-entry is needed prior to a patient's transport to the OR. Just as in other bleeding scenarios, permissive hypotension is appropriate in this setting, allowing for the lowest blood pressure associated with clinical perfusion. If hypotension is severe and demands intervention prior to readiness of the surgical team, the use of vasoactive medications should be strictly avoided. Instead, the patient should be treated with volume resuscitation (with blood products whenever available).

A more common clinical scenario involves postoperative bleeding that exceeds the expected/acceptable rate but where there is no indication for immediate re-exploration. The decision for non-operative management must be individualized and must involve communication with the attending cardiac surgeon but is typified by a patient with transiently high drain output but generally acceptable hemodynamics and adequate end-organ perfusion. Non-operative management is also the initial treatment of choice in the setting of bleeding with a severe coagulopathy and when chest drain output is steadily downtrending (without clinical evidence of tamponade).

Elements of care for the non-operative management of bleeding after cardiac surgery can be remembered using the "P's" pneumonic (Fig. 13.4):

Fig. 13.4 Management of "nonsurgical" bleeding after cardiac surgery

Plasma for INR > ~1.3 or as driven by point of care testing; supplement with cryoprecipitate if fibrinogen level < 100 - 150 mg/dL	**Platelets** if platelet count below 80 - 100,000/uL or evidence of functional platelet deficit; consider IV desmopressin acetate if renal failure/uremia
Protamine if Activated Clotting Time above 120 – 140 sec or Partial Thromboplastin Time > ~40 sec	**Positive End Expiratory Pressure (PEEP)** increased to 8 – 10 cmH_2O
Poikilothermia (aka hypothermia) treated aggressively	**Packed** red blood cell transfusion considered with lower than normal threshold for transfusion
Pressure (Blood) goal of lowest possible pressure to support adequate clinical perfusion (typically systolic pressures 80s to 90s mmHg)	**Prothrombinase** concentrate (off-label) or activated recombinant factor VIIa can be considered, particularly in setting of refractory coagulopathy
Partners consulted for input	**Prolene** (surgical intervention) may be needed if bleeding does not abate with other "Ps" or if clinical decline

- *P*lasma should be administered for any significant elevation in the international normalized ratio (INR) of a bleeding patient (or as driven by point-of-care functional testing). In a bleeding patient, fibrinogen level should be assessed. If the fibrinogen level is less than 100–150 mg/dL in this setting, 6–10 units of cryoprecipitate (which contains fibrinogen and clotting factors, particularly factor VIII) should be administered.
- *P*latelets should be administered for a bleeding patient with a platelet count below 80–100,000/uL, where there is TEG or ROTEM evidence of a functional platelet deficit or where there is clinical suspicion of such a deficit (as might occur in the setting of a prolonged cardiopulmonary bypass time or the preoperative administration of antiplatelet therapy). IV desmopressin acetate (DDAVP) may have some benefit in alleviating platelet dysfunction, is typically dosed at 0.3 mg/kg in this setting, and may be particularly indicated for a bleeding patient with renal failure/uremia [24, 50].
- *P*rotamine is indicated to reverse any residual heparin, as evidenced by an activated clotting time (ACT) above 120–140 s or a significantly prolonged partial thromboplastin time (PTT). Typically, a dose of 10–25 mg is adequate (and should be administered slowly to minimize associated hypotension). Excessive protamine administration is contraindicated, as this may actually lead to coagulopathy and platelet dysfunction [51].
- *P*ositive end-expiratory pressure (PEEP) is thought to have a favorable effect on chest wall bleeding by promoting contact between the lungs and the chest wall (typically increasing PEEP to 8–10 cmH_2O), although the use of increased PEEP in this setting is not supported by strong evidence.
- *P*oikilothermia (aka hypothermia) must be treated aggressively with active rewarming (Bair Hugger, fluid warmer, etc.).
- *P*acked red blood cell transfusion may be indicated with a lower threshold for transfusion, recognizing that in the setting of ongoing bleeding, laboratory hemoglobin values do not reflect actual equilibrated levels.
- *P*ressure (blood) management is critical, including the strict avoidance of HTN and a target blood pressure of the lowest possible pressure associated with adequate clinical perfusion (typically systolic pressures in the 80s to 90s mmHg).
- *P*rothrombinase concentrate (off-label use) or activated recombinant factor VIIa can be considered, particularly in the setting of refractory coagulopathy. There is retrospective evidence suggesting that either of these medications may have therapeutic value in patients with excessive bleeding after cardiac surgery. However, because there are reports of thrombotic complications (including stroke and coronary graft thrombosis) with the use of these adjuncts, and because these medications are costly, the decision for their use should always involve discussion with the patient's cardiac surgeon [52].
- Never hesitate to seek assistance from your experienced clinical *P*artners, as clinical decision-making for patients in this scenario may be complex and dynamic.
- Finally if all else fails, the "last P" in the algorithm (other than the less reliable modalities of *P*rayer and *P*anic) is *P*rolene – indicating the need for surgical re-exploration.

One should never hesitate to reoperate for bleeding if there is not a prompt response to other treatments, as it is far better to have a "negative" re-exploration (absence of a clear, focal surgical bleeding source) than to allow for protracted end-organ malperfusion from bleeding and/or the effects of massive blood product transfusions.

When pursuing non-operative therapy for bleeding after cardiac surgery, one most always remain cognizant that the cessation of bleeding should not normally be accompanied by deteriorating hemodynamics and perfusion. This constellation of findings is highly suggestive of tamponade (the diagnosis and management of which is described below).

Specific Management: Cardiac Tamponade

Cardiac tamponade occurs in a small proportion of patients undergoing cardiac surgery, with an incidence of <0.5% after isolated CABG, an intermediate incidence after valve surgery, and an incidence of up to 8% after cardiac transplantation [53]. Tamponade most often occurs in patients with excessive bleeding in the OR and/or in the early postoperative period. Tamponade occurring within the first 24 hrs is most commonly related to postoperative bleeding, but late tamponade (>10 days post-procedure) is likely multifactorial [54].

The primary pathological mechanism of shock in the setting of tamponade is compromised venous return to the left heart (preload). Unlike medical causes of tamponade, most postoperative cases result from compression of a single cardiac chamber (most commonly the right atrium) by focal hematoma or fluid collection(s) [53, 54].

The diagnosis of tamponade after cardiac surgery can be challenging in some cases, as the presentation of tamponade may share clinical features with those associated with post-cardiopulmonary bypass LV dysfunction, inflammatory response, prosthetic valve dysfunction, or inappropriate volume loading. It typically manifests as hypotension, tachycardia, and a low output state, most commonly the result of cardiac chamber compression and associated LV under-filling. However, the clinical manifestations of postoperative tamponade are highly variable and nonspecific, particularly in the setting of single-chamber compression. Pulsus paradoxus and equalization of right and left heart pressures are seen in a minority of cases, and CVP elevation is not a consistent finding [55]. A CXR demonstrating marked interval enlargement of the cardiomediastinal silhouette (and/or pleural space opacification, if the pleural spaces were opened at surgery) relative to the patient's previous postoperative study certainly supports the diagnosis of tamponade in the appropriate clinical setting.

Because compression of a single cardiac chamber may not affect normal function of the remaining chambers, the typical echocardiographic features of medical tamponade are not reliably present in patients after cardiac operations. Transthoracic echocardiography (TTE) may be diagnostic in some patients, revealing a hyperdynamic but empty left ventricle, diastolic collapse of the right atrium/ventricle, and possibly direct visualization of cardiac chamber compression due to hematoma. However, TTE is often technically unsatisfactory in the early postoperative period due to air in the pericardium, limitations in positioning, or interference from dressings and monitoring devices [56]. Although TEE is a reliable diagnostic modality for clinically suspected tamponade [56], it is rarely immediately available in the ICU.

Cardiac tamponade must be high in the differential diagnosis for any patient with a persistent low cardiac output state or persistent hypotension after cardiac surgery. In the "classic" scenario of a patient with decreased blood pressure and malperfusion after the cessation of previously excessive chest tube output, no further diagnostic testing is indicated prior to surgical re-exploration. However, the presentation of tamponade after cardiac surgery is often not so straightforward, as it can coincide with continued excessive chest tube output and may initially respond to volume resuscitation. If there is clinical concern for tamponade in a relatively stable patient and TEE is immediately available, then this is the diagnostic modality of choice. Otherwise, the best diagnostic means for suspected tamponade is surgical re-exploration.

Although many cases of late tamponade (after 1 week) can be managed percutaneously, immediate surgical intervention represents the only consistently effective management of tamponade early after cardiac surgery [53, 55]. While mobilizing appropriate resources, one must specifically avoid the administration of either vasopressors or inotropes for a patient with suspected tamponade, as these agents will only further negatively affect cardiac output and myocardial oxygen consumption. The only appropriate temporizing measure is IV resuscitation (with blood products or fluid). Discontinuing PEEP and reducing tidal volumes may help transiently improve preload.

If a patient with suspected tamponade manifests cardiopulmonary arrest or hemodynamic instability that would preclude safe transport to the OR, immediate bedside ICU exploration is indicated, the steps in which have been outlined previously in this chapter. In the case of tamponade, generally the removal of sternal wires and placement of a sternal retractor allow for restoration of adequate preload to significantly improve a patient's hemodynamics. In the scenario where sternal re-entry alone stabilizes a patient, it is best to defer further interventions until the patient is transported to the OR for definitive care by the cardiac surgical team. If retractor placement alone does not lead to immediate hemodynamic improvement, further exploration and/or open cardiac massage may be necessary. Of note, in the rare case of a patient presenting with tamponade and cardiac arrest more than 10 days after cardiac surgery, bedside re-exploration is ill advised due to the likely presence of significant adhesions [49].

After placing the sternal retractor, the next step is visualization of the surgical field, with specific attention to the presence of obvious hematoma and/or bleeding, and assessment of cardiac activity. Specifically, because the pericardium is opened at the time of cardiac surgery, the right ventricle should be immediately apparent after sternal retraction. Any obvious hematoma should be carefully extracted manually with adjunctive suctioning. If the patient remains profoundly hypotensive at this stage and particularly if right ventricular activity is minimal or absent, open cardiac massage is necessary.

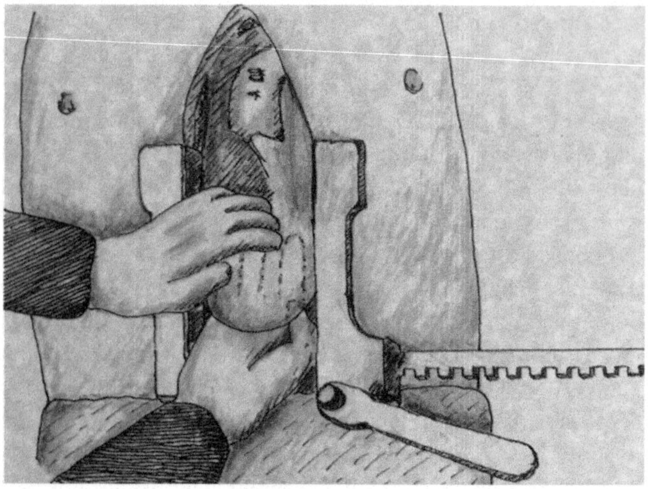

Fig. 13.5 Proper technique for two-handed open cardiac massage via median sternotomy; if standing on the patient's right, the right hand is slid along the diaphragm to a point posterior to the heart (to avoid injuring any coronary grafts); the fingers on both hands remain opposed to avoid digital cardiac injury

Safe open cardiac massage necessitates a two-handed technique with opposed fingers, to avoid digital perforation of a cardiac chamber (Fig. 13.5). The location and angle of compression should be adjusted to optimize blood pressure based on invasive arterial monitoring, when available. If coronary grafts are present, avoiding graft injury or avulsion is of paramount importance; as without the immediate bedside presence of a cardiac surgeon, this likely represents a terminal event. The safest means to introduce one's hand into the posterior pericardium for two-handed massage (from the patient's right side) is to slide the fingers of the right hand immediately along the diaphragm (to avoid graft avulsion). Gently sweeping the right hand so that it is located immediately posterior to the heart should avoid direct compression of any typical suture lines.

Specific Management: Low Cardiac Output State

As described previously, the determination of a low cardiac output state is based on clinical assessment rather than a specific numeric value. If a cardiac output and index are available, most patients with a low cardiac output state have a cardiac index below 2–2.2 L/min/m^2. Although a cardiac index above this level is a reassuring piece of information, it should be supported by an adequate mixed venous oxygen saturation, normal or downtrending serum lactate, well-perfused extremities, adequate urine output, etc.

When there is clinical evidence of a low cardiac output state, one should always first assess for significant bleeding, cardiac tamponade, and myocardial ischemia, as these are conditions that often require immediate intervention for effective treatment. Only after these surgical emergencies have been ruled out (to the extent possible) should management proceed otherwise. One approach to low cardiac output is to assess and treat the following variables affecting cardiac output in series: RATE, RHYTHM, PRELOAD, AFTERLOAD, and CONTRACTILITY. As with other aspects of management for cardiac surgical patients, it is important to avoid making multiple interventions simultaneously (outside of a cardiac arrest scenario). Rather, one should be able to make a targeted intervention and assess for effect, as the presence or absence of a favorable response will guide further management (Fig. 13.6).

As described previously, pacing at a higher rate (ideally utilizing atrial or dual pacing) will significantly augment cardiac output for most patients. Certainly, the restoration of sinus rhythm (where possible) in patients with atrial arrhythmias and low cardiac output will have a favorable effect on clinical perfusion. With regard to assessment for preload, PA pressures and CVP assessment provide the highest reliability when reviewed over time and when assessed relative to changes after fluid administration. Regardless of the cause of low cardiac output, with the possible exception of a patient with advanced right ventricular dysfunction/failure, volume administration (albumin, crystalloid, or blood products where appropriate) is a safe early move in the management of low cardiac output. Fluid administration may be both therapeutic and diagnostic; as if it is followed by significant improvement in cardiac output, it is very likely that the patient has inadequate intravascular volume/preload. Afterload reduction with IV vasodilator medications may be appropriate in a patient with reduced cardiac output and elevated systemic vascular resistance. Augmenting cardiac contractility (with inotropic medications) is typically employed only after addressing rate, rhythm, preload, and afterload, as all inotropic medications have the potential for significant deleterious secondary effects. Finally, mechanical support (IABP placement or in advanced cases the initiation of ventricular assist device [VAD] or extracorporeal membrane oxygenation [ECMO] support) may be necessary if the above interventions fail to restore adequate cardiac output to support end-organ perfusion.

Specific Management: Management of the Open Chest

In rare circumstances, primary sternal closure is either not attempted or is aborted at the time of a cardiac surgical procedure. Scenarios where this management strategy may be applied include extremely protracted cardiac surgical procedures (where edema precludes safe closure), severe coagulopathic bleeding (with anticipated need for return/washout),

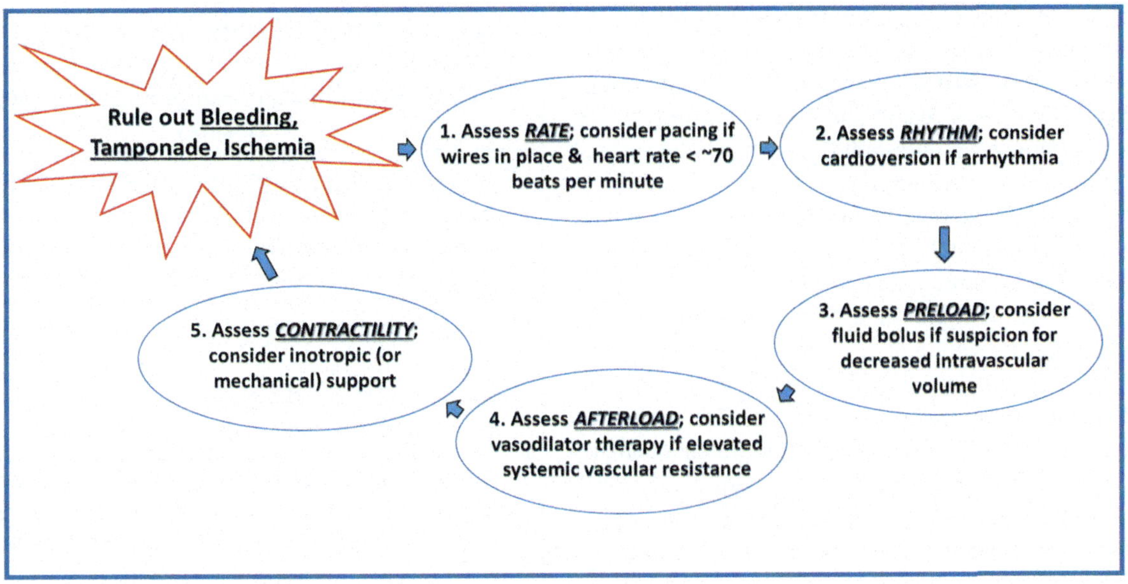

Fig. 13.6 Algorithm for the management of low cardiac output after cardiac surgery

and when a patient requires mechanical support (VAD or ECMO) to leave the OR. In these cases, the sternum will remain open, and the chest will be temporarily closed with either a vacuum sponge dressing, gauze, occlusive iodine-impregnated drape, or some combination of the above.

The management of a patient with an open chest does not differ a great deal from that of a typical postoperative patient, keeping in mind that by definition a patient requiring temporary closure will be acutely ill and unstable. It is important to realize that a temporary sternal closure does not preclude the development of tamponade. Visible bulging of a clear, occlusive dressing or wound vac dressing can be a sign of extensive clot formation in the chest. If tamponade is suspected in a patient with a temporary closure, therapy is relatively straightforward and simply entails removal of the temporary closure to allow for assessment and treatment (either in the OR or in the ICU for a particularly unstable patient).

The timing for return to the OR for washout and possible closure will vary based on the reason for temporary closure and a patient's course/condition. It is rare to plan return to the OR before the first postoperative day, unless needed to manage bleeding or tamponade. If closure was aborted due to edema, aggressive diuresis should be initiated once a patient's condition will tolerate it. Most surgeons would return to the OR around the second postoperative day in this setting, realizing that conditions at that time may still not be satisfactory for closure, but that this would at least allow for a washout and reassessment of conditions in the operative field. If chest closure was aborted due to coagulopathy and bleeding, most surgeons would return to the OR sooner than the second postoperative day, in the hopes of performing washout and closure at that time (assuming bleeding and coagulopathy have resolved). In the setting of an open chest with ongoing mechanical circulatory support, plans to return to the OR will vary widely depending on the scenario and a patient's ICU course.

Specific Management: Oliguria/Renal Failure

The management of oliguria and/or new renal dysfunction after cardiac surgery is similar to that in other surgical ICU patients. As in all cases, bladder ultrasound and flushing the bladder catheter are important initial measures in an oliguric patient. Determining the exact prevalence of acute kidney injury (AKI) after cardiac surgery is limited by widely variable definitions of AKI. Regardless of definition, AKI complicates a substantial proportion of cardiac surgical procedures [57]. One to three percent of cardiac surgery patients develop a new postoperative dialysis requirement (which is associated with a new permanent dialysis requirement in the majority of cases), with the strongest predictor being abnormal baseline renal function [57].

Although new renal dysfunction is associated with a significantly greater risk for other major complications and mortality, no perioperative strategies have demonstrated consistent success in preventing this complication [58]. Regardless, fundamental principles of optimal postoperative cardiac surgical care, such as minimizing vasopressor use, maintaining adequate intravascular volume and cardiac output, and minimizing exposure to nephrotoxic medications, will all reduce the likelihood of renal injury. Cardiac tamponade can on occasion present with isolated oliguria and renal insufficiency, particularly when it occurs beyond the early postoperative period. Therefore, in addition to the standard clinical evaluation for patients with new renal failure (urine electrolyte and microscopy studies, renal ultrasound), an echocardiogram is appropriate for post-cardiac surgical patients.

As in any patient with renal failure, all nephrotoxic medications must be immediately discontinued and other medication dosages adjusted appropriately. Although not explicitly a renal toxin, any ACE inhibitor and ARB medications should be discontinued in the setting of new renal insufficiency [59]. As in other ICU populations, low-dose dopamine has no role in the treatment (or prevention) of renal insufficiency after cardiac surgery [60]. Medications such as fenoldopam (a selective DA-1 dopamine receptor agonist), carperitide (atrial natriuretic peptide), and nesiritide (human B-type natriuretic peptide) have been studied for the prevention and treatment of renal failure after cardiac surgery with inconclusive results to date. Because the administration of these medications can cause significant hypotension, their routine use after cardiac surgery cannot be recommended at this time. As with other populations with renal failure, there is no evidence that loop diuretics or mannitol affects the likelihood of renal recovery or the overall prognosis in cardiac surgical patients.

Specific Management: Right Ventricular Dysfunction and Pulmonary Hypertension

Cardiac surgical patients with significant right ventricular (RV) dysfunction can present extreme management challenges in the postoperative setting. In some cases, patients may have preexisting RV dysfunction, whereas other patients may develop new RV dysfunction at the time of surgery. The latter scenario carries a particularly high risk for mortality [61].

Preexisting RV dysfunction in cardiac surgical patients is most often secondary to chronic left-sided heart failure and/or cardiac valvular disease (particularly with mitral stenosis, tricuspid regurgitation, or advanced mitral regurgitation). It can also occur secondary to RV myocardial infarction, severe chronic lung disease ("cor pulmonale"), chronic pulmonary hypertension, or from congenital heart disease.

New RV dysfunction after cardiac surgery may result from inadequate myocardial protection during the period of ischemic arrest. Right coronary artery (RCA) occlusion and associated RV ischemic dysfunction can occur after CABG if there is a technical anastomotic error or coronary dissection at the time of RCA grafting. An aortic valve prosthetic can occlude the RCA ostium during aortic valve replacement, or the RCA can be kinked due to excessive redundancy after reimplantation during an aortic root replacement ("modified Bentall" procedure). Coronary air embolism is very common in the immediate period after separation from

ASSESS/TREAT ANY POTENTIALLY CORRECTABLE PATHOLOGY (surgical coronary obstruction, massive pulmonary embolism, compromise from sternal closure)

OPTIMIZE RIGHT VENTRICULAR PRELOAD; unless obvious fluid overload, initiate cautious volume loading with continuous monitoring of filling pressures, cardiac output, hemodynamics

AVOID SECONDARY INSULT to right ventricular function; aggressively treat hypoxia, acidosis, hypercapnia; avoid high airway pressures; correct arrhythmias, systemic hypotension

APPROPRIATE SUPPORTIVE THERAPY; if elevated pulmonary pressures, consider inhaled pulmonary vasodilator therapy; initiate inotropic/mechanical support if needed

Fig. 13.7 Overview of the management of new right ventricular dysfunction/failure after cardiac surgery

bypass and most often embolizes into the right coronary circulation [61]. However, it is rare that RV dysfunction from air embolism would persist through transport to the ICU or occur de novo after ICU transfer. Massive pulmonary embolism (PE) is very uncommon after cardiac surgery but should always be considered in a patient with new significant RV dysfunction, particularly when there is no obvious alternative etiology. RV failure may occur after cardiac transplantation or LVAD placement. Inappropriate sternal closure after a protracted cardiac surgery with extensive tissue edema (particularly in an obese patient) may lead to compromise of RV function postoperatively. A "type III" protamine reaction may manifest as transient RV dysfunction with elevated PA pressures shortly after protamine exposure, although most often this condition will present in the OR and will have resolved with supportive therapy by the time of ICU arrival. Finally, for cardiac surgical patients with a complex or protracted course, sepsis and acute respiratory distress syndrome may contribute to new RV dysfunction.

RV dysfunction can contribute to low overall cardiac output due to RV systolic dysfunction and/or diastolic dysfunction, both of which impair the delivery of blood to the left cardiac circulation. Tricuspid regurgitation (TR), which may be either the result or the cause of RV dysfunction, will further decrease effective preload. The treatment of RV dysfunction after cardiac surgery should begin with correction of any apparent reversible cause, optimization of RV preload, and appropriate supportive therapy to avoid secondary RV insult (Fig. 13.7).

Volume optimization in patients with RV dysfunction/failure can be very difficult – while intravascular hypovolemia will reduce RV preload and overall cardiac output, excessive volume loading may paradoxically decrease LV preload by increasing pericardial constraint. If there is obvious clinical fluid overload in a patient with RV dysfunction (as may occur in the setting of biventricular failure), progressive diuresis is indicated. Otherwise, cautious volume loading is indicated, with continuous monitoring of CVP, cardiac output, and hemodynamics.

Potentially reversible causes of new RV dysfunction after cardiac surgery include surgical RCA occlusion from an intraoperative technical error (which would most often mandate immediate surgical re-intervention). Acute massive PE may be treatable with anticoagulation and thrombolysis or surgical thrombectomy (particularly when associated with hemodynamic instability, in addition to RV dysfunction). If primary sternal closure in an edematous patient has resulted in functional RV compromise, return to the OR for conversion to temporary closure will be therapeutic.

In order to optimize RV function, hypoxia, acidosis, and hypercapnia must be treated aggressively, as these conditions will increase RV afterload and exacerbate RV dysfunction. The optimization of pH, pO2, and pCO2 may require continued mechanical ventilation. Every effort must be made to avoid high mean airway pressures (and high PEEP), which can further compromise RV preload. Toward this end, a short inspiratory time to expiratory time ratio should be used, and deep sedation (or even paralysis) may be needed. Any significant pleural effusion should be drained to optimize oxygenation and ventilation. Atrial tachyarrhythmias are poorly tolerated in patients with significant RV dysfunction and should be treated with immediate direct current cardioversion (DCCV) whenever possible. Systemic hypotension must be avoided; as in addition to its other untoward effects, hypotension may exacerbate RV dysfunction by contributing to RV ischemia.

If the optimization of a patient's volume status, correction of any reversible etiology, and optimal systemic support fail to result in adequate overall cardiac output and clinical perfusion in a patient with RV dysfunction after cardiac surgery, then the addition of RV afterload reduction and/or RV inotropic support may be needed.

When RV dysfunction coincides with significant pulmonary arterial hypertension (PAH), a reduction in PA pressures to reduce RV work may be achieved with inhaled nitric oxide (iNO), inhaled epoprostenol, or using certain inotropic medications. Although nonspecific vasodilators (such as sodium nitroprusside or nitroglycerin) may reduce pulmonary resistance, because they also reduce systemic pressures, these medications have little specific role in the management of RV dysfunction. Of the approved options to reduce PAH, inhaled agents (where available) represent the optimal treatment, as they do not affect systemic blood pressure (nor do they preclude the use of systemic vasopressors when needed). iNO is very costly, but for patients with significant PAH in the setting of moderate or severe postoperative RV dysfunction, it is often very effective. It is generally started at a dose of 10 ppm (through the ventilator circuit) and can be advanced slowly up to 40 ppm as needed for effect. After a patient's condition has stabilized, iNO can be gradually weaned off, can be transitioned to lower-dose therapy via face mask administration, or may be transitioned to oral sildenafil therapy. While less potent than iNO as a pulmonary vasodilator, inhaled prostacyclin has similar effects, can also be given via the ventilator circuit or via face mask/tent, and is less costly. The usual effective dose of inhaled prostacyclin is 30 ng/kg/min. When inhaled agents are unavailable or when inotropic support is otherwise needed, milrinone and dobutamine both have favorable effects on PAH (although due to their systemic vasodilatory effects, the use of either of these agents may require additional systemic vasopressor support).

When RV inotropic support is needed in the absence of significant PAH, the most appropriate inotropic medications for RV dysfunction are isoproterenol, milrinone, dobutamine, dopamine, and epinephrine. IV isoproterenol infusion can be very effective in augmenting RV contractility, but its effectiveness may be limited by significant tachycardia. Milrinone infusion will typically augment both RV and LV contractility and will improve RV diastolic function, although systemic vasodilator effects may limit its use. A low- to moderate-dose dobutamine infusion will generally augment RV contractility and increase cardiac output through both direct inotropic effects and improvement in RV filling/preload. If RV dysfunction coexists with severe systemic hypotension, dopamine or epinephrine infusion therapy may be most appropriate.

When all of the above measures fail to achieve adequate perfusion in a patient with postoperative RV failure, the only remaining treatments involve mechanical circulatory support. IABP counterpulsation is generally not of much value for RV failure [62]. However right ventricular assist device (RVAD) support may be used as a bridge to transplantation or to recovery (particularly for patients with RV failure after the institution of LVAD support). ECMO support may be the only treatment option if a patient has the combination of refractory RV failure and refractory hypoxia.

PAH may be present in cardiac surgery patients in the absence of RV dysfunction, particularly for patients undergoing surgery for mitral or tricuspid valve disease, or in patients with advanced ischemic LV dysfunction [63]. PA catheter monitoring should be standard for any patient with known PAH and for any patient undergoing mitral or tricuspid valvular intervention. PAH will improve after valve surgery in the majority of patients [64]. The management of PAH after cardiac surgery in the setting of preserved RV function generally involves standard postoperative monitoring and goal-directed care, including avoidance of hypercapnia, hypoxia, acidosis, and high ventilator pressures. If inotropic support is needed, the use of milrinone is likely preferred over other agents [65]. As with patients with PAH and compromised RV function, inhaled therapy with iNO or prostacyclin may be beneficial to stabilize patients with very advanced PAH.

When a patient without significant preoperative PAH develops new PAH in the postoperative period, this can be the result of a surgical complication (e.g., severe patient-prosthetic valve sizing mismatch), pulmonary reperfusion syndrome (related to cardiopulmonary bypass), blood transfusion effects, a severe protamine reaction, hypercarbia, hypoxia, or acute massive pulmonary embolism. Therapy should include the prompt diagnosis and correction of any reversible contributing conditions and targeted supportive care as outlined above.

Specific Management: Atrial Arrhythmias

Transient atrial arrhythmias, most commonly atrial fibrillation (Afib) or atrial flutter (Aflutter), occur during the early postoperative period in at least 30% of cardiac surgical patients, with a peak incidence on the second–third postoperative days. The strongest risk factors include prior atrial arrhythmias, older age, long-standing HTN, and mitral valve surgery. While generally not immediately life-threatening, atrial arrhythmias after cardiac surgery are associated with an increased risk of stroke, increased mortality risk, and increases in average length of stay, costs of care, and rates of hospital readmission [66, 67].

The first priority with new-onset postoperative Afib or Aflutter is the assessment of hemodynamic stability and perfusion. Atrial arrhythmias may cause profound hypotension and instability, most often when associated with extremes of rapid ventricular response (RVR) and/or when they occur in patients with marginal LV/RV function. In addition, patients with severe LV hypertrophy (from aortic stenosis or long-standing HTN) may decompensate with Afib/Aflutter even in the absence of a very high ventricular rate, as such patients are more dependent on atrial function and require more time for diastolic filling. If a cardiac surgery patient develops new-onset Afib/Aflutter with significant hypotension, immediate synchronized DCCV is indicated. When DCCV is used for atrial arrhythmias, an anterior-posterior patch orientation is most effective, and typical biphasic waveform energy is set at 120 or 200 J for Afib and 50 or 100 J for Aflutter [68, 69]. In cases where a wake patient has marginal blood pressure and is clearly symptomatic, judicious IV sedation should be considered prior to cardioversion.

Once determining that a patient with new-onset Afib/Aflutter is stable and does not require immediate cardioversion, the next priority is rate control. A sustained heart rate above 100–110 bpm can greatly increase the metabolic demands of the heart, which is certainly not a desirable scenario in the early period after cardiac surgery. In addition, long-standing tachycardia may induce a cardiomyopathy than can persist even after rate control and/or DCCV [70]. Rate control for an ICU patient with new-onset Afib and RVR is generally most readily achieved with IV metoprolol, given in 2.5–5 mg increments, administered over several minutes (up to a dose of 10–15 mg total dose). IV metoprolol obviously has the potential to cause vasodilation and hypotension, but generally the improvement in diastolic filling time associated with reduction in heart rate will prevent significant hypotension from its use in this setting. Other options for immediate rate control include diltiazem (IV bolus and infusion) or digoxin (IV load) therapy. In addition to IV therapy, oral agents should be administered concomitantly (or dose-adjusted) to facilitate more long-standing rate control.

After initial rate control, treatment should focus on correcting/alleviating factors that may be driving a patient's new atrial arrhythmia. Hypokalemia and hypomagnesemia should be treated aggressively (with general goals of a potassium level above 4.2 mEq/L and a magnesium level above 2.2 mEq/L). Adrenergic stimulation due to uncontrolled postoperative pain will predispose atrial arrhythmias and will make rate control more challenging. Atrial stretch due to intravascular fluid overload is likely also a contributing factor to atrial arrhythmias. As such, diuretics should be continued in patients with Afib/Aflutter. Neither Afib nor Aflutter is a sign of myocardial ischemia. Unless there is other evidence of ischemia, cardiac enzymes and echocardiography have no role in the workup for postoperative atrial arrhythmias.

Once adequate rate control has been achieved and potential exacerbating factors are addressed, the focus should be on the restoration of sinus rhythm. Although not FDA approved for atrial arrhythmias, amiodarone is first-line treatment at most centers for atrial fibrillation after cardiac surgery [71]. In addition to facilitating cardioversion, amiodarone has beta-blocker effects that will usually improve rate control. A typical IV load regimen would entail 150 mg over 10 min, followed by 1 mg/min for 6 h, and then 0.5 mg/min for 18 h (to complete a 24-h 1 g load). After completion of IV loading, most patients are started on oral maintenance therapy at 100–200 mg twice daily. Initial IV amiodarone administration may lead to hypotension (which is usually transient and easily managed). Daily ECGs are needed to monitor for QT-interval prolongation, which can be a sign of amiodarone toxicity. As amiodarone inhibits the cytochrome P-450 enzyme pathway, there are many potential interactions with other medications. Patients taking this medication over longer periods should be monitored for hepatic, pulmonary, and thyroid toxicity [72]. Alternatives to amiodarone for pharmacologic rhythm control in patients with postoperative Afib or Aflutter include digoxin (IV or oral) and sotalol.

Postoperative Afib/Aflutter tends to have a pattern of paroxysms, interspersed with periods of sinus rhythm. When a patient is experiencing intermittent Afib/Aflutter, there is no role for DCCV in the absence of hemodynamic compromise. For patients with Afib/Aflutter persisting beyond 24–48 h, synchronized DCCV (generally under sedation) is perfectly appropriate. The likelihood of successful/sustained restoration of sinus rhythm is increased if antiarrhythmic medications (amiodarone, digoxin, sotalol) are on board at the time of DCCV [68]. If sustained Afib/Aflutter has been present for more than 48 h, TEE is recommended at the time of DCCV to assess for left atrial thrombus [68].

As an alternative to DCCV, ibutilide (10 mg IV over 10 min) is specifically approved for use in both Afib and Aflutter and may be used for immediate cardioversion. Ibutilide should be administered in an ICU setting with a defibrillator immediately available, as there is a 4% risk of inducing torsade de pointes, which can be mitigated in part by ensuring normal magnesium level prior to attempted cardioversion [73]. ICU monitoring should be continued for at least 4 h after administration.

The optimal means of anticoagulation for patients with Afib/Aflutter after cardiac surgery is controversial and complex, and the decision involves balancing the risks of secondary thromboembolic complications for a particular patient against the risks of bleeding complications with warfarin or with a newer-generation "novel oral anticoagulant" (dabigatran, apixaban, and rivaroxaban). The decision regarding anticoagulation in this patient group is generally beyond the scope of ICU care and should be deferred to the surgical team.

Some centers have adopted oral amiodarone prophylaxis for elective cardiac surgical procedures to reduce the incidence of postoperative atrial fibrillation [74]. When utilized, a typical regimen might entail amiodarone 10 mg/kg daily (divided BID or TID) for 6 days before and after surgery.

Specific Management: Ventricular Arrhythmias

Ventricular ectopy in the form of occasional premature ventricular complexes (PVCs) is very common in the early period after cardiac surgery and may be due to electrolyte disturbances, pH imbalance, the effects of inotropic medications, and the reperfusion of previously ischemic myocardium after CABG or may be the result of residual effects from cardioplegia/ischemic arrest. However, ventricular tachycardia (Vtach) is never a normal event in the postoperative period.

When not associated with pulselessness or shock (which would dictate need for immediate defibrillation), the evaluation of Vtach after cardiac surgery should begin by ensuring that the patient's rhythm is being interpreted correctly. Specifically, atrial (or junctional) tachycardia with aberrant conduction can be easily confused for Vtach (Fig. 13.8). Vtach should consistently be associated with both of the following features: wide QRS complexes in all leads and a clearly regular rate, generally in excess of 180 bpm [75].

Once the diagnosis of hemodynamically stable Vtach is confirmed, prior to any further assessment or treatment in a patient after cardiac surgery, PA catheter position should be assessed. Specifically, an RV location of the catheter tip is a common cause of intermittent Vtach after cardiac surgery and is suggested by an RV PA catheter trace, catheter distance at the skin of less than 40–45 cm, or coiling of the PA catheter on CXR. Assuming that PA catheter malposition has been ruled out and that a patient is hemodynamically stable, an assessment of readily correctable causes should ensue – specifically electrolytes and pH should be examined. Current inotrope requirements should be evaluated, as all inotropic medications are arrhythmogenic to some degree and should be reduced to the minimum necessary level of support in the setting of a new ventricular arrhythmia. In the absence of another etiology, an evaluation for potential ischemia should ensue, including an ECG and bedside TTE (for wall motion assessment) at a minimum.

Once active ischemia has been ruled out, a cardiology consult is appropriate to direct further therapy, which may consist of IV procainamide, sotalol, or amiodarone therapy (preferred if abnormal LV function), or synchronized DCCV for refractory cases.

Given pulseless Vtach or ventricular fibrillation (Vfib) after cardiac surgery, management should follow most advanced cardiac life support (ACLS) principles, with several important exceptions [49]. Bolus doses of epinephrine or vasopressin should generally be avoided (unless specifically directed by the surgical team) as excessive HTN in the early postoperative period can have disastrous consequences. In the absence of prompt return of circulation with defibrillation, prolonged chest compressions are not appropriate in a patient who is within 1 week of cardiac surgery. Instead, emergent bedside sternal re-entry should be carried out, for open cardiac massage and internal defibrillation. The technique for open cardiac massage in a postoperative patient is described earlier in this chapter. For defibrillation after emergent sternal re-entry, internal paddles can be used as follows: one paddle is carefully placed between the cardiac apex and the diaphragm and moved firmly against the posterior aspect of the heart (typically the left atrium); the second paddle is placed firmly on the anterior aspect of the heart (Fig. 13.9).

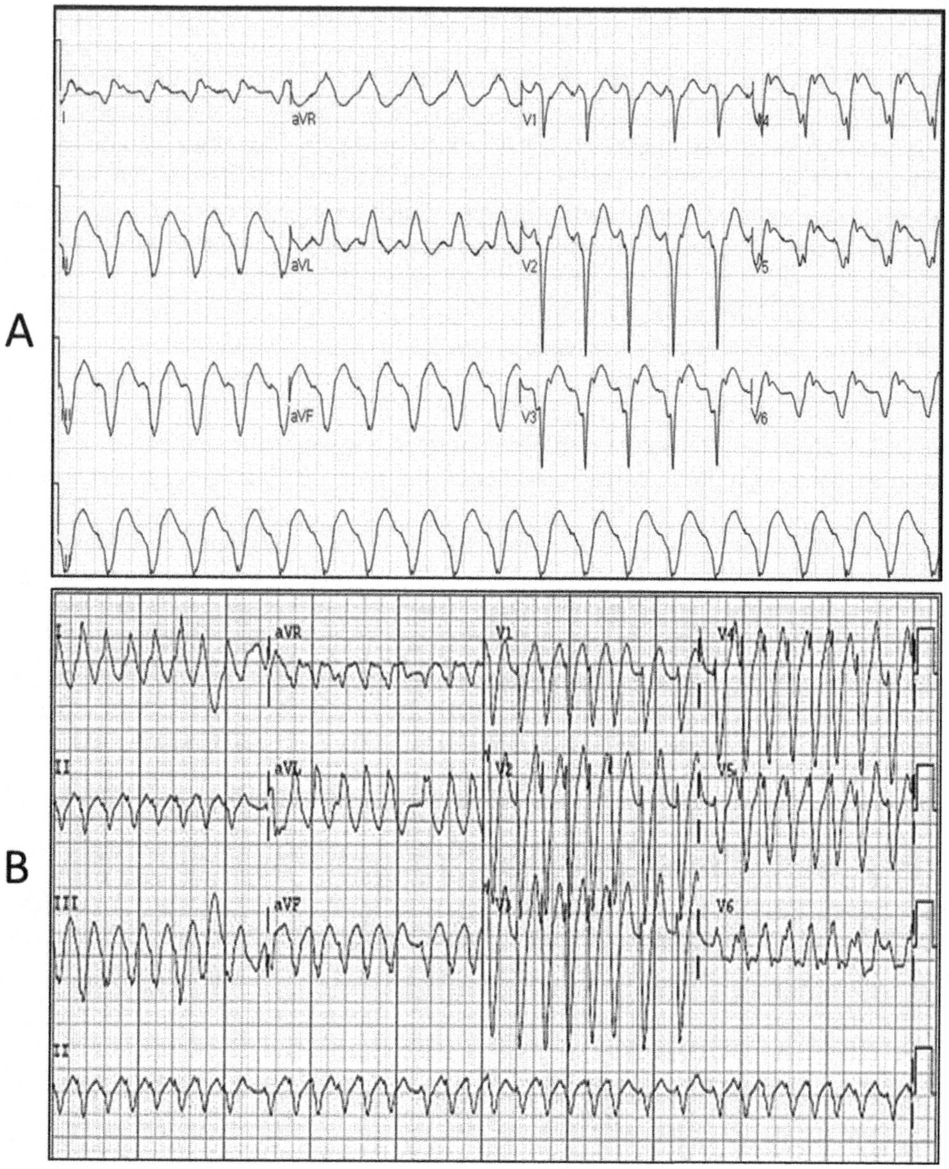

Fig. 13.8 Differentiating ventricular tachycardia (Vtach) from atrial fibrillation/flutter with aberrant conduction can be challenging after cardiac surgery. A, Top image shows findings typical for monomorphic Vtach – regular morphology, wide complexes in all leads, and a regular rate; B, bottom image shows findings typical for atrial fibrillation with aberrant conduction, including variable QRS morphology and rate

Specific Management: Bradycardia

When symptomatic or hemodynamically significant bradycardia occurs in the early postoperative period and functional temporary epicardial pacemaker leads are in place, management is straightforward. As described earlier in this chapter, synchronous atrial or dual-chamber pacing is preferred. When epicardial pacing leads are not in place, heart rate can be augmented pharmacologically. Options include IV atropine (generally of only transient benefit) or the IV infusion of isoproterenol (preferred if available), dopamine, or epinephrine. If persistent, bradycardia may require cardiology consultation for placement of a transvenous pacer system.

Temporizing measures while awaiting cardiology engagement include transcutaneous pacing or bedside placement of a temporary pacing lead or pacing PA catheter. If a patient still has a large-bore (8 Fr) internal jugular (or subclavian) catheter in place, placement of a temporary transvenous ventricular pacer lead or a dual-pacing PA catheter is usually straightforward. If available at your institution, temporary transesophageal atrial pacing (which requires a sedated patient and an intact conduction system) may be an additional option for short-term support.

Specific Management: Concern for Myocardial Ischemia

ECG changes are extremely common after cardiac surgery. In particular, some degree of interventricular conduction delay is often present after valve procedures, and changes in T-wave and ST-segment morphology are the norm after CABG (presumably related to reperfusion and changes in

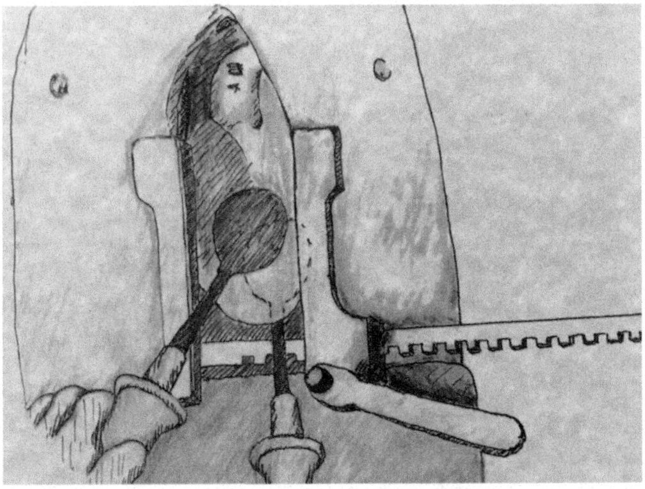

Fig. 13.9 Internal defibrillation via median sternotomy (with operator standing on the patient's right side); the right-handed paddle is slid along the diaphragm to a position posterior to the heart; the left-handed paddle is placed directly anteriorly on the heart (typically on the right ventricular surface)

coronary blood flow dynamics). In the absence of clinical evidence of ischemia (hemodynamic instability, ventricular arrhythmias), most T-wave or ST-segment changes on an immediate postoperative ECG are of no clinical importance. However, ST-segment elevation in a regional pattern with malignant morphology can be an indication of graft failure after CABG or a technical complication after valve surgery (e.g., RCA occlusion from aortic valve replacement or left circumflex coronary artery injury during mitral valve replacement). Transient ischemia may occur after CABG due to vasospasm of the native coronary arteries or arterial graft conduit(s). Diffuse ST-segment elevation, particularly when associated with concave morphology and PR-segment depression, is more suggestive of pericarditis than myocardial ischemia. Although ECG evidence of pericarditis would be unexpected on an initial ECG after arrival from the OR, pericarditis is a very common cause of ECG changes thereafter (Fig. 13.10).

Several studies have attempted to define "typical" or expected cardiac enzyme levels after uncomplicated cardiac surgery, based on procedure type and interval from surgery [76]. Certainly, dramatically high enzyme levels (more than 5–10 times the upper limits of normal) might suggest ongoing ischemia/infarction. In general, cardiac enzymes have limited value in assessment after cardiac surgery, although marked elevation may be associated with increased multifactorial morbidity [77].

If there are concerns for ischemia, an echocardiogram may be very useful, as the demonstration of stable/normal LV function and wall motion provides reassurance that transmural ischemia/infarction in a significant myocardial territory is unlikely [78]. If there is a high level of clinical concern (e.g., anterior ST-elevation in a CABG patient with ventricular arrhythmias and/or a high-level vasopressor requirement), the cardiac surgical team should be contacted immediately. Pending discussion with the surgical team, emergent cardiology consultation, and cardiac catheterization may be appropriate.

Specific Management: Metabolic Acidosis

Metabolic acidosis is extremely common in the immediate period after cardiac surgery, usually the result of lactate washout after separation from cardiopulmonary bypass and/or from high-volume crystalloid infusion during surgery (which will lead to a hyperchloremic acidosis in many patients) [79]. Although IV sodium bicarbonate is rarely used for most other postsurgical patients, it is very appropriate to administer this medication for cardiac surgical patients with a significant hyperchloremic metabolic acidosis (associated with base deficit of less than −6 to −8, or pH less than 7.30). Otherwise, acidosis may increase a patient's susceptibility to arrhythmias, contribute to altered enzyme function and coagulation, or may reduce the efficacy of vasoactive medications.

Unlike hyperchloremic metabolic acidosis (which is associated with a normal anion gap and is generally benign), significant lactic acidosis in a patient after cardiac surgery can be a sign of a catastrophic complication (such as gut or limb ischemia). A mild lactic acidosis (lactate <4–5 mmol/L) on initial ICU arrival should prompt the ICU team to ensure adequate clinical perfusion and intravascular volume (including red blood cell transfusion where appropriate), to reduce vasopressor doses as much as possible and to closely follow serial lactate levels. If lactate levels trend steadily downward (and normalize within ~12 h), no further evaluation or treatment is indicated. If, however, serum lactate is markedly elevated upon a patient's ICU arrival or continues to trend upward, there should be a high index of suspicion for a causative event. In addition to the above measures, the ICU team must evaluate for a secondary surgical complication. Specific emphasis should be on the abdominal examination and examination of the extremities.

Specific Management: Delirium and Neurological Deficits

Neurological complications of some form occur in up to 30% of patients after cardiac surgery [80], ranging from transient, self-limiting delirium to debilitating stroke or hypoxic encephalopathy. Transient or permanent neurological deficits can occur after cardiac surgery as a result of microemboli during surgery, cerebral hypoperfusion due to low flow, underlying cerebrovascular disease, intracranial hemorrhage

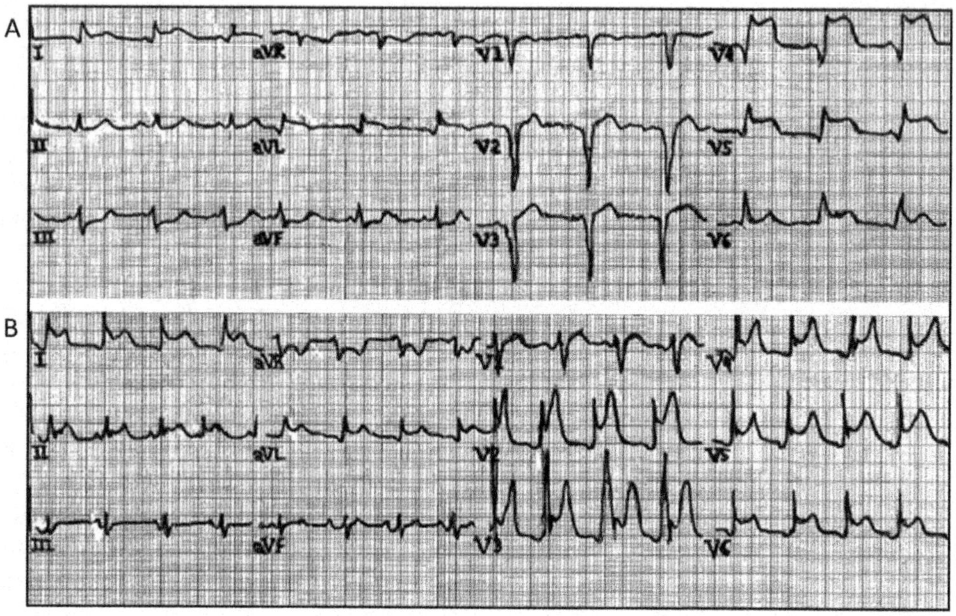

Fig. 13.10 (**a**) ECG shows findings typical of acute ST-segment elevation myocardial infarction, in the form of focal ST-elevation (most pronounced in leads V4 and V5) with reciprocal ST-segment depression (most pronounced in leads III and aVF); (**b**) ECG shows findings more typical of acute pericarditis – relatively diffuse ST-segment elevation with a concave morphology and with PR-segment depression

related to anticoagulation, air embolism, or macroscopic embolic events. A review of the comprehensive evaluation and management of these conditions is beyond the scope of this text. However, a brief overview of neurologic complications in cardiac surgical patients within the context of ICU care is presented below.

Stroke complicates between 1 and 2% of isolated CABG procedures and is slightly more common after cardiac surgery involving valve replacement or repair. Aortic arch surgery involving the use of circulatory arrest is associated with stroke rates as high as 7% [80]. Thirty to forty percent of strokes are thought to occur intraoperatively, with the vast majority of the remainder presenting in the first 24–48 h after surgery [80]. In the setting of a new focal neurological deficit (sensorimotor, visual, or language deficit) after cardiac surgery, brain imaging should be obtained as soon as possible.

Diffusion-weighted brain magnetic resonance imaging (MRI) is clearly the study of choice for the early detection and characterization of stroke [81]. There are limitations in available monitoring and care during the extended period needed to complete this study, and therefore MRI should not be obtained in an unstable patient. Of note, sternal wires and surgical clips are MRI compatible. Although not explicitly MRI "approved," there is no evidence that temporary epicardial pacemaker leads preclude safe MRI imaging [82]. Noncontrast computed tomography (CT) of the brain is a more readily available and more rapid imaging modality compared with brain MRI but has very limited sensitivity for the early detection of stroke [81].

The timing of a focal neurological deficit can have important management implications. If noted upon a patient's emergence from sedation after cardiac surgery, it is less likely that a patient would be in the 6-h window for potential interventional therapy. In contrast, for a patient who is initially apparently neurologically intact but later develops a focal deficit, there may be options for therapeutic intervention. In addition, in this latter scenario, there may be greater potential for recurrent events due to ongoing risk factors (e.g., atrial fibrillation, intracardiac thrombus), as opposed to stroke from intraoperative embolization or low flow [80].

IV systemic thrombolytic therapy is absolutely contraindicated after cardiac surgery. However, where available expertise exists, neurointerventional procedure (catheter thrombectomy, local directed thrombolytic administration) may be an option when it can be determined with confidence that an ischemic neurological deficit has not been present for longer than 6 h in a cardiac surgical patient [83].

Supportive therapy for stroke after cardiac surgery is similar to that for other ICU populations – including permissive HTN (to the extent deemed acceptable by the surgical team), and strict avoidance of hypotension, hypoxia, hyperglycemia, and fever. There is no proven role for anticoagulation beyond antiplatelet therapy in the absence of another indication (e.g., atrial arrhythmia or mechanical prosthetic valve) [84]. In the rare circumstance of significant cerebral air embolism, there may be some benefit from hyperbaric oxygen therapy [85].

When a cardiac surgery patient presents with a non-focal neurological deficit, such as confusion/delirium, seizures, reduced level of responsiveness, or coma, evaluation and treatment may differ slightly relative to that for a focal deficit. Delirium occurs more often in patients with preexisting dementia or prior stroke, elderly patients, and those with known cerebrovascular disease. It may often simply be the consequence of residual effects from anesthetic agents, sedatives, and narcotics. Therefore, initial management usually consists of observation, avoidance of any CNS-depressant medications, and care to avoid aspiration or other secondary complications from reduced sensorium. If delirium does not improve/resolve with these measures alone, the ICU team should evaluate for metabolic causes (thyroid disease, renal failure, liver failure) and consider neurology consultation. The neurology consultant will typically facilitate an electroencephalogram and request a brain MRI in this setting.

Seizures are unusual after cardiac surgery and may be the result of electrolyte alterations, drug toxicity, or stroke. Coma may result from global anoxic brain injury, a large stroke, nonconvulsive status epilepticus, or severe metabolic derangements [86]. Less severe disturbances in higher cognitive function (memory, attention, etc.) are very common after cardiac surgery, particularly when assessed by formal neuropsychiatric testing. Such deficits usually resolve over time, with little relevance for a patient's ICU course.

One neurological complication specific to aortic surgery (particularly descending thoracic or thoracoabdominal aneurysm repair) is lower extremity paralysis. Refinements in anesthetic and surgical technique have significantly reduced the incidence of this complication to below 5% in most series [87]. Postoperative adjuncts to minimize the risk of paralysis include permissive HTN and continued cerebrospinal fluid (CSF) drainage for select patients through the second or third postoperative day [88].

Specific Management: Thrombocytopenia

Thrombocytopenia is a normal consequence of surgery with the use of CPB. In spite of numerous advances in bypass circuitry, filter design, and the conduct of bypass, CPB leads to predictable platelet deformity and destruction. Thrombocytopenia (as defined by postoperative platelet count <150,000 cells/μL) occurs in over one third of patients, with the effects of CPB (platelet consumption and hemodilution) being the predominant etiology [89]. Platelet counts from CPB-related thrombocytopenia tend to nadir on the second or third postoperative day, after which there is steady normalization over the next several weeks, and associated bleeding complications are rare [90]. The most common challenge related to thrombocytopenia after cardiac surgery centers around the potential for heparin-induced thrombocytopenia (HIT). Unlike CPB-related thrombocytopenia, HIT represents a life-threatening condition. Additional less common causes of thrombocytopenia in cardiac surgical patients mirror those encountered in other ICU populations, including medication effects, sepsis, or multi-organ failure.

HIT, which has an estimated 2% incidence after cardiac surgery, is classified into direct interaction between heparin and platelets (Type I) and an IgG-related immunologic form, characterized by antibodies to the heparin-platelet factor 4 complex (Type II). Type I HIT appears early after surgery (within the first 1–3 days) and is typically characterized by uneventful resolution within several days. In contrast, Type II HIT most often occurs 5–10 days after surgical heparin exposure. In cases where a patient with HIT has received heparin within the preceding 3 months of a cardiac surgical procedure, Type II HIT can present much more immediately after surgery due to the presence of existing antibodies [91].

Type II HIT is associated with a high risk of thrombotic complications (40–75%) and carries a mortality of at least 25% in cardiac surgical patients [92, 93]. Therefore, early recognition and treatment are critical in this population. HIT must be considered in any cardiac surgical patient with a drop in platelet count of more than 50% after surgery, a reduction of 30% or greater to <100,000 cells/μL, or any thrombotic event within a month of surgery.

There are two available types of diagnostic testing for HIT: enzyme immunoassay for the detection of platelet factor 4-reactive HIT antibodies and "functional" testing to measure platelet activity in the presence of the patient's serum and heparin (most often a "serotonin release assay" or a "heparin-induced platelet activation assay"). Functional testing has greater specificity but can be difficult to perform [94]. Because no single assay has 100% sensitivity and specificity for the diagnosis of HIT, functional and immune assays are best submitted in combination [94]. However, most institutions rely on reference laboratory testing for these studies, and there is a typical delay of at least several days before results are available.

When HIT is strongly suspected (fall in platelet count of more than 50% at an interval between 5 and 10 days after cardiac surgery), diagnostic studies should be sent, but treatment should not be delayed for results. Effective treatment for HIT mandates the immediate discontinuation of all heparin-based medications (including heparin flushes, subcutaneous microdose heparin, and LMWH) and should ideally entail anticoagulation with an alternative medication class to mitigate the risk of thrombotic complications. Heparin alternatives include the IV direct thrombin inhibitors – argatroban (hepatic excretion), lepirudin (renal excretion), or bivalirudin. Platelet transfusion should be avoided in the absence of clinical bleeding (which is rare in HIT). IV anticoagulation should be transitioned to oral anticoagulation (with warfarin) after platelet counts have substantially recovered. Finally, close monitoring for thrombotic complications (some of which may require surgical therapy) is critical [95].

On rare occasion, a patient with a known history of HIT requires cardiac surgery. If the patient's HIT predated the planned surgical procedure by at least 100 days, a single heparin re-exposure immediately prior to the institution of CPB is generally safe. Ideally, the absence of HIT antibodies should be confirmed prior to surgery. Thereafter, no heparin products should be utilized in these patients during the postoperative period. In the setting of urgent or emergent cardiac surgery within 100 days of a known episode of HIT (or particularly when there are still significant serum antibodies present), the surgical team must choose to either utilize an alternative anticoagulant for CPB (argatroban, bivalirudin, or lepirudin, none of which are FDA approved for this indication) or to risk a significant (but poorly defined) likelihood of complications with early heparin re-exposure for CPB.

Specific Procedures: CABG

The radial artery is used as a graft conduit in a small proportion of CABG procedures in the USA, most often in the setting of all-arterial grafting (with one or both internal mammary arteries). Radial artery grafts have a strong propensity for vasospasm [96]. Although specific institutional protocols vary, essentially all patients receiving a radial graft for CABG should be placed on a low-dose nitroglycerin or diltiazem IV infusion for the first 24 h (irrespective of systemic blood pressure), after which IV therapy can generally be transitioned to an oral long-acting nitrate or diltiazem formulation [96].

The care of patients undergoing off-pump coronary artery bypass (opCAB) is not dramatically different from the standard care of other cardiac surgical patients. opCAB patients are generally less prone to coagulopathy and bleeding, although they may also be more prone to thrombotic complications [97]. Relative to CABG with CPB, opCAB patients less often experience issues with heart rate or rhythm after surgery and may not have epicardial pacemaker wires placed at surgery. Because opCAB patients are not "rewarmed" using the CPB heater-cooler unit, they may be more prone to hypothermia in the ICU. Finally, because the heart is not subjected to a period of ischemic arrest from aortic cross-clamping, opCAB patients may not experience the transient postsurgical decline in LV function that is often seen after cardiac surgical procedures utilizing CPB.

Specific Procedures: Mitral Valve Repair

A relatively unique aspect of postoperative care after mitral valve repair is the risk of systolic anterior motion (SAM) of the mitral valve. SAM refers to displacement of the anterior mitral valve leaflet and/or subvalvular apparatus into the left ventricular outflow tract in systole, where it can lead to dynamic outflow obstruction (Fig. 13.11). Patients with degenerative/myxomatous mitral valve disease are both the most common patients to undergo mitral repair and are the most prone to SAM physiology (due to redundant leaflet tissue and elongated mitral valve chords). In addition to myxomatous mitral disease with redundant valve tissue, excessive "downsizing" of the mitral valve annulus (with an "annuloplasty" ring or band) at the time of mitral repair can contribute to SAM.

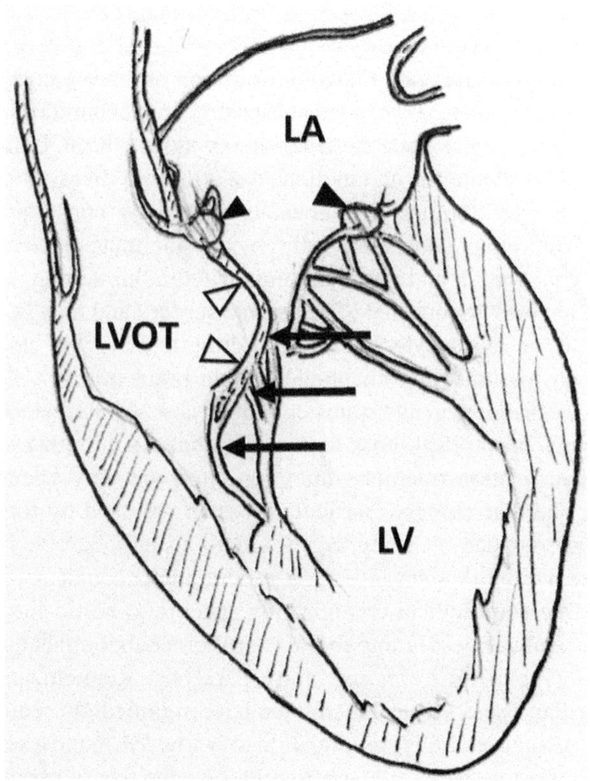

Fig. 13.11 Systolic anterior motion (SAM) of the anterior leaflet (open arrowheads) and subvalvular structures of the mitral valve after mitral repair with an annuloplasty ring (arrowheads); displacement in an anterior direction (denoted by arrows) can lead to obstruction of flow through the left ventricular outflow tract (LVOT); LA, left atrium; LV, left ventricle

SAM typically presents as a low cardiac output state and can coexist with recurrent significant mitral valve regurgitation after a previously competent mitral repair. SAM should be a diagnostic consideration in any mitral repair patient who develops new hypotension and/or malperfusion after surgery and can be documented on a bedside TTE study. In most cases, SAM is medically manageable – through aggressive volume resuscitation, avoidance of tachycardia, avoidance of inotropic medications, and actively increasing systemic afterload. Rarely, SAM may require return to the OR for revision of repair (or conversion to mitral valve replacement).

Specific Procedures: Aortic Valve Replacement

Aortic valve replacement (AVR) is most commonly performed for aortic stenosis (AS). Although transcatheter valve replacement is being used with increasing frequency in lieu of surgical AVR, AVR remains the second most common elective cardiac surgical procedure in the USA [98]. Patients with severe AS characteristically have significant left ventricular hypertrophy (LVH) and diastolic dysfunction, similar to those with long-standing/poorly controlled systemic hypertension.

Severe LVH is associated with reduced ventricular compliance, which leads to a need for higher left ventricular end-diastolic pressure to achieve an adequate left ventricular volume (or preload). After successful AVR, LVH will regress over time but is obviously still present in the early postoperative period. AS patients will generally be dependent on higher preload/intravascular volume and may manifest severe lability when intravascular volume is low. AS patients also may have more stable hemodynamics and better perfusion with lower heart rates, which allow for greater proportional time for diastolic filling. Because of reduced LV compliance, AS patients may be more dependent on active atrial contraction (relative to passive LV filling) and therefore may be more susceptible to hypotension and malperfusion in the setting of a postoperative atrial arrhythmia.

Significant perivalvular leak is a rare technical complication of surgical AVR. In severe cases, a perivalvular leak may lead to reduced cardiac output and/or hemodynamic instability due to reduced effective forward blood flow. In cases where a perivalvular leak has a high velocity, it can be associated with red cell hemolysis [99]. In the setting of reduced cardiac output or suspected hemolysis (anemia with schistocytes on a peripheral smear, reduced serum haptoglobin level, and/or increased indirect serum bilirubin level), an echocardiogram in the ICU is appropriate to assess for perivalvular leak.

Coronary obstruction can rarely occur after surgical AVR, generally because of the prosthetic device occluding one or both coronary ostia. This complication will generally manifest in the immediate period during/after separation from CPB and mandates immediate surgical correction (either revision of the AVR or addition of CABG). However, right coronary artery (RCA) obstruction after AVR may be overlooked in the OR and may manifest in the form of ECG changes and/or arrhythmias in the ICU. Any patient with new inferior ST-segment changes after AVR (particularly in association with arrhythmias or hemodynamic derangements) should be evaluated by the surgical team for possible RCA obstruction.

Heart block may occur after AVR due to direct injury of the conduction system (located in the membranous septum, just below the aortic annulus) or due to edema. Permanent pacemaker implantation, which is required in about 7% of patients after AVR, should generally be performed if a patient remains pacer-dependent beyond 5–7 days after surgery [100].

Anticoagulation is indicated after all mechanical AVR procedures and is used on a temporary basis by some surgeons after bioprosthetic AVR (particularly for patients with significant LV dysfunction or a history of atrial arrhythmias). Most surgeons will initiate oral warfarin therapy on the first or second day after mechanical AVR. The use of a heparin "bridge" while awaiting a therapeutic INR (2–3 for most mechanical aortic valve prosthetics) is variable between institutions and surgeons and balances the small risk of valve thrombosis/thromboembolism during the interval prior to a therapeutic warfarin level against the risk of late surgical bleeding from anticoagulation. Many surgeons will start either low-dose IV heparin or subcutaneous LMWH if a patient with a new mechanical aortic valve is not fully anticoagulated by 3–4 days after surgery.

Specific Procedures: Mitral Valve Replacement

Just as with AVR, patients undergoing mitral valve replacement (MVR) may develop reduced cardiac output and/or hemolysis in the setting of a significant perivalvular leak. When suspected, the presence or absence of a perivalvular leak can be determined by an echocardiogram in the ICU. However, adequate visualization of the mitral valve in a patient in the early period after cardiac surgery may necessitate the use of TEE.

A rare complication after MVR (or mitral repair) is surgical injury to the left circumflex coronary artery, which might manifest with new lateral or inferolateral ECG changes, hemodynamic effects (in the setting of complete occlusion of a large/dominant circumflex), or subjective complaints (persistent non-incisional chest discomfort, nausea, etc.). If there is clinical concern for a circumflex injury after MVR, the surgical team should be consulted immediately to determine appropriate evaluation.

Just as with mechanical AVR, all patients with a mechanical mitral prosthetic valve will require lifelong anticoagulation. Also as with AVR, some surgeons will place bioprosthetic MVR patients on anticoagulation for several months after surgery. Conduction system injury may occur with mitral valve surgery, but permanent pacemaker placement is less common than after AVR [101].

Specific Conditions/Procedures: Atrial Arrhythmia Surgery

Surgical treatment for atrial arrhythmias may consist of either a "Cox maze" procedure or pulmonary vein electrical isolation (PVI), both of which utilize energy sources such as radiofrequency or cryo-treatment. Either a maze procedure or PVI may be performed at the time of another cardiac surgical procedure or less commonly as a "stand-alone" intervention. Because of the strong association between mitral valve disease and atrial arrhythmias, arrhythmia surgery is most often performed as an adjunct to mitral valve surgery

[102]. Rhythm disturbances are the norm after the maze procedure or PVI. A substantial proportion of patients require temporary postoperative pacing for either sinoatrial node dysfunction or heart block after a complete maze procedure, and 10–15% may require "permanent" endocardial pacemaker lead placement [103].

Because the modalities utilized for the surgical treatment of arrhythmias are not consistently transmural until several months after surgery, transient atrial arrhythmias are present in the majority of patients in the early postoperative period [102]. Antiarrhythmic medications such as amiodarone, beta-blockers, or sotalol may be initiated in the early postoperative period, but due to the potential for sinus node dysfunction and/or heart block in this patient population, these medications should be initiated with caution.

Due to the effect of atrial energy sources (and possibly due to a reduction in atrial natriuretic peptide levels) after a maze procedure, fluid retention and edema are common. Patients should be treated with active diuresis in the early postoperative period.

Specific Procedures: Aortic Procedures

Aggressive control of postoperative hypertension is of particular import after aortic surgery, which is often associated with multiple suture lines under systemic pressure. In addition, the extended CPB duration required for complex aortic surgical interventions and the need for more pronounced systemic cooling in some cases make coagulopathic bleeding more common than after isolated CABG or valve replacement.

Surgical procedures involving the aortic arch require the use of hypothermic circulatory arrest (HCA) techniques – or a period during which the need for direct surgical access to the aortic arch necessitates transient discontinuation of CPB. Although aortic arch procedures are often supplemented with surgical strategies for neuroprotection, the use of HCA during a cardiac surgical procedure is still associated with an increase in the risk of stroke [104].

Although increasingly being supplanted by endovascular techniques, surgery on the descending thoracic or thoracoabdominal aorta is associated with a risk for paraplegia due to spinal cord ischemia in the perioperative period. Paralysis may present in a delayed fashion after descending aortic surgery, most often during/after a period of relative hypotension or hypoperfusion. In addition to intraoperative surgical strategies to reduce the incidence of paraplegia (e.g., assisted circulation, intercostal artery reimplantation), there are important postoperative measures intended to reduce the likelihood of this catastrophic complication. It is critical to maintain adequate systemic perfusion. Depending on the surgeon's comfort with surgical hemostasis, some will employ a strategy of "permissive hypertension" in the ICU. By targeting MAPs as high as 80–90 mmHg, the risk for spinal cord ischemia is reduced. Lumbar CSF drainage is used by many surgeons and many centers for surgical procedures involving the descending thoracic aorta and is intended to augment relative spinal cord perfusion pressures. CSF drainage is typically initiated preoperatively or intraoperatively and is continued for several days after surgery, generally targeting a CSF pressure of <10 mmHg [105].

Specific Procedures: Ventricular Assist Device Placement

Placement of a temporary VAD may be required during cardiac surgery when the typical means for support (inotropes, vasopressors, IABP counterpulsation) do not allow for a patient's successful separation from CPB. The scenario of a "post-pericardiotomy" VAD requirement most often occurs after an extensive/extended cardiac surgical procedure in a patient with severe preexisting cardiac dysfunction, when cardiac surgery is performed in the setting of a recent or ongoing large myocardial infarction, or when there are major intraoperative technical complications. In all of these settings, it is hoped that VAD support for a period of between several days and 1 week might allow for adequate cardiac recovery to facilitate a transition back to effective native perfusion. In some cases, VAD support after surgery may provide a "bridge" to urgent cardiac transplantation or for the placement of a longer-term cardiac assist device. In reality, the mortality for any patient with a need for VAD support to separate from CPB is approximately 50% under any circumstance [106]. VAD patients have very high rates of bleeding requiring reoperation and high rates of nosocomial infection. All VAD devices require some [variable] degree of anticoagulation during use (typically IV heparin).

An LVAD can reduce LV stress by 80% and reduce LV myocardial oxygen demand by nearly 40% [103]. LVAD implantation requires the surgical placement of a VAD "inflow" cannula in the left atrium or LV apex and a VAD "outflow" cannula in the ascending aorta (Fig. 13.12). After LVAD cannula placement and initiation of LVAD support, temporary sternal closure is achieved. Great care must be taken by the surgical team to adequately secure all VAD cannulae; as if a cannula is dislodged in the ICU, nearly immediate exsanguination will ensue (in addition to the immediate cessation of device function). Similarly, transport of any patient with a VAD in place represents a high-risk activity that demands adequate staffing and careful attention.

LVAD support is typically initiated in the OR at a flow rate of 2.2 L/min/m2, after which time flow rates are adjusted to support adequate systemic perfusion (and based on left atrial filling pressures). The specific management and troubleshooting of an LVAD circuit require an experienced perfusionist and/or cardiac surgeon. However, it is useful for the critical

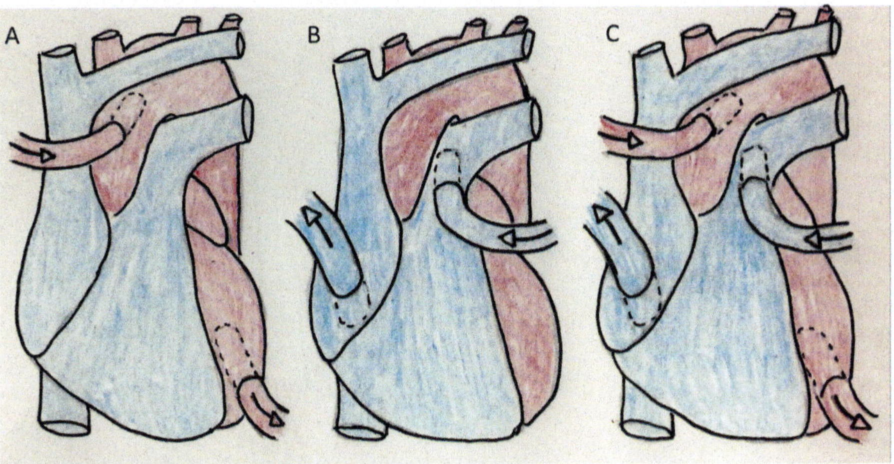

Fig. 13.12 (**a**) Left image shows typical cannulation for a left ventricular assist device, with drainage from left ventricular apex and return into the ascending aorta (alternate site for drainage is the left atrium, via the pulmonary vein); (**b**) center image shows typical cannulation for a right ventricular assist device, with drainage from the right atrium and return into the main pulmonary artery; (**c**) right image shows typical cannulation for biventricular assist device support. Blue area, right atrium/ventricle; red area, left atrium/ventricle and aortic arch

care team to understand the most common reasons for inadequate VAD flow, which include hypovolemia, cardiac tamponade, and cannula/device malposition or occlusion. Therefore, the initial approach to an unexpected decrease in LVAD flow rate entails an assessment of a patient's volume status, assessment for bleeding/tamponade, and comprehensive device interrogation by the cardiac surgical team.

In a patient with established LVAD support, LV function should be reassessed at regular intervals (typically 24–48 h), and if there is evidence of myocardial recovery, LVAD flow rates can be gradually reduced to "wean" the patient from mechanical support. If a patient is successfully liberated from LVAD support, return to the OR will be necessary for decannulation and chest closure. If a patient cannot be weaned from LVAD support within a week, more definitive means for support (transplantation or longer-term assist device) or withdrawal of care must be considered.

RVAD support requires the surgical placement of cannulae in the right atrium and pulmonary artery (Fig. 13.12). Postsurgical RVAD support may be required for refractory RV failure in the setting of a large inferior myocardial infarction or due to surgical complications related to RV myocardial protection and/or perfusion. More commonly, RVAD support must be initiated in a patient with an LVAD in place. One third of patients with LVAD support manifest or develop biventricular failure, requiring the addition of an RVAD [103]. The combined use of LVAD and RVAD support is known as a "biventricular assist device" (BiVAD; Fig. 13.12). A BiVAD will support both the systemic and pulmonary circulations, but unlike ECMO support does not provide for oxygenation. RVAD support is initiated and weaned in a fashion similar to that for LVAD support.

Specific Procedures: Extracorporeal Membrane Oxygenator Support

ECMO support may rarely be required in the early postoperative period after cardiac surgery. Unlike VAD support, an ECMO circuit includes an oxygenator. Criteria for the initiation of ECMO support after cardiac surgery are similar to those for VAD support, except that ECMO is the preferred modality in a patient with refractory hypoxia. Depending on whether a patient has isolated refractory respiratory failure or coexisting respiratory failure and inadequate systemic perfusion, an ECMO circuit may be designed to support the pulmonary circulation alone (venovenous or "VV" ECMO) or to support both the systemic and pulmonary circulations (venoarterial or "VA" ECMO).

When ECMO is utilized for a patient who cannot be weaned from CPB, it typically utilizes the existing surgical CPB cannulae (right atrial cannula for ECMO drainage and aortic cannula for ECMO infusion (Fig. 13.13). An additional ECMO drainage cannula may be placed into the left atrium or left ventricle to ensure adequate LV decompression during ECMO support. When ECMO support is initiated for a patient not in the OR, VA ECMO typically entails placement of an internal jugular or femoral venous cannula (directed into the right atrium) and a femoral arterial cannula (Fig. 13.13). For VV ECMO initiation, a femoral inflow cannula (tip in right atrium) may be used with an interval jugular catheter for ECMO outflow, or bilateral femoral venous cannulae may be used (with one of the cannulae being a long cannula extending into the inferior vena cava/right atrium; Fig. 13.13). More recently, the development of a multi-lumen internal jugular

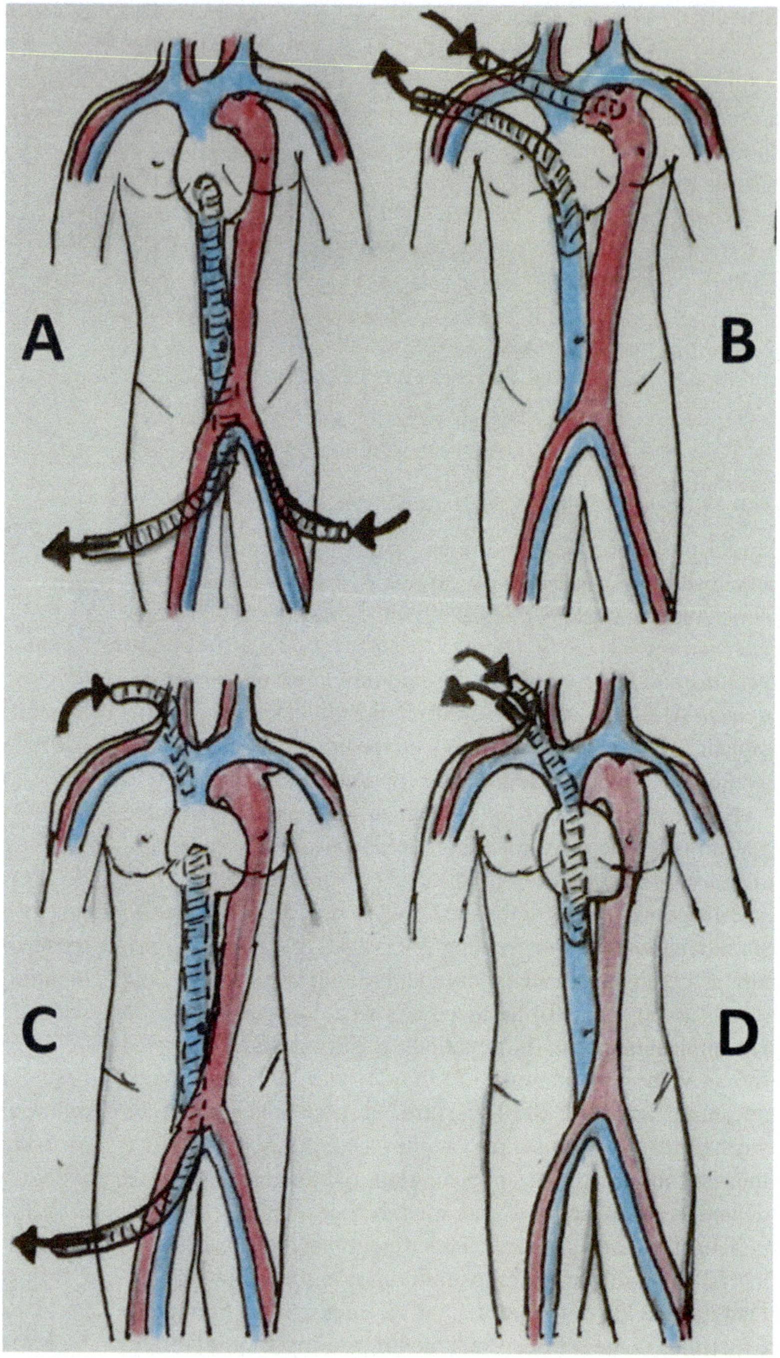

Fig. 13.13 Configurations for extracorporeal membrane oxygenation (ECMO); "A" depicts peripheral venoarterial ECMO cannulation utilizing a venous inflow cannula in the right atrium via the right femoral vein and a left femoral arterial outflow cannula; "B" depicts central ECMO cannulation (performed in the operating room, generally at the time of another cardiac surgical procedure), with the ECMO inflow cannula in the right atrium and inferior vena cava (IVC) and ECMO outflow via an aortic cannula; "C" depicts cannulation for venovenous ECMO using an inflow cannula in the right atrium/IVC and an outflow cannula in the right internal jugular (IJ) vein (contralateral femoral venous cannulation is an alternative for ECMO outflow); "D" depicts venovenous ECMO utilizing a dual-lumen catheter placed into the right atrium and IVC via the right IJ vein

venous cannula (Avalon Laboratories, Rancho Dominguez, USA) allows for VV ECMO using a single cannulation site.

In most cases, ECMO requires lower levels of heparin relative to VAD support [107] due to the use of a heparin-bonded circuit, although protocols for heparinization during ECMO vary widely. VA ECMO support, which is non-pulsatile, may be combined with IABP counterpulsation in some cases to augment coronary perfusion.

When a patient is on VA ECMO, ventilatory pressures and oxygen levels should be minimized. Vasopressor support will still generally be needed, but inotrope use should be minimized to allow for myocardial rest/recovery. As with VAD use after cardiac surgery, ECMO is only a means for temporary support. If a patient cannot be weaned from ECMO within 1 week after cardiac surgery, either the institution of more durable support or withdrawal of care is generally appropriate.

Specific Procedures: Cardiac Transplantation

Antirejection therapy and prophylaxis against early infection are critical priorities for the care of transplant patients but should be coordinated by the heart transplant team and are outside the scope of ICU care.

In spite of numerous advancements in surgical technique, myocardial preservation, and postoperative care, RV failure remains a significant complication in cardiac transplant recipients and constitutes a very common cause of early allograft failure [108]. Many heart transplant recipients have significant PA hypertension as a result of their advanced heart failure, presenting the donor heart with a sudden increase in afterload relative to the donor pulmonary circulation.

In addition to the risk of RV dysfunction, inadequate myocardial protection and/or prolonged allograft ischemic time may lead to biventricular dysfunction or failure after transplant. Accelerated or "hyperacute" rejection is an additional rare cause of early cardiac failure in this population. Together, these entities represent causes of primary graft failure (PGF), a syndrome in which the transplanted heart fails to meet the circulatory requirements of the recipient in the immediate posttransplant period after cardiac transplantation.

PGF manifests as persistent hypotension and low cardiac output in the early postoperative period, in spite of apparently adequate preload and filling pressures. RV failure should specifically be suspected with refractory hypotension, elevated central venous pressure, and a decrease in PA pressures. It is critical to rule out cardiac tamponade in this setting, as tamponade is not uncommon after transplant and may present with clinical findings similar to PGF [109]. The patient should also be assessed by the transplant team for hyperacute rejection in the setting of acute hemodynamic compromise early after cardiac transplant. The incidence of hyperacute rejection, which results from preformed antibodies, has been greatly reduced by the routine use of a pretransplant donor-recipient crossmatch (which may guide pretransplant plasmapheresis and/or immunoglobulin therapy). The only effective treatment for hyperacute rejection is re-transplantation.

In milder cases of primary allograft dysfunction, inotropic agents may be sufficient to restore myocardial contractility and hemodynamic stability. The management of isolated RV failure after transplantation is similar to that described in this chapter's section on RV failure in the general cardiac surgical population. This entails careful optimization of RV preload, ensuring adequate RV perfusion by maintaining adequate systemic blood pressure and avoiding secondary insult from hypoxia, acidosis, high ventilator pressures, or hypercapnia. In addition, PA hypertension should be managed aggressively, with a very low threshold to initiate iNO therapy.

With more severe cases of graft failure, mechanical circulatory support may be needed to maintain adequate perfusion until graft function improves. Depending on the specific circumstance, this might entail LVAD support, RVAD support, BiVAD support, or VA ECMO.

With the conversion from a "biatrial" to "bicaval" surgical technique for cardiac transplantation at the vast majority of centers, the incidence of sinus node dysfunction or complete heart block has been significantly reduced, with less than 10% of patients now requiring permanent pacemaker placement [110]. The transplant donor heart is completely denervated during transplantation. As a result, most transplant patients have higher than average resting heart rate. However, the period of cardiac graft ischemic time continues to predispose these patients to conduction system injury and sinus node dysfunction in the early postoperative period [111]. Bradycardia should be managed with temporary epicardial pacing until sinus rhythm returns. Permanent pacemaker implantation should generally be deferred for 2–3 weeks after transplant to allow for potential recovery of native rhythm [111]. Atrial arrhythmias are less common after cardiac transplantation than after most other cardiac surgical procedures [111]. When atrial arrhythmias do occur, the management strategy is similar to that described above for the general cardiac surgical population.

Because cardiac transplant patients have often had multiple prior cardiac surgical interventions and are often anticoagulated preoperatively, they are at an increased risk for bleeding complications after surgery. The small size of the donor heart relative to the recipient pericardium may allow for the collection of a relatively large volume of blood within the pericardium before there are clinical manifestations of tamponade.

References

1. Cohn LH, Rosborough D, Fernandez J. Reducing costs and length of stay and improving efficiency and quality of care in cardiac surgery. Ann Thorac Surg. 1997;64(6 Suppl):S58–60. discussion S80-2
2. Xu F, et al. Use of pulmonary artery catheter in coronary artery bypass graft. Costs and long-term outcomes. PLoS One. 2015;10(2):e0117610.
3. Whitener S, Konoske R, Mark JB. Pulmonary artery catheter. Best Pract Res Clin Anaesthesiol. 2014;28(4):323–35.
4. St Andre AC, DelRossi A. Hemodynamic management of patients in the first 24 hours after cardiac surgery. Crit Care Med. 2005;33(9):2082–93.
5. Baele PL, et al. Continuous monitoring of mixed venous oxygen saturation in critically ill patients. Anesth Analg. 1982;61(6):513–7.
6. Marik PE, Cavallazzi R. Does the central venous pressure predict fluid responsiveness? An updated meta-analysis and a plea for some common sense. Crit Care Med. 2013;41(7):1774–81.

7. Reddy PS, et al. Cardiac tamponade: hemodynamic observations in man. Circulation. 1978;58(2):265–72.
8. Stern DH, et al. Can we trust the direct radial artery pressure immediately following cardiopulmonary bypass? Anesthesiology. 1985;62(5):557–61.
9. Pauca AL, et al. Radial artery-to-aorta pressure difference after discontinuation of cardiopulmonary bypass. Anesthesiology. 1989;70(6):935–41.
10. Gravlee GP, et al. A comparison of radial, brachial, and aortic pressures after cardiopulmonary bypass. J Cardiothorac Anesth. 1989;3(1):20–6.
11. Herr DL, Sum-Ping ST, England M. ICU sedation after coronary artery bypass graft surgery: dexmedetomidine-based versus propofol-based sedation regimens. J Cardiothorac Vasc Anesth. 2003;17(5):576–84.
12. Ketorolac Medication Guide, R.L. Inc, Editor. Nutley, 2008. https://www.accessdata.fda.gov/drugsatfda_docs/label/2013/019645s019lbl.pdf
13. Oliveri L, Jerzewski K, Kulik A. Black box warning: is ketorolac safe for use after cardiac surgery? J Cardiothorac Vasc Anesth. 2014;28(2):274–9.
14. Wong WT, et al. Fast-track cardiac care for adult cardiac surgical patients. Cochrane Database Syst Rev. 2016;9:Cd003587.
15. Rafiq S, et al. Multimodal analgesia versus traditional opiate based analgesia after cardiac surgery, a randomized controlled trial. J Cardiothorac Surg. 2014;9:52.
16. Ucak A, et al. The effects of gabapentin on acute and chronic postoperative pain after coronary artery bypass graft surgery. J Cardiothorac Vasc Anesth. 2011;25(5):824–9.
17. Rodrigues RR, et al. Computed tomography assessment of lung structure in patients undergoing cardiac surgery with cardiopulmonary bypass. Braz J Med Biol Res. 2011;44(6):598–605.
18. Garcia-Delgado M, Navarrete-Sanchez I, Colmenero M. Preventing and managing perioperative pulmonary complications following cardiac surgery. Curr Opin Anaesthesiol. 2014;27(2):146–52.
19. Haverich A. Frequency, risk factors, and outcome of hyperlactatemia after cardiac surgery. J Thorac Cardiovasc Surg. 2003;123(5):1361–6.
20. O'Shaughnessy K. Adrenergic mechanisms and drugs. In: Clinical pharmacology. Edinburgh: Elsevier; 2012. p. 382–92.
21. Morales DL, et al. A double-blind randomized trial: prophylactic vasopressin reduces hypotension after cardiopulmonary bypass. Ann Thorac Surg. 2003;75(3):926–30.
22. Leyh RG, et al. Methylene blue: the drug of choice for catecholamine-refractory vasoplegia after cardiopulmonary bypass? J Thorac Cardiovasc Surg. 2003;125(6):1426–31.
23. Cotton BA, et al. Increased risk of adrenal insufficiency following etomidate exposure in critically injured patients. Arch Surg. 2008;143(1):62–7. discussion 67
24. Lexicomp. 2016. Wolters Kluwer. https://dailymed.nlm.nih.gov/dailymed/archives/fdaDrugInfo.cfm?archiveid=4086.
25. Ho KM, Bham E, Pavey W. Incidence of venous thromboembolism and benefits and risks of Thromboprophylaxis after cardiac surgery: a systematic review and meta-analysis. J Am Heart Assoc. 2015;4(10):e002652.
26. Dunning J, et al. Guideline on antiplatelet and anticoagulation management in cardiac surgery. Eur J Cardiothorac Surg. 2008;34(1):73–92.
27. Mathew JG, et al. Efficacy and safety of early parenteral anticoagulation as a bridge to warfarin after mechanical valve replacement. Thromb Haemost. 2014;112(6):1120–8.
28. Passaglia LG, de Barros GM, de Sousa MR. Early postoperative bridging anticoagulation after mechanical heart valve replacement: a systematic review and meta-analysis. J Thromb Haemost. 2015;13(9):1557–67.
29. Jain MK, Ridker PM. Anti-inflammatory effects of statins: clinical evidence and basic mechanisms. Nat Rev Drug Discov. 2005;4(12):977–87.
30. Mariscalco G, et al. Observational study on the beneficial effect of preoperative statins in reducing atrial fibrillation after coronary surgery. Ann Thorac Surg. 2007;84(4):1158–64.
31. Ozguler IM, et al. Rosuvastatin lowers systemic inflammatory response in coronary artery bypass graft accompanied by cardiopulmonary bypass surgery: a randomized controlled study. Clin Invest Med. 2015;38(4):E154–63.
32. Zheng Z, et al. Perioperative Rosuvastatin in cardiac surgery. N Engl J Med. 2016;374(18):1744–53.
33. Ker K, et al. Effect of tranexamic acid on surgical bleeding: systematic review and cumulative meta-analysis. BMJ. 2012;344:e3054.
34. Blommaert D, et al. Effective prevention of atrial fibrillation by continuous atrial overdrive pacing after coronary artery bypass surgery. J Am Coll Cardiol. 2000;35(6):1411–5.
35. Neto VA, et al. Temporary atrial pacing in the prevention of postoperative atrial fibrillation. Pacing Clin Electrophysiol. 2007;30(Suppl 1):S79–83.
36. Alpert JS, Petersen P, Godtfredsen J. Atrial fibrillation: natural history, complications, and management. Annu Rev Med. 1988;39:41–52.
37. Elmi F, Tullo NG, Khalighi K. Natural history and predictors of temporary epicardial pacemaker wire function in patients after open heart surgery. Cardiology. 2002;98(4):175–80.
38. Gordon RS, et al. Permanent cardiac pacing after a cardiac operation: predicting the use of permanent pacemakers. Ann Thorac Surg. 1998;66(5):1698–704.
39. Merin O, et al. Permanent pacemaker implantation following cardiac surgery: indications and long-term follow-up. Pacing Clin Electrophysiol. 2009;32(1):7–12.
40. Del Nido P, Goldman BS. Temporary epicardial pacing after open heart surgery: complications and prevention. J Card Surg. 1989;4(1):99–103.
41. van den Berghe G, et al. Intensive insulin therapy in critically ill patients. N Engl J Med. 2001;345(19):1359–67.
42. Hajjar LA, et al. Transfusion requirements after cardiac surgery: the TRACS randomized controlled trial. JAMA. 2010;304(14):1559–67.
43. van Straten AH, et al. Transfusion of red blood cells: the impact on short-term and long-term survival after coronary artery bypass grafting, a ten-year follow-up. Interact Cardiovasc Thorac Surg. 2010;10(1):37–42.
44. Hebert PC, et al. A multicenter, randomized, controlled clinical trial of transfusion requirements in critical care. Transfusion requirements in critical care investigators, Canadian critical care trials group. N Engl J Med. 1999;340(6):409–17.
45. Weitzel NS, et al. Platelet mapping as part of modified thromboelastography (TEG(R)) in patients undergoing cardiac surgery and cardiopulmonary bypass. Anaesthesia. 2012;67(10):1158–65.
46. White JM, Ruygrok PN. Intra-aortic balloon counterpulsation in contemporary practice - where are we? Heart Lung Circ. 2015;24(4):335–41.
47. Kogan A, et al. Heparin-free management of intra-aortic balloon pump after cardiac surgery. J Card Surg. 2012;27(4):434–7.
48. Choong CK, et al. Delayed re-exploration for bleeding after coronary artery bypass surgery results in adverse outcomes. Eur J Cardiothorac Surg. 2007;31(5):834–8.
49. Dunning J, et al. Guideline for resuscitation in cardiac arrest after cardiac surgery. Eur J Cardiothorac Surg. 2009;36(1):3–28.
50. Schulman S. Pharmacologic tools to reduce bleeding in surgery. Hematology Am Soc Hematol Educ Program. 2012;2012:517–21.

51. Bolliger D, et al. The anticoagulant effect of protamine sulfate is attenuated in the presence of platelets or elevated factor VIII concentrations. Anesth Analg. 2010;111(3):601–8.
52. O'Connell KA, et al. Thromboembolic adverse events after use of recombinant human coagulation factor VIIa. JAMA. 2006;295(3):293–8.
53. Carmona P, et al. Management of cardiac tamponade after cardiac surgery. J Cardiothorac Vasc Anesth. 2012;26(2):302–11.
54. Pepi M, et al. Pericardial effusion after cardiac surgery: incidence, site, size, and haemodynamic consequences. Br Heart J. 1994;72(4):327–31.
55. Tsang TS, Oh JK, Seward JB. Diagnosis and management of cardiac tamponade in the era of echocardiography. Clin Cardiol. 1999;22(7):446–52.
56. Price S, et al. 'Tamponade' following cardiac surgery: terminology and echocardiography may both mislead. Eur J Cardiothorac Surg. 2004;26(6):1156–60.
57. Vives M, et al. Cardiac surgery-associated acute kidney injury. Interact Cardiovasc Thorac Surg. 2014;18(5):637–45.
58. Shin SR, et al. Prediction and prevention of acute kidney injury after cardiac surgery. Biomed Res Int. 2016;2016:2985148.
59. Dreischulte T, et al. Combined use of nonsteroidal anti-inflammatory drugs with diuretics and/or renin-angiotensin system inhibitors in the community increases the risk of acute kidney injury. Kidney Int. 2015;88(2):396–403.
60. Zacharias M, et al. Interventions for protecting renal function in the perioperative period. Cochrane Database Syst Rev. 2013;9:Cd003590.
61. Itagaki S, Hosseinian L, Varghese R. Right ventricular failure after cardiac surgery: management strategies. Semin Thorac Cardiovasc Surg. 2012;24(3):188–94.
62. Vlahakes GJ. Right ventricular failure after cardiac surgery. Cardiol Clin. 2012;30(2):283–9.
63. Thunberg CA, et al. Pulmonary hypertension in patients undergoing cardiac surgery: pathophysiology, perioperative management, and outcomes. J Cardiothorac Vasc Anesth. 2013;27(3):551–72.
64. Zener JC, et al. Regression of extreme pulmonary hypertension after mitral valve surgery. Am J Cardiol. 1972;30(8):820–6.
65. Denault A, et al. Pulmonary hypertension in cardiac surgery. Curr Cardiol Rev. 2010;6(1):1–14.
66. Mathew JP, et al. Atrial fibrillation following coronary artery bypass graft surgery: predictors, outcomes, and resource utilization. MultiCenter study of perioperative ischemia research group. JAMA. 1996;276(4):300–6.
67. Mathew JP, et al. A multicenter risk index for atrial fibrillation after cardiac surgery. JAMA. 2004;291(14):1720–9.
68. Gowda SA, Shah A, Steinberg JS. Cardioversion of atrial fibrillation. Prog Cardiovasc Dis. 2005;48(2):88–107.
69. Risius T, et al. Comparison of antero-lateral versus antero-posterior electrode position for biphasic external cardioversion of atrial flutter. Am J Cardiol. 2009;104(11):1547–50.
70. Khasnis A, et al. Tachycardia-induced cardiomyopathy: a review of literature. Pacing Clin Electrophysiol. 2005;28(7):710–21.
71. Arsenault KA, et al. Interventions for preventing post-operative atrial fibrillation in patients undergoing heart surgery. Cochrane Database Syst Rev. 2013;1:Cd003611.
72. McDonald MG, Au NT, Rettie AE. P450-based drug-drug interactions of Amiodarone and its metabolites: diversity of inhibitory mechanisms. Drug Metab Dispos. 2015;43(11):1661–9.
73. Oral H, et al. Facilitating transthoracic cardioversion of atrial fibrillation with ibutilide pretreatment. N Engl J Med. 1999;340(24):1849–54.
74. Chatterjee S, et al. Timing and route of amiodarone for prevention of postoperative atrial fibrillation after cardiac surgery: a network regression meta-analysis. Pacing Clin Electrophysiol. 2013;36(8):1017–23.
75. Vereckei A. Current algorithms for the diagnosis of wide QRS complex tachycardias. Curr Cardiol Rev. 2014;10(3):262–76.
76. Califf RM, et al. Myonecrosis after revascularization procedures. J Am Coll Cardiol. 1998;31(2):241–51.
77. Domanski MJ, et al. Association of myocardial enzyme elevation and survival following coronary artery bypass graft surgery. JAMA. 2011;305(6):585–91.
78. Hauser AM, et al. Sequence of mechanical, electrocardiographic and clinical effects of repeated coronary artery occlusion in human beings: echocardiographic observations during coronary angioplasty. J Am Coll Cardiol. 1985;5(2 Pt 1):193–7.
79. Lobo DN, Awad S. Should chloride-rich crystalloids remain the mainstay of fluid resuscitation to prevent 'pre-renal' acute kidney injury?: con. Kidney Int. 2014;86(6):1096–105.
80. McKhann GM, et al. Stroke and encephalopathy after cardiac surgery: an update. Stroke. 2006;37(2):562–71.
81. Wityk RJ, et al. Diffusion- and perfusion-weighted brain magnetic resonance imaging in patients with neurologic complications after cardiac surgery. Arch Neurol. 2001;58(4):571–6.
82. Hartnell GG, et al. Safety of MR imaging in patients who have retained metallic materials after cardiac surgery. AJR Am J Roentgenol. 1997;168(5):1157–9.
83. Bush CK, et al. Endovascular treatment with stent-retriever devices for acute ischemic stroke: a meta-analysis of randomized controlled trials. PLoS One. 2016;11(1):e0147287.
84. Coull BM, et al. Anticoagulants and antiplatelet agents in acute ischemic stroke: report of the joint stroke guideline development Committee of the American Academy of neurology and the American Stroke Association (a division of the American Heart Association). Stroke. 2002;33(7):1934–42.
85. Muth CM, Shank ES. Gas embolism. N Engl J Med. 2000;342(7):476–82.
86. Gootjes EC, Wijdicks EF, McClelland RL. Postoperative stupor and coma. Mayo Clin Proc. 2005;80(3):350–4.
87. Acher CW, et al. Lexicomp a quantitative assessment of the impact of intercostal artery reimplantation on paralysis risk in thoracoabdominal aortic aneurysm repair. Ann Surg. 2016;248(4):529–40.
88. Coselli JS, et al. Cerebrospinal fluid drainage reduces paraplegia after thoracoabdominal aortic aneurysm repair: results of a randomized clinical trial. J Vasc Surg. 2002;35(4):631–9.
89. Ranucci M. Hemostatic and thrombotic issues in cardiac surgery. Semin Thromb Hemost. 2015;41(1):84–90.
90. Nader ND, et al. Blood product use in cardiac revascularization: comparison of on- and off-pump techniques. Ann Thorac Surg. 1999;68(5):1640–3.
91. Warkentin TE, Kelton JG. Temporal aspects of heparin-induced thrombocytopenia. N Engl J Med. 2001;344(17):1286–92.
92. Kerendi F, et al. Impact of heparin-induced thrombocytopenia on postoperative outcomes after cardiac surgery. Ann Thorac Surg. 2007;84(5):1548–53. discussion 1554-5
93. Wan C, et al. Clinical presentation, temporal relationship, and outcome in thirty-three patients with type 2 heparin-induced thrombocytopenia after cardiotomy. Ann Thorac Surg. 2006;82(1):21–6.
94. Warkentin TE, Sheppard JA. Testing for heparin-induced thrombocytopenia antibodies. Transfus Med Rev. 2006;20(4):259–72.
95. Greinacher A, Warkentin TE. Recognition, treatment, and prevention of heparin-induced thrombocytopenia: review and update. Thromb Res. 2006;118(2):165–76.
96. Kitamura T, et al. Vascular antispastic medication should take priority over other antihypertensives after coronary artery bypass grafting using a radial artery conduit. Interact Cardiovasc Thorac Surg. 2011;13(6):679–81.
97. Kon ZN, et al. Warm ischemia provokes inflammation and regional hypercoagulability within the heart during off-pump coronary artery bypass: a possible target for serine protease inhibition. Eur J Cardiothorac Surg. 2008;33(2):215–21.

98. Roger VL, et al. Heart disease and stroke statistics--2011 update: a report from the American Heart Association. Circulation. 2011;123(4):e18–e209.
99. Yoganathan AP, Woo YR, Sung HW. Turbulent shear stress measurements in the vicinity of aortic heart valve prostheses. J Biomech. 1986;19(6):433–42.
100. Matthews IG, et al. In patients undergoing aortic valve replacement, what factors predict the requirement for permanent pacemaker implantation? Interact Cardiovasc Thorac Surg. 2011;12(3):475–9.
101. Onalan O, et al. Determinants of pacemaker dependency after coronary and/or mitral or aortic valve surgery with long-term follow-up. Am J Cardiol. 2008;101(2):203–8.
102. von Oppell UO, et al. Mitral valve surgery plus concomitant atrial fibrillation ablation is superior to mitral valve surgery alone with an intensive rhythm control strategy. Eur J Cardiothorac Surg. 2009;35(4):641–50.
103. Bojar RM, et al. Manual of perioperative Care in Adult Cardiac Surgery the anticoagulant effect of protamine sulfate is attenuated in the presence of platelets or elevated factor VIII concentrations. Anesth Analg. 2011;111(3):601–8.
104. Kaneko T, et al. The safety of deep hypothermic circulatory arrest in aortic valve replacement with unclampable aorta in non-octogenarians. Interact Cardiovasc Thorac Surg. 2015;20(1):79–84.
105. Bilal H, et al. Is cerebrospinal fluid drainage of benefit to neuroprotection in patients undergoing surgery on the descending thoracic aorta or thoracoabdominal aorta? Interact Cardiovasc Thorac Surg. 2012;15(4):702–8.
106. Hernandez AF, et al. A decade of short-term outcomes in post cardiac surgery ventricular assist device implantation: data from the Society of Thoracic Surgeons' national cardiac database. Circulation. 2007;116(6):606–12.
107. Combes A, et al. Extracorporeal membrane oxygenation for respiratory failure in adults. Curr Opin Crit Care. 2012;18(1):99–104.
108. Klima U, et al. Severe right heart failure after heart transplantation. A single-center experience. Transpl Int. 2005;18(3):326–32.
109. Al-Dadah AS, et al. Clinical course and predictors of pericardial effusion following cardiac transplantation. Transplant Proc. 2007;39(5):1589–92.
110. Davies RR, et al. Standard versus bicaval techniques for orthotopic heart transplantation: an analysis of the united network for organ sharing database. J Thorac Cardiovasc Surg. 2010;140(3):700–8. 708.e1-2
111. Thajudeen A, et al. Arrhythmias after heart transplantation: mechanisms and management. J Am Heart Assoc. 2012;1(2):e001461.

Targeted Temperature Management After Cardiac Arrest

14

Cindy H. Hsu and Hasan B. Alam

Introduction

Cardiac arrest is one of the leading causes of death in the United States. Out-of-hospital cardiac arrests (OHCA) claim approximately 350,000 lives each year [15], while 209,000 people are treated for in-hospital cardiac arrest (IHCA) annually [83]. Globally, deaths from cardiovascular disease is the leading cause of death, claiming 17 million lives annually, out of which 40–50% are from sudden cardiac deaths [79]. Despite recent advancements in cardiopulmonary resuscitation, the survival rate of cardiac arrest remains low. Survival to hospital discharge for all OHCA was 10.6%, and survival with good neurologic function was only 8.6%. Survival to hospital discharge for IHCA was 23.8% [15].

Targeted temperature management (TTM), previously known as therapeutic hypothermia, is the active control of temperature at any target [24], which usually ranges from mild (34–35.9 °C) to moderate hypothermia (32–33.9 °C) during post-arrest arrangement. Previous studies have shown that TTM at 32–34 °C for 12–24 h in comatose cardiac arrest patients after shockable OHCA led to significant improvement in survival [60] and neurologic function [17, 60] when compared to standard therapy. In addition, TTM implementation has also been shown to associate with improved outcome after nonshockable cardiac arrests [91, 101, 122]. More recently, the TTM trial conducted by Nielsen et al. showed that target temperature of 33 °C did not offer additional survival benefit when compared to 36 °C in unconscious OHCA survivors [90]. This chapter will focus on the pathophysiology and practical considerations of TTM after adult non-traumatic cardiac arrest. The indications, implementation, and side effects of TTM are discussed here in order to assist readers in its application during post-arrest management.

Mechanisms

Post-cardiac arrest syndrome (PCAS) is defined as a complex syndrome consisting of brain injury, myocardial dysfunction, and systemic ischemia/reperfusion response after cardiac arrest [92]. TTM provides neuroprotection during PCAS through complex and multifactorial mechanisms. Hypothermia decreases cerebral blood flow and cerebral oxygen consumption approximately by 6–10% per 1 °C decrement [5, 41, 43, 54, 86, 96, 112, 121], thereby preventing secondary cerebral injury after the initial anoxic insult [81, 102]. However, reduction of metabolic rate is only one of the many mechanisms underlying the protective effects of hypothermia. It also leads to reduction in post-arrest endothelial dysfunction, decreased free radical production, blunting of the post-reperfusion inflammatory cascade [105], and prevention of cerebral edema caused by blood-brain barrier disruption and increased vascular permeability following ischemia-reperfusion injury [29, 64]. Finally, hypothermia also inhibits both intrinsic mitochondrial and extrinsic extracellular apoptotic cell death pathways [136].

Inclusion and Exclusion Criteria

Post-arrest TTM was initially implemented only for shockable OHCA. Its use has since expanded to include nonshockable OHCA and IHCA based on retrospective studies showing potential benefits in those patient cohorts [91, 101, 122]. Table 14.1 highlights the 2015 American Heart Association (AHA) recommendations for post-arrest TTM based on the AHA Class of Recommendation (COR) and

C. H. Hsu
Department of Emergency Medicine and Surgery, University of Michigan, Ann Arbor, MI, USA

H. B. Alam (✉)
Department of General Surgery, University of Michigan, Ann Arbor, MI, USA
e-mail: alamh@med.umich.edu

A. Salim et al. (eds.), *Surgical Critical Care Therapy*, https://doi.org/10.1007/978-3-319-71712-8_14

Table 14.1 Highlights from the 2015 American Heart Association recommendations for TTM after cardiac arrest [24]

1. Class I (strong) recommendations for
(a) TTM to treat comatose post-cardiac arrest patients suffering out-of-hospital VF/pulseless VT (LOE B-Randomized)
(b) TTM to treat comatose post-cardiac arrest patients suffering non-VF/pulseless VT (nonshockable) rhythms and IHCA (stronger recommendation than the 2010 guidelines) (LOE C-Expert Opinion)
(c) Selection and maintenance of a constant temperature within the range from 32 °C to 36 °C (LOE B-Randomized)
2. Class IIa (moderate) recommendation for TTM to be maintained for at least 24 h after reaching target temperature (LOE C-Expert Opinion)
3. Class IIb (weak) recommendation that it may be reasonable to actively prevent fever in comatose patients (LOE C-Limited Data)
4. Class III (moderate – no benefit) recommendation against routine prehospital cooling of patients after ROSC with the rapid infusion of cold intravenous fluids (LOE A)

For more information, visit https://eccguidelines.heart.org/wp-content/uploads/2015/10/2015-AHA-Guidelines-Highlights-English.pdf
Level of evidence (*LOE*), target temperature management (*TTM*), ventricular fibrillation (*VF*), ventricular tachycardia (*VT*), return of spontaneous circulation (*ROSC*)

Table 14.2 Recommended exclusion criteria for TTM

Do-not-resuscitate/do-not-intubate status
Terminal illness
More than 12 h since return of spontaneous circulation (ROSC)
Glasgow motor score >5
Minimal premorbid cognitive status
Other reason for coma such as intracranial pathology (i.e., intracranial hemorrhage, ischemic stroke), subarachnoid hemorrhage, or sedation
Sepsis as etiology for arrest
Uncontrollable bleeding or significant trauma

Level of Evidence (LOE) system. These recommendations originated from an extensive evidence review process by the International Liaison Committee on Resuscitation (ILCOR). The AHA provides Class I (strong) recommendation for the application of TTM by maintaining temperature between 32 °C and 36 °C (LOE B-Randomized) for comatose cardiac arrest patients who sustained an out-of-hospital shockable rhythm (LOE B-Randomized), nonshockable rhythm (LOE C-Expert Opinion), and IHCA (LOE C-Expert Opinion). Class IIa (moderate) recommendation was made for TTM maintenance for at least 24 h after reaching target temperature (LOE C-Expert Opinion), while Class IIb (weak) recommendation to actively prevent fever in comatose patients (LOE C-Limited Data) [24]. The absolute contraindications for TTM are more variable depending on institutional guidelines. Table 14.2 lists the common recommended TTM exclusion criteria.

Clinical Implementation

TTM consists of three key phases – induction, maintenance, and rewarming. The understanding of physiology during each phase is essential for the optimization of patient management. Figure 14.1 illustrates the three TTM phases with their respective temperature, range, and duration.

Induction

The induction phase starts from initiation of active cooling to when the patient reaches target temperature [100], which is typically between 32 °C and 36 °C. Rapid induction of hypothermia can be achieved by infusion of 30–40 cc/kg 4 °C isotonic fluid [108], providing that the patient does not have evidence of heart failure or pulmonary edema. Surface cooling tools such as ice packs or pre-refrigerated surface pads and external cooling device can also be applied. In addition, endovascular catheters can induce rapid core cooling but require the placement of invasive catheters. In a retrospective analysis of the TTM trial, endovascular and surface cooling were equally effective during induction of mild hypothermia. However, surface cooling was associated with less precision during the maintenance phase. There was no difference in adverse events, mortality, or poor neurologic outcomes between patients treated with endovascular and surface cooling devices [51]. Once induction has begun, an external cooling device is applied to maintain the patient at target temperature. All devices work via a feedback loop that adjusts the temperature of the water circulating through the cooling system to maintain a constant target core body temperature, which should be continuously monitored via an esophageal, bladder, or rectal temperature probe [8].

During the induction phase, the registered temperature will constantly lag behind actual core temperature, which means that the cooling device may continue to cool the patient when the target temperature has been reached. Faster cooling rate will cause greater lag time between registered and actual core temperature. Small overshoot of ≤1 °C is generally acceptable provided that core temperature is maintained above 30 °C [106].

Induction of hypothermia is generally easier in older patients than younger patients due to decreased ability to regulate body temperature, lower rate of metabolism, and lower body mass index associated with older age [38, 118]. Thus, the requirement of opiates and sedatives during TTM is generally higher for younger patients. Achieving hypothermia in obese patients also takes more time due to their larger body mass index [106]. Side effects such as hypovolemia, electrolyte derangement, hyperglycemia, hemodynamic instability, and shivering are generally greatest during

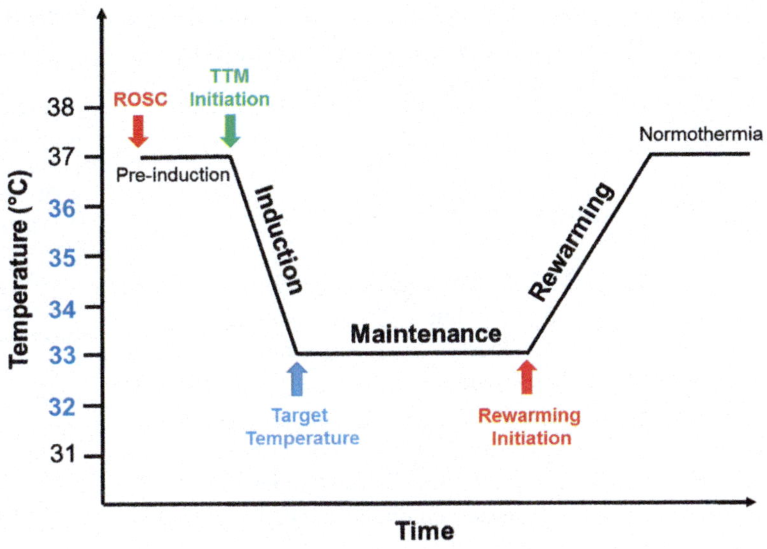

Fig. 14.1 Phases of targeted temperature management (TTM). A schematic diagram illustrating the first 72 h after return of spontaneous circulation (ROSC), assuming starting at normothermia and target temperature of 33 °C

induction phase [103, 104, 107]. This may be minimized by cooling the patients as rapidly as possible [106].

Animal studies have shown that earlier initiation of TTM and time to target temperature of within 4 h after return of spontaneous circulation (ROSC) can improve survival with good neurologic function [27]. In addition, the initiation of intra-arrest hypothermia may reduce brain injury [1, 67, 68, 93, 123, 138]. However, these findings have not been consistently observed in human subjects. In recent studies, shorter time to target temperature was associated with worse outcome [56, 80, 99, 133], likely due to more significant injury and impaired thermoregulation in the shorter time to target temperature group. In a randomized, non-blinded controlled trial, intra-arrest hypothermia was induced with intravenous cold saline and external cooling device for OHCA patients. There was no observed short-term survival or functional difference at 1 month between the intra-arrest hypothermia patients and those who received routine post-arrest TTM [39]. Another trial found an increase in pulmonary edema and rearrest among patients treated with a goal of prehospital infusion of 2 L cold fluid [66]. These observations illustrate the complex relationship between early neurologic damage and post-arrest thermoregulation. Given the conflicting data, the AHA recommends against routine prehospital cooling of patients after ROSC with the rapid infusion of cold intravenous fluids [24]. An ongoing randomized study (PRINCESS trial) plans to examine the efficacy of prehospital intranasal cooling.

Maintenance

The maintenance phase extends from the achievement of target temperature to the initiation of rewarming. During this time, the goal is to tightly control core temperature with small or no temperature variation (range of ≤0.2–0.5 °C). Patients generally achieve relative stability during this time due to minimal temperature variation.

The duration of maintenance phase remains an area of active investigation. Although the maintenance phase usually lasts 24 h, animal studies have shown that TTM for 48 h led to improved survival and functional outcome [27]. An upcoming prospective randomized trial will shed light on this topic by comparing the survival differences between OHCA patients who receive 24 versus 48 h of TTM (TTH48 study, NCT 01689077). Patient may stay in the maintenance phase for several days, particularly if there are cerebral edema or intracranial hypertension related issues [8].

Rewarming

Rewarming phase is the period during which patients are gradually rewarmed to normothermia. It is a dynamic and challenging phase due to side effects associated with increase in temperature. This is especially true for patients with cerebral edema, as they have higher risk of intracranial hypertension during rewarming. Furthermore, normalization of body temperature can cause systemic vasodilation and hypotension, thereby triggering cerebral vasodilation. In addition, warmer temperature will induce electrolyte extracellular shifts, making hyperkalemia a potential side effect.

In general, rewarming rate of no faster than 0.2–0.5 °C/h is recommended, and it can be reduced to 0.1 °C/h if there is intracranial hypertension. Rewarming should be performed under controlled fashion [8]. After rewarming, normothermia should be maintained to avoid pyrexia, which has been shown to associate with worse outcome after cardiac arrest [53, 70, 106]. The duration of normothermia varies, but most protocols suggest maintaining additional 48–72 h of normothermia after rewarming.

Core Temperature Measurement

A critical step in TTM is the accurate measurement of core body temperature. While pulmonary artery and jugular bulb catheters enable instantaneous and accurate measurement of core blood and brain temperature, respectively, they are invasive and thus seldom performed for the sole purpose of temperature measurement. Endovascular cooling catheters are able to simultaneously measure blood temperature at the catheter tip during temperature modulation. Esophageal temperature probe, when inserted to the distal 1/3 of the esophagus, can achieve the most accurate noninvasive measurement of core temperature and thus is preferred for continuous temperature measurement during TTM. Compared to bladder or rectal temperature probes, esophageal temperature probes have less lag time between registered temperature and measured core temperature and are therefore least likely to cause overshooting during the induction phase of TTM. Tympanic membrane and nasopharyngeal temperature probes may reflect brain temperature better than more distant sites. However, they have higher risks for probe displacement and bleeding [106].

TTM implementation is best performed with protocol-driven therapy [49, 125]. Table 14.3 provides a practical checklist for TTM implementation during each phase. For compilation of different institutional TTM protocols, please refer to the Penn Post-Cardiac Arrest Care/Therapeutic Hypothermia Resources website (https://www.med.upenn.edu/resuscitation/hypothermia/index.shtml).

Table 14.3 Practical checklist for TTM implementation

Induction and maintenance
Use an esophageal probe for core temperature measurement if possible. Temperature sensing bladder catheter is preferred over rectal probe if an esophageal probe is not feasible or contraindicated
Induce hypothermia with bolus 30–40 cc/kg cold intravenous fluid if there is no evidence of heart failure or pulmonary edema
Apply external cooling device or insert endovascular cooling catheter
Maintain target temperature of 32–36 °C for at least 24 h
If the patient becomes unstable or has increased bleeding risk, target temperature of 36 °C can be considered
Do not let core temperature fall below 30 °C
Avoid electrolyte derangements including hypokalemia, hypophosphatemia, hypomagnesemia
Avoid hypovolemia from cold diuresis
Avoid hyperglycemia
Control shivering
Initiate continuous EEG during induction if possible
Obtain head computerized tomography scan if intracranial pathology is of concern
Rewarming
Rewarm slowly (0.2–0.5 °C/h, 0.1 °C/h if concern for cerebral edema)
Adjust insulin dosage and avoid hypoglycemia
Monitor for hyperkalemia
Control shivering
Maintain normothermia for 48–72 h after rewarming
Overall
Provide good intensive care
Avoid hypotension. Recommend maintaining systolic blood pressure ≥90 mm Hg and mean arterial pressure ≥65 mm Hg
Avoid hypoxemia
Maintain normocarbia. Adjust ventilator settings by using temperature corrected arterial blood gases and continuous end tidal capnography
Avoid and treat infections
Monitor for bleeding and coagulopathy. Consider using thromboelastography measured at the appropriate temperature
Adjust medication dosage according to patient temperature and organ dysfunction
Do no prognosticate until at least 72 h after rewarming

Side Effects

Shivering

Shivering is the most common side effect of hypothermia. In conjunction with peripheral vasoconstriction, shivering provides hypothalamus-driven thermoregulation. In healthy humans, peripheral vasoconstriction is triggered at 36.5 °C and shivering at 35.5 °C [118]. Temperature threshold for vasoconstriction and shivering can be higher than normal in brain-injured [10] or febrile patients [105], thereby inducing these thermoregulatory responses at higher temperature. If left untreated, shivering can impede the cooling process and result in increased cerebral metabolic demand [9, 10], increased myocardial oxygen consumption from tachycardia [48], and excessive work of breathing [106]. Shivering is best managed by adequate monitoring and stepwise administration of medication specifically targeting shivering responses. Anti-shivering medications include fentanyl, meperidine, buspirone, dexmedetomidine, propofol, clonidine, magnesium, and neuromuscular blockers [106].

Electrolyte Derangements

Patients frequently develop low electrolytes during hypothermia due to combination of cellular shifts, renal tubular dysfunction, and cold diuresis [107]. Hypothermia induces electrolyte influx into the intracellular compartments, resulting in hypokalemia, hypomagnesemia, and hypophosphatemia [105]. However, these electrolytes are released into the extracellular spaces during rewarming. Thus, excessive potassium replacement should be avoided during the maintenance phase to avoid rebound hyperkalemia during rewarming [103]. The rate of rebound hyperkalemia is associated with rate of rewarming [8]. Hypomagnesemia can increase the risk of arrhythmias, brain injury, and myocardial infarction [2, 4, 28, 82, 109, 115, 129, 134]. Cold diuresis can cause hypovolemia particularly during the induction and maintenance phases.

Cardiac Function and Hemodynamics

At 33–35 °C, bradycardia and reduced myocardial contractility cause reduced cardiac output and blood pressure. Temperature below 32 °C can lead to atrial and ventricular tachycardia and fibrillation [8, 16, 103]. In addition, hypomagnesemia can further predispose cardiomyocytes to arrhythmias and myocardial infarction. Studies of patients after cardiac arrest have found that a systolic blood pressure less than 90 mm Hg [22, 125, 127] or a mean arterial pressure of less than 65 mm Hg is associated with higher mortality and diminished functional recovery [125]. Therefore, it is reasonable to avoid and immediately correct hypotension (systolic blood pressure <90 mmg Hg or mean arterial blood pressure <65 mm Hg) during post-arrest care, although optimal hemodynamic goals remain unclear and may be patient dependent (Class IIb, LOE C-Limited Data) [24].

Acid Base

Carbon dioxide becomes more soluble in colder temperature; thus the pCO_2 falls and pH rises during hypothermia. The reduction of metabolic rate during hypothermia further reduces oxygen consumptions and carbon dioxide production. Therefore, hyperventilation will occur if ventilator settings are left unchanged, leading to potential adverse consequences such as cerebral vasoconstriction [31, 32]. Patient's acid base status should be monitored with frequent arterial blood gases especially during induction period to make the appropriate ventilator setting changes. The interpretation of blood gas can either be maintained at 37 °C regardless of patient's actual temperature (alpha-stat management) or corrected to account for colder temperature (pH-stat management). There is substantial controversy regarding which management is preferable. Only one method should be used for consistent patient management [8]. Continuous end-tidal capnography is also helpful for the prevention of prolonged hyperventilation.

Insulin Resistance

Hypothermia leads to decreased insulin secretion and moderate insulin resistance. Hyperglycemia may require significant insulin infusion during hypothermia. Insulin resistance may be rapidly reversed during rewarming phase, leading to hypoglycemia if insulin dosage is not appropriately adjusted. Glucose levels should be monitored frequently during TTM [105, 106].

Impaired Immune Function

Hypothermia inhibits leukocyte migration, phagocytosis, and secretion of proinflammatory cytokines. It can increase the risk of infection due to reduced leukocyte function, peripheral vasoconstriction, and hyperglycemia [105]. Although hypothermia-associated infection has not correlated with worse outcome [106], care should be taken to prevent bedsores, monitor surgical wounds, and minimize catheter site infections.

Coagulation

The interplay between cardiac arrest-induced hypercoagulopathy and potential bleeding diathesis caused by hypothermia is complex. Cardiac arrest results in intravascular fibrin deposits and formation of microthromboses [36, 57]. Hypercoagulable state of cardiac arrest is thought to be triggered by stasis, acidosis, glycocalyx shedding, and endothelial release of clotting factors such as thrombin [46, 47, 50, 63, 88]. On the other hand, hypothermia during TTM may cause platelet dysfunction, increased fibrinolysis, and decreased coagulation enzymatic activities that can contribute to bleeding. However, clinically relevant bleeding in hypothermia occurs more frequently in trauma than medically induced hypothermia. Standard coagulation tests will not show abnormalities unless they are performed at the patient's actual core temperature [106]. Nevertheless, hypothermia does not affect platelet function until below 35 °C [84, 130], and clotting factors are affected below 33 °C [97, 128, 130]. Thus, TTM at 36 °C may be preferable for patients who are actively bleeding or at high risk for bleeding.

Drug Metabolism

The combination of decreased volume of distribution, cardiac output, and metabolism/ excretion of drugs during cardiac arrest and hypothermia result in higher plasma concentrations for most medications during TTM. The renal, hepatic, and biliary clearance of drugs administered during cardiac arrest and TTM are decreased [34]. Furthermore, hypothermia results in modifications of plasma protein-binding capacity to drugs. Lingering effects of sedatives may confound prognostication and even mimic brain death [131]. For example, studies have shown the decrease of propofol, remifentanil, and midazolam levels during rewarming, whereas no changes were observed for fentanyl concentration, indicating that pharmacokinetic changes to fentanyl occurs during induction and maintenance phases but persist during rewarming [19]. Some anti-shivering medications such as meperidine are longer acting, and their prolonged half-life during hypothermia may further interfere with prognostication.

Adjunct Therapies

Electroencephalography

Clinical seizures are common after cardiac arrest and predictive of poor neurologic outcome. A post hoc analysis of the TTM trial reported 29% prevalence of clinical seizures during days 1–7 after cardiac arrest [77]. Myoclonic seizures were the most common and predictive of poor outcome. The 2015 AHA Guidelines recommend that patients be monitored frequently or continuously with electroencephalography (EEG) during TTM to identify and promptly treat seizures (Class I, LOE C-Limited Data). The same anticonvulsants for the treatment of status epilepticus caused by other etiologies may be considered after cardiac arrest (Class IIb, LOE C-Limited Data) [24]. Routine use of prophylactic anticonvulsant is not recommended due to potential side effects and uncertain benefits.

Coronary Angiography

The indication for emergent cardiac catheterization after cardiac arrest remains an area of debate. For OHCA survivors whose cardiac arrest was due to suspected cardiac etiology with a post-arrest electrocardiography (ECG) showing ST elevation myocardial infarction (STEMI), emergent cardiac catheterization is recommended for prompt identification and recanalization of the culprit coronary lesions (Class I, LOE B-Nonrandomized) [24]. However, the initial rhythm and ECG findings of cardiac arrest survivors can be poor predictor of acute coronary artery occlusion. A recent meta-analysis demonstrated that as much as 32.2% of patients who had been successfully resuscitated from cardiopulmonary arrest without ST elevation on ECG had an acute coronary lesion that would benefit from emergent percutaneous coronary intervention [87].

The 2015 AHA Guidelines state that emergent coronary angiography is reasonable for select adult patients after OHCA of suspected cardiac origin but without ST elevation on EKG (Class IIa, LOE B-Nonrandomized) [24]. The decision to perform coronary angiography should not include consideration of neurologic status due to the unreliability of early prognostic signs. An ongoing prospective study plans to examine the mortality benefit of transfer of OHCA survivors with non-ischemic EKG to cardiac arrest center for urgent coronary catheterization versus receiving care at local hospitals (ARREST trial, ISRCTN96585404). Another study will compare emergent versus delayed coronary angiogram in OHCA survivors with no obvious non-cardiac cause of arrest (EMERGE trial, NCT02876458). These trials will hopefully provide further insights regarding the characteristics of OHCA patients who will benefit from emergent percutaneous coronary intervention.

Extracorporeal Cardiopulmonary Resuscitation (ECPR)

For a subset of patients with refractory cardiac arrest, extracorporeal cardiopulmonary resuscitation (ECPR) may provide temporary circulatory support until definitive treatment and myocardial recovery. Retrospective studies have reported that utilization of ECPR in refractory OHCA with survival rate ranging from 4% to 55% [6, 14, 30, 44, 45, 55, 62, 65, 69, 74, 78, 116, 124, 135]. However, there is currently insufficient evidence to recommend routine use of ECPR for patients with cardiac arrest. In settings where it can be rapidly implemented, ECPR may be considered for select patients for whom the suspected etiology of the cardiac arrest is potentially reversible during a limited period of mechanical cardiorespiratory support (Class IIb, LOE-C Limited Data) [24].

Prognostication

Post-arrest prognostication is a multimodal approach that consists of clinical examination, biomarkers, EEG, somatosensory evoked potentials (SSEP), and brain imaging to predict patient outcome [91]. The absence of motor movements, extensor posturing [18, 21, 35, 113, 114, 117], or myoclonus [18, 21, 33, 73, 94, 113, 114] should not be used alone to predict outcome due to their high false-positive rate. In comatose patients who are treated with TTM, the absence of pupillary reflex to light at 72 h or more after cardiac arrest is useful to predict poor neurologic outcome. Other clinical findings associated with poor neurologic outcome include the presence of status myoclonus during the first 72 h after cardiac arrest, the absence of the N20 SSEP cortical wave 24–72 h after cardiac arrest or after rewarming, the presence of a marked reduction of the gray-white ratio on brain computed tomography obtained within 2 h after cardiac arrest, extensive restriction of diffusion on brain magnetic resonance imaging at 2–6 days after cardiac arrest, persistent absence of EEG reactivity to external stimuli at 72 h after cardiac arrest, and persistent burst suppression or intractable status epilepticus on EEG after rewarming [24].

Taken together, the earliest time to prognosticate a poor neurologic outcome is 72 h after rewarming, and the interval should be extended longer if the residual effect of sedation and/or paralysis confounds the clinical examination. Recent retrospective studies have shown that TTM was associated with variable delay in awakening beyond 3 days after ROSC or rewarming [42, 52, 89, 98, 110, 137]. In addition to hypothermia, factors such as older age, renal insufficiency, and post-resuscitation shock were also independent predictors of delayed awakening after cardiac arrest [98, 110].

Other Considerations

Asphyxial and Hanging-Induced Cardiac Arrest

The effects of TTM for asphyxial and hanging-induced cardiac arrest remain unclear. Recent case reports [61, 72] and small retrospective studies [11, 20, 59, 71, 120, 132] have suggested that TTM may lead to good neurologic outcome for adult survivors who sustained asphyxial cardiac arrest. Furthermore, studies in animals and newborns have demonstrated beneficial effects of TTM in reducing hypoxic encephalopathy caused by asphyxia [7, 75]. Cardiac arrests caused by asphyxia or hanging are often unwitnessed, received no bystander CPR, and have more dismal outcome. Given the relative low side effect profile associated with TTM, it is reasonable to implement post-arrest TTM for these patients given their otherwise poor outcome.

Pregnant Patients

Cardiac arrest related to pregnancy is rare. TTM may be considered on an individual basis after cardiac arrest in a comatose pregnant patient. Few case reports [26, 37, 95] described the use of TTM for cardiac arrest during pregnancy, which led to mothers discharged with good neurologic outcome and variable fetal outcome. A comprehensive, team-based approach involving cardiologists, emergency physicians, intensivists, obstetricians, and neurologists should be used in evaluating and selecting pregnant patients who might benefit from TTM.

Traumatic Cardiac Arrest

No clinical trials have studied the effect of TTM on traumatic cardiac arrest. While induced TTM is protective through several different mechanisms in non-traumatic cardiac arrest, spontaneous hypothermia after traumatic injury and hemorrhagic shock is a marker for injury severity, greater transfusion requirement, and worse outcome [3, 76, 119]. Hypothermia, acidosis, and coagulopathy constitute the lethal triad of poor outcome in trauma patients [23, 58]. Unfortunately, the outcome of traumatic cardiac arrest remains dismal [111] despite prompt hemorrhagic control and balanced resuscitation.

The rapid induction of deep hypothermia (less than 15 °C) has been shown to improve the outcome of exsanguinating cardiac arrest in animals [25, 126] for up to 90 min no-flow time in canine models [12, 13]. The Emergency Preservation and Resuscitation for Cardiac Arrest from Trauma (EPR-CAT, NCT01042015) trial is an ongoing multicenter phase 2 study that examines the feasibility and outcome of deep hypothermia in penetrating traumatic cardiac arrest subjects. Inclusion criteria include those who sustained exsanguinating penetrating trauma and loss of pulse <5 min prior to arriving or in the emergency department and without immediate ROSC after aortic cross-clamp. An arterial catheter will be inserted into the descending thoracic aorta, and a large quantity of ice-cold saline will be infused as rapidly as possible into the aorta with the goal of cooling the brain (tympanic membrane temperature) to <10 °C. Once the subjects have been sufficiently cooled, bleeding will be controlled surgically. They will then be resuscitated and rewarmed with full cardiopulmonary bypass. The goal is to improve neurologically intact survival by inducing hypothermic preservation in trauma victims who have exsanguinated to cardiac arrest (https://clinicaltrials.gov/ct2/show/NCT01042015).

Conclusion

It has been over 15 years since the publication of two landmark studies demonstrating improved survival and functional outcome of TTM for OHCA patients. Despite established guidelines for the use of TTM in patients who suffer cardiac arrest [24], adoption of this practice has been low, especially for IHCA patients [85] and patients who had initial nonshockable rhythms [40]. Many topics such as the optimal target temperature, rate of induction, duration of maintenance phase, efficacy of intra-arrest cooling, and benefit of TTM for IHCA and nonshockable rhythms remain areas in need for further investigation. Ongoing and future prospective TTM-related trials are highlighted in Table 14.4 and can hopefully provide further guidance for the utilization of TTM in post-arrest management.

Table 14.4 Ongoing and planned TTM studies

Study name	Primary outcomes	Study status[a]
Mild induced hypothermia (33 °C) versus fever control (≤37.8 °C) only (TTM-2, NCT02908308)	Mortality at 6 months	Not yet recruiting
Targeted temperature management after nonshockable cardiac arrest: 32.5–33.5 °C versus 36.5–37.5 °C (NSE-HYPERION, NCT02722473)	NSE values between day 1 and day 3	Recruiting
Targeted temperature management after cardiac arrest for 24 versus 48 h (TTH48, NCT01689077)	Neurologic outcome at 6 months (CPC1–2)	Finished recruitment
Influence of Cooling Duration On Efficacy in Cardiac Arrest Patients (ICECAP, randomized adaptive trial)	Modified Rankin score at 90 days	Not yet recruiting
Prehospital Resuscitation Intra Nasal Cooling Effectiveness Survival Study (PRINCESS, NCT01400373)	Neurologically intact survival (CPC1–2) at 90 days after cardiac arrest	Recruiting

NSE Neuron-specific enolase, *CPC* cerebral performance category, *TTM* targeted temperature management
[a]As of April, 2017

References

1. Abella BS, Zhao D, Alvarado J, Hamann K, Vanden Hoek TL, Becker LB. Intra-arrest cooling improves outcomes in a murine cardiac arrest model. Circulation. 2004;109(22):2786–91. https://doi.org/10.1161/01.CIR.0000131940.19833.85.
2. Abraham AS, Eylath U, Weinstein M, Czaczkes E. Serum magnesium levels in patients with acute myocardial infarction. N Engl J Med. 1977;296(15):862–3. https://doi.org/10.1056/NEJM197704142961509.
3. Alam HB, Pusateri AE, Kindzelski A, Egan D, Hoots K, Andrews MT, Rhee P, Tisherman S, Mann K, Vostal J, Kochanek PM, Scalea T, Deal V, Sheppard F, Sopko G, HYPOSTAT workshop participants. Hypothermia and hemostasis in severe trauma: a new crossroads workshop report. J Trauma Acute Care Surg. 2012;73(4):809–17. https://doi.org/10.1097/TA.0b013e318265d1b8.
4. Altman D, Carroli G, Duley L, Farrell B, Moodley J, Neilson J, Smith D, Magpie Trial Collaboration G. Do women with pre-eclampsia, and their babies, benefit from magnesium sulphate? The Magpie Trial: a randomised placebo-controlled trial. Lancet. 2002;359(9321):1877–90.
5. Aoki M, Nomura F, Stromski ME, Tsuji MK, Fackler JC, Hickey PR, Holtzman DH, Jonas RA. Effects of pH on brain energetics after hypothermic circulatory arrest. Ann Thorac Surg. 1993;55(5):1093–103.
6. Avalli L, Maggioni E, Formica F, Redaelli G, Migliari M, Scanziani M, Celotti S, Coppo A, Caruso R, Ristagno G, Fumagalli R. Favourable survival of in-hospital compared to out-of-hospital refractory cardiac arrest patients treated with extracorporeal membrane oxygenation: an Italian tertiary care centre experience. Resuscitation. 2012;83(5):579–83. https://doi.org/10.1016/j.resuscitation.2011.10.013.
7. Azzopardi DV, Strohm B, Edwards AD, Dyet L, Halliday HL, Juszczak E, Kapellou O, Levene M, Marlow N, Porter E, Thoresen M, Whitelaw A, Brocklehurst P, Group TS. Moderate hypothermia to treat perinatal asphyxial encephalopathy. N Engl J Med. 2009;361(14):1349–58. https://doi.org/10.1056/NEJMoa0900854.
8. Badjatia N. Therapeutic hypothermia protocols. Handb Clin Neurol. 2017;141:619–32. https://doi.org/10.1016/B978-0-444-63599-0.00033-8.
9. Badjatia N, Strongilis E, Gordon E, Prescutti M, Fernandez L, Fernandez A, Buitrago M, Schmidt JM, Ostapkovich ND, Mayer SA. Metabolic impact of shivering during therapeutic temperature modulation: the Bedside Shivering Assessment Scale. Stroke. 2008;39(12):3242–7. https://doi.org/10.1161/STROKEAHA.108.523654.
10. Badjatia N, Strongilis E, Prescutti M, Fernandez L, Fernandez A, Buitrago M, Schmidt JM, Mayer SA. Metabolic benefits of surface counter warming during therapeutic temperature modulation. Crit Care Med. 2009;37(6):1893–7. https://doi.org/10.1097/CCM.0b013e31819fffd3.
11. Baldursdottir S, Sigvaldason K, Karason S, Valsson F, Sigurdsson GH. Induced hypothermia in comatose survivors of asphyxia: a case series of 14 consecutive cases. Acta Anaesthesiol Scand. 2010;54(7):821–6. https://doi.org/10.1111/j.1399-6576.2010.02248.x.
12. Behringer W, Prueckner S, Safar P, Radovsky A, Kentner R, Stezoski SW, Henchir J, Tisherman SA. Rapid induction of mild cerebral hypothermia by cold aortic flush achieves normal recovery in a dog outcome model with 20-minute exsanguination cardiac arrest. Acad Emerg Med. 2000;7(12):1341–8.
13. Behringer W, Safar P, Wu X, Kentner R, Radovsky A, Kochanek PM, Dixon CE, Tisherman SA. Survival without brain damage after clinical death of 60-120 mins in dogs using suspended animation by profound hypothermia. Crit Care Med. 2003;31(5):1523–31. https://doi.org/10.1097/01.CCM.0000063450.73967.40.
14. Bellezzo JM, Shinar Z, Davis DP, Jaski BE, Chillcott S, Stahovich M, Walker C, Baradarian S, Dembitsky W. Emergency physician-initiated extracorporeal cardiopulmonary resuscitation. Resuscitation. 2012;83(8):966–70. https://doi.org/10.1016/j.resuscitation.2012.01.027.
15. Benjamin EJ, Blaha MJ, Chiuve SE, Cushman M, Das SR, Deo R, de Ferranti SD, Floyd J, Fornage M, Gillespie C, Isasi CR, Jimenez MC, Jordan LC, Judd SE, Lackland D, Lichtman JH, Lisabeth L, Liu S, Longenecker CT, Mackey RH, Matsushita K, Mozaffarian D, Mussolino ME, Nasir K, Neumar RW, Palaniappan L, Pandey DK, Thiagarajan RR, Reeves MJ, Ritchey M, Rodriguez CJ, Roth GA, Rosamond WD, Sasson C, Towfighi A, Tsao CW, Turner MB, Virani SS, Voeks JH, Willey JZ, Wilkins JT, Wu JH, Alger HM, Wong SS, Muntner P, American Heart Association Statistics C, Stroke Statistics S. Heart disease and stroke statistics-2017 update: a report from the American Heart Association. Circulation. 2017;135(10):e146–603. https://doi.org/10.1161/CIR.0000000000000485.
16. Bergman R, Braber A, Adriaanse MA, van Vugt R, Tjan DH, van Zanten AR. Haemodynamic consequences of mild therapeutic hypothermia after cardiac arrest. Eur J Anaesthesiol. 2010;27(4):383–7. https://doi.org/10.1097/EJA.0b013e3283333a7d.
17. Bernard SA, Gray TW, Buist MD, Jones BM, Silvester W, Gutteridge G, Smith K. Treatment of comatose survivors of out-of-hospital cardiac arrest with induced hypothermia. N Engl J Med. 2002;346(8):557–63. https://doi.org/10.1056/NEJMoa003289.
18. Bisschops LL, van Alfen N, Bons S, van der Hoeven JG, Hoedemaekers CW. Predictors of poor neurologic outcome in patients after cardiac arrest treated with hypothermia: a retrospective study. Resuscitation. 2011;82(6):696–701. https://doi.org/10.1016/j.resuscitation.2011.02.020.

19. Bjelland TW, Klepstad P, Haugen BO, Nilsen T, Salvesen O, Dale O. Concentrations of remifentanil, propofol, fentanyl, and midazolam during rewarming from therapeutic hypothermia. Acta Anaesthesiol Scand. 2014;58(6):709–15. https://doi.org/10.1111/aas.12300.
20. Borgquist O, Friberg H. Therapeutic hypothermia for comatose survivors after near-hanging-a retrospective analysis. Resuscitation. 2009;80(2):210–2. https://doi.org/10.1016/j.resuscitation.2008.10.013.
21. Bouwes A, Binnekade JM, Kuiper MA, Bosch FH, Zandstra DF, Toornvliet AC, Biemond HS, Kors BM, Koelman JH, Verbeek MM, Weinstein HC, Hijdra A, Horn J. Prognosis of coma after therapeutic hypothermia: a prospective cohort study. Ann Neurol. 2012;71(2):206–12. https://doi.org/10.1002/ana.22632.
22. Bray JE, Bernard S, Cantwell K, Stephenson M, Smith K, Committee VS. The association between systolic blood pressure on arrival at hospital and outcome in adults surviving from out-of-hospital cardiac arrests of presumed cardiac aetiology. Resuscitation. 2014;85(4):509–15. https://doi.org/10.1016/j.resuscitation.2013.12.005.
23. Brohi K, Singh J, Heron M, Coats T. Acute traumatic coagulopathy. J Trauma. 2003;54(6):1127–30. https://doi.org/10.1097/01.TA.0000069184.82147.06.
24. Callaway CW, Donnino MW, Fink EL, Geocadin RG, Golan E, Kern KB, Leary M, Meurer WJ, Peberdy MA, Thompson TM, Zimmerman JL. Part 8: post-cardiac arrest care: 2015 American Heart Association guidelines update for cardiopulmonary resuscitation and emergency cardiovascular care. Circulation. 2015;132(18 Suppl 2):S465–82. https://doi.org/10.1161/CIR.0000000000000262.
25. Capone A, Safar P, Radovsky A, Wang YF, Peitzman A, Tisherman SA. Complete recovery after normothermic hemorrhagic shock and profound hypothermic circulatory arrest of 60 minutes in dogs. J Trauma. 1996;40(3):388–95.
26. Chauhan A, Musunuru H, Donnino M, McCurdy MT, Chauhan V, Walsh M. The use of therapeutic hypothermia after cardiac arrest in a pregnant patient. Ann Emerg Med. 2012;60(6):786–9. https://doi.org/10.1016/j.annemergmed.2012.06.004.
27. Che D, Li L, Kopil CM, Liu Z, Guo W, Neumar RW. Impact of therapeutic hypothermia onset and duration on survival, neurologic function, and neurodegeneration after cardiac arrest. Crit Care Med. 2011;39(6):1423–30. https://doi.org/10.1097/CCM.0b013e318212020a.
28. Chernow B, Bamberger S, Stoiko M, Vadnais M, Mills S, Hoellerich V, Warshaw AL. Hypomagnesemia in patients in postoperative intensive care. Chest. 1989;95(2):391–7.
29. Chi OZ, Liu X, Weiss HR. Effects of mild hypothermia on blood-brain barrier disruption during isoflurane or pentobarbital anesthesia. Anesthesiology. 2001;95(4):933–8.
30. Choi DS, Kim T, Ro YS, Ahn KO, Lee EJ, Hwang SS, Song SW, Song KJ, Shin SD. Extracorporeal life support and survival after out-of-hospital cardiac arrest in a nationwide registry: a propensity score-matched analysis. Resuscitation. 2016;99:26–32. https://doi.org/10.1016/j.resuscitation.2015.11.013.
31. Coles JP, Fryer TD, Coleman MR, Smielewski P, Gupta AK, Minhas PS, Aigbirhio F, Chatfield DA, Williams GB, Boniface S, Carpenter TA, Clark JC, Pickard JD, Menon DK. Hyperventilation following head injury: effect on ischemic burden and cerebral oxidative metabolism. Crit Care Med. 2007;35(2):568–78. https://doi.org/10.1097/01.CCM.0000254066.37187.88.
32. Coles JP, Minhas PS, Fryer TD, Smielewski P, Aigbirihio F, Donovan T, Downey SP, Williams G, Chatfield D, Matthews JC, Gupta AK, Carpenter TA, Clark JC, Pickard JD, Menon DK. Effect of hyperventilation on cerebral blood flow in traumatic head injury: clinical relevance and monitoring correlates. Crit Care Med. 2002;30(9):1950–9. https://doi.org/10.1097/01.CCM.0000026331.91456.9A.
33. Crepeau AZ, Rabinstein AA, Fugate JE, Mandrekar J, Wijdicks EF, White RD, Britton JW. Continuous EEG in therapeutic hypothermia after cardiac arrest: prognostic and clinical value. Neurology. 2013;80(4):339–44. https://doi.org/10.1212/WNL.0b013e31827f089d.
34. Crombez T, Hachimi-Idrissi S. The influence of targeted temperature management on the pharmacokinetics of drugs administered during and after cardiac arrest: a systematic review. Acta Clin Belg. 2017:1–7. https://doi.org/10.1080/17843286.2017.1291782.
35. Cronberg T, Rundgren M, Westhall E, Englund E, Siemund R, Rosen I, Widner H, Friberg H. Neuron-specific enolase correlates with other prognostic markers after cardiac arrest. Neurology. 2011;77(7):623–30. https://doi.org/10.1212/WNL.0b013e31822a276d.
36. Crowell JW, Sharpe GP, Lambright RL, Read WL. The mechanism of death after resuscitation following acute circulatory failure. Surgery. 1955;38(4):696–702.
37. De Santis V, Negri M, Nencini C, Fusari M. Successful use of targeted temperature management in pregnancy after out-of-hospital cardiac arrest. Am J Emerg Med. 2016;34(1):122 e123–4. https://doi.org/10.1016/j.ajem.2015.05.049.
38. De Witte J, Sessler DI. Perioperative shivering: physiology and pharmacology. Anesthesiology. 2002;96(2):467–84.
39. Debaty G, Maignan M, Savary D, Koch FX, Ruckly S, Durand M, Picard J, Escallier C, Chouquer R, Santre C, Minet C, Guergour D, Hammer L, Bouvaist H, Belle L, Adrie C, Payen JF, Carpentier F, Gueugniaud PY, Danel V, Timsit JF. Impact of intra-arrest therapeutic hypothermia in outcomes of prehospital cardiac arrest: a randomized controlled trial. Intensive Care Med. 2014;40(12):1832–42. https://doi.org/10.1007/s00134-014-3519-x.
40. Dumas F, Grimaldi D, Zuber B, Fichet J, Charpentier J, Pene F, Vivien B, Varenne O, Carli P, Jouven X, Empana JP, Cariou A. Is hypothermia after cardiac arrest effective in both shockable and nonshockable patients?: insights from a large registry. Circulation. 2011;123(8):877–86. https://doi.org/10.1161/CIRCULATIONAHA.110.987347.
41. Ehrlich MP, McCullough JN, Zhang N, Weisz DJ, Juvonen T, Bodian CA, Griepp RB. Effect of hypothermia on cerebral blood flow and metabolism in the pig. Ann Thorac Surg. 2002;73(1):191–7.
42. Eid SM, Albaeni A, Vaidya D, Nazarian SM, Llinas R, Chandra-Strobos N. Awakening following cardiac arrest: determined by the definitions used or the therapies delivered? Resuscitation. 2016;100:38–44. https://doi.org/10.1016/j.resuscitation.2015.12.017.
43. Erecinska M, Thoresen M, Silver IA. Effects of hypothermia on energy metabolism in mammalian central nervous system. J Cereb Blood Flow Metab. 2003;23(5):513–30. https://doi.org/10.1097/01.WCB.0000066287.21705.21.
44. Fagnoul D, Combes A, De Backer D. Extracorporeal cardiopulmonary resuscitation. Curr Opin Crit Care. 2014;20(3):259–65. https://doi.org/10.1097/MCC.0000000000000098.
45. Fagnoul D, Taccone FS, Belhaj A, Rondelet B, Argacha JF, Vincent JL, Backer DD. Extracorporeal life support associated with hypothermia and normoxemia in refractory cardiac arrest. Resuscitation. 2013;84(11):1519–24. https://doi.org/10.1016/j.resuscitation.2013.06.016.
46. Fischer M, Bottiger BW, Popov-Cenic S, Hossmann KA. Thrombolysis using plasminogen activator and heparin reduces cerebral no-reflow after resuscitation from cardiac arrest: an experimental study in the cat. Intensive Care Med. 1996;22(11):1214–23.
47. Fischer M, Hossmann KA. No-reflow after cardiac arrest. Intensive Care Med. 1995;21(2):132–41.

48. Frank SM, Beattie C, Christopherson R, Norris EJ, Perler BA, Williams GM, Gottlieb SO. Unintentional hypothermia is associated with postoperative myocardial ischemia. The Perioperative Ischemia Randomized Anesthesia Trial Study Group. Anesthesiology. 1993;78(3):468–76.
49. Gaieski DF, Band RA, Abella BS, Neumar RW, Fuchs BD, Kolansky DM, Merchant RM, Carr BG, Becker LB, Maguire C, Klair A, Hylton J, Goyal M. Early goal-directed hemodynamic optimization combined with therapeutic hypothermia in comatose survivors of out-of-hospital cardiac arrest. Resuscitation. 2009;80(4):418–24. https://doi.org/10.1016/j.resuscitation.2008.12.015.
50. Ge L, Zhou X, Ji WJ, Lu RY, Zhang Y, Zhang YD, Ma YQ, Zhao JH, Li YM. Neutrophil extracellular traps in ischemia-reperfusion injury-induced myocardial no-reflow: therapeutic potential of DNase-based reperfusion strategy. Am J Physiol Heart Circ Physiol. 2015;308(5):H500–9. https://doi.org/10.1152/ajpheart.00381.2014.
51. Glover GW, Thomas RM, Vamvakas G, Al-Subaie N, Cranshaw J, Walden A, Wise MP, Ostermann M, Thomas-Jones E, Cronberg T, Erlinge D, Gasche Y, Hassager C, Horn J, Kjaergaard J, Kuiper M, Pellis T, Stammet P, Wanscher M, Wetterslev J, Friberg H, Nielsen N. Intravascular versus surface cooling for targeted temperature management after out-of-hospital cardiac arrest - an analysis of the TTM trial data. Crit Care. 2016;20(1):381. https://doi.org/10.1186/s13054-016-1552-6.
52. Grossestreuer AV, Abella BS, Leary M, Perman SM, Fuchs BD, Kolansky DM, Beylin ME, Gaieski DF. Time to awakening and neurologic outcome in therapeutic hypothermia-treated cardiac arrest patients. Resuscitation. 2013;84(12):1741–6. https://doi.org/10.1016/j.resuscitation.2013.07.009.
53. Grossestreuer AV, Gaieski DF, Donnino MW, Wiebe DJ, Abella BS. Magnitude of temperature elevation is associated with neurologic and survival outcomes in resuscitated cardiac arrest patients with postrewarming pyrexia. J Crit Care. 2017;38:78–83. https://doi.org/10.1016/j.jcrc.2016.11.003.
54. Hagerdal M, Harp J, Nilsson L, Siesjo BK. The effect of induced hypothermia upon oxygen consumption in the rat brain. J Neurochem. 1975;24(2):311–6.
55. Haneya A, Philipp A, Diez C, Schopka S, Bein T, Zimmermann M, Lubnow M, Luchner A, Agha A, Hilker M, Hirt S, Schmid C, Muller T. A 5-year experience with cardiopulmonary resuscitation using extracorporeal life support in non-postcardiotomy patients with cardiac arrest. Resuscitation. 2012;83(11):1331–7. https://doi.org/10.1016/j.resuscitation.2012.07.009.
56. Haugk M, Testori C, Sterz F, Uranitsch M, Holzer M, Behringer W, Herkner H, Time to Target Temperature Study G. Relationship between time to target temperature and outcome in patients treated with therapeutic hypothermia after cardiac arrest. Crit Care. 2011;15(2):R101. https://doi.org/10.1186/cc10116.
57. Hekmatpanah J. Cerebral blood flow dynamics in hypotension and cardiac arrest. Neurology. 1973;23(2):174–80.
58. Holcomb JB, Jenkins D, Rhee P, Johannigman J, Mahoney P, Mehta S, Cox ED, Gehrke MJ, Beilman GJ, Schreiber M, Flaherty SF, Grathwohl KW, Spinella PC, Perkins JG, Beekley AC, McMullin NR, Park MS, Gonzalez EA, Wade CE, Dubick MA, Schwab CW, Moore FA, Champion HR, Hoyt DB, Hess JR. Damage control resuscitation: directly addressing the early coagulopathy of trauma. J Trauma. 2007;62(2):307–10. https://doi.org/10.1097/TA.0b013e3180324124.
59. Hsu CH, Haac B, McQuillan KA, Tisherman SA, Scalea TM, Stein DM. Outcome of suicidal hanging patients and the role of targeted temperature management in hanging-induced cardiac arrest. J Trauma Acute Care Surg. 2017;82(2):387–91. https://doi.org/10.1097/TA.0000000000001281.
60. Hypothermia after Cardiac Arrest Study G. Mild therapeutic hypothermia to improve the neurologic outcome after cardiac arrest. N Engl J Med. 2002;346(8):549–56. https://doi.org/10.1056/NEJMoa012689.
61. Jehle D, Meyer M, Gemme S. Beneficial response to mild therapeutic hypothermia for comatose survivors of near-hanging. Am J Emerg Med. 2010;28(3):390 e391–3. https://doi.org/10.1016/j.ajem.2009.07.022.
62. Johnson NJ, Acker M, Hsu CH, Desai N, Vallabhajosyula P, Lazar S, Horak J, Wald J, McCarthy F, Rame E, Gray K, Perman SM, Becker L, Cowie D, Grossestreuer A, Smith T, Gaieski DF. Extracorporeal life support as rescue strategy for out-of-hospital and emergency department cardiac arrest. Resuscitation. 2014;85(11):1527–32. https://doi.org/10.1016/j.resuscitation.2014.08.028.
63. Jordan JE, Zhao ZQ, Vinten-Johansen J. The role of neutrophils in myocardial ischemia-reperfusion injury. Cardiovasc Res. 1999;43(4):860–78.
64. Jurkovich GJ, Pitt RM, Curreri PW, Granger DN. Hypothermia prevents increased capillary permeability following ischemia-reperfusion injury. J Surg Res. 1988;44(5):514–21.
65. Kagawa E, Inoue I, Kawagoe T, Ishihara M, Shimatani Y, Kurisu S, Nakama Y, Dai K, Takayuki O, Ikenaga H, Morimoto Y, Ejiri K, Oda N. Assessment of outcomes and differences between in- and out-of-hospital cardiac arrest patients treated with cardiopulmonary resuscitation using extracorporeal life support. Resuscitation. 2010;81(8):968–73. https://doi.org/10.1016/j.resuscitation.2010.03.037.
66. Kim F, Nichol G, Maynard C, Hallstrom A, Kudenchuk PJ, Rea T, Copass MK, Carlbom D, Deem S, Longstreth WT Jr, Olsufka M, Cobb LA. Effect of prehospital induction of mild hypothermia on survival and neurological status among adults with cardiac arrest: a randomized clinical trial. JAMA. 2014;311(1):45–52. https://doi.org/10.1001/jama.2013.282173.
67. Kim T, Paine MG, Meng H, Xiaodan R, Cohen J, Jinka T, Zheng H, Cranford JA, Neumar RW. Combined intra- and post-cardiac arrest hypothermic-targeted temperature management in a rat model of asphyxial cardiac arrest improves survival and neurologic outcome compared to either strategy alone. Resuscitation. 2016;107:94–101. https://doi.org/10.1016/j.resuscitation.2016.07.232.
68. Kuboyama K, Safar P, Radovsky A, Tisherman SA, Stezoski SW, Alexander H. Delay in cooling negates the beneficial effect of mild resuscitative cerebral hypothermia after cardiac arrest in dogs: a prospective, randomized study. Crit Care Med. 1993;21(9):1348–58.
69. Le Guen M, Nicolas-Robin A, Carreira S, Raux M, Leprince P, Riou B, Langeron O. Extracorporeal life support following out-of-hospital refractory cardiac arrest. Crit Care. 2011;15(1):R29. https://doi.org/10.1186/cc9976.
70. Leary M, Grossestreuer AV, Iannacone S, Gonzalez M, Shofer FS, Povey C, Wendell G, Archer SE, Gaieski DF, Abella BS. Pyrexia and neurologic outcomes after therapeutic hypothermia for cardiac arrest. Resuscitation. 2013;84(8):1056–61. https://doi.org/10.1016/j.resuscitation.2012.11.003.
71. Lee BK, Jeung KW, Lee HY, Lim JH. Outcomes of therapeutic hypothermia in unconscious patients after near-hanging. Emerg Med J. 2012;29(9):748–52. https://doi.org/10.1136/emermed-2011-200493.
72. Legriel S, Bouyon A, Nekhili N, Tremey B, Abbosh N, Henry M, Troche G, Guezennec P, Bruneel F, Bedos JP. Therapeutic hypothermia for coma after cardiorespiratory arrest caused by hanging. Resuscitation. 2005;67(1):143–4. https://doi.org/10.1016/j.resuscitation.2005.05.001.
73. Legriel S, Hilly-Ginoux J, Resche-Rigon M, Merceron S, Pinoteau J, Henry-Lagarrigue M, Bruneel F, Nguyen A, Guezennec P, Troche G, Richard O, Pico F, Bedos JP. Prognostic value of electrographic postanoxic status epilepticus in comatose

cardiac-arrest survivors in the therapeutic hypothermia era. Resuscitation. 2013;84(3):343–50. https://doi.org/10.1016/j.resuscitation.2012.11.001.

74. Leick J, Liebetrau C, Szardien S, Fischer-Rasokat U, Willmer M, van Linden A, Blumenstein J, Nef H, Rolf A, Arlt M, Walther T, Hamm C, Mollmann H. Door-to-implantation time of extracorporeal life support systems predicts mortality in patients with out-of-hospital cardiac arrest. Clin Res Cardiol. 2013;102(9):661–9. https://doi.org/10.1007/s00392-013-0580-3.
75. Logue ES, McMichael MJ, Callaway CW. Comparison of the effects of hypothermia at 33 degrees C or 35 degrees C after cardiac arrest in rats. Acad Emerg Med. 2007;14(4):293–300. https://doi.org/10.1197/j.aem.2006.10.097.
76. Luna GK, Maier RV, Pavlin EG, Anardi D, Copass MK, Oreskovich MR. Incidence and effect of hypothermia in seriously injured patients. J Trauma. 1987;27(9):1014–8.
77. Lybeck A, Friberg H, Aneman A, Hassager C, Horn J, Kjaergaard J, Kuiper M, Nielsen N, Ullen S, Wise MP, Westhall E, Cronberg T, TT-t Investigators. Prognostic significance of clinical seizures after cardiac arrest and target temperature management. Resuscitation. 2017;114:146–51. https://doi.org/10.1016/j.resuscitation.2017.01.017.
78. Maekawa K, Tanno K, Hase M, Mori K, Asai Y. Extracorporeal cardiopulmonary resuscitation for patients with out-of-hospital cardiac arrest of cardiac origin: a propensity-matched study and predictor analysis. Crit Care Med. 2013;41(5):1186–96. https://doi.org/10.1097/CCM.0b013e31827ca4c8.
79. Mathers CD, Loncar D. Projections of global mortality and burden of disease from 2002 to 2030. PLoS Med. 2006 Nov;3(11):e442
80. Mattia AD, Pellis T, Gregori D, Nielsen N, Campanile V, Peratoner A, Brunetti I, Pelosi P, Kjaergaard J, Hassager C. Time to target temperature and outcome after out-of-hospital cardiac arrest. Circulation. 2015;132:A13943.
81. McCullough JN, Zhang N, Reich DL, Juvonen TS, Klein JJ, Spielvogel D, Ergin MA, Griepp RB. Cerebral metabolic suppression during hypothermic circulatory arrest in humans. Ann Thorac Surg. 1999;67(6):1895–9; discussion 1919–1821.
82. McIntosh TK, Vink R, Yamakami I, Faden AI. Magnesium protects against neurological deficit after brain injury. Brain Res. 1989;482(2):252–60.
83. Merchant RM, Yang L, Becker LB, Berg RA, Nadkarni V, Nichol G, Carr BG, Mitra N, Bradley SM, Abella BS, Groeneveld PW, American Heart Association Get With The Guidelines-Resuscitation I. Incidence of treated cardiac arrest in hospitalized patients in the United States. Crit Care Med. 2011;39(11):2401–6. https://doi.org/10.1097/CCM.0b013e3182257459.
84. Michelson AD, MacGregor H, Barnard MR, Kestin AS, Rohrer MJ, Valeri CR. Reversible inhibition of human platelet activation by hypothermia in vivo and in vitro. Thromb Haemost. 1994;71(5):633–40.
85. Mikkelsen ME, Christie JD, Abella BS, Kerlin MP, Fuchs BD, Schweickert WD, Berg RA, Mosesso VN, Shofer FS, Gaieski DF, American Heart Association's Get With the Guidelines-Resuscitation I. Use of therapeutic hypothermia after in-hospital cardiac arrest. Crit Care Med. 2013;41(6):1385–95. https://doi.org/10.1097/CCM.0b013e318287f2c4.
86. Milde LN. Clinical use of mild hypothermia for brain protection: a dream revisited. J Neurosurg Anesthesiol. 1992;4(3):211–5.
87. Millin MG, Comer AC, Nable JV, Johnston PV, Lawner BJ, Woltman N, Levy MJ, Seaman KG, Hirshon JM. Patients without ST elevation after return of spontaneous circulation may benefit from emergent percutaneous intervention: a systematic review and meta-analysis. Resuscitation. 2016;108:54–60. https://doi.org/10.1016/j.resuscitation.2016.09.004.
88. Mori E, del Zoppo GJ, Chambers JD, Copeland BR, Arfors KE. Inhibition of polymorphonuclear leukocyte adherence suppresses no-reflow after focal cerebral ischemia in baboons. Stroke. 1992;23(5):712–8.
89. Mulder M, Gibbs HG, Smith SW, Dhaliwal R, Scott NL, Sprenkle MD, Geocadin RG. Awakening and withdrawal of life-sustaining treatment in cardiac arrest survivors treated with therapeutic hypothermia. Crit Care Med. 2014;42(12):2493–9. https://doi.org/10.1097/CCM.0000000000000540.
90. Nielsen N, Wetterslev J, Cronberg T, Erlinge D, Gasche Y, Hassager C, Horn J, Hovdenes J, Kjaergaard J, Kuiper M, Pellis T, Stammet P, Wanscher M, Wise MP, Aneman A, Al-Subaie N, Boesgaard S, Bro-Jeppesen J, Brunetti I, Bugge JF, Hingston CD, Juffermans NP, Koopmans M, Kober L, Langorgen J, Lilja G, Moller JE, Rundgren M, Rylander C, Smid O, Werer C, Winkel P, Friberg H, Investigators TTMT. Targeted temperature management at 33 degrees C versus 36 degrees C after cardiac arrest. N Engl J Med. 2013;369(23):2197–206. https://doi.org/10.1056/NEJMoa1310519.
91. Nolan JP, Hazinski MF, Aickin R, Bhanji F, Billi JE, Callaway CW, Castren M, de Caen AR, Ferrer JM, Finn JC, Gent LM, Griffin RE, Iverson S, Lang E, Lim SH, Maconochie IK, Montgomery WH, Morley PT, Nadkarni VM, Neumar RW, Nikolaou NI, Perkins GD, Perlman JM, Singletary EM, Soar J, Travers AH, Welsford M, Wyllie J, Zideman DA. Part 1: executive summary: 2015 international consensus on cardiopulmonary resuscitation and emergency cardiovascular care science with treatment recommendations. Resuscitation. 2015;95:e1–31. https://doi.org/10.1016/j.resuscitation.2015.07.039.
92. Nolan JP, Neumar RW, Adrie C, Aibiki M, Berg RA, Bottiger BW, Callaway C, Clark RS, Geocadin RG, Jauch EC, Kern KB, Laurent I, Longstreth WT, Merchant RM, Morley P, Morrison LJ, Nadkarni V, Peberdy MA, Rivers EP, Rodriguez-Nunez A, Sellke FW, Spaulding C, Sunde K, Hoek TV. Post-cardiac arrest syndrome: epidemiology, pathophysiology, treatment, and prognostication. A scientific statement from the International Liaison Committee on Resuscitation; the American Heart Association Emergency cardiovascular Care Committee; the Council on Cardiovascular Surgery and Anesthesia; the Council on Cardiopulmonary, Perioperative, and Critical Care; the Council on Clinical Cardiology; the Council on Stroke. Resuscitation. 2008;79(3):350–79. https://doi.org/10.1016/j.resuscitation.2008.09.017.
93. Nozari A, Safar P, Stezoski SW, Wu X, Kostelnik S, Radovsky A, Tisherman S, Kochanek PM. Critical time window for intra-arrest cooling with cold saline flush in a dog model of cardiopulmonary resuscitation. Circulation. 2006;113(23):2690–6. https://doi.org/10.1161/CIRCULATIONAHA.106.613349.
94. Oddo M, Rossetti AO. Early multimodal outcome prediction after cardiac arrest in patients treated with hypothermia. Crit Care Med. 2014;42(6):1340–7. https://doi.org/10.1097/CCM.0000000000000211.
95. Oguayo KN, Oyetayo OO, Stewart D, Costa SM, Jones RO. Successful use of therapeutic hypothermia in a pregnant patient. Tex Heart Inst J. 2015;42(4):367–71. https://doi.org/10.14503/THIJ-14-4331.
96. Palmer C, Vannucci RC, Christensen MA, Brucklacher RM. Regional cerebral blood flow and glucose utilization during hypothermia in newborn dogs. Anesthesiology. 1989;71(5):730–7.
97. Patt A, McCroskey BL, Moore EE. Hypothermia-induced coagulopathies in trauma. Surg Clin North Am. 1988;68(4):775–85.
98. Paul M, Bougouin W, Geri G, Dumas F, Champigneulle B, Legriel S, Charpentier J, Mira JP, Sandroni C, Cariou A. Delayed awakening after cardiac arrest: prevalence and risk factors in the Parisian registry. Intensive Care Med. 2016;42(7):1128–36. https://doi.org/10.1007/s00134-016-4349-9.

99. Perman SM, Ellenberg JH, Grossestreuer AV, Gaieski DF, Leary M, Abella BS, Carr BG. Shorter time to target temperature is associated with poor neurologic outcome in post-arrest patients treated with targeted temperature management. Resuscitation. 2015a;88:114–9. https://doi.org/10.1016/j.resuscitation.2014.10.018.
100. Perman SM, Goyal M, Neumar RW, Topjian AA, Gaieski DF. Clinical applications of targeted temperature management. Chest. 2014;145(2):386–93. https://doi.org/10.1378/chest.12-3025.
101. Perman SM, Grossestreuer AV, Wiebe DJ, Carr BG, Abella BS, Gaieski DF. The utility of therapeutic hypothermia for post-cardiac arrest syndrome patients with an initial nonshockable rhythm. Circulation. 2015b;132(22):2146–51. https://doi.org/10.1161/CIRCULATIONAHA.115.016317.
102. Polderman KH. Application of therapeutic hypothermia in the ICU: opportunities and pitfalls of a promising treatment modality. Part 1: indications and evidence. Intensive Care Med. 2004a;30(4):556–75. https://doi.org/10.1007/s00134-003-2152-x.
103. Polderman KH. Application of therapeutic hypothermia in the intensive care unit. Opportunities and pitfalls of a promising treatment modality--part 2: practical aspects and side effects. Intensive Care Med. 2004b;30(5):757–69. https://doi.org/10.1007/s00134-003-2151-y.
104. Polderman KH. Induced hypothermia and fever control for prevention and treatment of neurological injuries. Lancet. 2008;371(9628):1955–69. https://doi.org/10.1016/S0140-6736(08)60837-5.
105. Polderman KH. Mechanisms of action, physiological effects, and complications of hypothermia. Crit Care Med. 2009;37(7 Suppl):S186–202. https://doi.org/10.1097/CCM.0b013e3181aa5241.
106. Polderman KH, Herold I. Therapeutic hypothermia and controlled normothermia in the intensive care unit: practical considerations, side effects, and cooling methods. Crit Care Med. 2009;37(3):1101–20. https://doi.org/10.1097/CCM.0b013e3181962ad5.
107. Polderman KH, Peerdeman SM, Girbes AR. Hypophosphatemia and hypomagnesemia induced by cooling in patients with severe head injury. J Neurosurg. 2001;94(5):697–705. https://doi.org/10.3171/jns.2001.94.5.0697.
108. Polderman KH, Rijnsburger ER, Peerdeman SM, Girbes AR. Induction of hypothermia in patients with various types of neurologic injury with use of large volumes of ice-cold intravenous fluid. Crit Care Med. 2005;33(12):2744–51.
109. Polderman KH, van Zanten AR, Girbes AR. The importance of magnesium in critically ill patients: a role in mitigating neurological injury and in the prevention of vasospasms. Intensive Care Med. 2003;29(7):1202–3. https://doi.org/10.1007/s00134-003-1787-y.
110. Ponz I, Lopez-de-Sa E, Armada E, Caro J, Blazquez Z, Rosillo S, Gonzalez O, Rey JR, Monedero Mdel C, Lopez-Sendon JL. Influence of the temperature on the moment of awakening in patients treated with therapeutic hypothermia after cardiac arrest. Resuscitation. 2016;103:32–6. https://doi.org/10.1016/j.resuscitation.2016.03.017.
111. Rhee PM, Acosta J, Bridgeman A, Wang D, Jordan M, Rich N. Survival after emergency department thoracotomy: review of published data from the past 25 years. J Am Coll Surg. 2000;190(3):288–98.
112. Rosomoff HL, Holaday DA. Cerebral blood flow and cerebral oxygen consumption during hypothermia. Am J Phys. 1954;179(1):85–8.
113. Rossetti AO, Carrera E, Oddo M. Early EEG correlates of neuronal injury after brain anoxia. Neurology. 2012;78(11):796–802. https://doi.org/10.1212/WNL.0b013e318249f6bb.
114. Rossetti AO, Oddo M, Logroscino G, Kaplan PW. Prognostication after cardiac arrest and hypothermia: a prospective study. Ann Neurol. 2010;67(3):301–7. https://doi.org/10.1002/ana.21984.
115. Rubeiz GJ, Thill-Baharozian M, Hardie D, Carlson RW. Association of hypomagnesemia and mortality in acutely ill medical patients. Crit Care Med. 1993;21(2):203–9.
116. Sakamoto T, Morimura N, Nagao K, Asai Y, Yokota H, Nara S, Hase M, Tahara Y, Atsumi T, Group S-JS. Extracorporeal cardiopulmonary resuscitation versus conventional cardiopulmonary resuscitation in adults with out-of-hospital cardiac arrest: a prospective observational study. Resuscitation. 2014;85(6):762–8. https://doi.org/10.1016/j.resuscitation.2014.01.031.
117. Samaniego EA, Mlynash M, Caulfield AF, Eyngorn I, Wijman CA. Sedation confounds outcome prediction in cardiac arrest survivors treated with hypothermia. Neurocrit Care. 2011;15(1):113–9. https://doi.org/10.1007/s12028-010-9412-8.
118. Sessler DI. Defeating normal thermoregulatory defenses: induction of therapeutic hypothermia. Stroke. 2009;40(11):e614–21. https://doi.org/10.1161/STROKEAHA.108.520858.
119. Shafi S, Elliott AC, Gentilello L. Is hypothermia simply a marker of shock and injury severity or an independent risk factor for mortality in trauma patients? Analysis of a large national trauma registry. J Trauma. 2005;59(5):1081–5.
120. Shin J, Lee H, Kim J, Kim J, Choi S, Jeung K, Cho I, Cha G, Kim G, Han C, Lee D, Park K, Suh G, Hwang S. Outcomes of hanging-induced cardiac arrest patients who underwent therapeutic hypothermia: a multicenter retrospective cohort study. Resuscitation. 2014;85(8):1047–51. https://doi.org/10.1016/j.resuscitation.2014.04.012.
121. Small DL, Morley P, Buchan AM. Biology of ischemic cerebral cell death. Prog Cardiovasc Dis. 1999;42(3):185–207.
122. Soar J, Callaway CW, Aibiki M, Bottiger BW, Brooks SC, Deakin CD, Donnino MW, Drajer S, Kloeck W, Morley PT, Morrison LJ, Neumar RW, Nicholson TC, Nolan JP, Okada K, O'Neil BJ, Paiva EF, Parr MJ, Wang TL, Witt J, Advanced Life Support Chapter C. Part 4: advanced life support: 2015 international consensus on cardiopulmonary resuscitation and emergency cardiovascular care science with treatment recommendations. Resuscitation. 2015;95:e71–120. https://doi.org/10.1016/j.resuscitation.2015.07.042.
123. Sterz F, Safar P, Tisherman S, Radovsky A, Kuboyama K, Oku K. Mild hypothermic cardiopulmonary resuscitation improves outcome after prolonged cardiac arrest in dogs. Crit Care Med. 1991;19(3):379–89.
124. Stub D, Bernard S, Pellegrino V, Smith K, Walker T, Sheldrake J, Hockings L, Shaw J, Duffy SJ, Burrell A, Cameron P, de Smit V, Kaye DM. Refractory cardiac arrest treated with mechanical CPR, hypothermia, ECMO and early reperfusion (the CHEER trial). Resuscitation. 2015;86:88–94. https://doi.org/10.1016/j.resuscitation.2014.09.010.
125. Sunde K, Pytte M, Jacobsen D, Mangschau A, Jensen LP, Smedsrud C, Draegni T, Steen PA. Implementation of a standardised treatment protocol for post resuscitation care after out-of-hospital cardiac arrest. Resuscitation. 2007;73(1):29–39. https://doi.org/10.1016/j.resuscitation.2006.08.016.
126. Tisherman SA, Safar P, Radovsky A, Peitzman A, Marrone G, Kuboyama K, Weinrauch V. Profound hypothermia (less than 10 degrees C) compared with deep hypothermia (15 degrees C) improves neurologic outcome in dogs after two hours' circulatory arrest induced to enable resuscitative surgery. J Trauma. 1991;31(8):1051–61; discussion 1061–1052.
127. Trzeciak S, Jones AE, Kilgannon JH, Milcarek B, Hunter K, Shapiro NI, Hollenberg SM, Dellinger P, Parrillo JE. Significance of arterial hypotension after resuscitation from cardiac arrest. Crit Care Med. 2009;37(11):2895–903; quiz 2904.

128. Valeri CR, MacGregor H, Cassidy G, Tinney R, Pompei F. Effects of temperature on bleeding time and clotting time in normal male and female volunteers. Crit Care Med. 1995;23(4):698–704.
129. van den Bergh WM, Algra A, van Kooten F, Dirven CM, van Gijn J, Vermeulen M, Rinkel GJ, Group MS. Magnesium sulfate in aneurysmal subarachnoid hemorrhage: a randomized controlled trial. Stroke. 2005;36(5):1011–5. https://doi.org/10.1161/01.STR.0000160801.96998.57.
130. Watts DD, Trask A, Soeken K, Perdue P, Dols S, Kaufmann C. Hypothermic coagulopathy in trauma: effect of varying levels of hypothermia on enzyme speed, platelet function, and fibrinolytic activity. J Trauma. 1998;44(5):846–54.
131. Webb AC, Samuels OB. Reversible brain death after cardiopulmonary arrest and induced hypothermia. Crit Care Med. 2011;39(6):1538–42. https://doi.org/10.1097/CCM.0b013e3182186687.
132. Wee JH, You YH, Lim H, Choi WJ, Lee BK, Park JH, Park KN, Choi SP, Korean Hypothermia Network I. Outcomes of asphyxial cardiac arrest patients who were treated with therapeutic hypothermia: a multicentre retrospective cohort study. Resuscitation. 2015;89:81–5. https://doi.org/10.1016/j.resuscitation.2014.11.001.
133. Wolff B, Machill K, Schumacher D, Schulzki I, Werner D. Early achievement of mild therapeutic hypothermia and the neurologic outcome after cardiac arrest. Int J Cardiol. 2009;133(2):223–8. https://doi.org/10.1016/j.ijcard.2007.12.039.
134. Woods KL, Fletcher S, Roffe C, Haider Y. Intravenous magnesium sulphate in suspected acute myocardial infarction: results of the second Leicester Intravenous Magnesium Intervention Trial (LIMIT-2). Lancet. 1992;339(8809):1553–8.
135. Yannopoulos D, Bartos JA, Martin C, Raveendran G, Missov E, Conterato M, Frascone RJ, Trembley A, Sipprell K, John R, George S, Carlson K, Brunsvold ME, Garcia S, Aufderheide TP. Minnesota Resuscitation Consortium's advanced perfusion and reperfusion cardiac life support strategy for out-of-hospital refractory ventricular fibrillation. J Am Heart Assoc. 2016;5(6):e003732. https://doi.org/10.1161/JAHA.116.003732.
136. Yenari MA, Han HS. Neuroprotective mechanisms of hypothermia in brain ischaemia. Nat Rev Neurosci. 2012;13(4):267–78. https://doi.org/10.1038/nrn3174.
137. Zanyk-McLean K, Sawyer KN, Paternoster R, Shievitz R, Devlin W, Swor R. Time to awakening is often delayed in patients who receive targeted temperature management after cardiac arrest. Ther Hypother Temp Manag. 2016;7(2):95–100. https://doi.org/10.1089/ther.2016.0030.
138. Zhao D, Abella BS, Beiser DG, Alvarado JP, Wang H, Hamann KJ, Hoek TL, Becker LB. Intra-arrest cooling with delayed reperfusion yields higher survival than earlier normothermic resuscitation in a mouse model of cardiac arrest. Resuscitation. 2008;77(2):242–9. https://doi.org/10.1016/j.resuscitation.2007.10.015.

15 Assessment and Management of Acute Respiratory Distress in the ICU

Bishwajit Bhattacharya and Kimberly Davis

Introduction

Respiratory failure is a common cause of ICU admission in the United States accounting for up to 30% of ICU admissions [1, 2]. In recent years there has been an increasing trend in the number of admissions due to respiratory failure, approaching nearly two million admissions in 2009 [3]. Concurrently, the economic burden of respiratory failure has increased from $30.1 billion to $54.3 billion over the same time period with a calculated cost of $15,900 per case [3]. Approximately 30–40% of patients requiring mechanical ventilation die before discharge [4]. Patients who survive after requiring mechanical ventilation for treatment of respiratory failure have lower life expectancies, higher readmission rates, and greater long-term disability compared to those who do not require mechanical ventilation [5, 6].

Etiology of Respiratory Distress

Acute respiratory distress is a common clinical scenario for the clinician to encounter in the intensive care unit (ICU) as it serves as the final common pathway for a variety of disease processes. There are several causes for respiratory distress. Correct identification of the underlying cause will aid the clinician in timely correction of the precipitating cause. Respiratory failure can also be divided into acute vs. chronic. Clinicians in the ICU will generally encounter acute respiratory failure which has developed acutely over minutes to hours.

Respiratory failure can be broadly subdivided into four types. Type 1 respiratory failure is hypoxemic, defined as an arterial oxygen tension less than 60 mmHg. Type 2 failure is hypercarbic, defined as arterial carbon dioxide tension greater than 50 mmHg. Type 1 respiratory failure is due to failure of oxygen exchange, whereas Type 2 failure is due to either an inability to adequately ventilate or the development of increased dead space ventilation. Type 3 respiratory failure is perioperative, and Type 4 respiratory failure is secondary to other underlying disease processes, generally resulting in cardiovascular instability [7]. The severity of ARDS is classified by the PaO_2/FiO_2 ratio (arterial oxygen partial pressure/fractional inspired oxygen) according to the Berlin criteria. A PaO_2/FiO_2 ratio of 200–300 mmHg is classified as mild ARDS, a PaO_2/FiO_2 ratio of 100–200 mmHg is indicative of moderate ARDS, and a PaO_2/FiO_2 ratio of less than 100 mmHg is severe ARDS. The term acute lung injury (ALI) has been discontinued and is referred to as mild ARDS [8].

Respiratory failure can be defined by its underlying cause or mechanism, including airway obstruction, intrinsic lung disease, and/or extrinsic causes. Airway obstruction can be caused by aspiration due to chronic dysphagia or altered mental status due to acute illness that does not permit normal clearing of secretions and protection of the airway. Airway obstruction can also occur due to trauma, inflammation, infection, or anaphylaxis. In such scenarios mechanically clearing the airway or securing a protected airway is essential.

Intrinsic lung disease results in a ventilation perfusion mismatch. Both intrinsic and extrinsic lung disease can result in worsening compliance of the lung tissues and poor gas exchange, resulting in respiratory failure. In cases of acute illness, the lung parenchyma can experience an inflammatory response resulting in acute respiratory distress syndrome (ARDS). This disease process may present on a spectrum of severity characterized by the severity of the inflammatory response which may be precipitated by a broad variety of insults (Table 15.1). This response leads to capillary leak, resulting in an exudative release into the lung parenchyma, ultimately causing fibrosis and impaired gas exchange [9]. ARDS is characterized by patchy bilateral infiltrates seen on chest CT scan or CXR in the setting of a precipitating factor in the preceding 7 days. Under the revised classification of

B. Bhattacharya · K. Davis (✉)
Section of General Surgery, Trauma and Surgical Critical Care, Department of Surgery, Yale School of Medicine, New Haven, CT, USA
e-mail: Kimberly.Davis@yale.edu

A. Salim et al. (eds.), *Surgical Critical Care Therapy*, https://doi.org/10.1007/978-3-319-71712-8_15

Table 15.1 Etiologies of ARDS

Direct injury or inflammation	Systemic ischemia-reperfusion injury
Intrinsic causes	Extrinsic causes
Pulmonary contusion	Multiple trauma
Pneumonia	Sepsis
Aspiration	Massive transfusion
Inhalational injury	Pancreatitis
	Post-cardiopulmonary bypass

ARDS, pulmonary edema seen on chest imaging does not have to be ruled out to be secondary to hypervolemia or heart failure as both entities may be present in a patient [8].

Acute lung injury may also be precipitated by an inflammatory reaction mediated by blood product transfusion (TRALI) [10]. There are ongoing discussions of renaming this entity as transfused ARDS [11]. A ventilation/perfusion mismatch can also occur following a pulmonary embolism where a blood clot migrates into the pulmonary vasculature resulting in increased dead space, i.e., a zone that is ventilated but not perfused.

Extrinsic factors that can compromise respiratory function include disease processes resulting in increased intra-abdominal pressure, decreasing diaphragmatic excursion. Traumatic mechanisms including pneumothorax that cause collapse of lung and chest wall pain limiting chest wall movement as seen in multiple rib fractures. Patients with traumatic brain injury or upper level spinal cord injuries may not be able to breath due to central nervous system failure. Trauma patients who present with a Glasgow Coma Scale (GCS) score of 8 or less should be intubated for airway protection [12].

Certain patients are at increased risk of postoperative respiratory failure requiring reintubation. Respiratory failure in such scenarios may be due to several reasons including, residual anesthesia, atelectasis, and/or operative pain limiting respiratory effort. Patients at the extremes of age undergoing prolonged procedures with greater comorbidities and undergoing thoracic procedures are at greatest risk of failing postoperative extubation [13].

Assessment

Respiratory distress can be assessed by several objective and clinical criteria in the ICU. On physical exam patients may have tachypnea, labored breathing, nasal flaring, and the use of accessory breathing muscles. Patients demonstrating respiratory distress need the underlying cause addressed immediately. If the cause for respiratory distress cannot be quickly identified or corrected, the patients should be provided respiratory support and possibly mechanical ventilation before complete respiratory collapse.

Respiratory distress can be rapidly assessed with chest radiography. Chest X-ray can reveal air space disease or space-occupying lesions. The easy availability of portable bedside chest X-rays has over time led to an excess of its utilization [14]. The practice of routine chest X-rays in all patient who mechanically ventilated has been revisited in recent years due to concerns regarding unnecessary radiation exposure and costs. Many studies have demonstrated the lack of utility in obtaining daily chest X-rays in the ICU for mechanically ventilated patients unless a change in clinical status dictates a need [15, 16].

CT scans can provide greater sensitivity in diagnosing chest disease but are not readily available and involve transport to another hospital location, which may be suboptimal for patients requiring close continuous monitoring. CT scans have become the modality of choice in diagnosing pulmonary embolisms and are more sensitive than chest X-ray in detecting rib fractures [17]. CT scans are also more sensitive than chest X-rays in detecting infiltrates [18].

In recent years, ultrasound imaging has become a useful and rapid tool to be used at the bedside to aid in the diagnosis of thoracic pathology without radiation exposure to the patient. Pneumonia in children and adults may be diagnosed by ultrasound [19, 20]. In the case of trauma patients, a pneumothorax can be can be easily identified by ultrasound and reassessed for resolution after intervention at the bedside. Similarly, the progression of a pleural effusion can be tracked using serial ultrasound examinations [19, 20].

An arterial blood gas can quantify arterial oxygenation levels and acid-base disturbances secondary to respiratory alterations. Arterial oxygen and carbon dioxide levels can be used in determining type and severity of respiratory failure and to gauge the effects of a given intervention. Noninvasive monitoring with pulse oximetry and capnography can continuously trend oxygenation saturation and carbon dioxide levels, but both have their limitations. Pulse oximetry measures oxygen saturation and not arterial oxygen tension. Along the oxygen dissociation curve, there may be large increases or decreases in arterial oxygen tension along the upper and lower parts of the horizontal portions of the sigmoid curve with little change in oxygen saturation (Fig. 15.1). Pulse oximetry may also not be reliable in low flow states as the sensor will have difficulty detecting a signal. Motion artifact and noninvasive blood pressure monitoring may also interfere with pulse oximetry readings [21]. Continuous capnography is useful in monitoring changes in carbon dioxide exhaled in mixed gas and is useful in verifying endotracheal tube position, assessing return of a perfusing rhythm during cardiopulmonary resuscitation and for evaluating changes in dead space. Capnography is affected by cardiac output and hypothermia and may be unreliable in the critically ill patient [21].

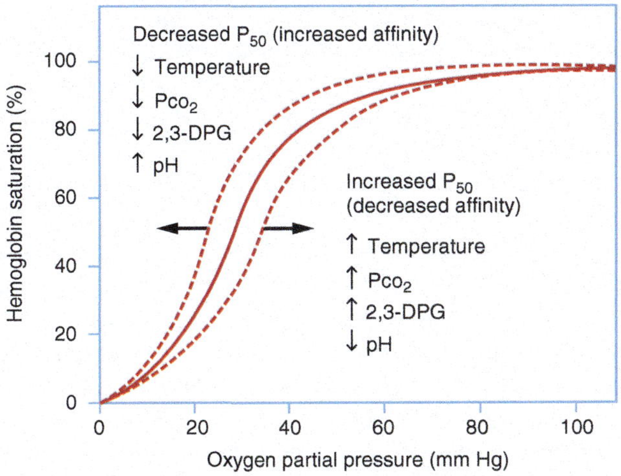

Fig. 15.1 Oxygen hemoglobin saturation curve (Reproduced with permission from Elsevier Books, Koeppen and Stanton [82])

Patients with hypoxia refractory to supplemental oxygen and/or hypercapnia not easily corrected, poor mental status, or anatomic injury that prevents the patient from protecting their airway are absolute indications for the initiation of mechanical ventilation. The plethora of objective data easily available to the clinician cannot be a substitute for good clinical judgment regarding the need for intubation and instituting mechanical ventilation. Sound clinical judgment is important to decide to initiate of mechanical ventilation before objective data reflect a state of extremis. It is preferable for the clinician to err on the side of caution and institute mechanical ventilation versus delay till the clinical situation deteriorates particularly in patients where a rapidly correctable etiology of respiratory failure is not quickly identified.

Management

Effective management of acute respiratory distress in the ICU requires recognizing the underlying cause and instituting treatment directed toward correcting the underlying pathology. Respiratory distress can be managed with interventions short of mechanical ventilation when the clinical situation is not dire and time is available to institute and assess the results of the therapeutic intervention. Airway obstruction resulting in physical obstruction of the airway can be managed with a digital sweep of the oropharynx or a jaw thrust to open the airway and allow for air passage. Upper airway obstruction can be temporarily relieved by the placement of nasal trumpets or an oral airway to relieve upper airway obstruction, which can then be supplemented with assisted ventilation to help with air exchange till a secure airway is established.

Respiratory distress resulting from intrinsic lung disease may be quickly correctable. In cases of pulmonary edema, intravascular volume reduction with the use of diuretics may quickly relieve distress. Similarly, cases of atelectasis may be opened with noninvasive ventilation. In such instances, invasive mechanical ventilation may be deferred as therapeutic interventions are given a chance to demonstrate efficacy. Some patients in such scenarios may benefit from noninvasive ventilation as a bridge till the underlying problem is corrected, if they have appropriate mental status, are hemodynamically stable, and do not have copious upper airway secretions or upper airway obstruction. The presence of recent upper GI surgery is a relative contraindication due to the potential gaseous distention on a recent anastomosis. Selected patients should be given a trail of 1–2 h for improvement in respiratory status beyond which they are likely to fail conservative management [22, 23]. In recent years there has been growing interest in the use of high-flow nasal cannula as an alternate noninvasive method of respiratory support. Studies suggest that it may be a more comfortable method of support with improved work of breathing. Its role in acute hypoxic respiratory failure is controversial as it may not prevent the need for mechanical ventilation [24, 25]. Its application may be more suitable in the setting of post-extubation support [26]. In other instances of intrinsic disease such as acute lung injury or pneumonia, the underlying pathology will take a longer course of treatment to resolve. Patients in respiratory distress in such circumstances warrant early institution of mechanical ventilation.

Certain extrinsic causes of respiratory failure can also be quickly addressed with rapid resolution. Pneumothorax resulting in pulmonary collapse and mediastinal shift causing decreased cardiac return and hypotension can be evaluated at the bedside by physical examination or with ultrasound. In an emergency, needle decompression of the tension pneumothorax with a large bore needle in the anterior chest along the midclavicular line in the second intercostal space will quickly release the tension until a thoracostomy tube can be placed. Similarly, large effusions causing pulmonary collapse can be relieved with tube thoracotomy or a pigtail catheter and can often be inserted under ultrasound guidance. Traditional teaching has advocated the use of large diameter tubes to drain suspected bloody fluid to prevent tube clogging. This dictum has been challenged in recent years, and smaller-sized tubes may also be adequate [27, 28]. Chest wall immobility may also cause respiratory failure. Rib fractures are commonly seen in emergency rooms and are associated with increasing mortality with the increasing number of fractures and age [29, 30]. Effective pain management is essential in such scenarios to allow adequate pulmonary effort to prevent atelectasis, pneumonia, and respiratory failure [31]. Other extrinsic causes of respiratory failure such as increased abdominal pressure will require operative intervention or percutaneous drainage for decompression and to address the underlying precipitating pathology.

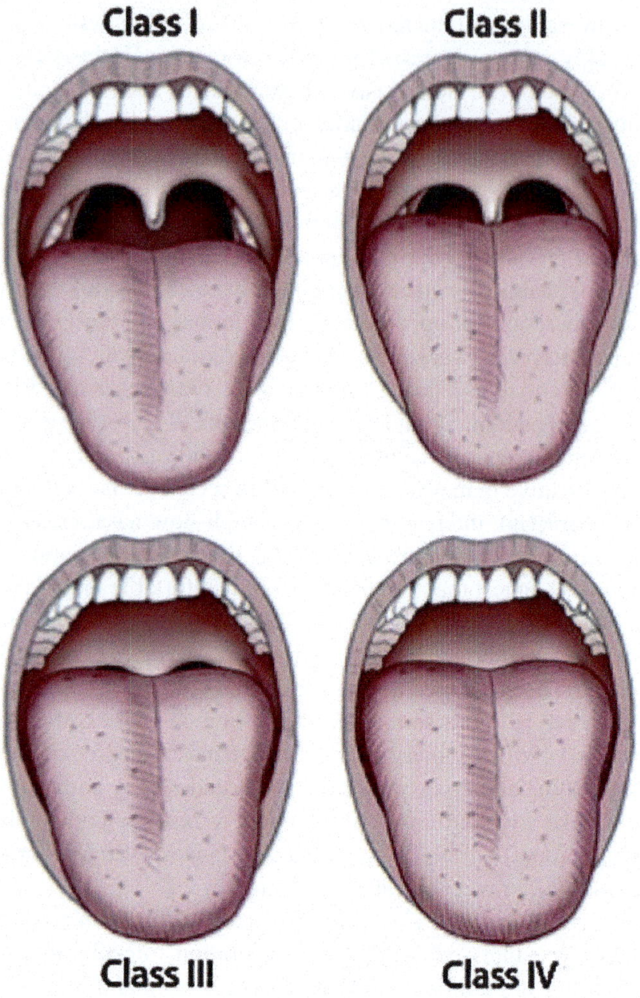

Fig. 15.2 Mallampati score. Mallampati classification: class I, the uvula and soft palate are fully visible; class II, the hard and soft palate and upper portion of the uvula are visible; class III, the soft and hard palate and base of the uvula are visible; class IV, only the hard palate is visible (Reproduced with permission from Elsevier Books, Islam et al. [83])

Intubation

If respiratory distress cannot be quickly corrected or if the patient is in extremis, mechanical ventilation will be required. Once the decision is made to institute mechanical ventilation, orotracheal intubation should be performed by an experienced clinician. The anticipated difficulty of intubation can be easily assessed using the Mallampati score by inspecting the oral airway view (Fig. 15.2). Patients with Mallampati scores of three or four have potentially difficult airways and predict sleep apnea [32, 33]. Many devices using video-assisted technology are now available to help optimize the visualization of the airway. However, the improved visualization during direct laryngoscopy does not necessarily increase the success of intubation [34, 35]. In cases where the airway is tenuous and sedation and relaxation may cause collapse of the airway, nasotracheal intubation may be performed over a bronchoscope while the patient is awake. The practice of holding cricoid pressure to decrease the risk of aspiration during rapid sequence intubation has not been supported by strong evidence [36].

In cases when an airway cannot be established with intubation and the patient is in extremis, a surgical airway will be required, generally a cricothyroidotomy. A vertical incision is made through skin over the cricothyroid membrane, and the membrane is transversely opened to gain entry into the airway. A horizontal incision runs the risk of lacerating the anterior neck veins and causes bleeding that will obscure the field. A smaller endotracheal tube can be placed in the airway till it is converted to a tracheostomy in a more controlled setting. Formal surgical sets may be available to perform the procedure, but if not available the procedure may be performed with a disposable scalpel. The back handle of the scalpel can be used to open the membrane by inserting the blunt end and twisting open the membrane to access to the airway and allow insertion of an endotracheal tube.

Mechanical Ventilation

Once the airway has been established, the clinician will have to choose a mode of ventilation. A basic understanding of mechanical ventilation physics will help the clinician make ventilator choices. Broadly speaking, a ventilator can be set to deliver a respiratory tidal volume based upon a preset volume setting (volume control) or can be set to deliver a respiratory tidal volume that is limited by airway pressure (pressure control). The stiffness of the lung, or lung compliance, is measured by change in volume divided by change in pressure. From a physics perspective, efforts at improving the function of the diseased lung are efforts in improving lung compliance. In volume control ventilation airway pressure is dependent upon the preset volume and compliance is constant. For the novice clinician setting, volume control settings may appear more intuitive. Minute ventilation can be directly set by choosing tidal volume and respiratory rate. Volume control mode ensures a guaranteed tidal volume and minute ventilation but does not take into account lung compliance and may result in barotrauma if airway pressure is not factored into the ventilator settings. In patients with low lung compliance, pressure control ventilation may be more appropriate. In both modes respiratory rate and fraction of inspired oxygen can be preset as well as positive end-expiratory pressure (PEEP). PEEP allows for alveoli to stay open at the end of expiration, augmenting functional residual capacity and thus permitting better gas exchange and oxygenation [37, 38]. Higher levels of PEEP however may impede cardiac venous return and contribute to hypotension [39].

In pressure control ventilation, the compliance is constant, and the pressure is set resulting in variable delivered volume. Pressure control ventilation may result in variable tidal volumes which may change with time as the lung compliance changes but prevents barotrauma. Pressure control ventilation may be more challenging to troubleshoot for the inexperienced clinician. Increasing PEEP and respiratory rate may attenuate ventilator difficulties. As PEEP is increased, the driving force between preset pressure and the PEEP decreases thus lowering the driving pressure which may result in lower delivered tidal volumes. Similarly increasing respiratory rate beyond a certain point may result in decreasing tidal volumes as an incomplete emptying between breaths will result in an auto-stacking. Because the system is set at a preset pressure setting, the stacking will not result in a rise of airway pressures but a decrease in driving pressure and hence in delivered volume [37, 38].

Excessive oxygen delivery resulting in hyperoxia can cause oxygen toxicity resulting in interstitial fibrosis, atelectasis, and tracheobronchitis [40, 41]. Systemically hyperoxia can cause vasoconstriction and the creation of toxic free radicals [42, 43]. Recent studies that setting FiO_2 at a lower level may have a survival benefit over higher oxygen settings. Patients targeted to maintain PaO_2 between 70 and 100 mmHg or arterial oxyhemoglobin saturation (SpO_2) between 94% and 98% versus a conventional approach achieving PaO_2 values up to 150 mmHg or SpO_2 values between 97% and 100% had lower ICU mortality and lower incidence of shock, liver failure, and bacteremia [44].

Mortality in severe ARDS can approach 40–50% [45–47]. The ARDSNET study demonstrated a survival benefit for patients with ARDS when ventilated with a lung-protective strategy. Patients placed on a lower tidal volume and higher respiratory rate have improved survival compared to patients placed on conventional settings [48]. The survival benefit is attributed to decreased barotrauma resulting in a decreased inflammatory cascades being created [49, 50].

Airway pressure release ventilation (APRV) is a lung-protective ventilation strategy that is a time-cycled pressure-controlled mode of ventilation. APRV is an open lung ventilation mode that works by cycling the ventilator cycle between a preset high (P_{high}) and low pressure (P_{low}) to avoid over- and under-distention of alveoli. The ventilator is cycled to be set preferentially to be spent at high pressure (T_{high}) at a significantly longer time relative to the low pressure setting (T_{low}) to prevent alveoli collapse and allow for recruitment through repetitive cycles [51, 52]. In essence, APRV is in effect inverse ratio ventilation, with the expiratory phase driven by the patient's chest recoil. APRV has many purported physiological benefits including increased cardiac return, improved oxygenation, decreased sedation requirements, and improved lung aeration [53–55]. However, APRV has not shown to have a survival benefit over ARDSNET protocol [56]. Patients on APRV ventilation may also take longer to be extubated compared to other conventional modes of ventilation. This increased time may be due to additional time taken to wean settings on this mode to prevent derecruitment of alveoli [57]. As patients are weaned from APRV, the P_{high} is lowered and compensated by an incremental increase in T_{high} so as to prevent collapse of alveoli that have been recruited. As the wean progresses, the mode approaches continuous positive airway pressure (CPAP) settings, and patients are extubated once low settings and standard criteria are achieved.

Another alternative to APRV mode of ventilation is to use high-frequency oscillatory ventilation (HFOV). HFOV first found clinical application in neonates, and its use has been expanded to adults in ARDS. HFOV is based upon the principle that high-frequency low tidal volumes can be used to achieve gas exchange thereby keeping the lung uniformly inflated over an extended period of time. In HFOV very small tidal volumes are delivered (2 ml/kg ideal body weight) with a relatively high constant mean airway pressure. In HFOV mode certain variables can be controlled including respiratory rate, the amplitude of ventilation, bias gas flow rate, inspiratory time, and FiO_2. The settings can be titrated based upon ABG results. The use of HFOV requires heavy sedation and paralytics to prevent ventilator dyssynchrony and to improve tolerance. HFOV mode can also be combined with the use of nitric oxide and prone positioning [58]. High-frequency oscillatory ventilation has not been shown to reduce 30-day mortality from ARDS compared to conventional mechanical ventilation and is not recommended as a first-line therapy [59].

In recent times the use of extracorporeal membrane oxygenation (ECMO) has expanded for use in patients in severe respiratory failure. Though not new technology, advances in critical care have made this modality a viable option in certain cases. Patients to be considered candidates for ECMO must have failed optimal treatment, have a reversible pathology, have an expectation to return to a functional state, be able to tolerate anticoagulation, and have an expectation to have good neurological outcome. An ECMO setup consists of four components: the cannula, a circuit, a pump, and a gas exchange device. ECMO can be performed via a venous-arterial (VA) route or a venous-venous (VV) route. VA ECMO is used to provide complete cardiopulmonary support. In most instances of respiratory failure, VV ECMO is utilized. VV access can be obtained by placing a catheter in the femoral vein and jugular vein or by placing a dual lumen catheter in the internal jugular vein with the distal end in the IVC and proximal port in the SVC. The system pump drives blood through the gas exchange membrane. Most gas exchange membranes consist of a tube with gas flowing through the tube, and blood flows outside the tube allowing for gas exchange by diffusion. The circuit tubing is coated to prevent blood adhesion and thrombus formation. The optimal ventilation mode while on ECMO has not been elucidated and varies by institutional policy [60]. Larger prospective studies are needed to determine the survival benefit of ECMO in the setting of severe respiratory failure [61].

There is also interest in the use of prone mechanical ventilation in severe respiratory failure. This strategy of lung recruitment places the patient in a prone position for prolonged periods of time during mechanical ventilation. This allows for recruitment of alveoli in the dorsal-dependent portions thereby allowing improved oxygenation. Prone positioning may result in derecruitment of ventral airspace, but this is compensated by greater recruitment of previously collapsed alveoli in the dorsal airspace [62]. Recent studies have demonstrated a survival advantage with prone ventilation in particular when used early in ARDS patients [63, 64]. Prone ventilation is not without its risks. Patients are at risk for developing pressure ulcers and unplanned extubation.

Ventilation Weaning

Weaning from mechanical ventilation is possible once the etiology of the respiratory failure has been treated. In recent years there has been greater understanding about ICU practice paradigms that can facilitate earlier liberation from mechanical ventilation. The traditional practice of placing mechanically ventilated patients on continuous sedation increases the incidence of delirium and prolongs ventilator time. Patients should be treated with intermittent narcotics as needed with a goal of achieving adequate analgesia and sedation without oversedation. Benzodiazepine exposure should be minimized as these drugs can contribute to delirium. Patients who require continuous sedation should have their sedation discontinued once a day to reassess to need for sedation [65–67]. This "sedation holiday" should be combined with a spontaneous breathing trial for a combined benefit of achieving earlier ventilator liberation [68]. Patients on mechanical ventilation benefit from a protocol-driven approach to ventilator liberation. Protocols that are not driven by physician discretion but parameter-guided respiratory therapist protocol lead to quicker ventilator liberation [69].

Many parameters can be obtained while a patient is on mechanical ventilation. The most sensitive and specific parameter to predict successful extubation is the rapid shallow breathing index. A breathing trial on minimal support for 30 min has a high sensitivity (0.97) for success and the best positive predictive value (0.78) for successful extubation compared to respiratory rate, minute ventilation, tidal volume, maximal inspiratory pressure, and static of dynamic compliance. Extending the trial to longer periods beyond 30 min does not improve sensitivity of the test as most patients who fail do so within the first 30 min [70, 71].

Patients will occasionally self-extubate resulting in unplanned discontinuation of mechanical ventilation. Approximately half of patients who self-extubate will succeed in remaining free of mechanical ventilation [72]. Unplanned extubation can result in increased rates of aspiration, pneumonia, and laryngeal edema. Some studies suggest self-extubation most commonly occurs during nursing shift changes. Younger surgical patients may be at higher risk for self-extubation as well as patients with lower levels of sedation and higher GCS scores [73].

Post-extubation Support

Respiratory support after extubation may improve success of remaining off mechanical ventilation with the most benefit being demonstrated among COPD patients. COPD patients electively placed on noninvasive ventilation post-extubation have decreased mortality, time on mechanical ventilation, ICU length of stay, and need for tracheostomy [74]. Among the general population, patients considered at high risk for reintubation (age >65, cardiac failure as cause if respiratory distress, APACHE score greater than 12 on day of extubation) have also been shown to benefit from elective noninvasive ventilator support after extubation, decreasing mortality [75]. Some patients are not candidates for noninvasive ventilator support due to increased secretions or concerns of foregut anatomy after surgical interventions. Another promising intervention to support extubated patients is the use of high-flow nasal cannula oxygen. Recent studies suggest this modality is non-inferior to noninvasive ventilation in preventing reintubation among high-risk patients. High-flow nasal cannula may be more apt for its use in post-extubation support compared to hypoxic respiratory failure [25, 26].

Chronic Respiratory Failure

Despite efforts to optimize a patient's respiratory function, some patients will not be successfully weaned off mechanical ventilation. Patients requiring long-term or permanent mechanical ventilation benefit from tracheostomy placement. It is debatable what the optimal practice paradigm is for tracheostomy placement in terms of which patient population benefits from early tracheostomy placement and what the definition is for early versus late tracheostomy timing. There has been conflicting data regarding the optimal practice [76–79]. Studies among trauma patients demonstrate decreased critical care utilization among early tracheostomy patients compared to delayed tracheostomy, a finding which may be applicable to other critically ill populations. Some studies have suggested a mortality benefit among trauma patients without brain injury and greater benefit to traumatic brain injury patients by decreasing mortality, ICU stay, ventilator time, and ventilator-associated pneumonia events [77, 78]. Other studies have shown no mortality benefit for early tracheostomy among critically ill patents [79]. However, a Cochrane review of critically ill patients only found suggestive evidence favoring early tracheostomy. Additional randomized controlled studies are needed among specific populations to better define the optimal practice paradigm [80].

Long-Term Outcomes

Many patients remain dependent on mechanical ventilation despite optimal medical treatment. Though a time period to define prolonged mechanical ventilation is not agreed upon, many studies have used a time period greater than 21 days [6]. Patients requiring prolonged ventilation have multiple transitions of care, persistent profound disability, and increased health-care costs approaching $3.5 million at the end of 1 year of survival [3]. Patients requiring prolonged mechanical ventilation have a higher 1-year mortality than those requiring shorter periods of mechanical ventilation. Among patients above 65 years of age, 1-year mortality can be 67%. Elderly patients who survive their critical illness have greater than expected disability based upon prior functional status compared to those who did not require mechanical ventilation. There is limited high-quality data to help identify prognostic factors to predict 6-month survival among those requiring long-term mechanical ventilation [3, 5, 6, 80]. A recent retrospective meta-analysis identified age, vasopressor use, thrombocytopenia, acute kidney injury/failure, pre-existing kidney disease, and inability to liberate from ventilation as strong predictors of 6-month mortality [81]. Patients and surrogate decision makers should be informed of long-term outcomes before embarking upon long-term mechanical ventilation treatment plans.

Conclusions

Respiratory distress is a common entity encountered in the ICU. Rapid diagnosis and intervention can help achieve optimal results. Evidence-based protocols for ventilator weaning and sedation result in decreased mechanical ventilation time. However, despite optimal treatment, many patients will not recover to their baseline function and will result in long-term ventilator dependence and disability. Establishing informed goals of care from patients and surrogate decision makers can help achieve goals compatible with the patient's wishes.

References

1. Esteban A, Anzueto A, Frutos F, et al. Characteristics and outcomes in adult patients receiving mechanical ventilation: a 28-day international study. JAMA. 2002;287:345–55.
2. Wunsch H, Linde-Zwirble WT, Angus DC, et al. The epidemiology of mechanical ventilation use in the United States. Crit Care Med. 2010;38:1947–53.
3. Unroe M, Kahn JM, Carson SS, Govert JA, Martinu T, Sathy SJ, et al. One-year trajectories of care and resource utilization for recipients of prolonged mechanical ventilation: a cohort study. Ann Intern Med. 2010;153(3):167–75.
4. Cooke CR. Economics of mechanical ventilation and respiratory failure. Crit Care Clin. 2012;28(1):39–55.
5. Barnato AE, Albert SM, Angus DC, Lave JR, Degenholtz HB. Disability among elderly survivors of mechanical ventilation. Am J Respir Crit Care Med. 2011;183(8):1037–42.
6. Cox CE, Carson SS, Lindquist JH, Olsen MK, Govert JA, Chelluri L, Quality of Life After Mechanical Ventilation in the Aged (QOL-MV) Investigators. Differences in one-year health outcomes and resource utilization by definition of prolonged mechanical ventilation: a prospective cohort study. Crit Care. 2007;11(1):R9.
7. Barjaktarevic I, Wang T. Acute respiratory failure. In: Textbook of critical care, vol. 9. Philadelphia: Elsevier; 2017. p. 33–7.
8. ARDS Definition Task Force, Ranieri VM, Rubenfeld GD, Thompson BT, Ferguson ND, Caldwell E, Fan E, et al. Acute respiratory distress syndrome: the Berlin Definition. JAMA. 2012;307(23):2526–33.
9. Bhargava M, Wendt CH. Biomarkers in acute lung injury. Transl Res. 2012;159(4):205–17.
10. Álvarez P, Carrasco R, Romero-Dapueto C, Castillo RL. Transfusion-related acute lung injured (TRALI): current concepts. Open Respir Med J. 2015;9:92–6.
11. Peters AL, Vlaar AP. Redefining transfusion-related acute lung injury: don't throw the baby out with the bathwater. Transfusion. 2016;56:2384–8.
12. ATLS Subcommittee, American College of Surgeons' Committee on Trauma, International ATLS working group. Advanced trauma life support ATLS student course manual. 9th ed. Chicago: American College of Surgeons; 2012.
13. Tillquist MN, Gabriel RA, Dutton RP, Urman RD. Incidence and risk factors for early postoperative reintubations. J Clin Anesth. 2016;31:80–9.
14. Hendrikse KA, Gratama JW, Hove W, Rommes JH, Schultz MJ, Spronk PE. Low value of routine chest radiographs in a mixed medical-surgical ICU. Chest. 2007;132(3):823–8.
15. Lakhal K, Serveaux-Delous M, Lefrant JY, Capdevila X, Jaber S, AzuRéa network for the RadioDay study group. Chest radiographs in 104 French ICUs: current prescription strategies and clinical value (the RadioDay study). Intensive Care Med. 2012;38(11):1787–99.
16. Ganapathy A, Adhikari NK, Spiegelman J, Scales DC. Routine chest x-rays in intensive care units: a systematic review and meta-analysis. Crit Care. 2012;16(2):R68.
17. Bhattacharya B, Fieber J, Schuster K, Davis K, Maung A. "Occult" rib fractures diagnosed on computed tomography scan only are still a risk factor for solid organ injury. J Emerg Trauma Shock. 2015;8(3):140–3.
18. Claessens YE, Debray MP, Tubach F, Brun AL, Rammaert B, Hausfater P, et al. Early chest computed tomography scan to assist diagnosis and guide treatment decision for suspected community-acquired pneumonia. Am J Respir Crit Care Med. 2015;192(8):974–82.

19. Ambroggio L, Sucharew H, Rattan MS, O'Hara SM, Babcock DS, Clohessy C, et al. Lung ultrasonography: a viable alternative to chest radiography in children with suspected pneumonia? J Pediatr. 2016;176:93–98.e7.
20. Xia Y, Ying Y, Wang S, Li W, Shen H. Effectiveness of lung ultrasonography for diagnosis of pneumonia in adults: a systematic review and meta-analysis. J Thorac Dis. 2016;8(10):2822–31.
21. Soubani AO. Noninvasive monitoring of oxygen and carbon dioxide. Am J Emerg Med. 2001;19(2):141–6.
22. Gray AJ, Goodacre S, Newby DE, et al. 3CPO Study Investigators. A multicentre randomized controlled trial of the use of continuous positive airway pressure and non-invasive positive pressure ventilation in the early treatment of patients presenting to the emergency department with severe acute cardiogenic pulmonary oedema: the 3CPO trial. Health Technol Assess. 2009;13:1–106.
23. Nava S, Gregoretti C, Fanfulla F, et al. Noninvasive ventilation to prevent respiratory failure after extubation in high-risk patients. Crit Care Med. 2005;33:2465–70.
24. Jones PG, Kamona S, Doran O, Sawtell F, Wilsher M. Randomized controlled trial of humidified high-flow nasal oxygen for acute respiratory distress in the emergency department: the HOT-ER study. Respir Care. 2016;61(3):291–9.
25. Frat JP, Thille AW, Mercat A, Girault C, Ragot S, Perbet S, et al.; FLORALI Study Group.; REVA Network. High-flow oxygen through nasal cannula in acute hypoxemic respiratory failure. N Engl J Med. 2015;372(23):2185–96.
26. Hernández G, Vaquero C, Colinas L, Cuena R, González P, Canabal A, et al. Effect of postextubation high-flow nasal cannula vs noninvasive ventilation on reintubation and postextubation respiratory failure in high-risk patients: a randomized clinical trial. JAMA. 2016;316(15):1565–74.
27. Inaba K, Lustenberger T, Recinos G, Georgiou C, Velmahos GC, Brown C, et al. Does size matter? A prospective analysis of 28-32 versus 36-40 French chest tube size in trauma. J Trauma Acute Care Surg. 2012;72(2):422–7.
28. Filosso PL, Sandri A, Guerrera F, Ferraris A, Marchisio F, Bora G, et al. When size matters: changing opinion in the management of pleural space-the rise of small-bore pleural catheters. J Thorac Dis. 2016;8(7):E503–10.
29. Battle CE, Evans PA. Predictors of mortality in patients with flail chest: a systematic review. Emerg Med J. 2015;32(12):961–5.
30. Shulzhenko NO, Zens TJ, Beems MV, Jung HS, O'Rourke AP, Liepert AE, et al. Number of rib fractures thresholds independently predict worse outcomes in older patients with blunt trauma. Surgery. 2016; pii: S0039–6060(16)30699–7.
31. Brasel KJ, Moore EE, Albrecht RA, deMoya M, Schreiber M, Karmy-Jones R, et al. Western trauma association critical decisions in trauma: management of rib fractures. J Trauma Acute Care Surg. 2017;82(1):200–3.
32. Hekiert AM, Mick R, Mirza N. Prediction of difficult laryngoscopy: does obesity play a role? Ann Otol Rhinol Laryngol. 2007;116(11):799–804.
33. Nuckton TJ, Glidden DV, Browner WS, Claman DM. Physical examination: Mallampati score as an independent predictor of obstructive sleep apnea. Sleep. 2006;29(7):903–8.
34. Sulser S, Ubmann D, Schlaepfer M, Brueesch M, Goliasch G, Seifert B, et al. C-MAC videolaryngoscope compared with direct laryngoscopy for rapid sequence intubation in an emergency department: a randomised clinical trial. Eur J Anaesthesiol. 2016;33(12):943–8.
35. Lewis SR, Butler AR, Parker J, Cook TM, Smith AF. Videolaryngoscopy versus direct laryngoscopy for adult patients requiring tracheal intubation. Cochrane Database Syst Rev. 2016;11:CD011136.
36. Algie CM, Mahar RK, Tan HB, Wilson G, Mahar PD, Wasiak J. Effectiveness and risks of cricoid pressure during rapid sequence induction for endotracheal intubation. Cochrane Database Syst Rev. 2015;11:CD011656.
37. Bone RC, Eubanks DH. The basis and basics of mechanical ventilation. Dis Mon. 1991;37(6):321–406.
38. Demling RH, Knox JB. Basic concepts of lung function and dysfunction: oxygenation, ventilation, and mechanics. New Horiz. 1993;1(3):362–70.
39. Versprille A. Basic mechanisms and clinical consequences of cyclic changes in pulmonary blood flow and blood volume during mechanical ventilation. Eur J Anaesthesiol. 1994;11(1):15–23.
40. Davis WB, Rennard SI, Bitterman PB, Crystal RG. Pulmonary oxygen toxicity: early reversible changes in human alveolar structures induced by hyperoxia. N Engl J Med. 1983;309(15):878–83.
41. Crapo JD. Morphologic changes in pulmonary oxygen toxicity. Annu Rev Physiol. 1986;48:721–31.
42. Reinhart K, Bloos F, König F, Bredle D, Hannemann L. Reversible decrease of oxygen consumption by hyperoxia. Chest. 1991;99(3):690–4.
43. Brueckl C, Kaestle S, Kerem A, et al. Hyperoxia-induced reactive oxygen species formation in pulmonary capillary endothelial cells in situ. Am J Respir Cell Mol Biol. 2006;34(4):453–63.
44. Girardis M, Busani S, Damiani E, Donati A, Rinaldi L, Marudi A, et al. Effect of conservative vs conventional oxygen therapy on mortality among patients in an intensive care unit: the oxygen-ICU randomized clinical trial. JAMA. 2016;316(15):1583–9.
45. Sloane PJ, Gee MH, Gottlieb JE, et al. A multicenter registry of patients with acute respiratory distress syndrome: physiology and outcome. Am Rev Respir Dis. 1992;146:419–26.
46. Doyle RL, Szaflarski N, Modin GW, Wiener-Kronish JP, Matthay MA. Identification of patients with acute lung injury: predictors of mortality. Am J Respir Crit Care Med. 1995;152:1818–24.
47. Zilberberg MD, Epstein SK. Acute lung injury in the medical ICU: comorbid conditions, age, etiology, and hospital outcome. Am J Respir Crit Care Med. 1998;157:1159–64.
48. The Acute Respiratory Distress Syndrome Network, et al. Ventilation with lower tidal volumes as compared with traditional tidal volumes for acute lung injury and the acute respiratory distress syndrome. The Acute Respiratory Distress Syndrome Network. N Engl J Med. 2000;342(18):1301–8.
49. Dreyfuss D, Saumon G, Hubmayr RD, editors. Ventilator-induced lung injury. New York: Taylor & Francis; 2006.
50. Villar J, Kacmarek RM, Pérez-Méndez L, Aguirre-Jaime A. A high positive end-expiratory pressure, low tidal volume ventilatory strategy improves outcome in persistent acute respiratory distress syndrome: a randomized, controlled trial. Crit Care Med. 2006;34:1311–8.
51. Varpula T, et al. The effects of ventilatory mode on lung aeration assessed with computer tomography: a randomized controlled study. J Intensive Care Med. 2009;24:122–30.
52. Frawley PM, Habashi NM. Airway pressure release ventilation: theory and practice. AACN Clin Issues. 2001;12:234–46.
53. Kaplan LJ, Bailey H, Formosa V. Airway pressure release ventilation increases cardiac performance in patients with acute lung injury/adult respiratory distress syndrome. Crit Care. 2001;5(4):221–6.
54. Fan E, et al. Sedation and analgesia usage with airway pressure release and assist-control ventilation for acute lung injury. J Intensive Care Med. 2008;23:376–83.
55. Walkey AJ, et al. Use of airway pressure release ventilation is associated with a reduced incidence of ventilator-associated pneumonia in patients with pulmonary contusion. J Trauma. 2011;70:E42–7.
56. Maxwell RA, et al. A randomized prospective trial of airway pressure release ventilation and low tidal volume ventilation in adult trauma patients with acute respiratory failure. J Trauma. 2010;69:501–11.
57. Maung AA, Schuster KM, Kaplan LJ, Ditillo MF, Piper GL, Maerz LL, et al. Compared to conventional ventilation, airway pressure release ventilation may increase ventilator days in trauma patients. J Trauma Acute Care Surg. 2012;73(2):507–10.

58. Stawicki SP, Goyal M, Sarani B. High-frequency oscillatory ventilation (HFOV) and airway pressure release ventilation (APRV): a practical guide. J Intensive Care Med. 2009;24(4):215–29.
59. Sud S, Sud M, Friedrich JO, Wunsch H, Meade MO, Ferguson ND, et al. High-frequency oscillatory ventilation versus conventional ventilation for acute respiratory distress syndrome. Cochrane Database Syst Rev. 2016;4:CD004085.
60. Bhatt N, Osborn E. Extracorporeal gas exchange: the expanding role of extracorporeal support in respiratory failure. Clin Chest Med. 2016;37(4):765–80.
61. Tramm R, Ilic D, Davies AR, Pellegrino VA, Romero L, Hodgson C. Extracorporeal membrane oxygenation for critically ill adults. Cochrane Database Syst Rev. 2015;1:CD010381.
62. Protti A, Chiumello D, Cressoni M, Carlesso E, Mietto C, Berto V, Lazzerini M, Quintel M, Gattinoni L. Relationship between gas exchange response to prone position and lung recruitability during acute respiratory failure. Intensive Care Med. 2009;35:1011–7.
63. Guérin C, Reignier J, Richard JC, Beuret P, Gacouin A, Boulain T, et al. Prone positioning in severe acute respiratory distress syndrome. N Engl J Med. 2013;368(23):2159–68.
64. Hu SL, He HL, Pan C, Liu AR, Liu SQ, Liu L, et al. The effect of prone positioning on mortality in patients with acute respiratory distress syndrome: a meta-analysis of randomized controlled trials. Crit Care. 2014;18(3):R109.
65. Anifantaki S, Prinianakis G, Vitsaksaki E, et al. Daily interruption of sedative infusions in an adult medical-surgical intensive care unit: randomized controlled trial. J Adv Nurs. 2009;65:1054–60.
66. de Wit M, Gennings C, Jenvey WI, et al. Randomized trial comparing daily interruption of sedation and nursing-implemented sedation algorithm in medical intensive care unit patients. Crit Care. 2008;12:R70.
67. Mehta S, Burry L, Martinez-Motta JC, Stewart TE, Hallett D, McDonald E, et al. A randomized trial of daily awakening in critically ill patients managed with a sedation protocol: a pilot trial. Crit Care Med. 2008;36(7):2092–9.
68. Juern JS. Removing the critically ill patient from mechanical ventilation. Surg Clin North Am. 2012;92(6):1475–83.
69. Kollef MH, Shapiro SD, Silver P, St John RE, Prentice D, Sauer S, et al. A randomized, controlled trial of protocol-directed versus physician-directed weaning from mechanical ventilation. Crit Care Med. 1997;25(4):567–74.
70. Yang KL, Tobin MJ. A prospective study of indexes predicting the outcome of trials of weaning from mechanical ventilation. N Engl J Med. 1991;324(21):1445–50.
71. Singh PM, Rewari V, Chandralekha, Arora MK, Trikha A. A retrospective analysis of determinants of self-extubation in a tertiary care intensive care unit. J Emerg Trauma Shock. 2013;6(4):241–5.
72. Whelan J, Simpson SQ, Levy H. Unplanned extubation. Predictors of successful termination of mechanical ventilatory support. Chest. 1994;105(6):1808–12.
73. Moons P, Sels K, De Becker W, De Geest S, Ferdinande P. Development of a risk assessment tool for deliberate self-extubation in intensive care patients. Intensive Care Med. 2004;30(7):1348–55.
74. Burns KE, Meade MO, Premji A, Adhikari NK. Noninvasive positive-pressure ventilation as a weaning strategy for intubated adults with respiratory failure. Cochrane Database Syst Rev. 2013;12:CD004127.
75. Ferrer M, Valencia M, Nicolas JM, Bernadich O, Badia JR, Torres A. Early noninvasive ventilation averts extubation failure in patients at risk: a randomized trial. Am J Respir Crit Care Med. 2006;173(2):164–70.
76. Keenan JE, Gulack BC, Nussbaum DP, Green CL, Vaslef SN, Shapiro ML, et al. Optimal timing of tracheostomy after trauma without associated head injury. J Surg Res. 2015;198(2):475–81.
77. McCredie VA, Alali AS, Scales DC, Adhikari NK, Rubenfeld GD, Cuthbertson BH, et al. Effect of early versus late tracheostomy or prolonged intubation in critically ill patients with acute brain injury: a systematic review and meta-analysis. Neurocrit Care. 2017;26(1):14–25.
78. Hyde GA, Savage SA, Zarzaur BL, Hart-Hyde JE, Schaefer CB, Croce MA, et al. Early tracheostomy in trauma patients saves time and money. Injury. 2015;46(1):110–4.
79. Mehta AB, Cooke CR, Wiener RS, Walkey AJ. Hospital variation in early tracheostomy in the United States: a population-based study. Crit Care Med. 2016;44(8):1506–14.
80. Andriolo BN, Andriolo RB, Saconato H, Atallah ÁN, Valente O. Early versus late tracheostomy for critically ill patients. Cochrane Database Syst Rev. 2015;1:CD007271.
81. Dettmer MR, Damuth E, Zarbiv S, Mitchell JA, Bartock JL, Trzeciak S. Prognostic factors for long-term mortality in critically ill patients treated with prolonged mechanical ventilation: a systematic review. Crit Care Med. 2017;45(1):69–74.
82. Koeppen B, Stanton BA. Oxygen and carbon dioxide transport. In: Berne & Levy physiology. London: Elsevier Mosby; 2010. p. 459–67.
83. Islam S, Selbong U, Taylor CJ, Ormiston IW. Does a patient's Mallampati score predict outcome after maxillomandibular advancement for obstructive sleep apnoea? Br J Oral Maxillofac Surg. 2015;53(1):23–7.

16 Noninvasive Ventilation

Eric Bui

Introduction

Noninvasive ventilation (NIV) is defined as a method of delivering ventilatory support to a patient without the use of an invasive airway such as an endotracheal, nasotracheal, or tracheostomy tube. Noninvasive ventilation can be provided with negative or positive pressure. In the early twentieth century, negative pressure ventilation was the predominant modality [1]. These large, tank-style ventilators enclosed a patient's entire thorax and created a negative pressure to help passively expand the patient's chest wall and lungs. Due to increased experience with the technique as well as improved ventilator technology, noninvasive positive pressure ventilation (NPPV) has now become the preferred method of NIV.

NPPV has been shown to be effective in treating chronic conditions such as obstructive sleep apnea and chronic obstructive pulmonary disease (COPD). As the use of NPPV has become more widespread and understood, the technique has been applied to a much wider spectrum of respiratory conditions and clinical scenarios, including those commonly seen in the critical care setting. The use of NPPV has been described in acute hypoxemic/hypercapnic respiratory failure, post-extubation failure, patients who are difficult to wean from the ventilator, and even acute respiratory distress syndrome (ARDS).

The appeal of NPPV is self-descriptive; it is noninvasive in nature. Many complications are associated with invasive ventilation. These include but are not limited to increased rates of hospital-acquired pneumonia, hospital days, ICU days, and mortality. Intubation itself is not a benign procedure and can cause direct trauma to airways and the oropharynx. Furthermore, patients who are endotracheally or nasotracheally intubated lose the ability to communicate verbally and eat normally. If these potential complications and limitations of traditional invasive ventilation can theoretically be prevented by the use of NPPV without jeopardizing patient safety, then the decision on which modality to use becomes clearer. The question becomes how to identify the patients that will benefit most from NPPV.

This chapter will discuss the practical applications of NPPV in the critical care setting, including appropriate indications and contraindications for its use.

Mechanism of Action

The physiology and theory of NPPV will be briefly addressed here. The principle of applying NPPV is similar to that of invasive positive pressure ventilation. The positive airway pressure provided forces air into the airways with the result of opening collapsed airways and alveoli. This recruits areas of under-ventilated or collapsed lung helping to correct ventilation/perfusion (*V*/*Q*) mismatch, leading to improvement in oxygenation and lung compliance. Increased lung compliance reduces the work of breathing for the patient. The delivered positive pressure also off-loads the muscles of respiration, contributing to improvement in respiratory mechanics. Other purported benefits include improvement of cardiac function in patients with congestive heart failure (CHF). The proposed mechanism of this is due to the increased intrathoracic pressure caused by the positive pressure delivered via NPPV. This increased intrathoracic pressure helps to decrease the venous return to the heart (decreased preload) and augment the ejection of blood by the left ventricle (decreased afterload).

There are many different ways that NPPV can be delivered, but the process essentially is distilled down into positive airway pressure being applied during a respiratory cycle. The two most common methods of delivering NPPV are continuous positive airway pressure (CPAP) and bi-level positive airway pressure (BPAP). Although some controversy exists as whether or not CPAP is truly a mode of NIV, for the purposes of this chapter, it will be included as such.

E. Bui (✉)
Department of Surgery, UCSF East Bay – Highland Hospital, Oakland, CA, USA
e-mail: ericbui@alamedahealthsystem.org

A. Salim et al. (eds.), *Surgical Critical Care Therapy*, https://doi.org/10.1007/978-3-319-71712-8_16

CPAP is a constant pressure that is delivered throughout both the inspiratory and expiratory phase of the respiratory cycle. It is often used in the treatment of sleep apnea, where the constant pressure provided prevents the upper airways from collapsing during sleep. This is the most rudimentary form of NPPV and requires the patient to initiate all breaths. Because the pressure does not change between the inspiratory and expiratory phases, it does not augment tidal volumes (i.e., it provides no pressure support).

BPAP provides separate inspiratory and expiratory positive airway pressures during the respiratory cycle. The inspiratory pressure is set higher than the expiratory pressure, and the difference between these two values (pressure support) is what augments tidal volume. The expiratory positive airway pressure is analogous to setting the PEEP for invasive mechanical ventilation. BPAP is a much more versatile mode of NPPV and does not necessarily require patient-initiated breaths, as a set "backup" rate can be dialed in. BPAP is the most commonly used mode of NPPV, and due to its flexibility, it is the preferred modality in the ICU.

Patient Selection

While noninvasive ventilation is an attractive option to provide ventilatory support with many potential upsides, it should never replace traditional invasive ventilation when that is what the clinical situation calls for. Table 16.1 lists contraindications to NPPV.

Patient selection is of the utmost importance when the decision is made to initiate NPPV, particularly in the ICU setting. The role of NPPV in critical care is still not well defined. Specific applications will be discussed later in the chapter. In general however, patients with the following characteristics generally will have greater success with NPPV application [2]:

- A rapidly reversible cause of hypoxemia
- Mild to moderate respiratory acidosis (pH 7.1–7.35)
- Moderate to severe dyspnea
- Tachypnea (greater than 24 breaths per minute for COPD, greater than 30–35 breaths per minute for hypoxemic respiratory failure)

The decision to initiate NPPV should be made early once a patient starts showing initial signs or symptoms of impending respiratory failure. Early application of NPPV will yield the highest rates of success. Waiting until a patient becomes too unstable or requires more advanced airway management before considering NPPV wastes a potential opportunity to circumvent such a scenario from occurring.

Table 16.1 Contraindications to NPPV

Cardiopulmonary arrest	Severe hypoxemia
Inability to protect airway	Airway obstruction
Hemodynamic instability	Massive hematemesis/hemoptysis
Severe acidosis	Facial trauma/burns
Inability to fit NPPV apparatus	Patient noncompliance
Recent upper GI surgery	

Specific Conditions

Chronic Obstructive Pulmonary Disease (COPD) and Cardiogenic Pulmonary Edema

The vast majority of studies pertaining to the use of NPPV have been in the treatment of respiratory failure related to COPD exacerbation and cardiogenic pulmonary edema.

Multiple randomized controlled studies and meta-analyses have shown marked benefits when using NPPV (generally BPAP) in the treatment of COPD exacerbation when compared to standard oxygen therapy and invasive mechanical ventilation [3–7]. Significant reductions in mortality, rate of intubation, and hospital length of stay have been demonstrated, although long-term outcome improvement has yet to be shown. A recent meta-analysis of NPPV in the acute care setting showed that its use reduces morality by almost half when compared to standard treatments [8]. NPPV appears to be more beneficial in moderate to severe cases of COPD exacerbation (defined as a baseline pH of <7.3) and thus is an appropriate modality for use in ICU patients who are admitted with respiratory failure due to COPD. NPPV is considered a first-line therapy in this patient population, with strong data to support its use [3–8].

Similar data exists for those who have respiratory failure secondary to cardiogenic pulmonary edema. NPPV has been shown to decrease rates of intubation and improve respiratory mechanics in this subset of patients [9–13]. The data regarding mortality is somewhat less compelling than that for COPD, though several reviews concluded that the use of NIV for cardiogenic pulmonary edema does improve overall survival [8, 14, 15]. Regardless, NPPV is considered a viable, first-line treatment for respiratory failure in these patients with high-quality evidence to support its use. It should be noted that the majority of studies done examining the use of NPPV in patients with acute cardiogenic pulmonary edema were done using CPAP as the primary modality. One RCT comparing CPAP to BPAP in these patients showed a higher incidence of myocardial infarction in the BPAP arm, but this may have been due to patient selection issues. Overall mortality between the two groups was no different [16].

Weaning from the Ventilator and Post-extubation Respiratory Failure

Early liberation of patients from the ventilator remains a priority of ICU care. Although invasive mechanical ventilation is frequently lifesaving and unavoidable, it is not a benign intervention, and prolonged intubation can lead to many detrimental (and some would say preventable) consequences.

Traditionally, ventilator-weaning trials are performed while the patient is still intubated. This may involve spontaneous breathing trials, pressure support modes, synchronized intermittent mechanical ventilation (SIMV), or other techniques. Regardless of the method, the patient is monitored, and a decision is made on whether or not the patient is ready for extubation. If the patient fails, they are left intubated on the ventilator, often for at least another 24 h until a subsequent weaning trial is performed.

The concept of using NIV to wean patients from the ventilator has appeal because the process of weaning occurs after the patient has been extubated. This may be a difficult concept to grasp at first. Some might assume that extubation equates to liberation from the ventilator; however, it would be remiss to forget that NPPV is still mechanical ventilation, only delivered without an invasive airway in place.

A 2013 Cochrane review examining NPPV as a weaning strategy for intubated patients contained 16 trials deemed to be of "moderate to good quality" concluded that weaning strategies that included NPPV "may reduce rates of mortality and ventilator-associated pneumonia without increasing the risk of weaning failure or re-intubation" [17]. The majority of patients in these studies (approximately two thirds of the total study population) were COPD patients with respiratory failure, so these results may be limited when applied to a broader patient population. Regardless, data exists that shows that NPPV could be a viable option to get patients extubated sooner.

The use of NPPV in post-extubation respiratory failure at first might seem similar to its use as a strategy to wean patients from the ventilator. However the key difference is in how this population is defined. NPPV has been described for use in patients who develop respiratory failure after extubation, presumably after passing a weaning trial while intubated, or immediately after extubation to circumvent the development of post-extubation respiratory failure. It is important to make this distinction because the data differs between these two groups.

A meta-analysis of 10 trials containing 1382 patients done in 2014 examined the efficacy of using NPPV to manage post-extubation respiratory failure. It concluded that in the subgroup of patients who developed respiratory failure after extubation, NPPV did not reduce the rate of re-intubation, nor did it reduce mortality [18]. In fact, there was a trend toward worse outcomes in this group. For those patients deemed to be at "high risk" for post-extubation respiratory failure (but are able to successfully pass a SBT during invasive ventilation), early application of NIV seems to show some benefit by reducing rates of re-intubation and mortality. The definition of "high risk" however is not uniform and subject to interpretation. Given the current evidence, the use of NPPV for the management of post-extubation failure should be done judiciously and only by clinicians with experience using it in the ICU setting. It should never delay re-intubation if clinically indicated.

Table 16.2 Risk factors for postoperative respiratory failure

Abdominal aortic aneurysm repair	Thoracic surgery
Neurosurgery	Upper abdominal surgery
Peripheral vascular surgery	Neck surgery
Emergent surgery	Albumin level < 30 g/L
Blood urea nitrogen level > 30 mg/dL	Dependent functional status
COPD	Age

Postoperative Respiratory Failure

Postoperative respiratory failure is a similar but distinct entity to post-extubation respiratory failure. It is defined as the continued need for mechanical ventilation immediately postoperatively or the need for re-intubation after postoperative extubation. Postoperative respiratory failure differs from other causes of respiratory failure in several ways. Surgery and general anesthesia lead to dysfunction of respiratory muscles, especially the diaphragm, resulting in impaired respiratory mechanics, atelectasis, hypoxia, hypoventilation, and the potential for subsequent respiratory failure. Additionally, the type of surgery and patient comorbidities often will contribute to the constellation of factors that lead to postoperative respiratory failure. A large multicenter Veterans Affairs (VA) study developed a model, which identified risk factors for postoperative respiratory failure (Table 16.2) [19].

A recent randomized clinical trial published in 2016 examined the effect of NIV on rates of tracheal re-intubation in patients with postoperative hypoxemic respiratory failure after undergoing abdominal surgery [20]. NIV was compared to oxygen delivered by mask at up to 15 L/min to maintain adequate saturation. NIV was shown in this population to significantly decrease the rates of re-intubation, ventilator days, and rates of nosocomial infection. No mortality benefit was observed. These results are similar to those found in a previous review on the subject, which included surgical patients of all disciplines and was not limited only to those receiving abdominal surgery [21].

The available data suggests that NIV may be a useful adjunct as both a prophylactic and therapeutic treatment for patients presenting with postoperative respiratory failure. Unfortunately many of the available studies are of low quality, and further research is required in order to make a stronger recommendation on its use in this specific population.

Hypoxemic Respiratory Failure

Hypoxemic respiratory failure encompasses a very large, heterogeneous population of patients, as the causes of this condition are numerous and varied. The definition of hypoxemic respiratory failure is not uniform but has been defined as hypoxemia ($SpO_2 < 90\%$ or PaO_2/FiO_2 ratio < 200) while breathing 50% supplemental oxygen via venturi mask [22, 23].

Many of the large meta-analyses that have been done reviewing the use of NPPV in the acute care setting include studies examining its use to treat respiratory failure from acute lung injury, trauma, ARDS, pneumonia, and other etiologies as well as the previously described conditions of COPD and cardiogenic pulmonary edema. The analyses conclude that overall in adult patients with acute respiratory failure, NPPV led to a lower intubation rate, shorter ICU length of stay, and lower rates of mortality when compared to conventional therapy [8, 18, 24].

The data supporting the use of NPPV for patients with respiratory failure due to COPD or cardiogenic pulmonary edema is quite robust. Fewer studies exist that have examined NPPV for treating hypoxemic respiratory failure in the absence of these two conditions. Data does exist however showing that NPPV can be effective in managing these patients. One study assigned patients with hypoxemic respiratory failure to receive either conventional invasive mechanical ventilation or NPPV via a standardized protocol. It was found that NPPV improved gas exchange just as effectively as invasive mechanical ventilation, measured as an improvement in the PaO_2/FiO_2 ratio. The NPPV arm also had significantly shorter stays in the ICU and fewer serious complications [22].

A randomized trial was subsequently done by a separate group examining the use of NPPV as a primary treatment for severe hypoxemic respiratory failure (the mean PaO_2/FiO_2 ratio of the study population was approximately 100 mmHg) and its effect on both survival and need for intubation [23]. Patients were randomized to receive either NPPV or high-concentration oxygen therapy. The study demonstrated that overall, patients treated with NPPV had a significantly lower need for intubation and had improved ICU and 90-day survival. These benefits were especially pronounced in patients with pneumonia. Conversely, in the subgroup of patients with respiratory failure due to ARDS, NPPV did not decrease rates of intubation or improve 90-day survival [23].

In 2013, an observational cohort study was published that looked to identify predictors of NPPV failure in patients with hypoxemic respiratory failure and determine the rates of failure when NPPV was used as a first-line treatment [24]. The patients included had hypoxemic respiratory failure in the absence of COPD and cardiogenic pulmonary edema. The study population was then divided into those who met clinical criteria for ARDS and those who did not. The ARDS group was further subdivided into those with mild, moderate, and severe ARDS based on the Berlin criteria. Similar to what was observed in the previously mentioned study, patients with ARDS had a significantly higher rate of intubation than those who did not. However those with no ARDS or mild ARDS had no difference in rates of intubation. Mortality was also higher in patients with ARDS. The authors identified that patients with active cancer, lower GCS scores, shock, moderate or severe ARDS, and lower levels of PEEP while on NPPV were predictive of failure [24].

It appears that NPPV does have a role in the treatment of hypoxemic respiratory failure not due to COPD or cardiogenic pulmonary edema and is especially effective for patients with pneumonia. Those with more severe disease such as ARDS or presenting in shock are still better served by invasive mechanical ventilation. The data seems to show that NPPV can be an effective strategy for hypoxemic respiratory failure, but selecting the appropriate patient will be a large determinant of its success.

Trauma

Respiratory failure in trauma patients is frequently multifactorial. Patients may have injuries to the chest wall such as rib fractures or sternal fractures that make breathing painful and alter respiratory mechanics, pulmonary contusions that cause impairment in gas exchange at the alveolar level, pneumothoraces, and other injuries that cause overall deconditioning of the patient. Because of this, trauma patients are a heterogeneous population by definition, and the use of NPPV is difficult to apply broadly. In 2002 the British Thoracic Society Standards of Care Committee gave a grade C (low) recommendation on the use of NPPV for patients with chest wall trauma who remain hypoxic despite the use of oxygen therapy and adequate analgesia, citing a lack of evidence [14]. Since this guideline was published, several studies and meta-analyses have been performed which suggest that in patients who have suffered chest trauma, NPPV can reduce rates of intubation, ICU length of stay, mortality, and overall complications when compared with high-flow oxygen therapy and invasive ventilation. It should be noted however, that many of these studies contain small sample sizes, the number of studies themselves is small, and the quality of the evidence is of low to moderate quality (few randomized controlled trials). A more recent clinical practice guideline published in 2011 by the Canadian Critical Care Society gave no recommendations on the use of NPPV in patients with chest trauma, citing a lack of strong evidence [15].

Given the lack of quality evidence to support the application of NPPV in trauma patients with hypoxemic respiratory failure, it is difficult to give a broad recommendation on its use in this population. NPPV should be used on a case-by-case basis for in appropriately selected trauma patients. Further studies on the use of NPPV in the trauma population are needed to better delineate the subset of patients that would benefit most from this modality.

Application of Noninvasive Ventilation

Once a patient has been identified that is a suitable candidate for NPPV, the next step is to initiate treatment as soon as possible. Early application of NPPV is one of the keys to its success.

NPPV is administered by face mask, and the two most common types are nasal masks and full face masks. Nasal masks are triangular-shaped devices that fit over the nose and form a seal over the face with an inflated cuff. The nasal mask is better tolerated over long periods of time due to a decreased sensation of claustrophobia and the ability to eat and converse normally. Nasal masks are more suited for chronic conditions. Full face masks are the preferred interface for delivering NIV in the acute setting [15]. They consist of a mask that covers both the nose and mouth, which leads to less air leakage through the mouth. A good mask fit is very important to the successful implementation of NPPV. Excessive air leak, especially when using ventilators that cannot compensate for it, will lead to suboptimal ventilatory support. If a mask is uncomfortable or a poor fit, patients will be less likely to tolerate noninvasive therapy and may require invasive mechanical ventilation.

There are many types of ventilators from different manufacturers that use proprietary nomenclature, but for all intents and purposes, BPAP is our preferred modality of NPPV for use in the critical care setting. Once the appropriate patient has been selected and a good mask fit established, initial ventilator settings are then selected. Selecting ventilator settings for NPPV is similar to doing so for invasive ventilation. An initial inspiratory positive airway pressure (IPAP) of 10 cm H_2O and an expiratory positive airway pressure (EPAP or PEEP) of 5 cm H_2O are a good starting point for most patients. FiO_2 is set at 100% and titrated down to the lowest number that provides the desired oxygen saturation on pulse oximetry. After a period of observation, adjustments can be made to achieve appropriate clinical endpoints. In general a tidal volume of 6–8 ml/kg should be targeted while watching the patient's respiratory rate. If desired, a backup respiratory rate can be dialed in for patients who have difficulty initiating spontaneous breaths. A summary of adjustments to the initial ventilator settings based on clinical picture can be found in Table 16.3.

Table 16.3 NIV adjustments

Hypercapnia	Increase IPAP in increments of 1–2 (max 25 cm H_2O)
Dyspnea	Increase IPAP in increments of 1–2 (max 25 cm H_2O)
Hypoxia	Increase EPAP in increments of 1–2 (max of 10–15 cm H_2O)

Once NPPV has been started, patients should be continuously monitored for clinical improvement and tolerance of the treatment. Blood gasses can be drawn as needed to track changes in gas exchange. Signs of recovery in respiratory status within 1–2 h after initiation of treatment tend to be predictive of success. If the patient does not appear to be improving and the clinician is confident that the interface is working appropriately and ventilator settings have been optimized, converting to traditional invasive ventilation should be strongly considered. Failure to do so can lead to unnecessary complications and even death.

Summary

Noninvasive ventilation provides many of the same benefits as traditional invasive ventilation while potentially mitigating the negatives that come with having an intubated patient. Thus it is understandable why there is so much interest in applying NIV to a broader spectrum of respiratory disorders. NIV has been proven in the literature to be extremely effective for the treatment of COPD exacerbation and respiratory failure attributed to cardiogenic pulmonary edema and should be considered a first-line strategy for these specific respiratory disorders.

What is less clear is the role of NIV in treating or preventing other causes of respiratory failure encountered in the critical care setting. The available data is promising and should encourage clinicians to incorporate it into their armamentarium for treatment of respiratory conditions they might encounter. The challenge at this moment appears to be identifying the patients will benefit the most from NIV and applying it early to get maximum benefit from its use. More high-quality studies will need to be done to help clarify this picture going forward.

References

1. Hill NS. Clinical applications of body ventilators. Chest. 1986;90(6):897–905.
2. McNeill GBS, Glossop AJ. Clinical applications of non-invasive ventilation in critical care. Contin Educ Anaesth Crit Care Pain. 2011;12(12):33–7.
3. Bott J, Carroll MP, Conway JH, et al. Randomised controlled trial of nasal ventilation in acute ventilatory failure due to chronic obstructive pulmonary disease. Lancet. 1993;341:1555–7.
4. Brochard L, Mancebo J, Wysocki M, et al. Noninvasive ventilation for acute exacerbations of chronic obstructive pulmonary disease. N Engl J Med. 1995;333:817–22.
5. Collaborative Research Group of Noninvasive Mechanical Ventilation for Chronic Obstructive Pulmonary Disease. Early use of non-invasive positive pressure ventilation for acute exacerbations of chronic obstructive pulmonary disease: a multicenter randomized controlled trial. *Chin Med J*. 2005;118:2034–40.
6. Ram FSF, Picot J, Lightowler J, et al. Non-invasive positive pressure ventilation for treatment of respiratory failure due to exacerbations of chronic obstructive pulmonary disease. *Cochrane Database Syst Rev*. 2004;3:CD004104.
7. Quon BS, Gan WQ, Sin DD. Contemporary management of acute exacerbations of COPD: a systematic review and metaanalysis. Chest. 2008;133:756–66.
8. Cabrini L, Landoni G, Oriani A, et al. Noninvasive ventilation and survival in acute care settings: a comprehensive systematic review and Metaanalysis of randomized controlled trials. Crit Care Med. 2015;43(4):880–8.
9. Masip J, Betbese AJ, Paez J, et al. Non-invasive pressure support ventilation versus conventional oxygen therapy in acute cardiogenic pulmonary oedema: a randomized trial. Lancet. 2000;356:2126–32.
10. Levitt MA. A prospective, randomized trial of BiPAP in severe acute congestive heart failure. J Emerg Med. 2001;21:363–9.
11. Kelly CA, Newby DE, McDonagh TA, et al. Randomised controlled trial of continuous positive airway pressure and standard oxygen therapy in acute pulmonary oedema. Eur Heart J. 2002;23:1379–86.
12. Nava S, Carbone G, DiBattista N, et al. Noninvasive ventilation in cardiogenic pulmonary edema: a multicenter, randomized trial. *Am J Resipr*. Crit Care Med. 2003;168:1432–7.
13. Park M, Sangean MC, Volpe M, et al. Randomized, prospective trial of oxygen, continuous positive airway pressure, and bilevel positive airway pressure by face mask in acute cardiogenic pulmonary edema. Crit Care Med. 2004;32:2407–15.
14. British Thoracic Society Standards of Care Committee. Non-invasive ventilation in acute respiratory failure. Thorax. 2002;57:192–211.
15. Keenan SP, Sinuff T, Burns KE, et al. Clinical practice guidelines for the use of noninvasive positive-pressure ventilation and noninvasive continuous positive airway pressure in the acute care setting. CMAJ. 2011;183:E195–214.
16. Mehta S, Jay GD, Woolard RH, et al. Randomized, prospective trial of bilevel versus continuous positive airway pressure in acute pulmonary edema. Crit Care Med. 1997;25:620–8.
17. Burns KEA, Meade MO, Premji A, et al. Noninvasive positive-pressure ventilation as a weaning strategy for intubated adults with respiratory failure. Cochrane Database Syst Rev. 2013;12:CD004127.
18. Lin C, Yu H, Fan H, et al. The efficacy of noninvasive ventilation in managing postextubation respiratory failure: a meta-analysis. Heart Lung. 2014;43(2):99–104.
19. Arozullah AM, Daley J, Henderson WG, et al. Multifactorial risk index for predicting postoperative respiratory failure in men after major noncardiac surgery. The National Veterans Administration Surgical Quality Improvement Program. Ann Surg. 2000;232:242–53.
20. Jaber S, Lescot T, Futier E. Effect of noninvasive ventilation on tracheal reintubation among patients with hypoxemic respiratory failure following abdominal surgery. JAMA. 2016;315(13):1345–53.
21. Chiumello D, Chevallard G, Gregoretti C. Non-invasive ventilation in postoperative patients: a systematic review. Intensive Care Med. 2011;37:918–29.
22. Antonelli M, Conti G, Rocco M, et al. A comparison of noninvasive positive-pressure ventilation and conventional mechanical ventilation in patients with acute respiratory failure. N Engl J Med. 1998;339:429–35.
23. Ferrer M, Esquinas A, Leon M, et al. Noninvasive ventilation in severe hypoxemic respiratory failure: a randomized clinical trial. Am J Respir Crit Care Med. 2003;168(12):1438–44.
24. Thille A, Contou D, Fragnoli C, et al. Non-invasive ventilation for acute hypoxemic respiratory failure: intubation rate and risk factors. Crit Care. 2013;17:R269.

Conventional Mechanical Ventilation

17

Elizabeth Warnack and Marko Bukur

Introduction

In 1670, John Mayow, an English scientist, developed the concept of external negative pressure ventilation that became widespread during the polio epidemic in the mid-twentieth century [20]. Negative pressure ventilation, or the "iron lung," developed by Drinker and Shaw in 1929, required the patient's body be enclosed within a tight box, with the head on the outside [11]. A pump evacuated gas creating negative pressure mimicking normal physiologic breaths. However, due to the cumbersome size of the containers and extensive maintenance requirements, this fell out of favor. The concept of positive pressure ventilation developed during the 1950's became the prevailing mode of ventilation that is currently used today. Supplemental pressure is given externally to the patient's airway, through an endotracheal or tracheostomy tube, and is greater than the pressure surrounding the rest of the patient's body; therefore air is forced into the lungs, expanding alveoli and improving oxygenation [15].

Mechanical ventilation is indicated when patients' spontaneous ventilation is inadequate to maintain aerobic cellular metabolism. Many different disease processes, including injury and major surgery, may lead to the need for mechanical ventilation. While the ventilator provides breathing assistance, it will not cure the underlying disease process. Therefore, the goal of mechanical ventilation is to support the majority of patients while treating the inciting condition.

E. Warnack · M. Bukur (✉)
Department of Surgery, Bellevue Hospital Center, New York, NY, USA

Division of Trauma and Surgical Critical Care, New York University School of Medicine, New York, NY, USA
e-mail: marko.bukur@nyumc.org

There are several different modes of mechanical ventilation. As every patient is different, there is not one perfect ventilation strategy that will fit every patient. Thus, physicians in the critical care setting should be familiar with all modes of conventional ventilation and know their limitations and drawbacks. This chapter focuses on ventilator strategies for acute respiratory failure using conventional techniques and is not meant to be an exhaustive review of the latest techniques. Rather, we hope to provide an evidence-based pragmatic approach to mechanical ventilation, based on our experience.

Physiology of Mechanical Ventilation and Acute Respiratory Failure

Normal Lung Physiology

In its most simplistic form, the function of the lungs is to absorb the cardiac output like a sponge and perform gas exchange between oxygen and carbon dioxide. Understanding a few key physiologic concepts will allow the reader to appreciate the rationale behind their manipulation through mechanical ventilation.

Gas exchange in the alveoli is defined by the alveolar gas equation:

$$PAO_2 = \left(FiO_2 \times \left[Patmos - PH_2O\right]\right) - \left(PaCO_2 / RQ\right)$$

where PAO_2 is alveolar O_2, Patmos is atmospheric pressure (760 mm Hg at sea level), PH_2O is water vapor pressure at 37 degrees (47 mm Hg), and RQ is the respiratory quotient, or the ratio of CO_2 eliminated divided by O_2 consumed. FiO_2, or fraction of inspired oxygen, is generally set at 21%, or 0.21. In a healthy patient at sea level, where FiO_2 is 0.21, Patmos is 760 mm Hg, PH_2O is 47 mm Hg, and RQ is 0.8, the normal PAO_2 is approximately 100 mm Hg. The A-a gradient is the difference between the alveolar and the arterial oxygen tension, or PAO_2-PaO_2. In a normal healthy patient, this ranges from 5 to 10. The A-a gradient increases with age and can

A. Salim et al. (eds.), *Surgical Critical Care Therapy*, https://doi.org/10.1007/978-3-319-71712-8_17

also be increased in *V*/*Q* (ventilation/perfusion) mismatch, or pulmonary shunting.

Normal systemic oxygen delivery depends on a variety of factors. The equation for oxygen delivery, or DO_2, delineates these factors:

$$DO_2 = CO \times CaO_2 \times 10\,\text{ml}/\text{min},$$

where CO is cardiac output and CaO_2 is the oxygen content in arterial blood. Arterial oxygen content largely depends on hemoglobin (Hgb) and oxygen saturation (SaO_2), as shown below:

$$CaO_2 = 1.34 \times \text{Hgb} \times SaO_2.$$

Therefore, the equation for oxygen delivery can be rewritten to substitute these values for CaO_2:

$$DO_2 = CO \times (1.34 \times \text{Hgb} \times SaO_2) \times 10.$$

Normal oxygen delivery ranges from 900 to 1100 ml/min. It follows that disease processes which cause anemia, a decrease in O_2 saturation or cardiac output, will decrease oxygen delivery to the rest of the body.

The minute ventilation is another important concept in lung physiology. Minute ventilation is defined as the volume of gas entering or leaving the lungs in a given amount of time. It is defined as the tidal volume (in liters) multiplied by the respiratory rate. For example, a tidal volume of 0.5 L and a respiratory rate of 12 breaths per minute, the minute ventilation would be 6 L/min, a value that is normally 80% of the cardiac output (i.e., *V*/*Q* of 0.8).

There are four zones of the lung, defined by West et al. in 1964 [23], that describe the anatomical relationship between ventilation and perfusion. These zones are defined by the relationships between alveolar pressure (PA), pulmonary artery pressure (Pa), pulmonary interstitial pressure (Pi), and pulmonary vein pressure (Pv). In zone I, the alveolar pressure is greater than the pulmonary artery pressure, which is greater than the venous pressure (PA > Pa > Pv). Zone I does not occur in the healthy human lung, as the arterial pressure is always greater than the alveolar pressure. This physiology is most commonly seen during positive pressure ventilation and results in ventilation exceeding perfusion which increases physiologic dead space (more on this topic later). In zone II, pulmonary artery pressure is greater than alveolar pressure, which is greater than venous pressure (Pa > PA > Pv). Zone III represents the area of highest blood flow in the lung. In this zone, arterial pressure is greater than venous pressure, which exceeds alveolar pressure (Pa > Pv > PA). The gradient between the arterial and venous flow therefore determines flow. Of note, Swan-Ganz catheters are placed in this region of the lung. Zone IV, the last zone, occurs when arterial pressure is greater than pulmonary interstitial pressure, which exceeds venous pressure, which exceeds alveolar pressure. In this zone, reduced blood flow occurs when pulmonary vascular resistance increases, which can be caused by disease processes such as pulmonary edema.

Understanding lung volumes is another important key to understanding mechanical ventilation (see Fig. 17.1).There are two essential volumes that must be understood to master mechanical ventilation. The first is the tidal volume, or the volume of air entering and exiting the lungs during a single inspiratory cycle. This is one of the key parameters set when initiating conventional mechanical ventilation. Inspiratory reserve volume is the amount of air that can be inhaled with maximal effort, in excess of the tidal volume. Expiratory reserve volume is the amount of air in excess of tidal expiration that can be exhaled with maximum effort. After a maximal expiration, the amount of air that remains in the lungs is termed residual volume. The functional residual capacity (FRC) is the other key summation of two volumes that can be manipulated through mechanical ventilation. FRC is the amount of air remaining in the lungs after normal tidal expansion. This therefore represents the residual volume plus the expiratory reserve volume. The FRC can be increased through the use of positive end-expiratory pressure (PEEP) or other increases in mean airway pressure which lead to improved oxygenation. The vital capacity is the amount of air that can be exchanged after maximal inspiration and expiration, a parameter that may be checked during the weaning process [24].

The compliance of the lung is another important topic in lung physiology as it is applied to ventilator settings. Compliance is defined as the change in lung volume over the change in transpulmonary lung pressure. A lower lung compliance means that greater pressure must be developed to produce the same level of lung expansion. Acute respiratory distress syndrome (ARDS) (see Fig. 17.2) is a classic example of a disease process that causes decreased compliance through lung inflammation. In patients ventilated using volume control, compliance can be quantified by taking the tidal volume and dividing this value over the change in plateau pressure and PEEP:

$$\text{Compliance} = \frac{\text{tidal volume}(\text{ml}/\text{cc})}{(\text{plateau pressure}(\text{cm}\,H_2O) - \text{PEEP}(\text{cm}\,H_2O))}.$$

The plateau pressure can be measured using an inspiratory pause at the end of inspiration on most modern ventilators. This formula represents the compliance of the lung when there is no air flow (i.e., at the end of inspiration), so it is termed "static compliance." Similarly, when the patient is being ventilated through a pressure-controlled cycle, the compliance can be determined by dividing the exhaled tidal volume by the airway pressure gradient:

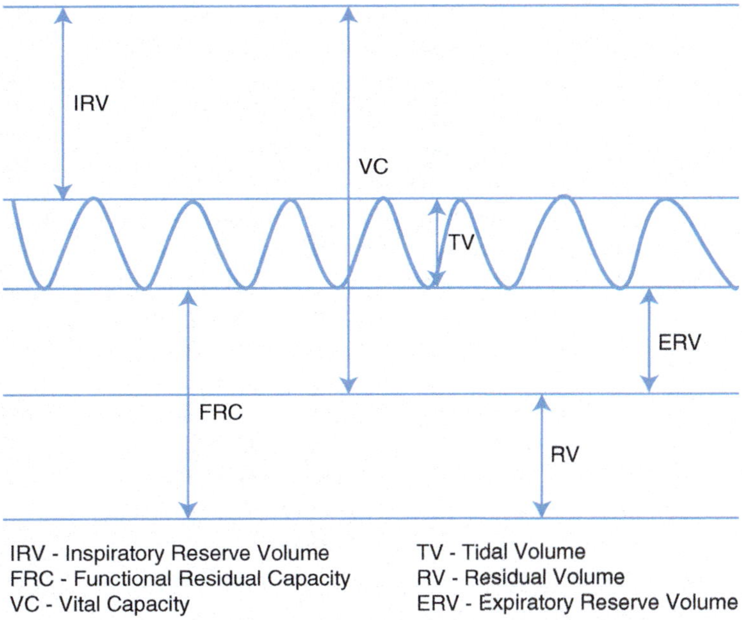

Fig. 17.1 Schematic of lung volumes. IRV inspiratory reserve volume, FRC functional residual capacity, VC vital capacity, TV tidal volume, RV residual volume, ERV expiratory reserve volume

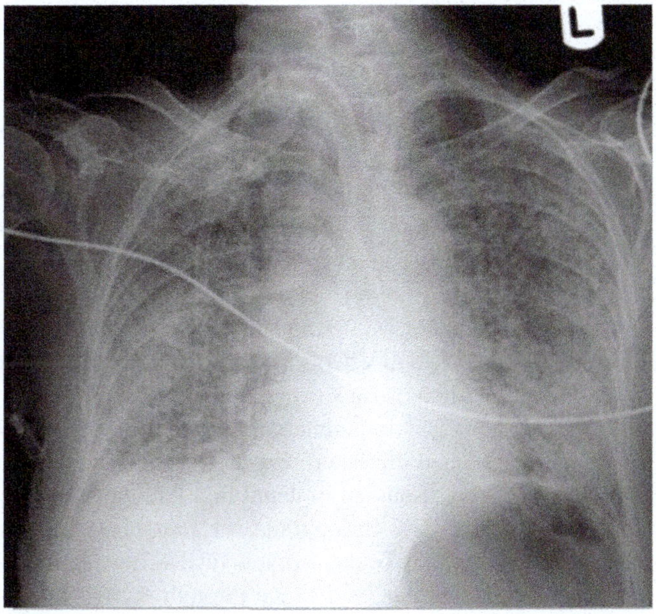

Fig. 17.2 Radiograph of acute respiratory distress syndrome

$$\text{Compliance} = \frac{\text{exhaled tidal volume}(\text{ml}/\text{cc})}{(\text{end inspiratory pressure}(\text{cm H}_2\text{O}) - \text{PEEP}(\text{cmH}_2\text{O}))}.$$

Normal values are 50–80 cc/cm H_2O, given a typical tidal volume of 500 cc over a change in pressure of 10 cm H_2O. Stiff, less compliant lungs are typically within the range of 10–20 cc/cm H_2O. Compliance should be checked daily in mechanically ventilated patients, as decreasing values can foreshadow worsening cardiopulmonary function, while improvements indicate better pulmonary mechanics.

One limitation to static compliance is that it can only be measured at just one lung volume. ARDS and other pathological states may affect some areas of the lung more severely than others, causing this compliance value to vary significantly within a range of lung volumes during each respiratory cycle.

Abnormal Lung Physiology

Acute respiratory failure can be caused by a variety of factors, such as hypoxia, hypercarbia, upper airway, and metabolic disease. All of these abnormalities can be supported by mechanical ventilation while the underlying cause is treated. Hypoxia can be caused by *V*/*Q* mismatch secondary to shunting and increased dead space. *V*/*Q* mismatch refers to the ratio of ventilation (*V*) compared to blood flow (*Q*) in the lungs. When the *V*/*Q* ratio is less than one, blood flow is excessive relative to ventilation. This is referred to as intrapulmonary shunting. This is most commonly secondary to inhaled gas that does not reach the alveoli in disease states such as pneumonia, pulmonary contusion, or ARDS. Shunts have a poor response to supplemental oxygen, particularly when the percentage of shunt is high. Actual calculation of shunt percentage requires a pulmonary artery catheter and is not frequently done. The *P*/*F* (PaO_2/FiO_2) ratio may be used as a simple surrogate. The normal *P*/*F* ratio is PaO_2 = 100 mmHg/21% O_2 (0.2) ~ 500 and when this value falls below 200 correlates with a shunt of >20% [5].

The inverse situation occurs when the *V*/*Q* ratio is greater than one, i.e., the ventilation is greater than blood flow. This leads to alveolar gas that does not participate in ventilatory exchange and is also referred to as dead space ventilation. It is important to remember that dead space also occurs physiologically in the large airways (trachea and bronchi) and can be estimated as 1 ml per centimeter of height. Dead space ventilation can also occur when the alveolar capillary interface is destroyed, such as in COPD or when alveoli are overdistended with excessive positive pressure ventilation or with large pulmonary emboli.

When there is *V/Q* mismatch, the A-a gradient is often elevated, and hypoxia occurs. Interestingly, the physiologic response to hypoxia in the lungs diverts blood away from alveoli with lower oxygen content. This phenomenon is called hypoxic pulmonary vasoconstriction. The pulmonary arteries constrict in the presence of hypoxia and redirect blood flow to alveoli that are better oxygenated. This is a compensatory measure to improve the *V/Q* ratio and increase the total area involved in oxygen exchange.

Other causes of acute respiratory failure include hypercarbia and upper airway disease processes. Hypercarbia can be caused by either increased CO_2 production or hypoventilation. Increased CO_2 production can be seen in carbohydrate overfeeding or in patients with severe lung disease that are ventilator dependent. Hypoventilation is seen most classically in patients with intoxication (i.e., narcotics or ethanol) but can also be seen in a variety of neuromuscular diseases, when respiratory muscles are too weak to appropriately ventilate CO_2. Upper airway causes such as neck trauma or inflammation and foreign body obstruction can also contribute to acute respiratory failure. Lastly, metabolic causes, such as sepsis, acidosis, or extensive burns, can lead increased physiological demands that need supportive mechanical ventilation.

Physiologic Changes that Occur with Positive Pressure Ventilation

Positive pressure ventilation alters the normal negative pressure environment that occurs physiologically in the pleural space. Preload volume tends to be reduced through two mechanisms. First, the pressure differential between the abdomen and thorax is decreased, leading to decreased venous return. Transmural pressure across the ventricular wall can also be affected, leading to decreased compliance and decreased filling. Additionally, medications frequently used for induction prior to intubation often lead to decreased vascular tone, leading to a drop in blood pressure in patients that have marginal volume status. Changes in afterload also occur with the addition of positive pressure. Though the added intrathoracic pressure impedes ventricular filling during diastole, it facilitates emptying during systole. As long as hypovolemia is avoided during positive pressure ventilation and excessive intrathoracic pressures are avoided, cardiac output will not change excessively.

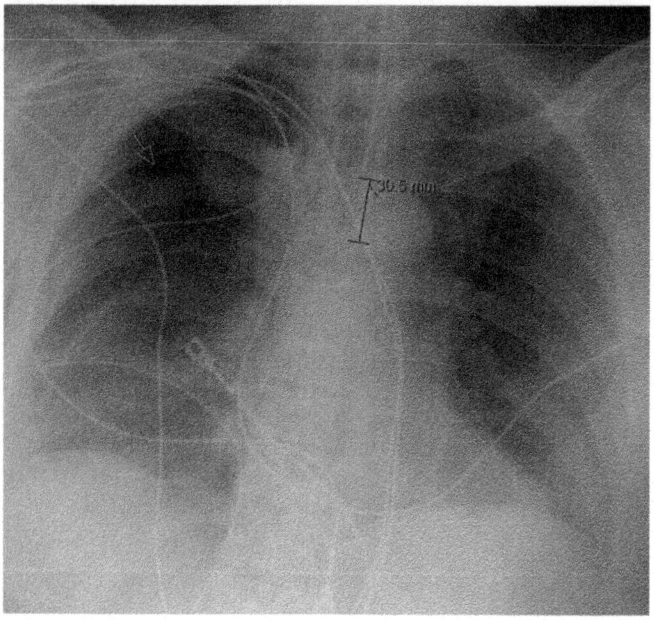

Fig. 17.3 Iatrogenic pneumothorax during mechanical ventilation. Arrow denotes the collapsed lung

Mechanical ventilation can cause pathologic changes in the lung itself. These changes are typically lumped together into a catchall category known as ventilator-induced lung injury or (VILI). There are several mechanisms by which VILI occurs, and they are most likely to manifest in patients with primary lung pathology but may occur in any mechanically ventilated patient. Volutrauma represents the most classic mechanism by which VILI is mediated and is due to high inflation volumes that cause alveolar overdistention with disruption and secondary inflammation. New ventilator protocols have heightened clinician awareness to this iatrogenic injury and will be discussed in detail in a later section (see Volume Control A/C). Barotrauma, or pressure-mediated damage to alveoli, may occur with low tidal volumes in noncompliant lungs and can be avoided through vigilant monitoring of inflation pressures. Barotrauma may also cause pneumothorax or pneumomediastinum (see Fig. 17.3). Overdistension and rupture of alveoli occur in as many as 5–25% of ventilator-dependent patients [22]. Underinflating alveoli can also be harmful secondary to atelectrauma. Through repeated opening and closing of lung units, this causes a mechanical shear type of injury. Application of PEEP is helpful in preventing this type of injury. Lastly, biotrauma is the process of cytokine release and neutrophil activation that occurs in the alveolar space secondary to VILI and can produce systemic manifestations that are similar to the systemic inflammatory response syndrome (SIRS).

Modes of Conventional Ventilation

The various types of conventional mechanical ventilation will be discussed below. Most variations share the same general principles. In controlled ventilation, either the pressure or the volume can be set by the physician, and the other ventilator parameters depend on these settings. For example, if volume is set, the other variable, pressure, cannot be controlled and is therefore a function of the compliance and resistance of the lungs themselves. This relationship between volume and pressure can be explained by the equation of motion:

$$\text{Muscle pressure} + \text{ventilator pressure} = (\text{volume} / \text{compliance}) + (\text{resistance} / \text{flow})$$

where, in mechanical ventilation, muscle pressure = 0, ventilator pressure = PEEP, volume = end-expiratory volume, and flow = 0. Compliance and resistance are constants, inherent properties of the lungs [3].

The relationship between pressure, volume, and flow is displayed graphically on the ventilator. Volume, pressure, and flow are tracked against time on the x axis (see Figs. 17.4 and 17.5). Positive flow values, above the x axis, correspond to inspiration, and negative flow values correspond to expiration. Units are liters (L) or milliliters (mL) for volume, cm H_2O for pressure, and L/s for flow. Time, on the x axis, is in seconds. In volume control, volume is a set, with the maximum volume representing tidal volume. Pressure is an upward linear line during inspiration as volume increases and drops to zero during expiration. The flow rate is a constant value in the volume control setting. The effects of decreased lung compliance are also depicted graphically and results in a higher airway pressure for a set tidal volume.

In pressure control, the pressure graph is a straight horizontal line as it is set at a constant value by the operator. The volume curve increases with inspiration and decreases with expiration, and flow is a function of this volume over time. Here decreased compliance is depicted by a lower tidal volume for a given set pressure.

Assist Control

Assist control (A/C), as suggested by its name, implies that breaths given by the ventilator can either be assisted (i.e., the ventilator assists a breath generated by the patient) or controlled (i.e., the ventilator gives a controlled breath independent of patient effort). This is a variant of controlled mechanical ventilation (CMV) in which all breaths are given by the ventilator. There are no unsupported breaths in A/C, either pressure or volume can be set by the physician, and the same volume or pressure will be given with each breath regardless of whether it is initiated by the patient or by the ventilator. The patient is allowed to initiate a mechanical breath by generating a trigger which is set by the physician. Overall, A/C is advantageous when patients cannot meet their own metabolic needs.

Triggers

A trigger may be set by either flow or pressure. Flow triggering allows the ventilator to sense changes in inspiratory flow to initiate delivered breaths. Flow triggering is generally the default method chosen for most mechanically ventilated patients. Typical flow sensitivity settings are between 1 and 10 L/min and are ventilator specific. If the flow setting is too low, auto-triggering may occur without a patient-initiated breath (i.e., movement of the patient or ventilator tubing), and this can lead to multiple breaths being delivered together. This can be corrected by increasing the flow trigger or switching to a pressure trigger.

When a pressure trigger is set, a decrease in airway pressure starts a mechanically generated breath. The sensitivity of the ventilator is the threshold that has to be met for the trigger variable to initiate inspiration and generally is 2–3 cm H_2O below the PEEP set on the ventilator. For example, with the conventional PEEP setting of 5 cm H_2O, the patient would need to reduce the airway pressure to 2 cm H_2O (assuming a pressure trigger setting of 3 cm H_2O). Using the pressure trigger becomes problematic in patients with disease states that impair the exhalation of gases from the lower airways (i.e., obstructive lung diseases or ARDS) which can lead to a phenomenon known as occult PEEP/auto-PEEP (see section on PEEP). When occult PEEP is present, this causes the patient to generate a greater negative inspiratory force for any set pressure trigger and leads to dyssynchrony between the patients initiating and receiving a breath. This can be detected by observing a delay between a patient's spontaneous respiratory effort and the breath delivered by the ventilator. In these cases, switching to a flow trigger may be more appropriate.

Respiratory Cycle and Inspiratory/Expiratory (*I*/*E*) Ratio

In addition to selecting a trigger in controlled mechanical ventilation, the respiratory cycle can also be adjusted through manipulation of the inspiratory/expiratory (*I*/*E*) ratio. Physiologically this ratio is normally 1:2–3, as inspiration is an active process and expiration a passive one. In obstructive airway pathology (i.e., COPD, acute asthma exacerbation), this may become even more prolonged and is an important consideration to remember when ventilating these patients to prevent the development of auto-PEEP. The *I*/*E* ratio can be made longer by increasing inspiratory flow or by decreasing either the respiratory rate or tidal volume. Inverting the normal 1:2 ratio to 2:1 (twice as much time spent in inspiration

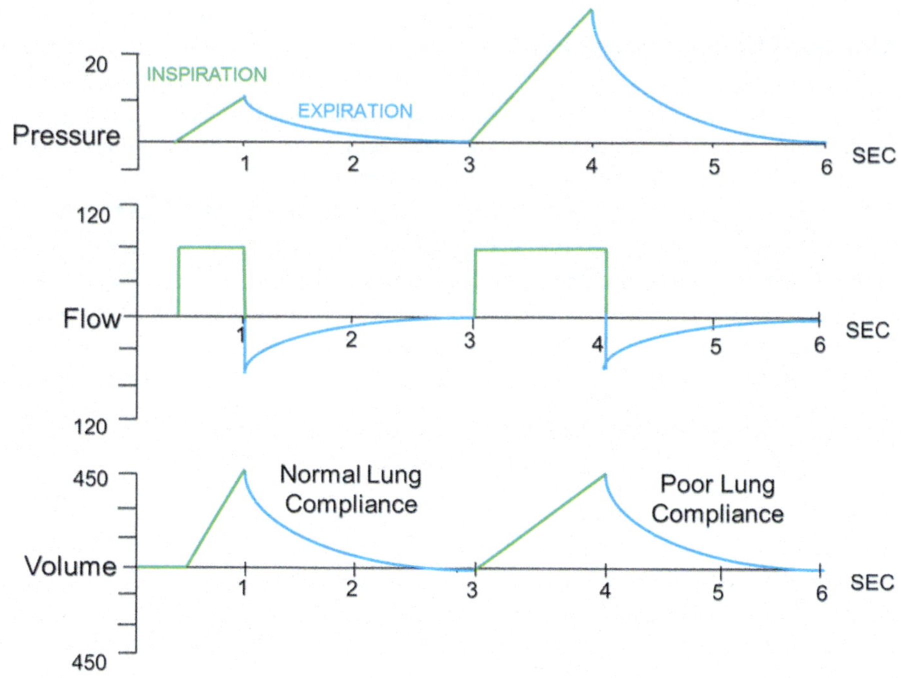

Fig. 17.4 Pressure, flow, and volume curves for volume control ventilation (Note the increased pressure for a given tidal volume when compliance is poor)

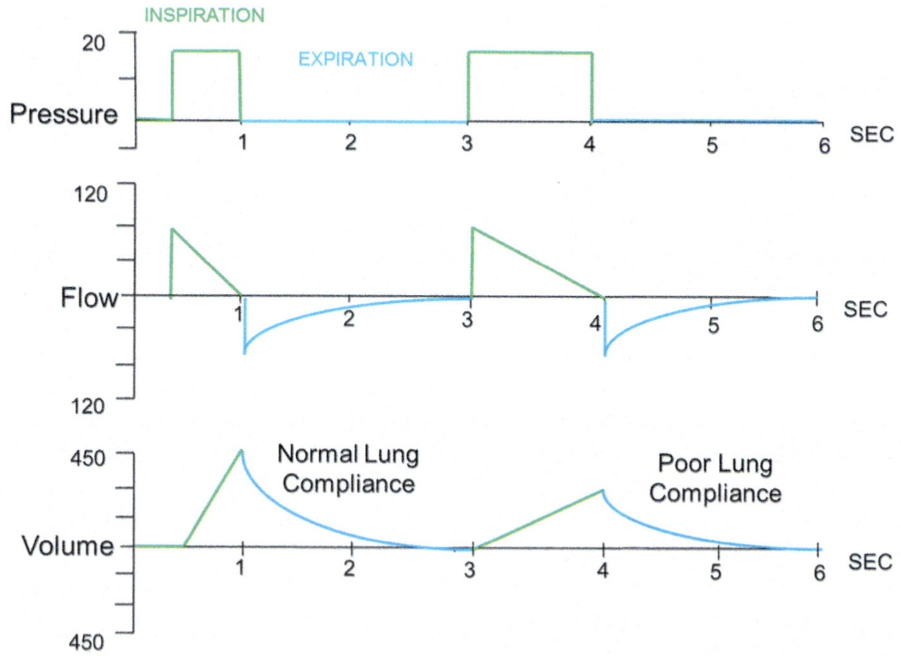

Fig. 17.5 Pressure, flow, and volume curves for pressure control ventilation (Note the decreased tidal volume for a given pressure when compliance is poor)

compared to expiration) is called inverse ratio ventilation (IRV). Prolonged inflation time prevents alveolar collapse and improves gas exchange. While this method increases PO_2, it may lead to increases in PCO_2 as well, due to decreased time for ventilation. This phenomenon, named permissive hypercapnia, is acceptable in some patients but should be avoided in patients with obstructive lung pathology and traumatic brain injury, where elevations in CO_2 can be detrimental to the patient. Generally, IRV requires sedation and paralysis, as alert patients will not tolerate this well.

Flow Rates and Patterns

The inspiratory flow rates and patterns that deliver the mechanically ventilated breaths are also ventilator parameters that physicians should be aware of. In most patients a flow rate of 60 L/min provides adequate gas exchange. However, in those that have "air hunger," or a minute ventilation ≥10 L/min, flow rates up to 100 L/min are not uncommon. Flow patterns are dependent on the type of breath being delivered (i.e., volume or pressure controlled). Figure 17.6 depicts a flow time curve that demonstrates the constant

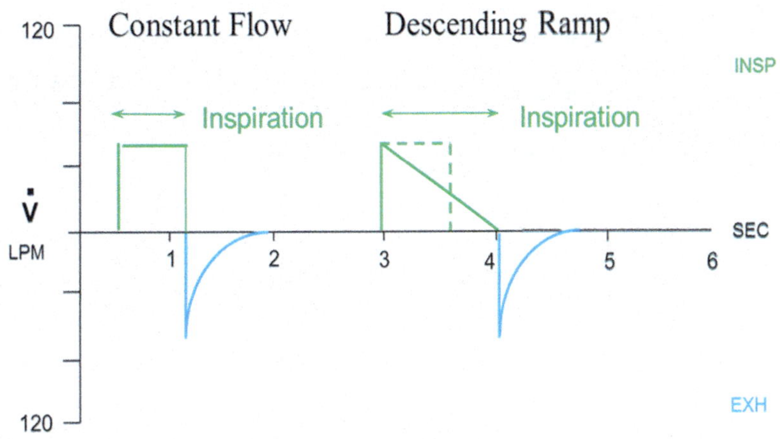

Fig. 17.6 Inspiratory flow patterns (Note longer inspiratory time with descending ramp pattern)

"square wave" shape in a volume-controlled breath, while a pressure-controlled breath follows a "descending ramp" shape. Note the effect that this change in flow rate has on inspiration. A descending ramp follow pattern increases inspiratory time. Most modern ventilators will allow selection of either flow pattern, even in the volume control setting. The relative benefit of the "descending ramp" pattern is that flow decreases throughout the breath and is therefore more comfortable, as opposed to the constant flow of the "square wave" pattern. Because the inspiratory time is longer in the "descending ramp" pattern, it must be used with caution in patients with obstructive lung pathology, as this can lead to auto-PEEP.

PEEP and Auto-PEEP

As previously mentioned, PEEP improves alveolar oxygenation by preventing alveolar collapse and increasing the FRC. However, PEEP can also reduce venous return and cardiac output when applied at high levels in those with impaired volume status or right ventricular function. Neurosurgeons are often concerned about the levels of PEEP applied in patients with respiratory failure due to potential increases in intracranial pressure. While this could occur in hypovolemic states, several clinical and animal studies have demonstrated that PEEP can be administered safely at levels exceeding 17 cm H_2O without compromising the cerebral perfusion pressure and jugular venous saturation or increasing the intracranial pressure [7, 10].

Pressure volume loops can help guide the operator to set the optimal PEEP for a given patient. A pressure volume curve sets pressure on the *x* axis and volume on the *y* axis (Fig. 17.7). Compliance is therefore represented by the slope of the line. To determine PEEP, examine the lower and upper inflection points of the pressure volume curve. The lower inflection point represents the point where the resistance of the patient's airways is overcome (with high resistance, this point shifts to the right). This is the critical opening pressure of the alveoli. At pressures below this level, there is a risk for atelectrauma, as previously described. Approaching the upper inflection point, alveoli continue to open and airway pressure rises, until alveoli reach their maximum volume. The upper inflection point represents the point at which the alveoli become maximally distended, and further pressure increases can lead to hyperinflation and predispose to volu−/barotrauma. The optimal PEEP setting is found between these two inflection points and can be calculated using the formulas described in the section on compliance. Further increases in PEEP are beneficial when both the compliance and *P*/*F* ratio improve. If these enhancements are not observed with additional PEEP, then ventilation is likely occurring at or beyond the upper inflection point. Additionally, the reader may find assistance in determining a starting level of PEEP for patients with hypoxemic respiratory failure (particularly ARDS) by consulting the ARDSNet and ALVEOLI PEEP tables published in the *New England Journal of Medicine* [17].

While PEEP is generally beneficial to patients, there are instances where it can be harmful. Exhalation is a passive process, and there is some collapse of the airways during this time. Airway collapse can become exaggerated in certain disease states (COPD and asthma being the most common), leading to complete closure of the airways. This leads to a state where the lungs are filled with air but are not allowed to evacuate, causing a buildup of pressure that can cause lung damage and have hemodynamic consequences. This condition has several synonymous names, i.e., *auto-PEEP*, *dynamic hyperinflation*, *occult PEEP*, and *intrinsic PEEP*. Patients that have this will often appear uncomfortable and will be unsynchronized with the ventilator, due to forceful exhalation in an attempt to empty inhaled gas. Wheezing will often be present.

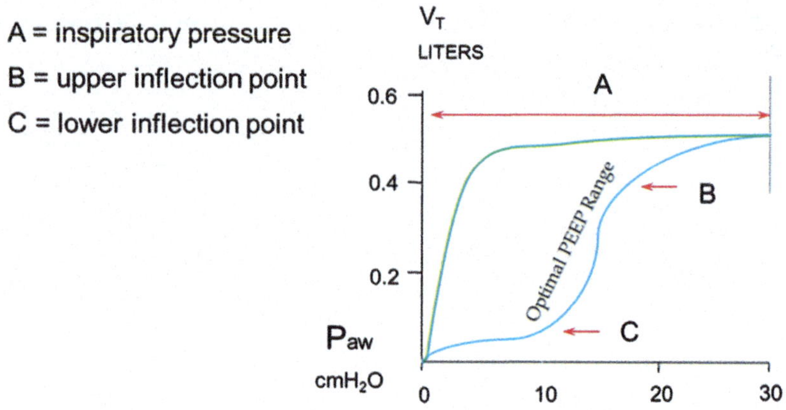

Fig. 17.7 Pressure volume loop. Point C represents the critical opening pressure, while point B represents the point of overdistention. A inspiratory pressure, B upper infection point, C lower infection point

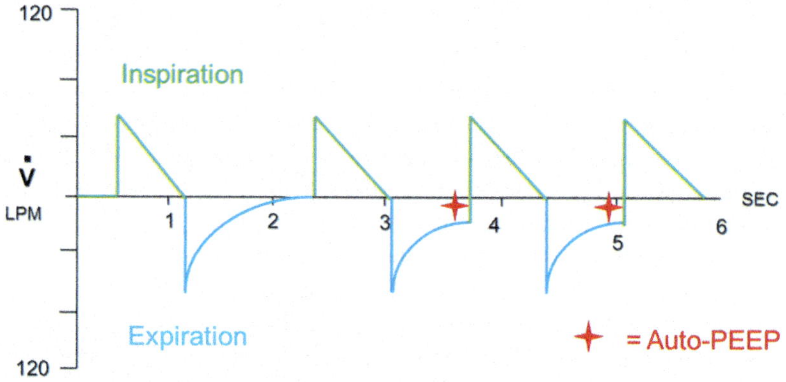

Fig. 17.8 Flow time waveforms for the detection of auto-PEEP (Note the failure of expiratory flow to return to zero when auto-PEEP is present)

The presence of auto-PEEP can also be detected by analyzing the flow/time waveforms on the ventilator as shown in Fig. 17.8. In patients with normal pulmonary physiology, expiratory flow will return to zero prior to the next inflation cycle. However, when auto-PEEP occurs, expiratory flow is still occurring when the ventilator is delivering its next breath. The amount of auto-PEEP present can be estimated by performing an expiratory pause at the end of expiration. An important caveat, auto-PEEP can only be quantified in this manner if the patient is not breathing spontaneously, due to the difficulty timing of the end of expiration. Note the difference between applied and auto-PEEP as shown in the pressure time diagram (Fig. 17.9). When auto-PEEP is present, the expiratory pressure does not return to zero or is greater than the PEEP level set on the ventilator.

Once the diagnosis of auto-PEEP is confirmed, adjustments in mechanical ventilator settings should be made. The goal should be to maximize the amount of time the patient has to expire in the respiratory cycle and can be accomplished by lowering tidal volumes, increasing inspiratory flow rates, and shortening inspiratory time. Reducing the patient's respiratory rate is also helpful and may require sedation and paralysis. Contrary to intuition, it is not helpful to remove all *applied* PEEP. If this is done, it would promote alveolar collapse in expiration and lead to further air trapping. Thus, the amount of applied PEEP should be set at a level that approximates the level of auto-PEEP measured. Since this is difficult to quantify in patients that are not paralyzed, the PEEP level can be set and titrated to a level that eliminates the end-expiratory flow observed on the flow time diagram in Fig. 17.8.

Modes of Assist Control (A/C) Ventilation

Volume Control A/C

If volume is chosen as the controlled variable, the tidal volume and inspiratory flow are set by the operator, and the airway pressure will be determined by the compliance and resistance of the lung. A compliant lung will therefore have low peak pressures. Respiratory rate (RR), PEEP, and FiO_2 are also chosen by the operator. RR is generally set at 10–12 breaths/minute and tidal volume at 6–8 ml/kg of predicted body weight. The equation for predicted body weight is based upon height and gender as shown below:

$$\text{PBW}(\text{females}): 45.5 + 2.3\left[\text{height}(\text{inches}) - 60\right]$$

$$\text{PBW}(\text{males}): 50 + 2.3\left[\text{height}(\text{inches}) - 60\right].$$

The patients' minute ventilation is based upon the product of RR and tidal volume and can be adjusted based upon the CO_2 noted on arterial blood gas. It is important to note again that the patient can breathe spontaneously in this setting, but once a breath is triggered, a fully supported breath will be given.

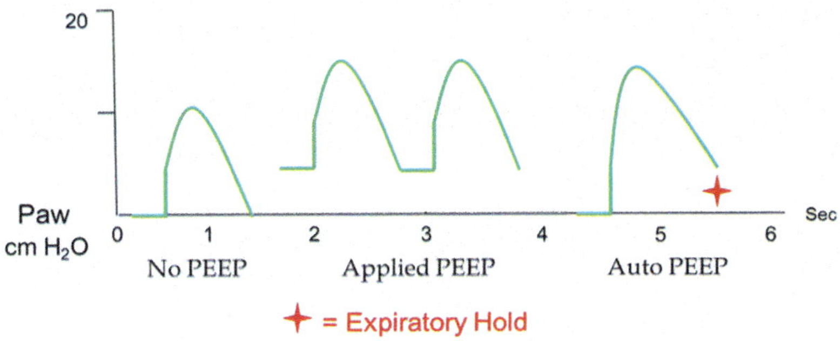

Fig. 17.9 Pressure time diagram illustrating differences in PEEP

Special considerations apply for ventilator settings in patients with ARDS. The ARDSNet trials set forth guidelines for lung protective strategies in patients with ARDS. The "ARDSNet paper" was published in *New England Journal of Medicine* in May 2000 and is the only trial to demonstrate a mortality benefit in ARDS [2]. This was a multicenter, randomized trial which took place at ten university center hospitals. Patients were randomized to be ventilated using two different tidal volume targets (12 ml/kg predicted body weight vs. 6 ml/kg). The primary outcome was death, and secondary outcome was number of days without ventilator use. The mortality was significantly lower in the group treated with lower volumes compared to the traditional volumes group (31% vs. 39.8%). In addition, the number of ventilator-free days was greater in the smaller tidal volume group.

To achieve optimal ventilator settings in patients with ARDS, the operator should set the tidal volume at 8 ml/kg of predicted body weight, and then adjust 1 ml/kg every 2 h until the goal tidal volume (6 ml/kg) is achieved. After setting tidal volume, the next step is to observe plateau pressure, which is determined by lung compliance. Plateau pressure is determined by pausing the ventilator at end inspiration and checking the pressure. The goal in ARDS is 35 cm H_2O or less, to avoid excessive barotrauma. If pressure is greater than 30 cm H_2O, the tidal volume is decreased 1 ml/kg until pressure is under 30 cm H_2O or the tidal volume reaches 4 ml/kg. Once plateau pressure is maximized and tidal volume is minimized, minute ventilation is generally adjusted through the respiratory rate. Arterial blood gases can be used to guide respiratory rate adjustments. In cases of severe ARDS, maintaining oxygenation (SpO_2 88–90%) and limiting tidal volumes/inflation pressures take precedence over normal ventilation (i.e., permissive hypercapnia). The FiO_2 should also be reduced to nontoxic levels (less than 60% if possible), to prevent free radical damage through application of PEEP to improve oxygenation. An excellent algorithm for this is provided on the ARDSNet website (www.ardsnet.org) which provides PEEP tables for given FiO_2 requirements. While the above strategy is useful, it should not be applied to certain subsets of patients. Traumatic brain injury is one subset in which the rise in PCO_2 can be detrimental, as this leads to cerebral vasodilation and elevation of intracranial pressure. Patients with obstructive airway disease may also tolerate permissive hypercapnia poorly, given that their baseline PCO_2 may be much greater, and these patients have reduced ability for renal compensation.

The main advantage of volume controlled A/C is the ability to control the tidal volume, independent of the mechanical properties of the lungs, which may vary greatly in critical illness. Disadvantages include the ability to generate high inspiratory pressures with changes in lung mechanics, as pressure cannot be controlled. Respiratory alkalosis is also common since all breaths are supported by the ventilator. This may cause patient-ventilator dyssynchrony and excessive work of breathing.

Pressure Control A/C

In this setting, the pressure is controlled instead of volume and is termed "pressure control." The operator sets the desired respiratory rate, inspiratory time, and target pressure. Dependent variables are therefore flow and volume. Some patients prefer this setting due to the higher initial flows delivered as compared with volume control. Pressure control settings also allow for the delivery of inverse ratio ventilation to improve oxygenation, but this often requires heavy sedation or paralysis. Advantages to this mode include the ability to control pressure settings and theoretically avoid barotrauma. Ideally the driving pressure should be set so peak pressure is 35 or less, and PEEP should be included in this calculation. In patients with ARDS or acute lung injury, the operator should also be mindful of the volumes the patient is receiving with the given driving pressure. These volumes should be in the 4–6 ml/kg range as per the ARDSNet guidelines. The major disadvantages of pressure control are the inability to control volume and minute ventilation, which can change insidiously depending on patients' disease state and lung compliance.

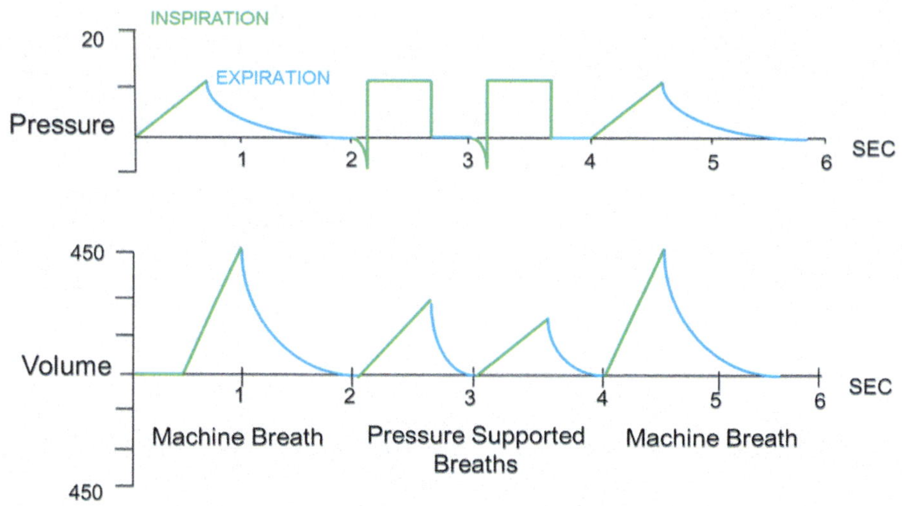

Fig. 17.10 Pressure and volume diagrams for a patient on SIMV (Note the variation in tidal volume for the pressure-supported breaths)

SIMV

Synchronized intermittent mandatory ventilation, or SIMV, is a common alternative to assist control. SIMV was initially introduced as a weaning tool and allows for independent patient breathing, or spontaneous breaths, which can be synchronized with mandatory breaths delivered by the ventilator. Like A/C, either pressure or volume can be controlled by the operator. Volume control IMV is often used for patients with relatively normal lung function recovering from critical illnesses, who are not ready for a spontaneous breathing trial.

In SIMV, the operator sets a mandatory breath rate, usually 10–12 breaths per minute. If the patient breathes more rapidly than the set rate, the patient is allowed to take "extra" spontaneous breaths that are only partially supported by the ventilator. A pressure support value can be set by the operator, usually at around 10 cm H_2O, to help overcome the resistance of the ventilator circuit. During these spontaneous breaths, the tidal volume generated depends upon the compliance of the patients' lungs and can vary breath to breath (see Fig. 17.10). The pressure support can be lowered as the patient's condition improves. On the other hand, if the patient does not initiate breaths, then all breaths are mechanically given, identical to controlled mechanical ventilation.

SIMV may be a more comfortable mode of ventilation for some patients who are able to generate spontaneous breaths, as opposed to getting fully supported breaths on assist control. This may be preferable for rapidly breathing patients with evidence of air trapping, as only a fraction of patient's inspiratory efforts will trigger a fully supported ventilator breath. The main disadvantage to this mode is that it is only useful when patients are pulling adequate tidal volumes on pressure-supported breaths; otherwise, there is a dramatic increase in the patient's work of breathing.

Pressure Support Ventilation

As mentioned above, pressure support can be used in conjunction with SIMV or can be used alone as the predominant mode of weaning from mechanical ventilation. In this mode, patients have complete control over their respiratory rate and inflation time. The pressure is set at a level high enough to overcome resistance to flow in the ventilator tubing, so that tidal volume is augmented during spontaneous breathing. The operator sets a starting inspiratory pressure and level of PEEP that is delivered in a decelerating flow pattern and controlled by patient effort. Unlike pressure control ventilation, where set pressure is continuous throughout the inspiratory cycle, this setting allows for a reduction in inspiratory flow (usually when inspiratory flow is <25% of the patient's peak effort) and switches the cycle to expiration. During inspiration, for example, the ventilator will deliver 12 cm H_2O of pressure, and during exhalation this pressure will drop to the set level of PEEP. The amount of tidal volume delivered will depend on the patient's lung compliance. If the compliance is 50 ml/cm H_2O, the delivered volume will be (12 × 50) 600 ml. The ability to overcome work of breathing is one of the advantages of pressure support. A disadvantage is the inability of a single pressure support value to meet the changing levels of patient demand. If the level is set too high, the patient may do very little work of breathing, and if set too low, the patient struggles and fatigues. Careful attention to this parameter is important when initiating weaning.

Daily Management of the Ventilated Patient

After determining initial ventilator settings, arterial blood gases are used to guide ventilator management. If the patient has low oxygen saturations or pO_2 on ABG, the FiO_2 may be increased as a temporizing measure, while the underlying cause is investigated. Increasing the functional residual capacity (FRC) through manipulation of the mean airway pressure should be the main strategy used to correct hypoxia. The mean airway pressure can be increased by increasing the PEEP or delta P on pressure-controlled modes or by adjusting the *I*/*E* ratio to lengthen the time spent in inspiration. Low CO_2 can be ameliorated by decreasing the respiratory rate or decreasing the set tidal volumes. For hypercapnia, increasing the respiratory rate may decrease CO_2 levels. However, if the patient is tachypneic, the hypercapnia may be due to increased dead space ventilation, and appropriate workup is required. Generally it is helpful to manipulate one ventilator variable at a time in most patients in response to an ABG. After an equalization period of approximately 30 min, a repeat ABG should be drawn to assess the efficacy of ventilator changes. If the ABG is acceptable at this point, monitoring the patient's SpO_2 and end-tidal CO_2 (if available) obviates the need for routine frequent ABGs. However, in patients with severe ARDS, changing lung compliance (particularly when ventilation occurs in a pressure control mode), or patients who are chemically paralyzed should be monitored more frequently.

Post intubation chest X-rays (CXRs) are essential to check endotracheal tube positioning, which should be no more than 5 cm above the carina. Right main stem intubation can occur when intubation occurs in the emergency setting or via migration of a previously well-placed tube leading to collapse of the left lung (Fig. 17.11). Traditional ICU management has dictated that a daily CXR be obtained for all intubated ICU patients. However there has been a trend to cut down on unnecessary costs associated with routine daily CXRs. A recent prospective observational study by Inaba et al. demonstrated that eliminating automatic daily CXRs decreased costs without affecting length of stay, morbidity, or mortality [18]. Interestingly, CXRs ordered based upon clinical changes had a greater frequency of new findings compared to those ordered routinely during the course of study.

An effort has also been made to cut down on unnecessary daily lab orders for intubated, critically ill patients. A paper by Ko, Murry et al. in 2015 applied a Lean Six Sigma approach to cut down on unnecessary lab draws in the SICU of a large academic medical center [12]. Daily checklists, staff educations, and visual reminders were employed to emphasize the importance of appropriate lab tests. This included the standardization of continuous capnography for ventilated patients. The number of complete blood counts, basic metabolic panels, and CXRs all significantly decreased. SICU mortality did not significantly change, but cost savings were estimated at $59,137/month, and estimated excess phlebotomy prevented was approximately 4 L blood per month. These findings have significant cost implications beyond the amount spent on routine bloodwork as phlebotomy accounts for up to 30% of anemia in the ICU and associated unnecessary transfusions.

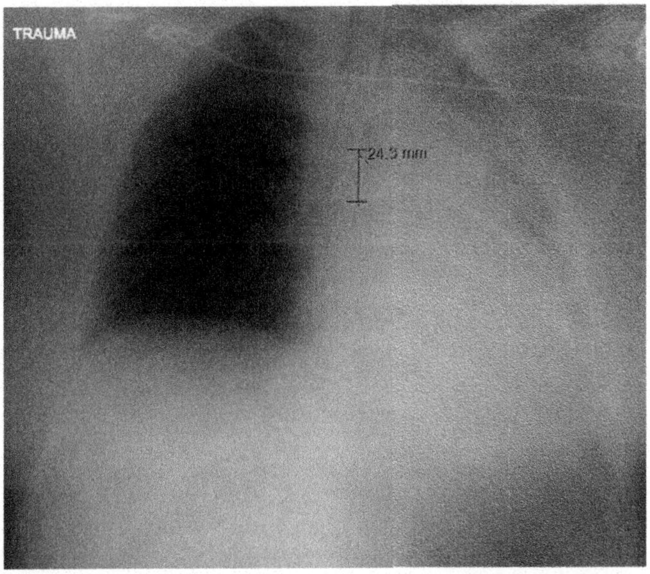

Fig. 17.11 Right mainstem intubation with collapse of the left lun (Note the tube is over 2 cm deep to the carina. The mediastinum has also shifted to the left from right lung hyperinflation)

Ventilator bundles can help decrease the rate of ventilator-associated pneumonia and have become a routine practice in many ICUs. A ventilator bundle includes the following: head-of-bed elevation, daily sedation vacations and assessment of readiness to extubate, peptic ulcer prophylaxis, DVT prophylaxis, and daily oral care with chlorhexidine [16]. Proper oral care is essential, as aspiration from the oropharynx is believed to be the inciting incident in most cases of ventilator-associated pneumonia. Continuous subglottic suctioning is available now on many endotracheal tubes and should be implemented where available. Bundles are most effective when followed in their entirety, and checklist implementation has been shown to assist with compliance as well as significant, sustainable reductions in ventilator-associated pneumonia and catheter-related blood stream infections [21].

In addition to oral care, intermittent suctioning may help clear respiratory secretions, particularly when these are thick and inspissated. Although frequently ordered, nebulized beta and anticholinergic agents are not effective means of "respiratory therapy." For thick secretions, mucolytics such as mucomyst may be directly injected into the airway to loosen secretions. Persistent thick secretions with elevations in peak inspiratory pressures are consistent with concretions in the endotracheal tube that can lead to ineffective ventilation and obstruction due to mucous plugging (see Fig. 17.12). Therapeutic bronchoscopy is indicated in cases such as these.

Sedation vacations, physical therapy, and early mobilization are helpful in weaning mechanically ventilated patients.

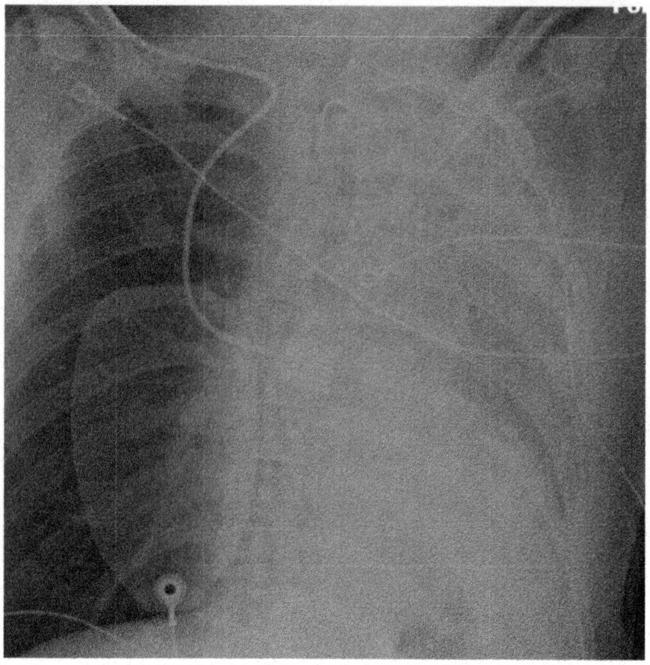

Fig. 17.12 Mucous plugging leading to collapse of the left lung

A randomized controlled trial by Kress et al. showed that daily interruption of sedative infusions in critically ill patients undergoing mechanical ventilation significantly improved outcomes. The study examined a control group in which sedative infusions were interrupted only at the discretion of ICU clinicians versus the intervention group, in which sedative infusions were interrupted until patients were awake, on a daily basis. The study found that daily interruption of sedative drugs decreased the duration of mechanical ventilation and ICU length of stay [14]. Therefore routine sedation interruption and reassessment of sedative requirements should be performed daily unless contraindications exist (i.e., malignant intracranial hypertension, chemical paralytic requirements, or *status epilepticus*).

The beneficial effects of early rehabilitation therapy on patients with mechanical ventilation have been well demonstrated [9]. These benefits include shorter duration of mechanical ventilation, shorter ICU and hospital length of stay, and improved physical function scores compared to controls. Several authors have demonstrated that early ambulation is feasible in mechanically ventilated patients [1]. Once patients are deemed medically stable by set criteria, progressive physical therapy sessions allow increased activity level, from sitting to standing to walking. Though highly beneficial to patients, these programs are highly labor and resource intensive, leading to poor widespread implementation. Development of such programs requires buy-in from multiple services (i.e., nursing, physical therapy, and respiratory therapy) and overcoming preconceived bias regarding the safety of activity in this critically ill cohort.

Troubleshooting

For any concerning status change in the ventilated patient in the ICU, the ABCs (airway, breathing, circulation) should be assessed first. Chest X-rays and arterial blood gases should also be considered as part of the initial ventilator troubleshooting workup, as they will be able to differentiate between many of the various respiratory pathologies listed below.

If there is a concern for airway patency, first ensure the ventilator tubing is free of kinks, obstructions, or condensation accumulation. ETT misplacement or dislodgement is always a possibility, and the patient's most recent chest X-ray should be assessed to determine the location of the endotracheal tube. Ventilator mode and settings should also be evaluated. For example, the patient may be tiring on spontaneous settings and may need to be switched to volume- or pressure-controlled modes. Evidence of cuff leak should also be assessed. Breath sounds should be checked to ensure that they are equal bilaterally. Respiratory rate and O_2 saturation should be assessed. If the patient is desaturating or becomes hemodynamically unstable, it is best to disconnect the patient from the ventilator and manually bag. Difficulty in bagging could signify an obstructed airway or increased lung resistance. If bagging ameliorates the problem, the issue is likely with the ventilator itself, and its settings should be adjusted. If this does not help, diagnoses such as excessive auto-PEEP and tension pneumothorax should be considered and appropriate action taken.

Ventilators are equipped with different pressure alarms, which may signify various issues with the airway or lungs. For example, an alarm for high airway pressure can signify endotracheal tube obstruction or simply that the patient is coughing and raising airway pressure. Low-pressure alarms may occur if the patient becomes disconnected from the vent or a leak in the system develops [6]. A high mean airway pressure alarm can be either due to issues with lung compliance or airway problems. The peak inspiratory pressure is obtained during inspiration and represents resistance to airflow, so an increase in peak inspiratory pressure relative to plateau pressure signifies an issue with the airway itself. The ventilator tubing may be kinked, or the patient may have developed upper airway obstruction secondary to increased secretions or bronchospasm. The plateau pressure is obtained during an inspiratory pause, eliminating airflow; therefore an elevation in plateau pressure relative to peak inspiratory pressure reflects an issue with compliance, in either chest wall or alveoli. Examples of causes of decreased compliance include pneumothorax, abdominal compartment syndrome, ARDS, pneumonia, and auto-PEEP dyssynchrony. Other ventilator alarms can refer to the input power, i.e., loss of electrical power or loss of pneumatic power, or issues with ventilator set volume or inspiratory/expiratory time [8].

Mechanical ventilation may be anxiety-inducing and thus the agitated patient is not uncommon. It is important to determine the underlying cause of patient discomfort. Pain, anxiety, and delirium may contribute to agitation, especially in the postoperative or post trauma setting, and the physician should not immediately sedate or paralyze the patient without first searching for a correctable underlying cause. Ventilator dyssynchrony can lead to patient agitation. The physician should check for synchrony between patient efforts and delivered breaths. If breathing is asynchronous, the type of flow trigger may need to be adjusted or the flow rate or pattern may be too low or inappropriate for the patient. Auto-PEEP may also be present if the patient is providing inspiratory effort but unable to initiate a mechanical breath from the ventilator.

Several agents may be employed to ameliorate anxiety. Benzodiazepines, which bind to GABA receptors, cause amnesia and sedation. Benzodiazepines work well for those patients with alcohol or drug withdrawal, but these drugs can rapidly accumulate and promote delirium, especially in elderly patients. Propofol, which also binds to GABA receptors, has amnestic and sedative effects but no analgesic properties. Advantages to propofol include its rapid onset of action and short half-life. However, it can cause respiratory depression and hypotension. Dexmedetomidine, an alpha 2 receptor agonist, has sedative, amnestic, and mild analgesic properties and causes cooperative sedation, meaning a patient can be aroused despite deep sedation levels and also does not impair respiratory drive. It causes less delirium compared with benzodiazepines and may hasten extubation. The main side effects of dexmedetomidine are bradycardia and hypotension due to its anti-adrenergic effects.

Weaning from Mechanical Ventilation

Readiness Criteria

Patients should be assessed daily for ability to wean from the ventilator. Each institution has its own set of readiness criteria, but some generally accepted parameters are described here. These criteria include respiratory, cardiovascular, and neurologic parameters. For the respiratory requirements, PaO_2/FiO_2 should be around 200, CO_2 should be within the normal range (or at baseline for COPD), and SpO_2 should be greater than 90 on PEEP <8 and FiO_2 < 40–50%. The patient should be hemodynamically stable, without active myocardial ischemia, and on minimal pressors to achieve normotension. The patient must also be arousable and able to initiate breaths and clear secretions with a strong cough. Comorbid conditions should be corrected if possible; and major signs of sepsis should not be present. Of note, several studies have demonstrated that weaning from mechanical ventilation using weaning protocol implemented by respiratory therapists is safe and can be more effective than physician-directed weaning. A randomized controlled trial by Kollef et al. randomly assigned patients to receive either protocol-directed or physician-directed weaning from mechanical ventilation [13]. The median duration of ventilation for patients in the protocol group was shorter, and hospital cost savings in protocol-directed group vs. physician-directed group were significant.

Weaning Parameters

Once the patient has met the above readiness criteria, weaning parameters can be used to determine who will be able to wean from a ventilator. This is generally accomplished while the patient is on a spontaneous breathing trial (see section below). These are physiologic tests which can be used as adjuncts to the readiness criteria above. There are multiple parameters that the clinician should be familiar with, as well as their associated limitations. No one parameter predicts success unequivocally, and clinician experience often outweighs any one given measurement. Minute volume was classically used to predict extubation outcome. Minute ventilation in healthy individuals at rest is 5–6 L/min, and this increases in mechanically ventilated patients in proportion to respiratory demand. A minute ventilation of greater than 10 L/min is often associated with an increased metabolic demand that spontaneous respiration is unlikely to support. This parameter may be skewed by patient anxiety during the breathing trial and therefore has a low negative predictive value. Tachypnea during the breathing trial is a common occurrence and can be from anxiety or weakness. Differentiating between the two can be particularly challenging. In general, those patients that are anxious will have normal or increased tidal volumes, while those that are weak or have insufficient reserve will have tidal volumes that progressively decline throughout the breathing trial.

Negative inspiratory force (NIF) is another weaning parameter that can be measured by asking the patient to maximally inspire and taking the pressure at the opening of the ETT. A large inspiratory force is expressed by a more negative number. A study by Sahn and Lakshminarayan demonstrated that 60% of patients with maximal inspiratory pressures less than −30 were successfully weaned, but all patients with NIF more than −20 failed [19]. This parameter may be underestimated in patients with head injury or language barriers, due to insufficient patient understanding and effort.

The rapid shallow breathing index (RSBI), otherwise known as the Tobin index, is the most commonly used weaning parameter. The RSBI is equal to the respiratory rate divided by the tidal volume in liters. In patients who do not tolerate weaning, breaths are often rapid and shallow, and these patients will therefore have a high RSBI. Given a normal respiratory rate of 10 and tidal volume of 500 ml, the normal RSBI is (10/0.5) 20. Using a cutoff ratio of 105, a value that is less than 105 has an 80% positive predictive value of successful extubation, while >105 has a negative predictive value of over 95%, making this the most "accurate" of the weaning parameters [26].

The cuff leak is another important parameter to check, particularly when patients have been intubated for more than 72 hours, due to the risk of laryngeal edema after extubation. To measure the cuff leak, the ETT cuff is deflated, and the volume of inhaled gas that escapes through the larynx is measured by placing the patient on a volume control setting and checking the measured amount of exhaled gas. For example, if a preset volume of 500 ml is chosen and 300 ml returns through the ventilator circuit, the calculated leak would be (200/500) 40%. A cuff leak of less than 30% is concerning for potential laryngeal edema. It is important to note that the methods for performing the leak test have not been standardized, and thresholds for determining leak vary. Therefore, this test may not be a reliable method for determining extubation success, but a positive test may be used as an indicator of increased vigilance at time of extubation. Laryngeal edema is a major cause of failed extubation and occurs in 5–22% of patients who have been intubated longer than 36 h [25]. When this occurs, it is the preference of the authors to give the patient three doses of 40 mg of methylprednisolone 6 h apart and attempt extubation at this point. This treatment regimen has been shown to result in subjectively less upper airway edema and lower rates of failed extubation [4].

Spontaneous Breathing Test

The spontaneous breathing test can determine which patients are ready for extubation. This is the "gold standard" method of weaning as the rate of success is greater than traditional SIMV and occurs about three times more quickly. In a spontaneous breathing trial (SBT), patients can either be connected to the ventilator or removed completely and attached to a T-piece. The SBT should last between 30 and 120 min but may be extended if patients have been ventilated for a prolonged period of time. To pass an SBT, the patient must maintain a hemodynamically stable state, without desaturation, and show no signs of increased respiratory effort such as marked diaphoresis or agitation. If the patients pass the SBT, they are then taken off the ventilator.

Pressure support ventilation at minimal settings can be used in an SBT to wean patients from the ventilator and is often the most common method used for weaning. Here the pressure support level is generally set at 5–8 cm H_2O, just enough to overcome the resistance of the ventilator circuit tubing. This small amount of support does not significantly alter the work of breathing imposed on the patient. This mode is advantageous because it allows for measurement of weaning parameters simultaneously during the trial.

When using the T-piece, the patient is disconnected from the vent and a T-shaped breathing circuit, which provides high-flow O_2 at a rapid rate and passes away expired CO_2, is connected to the patient. No single SBT method (i.e., low level of PSV or set at 5–8 cm H_2O or T-piece trial) is superior to the other, and the type of weaning method chosen should be dictated by local availability and clinician preference. Daily SBTs, regardless of method chosen, should be used to wean patient from the ventilator once the patient has met the aforementioned readiness criteria.

Once the patients have passed the SBT, they can be extubated. Generally, enteral nutrition is held for about 4 hours preceding extubation, the head of the bed is elevated, and suction is placed at bedside. The patient is suctioned, the ETT cuff is deflated, and the tube is removed. The patient is then placed on supplemental oxygen and monitored closely.

References

1. Bailey P, Thomsen GE, Spuhler VJ, et al. Early activity is feasible and safe in respiratory failure patients. Crit Care Med. 2007;35(1):139–45.
2. Brower R, Matthay M. Ventilation with lower tidal volumes as compared with traditional tidal volumes for acute lung injury and the acute respiratory distress syndrome. N Engl J Med. 2000;342(18):1301–8. https://doi.org/10.1056/nejm200005043421801.
3. Chatburn RL. Fundamentals of mechanical ventilation: a short course in the theory and application of mechanical ventilators. Cleveland Heights: Mandu Press; 2003.
4. Cheng K. Intravenous injection of methylprednisolone reduces the incidence of Postextubation stridor in intensive care unit patients. Surv Anesthesiol. 2007;51(6):281. https://doi.org/10.1097/sa.0b013e31815cofaf.
5. Covelli HD, Nessan VJ, Tuttle WK. Oxygen derived variables in acute respiratory failure. Crit Care Med. 1983;11(8):646–9. https://doi.org/10.1097/00003246-198308000-00012.
6. Dong Z. Effects of early rehabilitation therapy on patients with mechanical ventilation. World J Emerg Med. 2014;5(1):48. https://doi.org/10.5847/wjem.j.issn.1920-8642.2014.01.008.
7. Dries D. Effects of PEEP on the intracranial system of patients with head injury and subarachnoid hemorrhage: the role of respiratory system compliance. Yearb Crit Care Med. 2006:243–4. https://doi.org/10.1016/s0734-3299(08)70171-0.
8. Esteban A, Frutos F, Tobin MJ, Alía I, Solsona JF, Valverdu V, Blanco J. A comparison of four methods of weaning patients from mechanical ventilation. N Engl J Med. 1995;332(6):345–50. https://doi.org/10.1056/nejm199502093320601.
9. Gabrielli A, Layon AJ, Yu M, Civetta JM, Taylor RW, Kirby RR. Civetta, Taylor, & Kirby's critical care. Philadelphia: Lippincott Williams & Wilkins; 2009.
10. Huynh T, Messer M, Miles W, Jacobs D, Sing R, Thomason M. Positive end expiratory pressure alters intracranial and cerebral perfusion pressure in severe traumatic brain injury. J Trauma Inj Infect Crit Care. 1999;47(1):213. https://doi.org/10.1097/00005373-199907000-000.

11. Kenneth E, Behring Center. The iron lung and other equipment. Washington, DC: National Museum of American History; 2011.
12. Ko A, Murry JS, Hoang DM, Harada MY, Aquino L, Coffey C, Alban RF. High-value care in the surgical intensive care unit: effect on ancillary resources. J Surg Res. 2016;202(2):455–60. https://doi.org/10.1016/j.jss.2016.01.040.
13. Kollef MH, Shapiro SD, Silver P, John RE, Prentice D, Sauer S, Baker-Clinkscale D. A randomized, controlled trial of protocol-directed versus physician-directed weaning from mechanical ventilation. Crit Care Med. 1997;25(4):567–74. https://doi.org/10.1097/00003246-199704000-00004.
14. Kress J, Pohlman A. Daily interruption of sedative infusions in critically ill patients. N Engl J Med. 2000;343(11):814–5. https://doi.org/10.1056/nejm200009143431114.
15. Marino PL. The ICU book. Philadelphia: Wolters Kluwer Health/Lippincott Williams & Wilkins; 2014.
16. Munro N, Ruggiero M. Ventilator-Associated Pneumonia Bundle – AACN. 2016. Available via http://www.aacn.org/WD/CETests/Media/ACC4322.pdf. Accessed 15 Nov 2016.
17. No author. NHLBI ARDS Network. 2016. Available via www.ardsnet.org. Accessed 31 Dec 2016.
18. Resnick S, Inaba K, Karamanos E, Skiada D, Dollahite JA, Okoye O, Demetriades D. Clinical relevance of the routine daily chest X-ray in the surgical intensive care unit. Am J Surg. 2016. https://doi.org/10.1016/j.amjsurg.2016.09.059.
19. Sahn SA, Lakshminarayan S. Bedside criteria for discontinuation of mechanical ventilation. Chest. 1973;63:1002–5.
20. Schlager N. Science and its times: understanding the social significance of scientific discovery, Vol. 6: 1900–1950. Farmington Hills: Gale; 2000. p. 348.
21. Teixeira PG, Inaba K, Dubose J, Melo N, Bass M, Belzberg H, Demetriades D. Measurable outcomes of quality improvement using a daily quality rounds checklist. J Trauma Acute Care Surg. 2013;75(4):717–21. https://doi.org/10.1097/ta.0b013e31829d27b6.
22. Weg JG, Anzueto A, Balk RA, Wiedemann HP, Pattishall EN, Schork MA, Wagner LA. The relation of pneumothorax and other air leaks to mortality in the acute respiratory distress syndrome. N Engl J Med. 1998;338:341–6.
23. West J, Dollery C, Naimark A. Distribution of blood flow in isolated lung; relation to vascular and alveolar pressures. J Appl Physiol. 1964;19:713–24.
24. Widmaier EP, Raff H, Strang KT. Vander's human physiology: the mechanisms of body function. Boston: McGraw-Hill; 2006.
25. Wittekamp BH, van Mook WN, Tian DH, Zwaveling JH, Bermans DC. Clinical review: post-extubation laryngeal edema and extubation failure in critically ill adult patients. Crit Care. 2009;13(6):233. https://doi.org/10.1186/cc8142.
26. Yang KL, Tobin MJ. A prospective study of indexes predicting the outcome of trials of weaning from mechanical ventilation. N Engl J Med. 1991;324(21):1445–50.

Advanced Modalities and Rescue Therapies for Severe Respiratory Failure

18

Charles S. Parsons and Charles H. Cook

Overarching Concepts

Patients with severe ARDS who fail conventional ventilator strategies are a difficult clinical problem with an associated high mortality (35–40%) [1]. While the advent of mechanical ventilatory support has allowed clinicians to salvage many patients that were previously likely to expire, this capability has come at a price, and during the past 25 years, there has been increasing recognition of the harmful side effects of mechanical ventilation. In particular, three types of injury from positive pressure ventilation have been identified: (1) overdistention of alveoli and the related high-pressure changes at alveolar membranes (volutrauma/barotrauma), (2) injury caused by repeated cycles of recruitment and de-recruitment (atelectrauma), and (3) injury due to release of local inflammatory mediators (biotrauma). Collectively, these have been termed ventilator-induced lung injury (VILI) [2]. Many of the advanced techniques described in this chapter were advanced to try to minimize VILI, and understanding these mechanisms of VILI is central to optimal application of these techniques.

In 2000 the "ARDSNet" study underscored the importance of volutrauma. This study demonstrated improved mortality from 39.8% to 31.0% for patients with ARDS using a low tidal volume strategy ($V_T = 6$ mL/kg) when compared to conventional ventilation ($V_T = 12$ mL/kg) [3]. Low tidal volume ventilation has since become the standard of care for patients with ARDS. Interestingly, despite these data, a recent large observational database analysis (LUNG SAFE Trial) of 459 ICUs in 50 countries revealed that 35.1% of patients with ARDS receive tidal volumes greater than 8 mL/kg predicted body weight [1]. While low tidal volume ventilation may lack the excitement of a new ventilator modality or medical approach, its importance cannot be overemphasized.

In an attempt to minimize atelectrauma, there has been increased focus on the amount of positive end-expiratory pressure (PEEP) used to treat ARDS. Proponents of PEEP argue that it recruits collapsed or diseased lung to help with gas exchange and improves ventilation-perfusion (V/Q) mismatch while minimizing atelectrauma from cyclical opening and closure of recovering or damaged alveoli, which in turn may decrease resultant biotrauma. In the ARDSNet trial, PEEP was adjusted based on a pre-specified FiO_2-to-PEEP protocol [3]. Subsequent investigations have sought to elucidate the optimal amount of PEEP by a variety of methods. Talmor et al. studied the use of esophageal balloon manometry to titrate PEEP based on trans-pulmonary pressures in the thoracic cavity [4]. Numerous others have compared various high-PEEP strategies to low-PEEP strategies without a clear benefit [5–9]. Currently, no consensus exists as to the proper amount of PEEP to apply in ARDS; however most authors agree that in moderate-to-severe ARDS, higher levels of PEEP are likely beneficial, and work to confirm this is ongoing.

Incorporating these individual concepts into practice, there are several "strategies" that have emerged. The combination of low tidal volumes and high PEEP have been collectively referred to as the "open lung approach" (OLA) [10]. A similar strategy of low tidal volumes (V_T) and higher levels of PEEP that also seeks to minimize end-inspiratory plateau pressure has been termed lung protective ventilation (LPV) [11]. Broadly speaking, these strategies have become the foundation for ventilator management in ARDS.

In the event that these lung protective strategies are insufficient in achieving acceptable oxygenation, clinicians have

C. S. Parsons
Department of Surgery, Beth Israel Deaconess Medical Center, Harvard Medical School, Boston, MA, USA

C. H. Cook (✉)
Division of Acute Care Surgery, Trauma and Surgical Critical Care, Harvard Medical School, Boston, MA, USA
e-mail: chcook@bidmc.harvard.edu

A. Salim et al. (eds.), *Surgical Critical Care Therapy*, https://doi.org/10.1007/978-3-319-71712-8_18

several choices in two broad categories of intervention. First the clinician may consider the use of advanced ventilation strategies such as pressure-controlled ventilation (PCV) including airway pressure release ventilation (APRV) or high-frequency oscillatory ventilation (HFOV). In addition there are adjunctive treatments such as prone positioning, neuromuscular blockade, and selective pulmonary vasodilators that may be added. Finally, failing all of these, ECMO is emerging as a modality that can be used. It is notable that these choices are not mutually exclusive, and patients with unique ventilator strategies often concomitantly receive combinations of multiple therapies. In the chapter that follows, the reader will be provided more detailed descriptions of these "advanced" treatments for patients with severe ARDS.

Airway Pressure Release Ventilation (APRV)

Concept Background

Airway pressure release ventilation (APRV) was first described by Downs and Stock in 1987 as continuous positive airway pressure (CPAP) combined with a time-cycled expiratory release to allow ventilation of carbon dioxide [12, 13]. APRV is really an extension of inverse *I*:*E* ratio ventilation work published in the 1980s that had suggested improved oxygenation while maintaining lower peak inspiratory pressures (PIP) [14]. Unlike normal respiration that consists of a short inspiratory phase and prolonged expiratory phase, during APRV the majority of the respiratory cycle is spent with the lung inflated (T_{High}, 85–90% of respiratory cycle) at high mean airway pressures (P_{High}), with brief time-cycled releases (T_{Low}) or expiratory phase at low pressure (P_{Low}) (Fig. 18.1). During these releases, exhalation occurs, albeit very briefly. In this way, mean airway pressure (M_{AP}) is maintained at high levels to facilitate oxygenation. The concept of M_{AP} is important to understanding the purported benefits of APRV and is calculated as follows:

$$M_{\text{AP}} = \left(P_{\text{High}} \times T_{\text{High}}\right) + \left(P_{\text{Low}} \times T_{\text{Low}}\right) / \left(T_{\text{High}} + T_{\text{Low}}\right)$$

Thus as lungs spend the majority of every minute at high pressure (T_{H}) during APRV, the mean airway pressure is proportionally higher, translating into more time when the lung is open and available for gas exchange compared to the relatively short inspiratory duration during standard ventilation. This is thought to be most beneficial when lungs are stiff and noncompliant, as in ARDS.

Another important concept in APRV is that spontaneous inspiratory and expiratory cycles can occur independently from the time cycle set in APRV. In fact, during the high-pressure ($P_{\text{H}}/T_{\text{H}}$) phase in a spontaneously breathing patient, spontaneous respiration can continue while the lung is "open," decreasing work of breathing, enhancing gas exchange, and allowing further carbon dioxide removal [15]. Such breathing can therefore augment gas exchange that occurs during the airway release and APRV low-pressure phase ($P_{\text{L}}/T_{\text{L}}$) (Fig. 18.1).

After its description, there was considerable variability in how APRV was implemented, with most variability around duration of the CPAP high-pressure phase in relation to the airway release phase. A major obstacle to early APRV implementation was that ventilators during the era of its description did not yet offer the modality. Inclusion of APRV and its analogs as new modes in ventilators and popularization of a protocolized strategy by Habashi et al. during the mid-2000s further advanced the mode. This "Habashi protocol" recommended the use of prolonged T_{High} and very brief T_{Low} duration based on lung mechanics and slopes of expiratory flow curves [15]. The protocol also outlined initial settings and titrations according to dynamic physiologic parameters. This protocol for APRV continues to be one of the most commonly encountered formats of APRV in clinical practice.

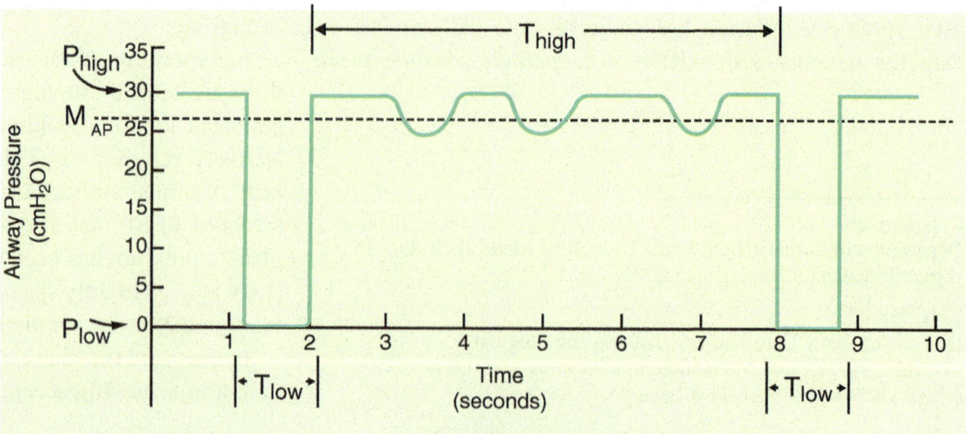

Fig. 18.1 Schematic of airway pressure and APRV settings [16]

Many of the benefits of APRV are thought to be a consequence of its use in spontaneously breathing patients. It allows patient-initiated ventilation during the high-pressure phase, while the lungs are maximally recruited, promoting decreased *V*/*Q* mismatch, preferential aeration of dependent lung adjacent to a functioning diaphragm, and decreased intrapulmonary shunting [17]. Numerous studies have also suggested that APRV also reduces the need for sedation and neuromuscular blockade when compared to standard modes of ventilation [18, 19]. This is thought to be consequent to better patient comfort as well as ease of weaning to conventional spontaneous modes of ventilation as the patient's status improves. Although spontaneous breathing is thought to offer an advantage, it is not "required," and in paralyzed or heavily sedated patients, APRV is really analogous to pressure-controlled ventilation [20].

Technique

Initial settings in APRV are a function of the underlying compliance of the lung. In many cases, patients may be on pressure-controlled modalities with high PEEP prior to transitioning to APRV. Static pressure volume curves are utilized to ensure that lung inflation is maximized at or near functional residual capacity (FRC). T_L should be minimized but still allow adequate exhalation (absence of flow) to prevent breath stacking and avoid auto-PEEP [20]. It is usually desirable to maintain M_{AP} at least at the level being used before transitioning to APRV. It is therefore important to note the M_{AP} in the preceding mode prior to choosing APRV settings (Table 18.1).

There is some debate about additional support for spontaneous breaths taken during APRV. Although additional pressure support can be added to aid spontaneous breathing during inspiration during P_{High}, APRV purists discourage this support, concerned about detrimental effects on airway pressure and alteration of physiologic sinusoidal flow during spontaneous breaths [20]. Many, however, will accept some form of tube compensation (when available) as it is not thought to contribute significantly to additional inspiratory pressures.

As patients recover and lung compliance improves, FiO_2 should be weaned to 40–60%. P_{High} is next gradually decreased and T_{high} increased, colloquially known as "dropping and stretching." Cessation of APRV usually occurs when the FiO_2 has reached a normal level (30–50%) and P_{High} is ≤16 cmH_2O, at which point patients can be transitioned to pressure support ventilation or CPAP that maintains similar M_{AP}. There are some enthusiasts, however, who will continue the modality much longer, at least until the "stretch" becomes impractical.

The safety of APRV has been well established in diverse populations, including post-cardiac surgery patients, vascular surgery patients, prone patients with ARDS, children, and even the morbidly obese [17, 21–24]. APRV must however be used with caution in select situations. Increasing mean airway pressure and intrathoracic pressure can potentially lead to hemodynamic instability due to impaired venous return, although numerous reports have suggested that APRV may actually have no effect or even favorably affect hemodynamic parameters, including cardiac output, oxygen delivery, and splanchnic blood flow [23–25]. Additionally, APRV is contraindicated in patients with severe obstructive lung disease and a prolonged expiratory time due to the short release phase and the risk of breath stacking and auto-PEEP [20]. Because of the pressures being applied, pneumothoraces can quickly develop tension physiology, so vigilance is required for patients undergoing APRV that experience sudden hemodynamic instability. Overall, the modality requires expertise and training at all levels, including respiratory therapists, residents, fellows, and faculty.

Proponents of APRV argue that high levels of continuous positive airway pressure inflate the lung for a prolonged period, facilitating recruitment of alveolar units and minimizing atelectrauma and ventilator-induced lung injury (VILI) from repeated opening and closure of the alveoli. If true, this suggests APRV as an ideal modality for the treatment of ARDS. However, as discussed below, human trials have not consistently shown a benefit of APRV in such patients.

Table 18.1 Settings in APRV

Setting	Abbreviation	Description	Initial setting
Time high	T_H	Time (seconds) at high pressure (CPAP)	4–6 s
Pressure high	P_H	Pressure (cmH_2O) maintained for T_H, equivalent to CPAP	20–30 cmH_2O (below upper inflection point of static PV curve)
Time low	T_L	Time (seconds) at low pressure	0.2–0.8 s
Pressure low	P_L	Pressure (cmH_2O) maintained for T_L, equivalent to low-pressure CPAP or PEEP	0–5 cmH_2O (above lower inflection point on static PV curve)

Evidence

There are multiple studies that show clear improvement in oxygenation with the use of APRV, but it remains unclear if these improvements translate to an effect on mortality, ICU stay, or other outcome measures [14, 17, 22, 26–28]. Varpula et al. have reported results from a randomized trial of APRV versus synchronized intermittent mechanical ventilation (SIMV) in patients with ARDS that showed decreased inspiratory pressures with APRV but no difference in physiologic parameters, ventilator-free days, or clinically significant outcomes including mortality [29]. Subsequently, Maxwell et al. reported results from their randomized control trial of APRV versus low tidal volume ventilation in trauma patients with ALI, also showing no significant differences in clinical outcomes [30]. Despite these results, a recent retrospective review by Andrews et al. in 2013 suggested that "early use of APRV reduced both incidence and mortality associated with ARDS as compared with …conventional mechanical ventilation for treatment of ARDS" [28]. The authors further suggest the intriguing possibility that early application of APRV may prevent development of ARDS [28]. If confirmed in future studies, APRV might be of benefit as a first-line modality, rather than a rescue approach for failing patients.

Complicating analysis of APRV outcomes is the variability in what has historically termed "APRV," as there is no consensus definition or protocol for the modality. Variability in trademarks used by ventilator manufacturers, such as "Bi-Level," "Bi-Vent," and "APRV/Biphasic," and differences in the application of APRV (e.g., 75% T_H:T_L vs 90% T_H:T_L ratio) further limit comparison [31]. Given this, it would be advantageous for future studies to utilize standard nomenclature to facilitate comparison of results.

As our cumulative experience approaches 30 years, APRV has been widely applied in a number of diverse patient populations. Despite clear evidence of a mortality benefit, APRV at least remains a useful adjunct in patients with severe hypoxia where conventional ventilation requires high peak inspiratory pressures. Future work should reveal if more widely adopted APRV can actually prevent some cases of ARDS. For now, APRV and the physiologic principles behind it are valuable to the clinician who favors an "open lung" strategy in caring for patients with severe respiratory failure.

High-Frequency Oscillatory Ventilation (HFOV)

Concept Background

High-frequency oscillatory ventilation (HFOV) utilizes an oscillator pump to rapidly deliver very small tidal volumes (1–4 mL/kg) at high frequency (3–15 Hz) around a set mean airway pressure (P_{AW} or mP_{AW}). The technique was initially developed in the early 1970s as an experimental model to limit hemodynamic consequences associated with conventional positive pressure ventilation [32–34]. Similar to APRV, HFOV seeks to maintain mean airway pressures at levels higher than those achieved in conventional ventilation. Alveolar units are recruited at high mean airway pressures near the maximum FRC, facilitating oxygenation and decreasing *V*/*Q* mismatch. By using relatively small tidal volumes, HFOV is thought to limit volutrauma and atelectrauma due to minimal opening and closing of alveolar units. In combination, this has been theorized to prevent the subsequent downstream inflammatory cascade (biotrauma).

Unlike other modalities, HFOV does not rely on physiologic tidal volumes for ventilation and gas exchange, with tidal volumes routinely chosen below the volume of anatomic dead space. Gas exchange during HFOV therefore occurs via a complex interplay of micro-ventilation and convective currents along the airways [35]. Several of these mechanisms have been summarized in Fig. 18.2 below, including turbulence of flow in the large airways that facilitates gas mixing; the pendelluft effect, whereby gas moves "between lung regions with different compliance and time constraints"; radial mixing based on venturi currents; longitudinal dispersion from rapid central jets of airflow; and augmented molecular diffusion as gas is absorbed at the alveolar-capillary membrane [36].

Technique

Initial settings for HFOV were a source of debate among trial authors that culminated in publication of a detailed protocol for implementation of HFOV by Fessler et al. [37]. Fundamental settings for HFOV include the mean airway pressure (mP_{AW}, usually 28–30 cmH_2O), inspired oxygen concentration (FiO_2), amplitude (ΔP = 90 cmH_2O), oscillatory frequency (usually 3–5 Hz), inspiratory/expiratory ratio (*I*:*E*, usually 1:2), and bias gas flow (usually 30–40 lpm). Recruitment maneuvers are frequently required during initiation of HFOV to facilitate lung expansion. Hypercapnia is tolerated down to a pH of 7.25, and in the event excessive respiratory acidosis develops, increasing ventilation is "achieved with frequency as the primary adjustment, rather than the oscillation pressure amplitude" [37]. Weaning of HFOV settings involves lowering FiO_2 and mean airway pressures as the lungs improve.

Proponents of HFOV argue that there is a clear improvement in oxygenation, at least in the first 24 h after initiation of HFOV [38, 39]. Low tidal volume ventilation, of which HFOV is an extension, has been suggested to decrease volutrauma and VILI in ARDS [3]. Furthermore, HFOV enables elevated positive mean airway pressure which in turn minimizes cyclic opening and collapse (atelectrauma) of lung units, as well as facilitating lung recruitment [35].

In contrast to other modes of ventilation, there are several obstacles to the use of HFOV. Currently, there are very few adult HFOV ventilators that are commercially available [34]. Like APRV, elevated mean airway pressures associated with

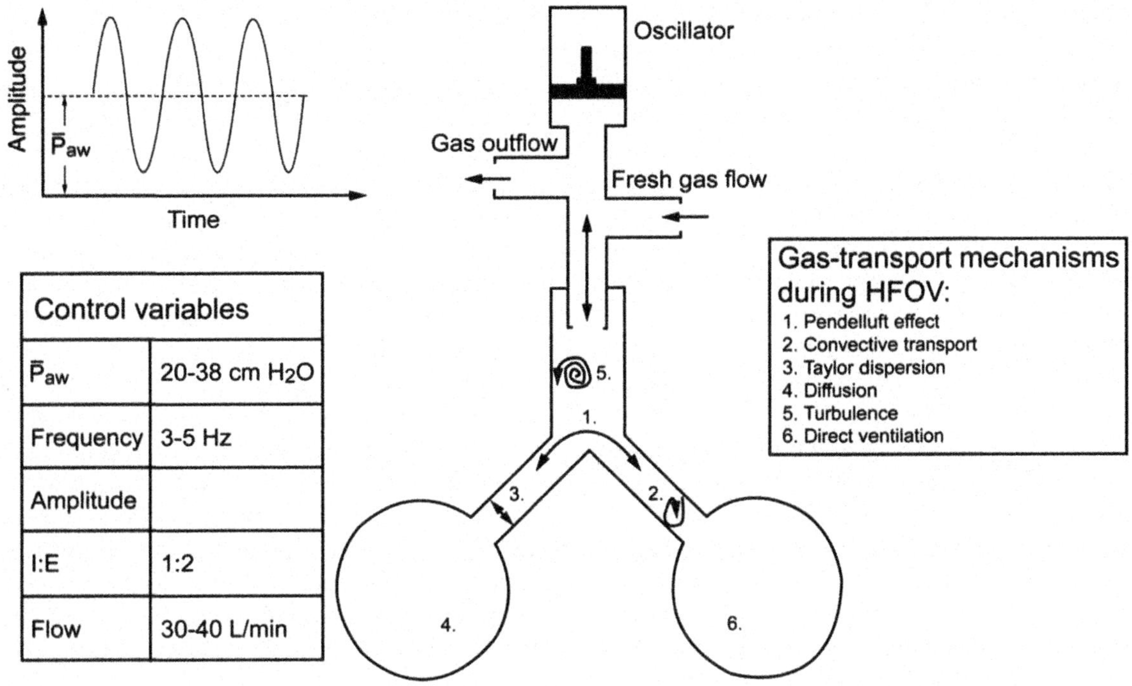

Fig. 18.2 HFOV, schematic representation of oscillator circuit, control variables, and mechanisms of gas exchange [35]

HFOV can have adverse hemodynamic consequences, requiring particular caution in patients receiving vasopressors or hemodynamic instability [37]. Similarly, obstructive airway disease is a contraindication to HFOV due to risk of breath stacking and auto-PEEP. Unlike PCV and APRV, HFOV requires heavy sedation and often paralysis due to patient intolerance and is therefore less desirable for spontaneously breathing patients.

Evidence

HFOV was initially applied enthusiastically to neonatal patients with respiratory distress syndrome of prematurity; however early trials showed mixed results. In 1989, the HIFI Study Group reported in a multicenter randomized trial that HFOV "did not reduce the incidence of bronchopulmonary dysplasia, did not produce more effective gas exchange, was not associated with decreased ventilator support, and did not reduce overall mortality" [40]. Importantly, it should be noted that this study preceded routine administration of exogenous surfactant for NRDS. A subsequent randomized trial by Johnson et al. in 2002 supported these findings, showing no significant difference in outcomes when comparing HFOV to conventional mechanical ventilation [41]. In contrast, Gerstmann et al. (1996) in a prospective randomized trial of 125 newborns showed a reduction in both acute and chronic lung injury when HFOV with surfactant and recruitment maneuvers was utilized when compared to conventional ventilation [42]. Numerous subsequent trials have been performed, with similarly mixed results [43].

In 1997 Fort et al. published the first case series of adult patients with ARDS who were rescued with HFOV [44]. This pilot study suggested that HFOV was both safe and effective in patients with ARDS that had failed conventional ventilation. Enthusiasm for the use of HFOV to treat adult patients with ARDS coincided with increasing understanding of the pathophysiology of ARDS and VILI, specifically the low tidal volume strategy suggested by ARDSNet. HFOV, which by design utilizes very low tidal volumes, seemed a logical extension of this philosophy and therefore garnered significant interest as a treatment for adult ARDS.

HFOV use was further bolstered by two subsequent studies. Derdak et al. published the first multicenter randomized controlled trial in 2002 comparing HFOV to conventional ventilation [38]. This study suggested that HFOV improves early oxygenation in ARDS, albeit without a statistically significant improvement in overall mortality. A similar randomized trial also suggested benefit of HFOV over conventional ventilation in more severe cases of ARDS, although it was stopped prematurely due to lack of enrollment [39]. During this period of enthusiasm, the chugging sound of the HFOV ventilators was heard more frequently in adult critical care units than ever before.

Following these promising results, two subsequent large, well-designed multicenter randomized trials, the OSCAR and OSCILLATE trials, brought into question the utility of

HFOV for treatment of adult ARDS. The OSCAR trial compared HFOV to usual-care controls in 795 patients and ultimately showed no significant difference in all-cause mortality at 28 days (41.7% in HFOV vs 41.1% in conventional ventilation, $p = 0.85$) [45]. Subsequently, the OSCILLATE trial of 548 patients with moderate-to-severe ARDS was stopped prematurely due to worsened mortality difference in the HFOV group (47% in HFOV vs 35% in low tidal volume/high PEEP) [46]. The OSCILLATE authors concluded that "early application of HFOV, as compared with a ventilation strategy of low tidal volume and high positive end-expiratory pressure, does not reduce, and may increase, in-hospital mortality" [46].

Following publication of these well-designed trials, numerous authors have questioned the use of HFOV in adult patients with moderate-to-severe ARDS [47, 48]. Despite initial enthusiasm for HFOV, at the current time, the use of HFOV has not been shown to offer any advantages to adult patients with ARDS when compared to low tidal volume ventilation and may even be deleterious, and therefore the use of HFOV in adult ARDS is currently not recommended [35, 49].

For neonatal ARDS, a recent Cochrane Review includes an updated meta-analysis of the 19 randomized trials to date comparing HFOV to conventional ventilation for acute pulmonary dysfunction in preterm infants. Their results suggest that HFOV may provide a "small reduction in chronic lung disease" in newborns, but the effect size was weak due to numerous inconsistent studies. They further noted that "most trials reporting long-term outcome" have not identified significant differences [43]. Despite this modest effect, HFOV is still routinely used in the neonatal setting.

Prone Positioning

Concept Background

The potential benefits of alternative positioning on lung aeration in ARDS were first suggested by Piehl et al. four decades ago [50]. The idea is to reposition patients to redistribute West zones and thereby improve ventilation-perfusion mismatch by recruiting atelectatic lung. For supine ventilated ICU patients, the biggest practical redistribution can occur by positioning them facedown (prone) for a specified period of time. Periodically placing patients prone was theorized to promote alveolar recruitment by constantly transitioning antedependent and dependent lung zones, thereby minimizing dependent atelectasis. This redistribution of ventilation to a more homogenous pulmonary system is thought to reduce overdistention (barotrauma) of the ventral alveolar units that are preferentially ventilated in the supine position, as well as decrease inflammatory responses due to atelectrauma in the dependent lung [51–53].

Technique

Placing patients in the prone position requires multiple personnel, ideally trained and experienced in the technique. As described by Guérin et al., the first step is to ensure that all lines and the ventilator circuit are of sufficient length, protected, and well secured prior to turning a patient. The patient must be adequately sedated and hemodynamically stable prior to placing in the prone position. Pressure points, including the knees, iliac crests, forehead, and thorax, are protected with adhesive skin protectors or other padding to prevent pressure sores, and the eyes are similarly protected by taping shut. At least three staff are required, one person at the head to ensure the endotracheal tube is secured and the head remains neutral and the other two on each side to slide and position the patient. The ipsilateral arm is tucked prior to turning the patient on their side, after which EKG electrodes are placed on the back, and then the patient is then fully turned to the prone position. Once in the prone position, the head is turned to either side ensuring adequate access to the endotracheal tube. Importantly, the head is positioned to alternating sides every 2 h to prevent pressure ulceration [54].

There have been a number of commercially available rotary beds designed specifically for prone positioning that in our experience do facilitate the process. These beds can simplify and expedite patient rotation, a feature particularly helpful in the case of emergencies such as cardiac arrhythmias or inadvertent extubation. However, as rightly pointed out by Gattinoni and others, prone positioning does not *require* such special equipment, with the caveat that it is performed by specifically trained personnel and undertaken with great care to minimize the risk of any potential life-threatening complications [53]. Limitations to the wide applicability of this technique include the added care requirements and training needed to safely perform this maneuver and the need for alternative management strategies for emergencies. Strict contraindications to prone positioning include spinal instability and elevated intracranial pressure; however there are a number of relative contraindications, including open abdominal wounds, unstable fractures, pregnancy, and hemodynamic instability, among others [53].

Evidence

In the late 1990s with increasing understanding of the pathophysiology of VILI, prone positioning became more popular as a possible treatment for ARDS [55]. This was based mostly upon several pilot studies that suggested prone positioning improves oxygenation in cases of severe hypoxemic respiratory failure (reviewed in [56]). However, until recently, high-quality data supporting a mortality benefit for proning patients with ARDS were lacking.

Since the late 1990s, five randomized controlled trials have been published evaluating prone positioning in moderate-to-severe ARDS [57–60]. The two earliest trials utilized short duration prone positioning (6–8 h/day for 4–5 days) in patients with mild-to-moderate ARDS (PaO_2:FiO_2 ratios 127–152) and found no difference in mortality [57, 58]. It is noteworthy that both protocols predated low tidal volume strategies and included patients with only moderate ARDS, which combined with short duration might in retrospect explain the lack of effect on mortality. Subsequently, Mancebo et al. reported work from their prematurely stopped trial (low enrollment) that suggested improved mortality with longer duration prone positioning in patients with moderate-to-severe ARDS using a volume-controlled strategy [59]. Unfortunately their sample size precluded statistical significance, a handicap shared by the similarly designed trial reported by Taccone et al. in 2009 [60]. Finally, the recent PROSEVA trial suggests that early prone positioning actually improves outcomes in patients with moderate-to-severe ARDS, by demonstrating significantly lower 28-day mortality (16.0% vs 32.8%, HR 0.39, $p < 0.001$), a difference that persisted at 90 days (23.6% vs 41.0%, $p < 0.001$) [54]. Interestingly, patients in this trial spent more time prone than they did supine (16 h/day) during the roughly 4-day-long intervention. It is also important to recognize that their strict selection criteria included only patients with moderate-to-severe ARDS, having the lowest average PaO_2:FiO_2 ratio on enrollment of 100, and all patients received a low tidal volume ventilation strategy ($Tv \leq 6$ mL/kg). To date, this is the strongest evidence that placing patients with severe ARDS prone improves mortality.

It is also critical to recognize the specific risks associated with prone positioning. By far the most common complication reported is that of pressure ulcers, with rates as high as 30% [56]. Perhaps the most fearsome complication in patients with moderate/severe ARDS is that of accidental extubation, which has been reported in almost 7% of patients [56]. As one might predict, there are also dislodgements of central venous catheter (4.8%) and thoracic drains (1.4%), as well as reports of pneumothorax (4.8%) [56]. It is therefore worth repeating the admonitions by Gattinoni and others that prone positioning in these critically ill patients be performed with great care.

In summary, prone positioning appears to provide some mortality benefit in patients with severe ARDS. It has therefore been endorsed as an adjunct to low tidal volume strategies in patients with advanced respiratory failure due to ARDS [61]. Although greatly facilitated by specialty beds, it is a simple maneuver that does not require such equipment, provided that staff are adequately trained. This technique can be performed safely in a wide variety of intensive care units; however providers must be aware of its attendant complications. Further study needs to be performed to see if this mortality benefit will persist in the era of "open lung" ventilation with high PEEP.

Neuromuscular Blocking Agents (NMBAs)

Concept Background

Neuromuscular blocking agents have been utilized for over 30 years in the management of severely ill patients on mechanical ventilation. In 1995, the Society of Critical Care Medicine (SCCM) published the first guideline that includes the use of NMBAs for ARDS in critically ill patients, and NMBAs are also included in subsequent guideline updates in 2002 and 2016 [62, 63]. A recent study on the current epidemiology and treatment of ARDS reported that NMBAs are used in approximately 38% of patients with severe ARDS [1].

Several putative mechanisms for the beneficial effect of NMBAs in severe respiratory failure have been proposed. NMBAs neutralize patient-ventilator dyssynchrony by paralyzing the diaphragm and intercostal musculature, minimizing the work of breathing. NMBAs have been theorized to decrease barotrauma and atelectrauma related to increased chest wall and lung compliance while also improving V/Q mismatch. Supporters of NMBA use point to improvements in oxygenation with continuous cisatracurium therapy [64]. In addition, the use of NMBAs has been shown to decrease inflammatory mediators when used in ARDS and by inference presumably biotrauma [65].

The main contraindications to NMBA use have historically been the associated risks of cardiac side effects, histamine release, and associated myopathy from continued use. Due to vagolytic activity of NMBAs, tachycardia is a frequent side effect of administration, which can exacerbate coronary disease and myocardial oxygen demand. Caution should be used in administration to patients with pre-existing tachycardia or known severe coronary disease. The use of steroid-based preparations such as vecuronium has been associated with increased rates of ICU-related myopathy and weakness [66–68]. It should be noted that cisatracurium does not typically cause histamine release and causes only mild tachycardia, thus favoring its use. Finally, the use of NMBAs also requires continuous sedation, which tends to be heavy to avoid the risk of recall. Heavy sedation has myriad side effects addressed elsewhere in this text.

Technique

Current guidelines support the use of cisatracurium as a continuous infusion for neuromuscular blockade in the ICU. In our practice, a single bolus dose of 0.15–0.2 mg/kg is given over 3–5 min, followed by a continuous infusion at 0.05–0.3 mg/kg/h. Prior to initiating neuromuscular blockade, a peripheral nerve stimulator (PNS) should be placed to monitor train-of-four (TOF) response. Importantly, PNS monitoring alone is inadequate to safely monitor response to NMBAs, and PNS monitoring must be accompanied by frequent advanced clinical assessments [63]. Concomitant physical therapy should be performed to mitigate the risk of myopathy due to immobility, and frequent turns with skin assessments are mandatory during NMBA therapy. Finally, NMBAs lack analgesic, sedative, or amnestic properties, and therefore adequate sedation *must* be ensured prior to initiating neuromuscular blockade. Such sedation is most commonly administered during neuromuscular blockade.

Evidence

To date, three large randomized multicenter trials have been published examining the role of NMBAs in ARDS, all from the Papazian group. In 2004, they found that patients with PaO_2:FiO_2 ratios <150 had improved oxygenation after administration of NMBA when compared to controls [64]. Subsequent work further supports the benefit of neuromuscular blockade for 48 h in the early treatment of severe ARDS (PaO_2:FiO_2 ratio <150) [69]. Although mortality did not significantly differ between the treatment groups, when groups were stratified based on severity of illness (APACHE II score), PaO_2:FiO_2 ratio, and plateau pressure, a significant improvement in mortality was suggested. Importantly, there was no difference in the incidence of ICU myopathy between the two groups in this study. Further studies are ongoing to solidify the role for NMBAs in the treatment of ARDS, with numerous authors currently supporting early use of NMBAs in the treatment of severe ARDS (P:$F \leq 150$) [63].

Selective Pulmonary Vasodilators (SPV)

Concept Background

Selective pulmonary vasodilators (SPV), including inhaled nitric oxide (iNO) and inhaled prostacyclins such as epoprostenol (iEPO), have been used extensively as adjunctive treatments for severe hypoxic respiratory failure. SPV cause pulmonary vascular vasodilation that improves perfusion to the ventilated lung (decreasing V/Q mismatch), thereby improving gas exchange. iEPO and other prostacyclins bind to endothelial cell prostaglandin receptors, while nitric oxide acts via soluble guanylate cyclase enzyme, both with the end result of causing smooth muscle relaxation in endothelial cells via a cAMP-mediated pathway. As inhaled agents with extremely short half-lives (45 s–3 min), both drugs have limited systemic side effects and upon inhalation act rapidly on the pulmonary vasculature [70].

Technique

iNO and iEPO are administered in-line with the ventilator circuit and require specialized training in their administration. Because it is cheaper and requires less equipment (simple nebulizer), iEPO is typically the first therapy used. Therapy can be initiated at 50 ng/kg/min and then weaned as tolerated. Numerous studies suggest that the optimal dose to yield clinically significant increase in PaO_2 and reduction in pulmonary artery pressures is 20–30 ng/kg/min in adults and 30 ng/kg/min in pediatric patients [70–72]. When therapy is no longer necessary, the dose is typically halved until ≤12.5 ng/kg/min and then stopped. Care must be taken not to wean iEPO too rapidly as rebound pulmonary hypertension can occur.

iNO administration requires specialized equipment that mixes and meters the gas into the ventilator circuit. For iNO, patients that respond will do so almost immediately with improved oxygenation and decreased pulmonary arterial pressures. Therapy is typically started at 5–10 ppm and over the course of 5 min titrated up to clinical effect or the maximum dose of 40 ppm. Given the significant costs associated with iNO, if substantial improvement in oxygenation or pulmonary hypertension/cardiac output is not observed, then iNO should be rapidly weaned and discontinued over the ensuing 5–10 min. In contrast, when patients manifest a favorable clinical response, therapy may be continued until their clinical condition allows discontinuation. In this setting, iNO is generally weaned 5–10 ppm/h as patients tolerate.

Evidence

Enthusiasm for the treatment of ARDS with inhaled nitric oxide coincided with work in the 1990s that showed pulmonary vasodilation, improved pulmonary vascular resistance, and improved oxygenation in patients with ARDS [73, 74]. Three early multicenter trials examined the benefit of nitric oxide in the treatment of ARDS and found that despite a clear improvement in oxygenation, there was no clear impact on mortality [75–77]. Subsequent work by Taylor et al. showed that low-dose nitric oxide therapy results in "short-term oxygenation improvements but has no substantial impact on the duration of ventilatory support or mortality" [78]. A recent Cochrane Systematic Review of inhaled nitric oxide suggests no significant benefit in overall mortality when patients with ARDS were treated with inhaled nitric oxide [79]. While oxygenation is consistently improved at 24 h of treatment, this benefit is not sustained and does not appear to translate into improvements in ventilator-free days. In addition, the review shows sufficient high-quality evidence to suggest a worrisome association between inhaled nitric oxide and acute renal failure when used for ARDS [79].

Data supporting the use of iEPO are significantly lacking. There are published data suggesting that iEPO and iNO improve oxygenation and PaO_2:FiO_2 ratios with near identical efficacy in patients with ARDS [70, 71]. Similar to iNO, there are no data showing improvement in outcomes. The single prospective iEPO trial, done in children with ALI, shows the now familiar improvement in oxygenation without improvement in 28-day mortality [72]. Accordingly, the most recent Cochrane for iEPO concluded that there is "no current evidence to support or refute the routine use of aerosolized prostacyclin for patients with ALI and ARDS" [80].

At this juncture it is unclear whether inhaled SPV should be routinely used for severe ARDS. While there are solid data showing improved oxygenation, no clear mortality benefit has been demonstrated. Questions of efficacy aside, the primary limitation of these agents is cost. Specifically, inhaled nitric oxide treatment is extremely expensive, often costing several thousand dollars per day of therapy. By comparison, iEPO has been shown to be substantially cheaper (4.5–17 times less) than iNO treatment [81]. Despite these costs, these agents are commonly used and are therefore included in the refractory hypoxemia pathway. For patients reaching this point in the algorithm, available data suggest that these agents may be removed from future pathways, going directly from other modality failures to extracorporeal support.

Extracorporeal Membrane Oxygenation (ECMO)

Concept Background

Robert Bartlett is commonly credited with developing ECMO and reported its first successes in children [82]. Successful prolonged extracorporeal membrane oxygenation (ECMO) for severe respiratory failure in an adult was first reported in 1972 by Hill et al. [83]. Despite initial enthusiasm, two early randomized prospective trials of veno-venous ECMO for severe hypoxic respiratory failure and carbon dioxide removal did not show a survival benefit [84, 85]. However, in the ensuing decades, technical advancements with ECMO circuits and cannulae, improvements in the understanding and treatment of severe ARDS, and persistent excellent outcomes in the neonatal population led to renewed interest in the use of ECMO for severe hypoxic respiratory failure and ARDS in adults. A turning point came in 2009 with the worldwide H1N1 influenza pandemic, during which numerous patients presented with severe hypoxemic respiratory failure, with up to 1/3 receiving ECMO as a life-saving salvage therapy for their refractory respiratory failure [86, 87]. Since the H1N1 pandemic, interest and research in ECMO have intensified, and ECMO has been expanded to a diverse array of indications, including the prehospital setting for cardiac arrest [88]. Numerous challenges still exist, most notably how to identify those patients most likely to benefit from this invasive and potentially morbid intervention.

Technique

In its simplest form, an ECMO circuit consists of large bore (27–31 Fr) inflow and outflow cannulae that circulate blood through an external membrane oxygenator via a centrifugal pump. During veno-venous ECMO (VV-ECMO), deoxygenated blood is diverted from the venous circulation by a percutaneous cannula. Blood oxygenation and gas exchange occur during circulation through a large surface area hollow-fiber membrane oxygenator. Oxygenated blood is then warmed and introduced into the circulation via the outflow cannula (Fig. 18.3a). Newer cannula designs have allowed diversion and return of deoxygenated/oxygenated blood through a single dual-lumen cannula as shown in Fig. 18.3b. In situations of mixed or combined pulmonary and cardiac failure, a venous-arterial ECMO (VA-ECMO) circuit or mixed (VVA-ECMO) circuit may be utilized with venous extraction and arterial return via an arterial outflow cannula (not shown). A related technique involves extracorporeal circulation with extraction of carbon dioxide with limited oxygenation (and no pump) and is termed extracorporeal CO_2 removal ($ECCO_2$-R).

Following cannulation and initiation of extracorporeal support, mechanical ventilation is continued at very low tidal volumes, a practice that has been termed "lung rest." Most authors suggest ultra-protective tidal volume ventilation with low tidal volumes, a respiratory rate of 4–5 bpm, low PEEP (10 cmH_2O), and PIP (<20 cmH_2O above PEEP), although no consensus exists [89].

While benefits of ECMO include temporary systemic oxygenation with lung rest that can lessen biotrauma and allow resolution of acute inflammation, there are numerous risks, and therefore patient selection remains tantamount to

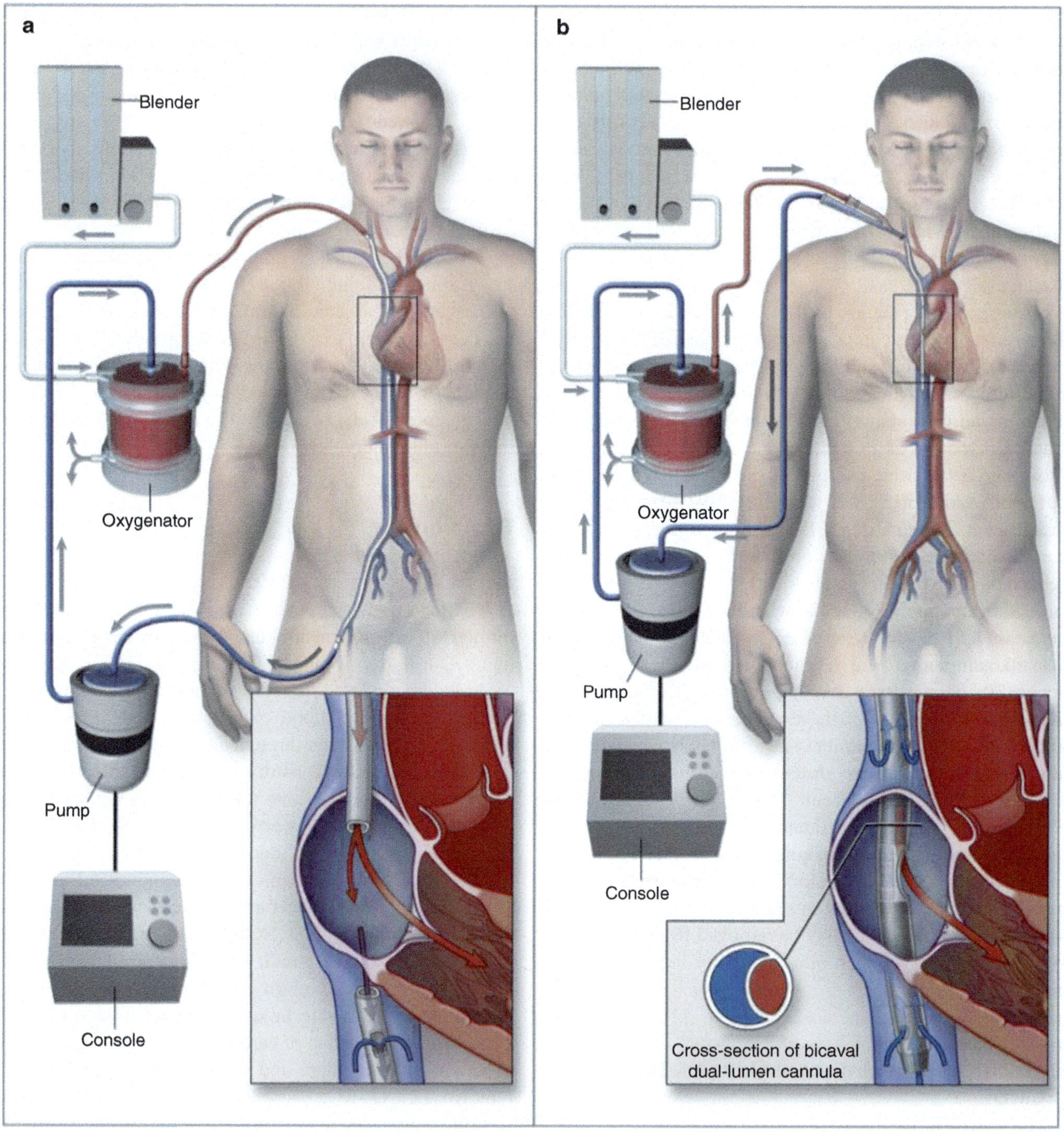

Fig. 18.3 2 Methods veno-venous extracorporeal oxygenation using (**a**) dual cannulae or (**b**) a single dual-lumen cannula [90]

success in those with severe ARDS. Indications include severe hypoxemia (PaO_2:FiO_2 ratio <80 mmHg on FiO_2 >0.9, despite aggressive PEEP), uncompensated hypercapnia (pH < 7.15), and prohibitively high end-inspiratory plateau pressures (>35–45 cmH_2O) [90]. Due to the risk of thrombosis and clotting of the ECMO circuit, systemic anticoagulation is necessary during ECMO therapy, so contraindications include recent or ongoing intracranial hemorrhage, severe bleeding, recent high-risk surgery, and other settings that preclude safe systemic anticoagulation. Relative contraindications to VV-ECMO include cases where there is not a reasonable expectation of near-term recovery of pulmonary function, including cases of severe underlying systemic disease. Several scoring systems have been developed to assess suitability for VV-ECMO, most recently the RESP-score which has been validated in adults with severe hypoxemia [91]. Because ECMO is an advanced therapy that requires 24-h supervision by highly trained specialists, most agree that its use should be limited to specialized centers that have achieved experience with the therapy [90, 92].

Evidence

To date, only three randomized trials have been published regarding the use of extracorporeal therapy in ARDS [84, 85, 92]. The two earliest trials did not show a significant benefit of extracorporeal therapy in ARDS [84, 85]. However, both studies predate modern advances in the treatment of ARDS, including the low tidal volume and high-PEEP "open lung" strategy, perhaps making the results poorly generalizable to modern VV-ECMO treatment.

The CESAR trial in 2009 brought renewed enthusiasm for extracorporeal support for adults with severe respiratory failure and ARDS [92]. CESAR was a prospective, randomized trial in the United Kingdom in which 180 patients were enrolled and randomly allocated to consideration for treatment by ECMO ($n = 90$) versus conventional management ($n = 90$). Although only 75% of the ECMO group ultimately received the treatment, 63% (57/90) of patients allocated to consideration for treatment by ECMO survived to 6 months without disability compared with only 47% (41/87) of those allocated to conventional management (relative risk 0.69; 95% CI 0.05–0.97, $p = 0.03$).

Despite these encouraging results, the outcomes for adult ECMO remain sobering. Reported mortality ranges from 25% in highly selected patients to as high as 60% [86]. A recent meta-analysis of VV-ECMO in ARDS reported a pooled mortality from 12 studies that was 37.7% (CI 95% = 31.8–44.1; $I^2 = 74.2\%$), with the best mortality in patients with H1N1 (24.8 vs 40.6%; $p = 0.027$) [93]. While these mortality rates might at first seem unreasonably high, it is important to remember that most of these patients were failing advanced conventional therapies and many faced near certain death.

The most recent variation of extracorporeal technology utilizes extracorporeal pumpless arteriovenous approaches that remove CO_2, also known as $ECCO_2$-R. When combined with low tidal volume ventilation, this technology has been shown to be effective at CO_2 removal associated with modest improvement in oxygenation [94]. A recent prospective trial of this strategy suggests potential benefit in patients with severe hypoxemia ($PaFiO_2:FiO_2 \leq 150$ mmHg) [95]. Importantly, mortality was low (16.5%), although this is undoubtedly a consequence of selection bias, as many of the sickest ARDS patients would not likely tolerate such therapy.

Any survival or outcome benefits must also be balanced by morbidities that can occur from ECMO. The most common complications are bleeding- and cannula-related complications [93]. A recent meta-analysis of VV-ECMO suggests bleeding complications in 20–40% of patients [93]. Cannula-related complications have been reported in as many as 1/3 of patients undergoing VA-ECMO and include both limb ischemia and hemorrhage [96]. Fortunately, these cannula-related complications do not appear to have a large impact on mortality, but they are nevertheless a considerable source of morbidity for these patients. Infections are another significant comorbidity, with 10–12% of patients undergoing ECMO experiencing hospital-acquired infections [97]. Finally, for patients undergoing VV-ECMO, a recent report suggests that 7% of these patients will suffer neurologic injury, with intracranial hemorrhage being the most common [98].

ECMO is slowly gaining more widespread adoption for the treatment of severe respiratory failure [99]. Given the limitations of the CESAR trial, it will be interesting to see whether their published benefits will be generalizable to other more heterogeneous health-care systems that provide ECMO therapy [100]. There is currently an ongoing large prospective randomized trial, the "Extracorporeal Membrane Oxygenation for Severe Acute Respiratory Distress Syndrome (EOLIA)" trial, that will hopefully further elucidate the benefits of ECMO therapy in patients with severe ARDS (clinicaltrials.gov, identifier: NCT01470703).

Refractory Hypoxemia Pathway

It is recommended to develop a stepwise approach to management of refractory hypoxemia. Figure 18.4 outlines one such approach, where PEEP with or without recruitment maneuvers is first used to improve hypoxemia. Next, alternate strategies including prone positioning, APRV or HFOV, or neuromuscular blockade may be attempted. Pulmonary vasodilators may also be trialed although evidence is admittedly limited for this intervention. Failing all of these modalities, VV- or VA-ECMO should be considered if the patient is an acceptable candidate.

Summary

This chapter has focused on several commonly used advanced therapies available for respiratory failure. Low tidal volumes (4–8 mL/kg predicted body weight) with lower inspiratory pressures (plateau pressure <30 cmH_2O), as well as prone positioning, are well-established interventions for ARDS. Current evidence does not support HFOV for treatment of

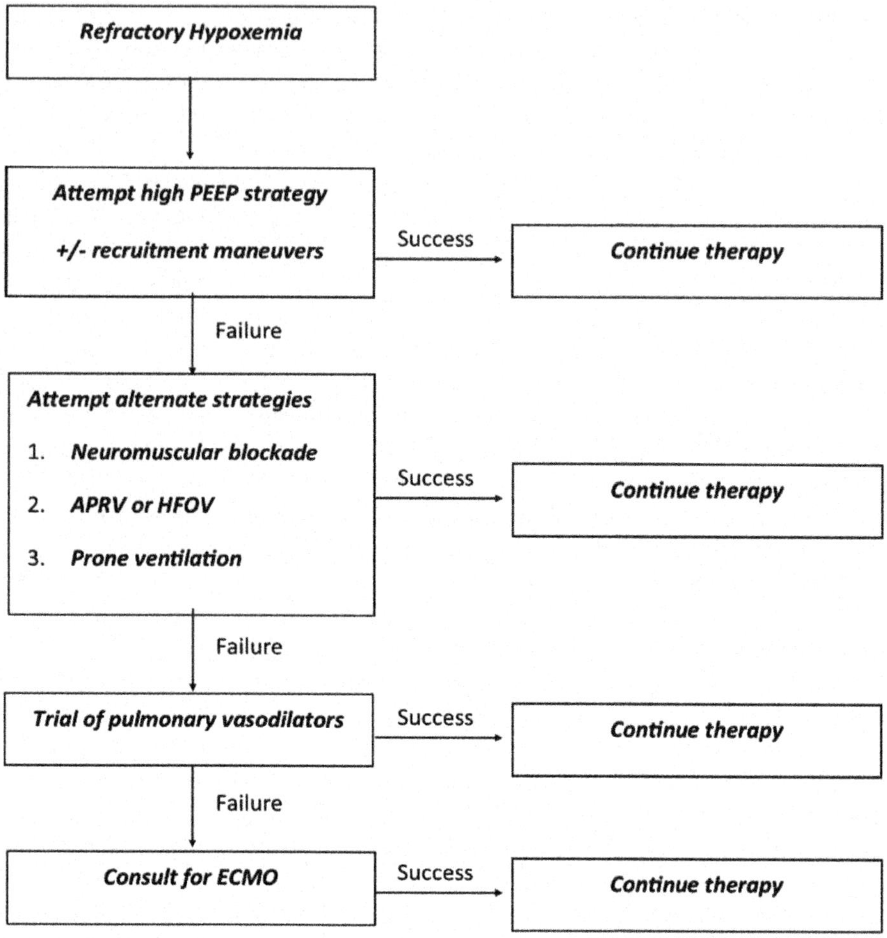

Fig. 18.4 Example of refractory hypoxemia pathway

adult ARDS. An "open lung" strategy with recruitment maneuvers or APRV as well as neuromuscular blockade may be helpful, particularly in severe ARDS. While inhaled pulmonary vasodilators showed initial physiologic promise, they have failed to deliver improvements in outcomes. Finally, VV-ECMO should be considered for suitable patients that experience hypoxemia that is refractory to advanced therapies.

References

1. Bellani G, et al. Epidemiology, patterns of care, and mortality for patients with acute respiratory distress syndrome in intensive care units in 50 countries. JAMA. 2016;315:788–800.
2. Hemmila MR, Napolitano LM. Severe respiratory failure: advanced treatment options. Crit Care Med. 2006;34:S278–90.
3. Acute Respiratory Distress Syndrome Network, et al. Ventilation with lower tidal volumes as compared with traditional tidal volumes for acute lung injury and the acute respiratory distress syndrome. N Engl J Med. 2000;342:1301–8.
4. Talmor D, et al. Mechanical ventilation guided by esophageal pressure in acute lung injury. N Engl J Med. 2008;359:2095–104.
5. Mercat A, et al. Positive end-expiratory pressure setting in adults with acute lung injury and acute respiratory distress syndrome: a randomized controlled trial. JAMA. 2008;299:646–55.
6. Santa Cruz R, Rojas JI, Nervi R, Heredia R, Ciapponi A. High versus low positive end-expiratory pressure (PEEP) levels for mechanically ventilated adult patients with acute lung injury and acute respiratory distress syndrome. Cochrane Database Syst Rev. 2013;(338):CD009098.
7. Meade MO, et al. Ventilation strategy using low tidal volumes, recruitment maneuvers, and high positive end-expiratory pressure for acute lung injury and acute respiratory distress syndrome: a randomized controlled trial. JAMA. 2008;299:637–45.
8. Villar J, Kacmarek RM, Pérez-Méndez L, Aguirre-Jaime A. A high positive end-expiratory pressure, low tidal volume ventilatory strategy improves outcome in persistent acute respiratory distress syndrome: a randomized, controlled trial. Crit Care Med. 2006;34:1311–8.
9. Brower RG, et al. Higher versus lower positive end-expiratory pressures in patients with the acute respiratory distress syndrome. N Engl J Med. 2004;351:327–36.
10. Kacmarek RM, et al. Open lung approach for the acute respiratory distress syndrome: a pilot, randomized controlled trial. Crit Care Med. 2016;44:32–42.
11. Fan E, et al. An official American Thoracic Society/European Society of Intensive Care Medicine/Society of Critical Care Medicine clinical practice guideline: mechanical ventilation in adult patients with acute respiratory distress syndrome. Am J Respir Crit Care Med. 2017;195:1253–63.
12. Downs JB, Stock MC. Airway pressure release ventilation: a new concept in ventilatory support. Crit Care Med. 1987;15:459–61.

13. Stock MC, Downs JB, Frolicher DA. Airway pressure release ventilation. Crit Care Med. 1987;15:462–6.
14. Gurevitch MJ, Van Dyke J, Young ES, Jackson K. Improved oxygenation and lower peak airway pressure in severe adult respiratory distress syndrome. Treatment with inverse ratio ventilation. Chest. 1986;89:211–3.
15. Habashi NM. Other approaches to open-lung ventilation: airway pressure release ventilation. Crit Care Med. 2005;33:S228–40.
16. Je.rrt. Airway pressure release ventilation graph. (Wikimedia Commons).
17. Putensen C, Mutz NJ, Putensen-Himmer G, Zinserling J. Spontaneous breathing during ventilatory support improves ventilation-perfusion distributions in patients with acute respiratory distress syndrome. Am J Respir Crit Care Med. 1999;159:1241–8.
18. Kallet RH. Patient-ventilator interaction during acute lung injury, and the role of spontaneous breathing: part 2: airway pressure release ventilation. Respir Care. 2011;56:190–203.– discussion 203–6.
19. Fan E, Khatri P, Mendez-Tellez PA, Shanholtz C, Needham DM. Review of a large clinical series: sedation and analgesia usage with airway pressure release and assist-control ventilation for acute lung injury. J Intensive Care Med. 2008;23:376–83.
20. Daoud EG. Airway pressure release ventilation. Ann Thorac Med. 2007;2:176–9.
21. Schultz TR, et al. Airway pressure release ventilation in pediatrics. Pediatr Crit Care Med. 2001;2:243–6.
22. Varpula T, Jousela I, Niemi R, Takkunen O, Pettilä V. Combined effects of prone positioning and airway pressure release ventilation on gas exchange in patients with acute lung injury. Acta Anaesthesiol Scand. 2003;47:516–24.
23. Kamath SS, Super DM, Mhanna MJ. Effects of airway pressure release ventilation on blood pressure and urine output in children. Pediatr Pulmonol. 2010;45:48–54.
24. Maung AA, Luckianow G, Kaplan LJ. Lessons learned from airway pressure release ventilation. J Trauma Acute Care Surg. 2012;72:624–8.
25. Hering Rudolf MD, et al. Effects of spontaneous breathing during airway pressure release ventilation on intestinal blood flow in experimental lung injury. Anesthesiology. 2003;99:1137–44.
26. Garner W, Downs JB, Stock MC, Rasanen J. Airway Pressure Release Ventilation (APRV). A human trial. Chest. 1988;94:779–81.
27. Navarrete-navarro P, Reynolds N, Rivera R, Chiu WC. Acute respiratory distress syndrome among trauma patients: trends in ICU mortality, risk factors, complications and resource utilization. Intensive Care Med. 2001;27:1133–40.
28. Andrews PL, et al. Early application of airway pressure release ventilation may reduce mortality in high-risk trauma patients: a systematic review of observational trauma ARDS literature. J Trauma Acute Care Surg. 2013;75:635–41.
29. Varpula T, et al. Airway pressure release ventilation as a primary ventilatory mode in acute respiratory distress syndrome. Acta Anaesthesiol Scand. 2004;48:722–31.
30. Maxwell RA, et al. A randomized prospective trial of airway pressure release ventilation and low tidal volume ventilation in adult trauma patients with acute respiratory failure. J Trauma. 2010;69:501–11.
31. Rose L, Hawkins M. Airway pressure release ventilation and biphasic positive airway pressure: a systematic review of definitional criteria. Intensive Care Med. 2008;34:1766–73.
32. Jonzon A, Oberg PA, Sedin G, Sjöstrand U. High-frequency positive-pressure ventilation by endotracheal insufflation. Acta Anaesthesiol Scand. 1971;43(Suppl 43):1–43.
33. Lunkenheimer PP, et al. Application of transtracheal pressure oscillations as a modification of "diffusing respiration". BJA Br J Anaesth. 1972;44:627.
34. Lall R, et al. A randomised controlled trial and cost-effectiveness analysis of high-frequency oscillatory ventilation against conventional artificial ventilation for adults with acute respiratory distress syndrome. The OSCAR (OSCillation in ARDS) study. Health Technol Assess. 2015;19:1–177.– vii.
35. Facchin F, Fan E. Airway pressure release ventilation and high-frequency oscillatory ventilation: potential strategies to treat severe hypoxemia and prevent ventilator-induced lung injury. Respir Care. 2015;60:1509–21.
36. Slutsky AS, Drazen JM. Ventilation with small tidal volumes. N Engl J Med. 2002;347:630–1.
37. Fessler HE, et al. A protocol for high-frequency oscillatory ventilation in adults: results from a roundtable discussion. Crit Care Med. 2007;35:1649–54.
38. Derdak S, et al. High-frequency oscillatory ventilation for acute respiratory distress syndrome in adults. Am J Respir Crit Care Med. 2012;166:801–8.
39. Bollen CW, et al. High frequency oscillatory ventilation compared with conventional mechanical ventilation in adult respiratory distress syndrome: a randomized controlled trial [ISRCTN24242669]. Crit Care. 2005;9:R430–9.
40. HIFI Study Group. High-frequency oscillatory ventilation compared with conventional mechanical ventilation in the treatment of respiratory failure in preterm infants. The HIFI Study Group. N Engl J Med. 1989;320:88–93.
41. Johnson AH, et al. High-frequency oscillatory ventilation for the prevention of chronic lung disease of prematurity. N Engl J Med. 2002;347:633–42.
42. Gerstmann DR, et al. The Provo multicenter early high-frequency oscillatory ventilation trial: improved pulmonary and clinical outcome in respiratory distress syndrome. Pediatrics. 1996;98:1044–57.
43. Cools F, Offringa M, Lm A. Elective high frequency oscillatory ventilation versus conventional ventilation for acute pulmonary dysfunction in preterm infants (Review). 2015. doi:https://doi.org/10.1002/14651858.CD000104.pub4.www.cochranelibrary.com.
44. Fort P, et al. High-frequency oscillatory ventilation for adult respiratory distress syndrome – a pilot study. Crit Care Med. 1997;25:937–47.
45. Young D, et al. High-frequency oscillation for acute respiratory distress syndrome. N Engl J Med. 2013;368:806–13.
46. Ferguson ND, et al. High-frequency oscillation in early acute respiratory distress syndrome. N Engl J Med. 2013;368:795–805.
47. Nguyen SQ, Divino CM. Surgical residents as medical student mentors. Am J Surg. 2007;193:90–3.
48. Ng J, Ferguson ND. High-frequency oscillatory ventilation: still a role? Curr Opin Crit Care. 2017;23:175–9.
49. Maitra S, Bhattacharjee S, Khanna P, Baidya DK. High-frequency ventilation does not provide mortality benefit in comparison with conventional lung-protective ventilation in acute respiratory distress syndrome: a meta-analysis of the randomized controlled trials. Anesthesiology. 2015;122:841–51.
50. PIEHL MA, BROWN RS. Use of extreme position changes in acute respiratory failure. Crit Care Med. 1976;4:13–4.
51. Broccard A, et al. Prone positioning attenuates and redistributes ventilator-induced lung injury in dogs. Crit Care Med. 2000;28:295–303.
52. Pelosi P, Brazzi L, Gattinoni L. Prone position in acute respiratory distress syndrome. Eur Respir J. 2002;20:1017–28.

53. Gattinoni L, Taccone P, Carlesso E, Marini JJ. Prone position in acute respiratory distress syndrome. Rationale, indications, and limits. Am J Respir Crit Care Med. 2013;188:1286–93.
54. Guérin C. Video: prone positioning in severe acute respiratory distress syndrome. N Engl J Med. 2013;368:2159–68.
55. Blanch L, et al. Short-term effects of prone position in critically ill patients with acute respiratory distress syndrome. Intensive Care Med. 1997;23:1033–9.
56. Sud S, Sud M, Friedrich JO, Adhikari NKJ. Effect of mechanical ventilation in the prone position on clinical outcomes in patients with acute hypoxemic respiratory failure: a systematic review and meta-analysis. CMAJ. 2008;178:1153–61.
57. Gattinoni L, et al. Effect of prone positioning on the survival of patients with acute respiratory failure. N Engl J Med. 2001;345:568–73.
58. Guérin C, et al. Effects of systematic prone positioning in hypoxemic acute respiratory failure: a randomized controlled trial. JAMA. 2004;292:2379–87.
59. Mancebo J, et al. A multicenter trial of prolonged prone ventilation in severe acute respiratory distress syndrome. Am J Respir Crit Care Med. 2006;173:1233–9.
60. Taccone P, et al. Prone positioning in patients with moderate and severe acute respiratory distress syndrome: a randomized controlled trial. JAMA. 2009;302:1977–84.
61. Beitler JR, et al. Prone positioning reduces mortality from acute respiratory distress syndrome in the low tidal volume era: a meta-analysis. Intensive Care Med. 2014;40:332–41.
62. Murray MJ, et al. Clinical practice guidelines for sustained neuromuscular blockade in the adult critically ill patient. Crit Care Med. 2002;30:142–56.
63. Murray MJ, et al. Clinical practice guidelines for sustained neuromuscular blockade in the adult critically ill patient. Crit Care Med. 2016;44:2079–103.
64. Gainnier M, et al. Effect of neuromuscular blocking agents on gas exchange in patients presenting with acute respiratory distress syndrome. Crit Care Med. 2004;32:113–9.
65. Forel J-M, et al. Neuromuscular blocking agents decrease inflammatory response in patients presenting with acute respiratory distress syndrome. Crit Care Med. 2006;34:2749–57.
66. Testelmans D, et al. Rocuronium exacerbates mechanical ventilation-induced diaphragm dysfunction in rats. Crit Care Med. 2006;34:3018–23.
67. Hermans G, Van den Berghe G. Clinical review: intensive care unit acquired weakness. Crit Care. 2015;19:274.
68. Price DR, Mikkelsen ME, Umscheid CA, Armstrong EJ. Neuromuscular blocking agents and neuromuscular dysfunction acquired in critical illness: a systematic review and meta-analysis. Crit Care Med. 2016;44:2070–8.
69. Papazian L, et al. Neuromuscular blockers in early acute respiratory distress syndrome. N Engl J Med. 2010;363:1107–16.
70. Zwissler B, et al. Inhaled prostacyclin (PGI2) versus inhaled nitric oxide in adult respiratory distress syndrome. Am J Respir Crit Care Med. 1996;154:1671–7.
71. Walmrath D, et al. Direct comparison of inhaled nitric oxide and aerosolized prostacyclin in acute respiratory distress syndrome. Am J Respir Crit Care Med. 1996;153:991–6.
72. Dahlem P, van Aalderen WMC, de Neef M, Dijkgraaf MGW, Bos AP. Randomized controlled trial of aerosolized prostacyclin therapy in children with acute lung injury. Crit Care Med. 2004;32:1055–60.
73. Rossaint R, Pison U, Gerlach H, Falke KJ. Inhaled nitric oxide: its effects on pulmonary circulation and airway smooth muscle cells. Eur Heart J. 1993;14(Suppl I):133–40.
74. Benzing A, Geiger K. Inhaled nitric oxide lowers pulmonary capillary pressure and changes longitudinal distribution of pulmonary vascular resistance in patients with acute lung injury. Acta Anaesthesiol Scand. 1994;38:640–5.
75. Payen D, Groupe d'Etude sur le NO inhale au cours de lARDS GENOA, Vallet B. Results of the French prospective multicentric randomized double-blind placebo-controlled trial on inhaled nitric oxide (NO) in ARDS. Intensive Care Med. 1999;25:S166.
76. Lundin S, Mang H, Smithies M, Stenqvist O, Frostell C. Inhalation of nitric oxide in acute lung injury: results of a European Multicentre Study. The European Study Group of Inhaled Nitric Oxide. Intensive Care Med. 1999;25:911–9.
77. Dellinger RP, et al. Effects of inhaled nitric oxide in patients with acute respiratory distress syndrome: results of a randomized phase II trial. Inhaled Nitric Oxide in ARDS Study Group. Crit Care Med. 1998;26:15–23.
78. Taylor RW, et al. Low-dose inhaled nitric oxide in patients with acute lung injury: a randomized controlled trial. JAMA. 2004;291:1603–9.
79. Gebistorf F, Karam O, Wetterslev J, Afshari A. Inhaled nitric oxide for acute respiratory distress syndrome (ARDS) in children and adults. Cochrane Database Syst Rev. 2016;(66):CD002787.
80. Afshari A, Brok J, Møller AM, Wetterslev J. Aerosolized prostacyclin for acute lung injury (ALI) and acute respiratory distress syndrome (ARDS). Cochrane Database Syst Rev. 2010;(32):CD007733.
81. Torbic H, et al. Inhaled epoprostenol vs inhaled nitric oxide for refractory hypoxemia in critically ill patients. J Crit Care. 2013;28:844–8.
82. Bartlett RH, et al. Extracorporeal membrane oxygenation (ECMO) cardiopulmonary support in infancy. ASAIO J. 1976;22:80–93.
83. Hill JD, et al. Prolonged extracorporeal oxygenation for acute post-traumatic respiratory failure (shock-lung syndrome). Use of the Bramson membrane lung. N Engl J Med. 1972;286:629–34.
84. Zapol WM, et al. Extracorporeal membrane oxygenation in severe acute respiratory failure. A randomized prospective study. JAMA. 1979;242:2193–6.
85. Morris AH, et al. Randomized clinical trial of pressure-controlled inverse ratio ventilation and extracorporeal CO2 removal for adult respiratory distress syndrome. Am J Respir Crit Care Med. 1994;149:295–305.
86. Australia and New Zealand Extracorporeal Membrane Oxygenation (ANZ ECMO) Influenza Investigators, et al. Extracorporeal membrane oxygenation for 2009 influenza A(H1N1) acute respiratory distress syndrome. JAMA. 2009;302:1888–95.
87. Holzgraefe B, et al. Extracorporeal membrane oxygenation for pandemic H1N1 2009 respiratory failure. Minerva Anestesiol. 2010;76:1043–51.
88. Choi DS, et al. Extracorporeal life support and survival after out-of-hospital cardiac arrest in a nationwide registry: a propensity score-matched analysis. Resuscitation. 2016;99:26–32.
89. Schmidt M, et al. Mechanical ventilation during extracorporeal membrane oxygenation. Crit Care. 2014;18:203.
90. Brodie D, Bacchetta M. Extracorporeal membrane oxygenation for ARDS in adults. N Engl J Med. 2011;365:1905–14.
91. Schmidt M, Hodgson C, Combes A. Extracorporeal gas exchange for acute respiratory failure in adult patients: a systematic review. Crit Care. 2015;19:99.

92. Peek GJ, et al. Efficacy and economic assessment of conventional ventilatory support versus extracorporeal membrane oxygenation for severe adult respiratory failure (CESAR): a multicentre randomised controlled trial. Lancet. 2009;374:1351–63.
93. Vaquer S, de Haro C, Peruga P, Oliva JC, Artigas A. Systematic review and meta-analysis of complications and mortality of veno-venous extracorporeal membrane oxygenation for refractory acute respiratory distress syndrome. Ann Intensive Care. 2017;7:51.
94. Bein T, et al. A new pumpless extracorporeal interventional lung assist in critical hypoxemia/hypercapnia. Crit Care Med. 2006;34:1372–7.
95. Bein T, et al. Lower tidal volume strategy (≈3 ml/kg) combined with extracorporeal CO2 removal versus 'conventional' protective ventilation (6 ml/kg) in severe ARDS: the prospective randomized Xtravent-study. Intensive Care Med. 2013;39:847–56.
96. Wong JK, et al. Cannulation-related complications on Veno-arterial extracorporeal membrane oxygenation: prevalence and effect on mortality. Artif Organs. 2017;65:e7.
97. Biffi S, et al. Infections during extracorporeal membrane oxygenation: epidemiology, risk factors, pathogenesis and prevention. Int J Antimicrob Agents. 2017;50:9–16.
98. Lorusso R, et al. Neurologic injury in adults supported with Veno-venous extracorporeal membrane oxygenation for respiratory failure: findings from the extracorporeal life support organization database. Crit Care Med. 2017;1. https://doi.org/10.1097/CCM.0000000000002502.
99. Thiagarajan RR, et al. Extracorporeal Life Support Organization Registry International Report 2016. ASAIO J. 2017;63:60–7.
100. Zwischenberger JB, Lynch JE. Will CESAR answer the adult ECMO debate? Lancet. 2009;374:1307–8.

Acute Respiratory Distress Syndrome (ARDS)

19

Trista D. Reid and David A. Spain

Introduction

Acute respiratory distress syndrome (ARDS) is one of the more challenging conditions faced by clinicians in the intensive care unit (ICU), affecting a significant portion of mechanically ventilated patients. The syndrome, an acute inflammatory lung injury characterized by diffuse alveolar damage and hypoxic respiratory failure, develops in approximately 10% of all ICU admissions and 23% of intubated patients [1]. The burden of disease is significant, with the incidence of ARDS cited as high as 86 per 100,000 person-years and with a mortality of 40–50% in patients who develop this disease process [1, 2]. Many ARDS survivors have significant physical and neuropsychological impairments that are difficult to quantify. The financial burden is more tangible; the costs incurred on the healthcare system from prolonged ICU stays are substantial, and the individual patients continue to have medical costs that average about $5000 to $6000 per year per patient, long after the acute insult has resolved. In addition, survival and discharge from the hospital are only partial victories; one third of these patients are discharged to nursing homes, and 40% are readmitted to the hospital within 2 years of discharge [3, 4]. Given the impressive morbidity and mortality associated with ARDS, a comprehensive understanding of this condition is a vital component in the ICU clinician's arsenal. This chapter will discuss in depth the causes of ARDS, the available diagnostic tools currently used, and the evidence-based management strategies to combat this disease process.

T. D. Reid
Division of General and Acute Care Surgery, UNC Department of Surgery, University of North Carolina at Chapel Hill, Chapel Hill, NC, USA

D. A. Spain (✉)
Department of Surgery, Stanford University, Stanford, CA, USA
e-mail: dspain@stanford.edu

Definition

As a syndrome rather than a discreet disease, ARDS is comprised of a collection of symptoms, inevitably leading to a very nuanced and complex definition. The syndrome was initially described in 1967, with an official definition proposed by the American-European Consensus Conference (AECC) in 1994 [5, 6]. The definition was recently changed in 2011 with the goal of developing a more precise classification to improve reliability and validity in predicting mortality. Known as the Berlin Definition, this updated designation describes ARDS as an acute, diffuse inflammatory lung injury that causes alveolar damage, leading to hypoxia, increased vascular permeability, and decreased lung compliance.

The criteria divide the degree of lung injury into three categories based on the arterial partial pressure of oxygen to fraction of inspired oxygen ratio (PaO_2/FiO_2 ratio). Mild ARDS is defined as a PaO_2/FiO_2 ratio of 200 mmHg to 300 mmHg with positive end-expiratory pressure (PEEP) or continuous positive airway pressure (CPAP) greater than or equal to 5. The mild subset of ARDS allows for PEEP provided by noninvasive positive pressure ventilation. Moderate ARDS is defined as a PaO_2/FiO_2 ratio of 100 mmHg to 200 mmHg with a PEEP greater than or equal to 5, while severe ARDS is defined as a PaO_2/FiO_2 ratio of less than or equal to 100 mmHg with a PEEP greater than or equal to 5. The Berlin Definition adds a component of timing to the syndrome, stipulating that the condition must develop within 1 week of a known clinical insult or new or worsening respiratory symptoms. The process must be associated with bilateral opacities on chest imaging (chest radiograph or computed tomography scan) that are not fully explained by effusions, lobar/lung collapse, nodules, cardiac failure, or fluid overload. If no risk factors are present, an objective assessment such as echocardiography must be done to exclude hydrostatic edema [7]. Of note, the previous pulmonary artery wedge pressure criterion was removed as part of the newer definition secondary to diminishing use of pulmo-

A. Salim et al. (eds.), *Surgical Critical Care Therapy*, https://doi.org/10.1007/978-3-319-71712-8_19

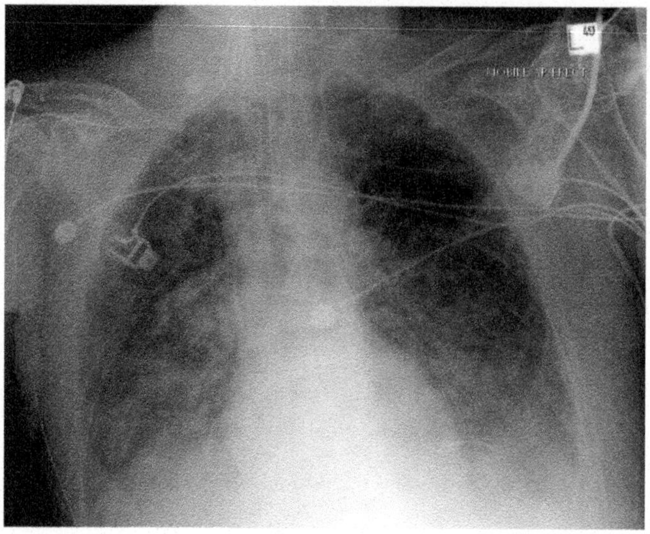

Fig. 19.1 Typical appearance of ARDS on chest radiography: heterogeneous bilateral patchy opacities *(Case courtesy of A.Prof Frank Gaillard, Radiopaedia.org, rID: 35985)*

nary artery catheters, as well as the understanding that concomitant fluid overload or cardiac failure may superimpose ARDS and thus these entities are not mutually exclusive. (Fig. 19.1, Table 19.1).

Causes

While 20% of ARDS cases do not have a discernable cause, most can be attributed to either direct lung injury or indirect damage provoked by systemic factors. The most common inciting events include aspiration and sepsis. Other provocations include bacterial and viral pneumonia, near drowning, smoke inhalation, pulmonary contusions, trauma in general, pancreatitis, blood transfusion, burns, medication overdose, cardiopulmonary bypass, and fat embolism. Additional risk factors for the development of ARDS include age, smoking, alcohol use, lactic acidosis, and hypoalbuminemia.

Diagnosis

As with most disease processes, diagnosis begins with the history and physical exam. Patients with ARDS develop dyspnea and hypoxic respiratory failure several hours to days after an inciting event. Physical exam may reveal fairly nonspecific findings of rales, tachypnea, tachycardia, and worsening oxygen requirements. Ruling out other treatable causes of dyspnea and hypoxia in the surgical patient is important. Tailored to each individual, a workup should consider the possibility of acute coronary syndrome, pulmonary embolism, postoperative intra-abdominal leak or infection, and pulmonary edema from volume overload, among others. Depending on the patient, this investigation may involve a full set of labs including complete blood count, complete metabolic panel, lipase, cardiac enzymes, cultures, brain natriuretic peptide, electrocardiogram, and imaging such as echocardiogram, plain films, or computed topography scan (CT). Blood gas analysis and radiographic confirmation of ARDS are inherent in the Berlin Definition and should be obtained. Regardless of whether or not ARDS has developed, correcting the underlying problem will expedite recovery.

Ultimately, the diagnosis of ARDS is dictated by the Berlin Definition guidelines. The calculated PaO_2/FiO_2 ratio is less than 300, and the severity is subdivided below this threshold as previously outlined. Diffuse or patchy bilateral pulmonary opacities develop on chest radiography (CXR) secondary to proteinaceous interstitial edema. Both CXR and CT are acceptable for diagnosis, although CT is a slightly better diagnostic tool. If the modality used is CT, consolidation is seen in the dependent regions of the lung early in the disease process, with a scattered background of ground-glass attenuation. Later, patchy reticular and ground-glass patterns can be seen, often in the nondependent areas of the lungs. This delayed presentation is often associated with pulmonary cysts or bullae. The imaging studies may completely normalize within 10–14 days; however as many as 76% of patients with ARDS will continue to have residual evidence of the syndrome on imaging [8, 9] (Figs. 19.2 and 19.3).

General Management Strategies

The management of ARDS is still in evolution. Because the syndrome is heterogeneous and provoked by disparate etiologies, not every patient is affected in the same way. Certain treatment regimens may work well in particular patient populations yet produce a limited response among others. As a result of this heterogeneity, some of the data available are contradictory or flawed, and many questions about treatment remain unanswered. The care is supportive at this point, focusing on allowing time for the damaged lungs to heal and addressing underlying correctable causes. The remainder of the chapter will focus on practical considerations in management and will discuss those evidence-based therapies that have been proven to reduce mortality, as well as some remedies that are in practice but have not yet demonstrated a mortality benefit.

Table 19.1 Berlin Definitions for ARDS

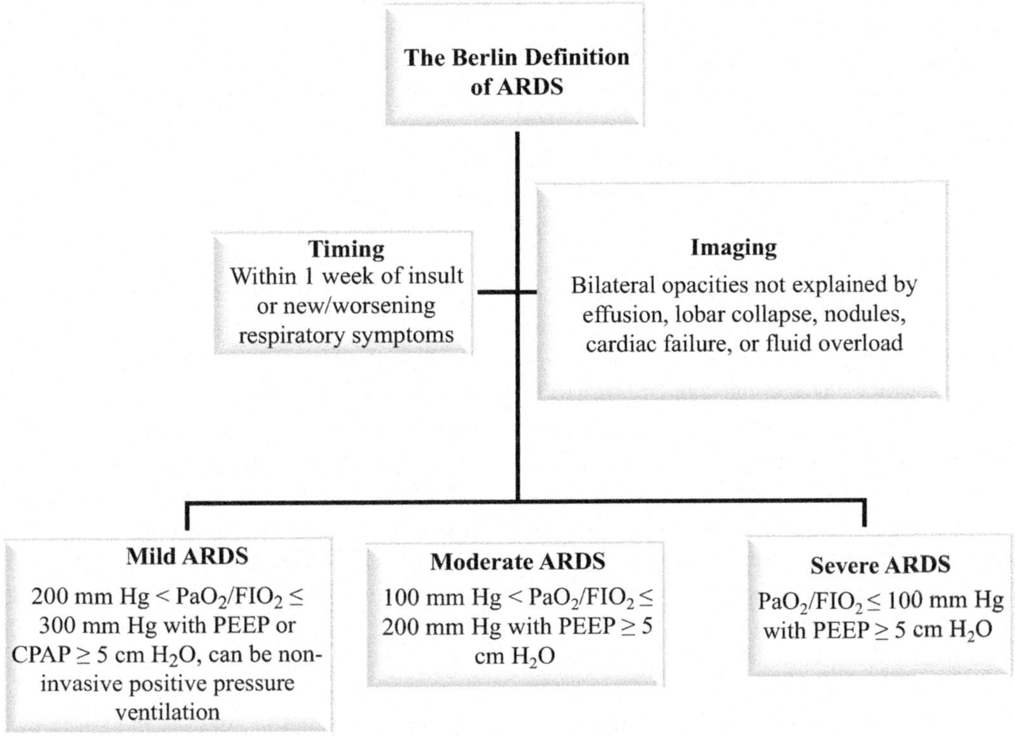

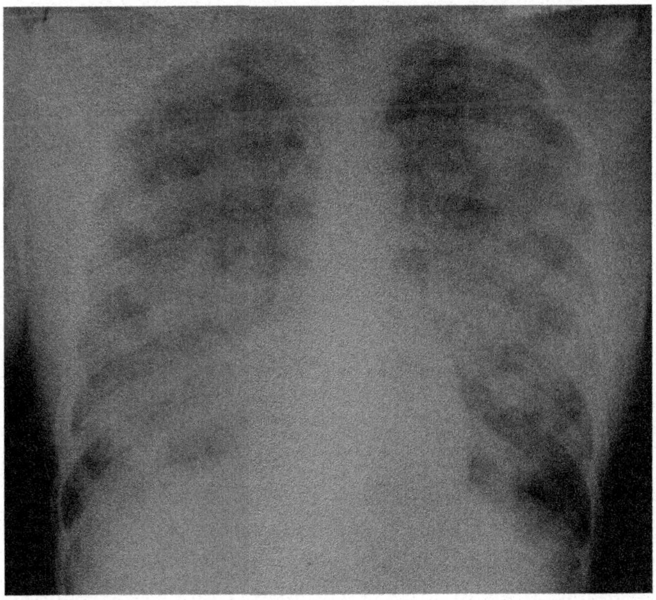

Fig. 19.2 Typical appearance of ARDS on chest radiograph: diffuse bilateral fluffy infiltrates *(Published with permission from learningradiology.com)*

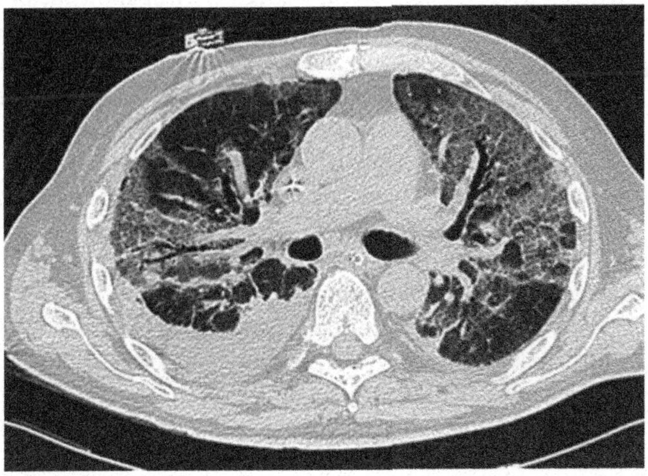

Fig. 19.3 Typical appearance of ARDS on CT: diffuse heterogeneous ground-glass opacities with thickened interlobular septa, more dense consolidation in dependent areas *(Courtesy of European Respiratory Review Dec 2014;23(134):519–30;* https://doi.org/10.1183/09059180.00001314*)*

Low Tidal Volume Ventilation

In 2000, the Acute Respiratory Distress Syndrome Network (ARDSNET) published results that revolutionized ventilator management in ARDS. A total of 861 patients from 10 US centers were randomized to traditional tidal volumes of 12 milliliters per kilogram (mL/kg) versus low tidal volumes of 6 mL/kg. The study determined that lower tidal volume ventilation reduced mortality from 39.8% to 31% and improved both ventilator-free days and days without non-pulmonary organ or system failure [10]. These findings are supported by several meta-analyses that have also shown decreased mortality with lower tidal volume ventilation; thus the low tidal volume strategy has become standard in ARDS management [11, 12]. Based on the goals in the ARDSNET trial, most centers aim for tidal volumes of 4–6 mL/kg and target plateau pressures less than or equal to 30 cm H_2O. The plateaus can be checked after any change to the ventilator or every 4 h. Plateau pressures greater than 30 may be adjusted by decreasing tidal volumes to as low as 4 mL/kg as needed.

Lower tidal volume ventilation may lead to a reduction in overall minute ventilation and resultant elevation in partial pressure of carbon dioxide (pCO_2). Termed "permissive hypercapnia," a certain amount of respiratory acidosis is conceded in order to prevent alveolar hyperinflation and is generally tolerated by the patients. Clinicians can minimize dead space in ventilator tubing and increase the respiratory rate to as high as 35 breaths per minute as needed to prevent excessive acidosis. However, most centers will allow the pH to fall to as low as 7.2 without correction, regardless of the pCO_2. While some might argue that even lower levels of pH could be tolerated, letting the pH drift below this threshold raises concerns for exacerbating arrhythmias, acute coronary syndrome, cerebral edema, seizures, and hypotension, among other deleterious sequelae [13].

Besides acidosis and hypercapnia, lower tidal volumes may provoke asynchrony and breath stacking. Higher respiratory rates used to counteract the reduction in minute ventilation can result in auto-PEEP. Tactics to alleviate breath stacking include increasing sedation levels or, if this approach fails, modestly increasing tidal volumes to 7–8 mL/kg while continuing to maintain a plateau airway pressure of less than 30 cm H_20. Although auto-PEEP is usually not a significant issue, when it occurs the ultimate solution may be to lower the respiratory rate and permit hypercapnia or alter the inspiratory-to-expiratory ratio to allow more time for expiration. If the problem is tachypnea produced by the patient over-breathing the set ventilator rate, escalating sedation may help.

Improving Oxygenation: PEEP and Other Strategies

In terms of oxygenation in ARDS, the objective is to titrate the FiO_2 below 0.7 while maintaining an arterial oxygen content greater than 55 mmHg and saturations of greater than 88%. The PEEP is set to at least 5 cm H_2O. Theoretically, a higher level of PEEP would prevent atelectrauma by reducing cyclical airway collapse and potentially homogenize ventilation, lessening ventilation perfusion mismatch. Increasing the PEEP will enhance oxygenation to help achieve these oxygenation goals; however currently the evidence does not support any improvement in mortality with changes in PEEP. A 2013 Cochrane review meta-analysis of 2565 patients with patients randomized to high versus low PEEP demonstrated better oxygenation in the high PEEP arm and no difference in mortality or ventilator-free days between the two groups. The researchers noted a trend toward improved mortality among the high PEEP group, without any indication of barotrauma caused by the augmented PEEP [14].

A 2010 meta-analysis demonstrated an improvement in oxygenation and ventilator-free days, as well as reduction in ICU mortality among patients treated with higher levels of PEEP. However, no appreciable change in hospital mortality was noted, and in subgroup analysis, only patients with a PaO_2/FiO_2 ratio of $\leq$200 mmHg truly seemed to benefit in terms of ICU mortality [15]. Considering these data, clinicians may use PEEP as needed to reduce FiO_2 and to preserve oxygenation targets, but the impetus to raise PEEP above these goals is uncertain.

In the subpopulation of patients with moderate to severe ARDS who are persistently hypoxemic, elevating the PEEP to as high as 22–24 cm H_2O may be advantageous, and in these cases, a higher PEEP strategy may be the answer. In the Assessment of Low Tidal Volume and Elevated End-Expiratory Volume to Obviate Lung Injury (ALVEOLI) trial, PEEP as high as 34 cm H_2O was employed in severely hypoxic patients [16]. Table 19.2 outlines the stepwise approach in escalating PEEP and FiO_2 developed in this trial and used by some centers to achieve oxygenation goals of PaO_2 55–80 mmHg and oxygen saturation of 88–95%. As discussed above, the higher PEEP approach can be instituted depending on individual patient characteristics.

In patients that are persistently hypoxic in spite of increasing levels of PEEP, some additional approaches are available. If the hypoxia is partially driven by dyssynchrony on the ventilator, deepening sedation, proning the patient, or addition of paralytics may be beneficial. Some of these

Table 19.2 ARDSNET use of low and high PEEP

Lower PEEP arm														
FiO_2	0.3	0.4	0.4	0.5	0.5	0.6	0.7	0.7	0.7	0.8	0.9	0.9	0.9	1.0
PEEP	5	5	8	8	10	10	10	12	14	14	14	16	18	18–24
Higher PEEP arm														
FiO_2	0.3	0.3	0.4	0.4	0.5	0.5	0.5–0.8	0.8	0.9	1.0				
PEEP	12	14	14	16	16	18	20	22	22	22–24				

Adapted from Browder et al. [33]

options are further discussed at length below. Increasing the inspiratory time may allow for additional alveolar recruitment and increased mean airway pressure, although this tactic may not be applied in every patient; the concomitant decrease in expiratory time can lead to worsening hypercapnia and acidosis, as well as auto-PEEP, air trapping, and barotrauma.

Open Lung Ventilation

While uncertainty surrounds the appropriate level of PEEP to use in ARDS patients, some studies have attempted to bundle ventilator interventions. Open lung ventilation is a combination of low tidal volume ventilation and higher PEEP to prevent overinflation while at the same time preventing cyclic alveolar collapse. A few smaller investigations have shown a decrease in mortality with this tactic, although methodological flaws have prevented the strategy from being fully accepted. The previously discussed meta-analyses that examined high versus low PEEP did use low tidal volumes in both groups and did not demonstrate a survival benefit. Further inspection of this technique is required.

Driving Pressure

Lung-protective mechanical ventilation strategies can have variable components that do not always work in concert. Often manipulation of one of these factors leads to unintended effects, such as elevation of the plateau pressure when the PEEP is increased or breath stacking or severe acidosis at lower tidal volumes. The proportion of lung available for ventilation is different for each patient; so, using a tidal volume based on predicted body weight could over- or underestimate ventilator needs.

Armato et al. looked at the ratio of tidal volume to respiratory system compliance as a way to indicate the functional size of the lung and to optimize lung-protective ventilation [17]. The researchers determined that this ratio, known as driving pressure (ΔP), was the variable most strongly associated with survival. Tidal volume and PEEP were not independently associated with survival unless they led to a decreased in ΔP. Although causality cannot be completely established based on the study, this evidence supports the hypothesis that variations in compliance and ΔP are relevant in lung-protective strategies. Additionally, these findings may explain why higher PEEP seems to be of benefit in patients with greater lung recruitability; elevations in PEEP may be effective only if an unchanged tidal volume is delivered at a lower driving pressure [17, 18]. Other data has revealed that ΔP, plateau pressure, and compliance are equally predictive of mortality; thus having knowledge of one or all three of these factors can help drive management [19].

Based on all the data accumulated on low tidal volumes, open lung ventilation, high vs low PEEP, and ΔP, lung-protective strategies focus on multiple variables and should be tailored to the individual patient. Keep the tidal volumes in the 4–6 mL/kg range if possible while reducing plateau pressures to less than or equal to 30. If using driving pressure, the aim is to maintain ΔP in the less than or equal to 13 cm H_2O range. Allow for hypercapnia, preserving a pH of greater than or equal to 7.2. Patients with severe ARDS who have greater lung recruitability may benefit from higher PEEP, and higher PEEP may be used to lower the FiO_2 below 0.7 while conserving a PaO_2 of greater than or equal to 55 and an oxygen saturation of greater than or equal to 88%. Even in individual patients, the disease process is dynamic, and having a protocol to adjust as compliance changes is beneficial. Of note, having a written procedure for ARDS management in the ICU has correlated with better compliance to lung-protective ventilation strategies [20].

Additional Management Adjuncts

Recruitment Maneuvers

Recruitment maneuvers assist in oxygenation by expanding collapsed alveoli through a transitory burst of continuous positive pressure at 30–40 cm H_2O for 40–60 s. Alternatively, the respiratory therapist can give three consecutive sighs per minute with a plateau pressure of 45 cm H_2O. These exercises have been shown to increase the PaO_2 but do not affect mortality in ARDS [21]. Although the tactic does not change mortality, it can be constructive in patients that have been briefly disconnected from the ventilator or experienced de-recruitment of some other form. Be aware that the maneuvers can cause hypotension secondary to transient decreased venous return, and repeated attempts can cause overinflation of the fragile alveolar sacs.

Prone Positioning

Another tool in the ICU clinician's armamentarium is prone positioning. A 2013 trial randomized 466 patients with severe early ARDS to supine versus prone positioning, which involved the patients being completely prone for at least 16 consecutive hours a day. The 28-day and 90-day mortality were significantly improved in the prone arm, without increase in adverse events such as cardiac arrest, unplanned extubation, or mainstemming of the endotracheal tube [22].

Several issues preclude this strategy's generalized use. Certain postsurgical patients such as patients with open abdomens, complex abdominal wall reconstructions, and large hernia repairs and morbidly obese patients may not be candidates for proning. Particularly in certain populations in the United States where the overall percentage of obese patients is higher, recruiting the manpower to prone an overweight patient may be logistically infeasible. Some centers do not have the personnel required to prone a large number of patients. That being said, in a poorly oxygenated patient with early severe ARDS and an appropriate body habitus, clinicians should consider proning if safe and resources are available to do so.

Neuromuscular Blockade

Neuromuscular paralysis is an available stratagem in ARDS, but this practice does have some limitations. A 2010 investigation performed in France evaluated patients diagnosed with severe ARDS within the previous 48 h and randomized them to either 48 h of cisatracurium or placebo. The cisatracurium arm demonstrated significantly improved 28-day and 90-day mortality, as well as increased ventilator-free days and organ-failure-free days [23]. The study had some flaws and was underpowered, yet some basic practical concerns also must be considered, including the potential development of critical illness polyneuromyopathy (CIPM). While the trial noted no significant difference in the development of ICU paresis with short-term paralysis versus placebo, neuromuscular blocking agents have been linked to CIPM, which has in turn been associated with increased mortality, length of stay in the ICU and hospital, and ventilator dependence.

In addition, patients who are paralyzed must also receive adequate levels of sedation, which can lead to hypotension and worsen delirium. Cisatracurium itself may cause bradycardia, hypotension, or flushing. Given these practical considerations, cisatracurium should be used judiciously and on an individualized basis. Unlike some neuromuscular blocking agents, cisatracurium can be used in renal and hepatic failure. In patients with early severe ARDS who are having issues with oxygenation or dyssynchrony on the ventilator, cisatracurium may be helpful. The patients that do undergo paralysis should be minimized to less than 48 h on the agent. If using train-of-four monitoring, the goal is one to two twitches out of four. If train-of-four monitoring is not available, clinical assessment alone may be acceptable; studies comparing train-of-four monitoring versus clinical assessment of neuromuscular blockade in the ICU have demonstrated mixed outcomes. As mentioned, deep sedation should be achieved before initiating blockade, and many centers employ bispectral index (BIS) monitoring.

Extracorporeal Membrane Oxygenation (ECMO)

Although not every center will have ECMO available, this salvage therapy can be considered in patients with persistent hypoxia in spite of maximal support. Initial studies of ECMO in ARDS did not look promising; however since the 1970s, ECMO techniques and protocols have been refined and selection criteria have changed. Veno-venous access is now used for pulmonary specific processes, lower levels of anticoagulation are employed, and the patients are rested on the ventilator with lung-protective strategies. The Conventional Ventilator Support Versus ECMO for Severe Adult Respiratory Failure (CESAR) randomized controlled trial looked at adult patients with potentially reversible severe respiratory failure as evidenced by a Murray score of more than three or pH of less than 7.2. The investigation noted survival without severe morbidity at 6 months to be significantly improved from 47% in the conventional group to 63% in the ECMO group [24]. Although the survival benefit could be attributable to ECMO, it may also have been secondary to transfer to a large ECMO center with protocols in place. Current trials are in progress to elucidate this question further.

Contraindications to ECMO include inability to be anticoagulated, metastatic cancer or other disease processes that are likely to significantly shorten the patient's lifespan, severe brain injury or intracranial hemorrhage, high pressure or high FiO_2 ventilation for greater than 7 days, or other irreversible lung conditions that are unlikely to improve with time. ECMO should be considered in patients with severe ARDS with PaO_2/FiO_2 ratios persistently less than 80 despite the application of high levels of PEEP, Murray score greater than three, hypercapnia with acidemia of pH less than 7.15 in spite of ventilator optimization, or excessive plateau pressures greater than 35–45 cm H_2O depending on the patient's body habitus.

Ventilator Modes

In general, the optimal ventilator mode is one that allows full support, such as assist control. Although volume limited ventilation facilitates clinician adherence to a low tidal volume strategy, pressure control is also adequate as long as the tidal volumes are stable within the target range. The choice may be driven by clinician familiarity with a particular mode.

Airway pressure release ventilation (APRV) is an inverse ratio, pressure-controlled, intermittent mandatory ventilation that allows spontaneous breathing and occasionally is used as a rescue therapy to recruit more alveoli in persistently hypoxic patients. While this mode enhances oxygenation temporarily, studies have not shown any benefit in mortality. No major harms have been noted; thus this setting may be used in ARDS. While smaller outdated studies had demonstrated potential promise in high-frequency oscillatory ventilation (HFOV) in ARDS management, a larger multicenter randomized controlled trial revealed that HFOV may actually augment mortality in early ARDS [25]. Based on these findings, HFOV is no longer recommended in adult ARDS patients.

Other Management Considerations

Inhaled Nitric Oxide

The pulmonary vasodilatory prowess of inhaled nitric oxide (iNO) is a well-described supplemental approach to enhancing oxygenation. Unfortunately, this medication will augment PaO_2 and oxygen saturations without any improvement in mortality. A 2004 trial of 385 patients with ARDS randomized the patients to 5 parts per million of iNO versus placebo and noted no change in any clinically relevant outcomes, including mortality. Institution of iNO did result in a temporary increase in PaO_2; however this difference did not last beyond 24–48 h [26]. In addition, the high costs of the drug are prohibitive; most centers have difficulty justifying $115–130 /hour for a medication that does not change outcomes in ARDS.

Steroids

Similarly, the use of steroids in ARDS is not indicated. Multiple trials of early corticosteroid administration in ARDS revealed no benefit in survival. Likewise, an ARDSNET trial looking at methylprednisolone therapy delivered 7 days or more after the onset of ARDS noted no improvement in mortality. Corticosteroids did improve the number of ventilator-free and shock-free days, as well as improved oxygenation, respiratory system compliance, and blood pressure; however in patients enrolled at least 14 days after the onset of ARDS, a significantly increased mortality was discovered [27].

Antiviral and Antibiotic Therapy

Although no data support the routine use of antiviral medications or antibiotics in all patients with ARDS, timely administration of antivirals in the case of H1N1 influenza infections (within 48 h) and antibiotics for bacterial pneumonia is recommended. Principally, in H1N1-induced ARDS, patients are more likely to have severe ARDS and require ECMO; thus current guidelines advocate for antivirals early in the disease course. Intravenous antibodies and other immune modulating therapies have no survival benefit in ARDS.

Esophageal Balloon and Transpulmonary Pressures

Particularly in obese patients, setting an appropriate level of PEEP is difficult, beyond the basic uncertainties surrounding proper PEEP levels in ARDS. Preferably, the ventilator should supply enough transpulmonary pressure (airway pressure–pleural pressure) to oxygenate the patient while preventing cyclic airway collapse. Measuring pressures via an esophageal balloon placed 40 cm from the incisors can be a surrogate for pleural pressure. A small randomized controlled trial used esophageal manometry to guide PEEP titration, noting higher levels of PEEP, improved PaO_2/FiO_2 ratios, and better compliance in the esophageal balloon arm with only a trend toward improved mortality [28]. Routine use of manometry is not indicated in ARDS based on these findings, although esophageal balloons may be useful in obese patients with hypoxia to help steer pressure goals. Larger trials may elucidate this issue further.

Fluid Management

Regarding fluid management in ARDS, a judicious approach is suggested while still treating septic shock adequately and maintaining urine output. To date, the data do not definitively support a reduction in mortality with conservative fluid management. In theory, a diminution in pulmonary edema should yield better gas exchange. The ARDSNET group looked at conservative versus liberal fluid management and did note an improvement in the oxygenation index and lung injury scores, as well as an increase in ventilator-free days. Conservative fluid management did not lead reduce mortality or augment non-pulmonary organ failures [29].

Nutrition

Early enteral nutrition is recommended as soon as feasible in mechanically ventilated patients. In 2012, the EDEN trial determined that a strategy of initial trophic enteral feeding for up to 6 days did not improve ventilator-free days, 60-day mortality, or infectious complications but was associated with less gastrointestinal intolerance compared to full enteral feeding [30]. Given the higher caloric demands on the body during states of stress, the clinician should initiate full enteral feeds if tolerated. Some evidence exists to support use of an inflammatory modulating formula rich in ω-3 fatty acids (eicosapentaenoic acid and gamma-linoleic acid) in ARDS; however more data are needed to verify these findings [31].

Mobilization

In general, early mobilization of ICU patients leads to improved functional outcomes and, in some studies, decreased length of ICU and hospital stay. In patients that have acutely decompensated, bedrest with head-of-bed elevation may be the only safe option initially. Therapists should still perform active and passive range of motion on these patients. Ultimately, mobilization may improve functional status in stable ARDS patients that are appropriate for this intervention [32].

Conclusions

ARDS remains a nuanced and complex disease process, and management must be tailored to the individual patient. Low tidal volume ventilation of 4–6 mL/kg is the mainstay of mechanical ventilator therapy, allowing for permissive hypercapnia and targeting plateau pressures of less than or equal to 30. The exact PEEP target is uncertain; however in patients that are experiencing hypoxia below a PaO_2 of 55 or oxygen saturations less than 88%, increasing levels of PEEP will improve oxygenation and may be beneficial in a subset of severe ARDS patients. Driving pressures and compliance should be taken into consideration, although more investigations are needed in these areas. Adjuncts such as proning and neuromuscular blockade are useful tools but may not be appropriate for every patient. The clinician should focus on maximum support on the ventilator initially, although a specific ventilator mode has not been identified to improve mortality. ECMO is an acceptable rescue strategy in populations that qualify.

Treating the underlying cause of the patient's decompensation is important, whether that care involves judicious fluid resuscitation, source control, and antibiotics for sepsis or stopping an offending medication causing pancreatitis. Early enteral nutrition and mobilization may be instituted when tolerated and safe based on clinical judgment. Finally, a written institutional protocol for ARDS ensures better compliance with the interventions that are known to improve mortality in ARDS. The intensive care clinician community is continuing to gain insight on how to combat this grave syndrome, and management strategies will hopefully become more refined as further studies are completed.

References

1. Bellani G, Laffey JG, Pham T, et al. for the LUNG SAFE Investigators and the ESICM Trials Group. Epidemiology, patterns of care, and mortality for patients with acute respiratory distress syndrome in intensive care units in 50 countries. JAMA. 2016;315(8):788–800.
2. Rubenfeld GD, Caldwell E, Peabody E, et al. Incidence and outcomes of acute lung injury. N Engl J Med. 2005;16:1685–93.
3. Herridge MS, Tansey CM, Matte A, et al. for the Canadian Critical Cares Trials Group. Functional disability 5 years after acute respiratory distress syndrome. N Engl J Med. 2011;364(14):1293–304.
4. Cheung AM, Tansey CM, Tomlinson G, et al. for the Canadian Critical Care Trials Group. Two year outcomes, health care use, and costs of survivors of acute respiratory distress syndrome. Am J Resp and Crit Care Med. 2006;174(5):538–44.
5. Ashbaugh DG, Bigelow DB, Petty TL, Levine BE. Acute respiratory distress in adults. Lancet. 1967;2(7511):319–23.
6. Bernard GR, Artigas A, Brigham KL, et al. The American-European consensus conference on ARDS: definitions, mechanisms, relevant outcomes, and clinical trial coordination. Am J Respir Crit Care Med. 1994;149(3 pt 1):818–24.
7. Ranieri VM, Rubenfeld GB, Thompson BT, et al. The ARDS definition task force. Acute respiratory distress syndrome the berlin definition. JAMA. 2012;307(23):2526–33.
8. Masclans JR, Roca O, Munoz X, et al. Quality of life, pulmonary function, and tomographic scan abnormalities after ARDS. Chest. 2011;139(6):1340–6.
9. Figueroa-Casas JB, Brunner N, Dwivedi AK, Ayyappan AP. Accuracy of the chest radiograph to identify bilateral pulmonary infiltrates consistent with the diagnosis of acute respiratory distress syndrome using computed tomography as reference standard. J Crit Care. 2013;28(4):352–7.
10. The Acute Respiratory Distress Syndrome Network. Ventilation with lower tidal volumes as compared with traditional tidal volumes for acute lung injury and the acute respiratory distress syndrome. N Engl J Med. 2000;342:1301–8.
11. Putensen C, Theuerkauf N, Zinserling J, et al. Meta-analysis: ventilation strategies and outcomes of the acute respiratory distress syndrome and acute lung injury. Ann Intern Med. 2009;151(8):566–76.
12. Petrucci N, De Feo C. Lung protective ventilation strategy for the acute respiratory distress syndrome. Cochrane Database Syst Rev. 2013;(2):CD003844.

13. Richecoeur J, Lu Q, Vieira SR, et al. Expiratory washout versus optimization of mechanical ventilation during permissive hypercapnia in patients with severe acute respiratory distress syndrome. Am J Respir Crit Care Med. 1999;160:77.
14. Santa Cruz R, Rojas JI, Nervi R, et al. High versus low positive end-expiratory pressure (PEEP) levels for mechanically ventilated adult patients with acute lung injury and acute respiratory distress syndrome. Cochrane Database Syst Rev. 2013;(6):CD009098.
15. Briel M, Meade M, Mercat A, et al. Higher vs lower positive end-expiratory pressure in patients with acute lung injury and acute respiratory distress syndrome: systematic review and meta-analysis. JAMA. 2010;303:865.
16. Browder RG, Lanken PN, MacIntyre N, et al. The National Heart, Lung, and Blood Institute ARDS Clinical Trials Network. Higher versus lower positive end-expiratory pressures in patients with the acute respiratory distress syndrome. NEJM. 2004;351(4):327–36.
17. Armato MB, Meade MO, Slutsky AS, et al. Driving pressure and survival in the acute respiratory distress syndrome. NEJM. 2015;372(8):747–55.
18. Grasso S, Fanelli V, Cafarelli A, et al. Effects of high versus low positive end expiratory pressures in acute respiratory distress syndrome. Am J Respir Crit Care Med. 2005;171:1002–8.
19. Guérin C, Papazian L, Reignier J, et al. Investigators of the Acurasys and Proseva trials. Effect of driving pressure on mortality in ARDS patients during lung protective mechanical ventilation in two randomized controlled trials. Crit Care. 2016;20(1):384.
20. Umoh NJ, Fan E, Mendez-Tellez PA, et al. Patient and intensive care unit organizational factors associated with low tidal volume ventilation in acute lung injury. Crit Care Med. 2008;36(5):1463–8.
21. Hodgson C, Keating JL, Holland AE, et al. Recruitment manoeuvres for adults with acute lung injury receiving mechanical ventilation. Cochrane Database Syst Rev. 2009;(11):CD006667.
22. Guérin C, Reignier J, Richard J, et al. Prone positioning in severe acute respiratory distress syndrome. NEJM. 2013;368(23):2159–68.
23. Papazian L, Forel J, Gacouin A, et al. Neuromuscular blockade in early acute respiratory distress syndrome. NEJM. 2010;363(12):1107–16.
24. Peek GJ, Mugford M, Tiruvoipati R, et al. CESAR trial collaboration. Efficacy and economic assessment of conventional ventilatory support versus extracorporeal membrane oxygenation for severe adult respiratory failure (CESAR): a multicentre randomised controlled trial. Lancet. 2009;374(9698):1351–63.
25. Ferguson ND, Cook DJ, Guyatt GH, et al. High frequency oscillation in early acute respiratory distress syndrome. NEJM. 2013;368(9):795–805.
26. Taylor RW, Zimmerman JL, Dellinger RP, et al. for the Inhaled Nitric Oxide in ARDS Study Group. Low-dose inhaled nitric oxide in patients with acute lung injury. A randomized controlled trial. JAMA. 2004;291(13):1603–9.
27. Steinberg KP, Hudson LD, Goodman RB, et al. National Heart, Lung, and Blood Institute Acute Respiratory Distress Syndrome Clinical Trials Network. Efficacy and safety of corticosteroids for persistent acute respiratory distress syndrome. NEJM. 2006;354(16):1671–84.
28. Talmor D, Sarge T, Malhotra A, et al. Mechanical ventilation guided by esophageal pressure in acute lung injury. NEJM. 2008;359(20):2905–104.
29. Wiedmann HP, Wheeler AP, Thompson BT, et al. National Heart, Lung, and Blood Institute Acute Respiratory Distress Syndrome Clinical Trials Network. Comparison of two fluid management strategies in acute lung injury. NEJM. 2006;354(24):2564–75.
30. Rice TW, Wheeler AP, Thompson BT, et al. National Heart, Lung, and Blood Institute Acute Respiratory Distress Syndrome Clinical Trials Network. Initial trophic vs full enteral feeding in patients with acute lung injury: the EDEN randomized trial. JAMA. 2012;307(8):795–803.
31. Pontes-Arruda A, Aragão AM, Albuquerque JD. Effects of enteral feeding with eicosapentaenoic acid, gamma-linoleic acid, and antioxidants in mechanically ventilated patients with severe sepsis and septic shock. Crit Care Med. 2006;34(9):2525–33.
32. Walsh CJ, Batt J, Herridge MS, Dos Santos CC. Muscle wasting and early mobilization in acute respiratory distress syndrome. Clin Chest Med. 2014;35(4):811–26.
33. Browder RG, Lanken PN, MacIntyre N, et al. The National Heart, Lung, and Blood Institute ARDS Clinical Trials Network. Higher versus lower positive end-expiratory pressures in patients with the acute respiratory distress syndrome. NEJM. 2000;352:1301–8.

Care of the Postoperative Pulmonary Resection Patient

20

John Kuckelman and Daniel G. Cuadrado

Indications for Admission to the ICU

Indication for Surgery

Lung cancer remains the predominate indication for pulmonary resection. Estimates from the American Cancer Society in the United States for 2017 report that 220,500 new cases of lung cancer will be diagnosed. Of these, only 10–15% present with disease that is potentially surgically curable. The same risk factors for the development of lung cancer place these patients at risk for other comorbid diseases such as coronary artery disease (CAD) and chronic obstructive pulmonary disease (COPD).

Anatomic pulmonary resection remains the gold standard treatment in medically operable patients with early-stage malignancies. Based on the NCCN guidelines, determination of resectability, surgical staging, and resection should be performed by a board-certified thoracic surgeon with patients undergoing a multidisciplinary evaluation.

Current recommendations guiding the preoperative evaluation of patients for pulmonary resection along with improved minimally invasive techniques will expand the number of patients that are offered pulmonary resection for non-small cell lung cancer (NSCLC) [1]. We can expect the number of patients who would have once been deemed physiologically inoperable to decrease. By increasing the number of early-stage diagnosis with low-dose CT scan (LDCT) lung cancer screening programs, we can expect an increasing population of higher-risk surgical candidates [2].

J. Kuckelman
Department of Surgery, Madigan Army Medical Center, Joint Base Lewis-McChord, Tacoma, WA, USA

D. G. Cuadrado (✉)
General and Thoracic Surgery, Department of Surgery, Madigan Army Medical Center, Tacoma, WA, USA
e-mail: daniel.g.cuadrado.mil@mail.mil

Admission Criteria: Planned Versus Unplanned

Routine postoperative admission to the ICU has been suggested for patients over the age of 70, ASA > II and preexisting fibrotic lung disease [3]. In general, ICU admission should be reserved for postoperative organ failure, high-risk patients, and complex surgical resections. Around 6.3–18% of patients undergoing pulmonary resection will require unplanned admission to intensive care postoperatively [4–7]. Table 20.1 lists the criteria for considering planned admission to intensive care.

Examination of the Society of Thoracic Surgeons (STS) database and other large series demonstrate that the perioperative mortality rate for all resections is around 2–4% [8, 9]. Independent predictors of mortality include pneumonectomy, bilobectomy, ASA, renal dysfunction, induction therapy, steroids, age, and urgent procedures [8]. Pneumonectomy in particular carries an inhospital and 90-day mortality rate of upward of 10% [8–10].

Patients undergoing diagnostic lung biopsy for interstitial lung disease represent a unique population deserving additional attention. A recent review of around 12,000 patients undergoing lung biopsy in the United States shows that these patients have a mortality of 1.7% for elective procedures [11]. This increases dramatically for nonelective procedures up to 16% [12].

Postoperative complications remain the main reason for admission to the ICU. Complications requiring reoperation are uncommon occurring in around 4% of cases. Bleeding represents the majority of these cases and is most often associated with technical issues or preoperative anticoagulants [13].

More than half of patients requiring salvage intensive care postoperatively require some degree of respiratory support. Those requiring mechanical ventilation, renal replacement therapy, or both have mortality rates upward of 70% [14].

Cardiopulmonary bypass is a well-established adjunct in allowing for extended thoracic resections [15, 16]. Extracorporeal membrane oxygenation (ECMO) as a means of salvage from cardiopulmonary failure may be an option in select institutions; however, long-term data in this population are lacking [17–19].

A. Salim et al. (eds.), *Surgical Critical Care Therapy*, https://doi.org/10.1007/978-3-319-71712-8_20

Table 20.1 Factors for consideration of planned postoperative admission to intensive care

Patient factors	Physiologic factors	Procedural factors
Pulmonary fibrosis	PPO FEV1/DLCO <30%	Pneumonectomy
Induction chemoradiotherapy	VO_2max <15 ml/kg/min	Carinal resection
Elevated ASA/poor performance status	Preoperative $PaCO_2$ >50 mmHg	Extended resection with cardiopulmonary bypass
Urgent/emergent surgery		Lung transplant
BMI > 40		

Functional Status

The preoperative physiologic assessment of patients being considered for pulmonary resection is performed using a systematic approach. As noted in the clinical practice guidelines published in Chest in 2013, age alone is not a factor, and it is recommended that all patients with resectable disease be evaluated for surgery [1].

The forced expiratory volume in 1 second (FEV1) and diffusing capacity for carbon monoxide (DLCO) are obtained during standard pulmonary function tests (PFTs) and provide a good noninvasive initial assessment. The predicted postoperative (PPO) FEV1 and DLCO can be calculated taking into account the number of bronchopulmonary segments to be resected. In patients in which PPO FEV1 and PPO DLCO are >60% predicted, no further testing is required prior to resection [1].

Low-technology exercises tests, such as the stair climb (>12 m), can be utilized in cases were either PPO FEV1 or DLCO is >30 but <60% predicted. Formal exercise testing with cardiopulmonary exercise testing (CPET) and a calculation of maximal oxygen consumption (VO_2 max) is reserved for patients with PPO FEV1/DLCO <30% predicted. A VO_2max <10 ml/kg/min or 35% predicted is a contraindication to major resection as it is associated with a high rate of mortality [1].

Patients with a preexisting cardiac disease, symptoms consistent with angina, heart failure, or the inability to climb two flights of stairs should receive a formal cardiology evaluation. As recommended in the Chest guidelines, smoking cessation, cardiac evaluation, and preoperative pulmonary rehabilitation are ways to mitigate poor outcomes in high-risk candidates.

Procedural Considerations

Surgical complexity varies greatly, and the resection needed depends on tumor size, adjacent organ involvement, prior ipsilateral operations, and proximity to the hilar vessels. The surgical approach may range from thoracotomy (posterolateral, axillary, muscle sparing), sternotomy, video-assisted thoracoscopic surgery (VATS), and robotic video-assisted thoracoscopic surgery (RVATS).

A recent review of the National Cancer Database examined patients undergoing surgery for stage I–IIIA NSCLC. During the 2-year time period from 2010 to 2012, 62,000 lobectomies were performed. The vast majority were performed via thoracotomy (73%) followed by VATS (21%) and robotic (6%) [20]. Other than a 1-day reduction in hospital stay, VATS and robotic lobectomy are equivalent in terms of morbidity, mortality, and long-term oncologic outcomes [21].

For patients undergoing anatomic lobectomy, segmentectomy, or non-anatomic resection, the rate of morbidity and mortality is low [8]. When comparing VATS to open lobectomy, patient undergoing VATS have a mortality and pulmonary morbidity rate of 2.5–26.2% compared to 7.8–45.5% with thoracotomy [22]. In patients with predicted postoperative FEV1 or DLCO <40%, mortality and complication rates are reduced by more than half with VATS over an open approach [23].

Extensive resections such as pneumonectomy or extrapleural pneumonectomy have higher rates of morbidity and mortality [8–10]. Sleeve resections are performed as a parenchymal sparing approach in anatomically favorable tumors but require bronchial anastomosis. Although more technically complex, sleeve resection offers better early- and long-term survival in large part due to preservation of lung function [12].

Neoadjuvant Therapy

Patients with locally advanced, but resectable, disease can be considered for surgery following either chemotherapy or concurrent chemoradiation. In reviewing patients that have undergone neoadjuvant therapy followed by resection, there was no difference between those who had completed neoadjuvant therapy with respect to morbidity and mortality [24]. The presence of neoadjuvant therapy alone is not an indication for elective ICU admission.

Timing of surgery after induction chemoradiotherapy is a common consideration given the deconditioning that occurs with the initial treatment. The majority of patients are taken to surgery between 3 and 6 weeks after chemoradiation. There is a significant drop in survival in patients that have a greater than 6 week break between chemoradiation and surgery [25].

Patients who have tumors that would require pneumonectomy for an R0 resection after induction therapy and restaging have been completed are considered a high-risk group. Based on the Intergroup 0139 trial, the operative mortality rate in this population was 27% for pneumonectomy [26]. Subsequent series have shown survival rates much higher for right-sided pneumonectomy than left (20% vs 9%) [27].

Failure to Rescue

Unplanned admission to the intensive care unit following pulmonary resection is an independent predictor of mortality [4, 5]. As previously stated, the leading admission diagnosis is respiratory failure, followed by cardiac, renal, and neurological events.

Failure to rescue patients from the before mentioned complications following lung resection ranges from 0.7% to 3.2% [28]. Farjah et al. noted in their study that variation between high- and low-mortality centers was present despite similar complication rates. Similar reviews have further illustrated this difference emphasizing the importance of the critical care management of this patient population [29].

This same difference in mortality holds true not only for lung cancer but also for cancers of the bladder, esophagus, colon, pancreas and stomach [30]. The commonality in these studies is that higher volume centers are better equipped to detect, manage, and rescue patients from there postoperative complications. Although a further discussion debating associated patient outcomes related to surgical volume is beyond the scope of this discussion, an emphasis on the common issues facing pulmonary resection patients is worth further review.

Common Issues

Respiratory

Single lung ventilation is required for the majority of pulmonary resections. This establishes an abnormal physiologic state that leads to decreases in oxygen partial pressure, activation of inflammatory processes, hypoxic pulmonary vasoconstriction, changes in cardiac output and barotrauma on the ventilated lung [31]. Measurements of cerebral oxygenation demonstrate significant decreases in cerebral saturation during single lung ventilation [32, 33].

Patients undergoing procedures requiring lung isolation have postoperative complication rates of 20% with evidence of acute lung injury (ALI) in anywhere from 4% to 15% depending on the extent of resection [34]. In fact, the leading cause of postoperative death in these patients is from ALI and ARDS [35, 36].

Atelectasis, surgical manipulation, and trauma occur on the operative lung, while the ventilated lung is exposed to baro- and volutrauma. Any preexisting underlying lung disease further exacerbates the effects of this insult. For example, patients with pulmonary fibrosis typically have noncompliant lungs, whereas patients with severe emphysema may have significant air trapping [37].

Intraoperative management of the ventilated lung is based on protective ventilation strategies. Tidal volumes (Vt) of 6 cc/kg are considered protective; however, reductions to 4–5 cc/kg may be required to minimize barotrauma [38]. Positive end-expiratory pressure (PEEP) is also routinely utilized for further protection of the lung [39].

Ventilator Management

Postoperative patients requiring continued mechanical ventilation as well as those intubated for respiratory failure require standard protective ventilation strategies [40]. Postoperative ARDS is an uncommon complication following pulmonary resection with an incidence of around 3% [41]. The incidence is higher among patients undergoing pneumonectomy (7.9%) when compared to lobectomy or a lesser resection (2.9%). As has been previously mentioned, the mortality rate is high and increases as the extent of the resection increases. Post-pneumonectomy ARDS has a mortality rate of 50–80% [38, 41].

Preventative strategies, such as noninvasive ventilation (NIV) for prevention of pulmonary complications, have had mixed results providing no overwhelming evidence for decreasing complication rates or mortality [42–44]. The early administration of NIV has been successful in some series with an overall success rate of 85.3% [45]. Underlying cardiac disease and lack of initial response to NIV were predictive of failure in this cohort.

ECMO utilization in ARDS following pulmonary resection is currently limited to case reports and small case series [46, 47]. Cardiopulmonary bypass is an intraoperative adjunct for complex resections of the trachea, tumors invading the heart, large mediastinal tumors, and lung transplant [15, 16, 18].

Postoperative Pneumonia

Postoperative pneumonia (POP) occurs in 2–30% of patients. Chronic obstructive pulmonary disease, male gender, and extent of resection are independent risk factor [48]. Among COPD patients, 19.% have positive bacterial cultures compared with 10.5% for patients without COPD [49]. As a result, these patients have a fivefold increase incidence of postoperative pneumonia (POP).

The bacteriology for postoperative pneumonias is most commonly community-acquired *Haemophilus* and *Streptococcus* species [48]. Appropriate preoperative antibiotics, early mobilization, good analgesia, and aggressive pulmonary toilet are keys to prevention as are smoking cessation. Liberal use of toilet bronchoscopy for management of retained secretions is standard practice for thoracic surgeons and should be employed as needed [50]. Minitracheostomy has been demonstrated to have a reduction in postoperative pneumonia but carries a complication rate of 5.6–57% [51].

Chest Tube Management

Few issues are as fraught with superstition, myth, and dogma as the management of chest tubes. The standard practice of connecting chest tubes to −20 cm H_2O suction should be reserved for cases in which drainage or apposition of the pleural space are critical such as pleurodesis or decortication [52]. Following pulmonary resection, resolution of an air leak is reduced on water seal when compared to continuous suction [53]. Patients who develop subcutaneous emphysema or large pneumothoraces on water seal will require a return to suction. Patients who have persistent air leaks on water seal can safely be discharged home with a chest tube in place to a Heimlich valve [54].

Early chest tube removal is an important part of postoperative recovery, removing a significant source of pain and allowing for better mobilization. In the absence of an air leak, chest tubes can be removed even with serous drainage of less than 500 cc/day [55]. Re-intervention rates for pleural space complications with this approach is less than 3%.

Mechanical ventilation is not a contraindication to the removal of a chest tube. In a study of mechanically ventilated trauma patients, 3% of patients required re-intervention for post-pull pneumothoraces [56]. The overall patient status, volume of drainage, and presence or absence of an air leak are the important factors when considering chest tube removal in the ventilated patient.

Fluid Management

Perioperative fluid administration in excess of 3 l over the first 24 h has been shown to increase the incidence of ALI [57, 58]. A significant decrease in the incidence of ALI has been seen with differences of intraoperative fluids administration of 1.2 l versus 1.6 l [7].

Strategies to minimize fluid administration without compromising end-organ perfusion are important. However, the rates of intraoperative fluid administration should not be in excess of 6 ml/kg/h [59].

Epidural analgesia, a common pain management tool for post-thoracotomy pain, can further complicate this due to hypotension. One must weigh the risks of fluid resuscitation for hypotension with the risks of impaired pulmonary toilet and mobilization by turning down the epidural infusion. Paravertebral catheters can ameliorate the need to treat hypotension with equivalent analgesia [60]. The use of peripheral infusion of phenylephrine often helps to bridge the gap between management of hypotension and the restriction of fluid resuscitation.

Acute kidney injury (AKI) is associated with an increase in pulmonary complications, hospital length of stay, and mortality [5, 61]. The risk appears to be decreased with VATS when compared to open thoracotomy. Fluid restriction, comorbidities, and overaggressive forced diuresis all contribute to the development of AKI.

Cardiac

The relationship between thoracic surgery and tachyarrhythmias has been well established [62]. Atrial fibrillation is the most common arrhythmia following noncardiac thoracic surgery with an incidence of 12.3–19% [63, 64]. Risks factors associated with the occurrence of atrial fibrillation include male sex, pneumonectomy, age >70 years, history of congestive heart failure (CHF), history of atrial fibrillation, and transfusion.

In isolation, atrial fibrillation is a relatively low-risk complication and a treatable arrhythmia. However, it is often a marker for the onset of further complications [64]. It is associated with an increased length of hospitalization and overall costs. As with all patients with atrial fibrillation, those with an elevated risk for stroke require anticoagulation unless contraindicated.

The etiology of postoperative atrial fibrillation (POAF) is multifactorial. It is typically seen on the second to fourth postoperative day and is usually self-limited with the majority of cases resolving by 6 weeks. Origination of the initiating aberrant foci is typically from the pulmonary veins [65]. While clearly surgical manipulation of the pulmonary veins during resection can be causative, local and systemic activation of the inflammatory cascade also plays a role [66]. In fact, stimulation of both the sympathetic and parasympathetic nervous system can initiate POAF [67].

Management of POAF following pulmonary resection is similar for any patient with POAF with one notable exception. A study published in Chest in 1994 illustrated the risk of the development of ARDS following pneumonectomy with a cumulative dose of amiodarone over 2150 mg [68]. As with all patients with atrial fibrillation, management of hemodynamically unstable patients with DC cardioversion is appropriate.

Prevention of atrial fibrillation has been often studied but is also often underutilized [69]. Beta-blocker withdrawal is a well-recognized cause of POAF, and beta-blocker therapy should be continued up to the time of surgery and immediately afterward [67]. Magnesium replacement through intravenous infusion should be used judiciously to maintain normal serum levels [70]. Statin therapy in statin naïve patients has been demonstrated to reduce not only atrial fibrillation but also overall complications [69, 71].

Lung Transplant

Critical care management of lung transplant patients deserves specific attention. Since the first reported series of lung transplants done in the 1980s, there have been significant improvements in outcomes for these patients. These advances are largely due to an improved understanding of what is required before, during, and after their operation [72]. Pulmonary transplant represents a formidable challenge when considering the complexities surrounding the human lung. Surgical technique is unique as is the immunologic and infectious implications of utilizing a colonized organ for transplantation. This section aims to briefly familiarize the reader with perioperative issues specific to lung transplant with the hopes of providing guidance for effective execution of critical care during their stay in the ICU.

Preoperative Considerations

Recipient selection is typically accomplished regionally by multidisciplinary teams at high-volume centers. The International Society for Heart and Lung Transplantation (ISHLT) provides guidelines on patient selection. Patients who have severe pulmonary pathology, which is refractory to medical management, and are likely to perish in less than 2 years typically qualify for transplantation. Ideally, recipients have minimal or no other organ dysfunction, no comorbidities, and an acceptable psych profile with adequate social support [73]. Transplant is absolutely contraindicated in patients with uncontrollable infections or those who have been diagnosed with a malignancy within the preceding 2 years. Candidates with a BMI >35 or any substance dependency to include smoking, alcohol, or illicit drug use are also disqualified. Lung transplant is typically avoided in patients older than 65 who have low physiologic reserve and patients colonized with particularly virulent or resistant pathogens as outcomes tend to be poor [73].

The most common indications for lung transplant include idiopathic pulmonary fibrosis (IPF), chronic obstructive pulmonary disease (COPD), interstitial lung disease (ILD), cystic fibrosis (CF), and bronchiectasis. Preoperative critical care may be active in some patients. Although ventilation dependence does portend poor outcomes, it does not preclude patients from transplantation. Further, venous-venous extracorporeal membrane oxygenation (ECMO) can be used as a bridge to transplant in some patients. One distinct advantage of using ECMO is that it allows patients to be off the ventilator and an active participant in preoperative preparations [74, 75].

The critical care team should also be familiar with appropriate preparation of lungs in potential donors. The perfect lung donor is young (age <55) and with physiologically normal lung tissue. However, liberalization of strict criteria has been accepted to increase the donor pool. Final decisions on prospective donor candidates are usually determined by the operating surgeon [75]. Potential donors from patients with brain death should be managed in such a way that their left ventricular ejection fraction remains above 45% and mean arterial pressure should be maintained at 60 mmHg with a central venous pressure and pulmonary capillary wedge pressure no higher than 8 and 12 mmHg, respectively. There is no level-one evidence to support a specific type of fluid over another; however, intuitively colloids may help minimize pulmonary edema. Acidosis should be corrected if pH is less than 7.2, and this may be accomplished with hyperventilation or the addition of bicarbonate solutions to resuscitative fluids. Most transplant surgeons prefer lung protective strategies for ventilation as this has been shown to increase donor eligibility [76]. Finally, donor lung function may be improved with the administration of methyl prednisone by way of decreasing pulmonary edema [77].

Pertinent Operative Aspects

Lung transplant may be accomplished by using single, bilateral or lobar transplantation with or without the use of cardiopulmonary bypass (CPB or v-v ECMO). Variations in the intraoperative technique used as well as the anesthesia care provided during the operation often have implications in the postoperative care. Every transplanted lung is accomplished with the creation of three separate anastomoses which include the bronchus, the pulmonary artery, and the pulmonary vein. The indication for transplant often dictates the length of the operation as it relates to the dissection needed for transplantation, type of transplant completed, and need for bypass. Each of these factors ultimately affects the clinical picture postoperatively.

Cardiopulmonary Bypass

Mechanical circulation is required in just under half of all patients undergoing lung transplant. Although CPB has been traditionally used, ECMO is now the modality of choice as it accomplishes the same bypass need for a lung operation as does CPB but has decreased postoperative morbidity and mortality [78]. Bypass is absolutely necessary in pediatric population as well as adults whom are undergoing transplant for pulmonary vascular disease. Patients with pulmonary fibrosis, pulmonary hypertension, and those bridged to transplant on ventilation or ECMO are more likely to require bypass. Patients who become hemodynamically unstable or hypoxic during the operation will often be converted mechanical circulation [79]. Patients returning to the ICU after bypass, particularly CPB, are at increased risk of bleeding and thus blood transfusions, primary graft dysfunction, delayed extubation, and renal failure [78, 80, 81]. It is imperative that any information related to CPB is communicated during the transition of care to the ICU team.

Type of Transplant

Bilateral transplant is the most commonly performed pulmonary transplant for all indications (75%) as it provides the best long-term outcomes. It is required for patients receiving transplant for pulmonary hypertension, infectious disease, and bronchiectasis [82]. It is typically performed using a transverse thoracosternotomy (clam shell). Single-lung ventilation is utilized first in the native lung then transitioned to the recently placed allograft, while each lung is removed and replaced sequentially.

Single-lung transplantation has the benefit of providing a greater number of individuals with lungs but is less commonly used as long-term outcomes are worse when compared to bilateral lung transplant. This operation is obviously less extensive and may be ideal in older or more debilitated patients. The choice to use single-lung transplant is center specific. This method may be more commonly utilized in patients with COPD. However, bilateral transplant still represents the vast majority of transplants completed for this population [82]. Single-lung transplant is accomplished through a posterior lateral thoracotomy, and the native lung is singly ventilated throughout the procedure. Hyperinflation of the native lung is a known postoperative issue, and in some cases overexpansion of the native lung may progress to compression of the newly transplanted lung, inhibiting respiration.

Lobar transplantation and live donor transplantation is rare in North America. It is typically only utilized as last resort in the small subset of patients who have located appropriate donor with regard to HLA serotyping and are also not likely to survive long enough for a cadaveric donor to become available.

Primary Graft Dysfunction

Primary graft dysfunction (PGD) due to reperfusion injury leading to diffuse alveolar damage is one of the most feared early complications of pulmonary transplantation. Despite prevention and treatment of this issue being an area of focus in the transplant community, it remains the leading cause of early death and is present in up to 25% of patients after lung transplant [82–84].

After the lung is transplanted, the effects of ischemia-reperfusion injury may be appreciated. Ischemia-reperfusion is a phenomenon that creates a physiologic environment that ultimately heralds tissue destruction. During times of no perfusion there is an upregulation of pro-inflammatory mediators causing thrombogenesis, cellular apoptosis/necrosis, complement activation, vasoconstriction, and immune-mediated destruction. In concern to leukocytes specifically, donor macrophages are first activated during ischemia, which is followed by attacks from recipient neutrophils and finally CD4+ T lymphocytes. The severity of this process is dependent on relative ischemic time and the state of the donor lung at the time of harvest [85–87].

Risk Factors

A number of factors are thought to contribute to the development of PGD. Generally, any change that induces or increases inflammation of the donor lung at any point throughout the entire transplantation process increases the risk of PGD. Many of the principles previously discussed for preparation of the donor lungs are aimed at preventing PGD. Protective lung strategies should be utilized when possible to prevent barotrauma from mechanical ventilation [76]. Further, hemodynamic regulation to maintain perfusion prior to procurement is critical. The administration of glucocorticoids prior to harvest may be beneficial in decreasing tissue insult due to inflammation [77]. During procurement, minimizing cold ischemia time is crucial in reducing the effects of oxidative stress, accumulation of intracellular sodium and calcium, and the release of cytokines such as tumor necrosis factor-a as well as various other pro-inflammatory molecules [88].

Independent risk factors have been identified that are related to both donor and recipient characteristics. Donor lungs that come from older females of African-American ethnicity seem to be at higher risk for PGD as do those that have a smoking history [89]. Increased risk for developing PGD has been identified in recipients who have pulmonary hypertension or patients receiving their lungs who have higher pulmonary artery pressures due to fibrosis, although it

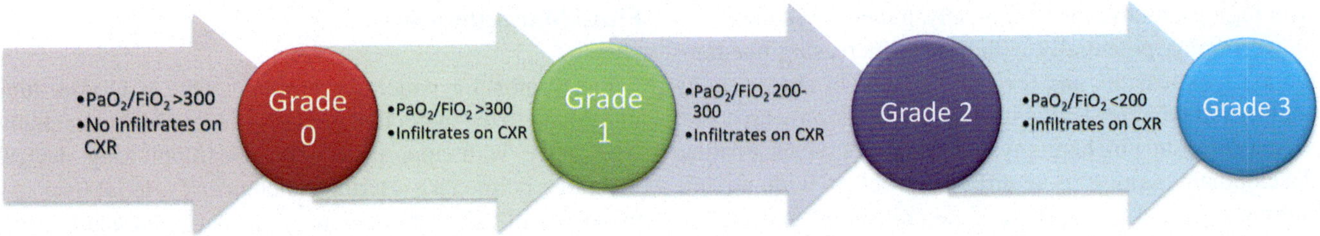

Fig. 20.1 International Society for Heart and Lung Transplant proposed primary graft dysfunction (PGD) severity grading scale. CXR chest X-ray, PaO_2 arterial oxygen, FiO_2 inspired oxygen

may be that these populations are more likely to need for CPB during their cases and thus are more likely to develop PGD as a sequelae of mechanical circulation. Innately, recipients with preformed autoantibodies are also at higher risk of developing PGD [89].

Diagnosis, Prevention, and Treatment

Primary graft dysfunction is ultimately a diagnosis of exclusion. It should be suspected in any patient with unexplained hypoxia and pulmonary infiltrates within the first 3 days following their transplant operation. Differential diagnoses to be ruled out include pulmonary edema, pneumonia, pulmonary embolism or thrombus, aspiration, and hyperacute rejection. Once the diagnosis has been made, a grading system shown in Fig. 20.1 has been proposed by the ISHLT and may help identify patients who will benefit from early aggressive management [90].

Prevention of PGD is geared to limiting the effects surrounding the pathophysiology. Minimizing the cold ischemia time is perhaps the most controllable variable and thus every effort should be made to prevent prolongation of the ischemic time. There is some data in animal models suggesting that slow reperfusion (over a 10-min period intraoperatively) decreases the effects of reperfusion injury. The addition of prostaglandins to preservative fluids may also be beneficial according to some animal models [91–93]. Although it has been suggested, the use of inhaled nitrous oxide (iNO) does not seem to have any preventative effects on the development of PGD.

Unfortunately, the treatment of PGD is mainly supportive. Strategies to improve oxygenation are similar to those used for acute respiratory distress syndrome (ARDS) using low tidal volumes and positive end-expiratory pressure (PEEP). Severe dysfunction (PGD Grade 3) may require treatment by decreasing the ventilation-perfusion mismatch with iNO. In addition to improved oxygenation, iNO decreases pulmonary artery pressures and has been shown to decrease the number of days mechanical ventilation is required. Methemoglobinemia is a common side effect of iNO. Prompt identification and treatment with methylene blue is necessary to reverse this complication. Recent and growing data suggests that ECMO should be initiated early (within 24 h) in patients with severe PGD and may be a lifesaving intervention in this subset of patients [92].

Airway Complications

The bronchial anastomosis is the operative element most susceptible to postoperative complications. As such, the surgical technique used for the creation of the bronchial anastomosis is an area that has been thoroughly evaluated for lung transplant. Currently, the preferred method involves an end-to-end anastomosis that no longer incorporates coverage with an omental flap or a bronchial artery anastomosis [94, 95]. This technique has led to the lowest reported airway complication rates in pulmonary transplant history, but airway complications still represent the most common postoperative complication with rates as high as 18%. Bronchial necrosis, due to a relative decrease in blood supply, is seen to some degree in nearly all post-op lung transplant patients. The effects of necrosis can range from sloughing of the mucosa to total anastomotic dehiscence [96].

Patients with necrosis limited to the mucosa are typically asymptomatic, while development of anastomotic dehiscence may present as a persistent air leak, dyspnea, or difficulty weaning from the vent. Necrosis and breakdown are often discovered after investigation with flexible bronchoscopy [96]. Asymptomatic necrosis confined to bronchial mucosa can be effectively managed conservatively with antibiotics and close observation. Patients who experience a small partial dehiscence may be managed with the temporary placement of an uncovered metallic stent with the hope the stent will induce granulation tissue [97]. Unfortunately stents have not been found to be consistently successful in the management of dehiscence and those who fail to improve with stent placement may benefit from primary repair with biologic glue products [98].

Bronchial necrosis may lead to local infection and abscess formation that can ultimately progress to fistulae development between the bronchus and surrounding spaces or vessels. Fistulae formation is uncommon but associated with high morbidity [96]. Clinically, patients will appear to be worsening, potentially with new or increasing pneumothorax, hypotension, and fever. A CT scan of chest usually confirms the diagnosis. Fistulae communication with a vessel may present with hemoptysis and signs of sepsis. Fistulae development represents a difficult problem with no one right answer. Drainage of any fluid collections and the initiation of appropriate antibiotics are imperative. Small fistulas may be managed with bronchoscopic application of fibrin glues or stent placement. Large fistulas frequently require surgical correction with either a surgical flap or reconstruction [96].

Bronchial necrosis and infection predispose lung transplant patients to airway stenosis. Though this is not typically an acute issue, it is the most common long-term airway complication seen, and regular surveillance, endoscopic dilation, and occasionally stent placement are required to prevent vanishing bronchus or complete occlusion of the airway [99, 100].

Standard Critical Care Management

Typical day-to-day intensive care of the postoperative lung transplant patient does not vary greatly from the care provided for patients undergoing major pulmonary resection as previously discussed in this chapter. However, there are a few salient points worth mentioning with regard to ventilator support and the management of fluids that should be more specifically addressed.

Mechanical Ventilation

The vast majority of patients will remain intubated after their transplant and be observed for a period in the intensive care unit prior to extubation. The typical post-op lung transplant patient will be able to wean quickly from mechanical ventilation, and early extubation is preferred whenever possible. When prolonged ventilator support is required, lung protective strategies using lower tidal volumes and positive end-expiratory pressure (PEEP) should be employed [101]. However, there are some caveats in lung transplant populations. Those receiving transplant for pulmonary hypertension should remain intubated for the first 24 h at minimum to best address any hypoxia or hemodynamic instability [101]. Minimal amounts limited to only physiologic levels of PEEP should be utilized in patients undergoing single-lung transplant. This is particularly true when transplant is performed for predominantly obstructive disease pattern as the use of PEEP can cause overinflation of the remaining native lung [101]. Hypoxia despite appropriate ventilator support should be swiftly evaluated keeping in mind that PGD is the most common cause of hypoxia post-lung transplant.

Fluid Management

It is common for patients returning to the ICU after lung transplant to be hemodynamically labile. Most recipients will arrive with appropriate invasive monitoring devices including pulmonary arterial catheters and arterial lines. All patients will arrive with some degree of pulmonary edema concomitantly due to loss of lymphatic drainage and inflammation driven vessel permeability. Resuscitation should strike a fine balance directed at maintaining tissue perfusion and cardiac output while avoiding fluid overload. There is not conclusive evidence advocating for one type of resuscitative fluid over another, but most centers prefer albumin colloid as it provides the theoretical advantage of promoting fluid shifts out of the interstitium.

Unexplained hypotension should be considered to be postoperative bleeding until proven otherwise which should be promptly investigated then treated with the appropriate intervention and product resuscitation. Systemic inflammation causing transient but severe vasoplegia leading to profound hypotension is not uncommon after transplantation particularly if CPB has been utilized. Vasoplegia may be resistant to standard vasopressors, and the use of methylene blue should be considered for refractory hypotension [102, 103].

Patients with high pulmonary artery pressures may present a formidable challenge postoperatively, and vigilant and decisive management of any lability should be employed. Management of these patients typically begins in the operating room by the anesthesia team with the monitoring of right heart function using transesophageal echocardiography. Right ventricular afterload can be effectively reduced by the use of pulmonary dilators such as milrinone or inhaled agents such as NO and prostacyclin [72, 104, 105]. These agents will usually be continued upon arrival to the ICU but should be weaned within the first 24–48 h as tolerated.

Immunosuppression

Postoperative management of immunotherapy is best approached with the aid of experienced pulmonologist and immunotherapy specialist. A full review of the methods and agents used are beyond the scope of this discussion. Issues pertinent to the critical care setting include induction immunosuppression, recognition, and management of hyperacute and acute rejections as well as a brief review of the opportunistic infections transplant patients are susceptible to.

Induction Immunotherapy

The use of induction immunotherapy has increased since 2001 and, according to the 2013 ISHLT registry, is currently

Table 20.2 Commonly used induction immunotherapy used in major pulmonary transplant centers

Drug	Dosing[a]	Mechanism	Adverse effects	Notes
Basiliximab	20 mg on DOS 20 mg on POD4	T-cell inhibition through CD25 inhibition and IL-2 inhibition	Well tolerated with few side effects	Used most commonly in transplant centers
Anti-thymocyte globulin	1.5 mg/kg (rabbit ab) or 7.5–15 mg/kg (horse ab) over 6 h on DOS and then every 24 h × 3 days	Nonspecific T-cell inhibition via polyclonal antibodies	Thrombocytopenia, leukocytopenia. Effects of polyclonal ab: Serum sickness, nephritis. Cytokine release syndrome	Requires premedication with steroids, acetaminophen and diphenhydramine 1 h prior to infusion
Alemtuzumab	30 mg over 2 h intraoperatively	T and B cell inhibition via CD52	Prolonged lymphopenia	Not well studied
Daclizumab	1 mg/kg on DOS then every 2 weeks × 5 doses	T-cell inhibition through CD25 inhibition and IL-2 inhibition	Well tolerated with few side effects	Not available in the USA
Muromonab-CD3 (OKT3)	2.5–5 mg/day × 7–14 days	T-cell depletion via CD3	Cytokine release storm	Not available in the USA

Note: References [106] and [107]

[a]There is no consensus on dosing. The dosing shown here are recommendations based on commonly used doses at transplant centers. DOS day of surgery, POD post-op day, USA United States

being used in over half of lung transplant patients [82]. Induction immunosuppression is the early use of potent agents to curb the effects of early T-cell mediated destruction. Arguably, this begins intraoperatively with the stress dosing of steroids administered just prior to perfusion of the new lung. Induction therapies are generally tailored on a patient-by-patient basis. The mechanism of action for these agents is by either inhibition of the effects of IL-2 or directly inhibition of T lymphocytes. A list of potential agents and associated side effects are listed in Table 20.2. There is no consensus on whether induction therapy should be routinely used and no conclusive studies supporting one agent over another. Some evidence does suggest a slight increase in survival in the first 2 weeks following transplant based on reports from the ISHLT looking at all transplants done in 2014 [82]. The same registry provides evidence that rejection within the first year may be lower in patients who received induction therapy when compared to no induction therapy (26% vs 34%, respectively) [82]. However, these positive outcomes do not account for confounders such as increased risk of infection or the resulting airway stenosis from early infection. Larger prospective randomized trials will need to be done before any solid recommendations can be made.

Rejection

Hyperacute or humoral rejection from preformed antibodies is exceedingly rare in the age of highly sensitive preoperative HLA antibody testing. Although case reportable, when it does occur, it presents within minutes to hours after transplant and can be devastating. Clinical indicators include profound hypoxia accompanied by pink frothy sputum, hypotension, and diffuse coagulopathy. If identified, early plasmapheresis and aggressive immunotherapy with allograft removal should be completed. Even with prompt and accurate treatment, prognosis is extremely poor [72].

Acute rejection typically occurs in the first 6 months following transplant, but there have been reports of presentation as early as a few weeks. When present during the acute postoperative period, it can prolong ICU stay, and aggressive immunotherapy may predispose patients to opportunistic infections and renal insufficiency. Immunotherapy may need to be curtailed to treat worsening infections or renal failure. It is evident that this back and forth can create the potential for a viscous cycle which may ultimately result in significant morbidity [72].

Infection

Lung transplant represents a unique cohort of transplant patients in that the transplanted organ is naturally colonized. This simple fact predisposes the transplanted environment to constant inoculation by bronchial organisms. Utilization of a multidisciplinary approach, involving transplant infectious disease specialist, is recommended. Prophylactic antibiotics that cover for common gram-positive and gram-negative nosocomial infections are given prior to incision and typically continued for at least 72 h postoperatively. Cultures should be obtained preoperatively from both the donor and recipient, and both prophylactic and treatment antibiotics should be tailored based on drug resistance data and local antibiograms. Prophylaxis with trimethoprim-sulfamethoxazole has the added benefit of covering multiple opportunistic pathogens such as *Pneumocystis jirovecii* in addition to strep species. A higher instance of multidrug-resistant flora may be seen in patients with cystic fibrosis and bronchiectasis specifically pseudomonas and rapidly growing nontuberculous mycobacteria, and treatment should be based on preoperative cultures in these populations [72]. Clinically significant viral infections are rare in the acute postoperative period, but recipients should be provided prophylaxis to the common influenza virus as well as cytomegalovirus (CMV).

References

1. Brunelli A, Kim AW, Berger KI, Addrizzo-Harris DJ. Physiologic evaluation of the patient with lung cancer being considered for resectional surgery. Diagnosis and management of lung cancer 3rd edition: American College of Chest Physicians Evidence-based Clinical Practice Guidelines. Chest. 2013;143(5 Supp):e166S–90S.
2. Aberle DR, Adams AM, Berg CD, et al. Reduced lung-cancer mortality with low-low dose computed tomographic screening. N Engl J Med. 2011;365(5):395–409.
3. Jordan S, Evans TW. Predicting the need for intensive care following lung resection. Thorac Surg Clin. 2008;18:61–9.
4. McCall PJ, Macfie A, Kinsella J, et al. Critical care after lung resection: CALor 1, a single-centre pilot study. Anaesthesia. 2015;70:1382–9.
5. Pilling JE, Martin-Ucar AE, Wallar DA. Salvage intensive care following initial recovery from pulmonary resection: is it justified? Ann Surg. 2004;77:1039–44.
6. Lim E, Baldwin D, Beckles M, et al. Guidelines on the radical management of patients with lung cancer. Thorax. 2010;65:1–27.
7. Licker M, de Perrot M, Spiliopoulos A, et al. Risk factors for acute lung injury after thoracic surgery for lung cancer. Anesth Analg. 2003;97:1558–65.
8. Kozower BD, Sheng S, O'Brien SM, et al. STS database risk models: predictors of morality and major morbidity for lung cancer resection. Ann Thorac Surg. 2010;90(3):875–83.
9. Rosen JE, Hancock JG, Kim AW, et al. Predictors of mortality after surgical management of lung cancer in the national cancer database. Ann Thorac Surg. 2014;98(6):1953–60.
10. Schneider L, Farrokhyar F, Schieman C, et al. Pneumonectomy: the burden of death after discharge and predictors of surgical mortality. Ann Thorac Surg. 2014;98(6):1976–82.
11. Hutchinson JP, Fogarty AW, McKeever TM, et al. In-hospital mortality after surgical lung biopsy for interstitial lung disease in the United States. 2000-2011. Am J Respir Crit Care Med. 2016;193(10):1161–7.
12. Ludwig C, Stoelben E, Olschewski M, et al. Comparison of morbidity, 30-day mortality, and long-term survival after pneumonectomy and sleeve lobectomy for non-small cell lung carcinoma. Ann Thorac Surg. 2005;79(3):968–73.
13. Foroulis CN, Kleontas A, Karatzopoulos A, et al. Early reoperation performed for the management of complications in patients undergoing general thoracic surgical procedures. J Thorac Dis. 2014;6(1):21–31.
14. Pilling JE, Martin-Ucar AE, Waller DA. Salvage intensive care following initial recovery from pulmonary resection: is it justified? Ann Thorac Surg. 2004;77:1039–44.
15. Byrne JG, Leacche M, Agnihotri AK, et al. The use of cardiopulmonary bypass during resection of locally advanced thoracic malignancies: a 10-year 2-center experience. Chest. 2004;125(4):1581–6.
16. Wiebe K, Baraki H, Macchiarini P, et al. Extended pulmonary resections of advanced thoracic malignancies with support of cardiopulmonary bypass. Eur J Cardiothorac Surg. 2006;29(4):571–7.
17. Peek GJ, Mugford M, Tiruvoipati R, et al. Efficacy and economic assessment of conventional ventilatory support versus extracorporeal membrane oxygenation for severe adult respiratory failure (CESAR): a multicentre randomised controlled trial. Lancet. 2009;374:1351–63.
18. Rosskopfova P, Perentes JY, Ris HB, et al. Extracorporeal support for pulmonary resection: current indications and results. World J Surg Oncol. 2015;14:25.
19. Redwan B, Ziegeler S, Freermann S, et al. Intraoperative veno-venous extracorporeal lung support in thoracic surgery: a single-centre experienced. Interact Cardiovasc Thorac Surg. 2015;21(6):766–72.
20. Rajaram R, Mohanty S, Bentrem DJ, et al. Nationwide assessment of robotic lobectomy for non-small cell lung cancer. Ann Thorac Surg. 2017;103(4):1092–100.
21. Louie BE, Wilson JL, Kim S, et al. Comparison of video-assisted thoracoscopic surgery and robotic approaches for clinical stage I and stage II non-small cell lung cancer using the Society of Thoracic Surgeons database. Ann Thorac Surg. 2016;102(3):917–24.
22. Zhang R, Ferguson MK. Video-assisted versus open lobectomy in patients with compromised lung function: a literature review and meta-analysis. PLoS One. 2015;10(7):e0124512.
23. Burt BM, Kosinski AS, Shrager JB, et al. Thoracoscopic lobectomy is associated with acceptable morbidity and mortality in patients with predicted postoperative forced expiratory volume in 1 second or diffusing capacity for carbon monoxide less than 40% of normal. J Thorac Cardiovasc Surg. 2014;148(1):19–28.
24. Siegenthaler MP, Pisters KM, Merriman KW, et al. Preoperative chemotherapy for lung cancer does not increase surgical morbidity. Ann Thorac Surg. 2001;71(4):1105–12.
25. Gao SJ, Corso CD, Wang EH, et al. Timing of surgery after neoadjuvant chemoradiation in locally advanced non-small cell lung cancer. J Thorac Oncol. 2017;12(2):314–22.
26. Uy KL, Darling G, Xu W, et al. Improved results of induction chemoradiation before surgical intervention for selected patients with stage IIIA-N2 non-small cell lung cancer. J Thorac. Cardiovasc Surg. 2007;134(1):188–93.
27. Kim AW, Faber LP, Warren WH, et al. Pneumonectomy after chemoradiation therapy for non-small cell lung cancer: does "side" really matter? Ann Thorac Surg. 2009;88(3):937–43.
28. Farjah F, Backhus L, Cheng A, et al. Failure to rescue and pulmonary resection for lung cancer. J Thorac Cardiovasc Surg. 2015;149(5):1365–71.
29. Grenda T, Revels SL, Yin H, et al. Lung cancer resection at hospitals with high vs low mortality rates. JAMA Surg. 2015;150(11):1034–40.
30. Wong SL, Revels SL, Yin H, et al. Variation in hospital mortality rates with inpatient cancer surgery. Ann Surg. 2015;261(4):632–6.
31. Hemmerling TM, Bluteau MC, Kazan R, et al. Significant decrease of cerebral oxygen saturation during single lung ventilation measured using absolute oximetry. Br J Anaesth. 2008;101(6):870–5.
32. Kazan R, Bracco D, Hemmerling TM. Reduced cerebral oxygen saturation measured by absolute cerebral oximetry during thoracic surgery correlates with postoperative complications. Br J Anaesth. 2009;103(6):811–6.
33. Tang L, Kazan R, Taddei R, et al. Reduced cerebral oxygen saturation during thoracic surgery predicts early postoperative cognitive dysfunction. Br J Anaesth. 2012;108(4):623–9.
34. Licker MJ, Widikker I, Robert J, et al. Operative mortality and respiratory complications after lung resection for cancer: impact of chronic obstructive pulmonary disease and time trends. Ann Thorac Surg. 2006;81:1830–7.
35. Licker M, Fauconnet P, Villiger Y, et al. Acute lung injury and outcomes after thoracic surgery. Curr Opin Anaesthesiol. 2009;22:61–74.

36. Fernandez-Perez ER, Sprung J, Afessa B, et al. Intraoperative ventilator settings and acute lung injury after elective surgery: a nested case control study. Thorax. 2009;64:121–7.
37. Ducros L, Moutafis M, Castelain MH, et al. Pulmonary air trapping during two-lung and one-lung ventilation. J Cardiothorac Vasc Anesth. 1999;13:35–9.
38. Della Rocca G, Coccia C. Acute lung injury in thoracic surgery. Curr Opin Anaesthesiol. 2013;26:40–6.
39. Ferrando C, Mugarra A, Gutierrez A, et al. Setting individualized positive end-expiratory pressure level with a positive end-expiratory pressure decrement trial after a recruitment maneuver improves oxygenation and lung mechanics during one-lung ventilation. Anesth Analg. 2014;118:657–65.
40. Bardoczky GI, Szegedi LL, d'Hollander AA, et al. Two-lung and one-lung ventilation in patients with chronic obstructive pulmonary disease: the effects of position and F(IO)2. Anesth Analg. 2000;90:35–41.
41. Dulu A, Pastores SM, Park B, et al. Prevalence and mortality of acute lung injury and ARDS after lung resection. Chest. 2006;130(1):73–8.
42. Auriant I, Jallot A, Herve P, et al. Noninvasive ventilation reduces mortality in acute respiratory failure following lung resection. Am J Respir Crit Care Med. 2001;165(7):1231–5.
43. Jaber S, Antonelli M. Preventive or curative postoperative noninvasive ventilation after thoracic surgery: still a grey zone? Intensive Care Med. 2014;40:280–3.
44. Lorut C, Lefebvre A, Planquette B, et al. Early postoperative noninvasive ventilation after major lung resection in COPD patients: a randomized controlled trial. Intensive Care Med. 2014;40(2):220–7.
45. Lefebrve A, Lorut C, Alifano M, et al. Noninvasive ventilation for acute respiratory failure after lung resection: an observational study. Intensive Care Med. 2009;35(4):663–70.
46. Dunser M, Hasibeder W, Reiger M, et al. Successful therapy of severe pneumonia-associated ARDS after pneumonectomy with ECMO and steroids. Ann Thorac Surg. 2004;78(1):335–7.
47. Martucci G, Panarello G, Bertani A. Veno-venous ECMO in ARDS after post-traumatic pneumonectomy. Intensive Care Med. 2013;39(12):2235–6.
48. Schlusser O, Alifano M, Dermine H, et al. Postoperative pneumonia after major lung resection. Am J Respir Crit Care Med. 2006;173(10):1161–9.
49. Yamada Y, Sekine Y, Suzuki H, et al. Trends of bacterial colonization and the risk of postoperative pneumonia in lung cancer patients with chronic obstructive pulmonary disease. Eur J Cardiothorac Surg. 2010;37(4):752–7.
50. Reilly J. Benefits of aggressive perioperative management in patients undergoing thoracotomy. Chest. 1995;6(supp):312S–5S.
51. Abdelaziz M, Naidu B, Agostini P. Is prophylactic minitracheostomy beneficial in high-risk patients undergoing thoracotomy and lung resection? Interact Cardiovasc Thorac Surg. 2011;12(4):615–8.
52. Coughlin SM, Emmerton-Coughlin HM, Malthaner R. Management of chest tubes after pulmonary resection: a systematic review and meta-analysis. Can J Surg. 2012;55(4):264–70.
53. Cerfolio RJ, Bryant AS. The management of chest tube after pulmonary resection. Thorac Surg Clin. 2010;20(3):399–405.
54. Royer A, Smith J, Miller A, Spiva M, et al. Safety of outpatient chest tube management of air leaks after pulmonary resection. Am Surg. 2015;81(80):760–3.
55. Bjerregaard LS, Jensen K, Petersen RH, et al. Early chest tube removal after video-assisted thoracic surgery lobectomy with serous fluid production up to 500 mL/day. Eur J Cardiothorac Surg. 2013;45(2):241–6.
56. Pizano LR, Houghton DE, Cohn SM, et al. When should a chest radiograph be obtained after chest tube removal in mechanically ventilated patients? A prospective study. J Trauma. 2002;53(6):1073–7.
57. Slinger PD. Perioperative fluid management for thoracic surgery: the puzzle of postpneumonectomy pulmonary edema. J Cardiothorac Vasc Anesth. 1995;9:442–51.
58. Moller AM, Pedersen T, Svendsen PE, et al. Perioperative risk factors in elective pneumonectomy: the impact of excess fluid balance. Eur J Anaesthesiol. 2002;19:57–62.
59. Arslantas MK, Kara HV, Tuncer BB, et al. Effect of the amount of intraoperative fluid administration on postoperative pulmonary complications following anatomic lung resections. J Thorac Cardiovasc Surg. 2015;149(1):314–21.
60. Ochroch EA, Gottschalk A, Augostides J, et al. Long-term pain and activity during recovery from major thoracotomy using thoracic epidural analgesia. Anesthesiology. 2002;97:1234–44.
61. Ishikawa S, Griesdale DE, Lohser J. Acute kidney injury after lung resection surgery: incidence and perioperative risk factors. Anesth Analg. 2012;114(6):1256–62.
62. Bailey C, Betts RH. Cardiac arrhythmias following pneumonectomy. N Engl J Med. 1943;229:356–9.
63. Vaporciyan AA, Correa AM, Rice DC, et al. Risk factors associated with atrial fibrillation after noncardiac thoracic surgery: analysis of 2588 patients. J Thorac Cardiovasc Surg. 2004;127(3):779–86.
64. Roselli EE, Murphy SC, Rice TW, et al. Atrial fibrillation complicating lung resection. J Thorac Cardiovasc Surg. 2005;130:438–44.
65. Haissaguerre M, Jais P, Shah DC, et al. Spontaneous initiation of atrial fibrillation by ectopic beats originating in the pulmonary veins. N Engl J Med. 1998;339:659–66.
66. Dixit S. Atrial fibrillation after major thoracic surgery: new insights into underlying mechanism. J Am Coll Cardiol. 2009;54(22):2049–51.
67. Fuster V, Ryden LE, Cannom DS, et al. 2011 ACCF/AHA/HRS focused updates incorporated into the ACC/AHA/ESC 2006 guidelines for the management of patients with atrial fibrillation: a report of the American College of Cardiology Foundation/American Heart Association Task Force on practice guidelines developed in partnership with the European Society of Cardiology and in collaboration with the European Heart Rhythm Association and the Heart Rhythm Society. J Am Coll Cardiol. 2011;57(11):e101–98.
68. Van Miegham W, Coolen L, Malysse I, et al. Amiodarone and the development of ARDS after lung surgery. Chest. 1994;105(6):1642–5.
69. Frendl G, Sodickson AC, Chung MK, et al. 2014 AATS guidelines for the prevention and management of perioperative atrial fibrillation and flutter (POAF) for thoracic surgical procedures. J Thorac Cardiovasc Surg. 2014;148(3):e153–93.
70. Terzi A, Furlan G, Chiavacci P, et al. Prevention of atrial tachyarrhythmias after non-cardiac thoracic surgery by infusion of magnesium sulfate. Thorac Cardiovasc Surg. 1996;44(6):300–3.
71. Amar D, Park B, Zhang H, et al. Beneficial effects of perioperative statins for major pulmonary resection. J Thorac Cardiovasc Surg. 2016;149(6):1532–8.
72. Lee JC, Diamond JM, Christie JD. Critical care management of the lung transplant recipient. Curr Respir Care Rep. 2012;1(3):168–76.
73. Weill D, Benden C, Corris PA, et al. A consensus document for the selection of lung transplant candidates: 2014 – an update from the Pulmonary Transplantation Council of the International Society for Heart and Lung Transplantation. J Heart Lung Transplant. 2015;34(1):1–15.
74. Fuehner T, Kuehn C, Hadem J, et al. Extracorporeal membrane oxygenation in awake patients as bridge to lung transplantation. Am J Respir Crit Care Med. 2012;185(7):763–8.
75. Fuehner T, Kuehn C, Welte T, et al. ICU care before and after lung transplantation. Chest. 2016;150(2):442–50.
76. Bhorade SM, Vigneswaran W, McCabe MA, et al. Liberalization of donor criteria may expand the donor pool without adverse consequence in lung transplantation. J Heart Lung Transplant. 2000;19(12):1199–204.

77. Mascia L, Pasero D, Slutsky AS, et al. Effect of a lung protective strategy for organ donors on eligibility and availability of lungs for transplantation: a randomized controlled trial. JAMA. 2010;304(23):2620–7.
78. Venkateswaran RV, Patchell VB, Wilson IC, et al. Early donor management increases the retrieval rate of lungs for transplantation. Ann Thorac Surg. 2008;85(1):278–86.
79. Machuca TN, Collaud S, Mercier O, et al. Outcomes of intraoperative extracorporeal membrane oxygenation versus cardiopulmonary bypass for lung transplantation. J Thorac Cardiovasc Surg. 2015;149(4):1152–7.
80. Ius F, Sommer W, Tudorache I, et al. Five-year experience with intraoperative extracorporeal membrane oxygenation in lung transplantation: indications and midterm results. J Heart Lung Transplant. 2016;35(1):49–58.
81. Bermudez CA, Shiose A, Esper SA, et al. Outcomes of intraoperative venoarterial extracorporeal membrane oxygenation versus cardiopulmonary bypass during lung transplantation. Ann Thorac Surg. 2014;98(6):1936–42.
82. Hoechter DJ, von Dossow V, Winter H. The Munich lung transplant group: intraoperative extracorporeal circulation in lung transplantation. Thorac Cardiovasc Surg. 2015;63(8):706–14.
83. Yusen RD, Edwards LB, Kucheryavaya AY, et al. The Registry of the International Society for Heart and Lung Transplantation: Thirty-second Official Adult Lung and Heart-Lung Transplantation Report--2015; focus theme: early graft failure. J Heart Lung Transplant. 2015;34(10):1264–77.
84. Christie JD, Sager JS, Kimmel SE, et al. Impact of primary graft failure on outcomes following lung transplantation. Chest. 2005;127(1):161–5.
85. King RC, Binns OA, Rodriguez F, et al. Reperfusion injury significantly impacts clinical outcome after pulmonary transplantation. Ann Thorac Surg. 2000;69(6):681–1685.
86. Black GE, Sokol KK, Shawhan RR, et al. Inducing metabolic suppression in severe hemorrhagic shock: pilot study results from the Biochronicity Project. J Trauma Acute Care Surg. 2016;81(6):1003–11.
87. Carden DL, Granger DN. Pathophysiology of ischaemia-reperfusion injury. J Pathol. 2000;190(3):255–66.
88. Fiser SM, Tribble CG, Long SM, et al. Lung transplant reperfusion injury involves pulmonary macrophages and circulating leukocytes in a biphasic response. J Thorac Cardiovasc Surg. 2001;121(6):1069–75.
89. Thabut G, Mal H, Cerrina J, et al. Graft ischemic time and outcome of lung transplantation: a multicenter analysis. Am J Respir Crit Care Med. 2005;171(7):786–91.
90. Christie JD, Kotloff RM, Pochettino A, et al. Clinical risk factors for primary graft failure following lung transplantation. Chest. 2003;124(4):1232–41.
91. Christie JD, Carby M, Bag R, et al. Report of the ISHLT Working Group on Primary Lung Graft Dysfunction part II: definition. A consensus statement of the International Society for Heart and Lung Transplantation. J Heart Lung Transplant. 2005;24(10):1454–9.
92. Pierre AF, DeCampos KN, Liu M, et al. Rapid reperfusion causes stress failure in ischemic rat lungs. J Thorac Cardiovasc Surg. 1998;116(6):932–42.
93. Chiang CH, Wu K, Yu CP, et al. Hypothermia and prostaglandin E(1) produce synergistic attenuation of ischemia-reperfusion lung injury. Am J Respir Crit Care Med. 1999;160(4):1319–23.
94. Shargall Y, Guenther G, Ahya VN, et al. Report of the ISHLT Working Group on Primary Lung Graft Dysfunction part VI: treatment. J Heart Lung Transplant. 2005;24(10):1489–500.
95. FitzSullivan E, Gries CJ, Phelan P, et al. Reduction in airway complications after lung transplantation with novel anastomotic technique. Ann Thorac Surg. 2011;92(1):309–15.
96. Hayanga JW, D'Cunha J. The surgical technique of bilateral sequential lung transplantation. J Thorac Dis. 2014;6(8):1063–9.
97. Santacruz JF, Mehta AC. Airway complications and management after lung transplantation: ischemia, dehiscence, and stenosis. Proc Am Thorac Soc. 2009;6(1):79–93.
98. Mughal MM, Gildea TR, Murthy S, et al. Short-term deployment of self-expanding metallic stents facilitates healing of bronchial dehiscence. Am J Respir Crit Care Med. 2005;172(6):768–71.
99. Maloney JD, Weigel TL, Love RB. Endoscopic repair of bronchial dehiscence after lung transplantation. Ann Thorac Surg. 2001;72(6):2109–11.
100. Yserbyt J, Dooms C, Vos R, et al. Anastomotic airway complications after lung transplantation: risk factors, treatment modalities and outcome-a single-centre experience. Eur J Cardiothorac Surg. 2016;49(1):e1–8.
101. Mulligan MS. Endoscopic management of airway complications after lung transplantation. Chest Surg Clin N Am. 2001;11:907–15.
102. Barnes L, Reed RM, Parekh KR, et al. Mechanical ventilation for the lung transplant recipient. Curr Pulmonol Rep. 2015;4:88–96.
103. Stawicki SP, Sims C, Sarani B, et al. Methylene blue and vasoplegia: who, when, and how? Mini Rev Med Chem. 2008;8(5):472–90.
104. Lenglet S, Mach F, Montecucco F. Methylene blue: potential use of an antique molecule in vasoplegic syndrome during cardiac surgery. Expert Rev Cardiovasc Ther. 2011;9(12):1519–25.
105. Castillo M. Anesthetic management for lung transplantation. Curr Opin Anaesthesiol. 2011;24(1):32–6.
106. Floreth T, Bhorade SM. Current trends in immunosuppression for lung transplantation. Semin Respir Crit Care Med. 2010;31(2):172–8.
107. McShane PJ, Garrity ER Jr. Minimization of immunosuppression after lung transplantation: current trends. Transpl Int. 2009;22(1):90–5.

Stress Gastritis and Stress Ulcers: Prevention and Treatment

21

Lisa M. Kodadek and Christian Jones

Introduction

Historical Perspective

Critically ill patients in intensive care unit (ICU) settings are at risk for stress-related gastrointestinal (GI) mucosal injury including stress gastritis and stress ulcers. These complications may occur quickly following severe physiologic insult such as traumatic injury, hemorrhage, sepsis, major surgery, or burns. Prior to widespread use of antisecretory agents such as histamine-2 receptor antagonists (H2RA) and proton pump inhibitors (PPI), operations for gastric bleeding were well known to the surgeons caring for critically ill patients [1]. One series published in 1971 reported hemorrhage from stress-related gastric ulcers in 300 patients, of whom 13% required operative intervention; mortality among those requiring an operation was 47% [2]. Operative intervention was not only associated with this high mortality but also with a high risk of rebleeding in 50–100% of patients following the procedure [1]. The difficulty of the problem was noted by Ferguson and Clarke in 1966 with this understatement: "Surgical therapy for acute hemorrhagic gastritis has not been entirely satisfactory" [3].

One of the earliest reports leading to the advent of medical prophylaxis of stress-related mucosal injury was published in 1969 [4]. This series examined 150 consecutive patients admitted to a surgical intensive care unit setting and found a 5% incidence of "lethal hemorrhage from acute stress ulceration of the stomach." The authors noted that these patients had acute gastric ulcers almost exclusively confined to the gastric fundus. This pattern of injury, distinct from chronic gastric ulcers which more commonly affected the antrum or antral-fundic junction, suggested a different pathogenesis than either chronic gastric or duodenal ulcer disease. Furthermore, this pattern of gastric injury was highly lethal: Seven of the eight patients in this series who developed gastric ulcers died from hemorrhage, respiratory failure, and sepsis for a mortality rate of 87.5%. A subsequent randomized controlled trial found that critically ill patients receiving antacid prophylaxis had a 4% incidence of gastric hemorrhage, but nearly 25% of patients receiving no prophylaxis experienced gastric hemorrhage [5]. A role for medical prophylaxis of stress-related mucosal hemorrhage was clear.

The first widely adopted approach to preventing stress-related GI mucosal bleeding, supported mainly by literature from the 1980s and early 1990s, was the administration of routine stress ulcer prophylaxis in all critically ill patients [6–9]. However, pharmacologic stress ulcer prophylaxis is not without risk, and the baseline rate of stress gastritis and stress ulcers appears to be decreasing over time [10]. This may be related to changing practices in the care of critically ill patients that emphasize the use of enteral nutrition when possible; some studies suggest that patients tolerating enteral nutrition may not require prophylaxis [10–13]. It remains unclear when the risks of prophylaxis treatment outweigh the benefits and thus in which critically ill patients stress ulcer prophylaxis is still needed. This chapter will briefly review the epidemiology and pathophysiology of stress-related GI mucosal injury but will primarily focus on the prevention of this complication as well as diagnosis and treatment. Current evidence and guidelines will be reviewed, and areas of ongoing investigation will be highlighted.

Epidemiology

It is difficult to determine the exact incidence of stress gastritis and stress ulcers since the patient populations at risk are heterogeneous and the findings or outcomes of interest are highly variable [14]. Most critically ill patients, 75–100% in available series, show evidence of stress gastritis or ulceration on endoscopy completed 24–72 h after onset of critical illness [15–19]. While changes to the gastric mucosa during critical illness are common, most of these changes are

L. M. Kodadek · C. Jones (✉)
Department of Surgery, Johns Hopkins University School of Medicine, Baltimore, MD, USA
e-mail: on-call@christianjones.md

A. Salim et al. (eds.), *Surgical Critical Care Therapy*, https://doi.org/10.1007/978-3-319-71712-8_21

probably not clinically significant and will heal without further sequelae [17]. Clinically important GI mucosal bleeding requiring blood transfusion or other interventions is uncommon among patients receiving stress ulcer prophylaxis. Studies from the 1990s noted an incidence of clinically important bleeding of 1.7–6% of ICU patients [20, 21], but this incidence appears to be decreasing over time. More recent studies suggest that the incidence of clinically important GI mucosal bleeding varies from 0.1 to 4% [11, 14, 22, 23]. This may be a result of changes in the approach to care of critically ill patients including improved resuscitation and nutrition [10, 14]. Finally, it is important to remember that some patients may have GI mucosal pathology that predates their critical illness but manifests only after they become critically ill; serious hemorrhage may occur in these patients and may not be modifiable by stress ulcer prophylaxis [16].

Pathophysiology

Stress-related GI mucosal injury includes stress gastritis, defined as diffuse superficial erosions limited to the gastric mucosa, and stress ulcers, which are focal lesions that erode deeper into the gastric submucosa. Stress ulcers have a higher risk of clinically important bleeding since these lesions are deeper and may involve larger blood vessels within the submucosa [24]. The pathophysiology of stress-related GI mucosal injury is complex, and it remains unclear whether stress gastritis is always a clear precursor for stress ulceration. However, it has been postulated that disruption of gastric mucosal integrity, as occurs in stress gastritis, with subsequent ischemia-reperfusion injury and/or failure of the glandular epithelium to protect and repair itself may then lead to more severe damage manifesting as a stress ulcer [25, 26].

Although *Helicobacter pylori* infection is an important cause of peptic ulcer disease, it has not been implicated in the pathogenesis of stress-related GI mucosal injury [25]. Instead, the basic pathophysiology of both stress gastritis and stress ulcers relates to impairment or loss of normal gastric mucosa defense mechanisms and resultant mucosal injury and ischemia. The gastric mucosa is constantly exposed to hydrochloric acid and pepsin which function to breakdown tissue as part of normal digestion. The mucosa maintains its structural integrity and function in this acidic environment through various defense mechanisms, including a pre-epithelial mucus-bicarbonate-phospholipid barrier, an epithelial barrier of cells connected by tight junctions, blood flow through mucosal microvasculature, and production of factors including prostaglandins and nitric oxide by epithelial cells [27]. Stress gastritis and ulcers result when these defenses are threatened or overwhelmed. Reduced mucosal blood flow secondary to splanchnic hypoperfusion is thought to be a major factor in the development of stress-related mucosal injury. Splanchnic hypoperfusion may result from any number of factors common in critical illness such as hypovolemia, decreased cardiac output, vasoconstriction, and pro-inflammatory cytokines [28]. This hypoperfusion may then lead to impaired production of protective bicarbonate, mucus, and prostaglandins and may also cause direct mucosal ischemia. Reduced blood flow may also decrease gastrointestinal motility, leading to prolonged exposure of gastric mucosa to acidic material. Reperfusion injury may also be involved in the pathogenesis of stress gastritis and stress ulcers; long periods of hypoperfusion followed by restoration of blood flow may cause elevated levels of nitric oxide synthase leading to hyperemia, an inflammatory response, and possible cell death. Stress gastritis and stress ulcers develop as a result of these changes, all common during critical illness.

Sequelae and Outcomes

Stress-related mucosal bleeding is divided into three classes: occult bleeding, overt bleeding, and clinically important bleeding [24]. Occult bleeding is heme-positive gastric aspirate or stool and may be of minimal consequence. Overt bleeding is hematemesis, melena, hematochezia, or "coffee ground" gastric aspirate. Clinically important bleeding is defined as overt bleeding complicated by hemodynamic changes, drop in hemoglobin by 2 or more g/dl, transfusion requirement of two or more units of blood within 24 h, and need for operative intervention [25]. Overt bleeding may occur in as many as 5% of ICU patients [24, 25]. However, only a small proportion of patients (0.1–4%) experience clinically important bleeding [11, 14, 22–25]. When clinically important bleeding does occur, it has a significant impact on patient outcomes [29]. Mortality is up to fourfold higher in those patients suffering from significant mucosal bleeding compared to patients without complications [30]. Furthermore, each episode of clinically important bleeding results in an increased length of ICU stay up to 8 additional days, an average of 7 additional lab tests, an average of 11 blood product transfusions, and an overall mean cost per episode of $12,000 [30].

Prevention

Risk Factors

A large observational study of 2252 ICU patients published in 1994 established respiratory failure and coagulopathy as the most important independent risk factors for clinically important stress-related mucosal bleeding [31]. A more recent international observational study published in 2015 examined risk factors for clinically important bleeding among 1034 patients from 97 ICUs in 11 countries [32]. This study determined that the following variables were independently associated with clinically important GI bleeding: three or more coexisting diseases, renal replacement therapy, coexisting coagulopathy, acute coagulopathy, and higher organ failure score. Additional major risk factors include traumatic brain injury and major burn (>35% total body surface area) [33]. Other risk factors have been established with less definitive evidence and include polytrauma with Injury Severity Score (ISS) greater than 15, sepsis, acute liver failure, high-dose corticosteroids, age greater than 50 years, and male gender [33, 34].

Prophylaxis with Enteral Feeding

Some data suggest patients tolerating enteral nutrition may not require stress ulcer prophylaxis (SUP) as they have much lower baseline rates of stress ulceration and hemorrhage [10–13]. Enteral feeds may serve as prophylaxis through direct cytoprotection of the GI mucosa and alkalinization of gastric contents [35, 36]. Current guidelines report that there is either insufficient evidence at this time to make any recommendation about enteral feeding and SUP or that enteral feeding alone may be insufficient as SUP [33, 37]. However, new data are challenging these recommendations. A recent study examined trauma ICU patients who received both mechanical ventilation and full enteral nutrition without administration of SUP [13]. The incidence of clinically important bleeding was very low at 0.50% in this population. The authors concluded that trauma patients at risk for stress-related mucosal bleeding did not benefit from continued pharmacologic SUP once they tolerated enteral nutrition. A 2010 systematic review and meta-analysis aimed to determine the benefit and risks of SUP and the moderating effect of enteral nutrition [10]. Seventeen studies (enrolling 1836 patients) were included. The authors found that SUP with H2RA reduced the risk of GI bleeding, but this treatment effect was noted *only* in the subgroup of patients who *did not* receive enteral nutrition. The authors concluded that SUP may not be required in patients receiving enteral nutrition. However, no randomized controlled trials to date have prospectively investigated the relationship between SUP and enteral nutrition, which limits the ability to make definitive recommendations.

Prophylaxis Regimens

Various pharmacologic treatments are available for preventing clinically important mucosal GI bleeding. Options for SUP include sucralfate and barrier medications, histamine-2 receptor antagonists (H2RA), and proton pump inhibitors (PPI). Antacids, however, are not considered appropriate prophylaxis secondary to concerns about side effects and labor-intensive dosing [33, 34]. Worldwide, PPI is prescribed by the majority of intensivists as the preferred SUP regimen [32].

Sucralfate and Barrier Medications

Sucralfate and other barrier medications function to protect the gastric mucosa by coating the mucosa, stimulating mucus and bicarbonate secretion, improving blood flow, and enhancing release of protective prostaglandins [34]. Sucralfate may be administered via nasogastric tube which may be of use in some patient populations. However, multiple daily doses are required (typically 1 g every 6 h), and NG tubes may become clogged by the medication [38]. Furthermore, sucralfate protects gastric mucosa without raising gastric pH. However, since sucralfate is not systemically absorbed, it may decrease absorption of other medications administered by mouth. Oral medications must be administered at least 2 h before sucralfate [34]. Other adverse effects of sucralfate include constipation and aluminum toxicity, especially in patients with renal failure or those patients receiving renal replacement therapy [33, 39].

A randomized controlled trial of 1200 patients showed sucralfate to be inferior to H2RA for the prevention of clinically important bleeding; rates of pneumonia, ICU stay, and mortality did not differ among the treatment groups [20]. However, two meta-analyses found sucralfate to be associated with lower rates of pneumonia when compared with antacids and H2RA [9, 40]. A recent retrospective cohort study also found lower rates of pneumonia among patients receiving sucralfate versus H2RA or PPI [41]. Although associated with lower rates of pneumonia, sucralfate is usually considered less effective than H2RA and PPIs in preventing clinically important bleeding. Sucralfate is not generally recommended for routine stress ulcer prophylaxis [20, 37, 42].

Histamine-2 Receptor Antagonists (H2RA)

Histamine-2 receptor antagonists (H2RA) function by reversible competitive inhibition of histamine H-2 receptors. Histamine, in addition to gastrin and acetylcholine, stimulates the gastric parietal cell hydrogen-potassium ATPase proton pump responsible for the secretion of acid. H2RA can substantially reduce the amount of acid secretion, but they are not capable of complete inhibition of acid production [43]. H2RA have been shown in meta-analysis to be better than placebo in reducing the incidence of clinically important stress-related mucosal GI bleeding [9]. H2RA have also been shown to be superior to sucralfate for SUP [20]. However, other studies have failed to show any significant difference in reduction of clinically important bleeding when comparing H2RA, placebo, and sucralfate [11, 44–46].

H2RA raise gastric pH, which has been associated with higher rates of pneumonia [9, 40, 41]. H2RA have been associated with development of tolerance, drug interactions, some neurologic complications, and thrombocytopenia. Tolerance to H2RA acid inhibition and rebound acid hypersecretion may occur as soon as 72 h after first administration [47, 48]. This effect is attributed to upregulation of the number of H2 receptors over time and does not respond to increased doses of the medication. Drug interactions may occur since H2RA inhibit cytochrome P-450 drug metabolism. This may lead to decreased clearance and associated toxicity of drugs such as warfarin, ketoconazole, theophylline, phenytoin, diazepam, and caffeine [49, 50]. Neurologic complications such as headache, confusion, delirium, slurred speech, and hallucinations have been reported, especially in elderly patients [51, 52]. H2RA is a known cause of thrombocytopenia, and this condition is reversible with discontinuation of the medication [53]. However, there are many other more common reasons ICU patients develop thrombocytopenia, so it is important to consider other explanations for this finding. If it is determined that thrombocytopenia is secondary to H2RA administration, an alternative antisecretory medication such as PPI should be prescribed.

Proton Pump Inhibitors (PPI)

Proton pump inhibitors (PPI) function to block the hydrogen-potassium ATPase proton pump, which is the final common step responsible for gastric acid secretion. For this reason, PPI provide the most potent acid inhibition available [54]. PPI are administered as prodrugs which remain inactive until the drug is taken up by parietal cells through the basolateral membrane. In the presence of acid, the prodrug is protonated and then undergoes a conformational change into the active form of the drug. Once active, the drug forms a covalent bond with cysteine residues on the hydrogen-potassium ATPase proton pump, thereby causing the pump to become inactivated [38]. PPI will only inactivate active proton pumps, and only about 70–80% of pumps are active at one time. Thus, it may take up to 3 or 4 days to realize the maximal acid inhibitory effect of PPI [38].

There have been a number of trials comparing PPI and H2RA [49, 55–57]. One of the earliest randomized controlled trials compared omeprazole and ranitidine in ICU patients at risk for stress-related GI mucosal bleeding [58]. This study found a statistically significant higher incidence of clinically important bleeding among patients prescribed H2RA (31%) as compared to PPI (6%). However, this trial was criticized since the incidence of clinically important bleeding was much higher than expected among those patients receiving H2RA, and the H2RA cohort had a higher number of risk factors than the PPI cohort. A trial comparing PPI, H2RA, sucralfate, and placebo found no difference among the treatment groups in terms of incidence of clinically important bleeding [45]. Another multicenter trial found PPI to be noninferior to H2RA when considering clinically important bleeding as the outcome of interest [59].

Several meta-analyses have compared PPI and H2RA, but the results are limited by aspects of methodology which differed substantially among the included trials and likely impacted outcomes [16, 55–57, 60, 61]. A meta-analysis published in 2013 included 14 trials enrolling 1720 patients [61]. This study found PPI to be more effective than H2RA at reducing clinically important bleeding and overt bleeding, but there were no differences between PPI and H2RA in risk of pneumonia, ICU mortality, or ICU length of stay. Two additional meta-analyses have found that PPI prophylaxis significantly decreased rates of clinically important bleeding compared to H2RA, again without any difference in pneumonia rates [55, 56]. However, a 2010 meta-analysis found no difference between PPI and H2RA in terms of incidence of clinically important bleeding, pneumonia, or mortality [57].

PPI are generally well-tolerated and have an acceptable safety profile. The neurologic changes, tolerance, and thrombocytopenia associated with H2RA have not been associated with PPI [38, 62]. Furthermore, there is less risk for drug interactions mediated by cytochrome p-450 enzymes with use of PPI [38]. Patients with significant thrombocytopenia ($<50{,}000\ mm^{-3}$) should probably be given PPI as opposed to H2RA [60]. PPI are more commonly associated with *Clostridium difficile* infection than H2RA [10, 38, 63, 64]. However, none of the trials included in a recent meta-analysis comparing PPI and H2RA reported on rates of *Clostridium difficile* infection [61].

Risks of Prophylaxis

Renewed interest in the topic of appropriate SUP prescription may be related to the risks of prophylaxis, which are not trivial. Each of the available SUP medications has unique risks, as previously discussed. In general, *Clostridium difficile* infection, ventilator-associated pneumonia, and thrombocytopenia are the most commonly recognized risks of SUP. Gastric acid is an important defense mechanism against bacterial colonization [65]. Administration of SUP causes acid inhibition, which leads to decreased gastric acidity. In an alkalinized environment, there may be overgrowth of bacteria, bacterial translocation, changes in gastrointestinal flora, and impairment of normal host defenses [66]. These changes are likely related to the increased incidence of *Clostridium difficile* infection among patients receiving SUP. A likely mechanism behind the increased risk of ventilator-associated pneumonia also relates to decreased gastric acidity. Since H2RA and PPI alkalinize the gastric contents, this may lead to bacterial overgrowth and oropharyngeal/airway colonization. Microaspiration of colonized bacteria may then lead to higher rates of pneumonia. A recent retrospective cohort study examined the causative organisms in cases of ventilator-associated pneumonia among patients receiving different types of SUP regimens [41]. In patients receiving sucralfate (which does not change the gastric pH), there was a lower rate of pneumonia, and the causative organisms were oropharyngeal flora. In patients receiving either PPI or H2RA (which raise gastric pH), there was a higher rate of pneumonia, and the causative organisms were *Pseudomonas* species, methicillin-resistant *Staphylococcus aureus*, and gram-negative bacilli. SUP regimens have an associated cost, and the benefits of such treatment, as well as the risks and associated costs of infectious complications from SUP therapy, must be carefully considered [16, 67]. For this reason, widespread and routine use of SUP in all critically ill patients is being reevaluated, and the safety of withholding SUP is being investigated [68, 69].

Guidelines for Prophylaxis

While it is agreed that critically ill patients who are at risk for clinically important stress-related mucosal GI bleeding should receive appropriate prophylaxis, more specific recommendations generate considerable debate. To this end, several organizations have published consensus guidelines with indications for stress ulcer prophylaxis and preferred regimens as summarized in Table 21.1. The most recently published 2014 guidelines from the Danish societies recommend *against* routine use of stress ulcer prophylaxis (SUP) in all critically ill patients [37]. When SUP is indicated, they recommend use of PPI as opposed to other types of SUP regimens. The 2012 Surviving Sepsis Guidelines offer similar recommendations: there is a strong recommendation for SUP using either PPI or H2RA for patients with bleeding risk factors, and there is a weak recommendation that patients without risk factors should *not* receive SUP [42]. Regarding a preferred SUP regimen, the Surviving Sepsis Guidelines make a weak recommendation based on lower-quality evidence that PPI should be used rather than H2RA [42]. The Eastern Association for the Surgery of Trauma (EAST) guidelines, published in 2008, recommend SUP for patients based on risk factors with varying levels of clinical certainty [33]. The highest level of certainty and strongest evidence support use of SUP in patients requiring mechanical ventilation and/or those patients with coagulopathy, traumatic brain injury, and major burn injury. SUP is recommended for patients with multi-trauma, sepsis, or acute renal failure with a moderate degree of clinical certainty. Patients with Injury Severity Score >15 and those being treated with high-dose corticosteroids should also receive SUP, but the degree of clinical certainty is not established. Finally, EAST does not distinguish at all between H2RA, PPI, and cytoprotective agents in terms of a preferred prophylaxis regimen.

While these guidelines reflect the currently available evidence, it is important to note that SUP is an active area of ongoing investigation. The Re-evaluating the Inhibition of Stress Erosions (REVISE) multicenter pilot trial in Canada, Saudi Arabia, and Australia has been designed to investigate the feasibility of a large randomized controlled trial to determine the safety and efficacy of withholding SUP by comparing administration of PPI versus placebo [68]. A similar

Table 21.1 Indications for stress ulcer prophylaxis and regimens from evidence-based guidelines

Organization, year of publication	Indications for stress ulcer prophylaxis (SUP)	Preferred prophylaxis regimen
Danish Society of Intensive Care Medicine and the Danish Society of Anesthesiology and Intensive Care Medicine, 2014 [37]	Recommend not using SUP routinely for adult critically ill patients in the ICU (GRADE 1C[a]) Insufficient evidence to make any recommendation on SUP and nutrition Insufficient evidence to make recommendations on SUP in specific ICU subpopulations such as trauma, burn, septic, or cardiothoracic patients	Recommend use of PPI when SUP is indicated in adult critically ill patients in the ICU (GRADE 2C[a])
Surviving Sepsis Campaign, 2012 [42]	Recommend SUP using H2RA or PPI for patients with septic shock who have bleeding risk factors (GRADE 1B[a]) Patients without risk factors should not receive SUP (GRADE 2B[a])	Recommend use of PPI rather than H2RA (GRADE 2C[a])
Eastern Association for the Surgery of Trauma, 2008 [33]	SUP recommended for patients with mechanical ventilation, coagulopathy, traumatic brain injury, or major burn injury (Level I[b]) SUP recommended for patients with multi-trauma, sepsis, or acute renal failure (Level II[b]) SUP recommended for patients with injury severity score >15 or high-dose steroid treatment (Level III[b]) In selected populations, no SUP is necessary (Level III[b])	No difference between H2RA, cytoprotective agents, and PPI (Level I[b]) Antacids are not recommended (Level I[b]) Aluminum-containing agents should not be used in patients on dialysis (Level II[b]) Enteral feeding alone may be insufficient (Level III[b])

SUP stress ulcer prophylaxis, *ICU* intensive care unit, *PPI* proton pump inhibitor, *H2RA* histamine-2 receptor antagonist

[a]GRADE: Grading of Recommendations Assessment, Development and Evaluation (Quality of evidence ranges from high (A) to very low (D), and strength of recommendation is either strong (1) or weak (2).)

[b]Level I, strongest evidence for effectiveness and represent principles of patient management that reflect a high degree of clinical certainty; Level II, moderate degree of clinical certainty; Level III, degree of clinical certainty is not established

randomized controlled trial in Europe, Stress Ulcer Prophylaxis in the Intensive Care Unit (SUP-ICU), will also examine outcomes among patients randomized to either PPI or placebo [69]. The primary outcome of interest is 90-day mortality, and secondary outcomes include proportion of patients with clinically important bleeding, pneumonia, and *Clostridium difficile* infection. As these and other trials provide new data, guideline revisions may be necessary to ensure the highest-quality evidence-based care is provided to critically ill patients.

Routine Prophylaxis Recommendations

A practical approach to prevention of clinically important stress-related GI bleeding should utilize published guidelines but must also recognize limitations in currently available scientific evidence. There is no SUP regimen that is clearly or definitively superior to others. *Typical SUP regimens include:*

- *Pantoprazole 40 mg intravenous once daily (PPI)*
- *Famotidine 20 mg intravenous twice daily (H2RA)*

There are several risk factors that are clearly linked with development of stress gastritis and stress ulcers. *Critically ill patients being cared for in the ICU setting with one of more of the following indications should receive SUP:*

- *Respiratory failure (Expected mechanical ventilation >48 h)*
- *Coagulopathy (platelets < 50,000 mm*$^{-3}$*, INR > 1.5, or aPTT > 2 times control)*
- *Traumatic brain injury*
- *Major burn injury (>35% total body surface area)*

Discontinuation of SUP should be considered if patients are no longer at risk for clinically important bleeding or no longer critically ill. Although the scientific evidence is inconclusive, discontinuation of SUP may also be considered in select mechanically ventilated patients once full enteral nutrition is tolerated.

Diagnosis and Treatment

Signs and Symptoms

As noted above, signs of stress gastritis and stress ulcers may include new occult or overt bleeding. Additionally, anemia of uncertain origin may be an initial indication of upper GI bleeding, but diseases with this finding are widespread in the surgical ICU; consideration for stress gastritis or ulceration may occur later than concern for surgical site bleeding or traumatic hemorrhage. Alternatively, significant bleeding may be associated with hemodynamic changes or an acute drop in hematocrit [25]. While frank perforation resulting in peritonitis and sepsis is possible, in the stress gastropathy patient, this is seldom the first sign.

Definitive Diagnosis

Radiographic imaging is rapid, and surgeons are accustomed to evaluating radiographic images themselves, but imaging has limited utility in evaluating stress gastropathy. In the absence of perforation, CT and X-ray are unlikely to demonstrate any abnormality. Angiography is useful for an intervention in the patient with significant bleeding but is prudent for diagnosis only in the patient who has previously undergone intervention and appears to be rebleeding. On the other hand, esophagogastroduodenoscopy (EGD) is both diagnostic and potentially therapeutic and should be performed urgently on any critically ill patient with suspected upper GI bleeding. On endoscopy, stress-related gastritis is identified by multiple subepithelial petechiae. These lesions may progress to erosions or discrete ulcerations, often in the gastric fundus. Lesions do not usually perforate and more often cause focal loss of superficial epithelium, coagulative necrosis of the mucosa, and bleeding from superficial mucosal capillaries [28].

Treatment Options

Medical

Little direct intervention is indicated for uncomplicated stress gastritis. Normal stress ulcer prophylaxis is appropriate, and gastric feeding may improve irritation. Gastric lavage with ice-cold saline or Ringer's lactate is often suggested as effective treatment [70] but has little supporting evidence and should not be performed [71]. Principles of urgent management for stress-related GI mucosal injury are nearly identical to those for any significantly bleeding patient, including resuscitation with fluid and blood products, correction of acidosis, correction of coagulopathy, and restoration or maintenance of normothermia. Additionally, nasogastric or orogastric tube placement is indicated for gastric decompression and removal of gastric contents and blood products; overdistension may potentiate mucosal irritation and injury. Intravenous PPI should be administered as a continuous drip until bleeding is controlled. In patients who manifest signs of sepsis, broad-spectrum antibiotics should be administered.

Endoscopic

Critically ill patients suspected of having upper gastrointestinal bleeding, even minor or occult, should undergo urgent endoscopic evaluation. Should an isolated location of bleeding be observed, electrocautery, hemoclips, or injections of vasopressin or epinephrine can be administered in an attempt to control the bleeding. Even with initial control of bleeding, the need for re-intervention remains high but is without major additional risk; serial endoscopy with intervention is nearly always preferred to surgery for the hemodynamically stable patient with a bleeding stress ulcer. Once bleeding is controlled, there is little benefit to continuous infusion of PPI; twice-daily dosing is appropriate. In cases of hemorrhagic gastritis, which is not usually associated with a discrete lesion, endoscopic therapy is unlikely to be successful.

Angiographic

Angiographic embolization is useful for the hemodynamically stable patient with apparent ongoing bleeding after EGD, either due to inability to visualize the bleeding endoscopically or inability to control it via endoscopic intervention. As with endoscopy, rebleeding is common, and repeated attempts at angioembolization and endoscopic intervention are appropriate as long as the patient remains stable. In cases of bleeding from diffuse stress gastritis, the rich blood supply to the stomach results in variable control of bleeding with interventional radiographic embolization of a single vessel. Selective intra-arterial infusion of vasoconstrictors may be effective in controlling more diffuse bleeding [72].

Surgical

Indications for operative intervention include bleeding with hemodynamic instability, ongoing transfusion requirements, and suspected gastric ulcer perforation. Patients with associated gastric perforation require definitive surgical management to control abdominal contamination and sepsis. Surgical management of stress gastritis and stress ulcers presents a major challenge, because patients who require surgical intervention are typically in acute hemorrhage shock and/or acutely septic. A "damage-control" staged operative approach may be necessary in some settings [73]. While operative intervention is similar to surgery for perforated peptic ulcers, patients with stress ulcers who develop perforation may have more injury to surrounding gastric mucosa and thus may require a more extensive surgical resection; examination of the mucosa surrounding the perforation is critical.

The surgical approach to control of hemorrhage may include anterior gastrotomy and oversewing of bleeding vessels or gastric resection. Depending on the location of hemorrhage, partial gastrectomy or subtotal gastrectomy may be necessary. Vagotomy and pyloroplasty were a common approach prior to the advent of prophylaxis medications and are still commonly used in the rare circumstance that operative intervention is required for stress ulcer management [74, 75]. In the event of life-threatening diffuse hemorrhagic gastritis, only total gastric devascularization has demonstrated significant success in controlling bleeding while retaining the stomach. However, the mortality of patients requiring this procedure remains high [76, 77]. The most extreme intervention, reserved for immediately life-threatening hemorrhage, is total gastrectomy.

Summary

Gastric mucosal changes related to the stress of critical illness are common in patients treated in the surgical ICU, but the incidence of clinically significant bleeding from stress gastritis and stress ulcers is dramatically lowered with prophylactic administration of PPI or H2RA. Judicious use of these medications in only those patients at high risk for bleeding may help prevent complications such as ventilator-associated pneumonia, *Clostridium difficile* colitis, thrombocytopenia, and poor uptake of enteric medications. Should bleeding from stress gastritis or stress ulcers occur, urgent endoscopy is indicated for diagnosis and potential therapy, with angiographic embolization considered a second-line option if this fails. Surgery is reserved for the hemodynamically unstable patient with unabated hemorrhage, with total gastrectomy having the highest rate of success but resulting in considerable mortality.

References

1. Menguy R, Gadacz T, Zajtchuk R. The surgical management of acute gastric mucosal bleeding. Arch Surg. 1969;99:198–206.
2. Lucas CE, Sugawa C, Riddle J, Rector F, Rosenberg B, Walt AJ. Natural history and surgical dilemma of "stress" gastric bleeding. Arch Surg. 1971;102(4):266–73.
3. Ferguson HL, Clarke JS. Treatment of hemorrhage from erosive gastritis by vagotomy and pyloroplasty. Am J Surg. 1966;112:739–42.
4. Skillman JJ, Bushnell LS, Goldman H, et al. Respiratory failure, hypotension, sepsis and jaundice. A clinical syndrome associated with lethal hemorrhage from acute stress ulceration of the stomach. Am J Surg. 1969;117:523–30.
5. Hastings PR, Skillman JJ, Bushnell LS, et al. Antacid titration in the prevention of acute gastrointestinal bleeding: a controlled, randomized trial in 100 critically ill patients. N Engl J Med. 1978;298:1041–5.
6. Basso N, Baragani Materia A, et al. Cimetidine and antacid prophylaxis of acute upper gastrointestinal bleeding in high risk patients. Am J Surg. 1981;141:339–41.
7. Friedman CJ, Oblinger MJ, Surrat PM, et al. Prophylaxis of upper gastrointestinal hemorrhage in patients requiring mechanical ventilation. Crit Care Med. 1982;10:316–9.
8. Cook DJ, Witt LG, Cook RJ, et al. Stress ulcer prophylaxis in the critically ill: a metaanalysis. Am J Med. 1991;91:519–27.
9. Cook DJ, Reeve BK, Guyatt GH, et al. Stress ulcer prophylaxis in critically ill patients. Resolving discordant meta-analyses. JAMA. 1996;275:308–14.
10. Marik PE, Vasu T, Hirani A, Pachinburavan M. Stress ulcer prophylaxis in the new millennium: a systematic review and meta-analysis. Crit Care Med. 2010;38:2222–8.

11. Faisy C, Guerot E, Diehl JL, et al. Clinically significant gastrointestinal bleeding in critically ill patients with and without stress ulcer prophylaxis. Intensive Care Med. 2003;29:1306–13.
12. Pingleton SK, Hadzima SK. Enteral alimentation and gastrointestinal bleeding in mechanically ventilated patients. Crit Care Med. 1983;11(1):13–6.
13. Palm NM, McKinzie B, Ferguson PL, et al. Pharmacologic stress gastropathy prophylaxis may not be necessary in at-risk surgical trauma ICU patients tolerating enteral nutrition. J Intensive Care Med. 2016; epub ahead of print. doi:10.1177/0885066616678385.
14. Krag M, Perner A, Wetterslev J, Moller MH. Stress ulcer prophylaxis in the intensive care unit: is it indicated? A topical systematic review. Acta Anaesthesiol Scand. 2013;57(7):835–47.
15. Brett S. Science review: the use of proton pump inhibitors for gastric acid suppression in critical illness. Crit Care. 2005;9:5–50.
16. Barletta JF, Bruno JJ, Buckley MS, Cook DJ. Concise definitive review: stress ulcer prophylaxis. Crit Care Med. 2016;44(7):1395–405.
17. Ali T, Harty RF. Stress-induced ulcer bleeding in critically ill patients. Gastroenterol Clin N Am. 2009;38(2):245–65.
18. Eddleston JM, Pearson RC, Holland J, Tooth JA, Vohra A, Doran BH. Prospective endoscopic study of stress erosions and ulcers in critically ill adult patients treated with either sucralfate or placebo. Crit Care Med. 1994;22(12):1949–54.
19. Martin LF. Stress ulcers are common after aortic surgery. Endoscopic evaluation of prophylactic therapy. Am Surg. 1994;60(3):169–74.
20. Cook D, Guyatt G, Marshall J, Leasa D, Fuller H, Hall R, et al. A comparison of sucralfate and ranitidine for the prevention of upper gastrointestinal bleeding in patients requiring mechanical ventilation. Canadian Critical Care Trials Group. N Engl J Med. 1998;338(12):791–7.
21. Fabian TC, Boucher BA, Croce MA, Kuhl DA, Janning SW, Coffey BC, et al. Pneumonia and stress ulceration in severely injured patients. A prospective evaluation of the effects of stress ulcer prophylaxis. Arch Surg. 1993;128(2):185–91. 191–2
22. Choung RS, Talley NJ. Epidemiology and clinical presentation of stress-related peptic damage and chronic peptic ulcer. Curr Mol Med. 2008;8:253–7.
23. Andersson B, Nilsson J, Brandt J, Hoglund P, Andersson R. Gastrointestinal complications after cardiac surgery. Br J Surg. 2005;92:326–33.
24. Fennerty MB. Pathophysiology of the upper gastrointestinal tract in the critically ill patient: rationale for the therapeutic benefits of acid suppression. Crit Care Med. 2002;30(Suppl):S351–5.
25. Reilly J, Fennerty MB. Stress ulcer prophylaxis: the prevention of gastrointestinal bleeding and the development of nosocomial infections in critically ill patients. J Pharm Pract. 1998;11:418–32.
26. Hurt RT, Frazier TH, McClave SA, et al. Stress prophylaxis in intensive care unit patients and the role of enteral nutrition. JPEN J Parenter Enteral Nutr. 2012;36(6):721–31.
27. Laine L, Takeuchi K, Tarnawski A. Gastric mucosal defense and cytoprotection: bench to bedside. Gastroenterology. 2008;135(1):41–60.
28. Stollman N, Metz DC. Pathophysiology and prophylaxis of stress ulcer in intensive care unit patients. J Crit Care. 2005;20(1):35–45.
29. Heyland D, Gafni A, Griffith L, et al. The clinical and economic consequence of clinically important gastrointestinal bleeding in critically ill patients. Clin Intensive Care. 1996;7:121–5.
30. Cook DJ, Griffith LE, Walter SD, et al. The attributable mortality and length of intensive care unit stay of clinically important gastrointestinal bleeding in critically ill patients. Crit Care. 2001;5(6):368–75.
31. Cook DJ, Fuller HD, Guyatt GH, et al. Risk factors for gastrointestinal bleeding in critically ill patients. Canadian Critical Care Trials Group. N Engl J Med. 1994;330(6):377–81.
32. Krag M, Perner A, Wetterslev J, et al. SUP-ICU co-authors: prevalence and outcome of gastrointestinal bleeding and use of acid suppressants in acutely ill adult intensive care patients. Intensive Care Med. 2015;41:833–45.
33. Guillamodegui OD, Gunter OL, Bonadies JA, Coates JE, Kurek SJ, De Moya MA, et al. Practice management guidelines for stress ulcer prophylaxis. Chicago: Eastern Association for the Surgery of Trauma (EAST); 2008.
34. Quenot JP, Thiery N, Barbar S. When should stress ulcer prophylaxis be used in the ICU? Curr Opin Crit Care. 2009;15(2):139–43.
35. McLaren R, Jarvis CL, Fish DN. Use of enteral nutrition for stress ulcer prophylaxis. Ann Pharmacother. 2001;35:1614–23.
36. Bonten MJ, Gaillard CA, Van Tiel FH, Van der Geest S, Stobberingh EE. Continuous enteral feeding counteracts preventive measures for gastric colonization in ICU patients. Crit Care Med. 1994;22:939–44.
37. Madsen KR, Lorentzen K, Clausen N, et al. Danish Society of Intensive Care Medicine; Danish Society of Anesthesiology and Intensive Care Medicine: guideline for stress ulcer prophylaxis in the intensive care unit. Dan Med J. 2014;61:C4811.
38. Welage LS. Overview of pharmacologic agents for acid suppression in critically ill patients. Am J Health Syst Pharm. 2005;62(10 Suppl 2):S4–S10.
39. Mulla H, Peek G, Upton D, et al. Plasma aluminum levels during sucralfate prophylaxis for stress ulceration in critically ill patients on continuous venovenous hemofiltration: a randomised, controlled trial. Crit Care Med. 2001;29:267–71.
40. Tryba M. Sucralfate versus antacids or H2-antagonists for stress ulcer prophylaxis. A meta-analysis on efficacy and pneumonia rate. Crit Care Med. 1991;19:942–9.
41. Grindlinger GA, Cairo SB, Duperre CB. Pneumonia prevention in intubated patients given sucralfate versus proton-pump inhibitors and/or histamine II receptor blockers. J Surg Res. 2016;206(2):398–404.
42. Dellinger RP, Levy MM, Rhodes A, et al. Surviving Sepsis Campaign Guidelines Committee Including the Pediatric Subgroup: Surviving sepsis campaign: international guidelines for management of severe sepsis and septic shock: 2012. Crit Care Med. 2013;41:580–637.
43. Wolfe MM, Soll AH. The physiology of gastric acid secretion. N Engl J Med. 1988;319:1707–15.
44. Messori A, Trippoli S, Gorini M, Corrado A. Bleeding and pneumoniae in intensive care patients given ranitidine and sucralfate for prevention of stress ulcer: meta-analysis of randomised controlled trials. BMJ. 2000;321:1103–6.
45. Kantorova I, Svoboda P, Scheer P, et al. Stress ulcer prophylaxis in critically ill patients: a randomized controlled trial. Hepato-Gastroenterology. 2004;51:757–61.
46. Ben-Menachem T, Fogel R, Patel RV, et al. Prophylaxis for stress-related gastric hemorrhage in the medical intensive care unit. Ann Intern Med. 1994;121:568–75.
47. Gillen D, McColl KE. Problems related to acid rebound and tachyphylaxis. Best Pract Res Clin Gastroenterol. 2001;15:487–95.
48. Spirt MJ, Stanley S. Update on stress ulcer prophylaxis in critically ill patients. Crit Care Nurse. 2006;26:18–29.
49. Tryba M, Cook D. Current guidelines on stress ulcer prophylaxis. Drugs. 1997;54:581–96.
50. American Society of Health-System Pharmacists Commission on Therapeutics. ASHP therapeutic guidelines on stress ulcer prophylaxis. Am J Health Syst Pharm. 1999;56:347–79.
51. Harty RF, Ancha HB. Stress ulcer bleeding. Curr Treat Options Gastroenterol. 2006;9:157–66.
52. Schentag JJ, Cerra FB, Calleri G, et al. Pharmacokinetic and clinical studies in patients with cimetidine-associated mental confusion. Lancet. 1979;1:177–81.

53. Wade EE, Rebuck JA, Healey MA, et al. H(2) antagonist-induced thrombocytopenia: is this a real phenomenon? Intensive Care Med. 2002;28:459–65.
54. Spirt MJ. Stress-related mucosal disease: risk factors and prophylactic therapy. Clin Ther. 2004;26:197–213.
55. Barkun AN, Bardou M, Pham CQ, et al. Proton pump inhibitors vs. histamine 2 receptor antagonists for stress-related mucosal bleeding prophylaxis in critically ill patients: a meta-analysis. Am J Gastroenterol. 2012;107:507–20.
56. Pongprasobchai S, Kridkratoke S, Nopmaneejumruslers C. Proton pump inhibitors for the prevention of stress-related mucosal disease in critically ill patients: a meta-analysis. J Med Assoc Thail. 2009;92:632–7.
57. Lin PC, Chang CH, Hsu PI, et al. The efficacy and safety of proton pump inhibitors vs histamine-2 receptor antagonists for stress ulcer bleeding prophylaxis among critical care patients: a meta-analysis. Crit Care Med. 2010;38:1197–205.
58. Levy MJ, Seelig CB, Robinson NJ, et al. Comparison of omeprazole and ranitidine for stress ulcer prophylaxis. Dig Dis Sci. 1997;42:1255–9.
59. Conrad SA, Gabrielli A, Margolis B, et al. Randomized, double blind comparison of immediate-release omeprazole oral suspension versus intravenous cimetidine for the prevention of upper gastrointestinal bleeding in critically ill patients. Crit Care Med. 2005;33:760–5.
60. Somberg L, Morris J Jr, Fantus R, et al. Intermittent intravenous pantoprazole and continuous cimetidine infusion: effect on gastric pH control in critically ill patients at risk of developing stress-related mucosal disease. J Trauma. 2008;64:1202–10.
61. Alhazzani W, Alenezi F, Jaeschke RZ, et al. Proton pump inhibitors versus histamine 2 receptor antagonists for stress ulcer prophylaxis in critically ill patients: a systematic review and meta-analysis. Crit Care Med. 2013;41:693–705.
62. Wolfe MM, Sachs G. Acid suppression: optimizing therapy for gastroduodenal ulcer healing, gastroesophageal reflux disease, and stress-related erosive syndrome. Gastroenterology. 2000;118(2suppl 1):S9–31.
63. Cunningham R, Dale B, Undy B, et al. Proton pump inhibitors as a risk factor for *Clostridium difficile* diarrhoea. J Hosp Infect. 2003;54:243–5.
64. Dial S, Alrasadi K, Manoukian C, et al. Risk of *Clostridium difficile* diarrhea among hospital inpatients prescribed proton pump inhibitors: cohort and case-control studies. Can Med Assoc J. 2004;171:33–8.
65. Howden CW, Hunt RH. Relationship between gastric secretion and infection. Gut. 1987;28:96–107.
66. Dial MS. Proton pump inhibitor use and enteric infections. Am J Gastroenterol. 2009;104(Suppl 2):S10–6.
67. Barletta JF, Sclar DA. Use of proton pump inhibitors for the provision of stress ulcer prophylaxis: clinical and economic consequences. Pharmacoeconomics. 2014;32:5–13.
68. Alhazzani W, Guyatt G, Marshall JC, et al. Re-evaluating the inhibition of stress erosions (REVISE): a protocol for pilot randomized controlled trial. Ann Saudi Med. 2016;36(6):427–33.
69. Krag M, Perner A, Wetterslev J, et al. Stress ulcer prophylaxis with a proton pump inhibitor versus placebo in critically ill patients (SUP-ICU trial): study protocol for a randomised controlled trial. Trials. 2016;17:205.
70. Tryba M, May B. Conservative treatment of stress ulcer bleeding: a new approach. Scand J Gastroenterol Suppl. 1992;191:16–24.
71. Leather RA, Sullivan SN. Iced gastric lavage: a tradition without foundation. CMAJ. 1987;136(12):1245–7.
72. Athanasoulis CA, Brown B, Shapiro JH. Angiography in the diagnosis and management of bleeding stress ulcers and gastritis. Am J Surg. 1973;125(4):468–73.
73. Waibel BH, Rotondo MF. Damage control for intra-abdominal sepsis. Surg Clin North Am. 2012;92(2):243–57.
74. Sullivan RC, Waddell WR. Accumulated experience with vagotomy and pyloroplasty for surgical control of hemorrhagic gastritis. Am J Surg. 1968;116:745.
75. Zarzaur BL, Kudsk KA, Carter K, et al. Stress ulceration requiring definitive surgery after severe trauma. Am Surg. 2001;67(9):875–9.
76. Richardson JD, Aust JB. Gastric devascularization: a useful salvage procedure for massive hemorrhagic gastritis. Ann Surg. 1977;185(6):649–55.
77. Hubert JP Jr, Kiernan PD, Welch JS, et al. The surgical management of bleeding stress ulcers. Ann Surg. 1980;191:672.

Nutritional Support in the Surgical Critical Care Patient

22

Matthew J. Martin, Joseph V. Sakran, and Robert G. Martindale

Introduction

A well-nourished 55-year-old female with a past medical history of hypertension, hypercholesterolemia, and major depression is admitted to the surgical intensive care unit (SICU) of a tertiary care hospital following an emergent laparotomy with Hartmann's procedure for sigmoid volvulus causing sigmoid perforation and fecal peritonitis. Upon arrival to the ICU, she is in septic shock requiring vasopressors. She is undergoing mechanical ventilation with the use of low tidal volumes and positive end-expiratory pressure (PEEP). Analgesia is provided by a continuous fentanyl infusion. The patient is found to have generalized oozing around arterial and central venous catheter insertion sites. This is most likely due to low-grade disseminated intravascular coagulation and does not currently merit any specific treatment other than supportive care and holding chemical venous thromboembolism (VTE) prophylaxis.

What approach would you use to provide initial nutrition support (if any) for this patient?

Optimal nutritional support is fundamental to modern intensive care unit (ICU) care, as critically ill patients often exhibit a catabolic stress state that is associated with increased morbidity and mortality. Historically one of the main problems with providing high-quality ICU nutrition was the lack of a robust and high-quality evidence base, with very few large randomized trials conducted. However, over the past two decades, there has been an explosion of outstanding nutrition research including multiple large and multicenter randomized trials. The problem faced by the modern ICU physician now is not the lack of an evidence base, but rather the difficulty in parsing the continually increasing body of literature on this topic. In addition, despite the recent decades of experience and research, the evidence for deciding who needs support, how much and when to deliver it, the optimal route and contents, and the underlying pathophysiologic mechanisms remain heavily debated. Accordingly, there exists widespread variation in enteral (EN) and total parenteral nutrition (TPN) utilization across all ICUs. Fortunately, there are several high-quality sources for ICU nutritional information, guidelines, and detailed synthesis and analysis of the existing literature. The first are the joint American Society of Parenteral and Enteral Nutrition (ASPEN)/Society of Critical Care Medicine (SCCM) nutrition guidelines, most recently updated and published in 2016 [1]. The second are the Canadian Critical Care Nutrition (CCCN) guidelines, last updated and published in 2015 [2]. In addition to the published literature review and guidelines, the Canadian group has an outstanding website dedicated to ICU nutrition (www.criticalcarenutrition.com) that includes nutrition and feeding guides and calculators, protocols, slide presentations, and educational materials. A third useful reference is the European Society of Parenteral and Enteral Nutrition (ESPEN) Guidelines for Surgery that were recently released in 2017 (www.espen.org/education/espen-guidelines).

Recent data has demonstrated that nutritional support protocols can result in significantly improved patient outcomes when they incorporate best practices and are appropriately tailored to the patient [3]. Some of the most common primary benefits include a decrease in local and systemic infections, attenuation of systemic inflammation, and improved metabolic/physiologic profiles. Of note, these benefits observed with early nutritional therapy do not appear directly correlated with the dose (both volume and caloric) of delivered nutrition. These findings suggest that nutritional therapy in the critically ill patient serves as a proactive

M. J. Martin (✉)
Trauma and Emergency Surgery Service, Legacy Emanuel Medical Center, Portland, OR, USA

J. V. Sakran
Division of Acute Care Surgery, Emergency General Surgery, The Johns Hopkins University, Baltimore, MD, USA

R. G. Martindale
Department of Surgery, Oregon Health & Science University, Portland, OR, USA

A. Salim et al. (eds.), *Surgical Critical Care Therapy*, https://doi.org/10.1007/978-3-319-71712-8_22

Top 10 Nutritional Practices to Avoid or Change:

1. Over-feeding based on erroneous assumptions about increased metabolism and increasing delivered calories based on "stress-factors"
2. Delivering supplemental nutrition in patients with minimal illness and expected to resume regular oral intake within several days
3. Delaying nutritional support in critically ill patients with existing malnutrition or who are at high nutritional risk
4. Failing to consider the dynamic changes in physiology, metabolism, nutritional needs, and ability to properly process nutrient loads that occurs in ICU patients over the course of an acute illness and recovery
5. Routine use of glutamine supplementation in ICU patients, or other "immune-enhancing" formulas in unselected critically ill patients
6. With-holding enteral feedings for prolonged periods based on presumed postoperative or medical "ileus", or using low volume thresholds (100-200 cc) for gastric residual
7. Failure to attempt post-pyloric feeding and prokinetics before switching to TPN for "enteral intolerance" to gastric feeds
8. Aggressive attempts at initiating enteral feeding and increasing rapidly to a "goal" rate in the presence of hemodynamic instability, moderate to high dose pressor dependence, rapidly declining renal/hepatic function, or the open abdomen with major ileus/bowel distension
9. Inadequate glucose control with prolonged/persistent intermittent blood glucose > 180 mg/dl
10. Performing non-urgent major surgical procedures in patients with pre-existing moderate to severe malnutrition without attempts at preoperative nutritional optimization

Fig. 22.1 Top 10 nutritional practices to avoid or change

therapeutic strategy to ameliorate or modulate the immune response, maintain gastrointestinal integrity and physiology, and ultimately alleviate the severity of the underlying disease process. One of the most important concepts to understand is that the critically ill patient does not resemble a normal healthy patient physiologically or metabolically and thus should not be fed like one [4]. Although it is often thought of as a positive and benign intervention, the improper delivery of nutritional therapy can result in multiple significant adverse effects that can nullify any positive effects and result in unnecessary added morbidity. Figure 22.1 outlines a "top 10 list" of ICU nutritional practices to avoid of change based on the most current evidence and experience.

Nutritional Assessment

Identifying whether a critically ill patient will benefit from nutritional therapy requires a thorough understanding of several patient factors and the interactions between these patient factors. By carefully evaluating these factors, a multidisciplinary team can then seek to estimate the patient's likelihood of receiving some or all of the benefits from nutritional therapy. These benefits should then be weighed against the potential risks and adverse effects of the nutritional intervention. This evaluation, however, does not automatically default to a favorable risk to benefit profile for all critically ill patients; there are myriad circumstances where nutritional

Table 22.1 Variables to consider prior to nutritional intervention

Key patient and disease factors	Potential risks of EN or TPN
Baseline nutritional status	Volume overload syndromes
Weight loss, laboratory markers, cross-sectional imaging	Hyperglycemia
Anthropometric measurements	Glucose shunting to lactate production
Age	Lipogenesis
Existing comorbidities	Protein shunting to nitrogenous waste, urea
Current diagnosis/cause of critical illness	Azotemia (rising BUN)
Severity of illness	Increased CO2 production, impaired ventilator weaning
APACHE, SAPS, ISS, MELD	Central line-associated infections
Vasopressor dependent and dose required	Fungal infections
Length of critical illness	Emesis and aspiration
Gut integrity, function, surgical interventions	Pro-inflammatory (TPN/lipids)
Estimated duration until able to resume oral intake	Bowel distension, edema, abdominal pain
Need for additional procedures or interventions	Electrolyte abnormalities
Available routes for feeding access or delivery	Bowel ischemia (rare)

Table 22.2 Nutrition Risk in Critically Ill (NUTRIC) score [6]

Variables	Range	Points
Age	<50	0
	50–75	1
	>75	2
APACHE II	<15	0
	15–19	1
	20–28	2
	≥28	3
SOFA	<6	0
	6–9	1
	≥10	2
Comorbidity (#)	0–1	0
	≥2	1
Hospital to ICU Admission (days)	0–1	0
	≥1	1
IL-6	<400	0
	≥400	1

Low score (0–5) = patients with low risk of malnutrition
High score (6–10) = patients with high risk of malnutrition

supplementation might not be beneficial, such as EN infusion on patients with escalating vasopressors or TPN in patients with fungemia. The following illustration (Table 22.1) provides several important factors, both positive and negative, that should be considered in weighing the risk to benefit analysis prior to implementation:

After reviewing the factors in Table 22.1 within a specific patient, the team should make a purposeful decision regarding the patient's nutritional risk status, the importance of starting supplementation, and if required, the optimal route for delivery. To address the large number of variables that go into this often complex decision, as well as the frequent non-linear interactions and correlations between variables, several standardized and validated scoring systems have emerged for guiding the team with estimating nutritional risk in a critically ill patient. One of the more commonly utilized methods is the Nutrition Risk in Critically Ill (NUTRIC) assessment tool [5]. The NUTRIC is calculated from a simple assignment of 0–3 points for each of the following six variables: age, Acute Physiology and Acute Chronic Health Evaluation (APACHE) II score, the Sequential Organ Failure Assessment (SOFA), number of comorbidities, days from hospital to ICU admission, and IL-6 level (Table 22.2). A score above five identifies individuals at high risk of major nutritional deficiency, prolonged mechanical ventilation, and mortality [6]. Because IL-6 is not readily available in most ICUs, the score may be modified by omitting the IL-6 component or by substituting it with the C-reactive protein (CRP) biomarker. Patients with a high NUTRIC score of 6–10, indicating a high risk of malnutrition, may benefit from early enteral therapy or immediate initiation of total parenteral nutrition (TPN) if they are unable to receive enteral feeding [3, 6]. While the NUTRIC score has been validated as a predictor of nutritional deficiency and adverse outcomes, it should be used as a tool that expands the clinician's armamentarium, and not in isolation as an absolute determinant for the timing or volume of nutritional support one should deliver. One critically important thing to understand is that a higher NUTRIC score does not necessarily mean that a patient needs more calories and should not reflexively be interpreted as an urgency to deliver higher than normal protein or calories.

One of the first steps in initiating nutritional support in the ICU is calculating or estimating the caloric and protein requirements. Although this would seem to be a relatively straightforward issue, there remains no consensus on the method of assessment or the caloric targets that should be utilized. The 2016 ASPEN/SCCM guidelines recommend the use of indirect calorimetry to measure the energy requirements when available, and providing there are no contraindications. However, the evidence behind this recommendation is rated as "very low," and there are multiple relatively common ICU factors that can compromise the accuracy of this test. If indirect calorimetry (IC) is utilized, the ICU physician must be aware of the limitations and confounders for this study. IC has been demonstrated to generally overestimate caloric requirements compared to predictive equations and can be confounded by factors such as diet-induced thermogenesis if the study is performed while the patient is being fed. The alternatives, if IC is not available or in the presence of factors that impact its reliability, are predictive equations or simplistic weight-based equations. Neither has shown superiority, although predictive equations derived from healthy volunteers (like the Harris-Benedict equations) are generally less accurate than those derived from hospitalized cohorts (like the Penn State equation) [1]. We would recommend use of the more simplified weight based calculations, particularly for calculating the initial energy requirements and caloric goals for an ICU patient. Full caloric feeding is generally between 25 kcal/kg and 35 kcal/kg, and lower-calorie targets (such as permissive underfeeding) can then be taken as percentages of this initial caloric goal calculation. For patients with large weight changes (massive fluid overload, edema, anasarca), the original body weight should be utilized. For obese patients, an ideal body weight should be calculated and used in the equation. Finally, do not forget to take into account the calories that are already being delivered to the patient in the form of dextrose-containing solutions, lipid-based medications such as propofol, and any ongoing enteral or parenteral feeding.

Initiating Nutrition

The two most common areas of contention and debate surrounding nutrition in the critically ill patient involve (1) the optimal timing for starting supplemental nutrition and (2) the benefits or disadvantages of EN versus TPN. The specific population of interest for providing either form of nutrition focuses on critically ill adult patients who have expected ICU stays of greater than 2–3 days. For the patient who is not critically ill, with no pre-existing malnutrition, and who is expected to resume oral intake within several days, there have been no demonstrated benefits of either aggressive EN or TPN support. We can reasonably assume that this patient population would derive very few (if any) potential benefits of EN or TPN but would still be at risk for the potential adverse effects and complications associated with caloric supplementation. For the remainder of the critically ill population, we can safely assume that any patient with an active illness requiring high levels of care is at a high risk for either having or developing both macro- and micronutrient deficiencies and a so-called caloric deficit. In addition, identifying patients with pre-existing malnutrition (body mass index <19, history of poor oral intake, weight loss >10–15% of baseline, pre-illness albumin <3, cancer with known cachexia) should prompt initiation of nutritional supplementation at the earliest possible time. These factors are already considered in the validated nutritional risk scoring systems such as the NRS and NUTRIC, and we would recommend automatically calculating one or both on every ICU admission [7–10].

Although there is no universal agreement for when to initiate feeding in all ICU patients, there is a general consensus to start enteral feedings early for optimal care, defined as within 24–48 h in the critically ill patient who is unable to maintain volitional intake unless there is some absolute contraindication [2, 3]. Studies have consistently demonstrated that early enteral feedings confer benefits in reduced infections, organ failure, decreased length of stay, and possible reduction in mortality rates, when compared to delayed initiation of enteral feeding or the use of TPN. Interestingly, these benefits of early EN appear to be relatively independent to the actual nutritional dose (amount of calories delivered) but are likely related more to the non-nutritional benefits such as minimizing adverse changes in gut permeability, minimizing immunosuppression, or even positively impacting the gut microbiome [11, 12]. Therefore, it is more important to have some level of enteral feeding delivered early in the hospital course of the critically ill patient in order to achieve at least minimal caloric targets and minimize morbidity. EN feeds can be initiated through the stomach or the lower gastrointestinal tract. Of note, while initiating through the small bowel is associated with a reduced risk of pneumonia, the benefit of early EN through the stomach outweighs its associated risks. It is therefore acceptable to begin EN feeds in the stomach until infusion can be diverted to the lower gastrointestinal tract [3, 13].

For the subset of patients that require TPN due to either complication or contraindication to EN, there is unfortunately a paucity of evidence associated with the benefit of early administration. Clinicians should consider the pre-existing nutritional status of the critically ill patient. If no evidence of significant malnutrition or elevated nutrition risk (by NRS or NUTRIC score) exists, then TPN should be considered after 5–7 days of inability to initiate or tolerate EN. However, if there are signs that point toward protein/calorie malnutrition upon admission or those deemed high risk for nutritional deficiency, TPN should be started immediately. For patients scheduled to undergo major surgery and with evidence of current malnutrition, then nutritional supplementation with EN (or TPN if enteral contraindicated or not tolerated) should be administered preoperatively for at least 5–7 days if possible.

The other aspect that is often discussed is the whether one should wait for return of bowel function prior to initiation. A significant proportion of critically ill patients, 30–70%, can have gastrointestinal dysfunction based on a variety of factors [14]. However, current literature and consensus guidelines suggest that return of bowel function (i.e., bowel sounds, flatus, bowel movement) is not necessary for initiation of EN [3]. For patients who have undergone gastrointestinal surgery, it is still important that a collaborative decision is reached between the multidisciplinary team that is caring for the patient.

Intensivists are also often faced with the critically ill patient requiring vasopressors. While clinicians have traditionally steered away from beginning EN in patients on vasopressors due to the ischemia and/or reperfusion injury risk, the literature has supported the early delivery of EN in patients who are on stable and low doses of vasopressors [12, 15]. However, one should be cautious in the hemodynamically unstable patient requiring an escalation of vasopressors or those maxed out on multiple high-dose vasopressors. In addition to being unlikely to tolerate enteral nutrition, there is a risk of bowel-related complications such as ischemia, dilation with perforation, or anastomotic breakdown with aggressive attempts at forcing enteral nutrition.

Enteral Versus Parenteral

The debate over the indications, benefits, and risks of enteral versus total parenteral delivery of nutritional support has raged for decades and continues to be a focus of scientific investigation. Although the enteral route is the seemingly more "natural" and common sense method of delivery, it does have significant limitations and unwanted side effects in many critically ill patients, particularly surgical patients. Accordingly, after landmark reports described using parenteral nutrition to successfully support infants with short gut syndrome, adult intensivists widely embraced TPN as a simpler and equally effective alternative to EN. However, as more experience with TPN was gained and multiple controlled trials were performed, there were consistent findings of worse outcomes in the TPN cohorts, prompting the pendulum to swing back to EN as the clearly superior route. It is important to note that these adverse outcomes were primarily infectious complications, including central line-associated infections and pneumonia, and were used to justify recommendations to avoid using TPN if at all possible. Currently, there is still general support for the superiority of EN over TPN among patients who are able to receive and tolerate enteral feeding, particularly in terms of a reduction in infectious complications. However, the pendulum is again swinging back to a more balanced perspective and greater acceptance of TPN as a viable option in the critically ill patient. This increasing acceptance is due to multiple factors, most notably that complications formerly associated with TPN such as central line-associated infections and ventilator-associated pneumonia have been drastically reduced with modern ICU care. This has been demonstrated in several recent prospective randomized trials that have shown no increased incidence of infections or other adverse outcomes among patients randomized to receive TPN [16, 17]. Other factors include the current focused attention on glycemic control and the current availability of a mixed lipid emulsion including fish oil, MCT, olive oil and soy oil that became available in teh USA in 2016. In addition, a very recent meta-analysis of studies of enteral versus TPN demonstrated that there was no difference in mortality between the two routes, but there was a decrease in infectious complications and length of stay associated with enteral feeding [18]. However, this difference appears to be attributable to studies where the TPN groups were given significantly more average caloric intake versus enteral feeding. When caloric delivery was equal between enteral and TPN, there was no difference in either mortality or morbidities [18].

The other proposed advantage of EN over TPN is the maintenance of gut mucosal integrity and the prevention of bacterial translocation across the gut wall and into the lymphatic and systemic circulation. These benefits from EN relative to TPN have been validated in animal models. Furthermore, while there is little to no direct evidence linking short- to medium-term TPN use (less than 4–6 weeks) with gut mucosal atrophy/breakdown or bacterial translocation, there are multiple serious adverse effects when TPN is used for prolonged periods of months to years (>4–6 weeks). These adverse effects include vascular access complications (infection, thrombosis), cholestasis and hepatocellular injury, glucose and electrolyte disturbances, and gut mucosal disuse atrophy. In addition, there is a growing body of literature that implicates the gut as a primary driver of local and distant organ injury in critical illness and that changes to the normal endogenous bacterial gut flora (aka "the microbiome") might be one of the primary factors in this process [19, 20]. In these situations where a patient is on prolonged TPN, aggressive attempts at initiating EN or improving tolerance to EN are warranted in order to avoid the severe potential complications with long-term TPN use.

Several factors have been found to improve the delivery of higher volumes/calories of EN and are recommended for all ICU patients. These include (1) the initiation of EN at a slow rate (10–20 cc/h) and then slow advancement to the calculated "goal" rate, (2) the use of prokinetic agents, (3) the use of higher thresholds of gastric residual volumes (>500), and (4) the post-pyloric feeding if there are persistent high gastric residuals/emesis/distension or in patients who are at high risk for aspiration. The optimal method to ensure maximized use of adequate nutritional support is having all the above included in a local protocol or algorithm using best-practice and evidence-based guidelines [21, 22]. However, suboptimal caloric delivery is unfortunately more the rule rather than the exception in most ICUs, due to interruption of feedings for procedures, trips for imaging studies, and high gastric residuals or other signs of feeding intolerance. The most effective proven system and protocols/practices to overcome these daily realities of modern ICU care have been elaborated in the PEP uP studies [21–23]. These include a nurse-driven "top-down" feeding approach that targets a daily volume of feeding (or calories) rather than a set hourly rate. Following any interruptions of feedings, the bedside nurse is empowered to calculate the new feeding rate to achieve the daily caloric goal using the formula: [new feeding rate = (daily volume goal - volume delivered)/hours remaining in day. This has been consistently shown to result in improved delivery of total calories and improved rates of achieving 100% delivery of daily caloric feeding goals [21–23]. Once again the pendulum has started to swing back to starting slow with EN to obtain those non-nutritional benefits, then over 4 to 5 days attempting to progress to goal rather than the rapid push to attain goals.

When to Use TPN

The previous sections have summarized the benefits of using EN over TPN whenever appropriate for patients. However, there will be times where patients should not undergo EN for various contraindications and may subsequently instead require TPN. Unfortunately, there is currently less of a consensus regarding the utilization and timing of TPN in the critically ill patient. This is mostly because the risk to benefit ratio does not appear to be as strong or as clearly demonstrated for TPN compared to EN nutrition.

An objective approach to decision-making with respect to TPN utilization and timing begins with determining the nutritional status of the patient. As described earlier, the NUTRIC score is one method to help identify if a patient is at low or high risk for nutritional deficiency [2]. The literature supports delaying TPN for the first week in patients who are at low risk for nutritional deficiency [24]. In fact, studies have demonstrated that early TPN in this subset of critically ill patients has been associated with increased morbidity [25]. However, for those found to be at high risk of nutritional deficiency, the recommendation is to begin TPN immediately upon ICU admission if EN is not feasible. A meta-analysis specifically evaluating malnourished patients in the ICU found a significant decrease in complications when TPN was initiated early [26, 27]. While the exact timing of TPN is not always clear, expert consensus recommends beginning TPN after 7–10 days regardless of nutritional status in patients who are not in the high-risk category by the initial risk assessment [1, 2].

During the initiation of TPN, it is important to consider the dosing of PN, especially in those patients who are found to be malnourished or at high risk for nutritional deficiency. Studies have found that minimizing excess energy intake early in the ICU stay may reduce morbidity (i.e., infection, hospital LOS) [28]. The SCCM/ASPEN and Canadian guidelines both recommend that during the initial administration of TPN, hypocaloric dosing (≤20 kcal/kg/d or 80% of estimated energy needs) with adequate protein (≥1.2 g protein/kg/d) should be delivered [1, 2].

Estimating Caloric Requirements and Selecting the Optimal Dose

Although determining the optimal dose of PN or EN to deliver to a critically ill patient may seem relatively straightforward, in practice this remains poorly understood, widely debated, and highly complex. The traditional teaching on this subject has almost exclusively focused on estimating the "caloric needs" of the ICU patient. Much less consideration has been given to estimating their physiologic and metabolic readiness and their ability to tolerate a caloric load. It is critical to understand that critical illness-induced catabolism is entirely different than simple protein/calorie malnutrition (or "starvation") and leads to disruption and dysfunction of the host's intrinsic nutrition processing capacity and antioxidant defense systems. As a result, nutritional supplementation is not just a matter of supplying adequate calories and nutritional substrates. For example, the critical illness response will primarily shuttle these nutrients into maladaptive and inefficient pathways that result in energy expenditure and the creation of useless or even harmful by-products such as lactate, urea, nitrogenous waste products, oxidative agents, and fat mass. Thus, initiating early feeding in these patients, particularly high-calorie feeding during peak periods of illness, may have the paradoxical effect of inducing cellular, tissue, and organ injury, without providing any substantive nutritional benefit. This is supported by numerous lines of evidence detailing the ultimate fate of supplied nutrients, the adverse effects of overfeeding in the ICU, and the consistently equivalent outcomes between patients receiving lower amounts of calories versus moderate and higher amounts. The best and most appropriate methods of nutritional support in the ICU patient must consider both sides of this equation, with equal attention paid to nutritional needs and to nutritional readiness or tolerance.

There are many available options and widely varying practices between providers in estimating the caloric requirements and calculating the optimal caloric dose of enteral or parenteral nutrition to deliver to the critically ill patient. The three main methods that are utilized in the majority of ICUs are (1) indirect calorimetry, (2) predictive equations, and (3) simplified weight-based calculation. There is a paucity of level 1 evidence examining the optimal method for estimating caloric needs and for guiding the delivered doses of supplemental nutrition. A review of two randomized trials comparing indirect calorimetry to predictive equation or weight-based calculation demonstrated no effect on mortality, but there were concerns that indirect calorimetry-guided strategy resulted in increased infections and longer ICU lengths of stay [29]. Using indirect calorimetry-guided dosing did result in an increased average daily caloric delivery, but this is not necessarily a beneficial outcome and in some cases could contribute to a higher complication profile. There

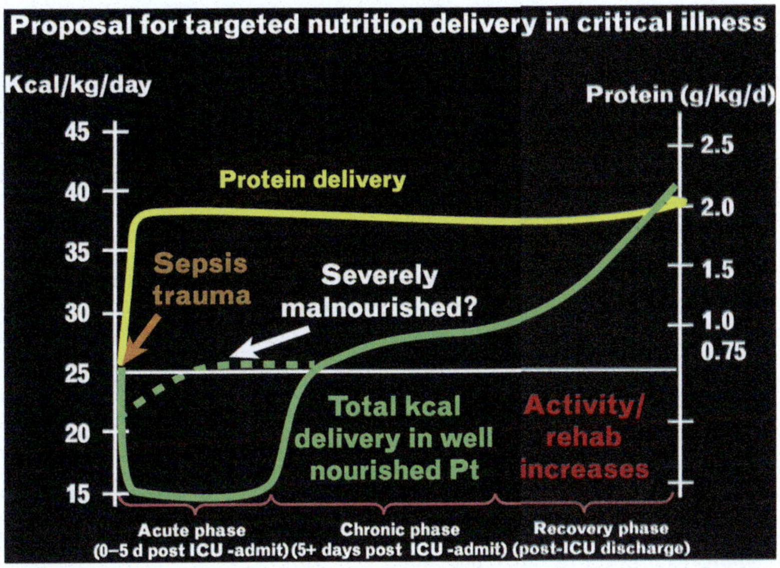

Fig. 22.2 Graph demonstrating targeted or "personalized" nutrition delivery in a standard ICU patient as they progress through the standard phases of critical illness and that also considers the disease severity and the presence of pre-existing severe malnutrition (Reproduced with permission from Wischmeyer [4])

has been no demonstrated evidence that the more complex predictive equations have any benefit over simple weight-based approaches, and a general range of 20–35 kcal/kg/day of nonprotein calories is widely accepted and utilized. For initiation of feeding or for feeding in the severely ill or acutely worsening patient, a lower caloric target may be chosen, with subsequent adjustment based on the patients overall clinical status, trajectory of disease, and response to nutrition therapy. It is also important to understand that the ICU patient is not static and will have significantly changes in the degree of illness, underlying metabolism and physiology, and metabolic response to nutrition over the course of their stay. Therefore, the nutritional assessment and calculation of caloric goals should not be a onetime only effort and should be frequently reevaluated and recalculated to take into account the dynamic nature of critical illness and the return to more normal physiology and nutritional requirements/tolerance in patients recovering from major insults (Fig. 22.2) [4].

Finally, there has been great interest in evaluating the independent effects of the primary nutrient sources (fat, protein, carbohydrates) and the numerous added supplements, as well as varying ratios and combinations of these components. Some of the current recommendations regarding the composition of TPN and EN, as well as the role of various additives and supplements, are listed in Table 22.3. A complete description of this topic is beyond the scope of this chapter, but several key summary points are as follows:

1. Carbohydrate, protein, and fats/lipids are the backbone nutritional components, and there appears to be no evidence for very low or very high protein or carbohydrate/fat ratio strategies, although there is some evidence supporting higher early protein delivery as beneficial.
2. Intravenous lipids, particularly soybean oil-based compounds (currently used in the USA), have many pro-inflammatory effects and have been associated with adverse outcomes in ICU patients. Interval and lower dosing of these lipids to avoid essential fatty acid deficiency is adequate in most patients. A mixed intravenous lipid emulsion is now available in the USA and should be considered in these hyperdynamic patients.
3. "Immune-enhancing" formulas have no proven benefit in unselected ICU patient populations and may be associated with worse outcomes in certain subpopulations (i.e., sepsis). There is some evidence that specific formulas containing fish oils, borage oils, and antioxidants are beneficial in patients with acute lung injury or ARDS, although most of this benefit has been proven in medical patients rather than surgical populations.
4. Glutamine supplementation by parenteral or enteral routes should *not* be routinely used in critically ill patients, and particularly in patients with shock or multiple organ failure. There may be some benefit in the burn patient population, but further study results (ongoing RE-ENERGIZE trial) are needed to clarify the safety vs benefit profile.

Trophic Feeding, Hypocaloric Feeding, and Permissive Underfeeding

As noted previously in this chapter, there have been multiple studies that have suggested that many of the benefits of ICU nutrition are not dependent on the overall amount of delivered calories or the aggressiveness of achieving 100% of the target or goal calories. There has also been evidence suggesting several potential adverse effects of delivering higher caloric content, including volume overload, hyperglycemia,

Table 22.3 Summary of the 2015 Canadian Critical Care Nutritional guidelines as compared to the previous (2013) guidelines. Changes from previous are highlighted in bold [2]

Topic	Recommendation	Change	Reason for rec or change
EN versus TPN	**Recommend use of EN over TPN if GI tract intact and functional**	**Downgrade**	**Downgraded from "strongly recommend" due to better outcomes in more recent TPN trials**
Timing of EN	Start early EN within 24–48 h	No change	Strong evidence for benefit
Timing of TPN	Early TPN not indicated in nutritionally low-risk patients, insufficient data for others	No change	For high-risk patients or not tolerating EN, decision of when to start TPN made on case-by-case basis
Determining energy/calorie needs	Insufficient data to support indirect calorimetry versus predictive equations for est. caloric need	No change	
Hypocaloric EN	**Hypocaloric feeding should be considered in patients at low nutrition risk**	**Upgrade**	**Several new PRCT showing identical outcomes and improved tolerance with hypocaloric feeds**
Arginine supplemented EN	Do not recommend arginine supplementation in ICU population	No change	No proven benefit in PRCT
Fish oils, borage oil, and antioxidant supplemented EN	Should be considered in patients with ALI or ARDS	No change	Improved pulmonary and overall outcomes in PRCTs in ALI/ARDS population
Glutamine supplement: EN	**Recommend that glutamine not be used in ICU patients**	**Downgrade**	**Evidence of harm among patients with shock, MSOF**
Glutamine supplement: TPN	**Recommend that glutamine not be used in ICU patients**	**Downgrade**	**Evidence of harm among patients with shock, MSOF**
High fat/low CHO or low fat/high CHO EN	Insufficient data to recommend in ICU patients	No change	
High protein vs low protein EN	Insufficient data to recommend in ICU patients	No change	
Use of motility agents for EN	Recommend the use of metoclopramide if EN intolerance	No change	Erythromycin not recommended due to safety concerns
Small bowel vs gastric feeding	Small bowel feeding may be assoc. with decreased pneumonia; small bowel feeding indicated in high risk for gastric intolerance or demonstrated gastric intolerance	No change	Based on 11 level 2 studies, including 1 new PRCT. Rec small bowel feeding tube placement if local logistics facilitate; otherwise, reserve for gastric intolerant patients
Gastric residuals: threshold and timing of residual checks	**Threshold of 250 to 500 cc checked every 4 or 8 h should be considered to optimize delivery of EN**	**Upgrade**	**Data demonstrating lower thresholds (<250 cc) have no benefit in preventing emesis/aspiration and serve to decrease caloric delivery**
Combined TPN + EN	Recommend against combined EN + TPN. Consider on a case-by-case basis if not tolerating adequate EN and all strategies to improve EN delivery exhausted	No change	
TPN vs standard care	**TPN should not be used routinely but should be considered for nutritionally high-risk pts. with contraindication to early EN**	**Upgrade**	**Based on improved complication profile in recent TPN studies and evidence of benefit in malnourished subgroups**
Lipids with TPN	Withholding lipids high in soybean oil should be considered in pts. who are not malnourished, are tolerating some EN, or require TPN < 10 days; insufficient evidence for all others	No change	Large reductions seen when withholding soybean oil lipids in infectious complications; trends toward reduced mortality, LOS, and mech ventilation

metabolic stress, renal injury, immunosuppression (primarily from lipids), and increased respiratory expenditures. This has led to significant debate about the correct targets for total calories and for protein delivery in the critically ill patient, particularly in the early acute phase of illness. In these patients we must balance the need for nutritional delivery to provide critical organ support versus the potential for delivered nutrients to fail to be utilized for energy needs, or even to result in harmful metabolic by-products. This has led to multiple recent prospective randomized studies evaluating alternative lower-calorie feeding strategies in general ICU patients or in select ICU subpopulations. These "permissive underfeeding" strategies generally provide a significantly lower volume of initial feeding that is then slowly increased based on some time schedule or on the patient's response and illness acuity. These approaches can generally be grouped into one of two categories: trophic or hypocaloric.

The trophic feeding strategy is exemplified by the EDEN trial, a multicenter randomized study conducted in ICU patients with acute lung injury [30]. The trophic strategy involved initiating enteral feeding at 20 cc/h for 6 days, and then advanced to full caloric goals after 6 days. This was compared to the "full" nutritional support group who received enteral feeds targeted to 25–30 kcal/kg/day of non-protein calories and 1.2–1.6 g/kg/day of protein. Therefore, the trophic strategy delivered significantly lower amounts of both calories and protein. Of interest, there were no differences in outcome measures between the two groups, and the trophic strategy causes less gastrointestinal intolerance than the full feeding approach. In addition, there were no significant differences noted in longer-term (1 year) survival or physical functioning [31]. Critics of this approach cite the extremely low amounts of protein delivered in the early phase of acute illness and argued for the potential superiority of a strategy delivering lower total calories but maintaining full protein delivery. This "hypocaloric" approach was studied in the PERMIT trial, where 894 patients were randomized to receive 50% of calculated goal calories plus full protein, versus standard feeding at 100% of calculated goals [32]. There was no identified difference in any primary outcome measure between the two groups, although the hypocaloric group had significantly less hyperglycemia and lower insulin requirements. A post hoc analysis that compared results when patients were categorized as either low or high baseline nutritional risks again showed no difference in outcomes by the assigned feeding strategy [33]. Similar results have also been demonstrated in a smaller study of surgical ICU patients [34]. As shown in Tables 22.3 and 22.4, both the ASPEN/SCCM and Canadian Critical Care Nutrition guidelines have now incorporated hypocaloric and trophic feeding strategies as acceptable alternatives for patients who are not deemed to be at high nutritional risk by the NRS or NUTRIC score. However, some have argued that there may be longer-term deficits in outcomes and physical functioning if we underfeed high-risk ICU patients, and several retrospective or secondary analyses have supported this concern [6, 22, 35]. This remains an area of current debate, with some arguing to feed every ICU patient at full goal rates, while others support selective use of hypocaloric feeding strategies as safe and less complicated for most ICU patients. Our bias is to initially use a hypocaloric feeding approach (50% calculated calories but full protein delivery) for initial feeding of most ICU patients, with targeted increase to 100% caloric delivery based on the patients underlying risk, disease severity, and course of illness.

Trauma/Burns

Trauma patients comprise an important subset of the critically ill patient. These patients are often complex and can present with a variety of factors that might make early nutrition delivery difficult. In fact, the significant metabolic response associated with trauma results in the breakdown of lean body mass unlike what is seen during starvation. This change in metabolism is compounded by a variety of other factors such as the immobility of trauma patients and the subsequent difficulty in providing adequate nutritional therapy. Similar to other critically ill patients, starting nutrition early within the first 24–48 h after resuscitation has been found to improve outcomes [36, 37]. A meta-analysis demonstrated a reduction in mortality with early feeding in trauma patients [36]. Clinicians should consider lower energy provision during the initial phases with a plan to ramp up to goals that range in the neighborhood of 20–35 kcal/kg/d. The amount of protein sits on the higher end of the range from 1.2 to 2 g protein/kg/d.

Traumatic brain injury (TBI) has been a widely discussed topic among this subset of patients. Like other trauma patients, those with TBIs can have greatly improved outcomes with early feeding (reference). While some evidence suggests that the benefit of early nutrition does not depend on the route of admission (EN vs TPN), expert consensus still recommends EN if possible as the first line of nutritional therapy. These patients can have a measured energy expenditure that is 100–200% of the predicted baseline resting energy expenditure (REE) [38]. There is also some data that suggests the utilization of arginine-containing immune-modulating formulations to supplement standard enteral formulas; however, at this point, it has not been extensively studied to make any strong evidence-based recommendations [39].

The other important group of patients we often seen are those with an open abdomen. Contrary to popular belief, the open abdomen patient can and should be started on early nutrition with the caveat that no bowel injury is present or that bowel continuity has been restored [40]. In addition, due to the significant exudative volume that is emitted from an open abdomen, adding 15–30 g of protein per liter should be considered. It is critical that the plan for initiating enteral feeding in the open abdomen patient be discussed with the responsible managing surgeon, and that the patient be closely monitored for signs of intolerance, worsening distension, or any other complication. This is particularly critical in the presence of newly formed anastomoses, which can become devastating entero-atmospheric fistulae if there is a leak caused by significant bowel distension due to aggressive enteral feeding.

Burn injury patients have also been found to require a significant amount of nutritional requirement. It can be difficult to estimate the exact energy needs, and expert consensus recommends measuring this via indirect calorimetry, as this is the most accurate method for doing so. Similar to trauma, patients with burn injuries require a higher level of protein ranging from 1.5 to 2 g/kg/d, which is recommended by the

Table 22.4 Summary of the new 2016 SCCM/ASPEN guidelines [1]

Nutrition assessment	Risk assessment should be performed (using NRS or NUTRIC) to identify "high-risk" patients
Determine energy requirements	Indirect calorimetry if available; equation or simple weight-based calculations if not
Initiation of feeding	1. Early EN within 24–48 h of ICU admission is preferred 2. Post-pyloric feeding if aspiration risk or gastric intolerance 3. If unstable, EN withheld until hemodynamically stable
Dosing of enteral nutrition	1. Either trophic or full feeding is appropriate in ARDS or expected vent >72 h 2. For high nutrition risk or severely malnourished, advance to goal (>80% of estimated calories) over 24–48 h 3. With either trophic or full, provide full protein (1.2–2 g/kg/day)
Use of specialized EN formulations	1. Should *not* be used routinely in unselected ICU patients 2. Immune enhancing reserved for TBI and major gastrointestinal surgery patients perioperatively 3. No rec regarding immune formula (omega-3 + borage oils) in ARDS/ALI patients[a]
Total parenteral nutrition (TPN)	1. No TPN until day 7 in low-risk patients not tolerating EN 2. Immediate TPN in high risk or malnourished who cannot tolerate EN 3. Supplemental TPN after 7 days if unable to deliver >60% energy and protein requirements by enteral route
Dosing of TPN	1. Hypocaloric (<20 kcal/kg/day) with full protein be considered in high risk or malnourished for first week of nutrition
Composition of TPN	1. Withhold or limit soybean oil lipids over first week 2. Alternative lipids be used when they become available in the USA
Glutamine supplementation	1. Rec against enteral glutamine supplementation in the ICU 2. Rec against parenteral glutamine supplementation in the ICU
Acute pancreatitis	1. Early enteral feeding at trophic rate in mod/severe pancreatitis 2. Use either gastric or jejunal route (no difference in outcomes) 3. TPN after 1 week if EN not feasible or tolerated
Trauma	1. Early EN with high protein within 24–48 h of injury 2. Immune formula with fish oils and arginine be considered in severe trauma and in TBI patients 3. Open abdomen give early EN if no bowel injury 4. Additional protein (15–30 g/liter of exudate) for fluid output
Sepsis	1. Early enteral nutrition once hemodynamically stabilized 2. Enteral preferred over parenteral route 3. No use of TPN in early phase of septic shock or severe sepsis 4. Trophic feeds for the initial phase of sepsis, advance to full feeds over the first week 5. Immune-modulating formulas NOT be used
Obesity	1. Hypocaloric, full protein feeding strategy be utilized initially 2. Goal should not exceed 65–70% of estimated calories 3. If calorimetry not available, use 11–14 kcal/kg *actual* body weight for BMI 30–50 and 22–25 kcal/kg/day of *ideal* body weight for BMI >50 4. Protein should be given at 2–2.5 g/kg/day *ideal* body weight

[a]Differs from Canadian Critical Care Nutrition guideline rec for the use of these formulas in ARDS/ALI

numerous guidelines including the American Burn Association [41]. As with other critically ill patients, EN compared with TPN has been associated with a reduction in morbidity and mortality [42], and early initiation (within 4–6 h of injury) of EN may be associated with a lower incidence of complications [43, 44]. Table 22.4 shows a summary of the ASPEN/SCCM nutrition guidelines that includes recommendations for special subpopulations including trauma, sepsis, obesity, and acute pancreatitis.

Parting Thoughts

Nutritional support in the intensive care unit or critically ill patient may be a key factor in determining both the short- and longer-term outcomes and the risk of major morbidity or mortality. The choice of the best route of feeding, dose, composition, supplementation, and adjustment strategy will vary highly, and the complex decision-making requires the understanding of multiple patient and disease factors and their interactions within each other. Simplistic policies that take a universal approach and attempt to provide full caloric support regardless of the patient status and disease severity will often result in overfeeding and have no benefit (or even harm) to the patient. For additional information and for much more in-depth analyses and evidence-based recommendations, we would recommend the Canadian Critical Care Nutrition guidelines (www.criticalcarenutrition.com), which have just been updated in 2015, as well as the ASPEN/SCCM nutrition guidelines, which were published in 2009 and have a newly released 2016 update [1–3, 29].

References

1. Taylor BE, McClave SA, Martindale RG, et al. Guidelines for the provision and assessment of nutrition support therapy in the adult critically ill patient: Society of Critical Care Medicine (SCCM) and American Society for Parenteral and Enteral Nutrition (A.S.P.E.N.). Crit Care Med. 2016;44(2):390–438.
2. Committee CCPG. The 2015 Canadian Critical Care Nutrition Clinical Practice guidelines. 2015. http://www.criticalcarenutrition.com/.
3. McClave SA, Martindale RG, Vanek VW, et al. Guidelines for the provision and assessment of nutrition support therapy in the adult critically ill patient: Society of Critical Care Medicine (SCCM) and American Society for Parenteral and Enteral Nutrition (A.S.P.E.N.). JPEN J Parenter Enteral Nutr. 2009;33(3):277–316.
4. Wischmeyer PE. Are we creating survivors...or victims in critical care? Delivering targeted nutrition to improve outcomes. Curr Opin Crit Care. 2016;22(4):279–84.
5. Rahman A, Hasan RM, Agarwala R, Martin C, Day AG, Heyland DK. Identifying critically-ill patients who will benefit most from nutritional therapy: further validation of the "modified NUTRIC" nutritional risk assessment tool. Clin Nutr. 2016;35(1):158–62.
6. Heyland DK, Dhaliwal R, Jiang X, Day AG. Identifying critically ill patients who benefit the most from nutrition therapy: the development and initial validation of a novel risk assessment tool. Crit Care. 2011;15(6):R268.
7. Bachmann J, Muller T, Schroder A, et al. Influence of an elevated nutrition risk score (NRS) on survival in patients following gastrectomy for gastric cancer. Med Oncol. 2015;32(7):204.
8. Kalaiselvan MS, Renuka MK, Arunkumar AS. Use of nutrition risk in critically ill (NUTRIC) score to assess nutritional risk in mechanically ventilated patients: a prospective observational study. Indian J Crit Care Med. 2017;21(5):253–6.
9. Reilly HM, Martineau JK, Moran A, Kennedy H. Nutritional screening–evaluation and implementation of a simple nutrition risk score. Clin Nutr. 1995;14(5):269–73.
10. Zhang B, Zhang Z. Association between nutrition risk in critically ill score and mortality may be mediated by nutritional therapy. J Crit Care. 2017;37:248.
11. Jabbar A, Chang WK, Dryden GW, McClave SA. Gut immunology and the differential response to feeding and starvation. Nutr Clin Pract: Off Publ Am Soc Parenter Enteral Nutr. 2003;18(6):461–82.
12. Khalid I, Doshi P, DiGiovine B. Early enteral nutrition and outcomes of critically ill patients treated with vasopressors and mechanical ventilation. Am J Crit Care. 2010;19(3):261–8.
13. Davies AR, Morrison SS, Bailey MJ, et al. A multicenter, randomized controlled trial comparing early nasojejunal with nasogastric nutrition in critical illness. Crit Care Med. 2012;40(8):2342–8.
14. Stechmiller JK, Treloar D, Allen N. Gut dysfunction in critically ill patients: a review of the literature. Am J Crit Care. 1997;6(3):204–9.
15. McClave SA, Chang WK. Feeding the hypotensive patient: does enteral feeding precipitate or protect against ischemic bowel? Nutr Clin Pract: Off Publ Am Soc Parenter Enteral Nutr. 2003;18(4):279–84.
16. Heidegger CP, Berger MM, Graf S, et al. Optimisation of energy provision with supplemental parenteral nutrition in critically ill patients: a randomised controlled clinical trial. Lancet. 2013;381(9864):385–93.
17. Wan X, Gao X, Tian F, Wu C, Wang X. Early parenteral nutrition alone or accompanying enteral nutrition in critically ill patients: a systematic review and meta-analysis. Asia Pac J Clin Nutr. 2015;24(2):227–33.
18. Elke G, van Zanten AR, Lemieux M, et al. Enteral versus parenteral nutrition in critically ill patients: an updated systematic review and meta-analysis of randomized controlled trials. Crit Care. 2016;20(1):117.
19. Alverdy JC, Krezalek MA. Collapse of the microbiome, emergence of the pathobiome, and the immunopathology of sepsis. Crit Care Med. 2017;45(2):337–47.
20. Meng M, Klingensmith NJ, Coopersmith CM. New insights into the gut as the driver of critical illness and organ failure. Curr Opin Crit Care. 2017;23(2):143–8.
21. Heyland DK, Dhaliwal R, Lemieux M, Wang M, Day AG. Implementing the PEP uP protocol in critical care units in Canada: results of a multicenter, quality improvement study. JPEN J Parenter Enteral Nutr. 2015;39(6):698–706.
22. Heyland DK, Cahill NE, Dhaliwal R, et al. Enhanced protein-energy provision via the enteral route in critically ill patients: a single center feasibility trial of the PEP uP protocol. Crit Care. 2010;14(2):R78.
23. Lee ZY, Barakatun-Nisak MY, Noor Airini I, Heyland DK. Enhanced protein-energy provision via the enteral route in critically ill patients (PEP uP protocol): a review of evidence. Nutr Clin Pract: Off Publ Am Soc Parenter Enteral Nutr. 2016;31(1):68–79.
24. Braunschweig CL, Levy P, Sheean PM, Wang X. Enteral compared with parenteral nutrition: a meta-analysis. Am J Clin Nutr. 2001;74(4):534–42.
25. Casaer MP, Mesotten D, Hermans G, et al. Early versus late parenteral nutrition in critically ill adults. N Engl J Med. 2011;365(6):506–17.
26. Heyland DK, MacDonald S, Keefe L, Drover JW. Total parenteral nutrition in the critically ill patient: a meta-analysis. JAMA. 1998;280(23):2013–9.
27. Heyland DK, Montalvo M, MacDonald S, Keefe L, XY S, Drover JW. Total parenteral nutrition in the surgical patient: a meta-analysis. Can J Surg. 2001;44(2):102–11.
28. McCowen KC, Friel C, Sternberg J, et al. Hypocaloric total parenteral nutrition: effectiveness in prevention of hyperglycemia and infectious complications--a randomized clinical trial. Crit Care Med. 2000;28(11):3606–11.
29. Dhaliwal R, Cahill N, Lemieux M, Heyland DK. The Canadian critical care nutrition guidelines in 2013: an update on current recommendations and implementation strategies. Nutr Clin Pract: Off Publ Am Soc Parenter Enteral Nutr. 2014;29(1):29–43.
30. National Heart L, Blood Institute Acute Respiratory Distress Syndrome Clinical Trials N, Rice TW, et al. Initial trophic vs full enteral feeding in patients with acute lung injury: the EDEN randomized trial. JAMA. 2012;307(8):795–803.
31. Needham DM, Dinglas VD, Bienvenu OJ, et al. One year outcomes in patients with acute lung injury randomised to initial trophic or full enteral feeding: prospective follow-up of EDEN randomised trial. BMJ. 2013;346:f1532.
32. Arabi YM, Aldawood AS, Haddad SH, et al. Permissive underfeeding or standard enteral feeding in critically ill adults. N Engl J Med. 2015;372(25):2398–408.
33. Arabi YM, Aldawood AS, Al-Dorzi HM, et al. Permissive underfeeding or standard enteral feeding in high- and low-nutritional-risk critically ill adults. Post hoc analysis of the permiT trial. Am J Respir Crit Care Med. 2017;195(5):652–62.
34. Charles EJ, Petroze RT, Metzger R, et al. Hypocaloric compared with eucaloric nutritional support and its effect on infection rates in a surgical intensive care unit: a randomized controlled trial. Am J Clin Nutr. 2014;100(5):1337–43.
35. Compher C, Chittams J, Sammarco T, Nicolo M, Heyland DK. Greater protein and energy intake may be associated with improved mortality in higher risk critically ill patients: a multicenter, multinational observational study. Crit Care Med. 2017;45(2):156–63.
36. Doig GS, Heighes PT, Simpson F, Sweetman EA. Early enteral nutrition reduces mortality in trauma patients requiring intensive care: a meta-analysis of randomised controlled trials. Injury. 2011;42(1):50–6.

37. Doig GS, Heighes PT, Simpson F, Sweetman EA, Davies AR. Early enteral nutrition, provided within 24 h of injury or intensive care unit admission, significantly reduces mortality in critically ill patients: a meta-analysis of randomised controlled trials. Intensive Care Med. 2009;35(12):2018–27.
38. Foley N, Marshall S, Pikul J, Salter K, Teasell R. Hypermetabolism following moderate to severe traumatic acute brain injury: a systematic review. J Neurotrauma. 2008;25(12):1415–31.
39. Falcao de Arruda IS, de Aguilar-Nascimento JE. Benefits of early enteral nutrition with glutamine and probiotics in brain injury patients. Clin Sci (Lond). 2004;106(3):287–92.
40. Burlew CC, Moore EE, Cuschieri J, et al. Who should we feed? Western Trauma Association multi-institutional study of enteral nutrition in the open abdomen after injury. J Trauma Acute Care Surg. 2012;73(6):1380–7; discussion 1387–1388.
41. Gibran NS, Committee on O, Delivery of Burn Care ABA. Practice guidelines for burn care, 2006. J Burn Care Res. 2006;27(4):437–8.
42. Rousseau AF, Losser MR, Ichai C, Berger MM. ESPEN endorsed recommendations: nutritional therapy in major burns. Clin Nutr. 2013;32(4):497–502.
43. Peng YZ, Yuan ZQ, Xiao GX. Effects of early enteral feeding on the prevention of enterogenic infection in severely burned patients. Burns. 2001;27(2):145–9.
44. Vicic VK, Radman M, Kovacic V. Early initiation of enteral nutrition improves outcomes in burn disease. Asia Pac J Clin Nutr. 2013;22(4):543–7.

Intra-abdominal Hypertension and Abdominal Compartment Syndrome

23

Javid Sadjadi and Gregory P. Victorino

Interest in intra-abdominal hypertension and abdominal compartment syndrome has intensified in recent years as the recognition of this condition has increased, thereby providing a potential therapeutic target to improve outcomes for critically ill patients [17]. According to a recent systematic review, the incidence of abdominal compartment syndrome varies between 0.5% and 36.4% of trauma patients, mortality is nearly universal if untreated, and for treated patients, overall survival is improved across all study cohorts, though survival rates range widely, from 25% to 75% [23].

Definition and Grading

Increased intra-abdominal pressure can result from multiple causes, such as volume occupying lesions, hemorrhage, ascites, overwhelming infection, and surgical packing. Definitions and a grading system have been developed by the World Society of the Abdominal Compartment Syndrome in an attempt to standardize the approach to intra-abdominal hypertension both clinically and in research. A normal intra-abdominal pressure is 2–7 mm Hg [19]. Intra-abdominal hypertension is the condition in which the patient has an elevated intra-abdominal compartment pressure, typically defined at a level of 12–15 mm Hg [19]. If untreated, the condition may progress to abdominal compartment syndrome, which occurs at an intra-abdominal pressure of greater than 20 mm Hg and is associated with end-organ dysfunction [19]. The grades of intra-abdominal hypertension and the associated intra-abdominal pressures are as follows:

Grade I:	12–15 mm Hg
Grade II:	16–20 mm Hg
Grade III:	21–25 mm Hg
Grade IV:	>25 mm Hg

An additional parameter that has been suggested as an endpoint of resuscitation is the abdominal perfusion pressure (APP). Abdominal perfusion pressure is calculated by subtracting the intra-abdominal pressure (IAP) from the mean arterial pressure (MAP): APP = MAP – IAP. An APP equal to or greater than 50 mm Hg has been demonstrated to be a good indicator of survival in patients with intra-abdominal hypertension or abdominal compartment syndrome [6].

Several risk factors for the development of abdominal compartment syndrome have been identified, including high-volume resuscitation, hypothermia, acidosis, ileus, and multisystem organ dysfunction [12, 13].

Measurement of Intra-abdominal Pressure

Intra-abdominal compartment pressure is typically measured in the intensive care setting, but because it is fairly straightforward to do, it can easily be measured anywhere in the inpatient setting. The technique involves measuring the pressure within the bladder in a supine patient at end expiration with a relaxed abdominal wall [21]. Fifty milliliters of saline are introduced into the bladder via the urinary drainage catheter, which is then clamped. The patient is placed in a level supine position, and the resulting pressure within the bladder is transduced at a height level to the patient's bladder [25]. Elevation of the head can result in artificially elevated values and thus should be avoided. Intra-vesicular pressure can then be transduced using a number of techniques. These include the use of an interposition T-piece, direct cannulation of the urinary catheter using a transducer-based needle, or the insertion of a continuous transduction method using a three-way Foley catheter. Perhaps the simplest technique was

J. Sadjadi · G. P. Victorino (✉)
Department of Surgery, University of California San Francisco East Bay, Oakland, CA, USA
e-mail: gregory.victorino@ucsfmedctr.org

A. Salim et al. (eds.), *Surgical Critical Care Therapy*, https://doi.org/10.1007/978-3-319-71712-8_23

described by Harrahill [11]. In this technique, after the 50 milliliters of saline is infused in the bladder, the column of urine generated in the Foley catheter that is raised straight up is measured in centimeters. This measurement correlates with intra-abdominal pressure. It should be remembered that this measurement is in cm H_2O, and the units defined in the grading system are in mm Hg. To convert from cm H_2O to mm Hg, multiply the value in cm by 0.74 [11]. A few additional key conversions to remember are that 16 cm H_2O is equal to 12 mm Hg and 27 cm H_2O is equal to 20 mm Hg.

Screening

Intra-abdominal hypertension and/or abdominal compartment syndrome is difficult to identify through physical examination alone. Recommendations from the International Conference of Experts on Intra-abdominal Hypertension and Abdominal Compartment Syndrome have identified patients who should be screened and/or surveilled for IAH or ACS.

These criteria include the following:

1. New intensive care unit admission
2. Evidence of clinical deterioration
3. Any two risk factors (listed in Table 23.1)

In patients who meet these criteria, bladder pressures should be monitored. However, the optimal frequency of pressure measurements is still unknown. Our usual practice is to check serial intra-abdominal pressures using the bladder pressure measurement technique every 4 h as long as the patient has one or more risk factors for the development of abdominal compartment syndrome.

Pathophysiology

Several mechanisms can lead to intra-abdominal hypertension and abdominal compartment syndrome. Primary intra-abdominal hypertension may develop as a result of retroperitoneal hemorrhage and infection. Secondary intra-abdominal hypertension, which is more common, refers to intra-abdominal hypertension developing in the setting of extra-abdominal or extrapelvic pathology. Secondary intra-abdominal hypertension develops when a large volume of resuscitation fluid (either crystalloid and/or blood products) is required to treat septic shock or hemorrhagic shock [24]. No matter the cause of shock, the pathophysiologic response is similar. Shock leads to the development of capillary leak. This capillary leak, combined with volume resuscitation, leads to extravasation of fluid from the intravascular space into the interstitial space. The release of inflammatory mediators leads to worsening of the condition, which develops into "intestinal distress syndrome" [20]. The increase in volume in the interstitial compartment leads to generalized edema throughout the body. Although commonly seen in the subcutaneous tissue, this process also occurs with the intra-abdominal viscera and the contents of the retroperitoneal space. This then leads to increased intra-abdominal pressure as the abdominal contents take on more fluid and increase volume, although the fascia of the abdominal wall does not increase in compliance. Under the constraints of a relatively non-compliant abdominal wall fascia, the volume of the intra-abdominal contents reaches a maximum, after which the intra-abdominal pressure begins to increase.

Table 23.1 Risk factors for intra-abdominal hypertension and/or abdominal compartment syndrome

Acute respiratory failure with increased intrathoracic pressures	Major trauma and/or burns
Gastroparesis	Ileus
Colonic pseudo-obstruction (Ogilvie's syndrome)	Ascites
Hemoperitoneum	Acidosis
Hypotension	Hypothermia
Massive transfusion [12]	Large volume resuscitation
Oliguria	Sepsis

Tertiary abdominal compartment syndrome occurs when the syndrome develops after initial treatment for abdominal compartment syndrome. In other words, it develops after the abdominal cavity has already been decompressed. This is occasionally referred to as chronic abdominal compartment syndrome. Repeated massive fluid resuscitation may result in an increased inflammatory response, bowel edema, and ascites. This can result in an abdominal compartment syndrome requiring further opening of the abdominal cavity and placement of a possibly less restrictive abdominal dressing [2].

Quaternary abdominal compartment syndrome occurs when the syndrome develops in the setting of hernia repair or abdominal wall closure. The greater use of abdominal wall reconstruction techniques, rather than "hole patch" incisional hernia repairs, understandably leads to an increased volume of viscera contained within the abdominal cavity. This has resulted in the recognition of a quaternary abdominal compartment syndrome which develops following the abdominal wall reconstruction [18].

Effects on Organ Systems

Cardiac

Intra-abdominal hypertension results in decreased cardiac output and decreased overall cardiac function. This is manifested clinically as hypotension, one of the hallmarks of abdominal compartment syndrome. Cardiac function is dependent upon preload, contractility, and afterload, and intra-abdominal hypertension affects all of these components of cardiac function in different ways [5].

Preload: Intra-abdominal hypertension leads to cephalad displacement of the diaphragm into the thoracic cavity. This increase in intra-abdominal pressure is transmitted to the thoracic cavity and pleural spaces. Besides the direct compression of the inferior vena cava (IVC) by the increased intra-abdominal pressure, the transmitted increase in intrathoracic pressure also reduces IVC blood flow. With marked flow reduction through the IVC, venous return is reduced and subsequently, so is preload. Additionally, measurements of preload via vascular catheters become inaccurate.

Contractility: Increased intrathoracic pressure and displacement of the diaphragm affect cardiac contractility. Direct cardiac compression from the increase in intrathoracic pressure decreases cardiac contractility. Additionally, the increase in intrathoracic pressure leads to in an increase in pulmonary vascular resistance that detrimentally affects right and left ventricular function. Together, both of these mechanisms decrease cardiac contractility.

Afterload: As cardiac output decreases due to decreased preload, peripheral vascular resistance will increase in compensation in order to maintain mean arterial pressure. Additionally, the relative under perfusion of the kidney leads to derangements in the renin angiotensin system, which also increases peripheral vascular resistance. The increase in peripheral vascular resistance increases afterload and thereby diminishes cardiac output.

Pulmonary

As the diaphragm becomes displaced into the thoracic cavity, several changes occur that affect the pulmonary system. The decreased compliance of the abdominal wall increases intra-abdominal pressure, which is distributed throughout the abdominal cavity, including against the diaphragm. This direct pressure on the diaphragm not only decreases the size of the thoracic cavity but also inhibits the excursion ability of the diaphragm, impacting pulmonary function [22].

Ventilation: As the diaphragm is pushed into the thoracic cavity, the size of the thoracic cavity decreases, and chest wall compliance decreases. The changes in chest wall compliance are often compounded by the effects of interstitial edema. Tidal volume decreases, impacting ventilation, which leads to a subsequent rise in airway pressures [15]. Clinically, one hallmark of abdominal compartment syndrome is elevated peak airway pressures.

Oxygenation: A decrease in size of the thoracic cavity due to increased pressure against the diaphragm also leads to a reduction in functional residual capacity. Atelectasis develops in response to increased intrathoracic pressure and can lead to pulmonary vascular shunting and ventilation perfusion mismatch. All of these mechanisms lead to the inability to oxygenate. Another hallmark of abdominal compartment syndrome is decreasing oxygen saturation.

Renal

Intra-abdominal hypertension has direct effects on renal vasculature, specifically compression of the renal veins and renal arterioles. These compressive effects lead to increased vascular resistance in the kidney, thereby compromising renal blood flow. This is especially true of the renal veins where the intravascular pressure is much less than in the renal arteries. The resultant decrease in relative perfusion can lead to renal failure from a prerenal cause [26]. If acute tubular necrosis develops, a patient could potentially develop anuric renal failure, which is linked to worse outcomes in critically ill patients. Relative hypoperfusion of the nephron leads to upregulation of the renin angiotensin system and aldosterone. The activation of this hormonal axis leads to further increases in vascular vasoconstriction together with systemic effects of increased afterload. Increased levels of angiotensin II will lead to increased renal vascular resistance and contribute to a decreased glomerular filtration rate, manifested as impaired renal function, further worsening renal circulation.

Gastrointestinal

It has been postulated that elevated intra-abdominal pressure could affect perfusion of organs [14]. Specifically, an IAP of 20 mm Hg leads to a reduction of flow of up to 25% in the portal vein. Reduction of blood flow may also affect capillary circulation to the mucosa of the gastrointestinal tract. Subsequent reperfusion injury may increase systemic inflammation and worsen intra-abdominal hypertension [14].

Central Nervous System

A relationship between intra-abdominal pressure and intracranial pressure has been described [4]. Specifically, intracranial pressure drops by 10 mm Hg after decompressive laparotomy in patients with abdominal compartment syndrome. This may be a result of relieving direct impedance to cerebral venous drainage or by modifying inflammatory mediators which contribute to intracranial pressure. These findings have opened up the possibility for decompressive laparotomy as an adjunct to treatment of refractory elevated intracranial pressure. The specific indications and role for this procedure in patients with elevated intracranial pressure are controversial and have not been clearly determined currently [16].

Management of Intra-abdominal Hypertension and the Abdominal Compartment Syndrome

There is a continuum of therapy for intra-abdominal hypertension and abdominal compartment syndrome, which culminates in decompressive laparotomy. The first steps involve decreasing the volume of the abdominal compartment (Table 23.2). This can be accomplished in several ways. The use of a nasogastric tube to decompress the stomach can decrease intra-abdominal pressure. If there are space-occupying lesions such as ascites, cysts, or abscesses, these can often be addressed with percutaneous drainage to decrease the intra-abdominal volume they occupy. If these measures do not accomplish a decrease in intra-abdominal pressure and/or result in an abdominal perfusion pressure of more than 50 mm Hg, the compliance of the abdominal wall can be increased pharmacologically to reduce intra-abdominal pressure. This approach is typically used in the intubated and mechanically ventilated patient and can be accomplished via neuromuscular blockade or by increasing sedation. These measures should be considered carefully because in critically ill patients, neuromuscular blockade can have adverse effects, including secondary infections and critical illness neuromyopathy, resulting in increased costs and length of stay [1] (Table 23.3).

Table 23.2 Nonoperative management of intra-abdominal hypertension and abdominal compartment syndrome

1. Evacuate intraluminal contents
2. Evacuate intra-abdominal space-occupying lesions
3. Optimize abdominal wall compliance
4. Optimize fluid administration
5. Optimize systemic and& regional perfusion

Table 23.3 Goals of managing the open abdomen

Cover and protect abdominal contents
Prevent evisceration
Prevent or treat ACS
Protect the fascia
Minimize loss of domain
Facilitate reoperation
Keep the patient warm and dry
Prevent hypothermia
Prevent adhesion formation
Remove infectious material

Decompressive Laparotomy

If medical therapy does not result in physiologic normalization in patients with suspected abdominal compartment syndrome, surgery is the sole remaining treatment. As such, the extreme end of the treatment spectrum is decompression of the abdominal cavity via laparotomy. Decompressive laparotomy entails opening the abdominal wall from the xiphoid to the pubic symphysis. This allows maximal decompression and leaves the patient with an open abdomen [3]. Particularly important is to ensure that adequate volume resuscitation has occurred before the abdominal cavity is opened. Endpoints of resuscitation, including central venous pressure and urinary output, may be artificially suppressed in a patient with intra-abdominal hypertension and abdominal compartment syndrome [14].

Decompressive laparotomy is effective at decreasing intra-abdominal pressure, but intra-abdominal hypertension persists in most patients [8, 9]. Mortality remains high—between 37% and 49% [8, 9]. Survival is highest when organ dysfunction is reversed, which suggests that timing of decompressive laparotomy may be important, thus reinforcing the importance of monitoring intra-abdominal pressures in critically ill patients. However, the effect of decompressive laparotomy on organ function is not uniform, and some studies found that decompressive laparotomy did not affect organ function [9]. Improvement in oxygenation and urinary output was the most pronounced effects of decompressive laparotomy [8].

Published case reports describe the use of decompressive laparotomy as a salvage maneuver in the intensive care unit [10]. However, in this scenario, which involves a patient who is severely critically ill, rapidly decompensating, and unable to tolerate transport to the operating room, anesthesia and perioperative care are understandably challenging. Decompressive laparotomy under these circumstances can be extremely challenging and fraught with complications.

References

1. Annane D. What is the evidence for harm of neuromuscular blockade and corticosteroid use in the intensive care unit? Semin Respir Crit Care Med. 2016;37:51–6.
2. Ball CG, kirkpatrick AW, karmali S, Malbrain ML, Gmora S, Mahabir RC, Doig C, Hameed SM. Tertiary abdominal compartment syndrome in the burn injured patient. J Trauma. 2006;61:1271–3.
3 Beckman M, Paul J, Neideen T, Weigelt JA. Role of the open abdomen in critically ill patients. Crit Care Clin. 2016;32:255–64.
4 Bloomfield GL, Ridings PC, Blocher CR, Marmarou A, Sugerman HJ. A proposed relationship between increased intra-abdominal, intrathoracic, and intracranial pressure. Crit Care Med. 1997;25:496–503.
5 Cheatham ML. Abdominal compartment syndrome: pathophysiology and definitions. Scand J Trauma Resusc Emerg Med. 2009;17:10.

6 Cheatham ML, White MW, Sagraves SG, Johnson JL, Block EF. Abdominal perfusion pressure: a superior parameter in the assessment of intra-abdominal hypertension. J Trauma. 2000;49:621–6; discussion 626–7.
7 Cotton BA, Gunter OL, Isbell J, Au BK, Robertson AM, Morris JA Jr, St Jacques P, Young PP. Damage control hematology: the impact of a trauma exsanguination protocol on survival and blood product utilization. J Trauma. 2008;64:1177–82; discussion 1182–3.
8 De Waele J, Desender L, De Laet I, Ceelen W, Pattyn P, Hoste E. Abdominal decompression for abdominal compartment syndrome in critically ill patients: a retrospective study. Acta Clin Belg. 2010;65:399–403.
9 De Waele JJ, Hoste EA, Malbrain ML. Decompressive laparotomy for abdominal compartment syndrome–a critical analysis. Crit Care. 2006;10:R51.
10 De Waele JJ, Kimball E, Malbrain M, Nesbitt I, Cohen J, Kaloiani V, Ivatury R, Mone M, Debergh D, Bjorck M. Decompressive laparotomy for abdominal compartment syndrome. Br J Surg. 2016;103:709–15.
11 Harrahill M. Intra-abdominal pressure monitoring. J Emerg Nurs. 1998;24:465–6.
12 Hecker A, Hecker B, Hecker M, Riedel JG, Weigand MA, Padberg W. Acute abdominal compartment syndrome: current diagnostic and therapeutic options. Langenbeck's Arch Surg. 2016;401:15–24.
13 Holodinsky JK, Roberts DJ, Ball CG, Blaser AR, Starkopf J, Zygun DA, Stelfox HT, Malbrain ML, Jaeschke RC, Kirkpatrick AW. Risk factors for intra-abdominal hypertension and abdominal compartment syndrome among adult intensive care unit patients: a systematic review and meta-analysis. Crit Care. 2013;17:R249.
14 Hunter JD, Damani Z. Intra-abdominal hypertension and the abdominal compartment syndrome. Anaesthesia. 2004;59:899–907.
15 Jensen KK, Backer V, Jorgensen LN. Abdominal wall reconstruction for large incisional hernia restores expiratory lung function. Surgery. 2017;161(2):517–24.
16 Joseph DK, Dutton RP, Aarabi B, Scalea TM. Decompressive laparotomy to treat intractable intracranial hypertension after traumatic brain injury. J Trauma. 2004;57:687–93; discussion 693–5.
17 Khan S, Verma AK, Ahmad SM, Ahmad R. Analyzing intra-abdominal pressures and outcomes in patients undergoing emergency laparotomy. J Emerg Trauma Shock. 2010;3:318–25.
18 Kirkpatrick AW, Nickerson D, Roberts DJ, Rosen MJ, Mcbeth PB, Petro CC, Berrevoet F, Sugrue M, Xiao J, Ball CG. Intra-abdominal hypertension and abdominal compartment syndrome after abdominal wall reconstruction: quaternary syndromes? Scand J Surg. 2016;106:97–106.
19 Kirkpatrick AW, Roberts DJ, Jaeschke R, De Waele JJ, De Keulenaer BL, Duchesne J, Bjorck M, Leppaniemi A, Ejike JC, Sugrue M, Cheatham ML, Ivatury R, Ball CG, Reintam Blaser A, Regli A, Balogh Z, D'amours S, De Laet I, Malbrain ML. Methodological background and strategy for the 2012–2013 updated consensus definitions and clinical practice guidelines from the abdominal compartment society. Anaesthesiol Intensive Ther. 2015;47 Spec No:s63–77.
20 Malbrain ML, Vidts W, Ravyts M, De Laet I, De Waele J. Acute intestinal distress syndrome: the importance of intra-abdominal pressure. Minerva Anestesiol. 2008;74:657–73.
21 Maluso P, Olson J, Sarani B. Abdominal compartment hypertension and abdominal compartment syndrome. Crit Care Clin. 2016;32:213–22.
22 Regli A, Chakera J, De Keulenaer BL, Roberts B, Noffsinger B, Singh B, Van Heerden PV. Matching positive end-expiratory pressure to intra-abdominal pressure prevents end-expiratory lung volume decline in a pig model of intra-abdominal hypertension. Crit Care Med. 2012;40:1879–86.
23 Strang SG, Van Lieshout EM, Van Waes OJ, Verhofstad MH. Prevalence and mortality of abdominal compartment syndrome in severely injured patients: a systematic review. J Trauma Acute Care Surg. 2016;81:585–92.
24 Sugrue M. Abdominal compartment syndrome. Curr Opin Crit Care. 2005;11:333–8.
25 Sugrue M, De Waele JJ, De Keulenaer BL, Roberts DJ, Malbrain ML. A user's guide to intra-abdominal pressure measurement. Anaesthesiol Intensive Ther. 2015;47:241–51.
26 Sugrue M, Jones F, Deane SA, Bishop G, Bauman A, Hillman K. Intra-abdominal hypertension is an independent cause of postoperative renal impairment. Arch Surg. 1999;134:1082–5.

Acute Liver Failure

24

Amar Gupta and Chad G. Ball

Definition

The term "acute liver failure" (ALF) describes the clinical consequence of a sudden injury to the liver, resulting in massive hepatocyte dysfunction and/or necrosis. Clinical hallmarks of ALF include liver dysfunction as measured by biochemical values, coagulopathy, encephalopathy, and multi-organ dysfunction (Table 24.1) [1]. More recent definitions employ the time interval between the development of jaundice and encephalopathy to further stratify this disease entity into hyperacute, acute, and subacute phenotypes (Table 24.2) [2–4]. Typically, hyperacute and acute cases (which occur secondary to viral infection or acetaminophen toxicity) have improved outcomes when compared to subacute scenarios [5]. Although many causes of ALF may also be implicated in chronic liver disease and subsequent cirrhosis, the patient must be free of chronic liver dysfunction to cinch the diagnosis of ALF.

Causes

Viral

Infection with hepatitis A, B, and E viruses (HAV, HBV, and HEV, respectively) is the most common causes of both ALF and liver transplantation in developing countries. ALF secondary to viral hepatitis is much less predominant in the Western world as a result of vaccination and modern sanitation. Transmission of HAV and HEV occurs via a fecal-oral route, while HBV is transmitted through exposure to contaminated blood and bodily fluids [6, 7]. ALF secondary to HAV and HEV infections usually follows a hyperacute timeline [8, 9]. Acute infection with HBV results in ALF in less than 4% of patients; however, outcomes are inferior to cases caused by HAV and HEV [1]. Furthermore, reactivation of subclinical HBV infection, often seen in cases of immunosuppression, results in especially high mortality [1, 5]. Identification of these at-risk patients and viral prophylaxis is recommended for this population [10–12]. Although much less common, ALF secondary to viral infection with *Herpes simplex virus* (HSV), parvovirus, *Cytomegalovirus* (CMV), Epstein-Barr virus, and varicella zoster virus has been well documented [13].

Drug-Induced

The most common cause of ALF in the Western world is drug-induced liver injury, with acetaminophen as the most frequent culprit drug [14, 15]. ALF secondary to acetaminophen toxicity tends to be hyperacute, with rapid progression to multi-organ failure [16]. Acetaminophen toxicity occurs in dose-dependent fashion, requiring massive doses (15–20 g). As a result, ALF secondary to acetaminophen is often the result of a suicide attempt, although indeliberate toxicity is also seen, especially in patients with underlying liver disease. Even in patients utilizing medications known as hepatotoxins, ALF due to drugs other than acetaminophen is rare and often a diagnosis of exclusion.

Post-hepatectomy

Post-hepatectomy liver failure (PHLF) is a well-established cause of ALF and is the result of inadequate liver remnant function following major hepatectomy. It is widely accepted that a future liver remnant of at least 25% is required to avoid PHLF in healthy patients [17]. This number rises to 40% in patients with underlying liver disease or with prior extensive chemotherapy exposure [18]. Strategies) to mitigate this risk include associating liver partition and portal vein ligation for

A. Gupta
Department of General Surgery, Foothills Medical Center, Calgary, AB, Canada

C. G. Ball (✉)
Department of Surgery, University of Calgary, Foothills Medical Center, Calgary, AB, Canada

A. Salim et al. (eds.), *Surgical Critical Care Therapy*, https://doi.org/10.1007/978-3-319-71712-8_24

Table 24.1 Clinical manifestations of organ system dysfunction secondary to acute liver failure

Organ system	Clinical features
Neurologic	Hepatic encephalopathy Cerebral edema Intracranial hypertension
Cardiovascular	Hypotension
Respiratory	Late respiratory failure
Coagulation	Impaired procoagulant and anticoagulant pathways
Renal	Acute kidney injury
Metabolic	Hypoglycemia Increased metabolic demand
Immunologic	Functional immunosuppression

Table 24.2 Classification of acute liver failure based on time from jaundice to encephalopathy

	Time from jaundice to encephalopathy
O'Grady system	
Hyperacute	0–1 week
Acute	1–4 weeks
Subacute	4–12 weeks
Bernuau system	
Fulminant	0–2 weeks
Subfulminant	2–12 weeks
Japanese system	
Fulminant	
Acute	0–10 days
Subacute	10 days–8 weeks
Late-onset	8–24 weeks

staged hepatectomy (ALPPS) [19], percutaneous portal vein embolization (PVE) [20], parenchymal-sparing resections, and two-stage hepatectomies. Several clinical indices have been developed in an attempt to predict PHLF. The 50–50 criterion employs prothrombin time <50% and total bilirubin >50 umol/L on postoperative day 5 as an indicator of PHLF [21]. The International Study Group of Liver Surgery adopted a more generalized definition of PHLF describing increasing INR and serum bilirubin above locally accepted cutoff values on or after postoperative day 5 [22]. The model for end-stage liver disease (MELD) has also been used to try and anticipate PHLF with promising predictive sensitivity [23]. Despite these multiple indices for identifying patients at risk for PHLF, treatment options still remain limited.

Other Causes

Acute liver injury as the result of profound ischemia is an important condition often seen in critically ill surgical patients. Hypoxic hepatitis may progress to ALF if the magnitude of hepatocellular necrosis is severe enough [24]. Wilson's disease, Budd-Chiari syndrome, autoimmune hepatitis, and toxic mushroom ingestion remain quite rare causes of ALF. A significant number of ALF have no identifiable cause and remain a diagnostic challenge [5].

Management

Patients suspected of having ALF should be managed in an intensive care setting, ideally under the multidisciplinary care of intensivists, liver surgeons, and hepatologists. The expansive role that the liver plays in maintaining homeostasis is evident in patients with ALF as a wide variety of organ systems are affected. A thorough knowledge of the secondary complications associated with ALF will allow the intensivist to identify and treat potential life-threatening conditions early. These are summarized in Table 24.1.

Neurologic

The development of encephalopathy is central to the diagnosis of ALF and is often associated with cerebral edema in hyperacute cases. Although the pathogenesis of cerebral edema and encephalopathy is incompletely understood, impaired ammonia detoxification clearly plays an important part. In patients with grades 3–4 encephalopathy, ammonia levels >120 umol/L on admission have been shown to be associated with higher rates of mortality [25]. Pharmacologic treatments used for elevated ammonia in chronic liver disease are not generally recommended in ALF [26]. Cerebral edema and elevated intracranial pressure (ICP) are the leading cause of death from ALF and thus must be a central focus for the treating physician. Steps to prevent or decrease cerebral edema should include correction of hyponatremia, avoiding hypoxia and hypercapnia often requiring endotracheal intubation in cases of severe hepatic encephalopathy, and pharmacologic sedation. Severe cerebral edema may lead to life-threatening elevations in ICP. Elevated ICP may be diagnosed with CT, MRI, and transcranial Doppler when combined with clinical findings [26]. Patients with severe hepatic encephalopathy (grades 3–4) can also be considered for direct ICP monitoring to guide and assess response to therapy as persistently elevated ICP and decreased cerebral perfusion pressure (CPP) result in poor outcomes following liver transplantation [27]. A randomized, controlled trial (RCT) evaluating the effect of hypertonic saline on intracranial hypertension demonstrated a reduced incidence and severity of elevated ICP when hypertonic saline was administered to patients with grades 3–4 encephalopathy due to ALF [28]. Some animal studies and clinical studies have shown promising results for mild hypothermia to prevent intracranial hypertension in ALF [29]. However, a multicentered RCT in ALF patients with high-grade hepatic encephalopathy failed to demonstrate neither any reduction of intracranial hypertension as measured by direct ICP monitoring nor any reduction in mortality [30]. Thus, it cannot be recommended to induce hypothermia in ALF patients, even in cases of suspected intracranial hypertension.

Cardiovascular

Cardiovascular derangements are frequent in ALF and are often multifactorial in origin. Initial management does not differ from standard critical care algorithms. Intravascular volume is restored using isotonic crystalloids. Pulse pressure variation has been shown to be an effective modality at assessing fluid responsiveness in ALF patients [31]. If hypotension persists despite adequate fluid resuscitation, vasopressors may be required to maintain adequate mean arterial pressure (MAP). In patients with intracranial hypertension, vasopressors may be required to maintain a MAP allowing for CPP >60 mm Hg. Patients with refractory hypotension may have relative adrenal insufficiency and may benefit from hydrocortisone replacement therapy [32].

Respiratory

Respiratory dysfunction is uncommon in the early stages of ALF. Despite this, endotracheal intubation is often required given the severity of hepatic encephalopathy in these critically ill patients [5]. Furthermore, ventilator manipulation allows for deep sedation as well the prevention of hypercapnia, which is a vital maneuver in preventing cerebral edema and intracranial hypertension as discussed above.

Coagulopathy

Elevated INR is a hallmark of ALF, and as such, many patients are aggressively transfused with fresh frozen plasma, vitamin K, and other coagulation factors. There is a paucity of data to support correction of laboratory markers of coagulation in ALF patients without evidence of active bleeding. Furthermore, it should be noted that the synthesis of anticoagulant factors produced in the liver is also impaired in ALF. As a result, the true coagulation profile of the patient may be closer to equilibrium than laboratory values suggest [33, 34]. As a result, in the absence of active bleeding, transfusion of coagulation factors should be avoided.

Renal

Renal dysfunction is observed in the majority of patients with ALF and is thought to be the result of a general systemic inflammatory response [35]. Renal replacement therapy is often required in the ALF patient to maintain fluid balance, prevent acid-base disturbances, and help to clear serum ammonia. Continuous renal replacement therapy is the preferred modality of intermittent hemodialysis as it provides greater hemodynamic stability [36] and can provide effective ammonia clearance [37]. The renal dysfunction identified with ALF is usually self-limiting and in most cases resolves once liver function has been reestablished (either through regeneration or transplantation) [38, 39].

Metabolic

Metabolic derangements in ALF are multifactorial and require attention and prompt correction to ensure favorable clinical outcomes. Impaired hepatic glucose regulation, along with increased metabolic demands, often results in profound hypoglycemia. Infusion of high-concentration intravenous dextrose is often required to maintain adequate blood glucose levels [40]. Patients with severe hepatic encephalopathy will require nasoenteric feeding access to deliver nutrition, while parenteral should be avoided. Caloric and protein goals are 25–40 kcal/kg/day and 0.8–1.2 g/kg/day, respectively, to prevent protein catabolism and preserve immune function [5, 40]. Protein restriction should be avoided in the absence of worsening hyperammonemia attributed to protein intake [41].

Infectious

Patients with ALF are felt to be at higher risk of systemic infection secondary to functional immunosuppression [5], and as a result, the majority of centers caring for ALF patients administer prophylactic antibiotics [42]. The US Acute Liver Failure Study Group identified systemic infection as a significantly contributor to hepatic encephalopathy exacerbation [43]. However, the same group recently demonstrated no significant reduction in bloodstream infection or 21-day mortality with the use of prophylactic antibiotics in ALF [44]. Given the paucity of reliable data given in the antibiotic use and ALF, we reserve antibiotic administration to patients with positive admission or surveillance cultures and clinical manifestations of infection such as fever or worsening leukocytosis, grades 3–4 encephalopathy, actively listed for liver transplantation.

Disease-Specific

When the etiology of ALF is identifiable, cause-specific interventions may be of benefit, although robust RCT data for many of the following treatments is not available. The most widely studied disease-specific treatment is the administration of N-acetylcysteine (NAC). Intravenous NAC has been shown to decrease overall mortality in ALF caused by acetaminophen toxicity [45]. Furthermore, NAC administration early in the course of non-acetaminophen ALF provided a transplant-free survival benefits in patients with grades 1–2 hepatic encephalopathy [46]. As a result, NAC should be administered early in acetaminophen-induced ALF and in non-acetaminophen cases of ALF with grades 1–2 hepatic encephalopathy.

Lamivudine administration may improve HBV-associated ALF outcomes [47–49] although RCT data is scarce. Similarly, acyclovir and ganciclovir have been used as treatment adjuncts in HSV and CMV causes of ALF, respectively, although no reliable data exists. Autoimmune ALF has been treated with steroid administration in some centers, although there is no literature demonstrating improved outcomes. In fact, some authors have suggested infectious complications which may be exacerbated with steroid administration [50].

Liver Transplantation

All patients suspected of ALF should be evaluated early for liver transplantation. The decision to proceed with liver transplantation for ALF is a difficult one, as liver grafts are in considerably short supply. Thus, identifying which patients will regain adequate hepatic reserve, and which will not, is of paramount importance to ensure efficient usage of such a valuable resource. The King's College Criteria were developed as a predictive tool to identify patients at risk for high mortality without urgent liver transplantation. They include patients with acetaminophen-induced ALF who have either an arterial pH < 7.30 after adequate volume resuscitation or an INR >6.5 and serum creatinine >3.4 mg/dL with grades 3–4 encephalopathy. Patients with non-acetaminophen ALF must demonstrate either an INR >6.5 or any 3 of age <10 or >40, INR >3.5, bilirubin >17.6 mg/dL, encephalopathy developing 7 or more days after jaundice, and etiology other than HAV/HBV hepatitis (Table 24.3) [51]. The MELD score uses serum bilirubin, INR, serum creatinine, and the need for renal replacement therapy to develop a predictive score. A MELD score above 30 is widely accepted as criteria to pursue liver transplantation. Furthermore, the MELD score has been suggested as being a superior predictive tool when compared to the King's College Criteria [52].

Live-donor liver transplant (LDLT) has been suggested as a potential solution to the shortage of deceased-donor liver grafts. Unfortunately, due to the rigorous preoperative workup, potential danger to the donor, and technically demanding nature of LDLT, few centers have pursued this modality for ALF. Those specialized centers that have reported LDLT for ALF have enjoyed favorable results however [53–56].

Table 24.3 King's College Criteria for identification of acute liver failure patients requiring transplantation

Acetaminophen ALF
Arterial pH <7.3 after adequate fluid resuscitation
Or all of the following:
INR >6.5
Serum creatinine >3.4 mg/dL
Grades 3–4 encephalopathy
Non-acetaminophen ALF
INR >6.5
Or any 3 of the following:
Age <10 or >40
INR >3.5
Bilirubin >17.6 mg/dL
Encephalopathy developing 7 or more days after jaundice
Etiology other than HAV/HBV hepatitis

Liver Support Systems

Although still not in wide clinical use, liver support systems (LSS) offer an appealing possibility of short-term stabilization of ALF patients when liver transplantation is not available or contraindicated [57].

Albumin dialysis systems remove albumin-bound molecules as well as water-soluble substances and are the most studied systems. The molecular adsorbent reticulating system (MARS) plus standard medical treatment was evaluated in an RCT versus standard medical therapy alone and was found to impart no survival benefit in ALF patients [58]. The Prometheus system has shown no significant survival benefit in patients with acute-on-chronic liver failure and has yet to be evaluated by an RCT [59].

High-volume plasma (HVP) exchange involves 8–12 L of plasma with fresh frozen plasma daily [57]. A multicenter RCT comparing HVP plus standard medical treatment to standard medical therapy alone demonstrated a significant survival advantage in the HVP group [60]. Importantly, this studies recruitment period was 13 years, during which period critical care of ALF has markedly improved. To this day, HVP is not routinely employed for ALF.

The HepatAssist system filters patient plasma through a small pore membrane where it comes in contact with cultured porcine hepatocytes before being returned to the patient. A recent RCT of HepatAssist plus standard medical treatment versus standard medical treatment alone demonstrated no 30-day survival advantage in patients with ALF or primary non-function (PNF) following liver transplantation. This study initially included all patients, even those treated with liver transplantation within the 30-day study period. When the patients undergoing liver transplant and the PNF patients were controlled for, the HepatAssist group has a significant survival advantage over the control group [61]. Despite these results, the HepatAssist has yet to be used outside of an experimental setting.

References

1. Bernal W, et al. Acute liver failure. Lancet. 2010;376(9736):190–201.
2. Bernuau J, Rueff B, Benhamou JP. Fulminant and subfulminant liver failure: definitions and causes. Semin Liver Dis. 1986;6(2):97–106.
3. Mochida S, et al. Re-evaluation of the Guideline published by the Acute Liver Failure Study Group of Japan in 1996 to determine the indications of liver transplantation in patients with fulminant hepatitis. Hepatol Res. 2008;38(10):970–9.
4. O'Grady JG, Schalm SW, Williams R. Acute liver failure: redefining the syndromes. Lancet. 1993;342(8866):273–5.
5. Bernal W, Wendon J. Acute liver failure. N Engl J Med. 2013;369(26):2525–34.
6. Dalton HR, et al. Hepatitis E: an emerging infection in developed countries. Lancet Infect Dis. 2008;8(11):698–709.
7. Wasley A, Samandari T, Bell BP. Incidence of hepatitis A in the United States in the era of vaccination. JAMA. 2005;294(2):194–201.
8. Taylor RM, et al. Fulminant hepatitis A virus infection in the United States: incidence, prognosis, and outcomes. Hepatology. 2006;44(6):1589–97.
9. Patra S, et al. Maternal and fetal outcomes in pregnant women with acute hepatitis E virus infection. Ann Intern Med. 2007;147(1):28–33.
10. Katz LH, et al. Lamivudine prevents reactivation of hepatitis B and reduces mortality in immunosuppressed patients: systematic review and meta-analysis. J Viral Hepat. 2008;15(2):89–102.
11. Mindikoglu AL, Regev A, Schiff ER. Hepatitis B virus reactivation after cytotoxic chemotherapy: the disease and its prevention. Clin Gastroenterol Hepatol. 2006;4(9):1076–81.
12. Torres HA, Davila M. Reactivation of hepatitis B virus and hepatitis C virus in patients with cancer. Nat Rev Clin Oncol. 2012;9(3):156–66.
13. Ichai P, Samuel D. Etiology and prognosis of fulminant hepatitis in adults. Liver Transpl. 2008;14(Suppl 2):S67–79.
14. Katarey D, Verma S. Drug-induced liver injury. Clin Med (Lond). 2016;16(Suppl 6):s104–9.
15. Reuben A, et al. Drug-induced acute liver failure: results of a U.S. multicenter, prospective study. Hepatology. 2010;52(6):2065–76.
16. Bernal W, et al. Outcome after wait-listing for emergency liver transplantation in acute liver failure: a single centre experience. J Hepatol. 2009;50(2):306–13.
17. Schindl MJ, et al. The value of residual liver volume as a predictor of hepatic dysfunction and infection after major liver resection. Gut. 2005;54(2):289–96.
18. van den Broek MA, et al. Liver failure after partial hepatic resection: definition, pathophysiology, risk factors and treatment. Liver Int. 2008;28(6):767–80.
19. Schnitzbauer AA, et al. Right portal vein ligation combined with in situ splitting induces rapid left lateral liver lobe hypertrophy enabling 2-staged extended right hepatic resection in small-for-size settings. Ann Surg. 2012;255(3):405–14.
20. de Graaf W, et al. Increase in future remnant liver function after preoperative portal vein embolization. Br J Surg. 2011;98(6):825–34.
21. Balzan S, et al. The "50-50 criteria" on postoperative day 5: an accurate predictor of liver failure and death after hepatectomy. Ann Surg. 2005;242(6):824–8, discussion 828–9.
22. Rahbari NN, et al. Posthepatectomy liver failure: a definition and grading by the International Study Group of Liver Surgery (ISGLS). Surgery. 2011;149(5):713–24.
23. Rahbari NN, et al. The predictive value of postoperative clinical risk scores for outcome after hepatic resection: a validation analysis in 807 patients. Ann Surg Oncol. 2011;18(13):3640–9.
24. Waseem N, Chen PH. Hypoxic hepatitis: a review and clinical update. J Clin Transl Hepatol. 2016;4(3):263–8.
25. Niranjan-Azadi AM, et al. Ammonia level and mortality in acute liver failure: a single-center experience. Ann Transplant. 2016;21:479–83.
26. Kodali S, McGuire BM. Diagnosis and management of hepatic encephalopathy in fulminant hepatic failure. Clin Liver Dis. 2015;19(3):565–76.
27. Wang DW, Yin YM, Yao YM. Advances in the management of acute liver failure. World J Gastroenterol. 2013;19(41):7069–77.
28. Murphy N, et al. The effect of hypertonic sodium chloride on intracranial pressure in patients with acute liver failure. Hepatology. 2004;39(2):464–70.
29. Vaquero J, Rose C, Butterworth RF. Keeping cool in acute liver failure: rationale for the use of mild hypothermia. J Hepatol. 2005;43(6):1067–77.
30. Bernal W, et al. A multicentre randomized controlled trial of moderate hypothermia to prevent intracranial hypertension in acute liver failure. J Hepatol. 2016;65(2):273–9.
31. Audimoolam VK, et al. Predicting fluid responsiveness in acute liver failure: a prospective study. Anesth Analg. 2017;124(2):480–6.
32. Maheshwari R, Subramanian RM. On the brink of death: managing acute liver failure. Am J Gastroenterol. 2016;112(2):200–6.
33. Barton CA. Treatment of coagulopathy related to hepatic insufficiency. Crit Care Med. 2016;44(10):1927–33.
34. Lisman T, Leebeek FW, de Groot PG. Haemostatic abnormalities in patients with liver disease. J Hepatol. 2002;37(2):280–7.
35. Leithead JA, et al. The systemic inflammatory response syndrome is predictive of renal dysfunction in patients with non-paracetamol-induced acute liver failure. Gut. 2009;58(3):443–9.
36. Davenport A. Continuous renal replacement therapies in patients with liver disease. Semin Dial. 2009;22(2):169–72.
37. Slack AJ, et al. Ammonia clearance with haemofiltration in adults with liver disease. Liver Int. 2014;34(1):42–8.
38. Moore K. Renal failure in acute liver failure. Eur J Gastroenterol Hepatol. 1999;11(9):967–75.
39. O'Riordan A, et al. Acute kidney injury in patients admitted to a liver intensive therapy unit with paracetamol-induced hepatotoxicity. Nephrol Dial Transplant. 2011;26(11):3501–8.
40. Ramos Figueira ER, et al. Nutritional support for fulminant hepatitis. Nutr Hosp. 2015;32(6):2427–32.
41. Montejo González JC, et al. Guidelines for specialized nutritional and metabolic support in the critically-ill patient: update. Consensus SEMICYUC-SENPE: liver failure and liver transplantation. Nutr Hosp. 2011;26(Suppl 2):27–31.
42. Rabinowich L, et al. Clinical management of acute liver failure: results of an international multi-center survey. World J Gastroenterol. 2016;22(33):7595–603.
43. Vaquero J, et al. Infection and the progression of hepatic encephalopathy in acute liver failure. Gastroenterology. 2003;125(3):755–64.

44. Karvellas CJ, et al. Effects of antimicrobial prophylaxis and blood stream infections in patients with acute liver failure: a retrospective cohort study. Clin Gastroenterol Hepatol. 2014;12(11):1942–9.e1.
45. Keays R, et al. Intravenous acetylcysteine in paracetamol induced fulminant hepatic failure: a prospective controlled trial. BMJ. 1991;303(6809):1026–9.
46. Lee WM, et al. Intravenous N-acetylcysteine improves transplant-free survival in early stage non-acetaminophen acute liver failure. Gastroenterology. 2009;137(3):856–64, 864.e1
47. Kumar M, et al. A randomized controlled trial of lamivudine to treat acute hepatitis B. Hepatology. 2007;45(1):97–101.
48. Miyake Y, et al. Lamivudine treatment improves the prognosis of fulminant hepatitis B. Intern Med. 2008;47(14):1293–9.
49. Tillmann HL, et al. Safety and efficacy of lamivudine in patients with severe acute or fulminant hepatitis B, a multicenter experience. J Viral Hepat. 2006;13(4):256–63.
50. Ichai P, et al. Usefulness of corticosteroids for the treatment of severe and fulminant forms of autoimmune hepatitis. Liver Transpl. 2007;13(7):996–1003.
51. O'Grady JG, et al. Early indicators of prognosis in fulminant hepatic failure. Gastroenterology. 1989;97(2):439–45.
52. Flamm SL, et al. American Gastroenterological Association Institute guidelines for the diagnosis and management of acute liver failure. Gastroenterology. 2017;152(3):644–7.
53. Goldaracena N, et al. Live donor liver transplantation: a valid alternative for critically ill patients suffering from acute liver failure. Am J Transplant. 2015;15(6):1591–7.
54. Kaido T, et al. Liver transplantation in adults with acute liver failure: a single center experience over a period of 15 years. Hepato-Gastroenterology. 2015;62(140):937–41.
55. Kirnap M, et al. Liver transplant for fulminant hepatic failure: a single-center experience. Exp Clin Transplant. 2015;13(4):339–43.
56. Park SJ, et al. Emergency adult-to-adult living-donor liver transplantation for acute liver failure in a hepatitis B virus endemic area. Hepatology. 2010;51(3):903–11.
57. Gonzalez HC, Jafri SM, Gordon SC. Management of acute hepatotoxicity including medical agents and liver support systems. Clin Liver Dis. 2017;21(1):163–80.
58. Saliba F, et al. Albumin dialysis with a noncell artificial liver support device in patients with acute liver failure: a randomized, controlled trial. Ann Intern Med. 2013;159(8):522–31.
59. Rifai K, et al. Prometheus--a new extracorporeal system for the treatment of liver failure. J Hepatol. 2003;39(6):984–90.
60. Larsen FS, et al. High-volume plasma exchange in patients with acute liver failure: an open randomised controlled trial. J Hepatol. 2016;64(1):69–78.
61. Demetriou AA, et al. Prospective, randomized, multicenter, controlled trial of a bioartificial liver in treating acute liver failure. Ann Surg. 2004;239(5):660–7; discussion 667–70.

Acute Pancreatitis

25

Peter Fagenholz and Marc de Moya

Introduction

Acute pancreatitis encompasses a wide range of severity, from mild and self-limited to lethal. This chapter will focus on medical and surgical management of severe pancreatitis requiring intensive care unit admission. We address the most common clinical questions related to care of severe acute pancreatitis, such as which patients should receive antibiotics, the best method of nutrition, which patients require surgery, what is the optimal surgical approach, and others.

Epidemiology and Etiology

Acute pancreatitis is the most common gastrointestinal disorder requiring hospitalization in the United States with an estimated 274,000 hospitalizations in 2009, and its incidence appears to be increasing [1, 2]. The most common causes of acute pancreatitis are ethanol ingestion and gallstones. Less frequent causes include instrumentation of the bile or pancreatic ducts (endoscopic retrograde cholangiopancreatography [ERCP]), medications (especially diuretics, antiepileptics, and protease inhibitors), hypertriglyceridemia, hypercalcemia, congenital anatomic or genetic conditions (e.g., pancreas divisum or CFTR mutation), mumps, pancreatic neoplasm, and trauma or hypoperfusion. In 10–15% of cases, the cause is not identified, though evidence is increasing that a significant percentage of these cases may be due to occult biliary tract disease [3]. The overall mortality is 2–4%, though the mortality rate of patients requiring intensive care is significantly higher [2, 4].

P. Fagenholz
Division of Trauma/Acute Care Surgery, Massachusetts General Hospital, Harvard Medical School, Boston, MA, USA

M. de Moya (✉)
Division of Trauma, Acute Care Surgery, Medical College of Wisconsin, Froedtert Hospital, Milaukee, WI, USA
e-mail: mdemoya@mcw.edu

Pathophysiology

The pathophysiology of acute pancreatitis is poorly understood. The most common causes of acute pancreatitis can generally be broken down into mechanical (gallstones, ERCP) or systemic (alcohol, medications, hypercalcemia, hypertriglyceridemia). There are two suggested mechanisms whereby the mechanical causes result in acute pancreatitis: obstruction of the ampulla or bile reflux into the pancreatic ductal system. How systemic agents trigger acute pancreatitis is even less clear.

Most investigators agree that, whatever the inciting mechanism, acute pancreatitis results from activation of trypsin within the pancreatic acinar cells. The pancreas has mechanisms for preventing intracellular trypsin activation and counteracting low levels of activation, but when these mechanisms are overwhelmed, pancreatic autodigestion ensues, which can progress beyond the gland itself and into the surrounding peripancreatic tissues. This local injury can in turn activate a variety of local, regional, and systemic inflammatory mediators (complement, interleukins, phospholipase A2) which may be responsible for the systemic effects seen in severe acute pancreatitis [5]. For the intensivist, the relevance is that acute pancreatitis can trigger a profound SIRS response and septic shock-like physiology even in the absence of infection.

Diagnosis, Classification, and Severity

The diagnosis of acute pancreatitis is based on the identification of two of the following three criteria: (1) clinical (central upper abdominal pain, often with associated nausea and vomiting, and sometimes radiating to the back), (2) laboratory (serum amylase or lipase greater than three times the upper limit of normal), and (3) radiographic (imaging (usually CT or MRI) characteristic of acute pancreatitis). Imaging is rarely required to make the diagnosis of acute pancreatitis, which can usually be made on the basis of clinical and

A. Salim et al. (eds.), *Surgical Critical Care Therapy*, https://doi.org/10.1007/978-3-319-71712-8_25

biochemical parameters alone. Imaging should only be used acutely when the diagnosis is unclear and is typically more valuable later in the course of disease to better define local complications (discussed below). In critically ill patients in which the diagnosis is unclear, CT with intravenous contrast is highly sensitive and specific and can also assess for many critical alternative diagnoses such as perforated peptic ulcer, aortic pathology, or mesenteric ischemia. The etiology of any episode of pancreatitis should be sought, as it may allow prevention of recurrent episodes. When there is no obvious inciting factor such as heavy alcohol use or recent ERCP, abdominal ultrasound should be performed to evaluate for gallstones as a potential cause.

There have been several classification systems for acute pancreatitis severity through the years, each with its inherent strengths and weaknesses. In theory such systems are most practically useful to the intensivist for triage and early identification of patients at high risk of complications who might benefit from initial resuscitation in an ICU setting. The presence of SIRS or organ failure on presentation and at 48 h is considered the best predictor of severity of acute pancreatitis. Complex or pancreatitis-specific severity scoring systems (e.g., Ranson, Glasgow, Balthazar, APACHE II) do not perform better and need not be calculated [6, 7]. Overall, at least 80% of acute pancreatitis is mild, and 20% is severe or moderately severe.

Initial Management

Fluid Resuscitation Severe or moderately severe pancreatitis patients often manifest systemic signs of inflammation. Fluid resuscitation is required in the acute phase with a balanced electrolyte solution, e.g., Ringer's lactate [8]. The rate and total amount of fluid used during initial resuscitation can be difficult to predict. The consequences of under-resuscitation include end-organ damage, in particular renal failure. Over-resuscitation can be complicated by pulmonary edema, respiratory failure, and abdominal compartment syndrome. The "sweet spot" between under- and over-resuscitation can be difficult to identify. Studies have shown increased morbidity and mortality when initial resuscitation is undertaken with 10–15 mL/kg/hr. compared to 5–10 mL/kg/hr. We suggest initial resuscitation with Ringer's lactate solution at 5–10 mL/kg/hr. with continuous reassessment of the endpoints of resuscitation. Relevant endpoints include clinical (e.g., heart rate, blood pressure, urine output), invasive (e.g., stroke volume variation), and biochemical (e.g., base deficit, lactate) parameters [9].

Pancreatitis patients can typically be divided into responders and nonresponders to initial fluid resuscitation. Most responders will manifest signs of improvement clinically and in measured endpoints of resuscitation within the first 4 L of fluid administration. Those who do not respond after 2–4 L may need vasopressor support (i.e., norepinephrine, vasopressin) in addition to ongoing volume resuscitation. Many of the patients who do not respond to this early resuscitation may never respond favorably even to massive resuscitation. One pitfall is to persist with high-volume fluid resuscitation in the hopes of achieving endpoints (low HR, improved urine output, whatever it may be) that will never be achieved with any volume of fluid administration, due to the severity of the underlying inflammation. In these patients, the complications of fluid overload can accumulate without any concomitant improvement in perfusion or organ function. Ask yourself in patients who have not shown significant improvement after high-volume fluid administration (e.g., 6–8 L): what will the ninth or tenth liter of fluid accomplish that the first eight did not? Starting early aggressive fluid resuscitation is the cornerstone of medical therapy of severe acute pancreatitis and is simple but must be judicious in nature. Knowing when to stop is just as important but can be a more difficult and nuanced decision. A balance between fluid resuscitation to meet the needs of the capillary leak and the use of vasopressors to meet the needs of a dilated distributive shock state is important.

Nutrition In mild pancreatitis oral intake can be resumed as soon as abdominal pain and laboratory parameters are improving, often within the first 24 h after presentation. Neither needs to be completely resolved before resuming oral intake. Oral intake can be rapidly advanced to a full solid diet. Indeed, one randomized controlled trial showed that initial oral intake can be with a full solid diet [10, 11]. In patients with severe pancreatitis requiring nutritional supplementation, enteral feeding should be the primary therapy and initiated early (24–48 h after initiation of resuscitation). No specific formulation or immunonutrition has been shown to improve outcomes. Nasogastric feeding if tolerated is equivalent to nasojejunal feeding, acknowledging that it may be less well tolerated in pancreatitis patients than in other critically ill patients due to mechanical compression of the gastric outlet or relative gastric dysmotility induced by inflammation in the lesser sac, since the pancreas abuts the posterior gastric wall and the duodenum. Parenteral nutrition should only be used in patients who cannot reach nutritional goals with enteral nutrition within 5–7 days [12–15].

Prevention, Diagnosis, and Treatment of Infection About 20% of pancreatitis is associated with detectable necrosis of pancreatic or peripancreatic tissue. About 20–30% of the time, this necrosis is complicated by infection. This is the primary indication for mechanical intervention (drainage or debridement) in acute pancreatitis, which is discussed in more detail below. Preventing infection could reduce the need for intervention and any associated morbidity, while prompt diagnosis and treatment of infection can limit the morbidity when infection does occur.

A relatively large literature exists on the administration of intravenous antibiotics to patients with either predicted severe acute pancreatitis or radiographic evidence of necrosis for the purpose of preventing infection of the necrosis. A recent meta-analysis and review of 14 randomized controlled trials concluded that there is no evidence to support the routine use of antibiotics in patients with predicted severe pancreatitis. It remains possible that subgroups may be identified and could benefit from antibiotic prophylaxis, but current guidelines recommend against systemic antibiotic administration for prophylactic purposes. Systemic antibiotics should be reserved for the treatment (not the prophylaxis) of infected pancreatic and peripancreatic necrosis [16]. In observational studies, early enteral feeding, as discussed above, is associated with a reduced incidence of infected necrosis. The presumed mechanism is by reducing the permeability of the gut's mucosal barrier. This benefit has not been supported in randomized trials. Alternative methods of preventing infection include intra-arterial antibiotic administration [17]. There is some evidence that prophylactic selective digestive decontamination (SDD) with enteral antibiotics may be effective in reducing the rate of infected pancreatic necrosis, but this is not strong enough to make SDD a standard recommendation [18]. In one randomized trial, "probiotics" have been found to be harmful [19].

The incidence of infected necrosis increases over the early course of acute pancreatitis and probably peaks in the third and fourth weeks after the onset of the disease. Infected necrosis can be diagnosed definitively by the finding of air in an area of pancreatic necrosis on CT scanning or by gram stain and culture of a fine-needle aspirate of the necrosis. However, infected necrosis remains a clinical diagnosis. It is important to remember that FNA is only approximately 75–90% sensitive for the diagnosis of infection. Thus, patients who are clinically unwell with suspicion for infected necrosis should be treated as if they have infection, since there is no reliable means to exclude it. The common clinical scenario is a patient whose fever curve, leukocytosis, and systemic inflammatory response are improving but begin to return at 3–4 weeks.

When treatment is initiated, carbapenems comprise the best initial regimen based on evidence of effective pancreatic tissue penetration and an appropriate spectrum of antimicrobial activity [20]. Since fungal infection is not uncommon (25%), patients with persistently worsening clinical condition or with microbiologic evidence for fungal infection should be treated with antifungals. If cultures show *Candida albicans*, fluconazole is appropriate. Although good evidence on the optimal antifungal agents in pancreatitis are lacking, if the indication is severe sepsis, we recommend using broader spectrum antifungal agents until definitive culture and sensitivities are available.

Imaging CT is the most common imaging modality used for diagnosis of acute pancreatitis and its complications. It is highly sensitive and specific for acute pancreatitis and relevant complications but is overused in general. As noted above, CT is rarely needed to make the diagnosis of acute pancreatitis and should not be used routinely at the time of presentation but should be reserved for cases in which there is diagnostic uncertainty or clinical deterioration in spite of appropriate initial treatment [21–23]. Whenever possible, CT should be performed with oral and intravenous contrast. If CT is performed to assess for local complications and the severity of the pancreatitis, the optimal timing is 72–96 h after presentation, as CT scans performed in the first 72 h frequently underestimate the degree of pancreatic and peripancreatic necrosis. Even when early CT shows significant abnormalities, follow-up imaging is not recommended unless there is clinical deterioration or lack of improvement. A patient who continues to improve after an episode of acute pancreatitis, even a severe episode with documented necrosis, does not require serial imaging to monitor resolution. MRI can provide most of the same information as CT. Potential advantages include the lack of ionizing radiation and superiority in delineating liquid and solid components within peripancreatic necrosis. As noted above in the diagnosis section, early ultrasonography should also be used to assess for gallstones as the source of the pancreatitis episode if no other etiology is apparent.

ERCP ERCP with sphincterotomy and common bile duct stone extraction is most commonly used to relieve biliary obstruction in cases of gallstone pancreatitis associated with cholangitis. Since the vast majority of gallstones responsible for gallstone pancreatitis pass spontaneously out of the common bile duct, ERCP is usually not necessary. Routine ERCP for all cases of biliary pancreatitis increases the rate of complications, so ERCP should only be employed when there is ongoing biliary obstruction. Sphincterotomy has the added benefit of reducing the risk of recurrent biliary complications. Occasionally biliary obstruction may result later in the course of disease when inflammation or necrosis in the region of the pancreatic head compresses the common bile duct; this usually requires biliary stenting to relieve the obstruction.

Abdominal Compartment Syndrome

As noted above, abdominal compartment syndrome in acute pancreatitis is usually related to high-volume fluid resuscitation, through retroperitoneal mass effect from peripancreatic edema and bowel edema. Diagnosis in acute pancreatitis is as for ACS of other etiologies with intra-abdominal pressures estimated by transduction of bladder pressures. The difficulty in diagnosing ACS in acute pancreatitis is that even in the absence of intra-abdominal hypertension, acute pancreatitis can result in all the clinical hallmarks of ACS such as acute kidney injury, respiratory failure with high peak inspiratory pressures, hypotension, and a tense distended abdomen. When these signs and symptoms occur in a patient with severe pancreatitis, it can be difficult to know if they are a manifestation of the systemic inflammation induced by pancreatitis or if they are a direct result of the intra-abdominal hypertension and thus whether they will improve with treatment of the intra-abdominal hypertension. Treatment is as for ACS of any etiology usually beginning with nasogastric and rectal decompression, volume removal with diuresis or ultrafiltration, and sedation or neuromuscular blockade to increase abdominal wall compliance. Ascites is often a major contributor to intra-abdominal hypertension in acute pancreatitis patients with ACS, and if significant ascites is present, it should be percutaneously drained [24]. When all of these measures fail, surgical decompression of the abdomen is the last resort. If abdominal decompression is performed, pancreatic necrosectomy should not be undertaken. ACS typically occurs early in the course of pancreatitis when surgical necrosectomy increases mortality. Although tempting, do not perform necrosectomy "just because you are there." If the indication for surgery is ACS, then treat the ACS. After decompression, diuresis and staged closure should achieve a high rate (>90%) of primary fascial closure [25].

Intervention

Initial medical management for pancreatitis can be easily provided at most hospitals, but intervention requires a facility with a multidisciplinary team including at least surgeons, interventional radiologists, and gastroenterologists experienced in managing the disease [26]. The clearest consensus indication for intervention is infected pancreatic necrosis.

Once the diagnosis of infected necrosis is made, treatment is with the supportive care described above. When possible intervention should be delayed to 28 days or more from the onset of the pancreatitis episode. This may be impossible if patients are clinically unstable. Whenever the first intervention is undertaken, a minimally invasive percutaneous or endoscopic drainage procedure should be the initial procedure as the first step in a so-called "step-up" approach [27, 28]. Between 20% and 45% of patients with infected necrosis can be successfully treated with percutaneous drainage alone, though this may require several repeat drainage procedures. Drains should be placed taking into account the planned strategies for subsequent stages of the step-up approach. When possible, this may involve placing at least one drain into the area of infected necrosis via a retroperitoneal route to allow for video-assisted retroperitoneal debridement (VARD) along the drain tract. This involves a small subcostal flank incision, dissection along the drain tract into the necrosis cavity, and blunt debridement of the necrotic and infected fluid and tissue. Long retractors are used to expose the tract and cavity, and a standard laparoscope is used to improve visualization of the cavity, though there is typically no insufflation [29]. For patients with necrosis anatomically amenable to such a "step-up" approach, short-term benefits include the ability to avoid any surgery in a significant subset of the population and less new-onset organ failure. Long-term benefits include reduced incidence of diabetes mellitus and incisional hernia. For patients debrided entirely via an endoscopic route, there may also be a mortality advantage compared to open surgery without any preoperative drainage procedure [30]. When no retroperitoneal drainage route is available, sinus tract endoscopy can utilize even transperitoneal drain tracts for debridement of necrosis that does not resolve with percutaneous drainage. This technique involves dilation of the drain tract to allow introduction of a debriding instrument (rigid nephroscopes, flexible endoscopes, and laparoscopic instruments have all been used) into the necrosis cavity [31]. Rarely, some patients with infected pancreatic necrosis will not be amenable to endoscopic or retroperitoneal debridement, in which case laparotomy or laparoscopy may be used for transperitoneal debridement. Additionally, it must be noted that while minimally invasive drainage – either percutaneous or endoscopic – as a first step likely confers significant advantages, when surgery is subsequently required, the evidence is less compelling that any one surgical approach is superior to others. The general principles of delay beyond 4 weeks and preoperative drainage of some form should still be applied whatever the approach is. Tansabdominal debridement should involve removal of all or nearly all infected or necrotic pancreatic and peripancreatic tissue with closed suction drainage of the necrotic cavity. The use of different incisions (midline versus subcostal), approaches to the pancreas (transmesocolic, through the gastrocolic omentum, or retroperitoneal), and drainage (closed packing, closed suction alone, continuous lavage) is at the discretion of the surgeon [32].

Intervention is less often needed for sterile pancreatic necrosis. The most common indication is gastric outlet obstruction. Intervention can often be delayed longer, as this complication will often resolve with time. If patients with presumed sterile necrosis remain persistently unwell, the possibility of occult infection must be considered. Intervention can include surgical debridement or bypass.

Other complications that may prompt intervention in the acute setting include abdominal compartment syndrome (ACS), hemorrhage of a visceral artery (usually splenic artery) pseudoaneurysm, and bowel perforation or fistula. When these complications arise in the acute setting, they should, as a rule, be treated by the least invasive methods possible. The treatment of ACS is discussed above. Bleeding from a visceral artery pseudoaneurysm should be controlled endovascularly by angioembolization whenever possible as direct surgical control in a region of active or recent pancreatitis is extremely difficult [33]. Intestinal perforation is similarly difficult to manage. Contained perforations or controlled fistulas may be manageable with drainage or diversion. When there is bowel ischemia or uncontrolled enteric spillage, resection will likely be necessary.

Late Complications

Pancreatic fistulas and pseudocysts result from disruption of the pancreatic duct due to destruction of the surrounding parenchyma. Fistulas may result from severe pancreatitis or as a complication of pancreatic debridement, after which they are common. One advantage of endoscopic transluminal debridement may be that such leaks from the pancreatic duct drain internally, rather than forming external fistulas. Whatever the cause, when the fistula is controlled with percutaneous drains, it will usually close, though it may require many weeks. Pancreatic duct stenting, octreotide administration, and restriction of enteral nutrition have all been advocated to aid in fistula closure but are not routinely helpful and should be used very selectively. In the special situation of a disconnected distal pancreatic remnant in which a segment of the gland has been completely separated from any route of drainage into the gastrointestinal tract, spontaneous closure is impossible. Such patients may either be treated endoscopically by transluminal stenting to attempt to convert the external fistula into a controlled internal fistula or may be treated surgically by either Roux-en-Y jejunostomy to the distal pancreatic remnant or resection of the disconnected distal segment.

Pseudocysts form when the ductal disruption is walled off by the body into an organized collection of pancreatic juice encased by reactive inflammatory tissue – a process that occurs 4 weeks or more after damage to the pancreatic duct. Asymptomatic pseudocysts do not require intervention. The most common symptoms are early satiety and abdominal pain. Pseudocysts may also cause true gastric outlet obstruction, become infected, or lead to pseudoaneurysm formation. Internal drainage is the treatment of choice for pseudocysts requiring intervention. For pseudocysts closely opposed to the stomach or duodenum, endoscopic pseudocyst-gastrostomy or duodenostomy is the treatment of choice. For very large or endoscopically inaccessible pseudocysts, surgical cyst gastrostomy or Roux-en-Y cyst jejunostomy is necessary [34].

Vascular complications of pancreatitis include arterial pseudoaneurysm and venous thrombosis. These most commonly involve the splenic vessels, but in pancreatitis primarily affecting the head, pseudoaneurysms of the pancreaticoduodenal or gastroduodenal arteries may occur along with thrombosis of the superior mesenteric or portal veins. Pseudoaneurysms result from the action of pancreatic enzymes on the arterial wall. They may be identified incidentally on contrast-enhanced CT or can present with catastrophic hemorrhage. We recommend intervening even on asymptomatic pseudoaneurysms in most cases, since there is no reliable way to predict hemorrhage. As above, whether elective or emergent, they are best treated with angioembolization [33]. Splenic vein thrombosis due to pancreatitis can usually be observed. We occasionally anticoagulate if clot extends into the main portal vein. Even without anticoagulation the thrombus can resolve. If it does not, the most common late complication is gastric varices. If these result in gastrointestinal bleeding, they can be eliminated by splenectomy [35].

Efforts should be made to prevent recurrence after an episode of pancreatitis by cessation of ethanol abuse for alcoholic pancreatitis, treatment of the underlying condition in hypercalcemia and hypertriglyceridemia, and cessation of any offending medications in cases of medication-induced pancreatitis. In patients with gallstone pancreatitis, cholecystectomy during the same hospitalization is recommended for mild cases. In patients undergoing transperitoneal necrosectomy, cholecystectomy at the time of necrosectomy is safe and reduces recurrent biliary complications [36]. In patients with peripancreatic fluid collections, cholecystectomy should be delayed for 6 weeks. In especially poor operative candidates, ERCP with sphincterotomy reduces the risk of recurrent gallstone pancreatitis and can be considered as an alternative to cholecystectomy.

References

1. Peery AF, Dellon ES, Lund J, Crockett SD, McGowan CE, Bulsiewicz WJ, Gangarosa LM, Thiny MT, Stizenberg K, Morgan DR, Ringel Y, Kim HP, Dibonaventura MD, Carroll CF, Allen JK, Cook SF, Sandler RS, Kappelman MD, Shaheen NJ. Burden of gastrointestinal disease in the United States: 2012 update. Gastroenterology. 2012;143(5):1179–87.
2. Fagenholz PJ, Castillo CF, Harris NS, Pelletier AJ, Camargo CA Jr. Increasing United States hospital admissions for acute pancreatitis, 1988–2003. Ann Epidemiol. 2007;17(7):491–7.
3. Räty S, Pulkkinen J, Nordback I, Sand J, Victorzon M, Grönroos J, Helminen H, Kuusanmäki P, Nordström P, Paajanen H. Can laparoscopic cholecystectomy prevent recurrent idiopathic acute pancreatitis?: a prospective randomized multicenter trial. Ann Surg. 2015;262(5):736–41.
4. Frossard JL, Steer ML, Pastor CM. Acute pancreatitis. Lancet. 2008;371(9607):143–52.
5. Sarr MG, Banks PA, Bollen TL, Dervenis C, Gooszen HG, Johnson CD, Tsiotos GG, Vege SS. The new revised classification of acute pancreatitis 2012. Surg Clin North Am. 2013;93(3):549–62.
6. Singh VK, Wu BU, Bollen TL, Repas K, Maurer R, Mortele KJ, et al. Early systemic inflammatory response syndrome is associated with severe acute pancreatitis. Clin Gastroenterol Hepatol. 2009;7:1247e51.

7. Papachristou GI, Muddana V, Yadav D, O'Connell M, Sanders MK, Slivka A, et al. Comparison of BISAP, Ranson's, APACHE-II, and CTSI scores in predicting organ failure, complications, and mortality in acute pancreatitis. Am J Gastroenterol. 2010;105:435e41.
8. BU W, Hwang JQ, Gardner TH, Repas K, Delee R, Yu S, Smith B, Banks PA, Conwell DL. Lactated Ringer's solution reduces systemic inflammation compared with saline in patients with acute pancreatitis. Clin Gastroenterol Hepatol. 2011;9:710–7.
9. Working Group IAP/APA Acute Pancreatitis Guidelines. IAP/APA evidence-based guidelines for the management of acute pancreatitis. Pancreatology. 2013;13(4 Suppl 2):e1–15.
10. Eckerwall GE, Tingstedt BB, Bergenzaun PE, Andersson RG. Immediate oral feeding in patients with mild acute pancreatitis is safe and may accelerate recovery-a randomized clinical study. Clin Nutr. 2007;26:758–63.
11. Moraes JM, Felga GE, Chebli LA, Franco MB, Gomes CA, Gaburri PD, Zanini A, Chebli JM. A full solid diet as the initial meal in mild acute pancreatitis is safe and result in a shorter length of hospitalization: results from a prospective, randomized, controlled, double-blind clinical trial. J Clin Gastroenterol. 2010;44:517–22.
12. Al-Omran M, Albalawi ZH, Tashkandi MF, Al-Ansary LA. Enteral versus parenteral nutrition for acute pancreatitis. Cochrane Database Syst Rev. 2010;(1):CD002837.
13. Petrov MS, Loveday BP, Pylypchuk RD, McIlroy K, Phillips AR, Windsor JA. Systematic review and meta-analysis of enteral nutrition formulations in acute pancreatitis. Br J Surg. 2009;96:1243–52.
14. Eatock FC, Chong P, Menezes N, Murray L, McKay CJ, Carter CR, Imrie CW. A randomized study of early nasogastric versus nasojejunal feeding in severe acute pancreatitis. Am J Gastroenterol. 2005;100:432–9.
15. Kumar A, Singh N, Prakash S, Saraya A, Joshi YK. Early enteral nutrition in severe acute pancreatitis: a prospective randomized controlled trial comparing nasojejunal and nasogastric routes. J Clin Gastroenterol. 2006;40:431–4.
16. Wittau M, Mayer B, Scheele J, Henne-Bruns D, Dellinger EP, Isenmann R. Systematic review and meta-analysis of antibiotic prophylaxis in severe acute pancreatitis. Scand J Gastroenterol. 2010;46(3):261–70.
17. Piascik M, Rydzewska G, Milewski J, Olszewski S, Furmanek M, Walecki J, et al. The results of severe acute pancreatitis treatment with continuous regional arterial infusion of protease inhibitor and antibiotic: a randomized controlled study. Pancreas. 2010;39:863e7.
18. Luiten EJ, Hop WC, Lange JF, Bruining HA. Controlled clinical trial of selective decontamination for the treatment of severe acute pancreatitis. Ann Surg. 1995;222:57e65.
19. Besselink MG, Van Santvoort HC, Buskens E, Boermeester MA, van Goor H, Timmerman HM, et al. Probiotic prophylaxis in predicted severe acute pancreatitis: a randomised, double-blind, placebo-controlled trial. Lancet. 2008;371:651e9.
20. Dellinger EP, Tellado JM, Soto NE, et al. Early antibiotic treatment for severe acute necrotizing pancreatitis: randomized, double-blind, placebo-controlled study. Ann Surg. 2007;245:674–83.
21. Fleszler F, Friedenberg F, Krevsky B, Friedel D, Braitman LE. Abdominal computed tomography prolongs length of stay and is frequently unnecessary in the evaluation of acute pancreatitis. Am J Med Sci. 2003;325:251–5.
22. Spanier BW, Nio Y, van der Hulst RW, Tuynman HA, Dijkgraaf MG, Bruno MJ. Practice and yield of early CT scan in acute pancreatitis: a Dutch Observational Multicenter Study. Pancreatology. 2010;10:222–8.
23. Mortele KJ, Ip IK, BU W, Conwell DL, Banks PA, Khorasani R. Acute pancreatitis: imaging utilization practices in an urban teaching hospital--analysis of trends with assessment of independent predictors in correlation with patient outcomes. Radiology. 2011;258:174–81.
24. Radenkovic DV, Bajec D, Ivancevic N, Bumbasirevic V, Milic N, Jeremic V, Gregoric P, Karamarkovic A, Karadzic B, Mirkovic D, Bilanovic D, Scepanovic R, Cijan V. Decompressive laparotomy with temporary abdominal closure versus percutaneous puncture with placement of abdominal catheter in patients with abdominal compartment syndrome during acute pancreatitis: background and design of multicenter, randomised, controlled study. BMC Surg. 2010;10:22.
25. Boone B, Zureikat A, Hughes SJ, Moser AJ, Yadav D, Zeh HJ, Lee KK. Abdominal compartment syndrome is an early, lethal complication of acute pancreatitis. Am Surg. 2013;79(6):601–7.
26. Freeman ML, Werner J, van Santvoort HC, Baron TH, Besselink MG, Windsor JA, Horvath KD, vanSonnenberg E, Bollen TL, Vege SS, International Multidisciplinary Panel of Speakers and Moderators. Interventions for necrotizing pancreatitis: summary of a multidisciplinary consensus conference. Pancreas. 2012;41(8):1176–94.
27. van Santvoort HC, Besselink MG, Bakker OJ, Hofker HS, Boermeester MA, Dejong CH, van Goor H, Schaapherder AF, van Eijck CH, Bollen TL, van Ramshorst B, Nieuwenhuijs VB, Timmer R, Laméris JS, Kruyt PM, Manusama ER, van der Harst E, van der Schelling GP, Karsten T, Hesselink EJ, van Laarhoven CJ, Rosman C, Bosscha K, de Wit RJ, Houdijk AP, van Leeuwen MS, Buskens E, Gooszen HG, Dutch Pancreatitis Study Group. A step-up approach or open necrosectomy for necrotizing pancreatitis. N Engl J Med. 2010;362(16):1491–502.
28. van Santvoort HC, Bakker OJ, Bollen TL, Besselink MG, Ahmed Ali U, Schrijver AM, Boermeester MA, van Goor H, Dejong CH, van Eijck CH, van Ramshorst B, Schaapherder AF, van der Harst E, Hofker S, Nieuwenhuijs VB, Brink MA, Kruyt PM, Manusama ER, van der Schelling GP, Karsten T, Hesselink EJ, van Laarhoven CJ, Rosman C, Bosscha K, de Wit RJ, Houdijk AP, Cuesta MA, Wahab PJ, Gooszen HG, Dutch Pancreatitis Study Group. A conservative and minimally invasive approach to necrotizing pancreatitis improves outcome. Gastroenterology. 2011;141(4):1254–63.
29. van Santvoort HC, Besselink MG, Horvath KD, Sinanan MN, Bollen TL, van Ramshorst B, Gooszen HG, Dutch Acute Pancreatis Study Group. Videoscopic assisted retroperitoneal debridement in infected necrotizing pancreatitis. HPB (Oxford). 2007;9(2):156–9.
30. Bakker OJ, van Santvoort HC, van Brunschot S, Geskus RB, Besselink MG, Bollen TL, van Eijck CH, Fockens P, Hazebroek EJ, Nijmeijer RM, Poley JW, van Ramshorst B, Vleggaar FP, Boermeester MA, Gooszen HG, Weusten BL, Timmer R, Dutch Pancreatitis Study Group. Endoscopic transgastric vs surgical necrosectomy for infected necrotizing pancreatitis: a randomized trial. JAMA. 2012;307(10):1053–61.
31. Carter CR, McKay CJ, Imrie CW. Percutaneous necrosectomy and sinus tract endoscopy in the management of infected pancreatic necrosis: an initial experience. Ann Surg. 2000;232(2):175–80.
32. Mantke R, Lippert H, Buchler MW, Sarr MG. International practices in pancreatic surgery. Part IV, Surgery of acute pancreatitis. New York: Springer; 2013.
33. Kalva SP, Yeddula K, Wicky S, Fernandez del Castillo C, Warshaw AL. Angiographic intervention in patients with a suspected visceral artery pseudoaneurysm complicating pancreatitis and pancreatic surgery. Arch Surg. 2011;146(6):647–52.
34. Samuelson AL, Shah RJ. Endoscopic management of pancreatic pseudocysts. Gastroenterol Clin N Am. 2012;41(1):47–62.
35. Besselink MG. Splanchnic vein thrombosis complicating severe acute pancreatitis. HPB (Oxford). 2011;13(12):831–2.
36. Fong ZV, Peev M, Warshaw AL, Lillemoe KD, Fernández-del Castillo C, Velmahos GC, Fagenholz PJ. Single-stage cholecystectomy at the time of pancreatic necrosectomy is safe and prevents future biliary complications: a 20-year single institutional experience with 217 consecutive patients. J Gastrointest Surg. 2015;19(1):32–7.

Management of the Post-op Abdominal Catastrophe and Open Abdomen

26

Priya S. Prakash and Patrick M. Reilly

Introduction

The use of the open abdomen in the management of the critically ill surgical patient is born from the concept of damage control surgery. This is one of the major advances in the surgical management of patients in extremis over the past few decades, centering the abbreviated laparotomy on control of hemorrhage and contamination in patients presenting with life-threatening physiologic derangement [1, 2]. Initially reserved for the moribund trauma patient, principles of damage control laparotomy (DCL) were applied to the critically ill, non-traumatized patient after reports of increased survival in this group [3, 4]. This approach was grounded in the principle that the potential for augmenting survivorship takes precedence over increasing morbidity, redirecting the efforts of resuscitation away from completing the operation and rather toward the goal of preserving life [5, 6]. This paradigm shift refocused importance on the intensive care unit (ICU) as the ideal setting for resuscitation and correction of the "lethal triad" of acidosis, hypothermia, and coagulopathy that previously led to physiologic exhaustion in these patients (Fig. 26.1). Thus, the intensivist has come to play a crucial role in the resuscitation and management of the patient with an open abdomen.

P. S. Prakash
Department of Surgery, Division of Trauma and Acute Care Surgery, Pritzker School of Medicine, University of Chicago, Chicago, IL, USA

P. M. Reilly (✉)
Department of Surgery, Division of Trauma, Surgical Critical Care, and Emergency Surgery, Perelman School of Medicine, University of Pennsylvania, Philadelphia, PA, USA
e-mail: reillyp@uphs.upenn.edu

Indications for an Open Abdomen

Abdominal compartment syndrome (ACS) is one of the most common indications for the use of the open abdomen technique. This topic is covered in more detail elsewhere in the text, but, briefly, ACS is defined as intra-abdominal hypertension (IAH) that produces end-organ dysfunction secondary to increased intra-abdominal pressure [7]. Primary IAH/ACS is due to an intraperitoneal or retroperitoneal process such as bleeding from a ruptured abdominal aneurysm, infection from mesenteric ischemia, or inflammation from necrotizing pancreatitis. Secondary IAH/ACS is associated with extra-abdominal processes such as large-volume resuscitation that can lead to bowel edema or intraperitoneal fluid accumulation [7]. It is also important to remember that IAH and ACS can develop in patients already treated with an open abdomen who have a temporary abdominal closure (TAC) in place [8]. In these patients, the temporary closure should be released as soon as signs of ACS are detected.

Another indication for the open abdomen technique is a damage control operation, typically performed in the moribund trauma patient. Traditionally, the major tenants of damage control surgery have highlighted rapid control of bleeding and contamination, temporary abdominal closure, physiologic resuscitation, and delayed definitive operation [2, 6, 9]. The concept of DCL evolved from the recognition that mortality for patients in extremis was more likely due to physiologic exhaustion of the patient than from failure to complete operative repairs. After rapid control of bleeding and gross contamination is established in the operating room, the emphasis shifts to correction of physiologic derangements in the intensive care unit to avoid the "lethal triad" of coagulopathy, hypothermia, and metabolic acidosis. Once these physiologic derangements have been resolved, the patient is taken back to the operating room for definitive, reconstructive surgical intervention.

A. Salim et al. (eds.), *Surgical Critical Care Therapy*, https://doi.org/10.1007/978-3-319-71712-8_26

Fig. 26.1 Phases of damage control sequence

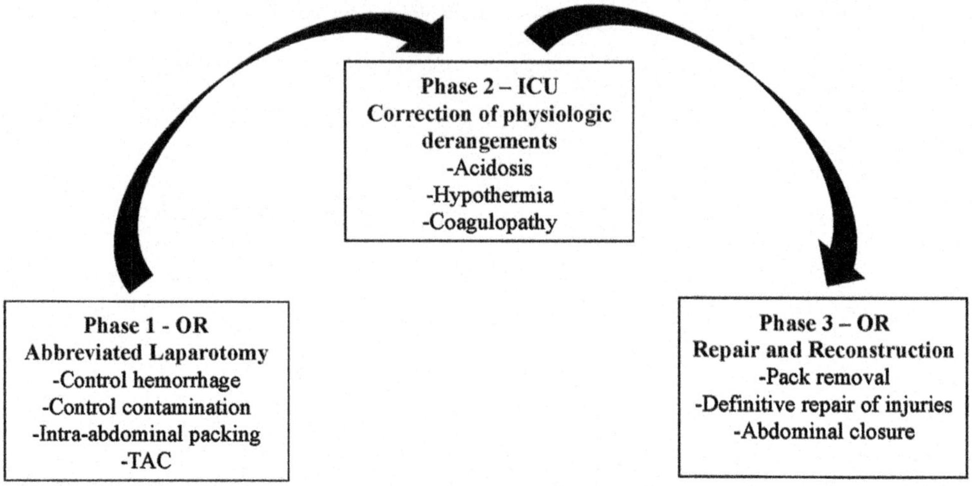

Intra-abdominal sepsis is another major condition that occasionally requires the application of the open abdomen technique. Ogilvie was the first to describe the open abdomen for the treatment of severe intra-abdominal sepsis [10]. The goal of treating intra-abdominal sepsis is to identify and control the source of infection. The abdomen may be left open to allow for a second-look operation to evaluate bowel viability, integrity of an anastomosis, or progression of an ischemic process. Alternatively, the abdomen is left open secondary to the large resuscitation that these patients often require, which can result in severe bowel edema, leading to IAH and secondary ACS.

Other indications to employ the open abdomen technique are the presence of multiple injuries within one body cavity or across multiple cavities, the time required for definitive repair of injuries exceeds the patient's physiologic reserve, transfusion requirements ≥10 units or total fluid replacement >12 L, and physiologic derangement as indicated by temperature <35 °C, pH < 7.20, persistent lactic acidosis, or coagulopathy as evidenced by ongoing nonsurgical bleeding or laboratory abnormalities [11–13] (Table 26.1). Regardless of the indication for use of the open abdomen technique, the main goal of the intensivist remains in reestablishing normal physiology in the patient prior to return to the operating room for definitive treatment.

Table 26.1 Indications for damage control laparotomy and open abdomen technique

Indications for an open abdomen	
Abdominal compartment syndrome	Hemodynamic instability
Damage control laparotomy	Acidosis (pH < 7.2)
Intra-abdominal sepsis	Hypothermia (T < 35 °C)
Multiple injuries ± multiple body cavities	Coagulopathy
Prohibitive operative time (>90 min)	Elevated lactate
Massive transfusion (≥10 units or >12 L IVF)	

Table 26.2 Techniques for temporary abdominal closure

Techniques for temporary abdominal closure (TAC)
Bogota bag
Towel-clip closure
Barker Vac Pac
Wittmann patch
Skin closure
Negative-pressure wound therapy

Technique for Temporary Abdominal Closure

A temporary abdominal closure (TAC) is required when the open abdominal technique is undertaken. Successful management of the open abdomen with a TAC is dependent on decreasing IAH, protecting the viscera, and reducing intra-abdominal complications such as fistulas and abdominal wall hernias. Historically, the Bogota bag was one of the first TAC techniques used in the open abdomen. A sterile saline bag sutured to the fascial edges functioned as a silo to cover the intra-abdominal contents and protect the exposed viscera from injury [14]. Another approach was the towel-clip closure, in which penetrating towel clips were placed on the skin 2–3 cm apart, to approximate the skin for the entire laparotomy. This has now largely been abandoned given the high rate of ACS, skin necrosis, and limited use when angiography is indicated.

There has been evolution in management of the open abdomen over the last few decades (Table 26.2). The Barker Vac Pac technique involves protection of the viscera with a perforated plastic covering, placement of suction devices in

Table 26.3 Advantages of negative-pressure wound therapy

Advantages of negative-pressure wound therapy
Covers wound
Protects the viscera
Reduces tissue edema
Decreases loss of abdominal wall domain
Decreases evaporative losses
Measures fluid loss accurately

surgical towels, and application of the system to wall suction [15]. Improved closure rates and decreased fistula rates have been reported with this technique. There are also commercially available devices that allow tension to be placed on the fascial edges, similar to the Wittmann Patch (http://www.starsurgical.com/wp.html), which employs a Velcro-like device that bridges the fascia and allows for easy access to the abdominal cavity. These devices range from trying to reapproximate the fascia to achieve dynamic closure of the abdomen to negative-pressure wound therapy devices that control peritoneal effluent and minimize abdominal wall retraction. Data suggest that negative-pressure wound therapy may be associated with better outcomes compared with other closure techniques [16, 17] (Table 26.3). In addition to wound coverage and protecting the viscera, negative-pressure wound therapy also reportedly reduces tissue edema and assists with fascial closure by decreasing loss of abdominal wall domain [18, 19]. A negative-pressure wound therapy device also helps decrease evaporative losses and allows accurate measurement of fluid loss through the wound [20, 21]. This allows for more precise replacement of fluid losses and minimization of hypovolemia. TAC dressings should be changed in the operating room or in the intensive care unit every 2–3 days. If the patient is not on antibiotics for other reasons, they are not indicated when using these devices.

ICU Management of the Open Abdomen

Resuscitation

Often patients who have an indication for an open abdomen require large volumes of fluid during their initial resuscitation, normally with crystalloid or blood product. These patients should have large-bore intravenous access and also often require invasive monitoring with a central line and arterial line catheters. Resuscitation is guided by reestablishing end-organ perfusion as indicated by adequate urine output, restitution of vital signs, and clearance of lactic acidosis (Fig. 26.2). Other resuscitation targets include an oxygen delivery index >600 mL/min/m2, oxygen consumption index >150 mL/min/m2, and lactate <2.5 mmol/L within 12 h [22, 23]. Lactic acid levels should be checked every 4 h until two consecutive measurements are less than or equal to 2 mmol/L [24]. If the lactic acidosis fails to clear after adequate fluid resuscitation, continued pathology such as ongoing bleeding, a missed injury, ACS, and intestinal ischemia should be considered. Failure to clear the lactate in a patient with an open abdomen may be an indication to return to the operating room for re-exploration. Vasoactive agents are also often required in this patient population but should not be used in lieu of appropriate volume resuscitation.

Hypothermia and Rewarming

Hypothermia impairs thrombin generation and contributes to platelet dysfunction. Correcting hypothermia and rewarming the patient assist in the resuscitative process by allowing cofactors in the clotting cascade to work, thereby decreasing blood loss and correcting acidosis [25, 26]. Terminating the procedure and providing a temporary closure of the abdomen are the first steps in the rewarming process for a patient with an abdominal catastrophe. The ICU room should be preheated to 29 °C. All wet clothing and linens should be removed, and the patient should be covered with warm blankets. Active external rewarming techniques should be used in patients with moderate hypothermia. These include the radiant warmer, electric blanket, forced warm-air blanket, and heating pads [27]. Active internal rewarming is used for moderate to severe hypothermia. This includes ventilation with humidified oxygen, warmed intravenous fluids, peritoneal lavage, and extracorporeal modalities such as dialysis, cardiopulmonary bypass, and extracorporeal life support [28]. These more invasive techniques are not without their disadvantages and should be used on a case-to-case basis.

Coagulopathy

As stated above, massive transfusion of blood products is often required during the first 24 h of a damage control surgery [29]. A 1:1:1 transfusion ratio of blood products is the favored approach to resuscitation as evidence suggests a lower overall fluid requirement and decreased blood utilization with this strategy [30, 31]. But large-volume resuscitation with both crystalloid and massive transfusion protocols is not without complications. Dilutional coagulopathy as a result of massive volume resuscitation should be addressed by the intensivist during the resuscitation phase of DCL. Blood products should be administered until the prothrombin time and partial thromboplastin time are less than 1.25 times normal, the platelet count is greater than 100,000/mm^3, and fibrinogen level is greater than 100 mg/dL [13]. In addition, calcium levels should be monitored closely and appropriately replaced in the setting of hypocalcemia secondary to massive transfusion.

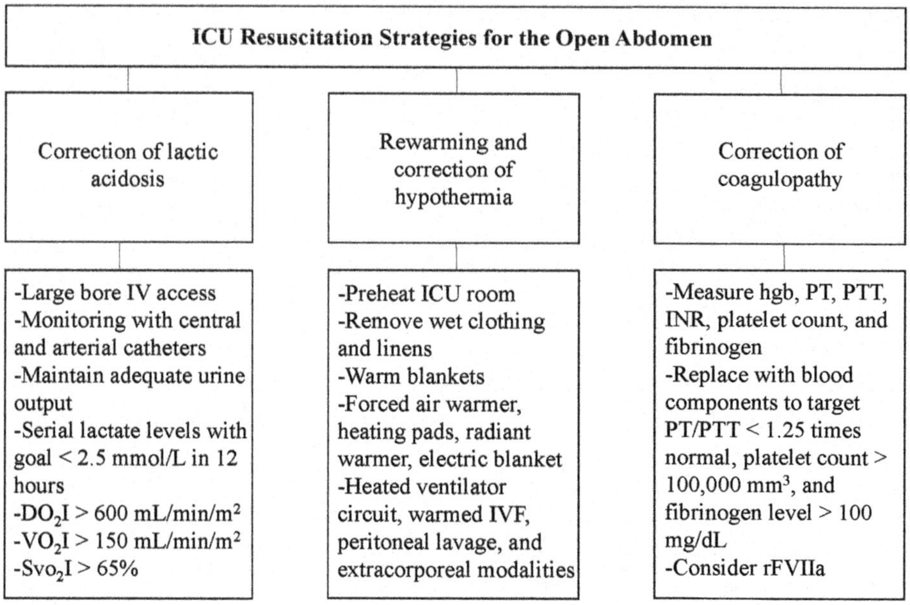

Fig. 26.2 ICU management strategies for the open abdomen

Recombinant factor VIIa (rFVIIa) is a prohemostatic agent that has been studied as an adjunct to hemorrhage control. Though there is a paucity of data from prospective controlled trials, case series suggest that the use of rFVIIa should be considered for lethal, nonsurgical hemorrhage during damage control resuscitation as it seems to reduce transfusion requirements and correct the coagulopathy profile, though mortality does not seem to improve with use [32–35].

Fluid and Electrolyte Management

Patients with an open abdomen are subject to ongoing insensible fluid losses due to large surface area of tissue defects and exposure of the peritoneal cavity. The large amount of protein losses across these wounds can also result in changes in oncotic pressure, contributing to further loss of volume into the interstitial space. The loss of hypotonic fluid from the wound and peritoneal cavity can result in hypovolemic hypernatremia. Choice of replacement fluid should be based on serum sodium and circulating volume status. In the hypovolemic patient, isotonic replacement fluids should be used until euvolemia is achieved.

Another challenge posed to the intensivist when managing an open abdomen is volume loss from an enteroatmospheric or enterocutaneous fistula, leading to hypovolemia, electrolyte disturbances, and malnutrition. Fistula output should be carefully estimated and replaced with the appropriate balanced salt solution. Replacement fluid should be based on the electrolyte composition and tonicity of the intestinal fluid losses. In the setting of a high-output fistula, re-feeding fistulous output can help to reduce fluid and electrolyte disturbances as well as increase caloric delivery.

There has been some evidence that suggests that the use of hypertonic saline (HTS) rather than standard isotonic fluids in the immediate postoperative period decreases time to fascial closure and increases overall rates of primary fascial closure [36]. HTS may be used as an adjunct to facilitate fascial closure in patients requiring DCL. Diuretics have also been utilized anecdotally to promote primary fascial closure. Though there has been an association between net negative fluid balance and higher primary closure rates, there is evidence to suggest that the addition of diuretics does not improve the rate or time to fascial closure [37].

Ventilation

Patients with an open abdomen who are otherwise hemodynamically normal can be extubated and sent to the floor without additional sedation. But those who require ongoing resuscitation and remain intubated are at high risk for the development of acute lung injury (ALI) and adult respiratory distress syndrome (ARDS) [38]. Factors that predispose the damage-controlled patient to ALI and ARDS include direct parenchymal lung injury, shock, and massive resuscitation volumes that the patient often receives during the first 24 h [38]. A large-volume resuscitation can lead to pulmonary edema and decreased chest wall compliance. In addition, abdominal packing and IAH increase intrathoracic pressure and decrease lung compliance by elevating the diaphragm.

The goal for ventilator strategy in the open abdomen patient should be to maintain oxygenation and ventilation while avoiding volutrauma and barotrauma (Table 26.4), which is usually achieved with the ARDSnet low-stretch protocol [39]. High levels of PEEP are frequently required to

Table 26.4 Ventilator strategies in patients with an open abdomen

Ventilator strategy	Goal of therapy
Low-stretch protocol (tidal volume ≤ 6 mL/kg)	Avoid volume and barotrauma
High PEEP	Maintain oxygenation
Reduced inspiration to expiration ratio (I:E)	Maintain oxygenation
Sedation/analgesia ± paralytics	Ventilator synchrony
Prone positioning	Decrease ventilation/perfusion mismatch
HFOV, APRV	Treat refractory hypoxia

maintain oxygenation in the patient with an open abdomen. Sometimes permissive hypercapnia due to reduction of the inspiration to expiration (I:E) ratio is required to maintain oxygenation. This is tolerated if the pH remains greater than 7.20. Sedation and analgesia, and sometimes a paralytic, are used to control the patient's discomfort and asynchrony on high ventilator settings. Despite these efforts, if the patient continues to have a severe ventilation/perfusion mismatch, prone positioning may be indicated. Other advanced modes of mechanical ventilation such as the oscillating ventilator or airway pressure release ventilation may also be required in the setting of refractory hypoxia.

It should also be recognized that patients with an open abdomen and TAC are also susceptible to developing ACS. This process occurs as the IAH pushes the diaphragm up, decreasing the intrathoracic volume. This is often first recognized by a change in pulmonary dynamics with a decrease in tidal volumes and increase in peak airway pressures, which can cause barotrauma and lead to ALI. Immediate release of the TAC is indicated in this situation.

Sedation/Analgesia/Neuromuscular Blockade

Patients who are extubated can often be managed with a standard postoperative regimen for analgesia and do not require additional sedation. But for those who remain intubated with an open abdomen, the optimal sedation and analgesia strategy is not well defined. Sedation and analgesia may be helpful in decreasing patient asynchrony with the ventilator when high levels of ventilator support are needed [40]. In addition, given that neuromuscular blockade has been successfully used as treatment for ACS, it has been suggested that it may be used to prevent abdominal wall retraction and improve primary fascial closure [41–43]. But when comparing neuromuscular blockade to sedation alone, the results are equivocal [44]. It is also important to recognize the complications associated with neuromuscular blockade, such as increased risk of infections, decubitus ulcers, and prolonged ICU neuropathy and myopathy.

Antibiotics

Standard perioperative prophylactic antibiotics should be administered and re-dosed intraoperatively if a large resuscitation or significant fluid shifts are anticipated [45–47] in the patient undergoing DCL or reoperation. Prophylactic antibiotics should not continue beyond 24 h in patients with an open abdomen [48]. The exception to this is the patient that is managed with DCL for intra-abdominal sepsis, in which broad spectrum antibiotics should be administered and then de-escalated according to culture results. Other indications for antibiotic use may be an intra-abdominal abscess or other ongoing infections such as ventilator-associated pneumonia. An open abdomen alone is not an indication for continued antibiotic therapy.

Nutrition

Because early administration of enteral nutrition has been shown to improve wound healing, reduce hospital and ICU lengths of stay, decrease infection rates, and improve survival after critical illness and injury [49–52], early enteral nutrition is the preferred route and should be initiated in the patient with an open abdomen when feasible. This may not be possible if the bowel is in discontinuity or the patient's hemodynamic status does not allow it. Parenteral nutrition may be required initially until physiologic status is normalized in patients presenting with overt signs of malnutrition [53]. In the well-nourished patient, nutrition should be initiated within 7 days. If full enteral nutrition cannot be achieved in this time period, parenteral nutrition should be used until enteral nutrition can be titrated and tolerated at goal rates.

Patients with an open abdomen require increased protein and caloric support given ongoing losses from large wounds. In general, most patients with an open abdomen will require 25–35 kcal/kg/d of nonprotein calories and 1.5–2.5 g of protein/kg/d. Estimation of nutritional requirements may be calculated from one of the many predictive equations for estimating basal energy expenditure, using indirect calorimetry with a metabolic cart or the establishment of a positive nitrogen balance. It is important to recognize that standard measures of anabolic metabolism will frequently be erroneous for patients with an open abdomen due to unmeasured protein losses across the large open abdomen [54]. Protein losses from these large wounds will be dependent on the daily volume of exudate, which can be estimated at approximately 2.9 g of protein/dL [55]. Weekly 24-h urine urea nitrogen levels should be followed and nutritional support adjusted based on these measurements. In addition, nitrogen balance should be calculated with the adjustment of 1 g of protein loss per 500 mL of fistula output [53] and 2.9 g of protein/dL of peritoneal exudate [55]. Failure to account for these unmeasured protein losses will lead to underfeeding and inadequate nutritional support in the patient with an open abdomen.

Options for nutritional access include a nasoenteric, gastrostomy, or jejunostomy tube. Post-pyloric nasoenteric feeding tubes offer potential for continued feeding in patients undergoing multiple trips to the operating room by minimizing the need for nutritional interruption. In addition, endoscopic placement of enteral access is an option, though this approach may not be as straightforward given the alterations in the abdominal wall and distortion of the anatomy. Surgical placement of a gastrostomy or jejunostomy tube is also an option and should be considered prior to definitive closure of the abdomen.

Definitive Reconstruction and Closure

The third phase of damage control surgery is definitive repair of injuries and abdominal wall reconstruction. This is undertaken once normal physiology has been restored in the patient, which is usually achieved within 12–24 h in the ICU but sometimes can take up to 72 h. During return to the operating room, abdominal packing is removed, all injuries are identified, and any ongoing bleeding is addressed. Intestinal continuity is reestablished at this time if the patient remains physiologically intact. Though the small intestine is usually put back in continuity, the colon still remains a point of contention. Anastomotic leak rates are significantly higher in the left colon compared to the right colon. Increased anastomotic leak rates are also associated with time to fascial closure greater than 5 days. Thus, colostomy should be considered in patients with left colon injuries and delay in time to fascial closure [56, 57].

Primary fascial closure is the goal for patients managed with an open abdomen. Closure may be addressed in an early or delayed fashion during the primary hospitalization. Early closure is defined as within 9 days of initial laparotomy and is associated with fewer complications. This is often more attainable in those with an open abdomen after trauma in comparison with those managed with an open abdomen for intra-abdominal sepsis [58, 59]. Often, daily trips to the operating room are required for incremental closure of the abdominal fascia. In situations where fascial closure is not possible due to ongoing visceral edema or loss of abdominal domain, the viscera is covered with a prosthetic or biological mesh material, which allows for formation of granulation tissue, which can eventually be skin grafted. Other options include skin-only closure over the viscera. These options result in a planned ventral hernia with delayed repair deferred to a subsequent hospitalization, usually in 6–12 months.

Consideration should be given to nutritional access prior to definitive closure of the abdomen. As mentioned above, surgical placement of a gastrostomy or jejunostomy tube should be considered if long-term enteral access is indicated. However, enteral access should not be placed until the patient is ready for definitive closure of the abdomen, as multiple repeat laparotomies can result in manipulation and movement of the enteral access site, leading to fistula formation.

Critical Care Challenges in the Open Abdomen

Wound Management

The TAC used to keep the intra-abdominal contents from eviscerating may fail (Table 26.5). Leakage of peritoneal effluent from the edge of the dressing is considered a minor failure of the dressing. This usually can be repaired by reinforcing the dressing with occlusive materials. Major dressing failure is considered complete evisceration of the bowel, which requires a reapplication of the entire dressing and possibly a different dressing all together, which is usually done in the operating room. Other reasons of dressing failure may include ongoing hemorrhage, poor patient sedation, and inadequate dressing placement initially.

Surgical Site Infections

Wound infections are common after an open abdomen. Lower rates of infection are reported when the skin is not closed compared with reports of skin closure at the time of fascial closure [58]. Polymicrobial wound colonization occurs while the abdomen is open, most commonly with

Table 26.5 Complications of an open abdomen and management strategies

Complication	Management
Leakage of effluent from TAC	Reinforcement with occlusive dressing
Evisceration of bowel	Return to OR, reapplication of TAC
Surgical site infection	Antibiotics, open wound
Intra-abdominal infection	Radiology-guided percutaneous drainage, reoperation, proximal diversion of intestinal flow
Enteroatmospheric fistula	Control sepsis, minimize and contain effluent, correction of fluid and electrolyte abnormalities, nutrition support, meticulous wound care
Ventral hernia	Complex abdominal wall reconstruction

enteric gram-negative and gram-positive bacilli from the skin. The median time to colonization is 2 days, with higher rates of colonization the longer the abdomen is left open [60]. After fascial closure, surgical site infection is decreased by leaving the skin open.

Intra-abdominal Infection

Dubose et al. reported a 20% incidence of intra-abdominal infection after closure of an open abdomen in trauma patients [61]. There may be an increase in intra-abdominal infection rates in patients with nontrauma indications for open abdomen, such as sepsis, but in recent prospective studies, the rates are similar, likely due to colonization of the abdomen during the take-back procedures [60]. Management typically consists of radiology-guided percutaneous drainage. Relative contraindications to percutaneous drainage include significant coagulopathy that cannot be reversed and lack of a safe access window for catheter placement [62]. If this technique is unsuccessful, reoperation may be required. If uncontrolled intra-abdominal infection is encountered as a result of a leak from a hollow viscous or from an anastomotic suture line, consideration must be given to operative intervention and diversion of the intestinal flow proximal to the leak.

Gastrointestinal Fistula

Because the fascia and skin are not approximated at the midline, the exposed bowel in an open abdomen is highly susceptible to injury and fistula formation. In addition, the longer it takes for fascial closure or wound coverage with skin grafting, the higher the rate of fistula formation [63]. Patients are at increased risk of fistula formation if the abdomen is open longer than 5–7 days. The incidence of enterocutaneous and enteroatmospheric fistulas is approximately 5% in the open abdomen [56, 61]. Injury to the intestines is the most common cause of fistulas. Other causes include anastomotic leak, distal obstruction, and injury to the intestines from suction from the TAC. Early fascial closure is the single best approach to reduce the rate of fistula formation [64].

Management of the enteroatmospheric fistula in the open abdomen can prove challenging. The main tenants in management of fistulas include control of ongoing sepsis, minimizing and containing fistula effluent, correction of electrolyte disturbances, nutritional support, and meticulous wound care [65]. The ultimate goal is surgical correction with fistula resection once the patient is ready for anterior abdominal wall reconstruction, usually 6–12 months after initial laparotomy [66].

Once an enteroatmospheric fistula has formed, minimizing effluent output and protecting the surrounding tissue and skin are of the utmost importance. If the fistula results in spillage of intestinal contents deep in the wound or intra-abdominally, sepsis can result. Proximal diversion of intestinal contents is one approach to controlling fistula output. If not possible, another approach is converting the enteroatmospheric fistula to an enterocutaneous fistula. If these two approaches are not feasible, controlling fistula effluent with strategic placement of suction drains under a vacuum-assisted dressing and isolation of the enteroatmospheric fistula as a "floating stoma" can be performed. There is some evidence that suggests octreotide increases the likelihood of fistula closure as well as reduces the time to fistula closure [67]. Other adjuncts used to decrease high fistula output include antimotility agents such as loperamide, diphenoxylate, and tincture of opium and antisecretory agents such as proton pump inhibitors. These may assist in minimizing electrolyte disturbances and volume depletion by turning a high-output fistula into a low-output fistula. In addition, enteral nutrition is better tolerated in patients with low-output fistulas [68], and wound care is more manageable.

Ventral Hernia

The most common late complication of an open abdomen is a ventral hernia, where 10% of people who undergo definitive abdominal closure develop a ventral hernia by 21 months [69]. Intra-abdominal sepsis, surgical site infection, fascial necrosis, and loss of domain as the abdominal muscles contract away from the midline are the most common causes of ventral hernias after an open abdomen. Fascial necrosis after closure occurs due to ischemia secondary to the tissue being under too much tension, followed by either dehiscence or evisceration. A second attempt at fascial closure results in further damage to the fascia. Sometimes primary closure of the fascia is not possible in an open abdomen, and prosthetic material is needed, which leads to a planned ventral hernia. Many of these patients will need complex abdominal wall reconstruction at a subsequent hospitalization.

Conclusion

Damage control laparotomy and the open abdomen are essential and lifesaving in treating the physiologically deranged patient requiring emergent laparotomy. The intensivist plays a key role in caring for this challenging patient population. Resuscitation, management of fluid and electrolyte disturbances, meticulous wound care, and optimizing nutritional support are essential to the successful outcomes in the patient with an open abdomen.

References

1. Diaz JJJ, Cullinane DC, Dutton WD, Jerome R, Bagdonas R, Bilaniuk JW, et al. The management of the open abdomen in trauma and emergency general surgery: part 1-damage control. J Trauma-Inj Infect Crit Care. 2010;68(6):1425–38.
2. Rotondo MF, Schwab CW, McGonigal MD, Phillips GR, Fruchterman TM, Kauder DR, et al. 'Damage control': an approach for improved survival in exsanguinating penetrating abdominal injury. J Trauma. 1993. discussion 382-3;35(3):375–82.
3. Stone HH, Strom PR, Mullins RJ. Management of the major coagulopathy with onset during laparotomy. Ann Surg. 1983;197(5):532–5.
4. Cinat ME, Wallace WC, Nastanski F, West J, Sloan S, Ocariz J, et al. Improved survival following massive transfusion in patients who have undergone trauma. Arch Surg. 1999. discussion 968-70;134(9):964–8.
5. Hirshberg A, Walden R. Damage control for abdominal trauma. Surg Clin North Am. 1997;77(4):813–20.
6. Rotondo MF, Zonies DH. The damage control sequence and underlying logic. Surg Clin North Am. 1997;77(4):761–77.
7. Kirkpatrick AW, Roberts DJ, De Waele J, Jaeschke R, Malbrain MLNG, De Keulenaer B, et al. Intra-abdominal hypertension and the abdominal compartment syndrome: updated consensus definitions and clinical practice guidelines from the World Society of the Abdominal Compartment Syndrome. Intensive Care Med. 2013;39(7):1190–206.
8. Ouellet J, Ball CG. Recurrent abdominal compartment syndrome induced by high negative pressure abdominal closure dressing. J Trauma. 2011;71(3):785–6.
9. Johnson JW, Gracias VH, Schwab CW, Reilly PM, Kauder DR, Shapiro MB, et al. Evolution in damage control for exsanguinating penetrating abdominal injury. J Trauma. 2001. discussion 269-71;51(2):261–9.
10. Kreis BE, de Mol van Otterloo AJ, Alexander JC, Kreis RW. Open abdomen management: a review of its history and a proposed management algorithm. Med Sci Monit. 2013;19:524–33.
11. Asensio JA, Petrone P, Roldán G, Kuncir E, Ramicone E, Chan L. Has evolution in awareness of guidelines for institution of damage control improved outcome in the management of the posttraumatic open abdomen? Arch Surg. 2004;139(2):209–14.
12. Asensio JA, McDuffie L, Petrone P, Roldan G, Forno W, Gambaro E, et al. Reliable variables in the exsanguinated patient which indicate damage control and predict outcome. Am J Surg. 2001;182(6):743–51.
13. Moore EE, Burch JM, Franciose RJ, Offner PJ, Biffl WL. Staged physiologic restoration and damage control surgery. World J Surg. 1998. discussion 1190-1;22(12):1184–90.
14. Kirshtein B, Roy-Shapira A, Lantsberg L, Mizrahi S. Use of the "Bogota bag" for temporary abdominal closure in patients with secondary peritonitis. Am Surg. 2007;73(3):249–52.
15. Barker DE, Kaufman HJ, Smith LA, Ciraulo DL, Richart CL, Burns RP. Vacuum pack technique of temporary abdominal closure: a 7-year experience with 112 patients. J Trauma. 2000. discussion 206-7;48(2):201–6.
16. Garner GB, Ware DN, Cocanour CS, Duke JH, McKinley BA, Kozar RA, et al. Vacuum-assisted wound closure provides early fascial reapproximation in trauma patients with open abdomens. Am J Surg. 2001;182(6):630–8.
17. Roberts DJ, Zygun DA, Grendar J, Ball CG, Robertson HL, Ouellet JF, et al. Negative-pressure wound therapy for critically ill adults with open abdominal wounds: a systematic review. J Trauma Acute Care Surg. 2012;73(3):629–39.
18. Miller PR, Thompson JT, Faler BJ, Meredith JW, Chang MC. Late fascial closure in lieu of ventral hernia: the next step in open abdomen management. J Trauma. 2002;53(5):843–9.
19. Suliburk JW, Ware DN, Balogh Z, McKinley BA, Cocanour CS, Kozar RA, et al. Vacuum-assisted wound closure achieves early fascial closure of open abdomens after severe trauma. J Trauma. 2003. discussion 1160-1;55(6):1155–60.
20. Caro A, Olona C, Jimenez A, Vadillo J, Feliu F, Vicente V. Treatment of the open abdomen with topical negative pressure therapy: a retrospective study of 46 cases. Int Wound J. 2011;8(3):274–9.
21. Schecter WP, Ivatury RR, Rotondo MF, Hirshberg A. Open abdomen after trauma and abdominal sepsis: a strategy for management. J Am Coll Surg. 2006;203(3):390–6.
22. Moore FA, Haenel JB, Moore EE, Whitehill TA. Incommensurate oxygen consumption in response to maximal oxygen availability predicts postinjury multiple organ failure. J Trauma. 1992. discussion 65-7;33(1):58–65.
23. Shoemaker WC, Appel PL, Kram HB. Tissue oxygen debt as a determinant of lethal and nonlethal postoperative organ failure. Crit Care Med. 1988;16(11):1117–20.
24. Abramson D, Scalea TM, Hitchcock R, Trooskin SZ, Henry SM, Greenspan J. Lactate clearance and survival following injury. J Trauma. 1993. discussion 588-9;35(4):584–8.
25. Hess JR, Brohi K, Dutton RP, Hauser CJ, Holcomb JB, Kluger Y, et al. The coagulopathy of trauma: a review of mechanisms. J Trauma. 2008;65(4):748–54.
26. Michelson AD, MacGregor H, Barnard MR, Kestin AS, Rohrer MJ, Valeri CR. Reversible inhibition of human platelet activation by hypothermia in vivo and in vitro. Thromb Haemost. 1994;71(5):633–40.
27. Scheck T, Kober A, Bertalanffy P, Aram L, Andel H, Molnar C, et al. Active warming of critically ill trauma patients during intrahospital transfer: a prospective, randomized trial. Wien Klin Wochenschr. 2004;116(3):94–7.
28. DelRossi AJ, Cernaianu AC, Vertrees RA, Fuller SJ, Costabile J, Yu Y, et al. Heparinless extracorporeal bypass for treatment of hypothermia. J Trauma. 1990;30(1):79–82.
29. Burch JM, Ortiz VB, Richardson RJ, Martin RR, Mattox KL, Jordan GLJ. Abbreviated laparotomy and planned reoperation for critically injured patients. Ann Surg. 1992. discussion 483-4;215(5):476–83.
30. Holcomb JB, Wade CE, Michalek JE, Chisholm GB, Zarzabal LA, Schreiber MA, et al. Increased plasma and platelet to red blood cell ratios improves outcome in 466 massively transfused civilian trauma patients. Ann Surg. 2008;248(3):447–58.
31. Holcomb JB, Tilley BC, Baraniuk S, Fox EE, Wade CE, Podbielski JM, et al. Transfusion of plasma, platelets, and red blood cells in a 1:1:1 vs a 1:1:2 ratio and mortality in patients with severe trauma: the PROPPR randomized clinical trial. JAMA. 2015;313(5):471–82.
32. Levi M, Peters M, Buller HR. Efficacy and safety of recombinant factor VIIa for treatment of severe bleeding: a systematic review. Crit Care Med. 2005;33(4):883–90.
33. Holcomb JB, Hoots K, Moore FA. Treatment of an acquired coagulopathy with recombinant activated factor VII in a damage-control patient. Mil Med. 2005;170(4):287–90.
34. Benharash P, Bongard F, Putnam B. Use of recombinant factor VIIa for adjunctive hemorrhage control in trauma and surgical patients. Am Surg. 2005;71(9):776–80.
35. Rizoli SB, Nascimento BJ, Osman F, Netto FS, Kiss A, Callum J, et al. Recombinant activated coagulation factor VII and bleeding trauma patients. J Trauma. 2006;61(6):1419–25.
36. Harvin JA, Mims MM, Duchesne JC, Cox CSJ, Wade CE, Holcomb JB, et al. Chasing 100%: the use of hypertonic saline to improve early, primary fascial closure after damage control laparotomy. J Trauma Acute Care Surg. 2013. discussion 431-2;74(2):426–30.

37. Webb LH, Patel MB, Dortch MJ, Miller RS, Gunter OL, Collier BR. Use of a furosemide drip does not improve earlier primary fascial closure in the open abdomen. J Emerg Trauma Shock. 2012;5(2):126.
38. Zielinski MD, Jenkins D, Cotton BA, Inaba K, Vercruysse G, Coimbra R, et al. Adult respiratory distress syndrome risk factors for injured patients undergoing damage-control laparotomy: AAST multicenter post hoc analysis. J Trauma Acute Care Surg. 2014;77(6):886–91.
39. Stewart TE, Meade MO, Cook DJ, Granton JT, Hodder RV, Lapinsky SE, et al. Evaluation of a ventilation strategy to prevent barotrauma in patients at high risk for acute respiratory distress syndrome. N Engl J Med. 1998;338(6):355–61.
40. Dutton WD, Diaz JJJ, Miller RS. Critical care issues in managing complex open abdominal wound. J Intensive Care Med. 2012;27(3):161–71.
41. Malbrain MLNG, Cheatham ML, Kirkpatrick A, Sugrue M, Parr M, De Waele J, et al. Results from the international conference of experts on intra-abdominal hypertension and abdominal compartment syndrome. I. Definitions. Intensive Care Med. 2006;32(11):1722–32.
42. Cheatham ML, Malbrain MLNG, Kirkpatrick A, Sugrue M, Parr M, De Waele J, et al. Results from the international conference of experts on intra-abdominal hypertension and abdominal compartment syndrome. II. Recommendations. Intensive Care Med. 2007;33(6):951–62.
43. Abouassaly CT, Dutton WD, Zaydfudim V, Dossett LA, Nunez TC, Fleming SB, et al. Postoperative neuromuscular blocker use is associated with higher primary fascial closure rates after damage control laparotomy. J Trauma. 2010;69(3):557–61.
44. Teixeira PGR, Salim A, Inaba K, Brown C, Browder T, Margulies D, et al. A prospective look at the current state of open abdomens. Am Surg. 2008;74(10):891–7.
45. Fabian TC. Infection in penetrating abdominal trauma: risk factors and preventive antibiotics. Am Surg. 2002;68(1):29.
46. Ericsson CD, Fischer RP, Rowlands BJ, Hunt C, Miller-crotchett P, Lawrence Reed I. Prophylactic antibiotics in trauma: the hazards of underdosing. J Trauma Acute Care Surg. 1989;29(10):1356–61.
47. Reed RL, Ericsson CD, Wu A, Miller-Crotchett P, Fischer RP. The pharmacokinetics of prophylactic antibiotics in trauma. J Trauma. 1992;32(1):21–7.
48. Goldberg S, Anand R, Como J, Dechert T, Dente C, Luchette F, et al. Eastern Association for the Surgery of Trauma. Prophylactic antibiotic use in penetrating abdominal trauma: an Eastern Association for the Surgery of Trauma practice management guideline. J Trauma Acute Care Surg. 2012;73(5 Suppl 4):S321–5.
49. Braunschweig CL, Levy P, Sheean PM, Wang X. Enteral compared with parenteral nutrition: a meta-analysis. Am J Clin Nutr. 2001;74(4):534–42.
50. Dabrowski GP, Rombeau JL. Practical nutritional management in the trauma intensive care unit. Surg Clin North Am. 2000;80(3):921–32.
51. Heyland DK. Nutritional support in the critically ill patients. A critical review of the evidence. Crit Care Clin. 1998;14(3):423–40.
52. Marik PE, Zaloga GP. Early enteral nutrition in acutely ill patients: a systematic review. Crit Care Med. 2001;29(12):2264–70.
53. Polk TM, Schwab CW. Metabolic and nutritional support of the enterocutaneous fistula patient: a three-phase approach. World J Surg. 2012;36(3):524–33.
54. Cheatham ML, Safcsak K, Brzezinski SJ, Lube MW. Nitrogen balance, protein loss, and the open abdomen. Crit Care Med. 2007;35(1):127–31.
55. Wade C, Wolf SE, Salinas R, Jones JA, Rivera R, Hourigan L, et al. Loss of protein, immunoglobulins, and electrolytes in exudates from negative pressure wound therapy. Nutr Clin Pract. 2010;25(5):510–6.
56. Burlew CC, Moore EE, Cuschieri J, Jurkovich GJ, Codner P, Crowell K, et al. Sew it up! A Western Trauma Association multi-institutional study of enteric injury management in the postinjury open abdomen. J Trauma. 2011;70(2):273–7.
57. Weinberg JA, Griffin RL, Vandromme MJ, Melton SM, George RL, Reiff DA, et al. Management of colon wounds in the setting of damage control laparotomy: a cautionary tale. J Trauma. 2009;67(5):929–35.
58. Miller RS, Morris JAJ, Diaz JJJ, Herring MB, May AK. Complications after 344 damage-control open celiotomies. J Trauma. 2005. discussion 1371-4;59(6):1365–71.
59. Tsuei BJ, Skinner JC, Bernard AC, Kearney PA, Boulanger BR. The open peritoneal cavity: etiology correlates with the likelihood of fascial closure. Am Surg. 2004;70(7):652–6.
60. Rasilainen SK, Juhani MP, Kalevi LA. Microbial colonization of open abdomen in critically ill surgical patients. World J Emerg Surg. 2015;10(1):25.
61. Dubose JJ, Scalea TM, Holcomb JB, Shrestha B, Okoye O, Inaba K, et al. Open abdominal management after damage-control laparotomy for trauma: a prospective observational American Association for the Surgery of Trauma Multicenter Study. J Trauma Acute Care Surg. 2013. discussion 1120-2;74(1):113–20.
62. Wallace MJ, Chin KW, Fletcher TB, Bakal CW, Cardella JF, Grassi CJ, et al. Quality improvement guidelines for percutaneous drainage/aspiration of abscess and fluid collections. J Vasc Interv Radiol. 2010;21(4):431–5.
63. Diaz JJJ, Dutton WD, Ott MM, Cullinane DC, Alouidor R, Armen SB, et al. Eastern Association for the Surgery of Trauma: a review of the management of the open abdomen--part 2 "Management of the open abdomen". J Trauma. 2011;71(2):502–12.
64. Demetriades D, Salim A. Management of the open abdomen. Surg Clin North Am. 2014;94(1):131–53.
65. Schecter WP. Management of enterocutaneous fistulas. Surg Clin North Am. 2011;91(3):481–91.
66. Latifi R, Joseph B, Kulvatunyou N, Wynne J, O'Keeffe T, Tang A, et al. Enterocutaneous fistulas and a hostile abdomen: reoperative surgical approaches. World J Surg. 2012;36(3):516–23.
67. Rahbour G, Siddiqui MR, Ullah MR, Gabe SM, Warusavitarne J, Vaizey CJ. A meta-analysis of outcomes following use of somatostatin and its analogues for the management of enterocutaneous fistulas. Ann Surg. 2012;256(6):946–54.
68. Joyce MR, Dietz DW. Management of complex gastrointestinal fistula. Curr Probl Surg. 2009;46(5):384–430.
69. Frazee RC, Abernathy S, Jupiter D, Davis M, Regner J, Isbell T, et al. Long-term consequences of open abdomen management. Trauma. 2013;16(1):37–40. 1460408613507686.

Acute Kidney Injury

27

Ian J. Stewart and Joseph J. DuBose

Introduction

Acute kidney injury (AKI) is a common complication in critically ill surgical patients, occurring in approximately 36% of admissions to the intensive care unit (ICU) and is strongly associated with subsequent mortality [1–3]. AKI has two major consequences. The first is an acute decline in renal function that impairs the ability to maintain homeostasis. This results in accumulation of nitrogenous waste products, electrolyte derangements, and hypervolemia. The second consequence of AKI is related to the kidney's response to injury. Damage to the kidneys results in elevations in a variety of cytokines (including interluekin-6 and tumor necrosis factor-α), which may increase the risk of other organ dysfunction, to include acute respiratory distress syndrome [4, 5]. In addition to the acute risk of death and multi-organ dysfunction, emerging evidence implicates an episode of AKI in poor outcomes years after the initial insult, including mortality [6], chronic kidney disease [7], and hypertension [8, 9]. Given the high prevalence and strong association of AKI with both adverse short- and long-term outcomes, an understanding of AKI is vital for the care of critically ill surgical patients.

Definitions

Early efforts to understand the impact of AKI on mortality in critically ill patients were hampered by a lack of consistent definitions for AKI. In an effort to define AKI for the purposes of research, the Risk, Injury, Failure, Loss, and End-stage kidney disease (RIFLE) criteria were proposed in 2004 [10]. RIFLE classified AKI on the basis of relative changes in serum creatinine and decreases in urine output. These criteria were subsequently updated by the AKI Network (AKIN) criteria in 2007 [11] and the Kidney Disease: Improving Global Outcomes (KDIGO) criteria in 2012 [12]. The most recent of these criteria, KDIGO, are summarized in Table 27.1.

The diagnosis of AKI can be made either by relative changes in serum creatinine or by decreases in urine output. If available, a known serum creatinine should be used for the "baseline." For example, say a patient has a creatinine measured prior to admission of 1.0 mg/dl. If this patient were then admitted to the ICU with a creatinine of 1.5 mg/dl, the patient would be diagnosed with stage 1 AKI. Alternatively, if this same patient had a creatinine of 1.0 mg/dl on admission, which subsequently increased to 1.3 mg/dl within 48 h, they would also be diagnosed with stage 1 AKI. It is important to note that the time cutoffs (7 days for the 1.5-fold rise and 48 h for the 0.3 mg/dl rise) apply only to the initial diagnosis of AKI. There is no time requirement for patients to transition to more severe stages. It should also be noted that when staging AKI, the higher stage from the creatinine and urinary output criteria is used. For example, if a patient has KDIGO stage 1 by creatinine criteria, but KDIGO stage 2 by the urine output criteria, the patient is classified as stage 2.

Epidemiology

Using the consensus definitions, AKI has been examined in a variety of populations. AKI occurs in 18% of hospitalized patients [13] and 36% of patients admitted to an ICU [1–3]. Furthermore, AKI and has been consistently associated with increased mortality. A variety of risk factors for AKI have been described. These include older age, African-American race, sepsis, burns, trauma, cardiac surgery, and comorbid conditions (e.g., hypertension, diabetes, and chronic kidney disease) [12, 14]. For patients undergoing surgery, the risk of AKI also seems to be impacted by the type of procedure performed. One study done in a population of veterans found

I. J. Stewart
Combat Casualty Care Research, Clinical Investigation Facility, David Grant USAF Medical Center, Travis AFB, CA, USA

J. J. DuBose (✉)
Division of Vascular Surgery, David Grant Medical Center, Travis AFB, CA, USA

A. Salim et al. (eds.), *Surgical Critical Care Therapy*, https://doi.org/10.1007/978-3-319-71712-8_27

Table 27.1 KDIGO criteria for the diagnosis of AKI

Stage	Serum creatinine	Urine output
1	1.5–1.9 times baseline[a] or ≥0.3 mg/dl increase[b]	<0.5 ml/kg/h for 6–12 h
2	2.0–2.9 times baseline	<0.5 ml/kg/h for ≥12 h
3	3.0 times baseline or increase in creatinine to >4 mg/dl or initiation of renal replacement therapy	<0.3 ml/kg/h for ≥24 h or complete anuria for ≥12 h

[a]Must occur, or be assumed to have occurred, within a 7-day time period
[b]0.3 mg/dl rise must occur within the first 48 h of hospitalization

Table 27.2 Differential diagnosis of acute kidney injury

Pre-renal	Intrinsic renal	Post-renal
Hemorrhage	Acute tubular necrosis	Prostatic hypertrophy
Hypovolemia	Thrombotic microangiopathy	Nephrolithiasis
Liver failure	Atheroembolic disease	Retroperitoneal lymphadenopathy
Heart failure	Glomerulonephritis	Retroperitoneal fibrosis
Vascular occlusion	Acute interstitial nephritis	Tumors

that AKI was most common after cardiac surgery [14]. The second highest risk was seen in general surgery patients, followed by thoracic, orthopedic, vascular, urologic, and ENT, respectively [14].

AKI is common in patients with burn injury, occurring in 25% of patients with an associated mortality of 35% [15]. Risk factors for AKI in burn patients include age, percentage of total body surface area burned, male gender, inhalation injury, catheter infection, and sepsis [5, 16]. In patients with trauma, AKI occurs in 12.5–26% of patients and is associated with a mortality rate of 13.1–32% [17–19]. Risk factors for AKI in trauma patients include amputations [17], injury severity score [17, 19], rhabdomyolysis [20, 21], African-American race [17, 22], and hemodynamic instability [17]. In cardiac surgery, AKI occurs in up to 42% of patients and is strongly associated with mortality in a dose response fashion [23]. Female sex, age, congestive heart failure, previous cardiac surgery, functional status, diuretic use, left main coronary stenosis >70%, and comorbidities (CKD, diabetes, and chronic obstructive pulmonary disease) have all been associated with AKI in patients undergoing cardiac surgery [24, 25]. Emergency surgery and the duration of cardiopulmonary bypass have also been associated with AKI [25]. Off-pump coronary artery bypass surgery has been associated with a decreased risk of AKI in some studies; however the evidence for this is conflicting [26–29].

In addition to poor short-term outcomes, AKI is increasingly recognized as a risk factor for poor long-term outcomes. This includes an increased risk for mortality, even years after the initial insult [6, 30]. An episode of AKI has also been associated with an increased risk of CKD, end-stage renal disease, and hypertension [7–9].

Causes of Acute Kidney Injury in the Surgical Patient

Classically, the differential diagnosis of AKI is divided into pre-renal, intrinsic renal, and post-renal etiologies (Table 27.2) [31]. Pre-renal insults result from renal hypoperfusion. While this can be seen in the setting of decreased effective circulating blood volume (cirrhosis or heart failure), the predominant cause in the majority of acutely ill surgical patients is hypovolemia (e.g., from hemorrhage or gastrointestinal losses). Intrinsic renal disease is damage to the kidneys themselves. This can be due to intrinsic medical diseases (such as glomerulonephritis) or acute tubular necrosis (ATN). ATN is the most common cause of AKI in the critical care setting and is caused by either ischemia (i.e., a prolonged pre-renal state from hypovolemia or hemorrhage) or nephrotoxins [31]. Toxins that can cause ATN include aminoglycosides, radiocontrast, and intratubular pigments (myoglobin and hemoglobin) [31]. Post-renal injury results from obstruction of the genitourinary tract. This can occur at any point: from the tubules (intravenous acyclovir), to the ureters (nephrolithiasis and retroperitoneal lymphadenopathy), to the bladder outlet (prostatic hypertrophy). If only one ureter is obstructed (e.g., from nephrolithiasis), AKI is uncommon because the non-obstructed kidney can usually make up for the loss in glomerular filtration rate. However, in a patient with a single or atrophic kidney, this can cause severe AKI.

In most critically ill patients, the etiology of AKI is ATN, often from a variety of ischemic and nephrotoxic causes [32]. However, there are several causes of AKI in the surgical setting that deserve further discussion. These include rhabdomyolysis, abdominal compartment syndrome (ACS), acute interstitial nephritis, and contrast-induced nephropathy.

Rhabdomyolysis

Rhabdomyolysis is the breakdown of skeletal muscle which results in the release of the intracellular contents into circulation [33]. This causes renal damage via three mechanisms. The first is that fluid is sequestered in the damaged muscle tissue, which results in renal vasoconstriction. The second mechanism is tubular damage induced by free-radical formation from myoglobin. The final mechanism is tubular obstruction, caused by myoglobin bound to Tamm-Horsfall protein, a process that is favored in acidic urine [33, 34].

While trauma is the most common cause of rhabdomyolysis, other etiologies include strenuous exertion, heat stroke, limb compression, artery occlusion, genetic defects, infections (influenza, legionella), medications (statins, fibrates, propofol), drugs (cocaine, alcohol, heroin), electrolyte disorders (hypokalemia, hypophosphatemia, hypocalcemia), and genetic disorders [33].

The classic triad of rhabdomyolysis includes muscle pain, weakness, and dark urine. Laboratory findings include elevated creatine kinase (CK), elevated myoglobin (in both the serum and the urine), hyperkalemia, hyperphosphatemia, hypocalcemia, hyperuricemia, and elevated creatinine. The reported incidence of AKI in the setting of rhabdomyolysis varies from 19% to 46% [20, 21, 35–38]. This wide range is due to differences in the patient populations and definitions used for both AKI and rhabdomyolysis. Despite this wide variation, AKI appears to be a common complication of rhabdomyolysis. While myoglobin is the presumed pathologic mechanism, CK is commonly used for diagnostic purposes given its longer half-life. Retrospective studies have demonstrated that a CK level >5000 U/L is the cutoff where AKI risk increases [20].

Since mortality appears to be driven by AKI [20, 21, 39, 40], the cornerstone of treatment for rhabdomyolysis is intravenous fluid therapy to prevent AKI. The goals of fluid administration are fourfold: to volume resuscitate the patient in the face of third spacing into damaged muscle tissue, to maintain renal perfusion, to increase urinary flow rate, and to increase potassium excretion. The goal urine output is 200–300 cc/hr and should be continued until myoglobinuria resolves. Solutions containing potassium (such as lactated Ringer's) should be avoided given the hyperkalemia that often accompanies rhabdomyolysis. As noted above, the precipitation of myoglobin with Tamm-Horsfall protein is favored in an acidic environment; therefore urinary alkalization is a theoretical treatment for rhabdomyolysis [34]. Additionally, alkalization inhibits reduction-oxidation cycling [41] and may inhibit myoglobin-induced vasoconstriction [42]. One theoretical disadvantage to akalinization is that it may further reduce the ionized calcium concentration. However, most authors suggest the use of urine alkalinization in the setting of rhabdomyolysis. This can be done by adding 50 meq of Na bicarbonate (one ampule) to 1 L of ½ normal saline. Alternatively, 100 meq of Na bicarbonate can be added to 1 L of D5W. Either solution that is used should be alternated liter by liter with normal saline. The goals of therapy are to achieve a urine pH of >6.5 while avoiding overt alkalemia (blood pH <7.5).

While some authors recommend mannitol, its use in the setting of rhabdomyolysis is controversial. While mannitol has a variety of theoretical benefits, including improved renal perfusion and acting as a free-radical scavenger, the primary benefit appears to be increasing urine flow [43]. The use of mannitol should be limited to patients that are volume replete and non-oliguric. If used, a test dose (60 mL of 20% solution) is recommended [44]. A positive response is defined as an increase in urine output by 30–50 cc per hour. If the patient has a positive response, mannitol can be added to the replacement fluid to achieve a dose of 5 g per hour. Patients given mannitol should be closely monitored and the therapy discontinued if (1) goal urine output cannot be achieved, (2) the osmolar gap is >55, or (3) the maximum dose is given (200 g per day or a total dose of 800 g).

Abdominal Compartment Syndrome

ACS remains a problematic complication of trauma resuscitation that can impede renal function through pre-renal, intrinsic renal, and post-renal effects [45–47]. From a pre-renal perspective, increased intra-abdominal pressure has the potential to decrease arterial renal blood flow. At the intrinsic level, the increased pressure can alter intra-renal pressure gradients and influence glomerular filtration and renal tubular function. Post-renal, increased extrinsic pressure impedes the ability of the urinary outflow tract to deliver urine to the bladder for excretion.

ACS should be considered in any patient who has received significant fluid resuscitation. Most at risk may be patients sustaining intra-abdominal trauma and burn victims. Whenever the diagnosis of ACS is entertained, bladder pressures should be promptly obtained. When obtaining these measurements, they are most reliable in the setting of paralytic utilization – as intrinsic abdominal and thoracic muscle contraction may artificially elevate intra-abdominal pressure and confound appropriate diagnosis. Any bladder pressure over 15 mm Hg should raise suspicion for the presence of ACS, with pressures in excess of 20 mm Hg being considered by most as diagnostic of this syndrome.

Once diagnosed, prompt treatment of ACS is required to avoid further progression of renal and multiple organ dysfunction. If significant ascites is visualized with ultrasound, paracentesis may prove useful in effectively lowering intra-abdominal pressure to safe levels. In the absence of free fluid, osmotic diuresis has been proposed as an adjunct to mitigate bowel edema – a potential cause of increased intra-abdominal pressure. Although these measures have the potential to assist in the treatment of ACS, strong consideration should be given to the expedient opening of the abdomen to definitively relieve intra-abdominal pressure – particularly in the postoperative patient. Inappropriate delay in relief of ACS will result in multi-organ dysfunction and potentially death.

Acute Interstitial Nephritis

Acute interstitial nephritis (AIN) is an inflammatory reaction in the kidney that can cause AKI. While AIN can be attributable to a variety of causes, the majority (71% of cases) are due to medications [48], many of which are commonly prescribed to surgical patients. These include antibiotics (penicillins, fluoroquinolones, cephalosporins, vancomycin, sulfonamides, rifampin, and imipenem [48]), proton pump inhibitors, and nonsteroidal anti-inflammatory drugs (NSAIDs).

In the absence of a renal biopsy, the diagnosis of AIN can be difficult. The classic triad of fever, rash, and eosinophilia is present in a minority of patients [49]. While the presence of eosinophils in the urine (as determined by Hansel's stain) was proposed as a sensitive and specific marker for the disease [50], recent evidence casts doubt on the utility of this test [51]. Common features of AIN include microhematuria, sterile pyuria (presence of leukocytes in the absence of infection) and non-nephrotic range proteinuria [49]. On analysis of urine microscopy, white blood cell casts may be seen.

The primary treatment for AIN is the discontinuation of the presumed offending agent. If renal function does not recover within 1 week, a renal biopsy should be done to confirm the diagnosis. Once confirmed, corticosteroid treatment should be considered. While the evidence for steroid treatment in AIN is conflicting [48, 52, 53], most authors recommend its use in the appropriate clinical setting. The typical dose is 1 mg/kg/day of prednisone which can be tapered off over 8–12 weeks. For severe disease, an initial course of methylprednisolone can be considered.

Contrast-Induced Nephropathy

Another potential cause of AKI in the surgical patient is contrast-induced nephropathy (CIN). CIN is postulated to be caused by two different mechanisms: [1] renal vasoconstriction with resultant decrease in renal blood flow and glomerular filtration rate [54] and [2] cytotoxic effects [55]. Risk factors for CIN include pre-existing chronic kidney disease, congestive heart failure, advanced age, concurrent nephrotoxic medications, diabetes, hypertension volume depletion, and hemodynamic instability [12]. Once established, there is no accepted treatment for CIN other than supportive care. Therefore, in patients at high risk for CIN, prophylactic therapy should be considered if possible. The KDIGO guidelines on AKI make recommendations for CIN prophylaxis [12]. These include using the lowest possible dose of contrast, avoiding high-osmolar contrast, volume administration (if appropriate), avoidance of concurrent nephrotoxins (e.g., NSAIDs), and administration of acetylcysteine. Fluid administration should be reserved for patients that are not volume overloaded and can be given as either normal saline or isotonic sodium bicarbonate (made by adding three 50 ml ampules of 1 mEq/mL solution to 850 mL of sterile water). Regardless of the fluid chosen, it should be administered at a rate of 1 cc/kg/h for 6–12 h pre- and post-contrast administration. While the evidence for acetylcysteine is mixed, the KDIGO guidelines recommend its use given its low cost and favorable side effect profile. The dose of acetylcysteine is 1200 mg twice daily for 2 days, with two doses given before and two doses given after the contrast load. Hemodialysis and diuretics are not indicated for CIN prevention.

Diagnosis

For patients with AKI, we suggest the initial workup detailed in Table 27.3. Examination of the urine under a microscope is useful for both diagnostic and prognostic purposes. For diagnosis, the presence of granular casts and renal tubular epithelial cells (RETCs) suggests ATN, the presence of red blood cell casts or acanthocytes suggests glomerulonephritis, and the presence of white blood cell casts suggests AIN. For prognosis in the setting of ATN, the number of granular casts and RTECs in the urine has been associated with the severity and likelihood of progression of AKI [56].

The fractional excretion of sodium (FENa) and the fractional excretion of urea (FEUrea) for patients taking diuretics are common tests used to differentiate pre-renal AKI from ATN or other intrinsic forms of AKI. The formula for FENa is calculated from the relative concentrations of sodium and creatinine in the serum and urine as shown in Fig. 27.1. A FENa of <1% means that almost all of the

Table 27.3 Suggested initial workup for patients with acute kidney injury

Laboratory measures	*History*
Chemistry with special attention to trends in creatinine Urine creatinine and electrolytes Complete blood count Urinalysis Urine microscopy	Review medications for known renal toxins Nonsteroidal anti-inflammatory medications Antibiotics Aminoglycosides AIN meds Urine output
Imaging	*Exam*
Renal sonogram Chest X-ray	Hemodynamic instability Assessment of volume status Edema Rales Elevated Jugular venous pressure

$$\text{FENa} = \frac{(\text{Urine Na})(\text{Serum Cr})}{(\text{Serum Na})(\text{Urine Cr})} \text{ x } 100$$

Fig. 27.1 Formula for the fractional excretion of sodium

sodium that is filtered at the glomerulus is reabsorbed, implying a pre-renal origin for AKI [57]. However, there are important limitations to this test. Firstly, it is only accurate in oliguric patients with a decreased glomerular filtration rate. Secondly, just because the FENa is low does not mean that volume repletion is required. For example, patients with heart or liver failure have a pre-renal physiology and will have a low FENa but are hypervolemic. Thirdly, patients on diuretics will have sodium wasting and thus an elevated FENa. In patients on diuretics, the FEUrea can be used instead [58]. The FEUrea can be calculated by replacing blood and urine sodium with blood and urine urea in Fig. 27.1. A value <35% implies a pre-renal etiology. Despite these limitations, the FENa and FEUrea can be of value in the workup of appropriate patients with AKI.

Management

There are no specific treatments for AKI, and management is primary supportive. This includes optimization of hemodynamics (with volume replacement and vasopressors as needed), treatment of underlying conditions (e.g., sepsis), and avoidance of nephrotoxic agents (e.g., NSAIDs, contrast, and aminoglycosides) [12]. Since many medications are renally cleared, medications should be reviewed and the doses adjusted as needed. Acutely, the most feared complication of AKI is hyperkalemia because it can result in cardiac arrhythmia and death. The medical treatment for hyperkalemia can be divided into three categories: stabilization of cardiac membranes, intracellular shifting of potassium, and potassium removal.

The first of these treatments is stabilization of the cardiac membranes. In the setting of hyperkalemia (defined as a potassium >6 meq/L), an EKG should be obtained. If the EKG demonstrates findings attributable to hyperkalemia (peaked T waves, widened QRS complex, or flattened P waves), calcium should be given to stabilize the cardiac membranes. This can be given as either calcium gluconate (one 10 ml ampule of 10% solution) or calcium chloride (one 10 ml ampule of 10% solution). Calcium gluconate can be given via a peripheral line; however calcium chloride should be given via a central line. Regardless of the calcium preparation used, the EKG should be reassessed 5 min and the dose repeated if EKG changes persist.

The second category is shifting of potassium intracellularly using either insulin or a beta-agonist [59]. Regular insulin should be given as an intravenous bolus of 10 units. Unless the patient's blood glucose is >250 mg/dl, one ampule (50 mL) of 50% dextrose should be given to avoid hypoglycemia. Albuterol is given via a nebulizer; however the dose used for hyperkalemia (10 mg) is higher than that used to treat bronchospasm (2.5 mg). Insulin/glucose and albuterol have an additive effect on hyperkalemia and can be used together to further reduce the serum potassium concentration [59].

It is important to understand that both cardiac membrane stabilization and intracellular shifting of potassium are temporizing measures. If potassium is not removed from the body, hyperkalemia will recur. The definitive method for potassium removal, renal replacement therapy (RRT), is discussed in a separate chapter. However, there are also medical methods that can be tried prior to initiating RRT. The first is a loop diuretic (e.g., furosemide). Furosemide increases the amount of sodium in the distal nephron, where it is exchanged for potassium, thus increasing potassium excretion. We suggest an initial dose of 40 mg intravenously. However, in the setting of AKI, with reduced glomerular filtration rate, much higher doses may be needed (up to 200 mg). The gastrointestinal tract can also be used to remove potassium. Classically, this has been accomplished using sodium polystyrene sulfonate. However, given questions as to its short-term efficacy and its association with intestinal necrosis [60], we discourage its use in surgical patients. We prefer the use of a recently approved medication, partiromer, which has been shown to significantly decrease potassium concentration within 7 h [61] and has not been associated with intestinal necrosis.

References

1. Bagshaw SM, George C, Dinu I, Bellomo R. A multi-centre evaluation of the RIFLE criteria for early acute kidney injury in critically ill patients. Nephrol Dial Transplant. 2008;23(4):1203–10. Available from: https://academic.oup.com/ndt/article-lookup/doi/10.1093/ndt/gfm744.
2. Ostermann M, Chang R, Riyadh ICU Program Users Group T. Correlation between the AKI classification and outcome. Crit Care. 2008;12(6):R144. Available from: http://www.ncbi.nlm.nih.gov/pubmed/19019254.
3. Ostermann M, Chang RWS. Acute kidney injury in the intensive care unit according to RIFLE. Crit Care Med. 2007;35(8):1837–43; quiz 1852. Available from: http://content.wkhealth.com/linkback/openurl?sid=WKPTLP:landingpage&an=00003246-200708000-00004.
4. Doi K, Ishizu T, Fujita T, Noiri E. Lung injury following acute kidney injury: kidney-lung crosstalk. Clin Exp Nephrol. 2011;15(4):464–70. Available from: http://link.springer.com/10.1007/s10157-011-0459-4.
5. Clemens MS, Stewart IJ, Sosnov JA, et al. Reciprocal risk of acute kidney injury and acute respiratory distress syndrome in critically ill burn patients*. Crit Care Med. 2016;44(10):e915–22. Available from: http://www.ncbi.nlm.nih.gov/pubmed/27340755.
6. Lafrance J-P, Miller DR. Acute kidney injury associates with increased long-term mortality. J Am Soc Nephrol. 2010;21(2):345–

52. Available from: http://www.jasn.org/cgi/doi/10.1681/ASN.2009060636.
7. Coca SG, Singanamala S, Parikh CR. Chronic kidney disease after acute kidney injury: a systematic review and meta-analysis. Kidney Int. 2012;81(5):442–8. Available from: http://linkinghub.elsevier.com/retrieve/pii/S0085253815553234.
8. Stewart IJ, Sosnov JA, Howard JT, et al. Retrospective analysis of long-term outcomes after combat injury: a hidden cost of war. Circulation. 2015;132(22):2126–33.
9. Hsu C-Y, Hsu RK, Yang J, Ordonez JD, Zheng S, Go AS. Elevated BP after AKI. J Am Soc Nephrol. 2016;27(3):914–23. Available from: http://www.ncbi.nlm.nih.gov/pubmed/26134154.
10. Bellomo R, Ronco C, Kellum JA, Mehta RL, Palevsky P. Acute Dialysis Quality Initiative workgroup. Acute renal failure - definition, outcome measures, animal models, fluid therapy and information technology needs: the Second International Consensus Conference of the Acute Dialysis Quality Initiative (ADQI) Group. Crit Care. 2004;8(4):R204–12. Available from: http://ccforum.biomedcentral.com/articles/10.1186/cc2872.
11. Mehta RL, Kellum JA, Shah SV, et al. Acute Kidney Injury Network: report of an initiative to improve outcomes in acute kidney injury. Crit Care. 2007;11(2):R31. Available from: http://ccforum.biomedcentral.com/articles/10.1186/cc5713.
12. Kellum JA, Lameire N, Aspelin P, et al. KDIGO clinical practice guideline for acute kidney injury. Kidney Int Suppl. 2012;2(1):1–138. Available from: http://www.pubmedcentral.nih.gov/articlerender.fcgi?artid=4089764&tool=pmcentrez&rendertype=abstract%5Cn http://www.pubmedcentral.nih.gov/articlerender.fcgi?artid=4089619&tool=pmcentrez&rendertype=abstract%5Cn http://www.pubmedcentral.nih.gov/articlerender.fcgi.
13. Uchino S, Bellomo R, Goldsmith D, Bates S, Ronco C. An assessment of the RIFLE criteria for acute renal failure in hospitalized patients. Crit Care Med. 2006;34(7):1913–7. Available from: http://content.wkhealth.com/linkback/openurl?sid=WKPTLP:landingpage&an=00003246-200607000-00008.
14. Grams ME, Sang Y, Coresh J, et al. Acute kidney injury after major surgery: a retrospective analysis of veterans health administration data. Am J Kidney Dis. 2016;67(6):872–80. Available from: http://www.ncbi.nlm.nih.gov/pubmed/26337133.
15. Brusselaers N, Monstrey S, Colpaert K, Decruyenaere J, Blot SI, Hoste EAJ. Outcome of acute kidney injury in severe burns: a systematic review and meta-analysis. Intensive Care Med. 2010;36(6):915–25. Available from: http://link.springer.com/10.1007/s00134-010-1861-1.
16. Coca SG, Bauling P, Schifftner T, Howard CS, Teitelbaum I, Parikh CR. Contribution of acute kidney injury toward morbidity and mortality in burns: a contemporary analysis. Am J Kidney Dis. 2007;49(4):517–23. Available from: http://linkinghub.elsevier.com/retrieve/pii/S0272638606019196.
17. Stewart IJ, Sosnov JA, Howard JT, Chung KK. Acute kidney injury in critically injured combat veterans: a retrospective cohort study. Am J Kidney Dis. 2016;68(4):564–70. Available from: http://www.ncbi.nlm.nih.gov/pubmed/27155727.
18. Bagshaw SM, George C, Gibney RTN, Bellomo R. A multi-center evaluation of early acute kidney injury in critically ill trauma patients. Ren Fail. 2008;30(6):581–9. Available from: http://www.tandfonline.com/doi/full/10.1080/08860220802134649%5Cnpapers3://publication/doi/10.1080/08860220802134649.
19. Bihorac A, Delano MJ, Schold JD, et al. Incidence, clinical predictors, genomics, and outcome of acute kidney injury among trauma patients. Ann Surg. 2010;252(1):158–65. Available from: http://www.pubmedcentral.nih.gov/articlerender.fcgi?artid=3357629&tool=pmcentrez&rendertype=abstract.
20. Brown CVR, Rhee P, Chan L, Evans K, Demetriades D, Velmahos GC. Preventing renal failure in patients with rhabdomyolysis: do bicarbonate and mannitol make a difference? J Trauma. 2004;56(6):1191–6. Available from: http://www.ncbi.nlm.nih.gov/pubmed/15211124.
21. Stewart IJ, Faulk TI, Sosnov JA, et al. Rhabdomyolysis among critically ill combat casualties. J Trauma Acute Care Surg. 2016;80(3):492–8. Available from: http://www.ncbi.nlm.nih.gov/pubmed/26670111.
22. Shashaty MGS, Meyer NJ, Localio AR, et al. African American race, obesity, and blood product transfusion are risk factors for acute kidney injury in critically ill trauma patients. J Crit Care. 2012;27(5):496–504. https://doi.org/10.1016/j.jcrc.2012.02.002.
23. Machado MN, Nakazone MA, Maia LN. Prognostic value of acute kidney injury after cardiac surgery according to kidney disease: improving global outcomes definition and staging (KDIGO) criteria. PLoS One. 2014;9(5):e98028. Available from: http://dx.plos.org/10.1371/journal.pone.0098028.
24. Chertow GM, Lazarus JM, Christiansen CL, et al. Preoperative renal risk stratification. Circulation. 1997;95(4):878–84. Available from: http://www.ncbi.nlm.nih.gov/pubmed/9054745.
25. Coleman MD, Shaefi S, Sladen RN. Preventing acute kidney injury after cardiac surgery. Curr Opin Anaesthesiol. 2011;24(1):70–6. Available from: http://content.wkhealth.com/linkback/openurl?sid=WKPTLP:landingpage&an=00001503-201102000-00014.
26. Nigwekar SU, Kandula P, Hix JK, Thakar CV. Off-pump coronary artery bypass surgery and acute kidney injury: a meta-analysis of randomized and observational studies. Am J Kidney Dis. 2009;54(3):413–23. Available from: http://linkinghub.elsevier.com/retrieve/pii/S0272638609004417.
27. Seabra VF, Alobaidi S, Balk EM, Poon AH, Jaber BL. Off-pump coronary artery bypass surgery and acute kidney injury: a meta-analysis of randomized controlled trials. Clin J Am Soc Nephrol. 2010;5(10):1734–44. Available from: http://cjasn.asnjournals.org/cgi/doi/10.2215/CJN.02800310.
28. Lamy A, Devereaux PJ, Prabhakaran D, et al. Off-pump or on-pump coronary-artery bypass grafting at 30 days. N Engl J Med. 2012;366(16):1489–97. Available from: http://www.nejm.org/doi/10.1056/NEJMoa1200388.
29. Reents W, Hilker M, Börgermann J, et al. Acute kidney injury after on-pump or off-pump coronary artery bypass grafting in elderly patients. Ann Thorac Surg. 2014;98(1):9–15. Available from: http://linkinghub.elsevier.com/retrieve/pii/S0003497514010388.
30. Hobson CE, Yavas S, Segal MS, et al. Acute kidney injury is associated with increased long-term mortality after cardiothoracic surgery. Circulation. 2009;119(18):2444–53. Available from: http://circ.ahajournals.org/cgi/doi/10.1161/CIRCULATIONAHA.108.800011.
31. Lameire N, Van Biesen W, Vanholder R. Acute renal failure. Lancet (Lond, Engl). 2005;365(9457):417–30. Available from: http://linkinghub.elsevier.com/retrieve/pii/S0140673605178313.
32. Mehta RL, Pascual MT, Soroko S, et al. Spectrum of acute renal failure in the intensive care unit: the PICARD experience. Kidney Int. 2004;66(4):1613–21. Available from: http://linkinghub.elsevier.com/retrieve/pii/S0085253815502329.
33. Bosch X, Poch E, Grau JM. Rhabdomyolysis and acute kidney injury. N Engl J Med. 2009;361(1):62–72. Available from: http://www.ncbi.nlm.nih.gov/pubmed/19571284.
34. Cervellin G, Comelli I, Lippi G. Rhabdomyolysis: historical background, clinical, diagnostic and therapeutic features. Clin Chem Lab Med. 2010;48(6):749–56. Available from: http://www.degruyter.com/view/j/cclm.2010.48.issue-6/cclm.2010.151/cclm.2010.151.xml.
35. Brown CVR, Rhee P, Evans K, Demetriades D, Velmahos G. Rhabdomyolysis after penetrating trauma. Am Surg. 2004;70(10):890–2.
36. He Q, Wang F, Li G, et al. Crush syndrome and acute kidney injury in the Wenchuan Earthquake. J Trauma. 2011;70(5):1213–8. Available from: http://www.ncbi.nlm.nih.gov/pubmed/21610435.

37. El-Abdellati E, Eyselbergs M, Sirimsi H, et al. An observational study on rhabdomyolysis in the intensive care unit. Exploring its risk factors and main complication: acute kidney injury. Ann Intensive Care. 2013;3(1):8. Available from: http://www.pubmedcentral.nih.gov/articlerender.fcgi?artid=3614462&tool=pmcentrez&rendertype=abstract.
38. Melli G, Chaudhry V, Cornblath DR. Rhabdomyolysis: an evaluation of 475 hospitalized patients. Medicine (Baltimore). 2005;84(6):377–85. Available from: http://www.ncbi.nlm.nih.gov/pubmed/16267412.
39. de Meijer AR, Fikkers BG, de Keijzer MH, van Engelen BGM, Drenth JPH. Serum creatine kinase as predictor of clinical course in rhabdomyolysis: a 5-year intensive care survey. Intensive Care Med. 2003;29(7):1121–5. Available from: http://link.springer.com/10.1007/s00134-003-1800-5.
40. Veenstra J, Smit WM, Krediet RT, Arisz L. Relationship between elevated creatine phosphokinase and the clinical spectrum of rhabdomyolysis. Nephrol Dial Transplant. 1994;9(6):637–41. Available from: http://www.ncbi.nlm.nih.gov/pubmed/7970089.
41. Moore KP, Holt SG, Patel RP, et al. A causative role for redox cycling of myoglobin and its inhibition by alkalinization in the pathogenesis and treatment of rhabdomyolysis-induced renal failure. J Biol Chem. 1998;273(48):31731–7. Available from: http://www.ncbi.nlm.nih.gov/pubmed/9822635.
42. Heyman SN, Greenbaum R, Shina A, Rosen S, Brezis M. Myoglobinuric acute renal failure in the rat: a role for acidosis? Exp Nephrol. 1997;5(3):210–6. Available from: http://www.ncbi.nlm.nih.gov/pubmed/9208280.
43. Zager RA, Foerder C, Bredl C. The influence of mannitol on myoglobinuric acute renal failure: functional, biochemical, and morphological assessments. J Am Soc Nephrol. 1991;2(4):848–55. Available from: http://www.ncbi.nlm.nih.gov/pubmed/1751788.
44. Sever MS, Vanholder R, RDRTF of ISN Work Group. Recommendations for the management of crush victims in mass disasters. Nephrol Dial Transplant. 2012;27(Suppl 1):i1. Available from: http://www.ncbi.nlm.nih.gov/pubmed/22467763.
45. Maerz L, Kaplan LJ. Abdominal compartment syndrome. Crit Care Med. 2008;36(4 Suppl):S212–5. Available from: http://content.wkhealth.com/linkback/openurl?sid=WKPTLP:landingpage&an=00003246-200804001-00012.
46. Shaheen AW, Crandall ML, Nicolson NG, et al. Abdominal compartment syndrome in trauma patients: new insights for predicting outcomes. J Emerg Trauma Shock. 2016;9(2):53–7. Available from: http://www.onlinejets.org/text.asp?2016/9/2/53/179452.
47. Shear W, Rosner MH. Acute kidney dysfunction secondary to the abdominal compartment syndrome. J Nephrol. 2006;19(5):556–65. Available from: http://www.ncbi.nlm.nih.gov/pubmed/17136682.
48. Muriithi AK, Leung N, Valeri AM, et al. Biopsy-proven acute interstitial nephritis, 1993–2011: a case series. Am J Kidney Dis. 2014;64(4):558–66. Available from: http://linkinghub.elsevier.com/retrieve/pii/S0272638614008270.
49. Praga M, González E. Acute interstitial nephritis. Kidney Int. 2010;77(11):956–61. Available from: http://linkinghub.elsevier.com/retrieve/pii/S0085253815541768.
50. Nolan CR, Anger MS, Kelleher SP. Eosinophiluria–a new method of detection and definition of the clinical spectrum. N Engl J Med. 1986;315(24):1516–9. Available from: http://www.nejm.org/doi/abs/10.1056/NEJM198612113152404.
51. Muriithi AK, Nasr SH, Leung N. Utility of urine eosinophils in the diagnosis of acute interstitial nephritis. Clin J Am Soc Nephrol. 2013;8(11):1857–62. Available from: http://cjasn.asnjournals.org/cgi/doi/10.2215/CJN.01330213.
52. Clarkson MR, Giblin L, O'Connell FP, et al. Acute interstitial nephritis: clinical features and response to corticosteroid therapy. Nephrol Dial Transplant. 2004;19(11):2778–83. Available from: https://academic.oup.com/ndt/article-lookup/doi/10.1093/ndt/gfh485.
53. González E, Gutiérrez E, Galeano C, et al. Early steroid treatment improves the recovery of renal function in patients with drug-induced acute interstitial nephritis. Kidney Int. 2008;73(8):940–6. Available from: http://linkinghub.elsevier.com/retrieve/pii/S0085253815531050.
54. Russo D, Minutolo R, Cianciaruso B, Memoli B, Conte G, De Nicola L. Early effects of contrast media on renal hemodynamics and tubular function in chronic renal failure. J Am Soc Nephrol. 1995;6(5):1451–8. Available from: http://www.ncbi.nlm.nih.gov/pubmed/8589322.
55. Heinrich MC, Kuhlmann MK, Grgic A, Heckmann M, Kramann B, Uder M. Cytotoxic effects of ionic high-osmolar, nonionic monomeric, and nonionic iso-osmolar dimeric iodinated contrast media on renal tubular cells in vitro. Radiology. 2005;235(3):843–9. Available from: http://pubs.rsna.org/doi/10.1148/radiol.2353040726.
56. Perazella MA, Coca SG, Hall IE, Iyanam U, Koraishy M, Parikh CR. Urine microscopy is associated with severity and worsening of acute kidney injury in hospitalized patients. Clin J Am Soc Nephrol. 2010;5(3):402–8. Available from: http://cjasn.asnjournals.org/cgi/doi/10.2215/CJN.06960909.
57. Espinel CH, Gregory AW. Differential diagnosis of acute renal failure. Clin Nephrol. 1980;13(2):73–7. Available from: http://www.ncbi.nlm.nih.gov/pubmed/7363517.
58. Diskin CJ, Stokes TJ, Dansby LM, Radcliff L, Carter TB. The comparative benefits of the fractional excretion of urea and sodium in various azotemic oliguric states. Nephron Clin Pract. 2010;114(2):c145–50. Available from: http://www.ncbi.nlm.nih.gov/pubmed/19887835.
59. Allon M, Copkney C. Albuterol and insulin for treatment of hyperkalemia in hemodialysis patients. Kidney Int. 1990;38(5):869–72. Available from: http://www.ncbi.nlm.nih.gov/pubmed/2266671.
60. Sterns RH, Rojas M, Bernstein P, Chennupati S. Ion-exchange resins for the treatment of hyperkalemia: are they safe and effective? J Am Soc Nephrol. 2010;21(5):733–5. Available from: http://www.jasn.org/cgi/doi/10.1681/ASN.2010010079.
61. Bushinsky DA, Williams GH, Pitt B, et al. Patiromer induces rapid and sustained potassium lowering in patients with chronic kidney disease and hyperkalemia. Kidney Int. 2015;88(6):1427–33. Available from: http://linkinghub.elsevier.com/retrieve/pii/S0085253815610584.

Renal Replacement Therapy: A Practical Approach

28

Craig R. Ainsworth and Kevin K. Chung

Epidemiology of Renal Replacement Therapy: Then and Now

Acute kidney injury (AKI) occurs during hospitalization in 39–57% of adult surgical patients [1, 2]. Among critically ill patients with AKI, 6–7% require some form of renal replacement therapy (RRT) with an associated mortality rate of 50–88% [3–7]. Among critically ill patients, even the mildest stage of AKI can result in worse clinical outcomes compared to patients who never have AKI [8–10]. Over the last decade, various diagnostic criteria have been proposed and validated in various populations, including surgical patients. These include the Risk, Injury, Failure, Loss, and End-stage renal failure (RIFLE) criteria, the Acute Kidney Injury Network (AKIN) criteria, and most recently the Kidney Disease: Improving Global Outcomes (KDIGO) criteria. The diagnosis and management of AKI in the critically ill surgical population are already discussed in another chapter in this textbook. The purpose of this chapter is to provide a practical review of RRT for the management of metabolic and fluid derangements encountered when caring for surgical patients who develop severe AKI.

Prior to the development of RRT, AKI was associated with a 90% mortality rate among trauma casualties in World War II [11]. Teschan and colleagues reported on their experience treating 51 combat casualties during the Korean War with a Brigham-Kolff artificial kidney (Fig. 28.1). These patients were referred for treatment at a special renal insufficiency center if they had a urine output less than 500 ml/24 h within 48 h of initial resuscitation and surgery [11]. Intervention with dialysis on these wounded service members during the Korean War reduced their mortality from 84% to 53% [12]. This led to Dr. Teschan advocating what he referred to as "prophylactic" dialysis, initiating dialysis in patients with AKI before the development of uremic symptoms. In 1960, Belding Scribner developed a Teflon-coated vascular access catheter that made it possible for patients to receive multiple, long-term dialysis treatments [13]. During the Vietnam War, Dr. John Conger used an Ultra-Flo 100 dialyzer to perform dialysis on 18 soldiers with traumatic injuries [14]. He randomized his patients to either aggressive dialysis (goal blood urea nitrogen (BUN) less than 70 mg/dl and serum creatinine less than 5 mg/dl) or less aggressive dialysis (therapy started if BUN >150 mg/dl or creatinine >10 mg/dl or refractory hyperkalemia, volume overload, or encephalopathy). The patients in the early aggressive arm had a 64% survival rate, whereas those in the less aggressive treatment arm had a 20% survival rate [14]. In 1972, the congress approved legislation that allowed dialysis treatment to be covered by Medicare which dramatically increased the availability of renal replacement therapy to the general public in the United States [13].

Kramer and colleagues first described a continuous arteriovenous hemofiltration (CAVH) technique in 1977 that could be used to manage AKI-associated metabolic disturbances and fluid overload [15]. This was followed in 1979 by the first use of continuous venovenous hemofiltration (CVVH) to treat AKI in a patient following cardiac surgery [16]. It wasn't until 1982 that CAVH was approved by the Food and Drug Administration for use in critically ill patients in the United States [13]. In 1984, Kaplan and colleagues described their experience treating 15 critically ill patients with CAVH [17]. They described the main benefit of this therapy over intermittent hemodialysis to be that it removed volume at a rate that was driven by the patient's blood pressure. Thus, it was thought to be more physiologic than machine-driven fluid removal. Additionally, since the therapy was continuous, it helped the patient avoid disequilib-

C. R. Ainsworth (✉)
Burn Intensive Care Unit, Burn Center, US Army Institute of Surgical Research, Brooke Army Medical Center, JBSA Fort Sam Houston, TX, USA

Uniformed Services University of the Health Sciences, Bethesda, MD, USA
e-mail: craig.r.ainsworth.mil@mail.mil

K. K. Chung
Department of Medicine, Brooke Army Medical Center, JBSA-Fort Sam Houston, TX, USA

Uniformed Services University of the Health Sciences, Bethesda, MD, USA

A. Salim et al. (eds.), *Surgical Critical Care Therapy*, https://doi.org/10.1007/978-3-319-71712-8_28

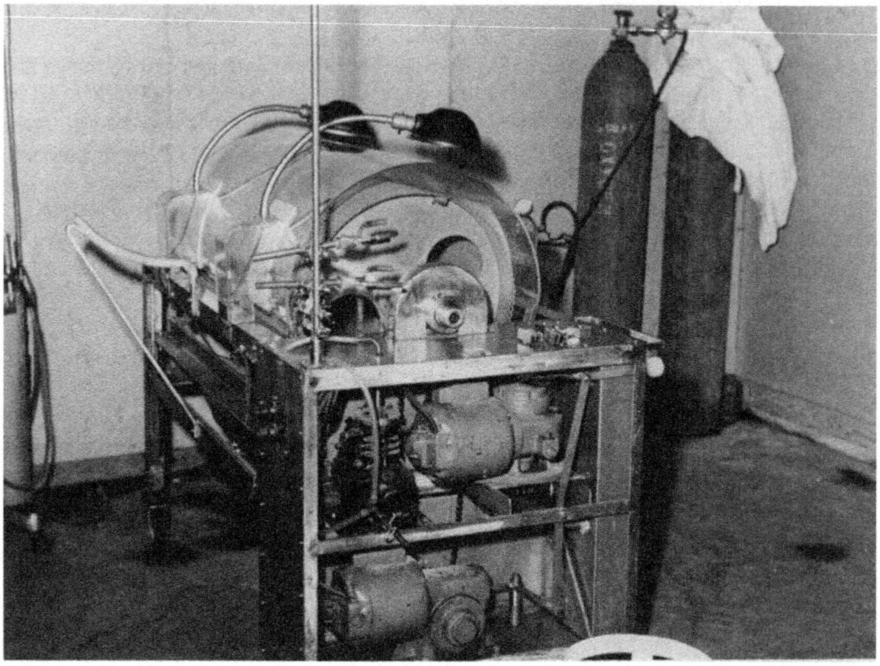

Fig. 28.1 Artificial kidney machine at the 11th Evacuation Hospital

rium syndrome caused by conventional dialysis. Finally, the therapy could be delivered without a specially trained dialysis technician. Over the next three decades, the acceptance and use of various modes of RRT became widespread due to the improvement in the RRT machines, vascular access catheters, hemofilters, replacement fluids, and anticoagulation methods.

RRT Modalities

Once a clinician has decided that a patient needs renal replacement therapy, the next determination to be made is whether or not an intermittent or continuous modality should be used. In order to understand these concepts, one should understand the anatomy of the hemofilter used in any mode of therapy (Fig. 28.2). The hemofilter consists of thousands of semipermeable, parallel, hollow fibers through which the blood passes. In between these hollow fibers is the interstitial space, and the entire hemofilter is encased in a cylindrical container with inflow and outflow ports at opposite ends.

Hemodialysis

Hemodialysis removes solutes by a process termed "diffusion." When a patient is receiving hemodialysis, the blood circulating through the hollow fibers is surrounded by a dialysate solution. Solutes diffuse down a concentration gradient (i.e., high to low) either from the blood through the semipermeable filter wall and into the dialysate or vice versa. Fresh dialysate is constantly being circulated through the interstitial space within the filter so that a concentration gradient can be maintained. The dialysis solution that contains the diffused metabolic waste from the patient's blood is drained from the system and is called effluent. Dialysis solutions typically do not come in direct contact with the patient's blood. These solutions can be produced real time or come in premixed solutions. Clearance via "diffusion" as it occurs during dialysis can efficiently remove smaller molecules from the blood that range in size from 10 to 100 kDa.

Hemofiltration

Hemofiltration, on the other hand, removes solute via a process known as "convection." During hemofiltration, a negative pressure is created in the interstitial space of the hemofilter, and solutes and water are pulled across the semipermeable hollow fibers by convection. Simultaneously, an electrolyte-balanced replacement fluid is added directly into the extracorporeal circuit or the patient's bloodstream. Given that replacement solution is infused directly into the patient's bloodstream (intra- or extracorporeal), it must be sterile. Due to its active nature, convective clearance can be used to clear larger "middle" molecules (10 to >10,000 kDa) from the blood which can impact clearance of various medications. Table 28.1 contains a list of molecules of various sizes and a description of which form of renal replacement therapy can be used to clear them from the circulation.

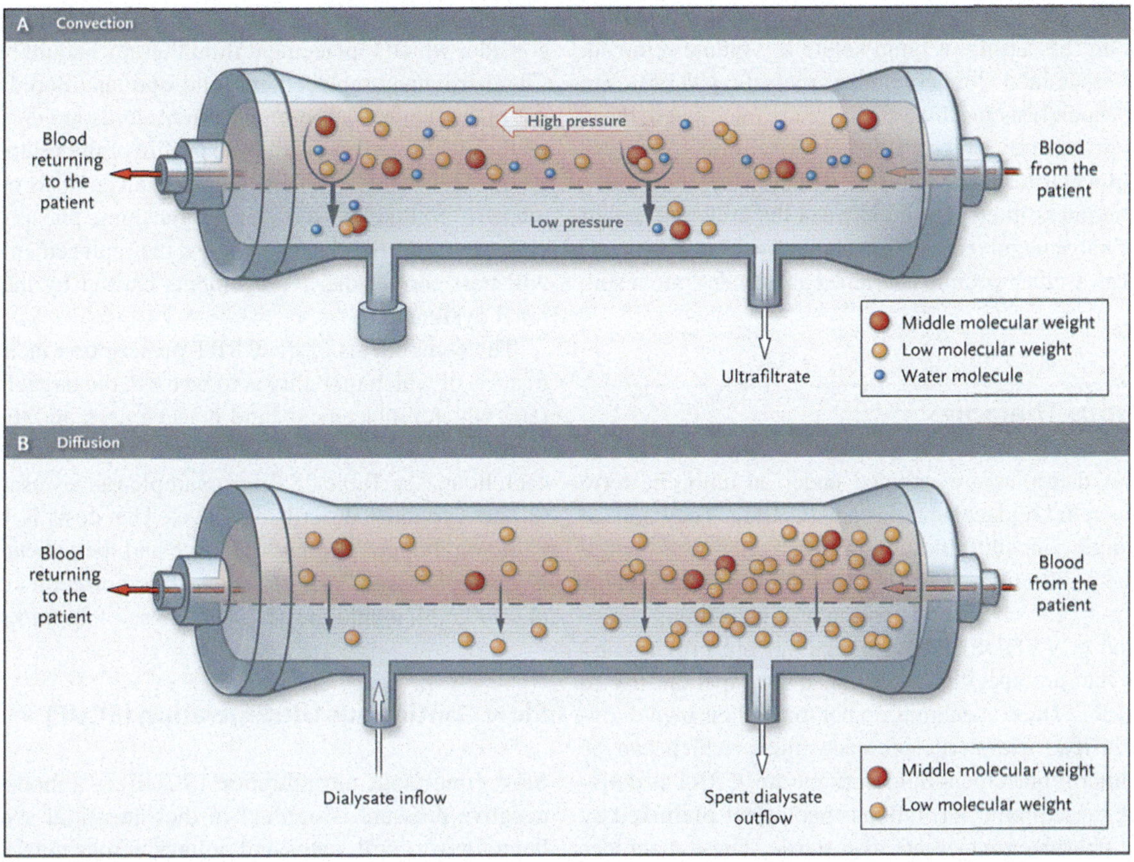

Fig. 28.2 Transport of solutes across a semipermeable membrane. As shown in panel A, convection occurs when solutes are transported across a semipermeable membrane with plasma water in response to a hydrostatic pressure gradient that is created on the blood side of the hemofilter. Convection enhances the removal of low- and middle-molecular-weight molecules. As shown in panel B, in diffusion, movement of solute across a semipermeable membrane is driven by a concentration gradient between the blood and the dialysate. Solutes move from the side with the higher concentration of particles to the side with the lower concentration. Diffusion is best for clearing low-molecular-weight solutes such as urea and creatinine (Used with permission) [50]

Table 28.1 Molecular size and clearance characteristics of common electrolytes and proteins

Biochemical	Molecular size and clearance
Sodium	23 Daltons cleared by hemodialysis or hemofiltration
Phosphorus	31 Daltons cleared by hemodialysis or hemofiltration
Potassium	35 Daltons cleared by hemodialysis or hemofiltration
Urea	60 Daltons cleared by hemodialysis or hemofiltration
Creatinine	113 Daltons cleared by hemodialysis or hemofiltration
Glucose	180 Daltons cleared only by hemofiltration
Vitamin B12	1,355 Daltons cleared only by hemofiltration
Inulin	5,200 Daltons cleared only by hemofiltration
Beta 2 microglobulin	11,800 Daltons cleared only by hemofiltration
Albumin	55,000–60,000 Daltons cleared only by hemofiltration

Intermittent Hemodialysis

Intermittent hemodialysis (IHD) is a renal replacement therapy based on diffusive clearance. The therapy is usually prescribed by a nephrologist either in an outpatient dialysis center or an inpatient hospital setting and requires the expertise of a dialysis technician. This therapy is usually delivered by a Fresenius® machine (Fresenius Medical Care, Waltham, Massachusetts) that produces dialysate real-time using a reverse osmosis system to purify tap water which is then mixed with electrolytes and buffers. An IHD therapy session is usually delivered over 2–4 h. Advantages of intermittent therapy include a short length of therapy, rapid clearance of solutes and fluid, and minimized interruptions in patient care activities as therapy can be delivered every other day. Solute clearance is much greater in IHD because of higher dialysate flow rates, and this may be of benefit to patients with severe electrolyte and metabolic derangements. One of the main disadvantages of this modality as applies to surgical critical care patients is that in can cause hemodynamic instability, especially in the setting of rapid solute or volume removal. IHD and sustained low-efficiency dialysis (SLED) are delivered via dialysis machines. As already mentioned, these machines do not rely on premade solutions; rather they use regular tap water to make dialysate which is then circulated through the interstitial space in between the hollow fibers of the filter. Dialysate mixed with metabolic waste products and excess intravascular volume is drained as effluent into a sink or drain.

Continuous Therapies

Continuous therapies are grouped under an umbrella term continuous renal replacement therapy (CRRT). They consist of slow continuous ultrafiltration (SCUF), continuous venovenous hemofiltration (CVVH), continuous venovenous hemodialysis (CVVHD), and continuous venovenous hemodiafiltration (CVVHDF). These modalities are provided by machines that are specifically designed for inpatient use to deliver CRRT. These machines do not make their own dialysate and instead use sterile premade fluids, which can be used as either replacement fluid or dialysate. CRRT is delivered using these premade solutions or solutions premixed by a hospital pharmacy which are also sterile. These machines can be operated by trained ICU nurses and do not require a dialysis technician. Two of the most commonly used machines to deliver CRRT are the Prismaflex® (Baxter International Inc., Deerfield, Illinois) and the NxStage System One® (NxStage Medical Inc., Lawrence, Massachusetts). The Prismaflex® uses five pumps for blood, dialysate, prefilter replacement fluid, post-filter replacement fluid, and effluent. This machine utilizes four scales for effluent and dialysate and two for replacement fluid, and these scales hold one 5-liter bag at a time. The Prismaflex® can perform SCUF, CVVH, CVVHD, CVVHDF, therapeutic plasma exchange, and hemoperfusion. The machine can deliver blood flow rates from 10 to 450 ml/min and can facilitate anticoagulation with citrate or heparin. It can deliver effluent up to 10 L/h and maximum ultrafiltration of 2 L/h. The NxStage System One® uses a disposable cartridge that contains all blood and fluid pathways so that the user can hang up to 29 L of replacement fluid at one time and connect effluent directly to a drain [16]. This minimizes replacement fluid bag changes and erases the need for effluent collection bags. The machine is configured to deliver SCUF, CVVH, CVVHD, and therapeutic plasma exchange. CVVHDF can be done on CVVHD mode with extra ultrafiltration that is replaced intravenously directly into the patient. The maximum blood flow rate is 600 ml/min, and the maximum replacement fluid rate is 12 L/h. It can remove up to 2.4 L/h of ultrafiltration.

Once a machine has been selected, the clinician should consider which replacement fluid therapy should be utilized. There are many replacement fluid options offered by different manufacturers. The replacement fluids are chosen based on the electrolyte and acid/base profile of the solution. Based on the goal of therapy, be it to correct an acidosis or derangement in potassium, sodium, magnesium, phosphorus, calcium etc., the clinician can choose the replacement fluid that will best correct the derangements caused by the patient's renal dysfunction.

The components of the CRRT prescription include specification of which modality is to be used, the target blood flow rate, which replacement fluid is to be used and the replacement fluid rate, and how much ultrafiltrate should be removed each hour. See Table 28.2 for example ranges used for each of the variables described above. The dose is calculated based on the replacement fluid rate and the patient's weight. For example, an 83-kg patient with a replacement fluid rate of 3000 ml/h would have a CRRT dose of 36 ml/kg/h.

Slow Continuous Ultrafiltration (SCUF)

Slow continuous ultrafiltration (SCUF) is a mode in which negative pressure is applied in the interstitial space of the hemofilter to pull water and solutes across the semipermeable membrane. This technique is most widely used in patients with diuretic-resistant volume overload as it removes volume and does not entail the use of any replacement fluid. SCUF was initially developed because acute ultrafiltration rates could remove intravascular volume faster than fluid refilling from the interstitial space could occur, causing harmful changes in circulating blood volume, peripheral perfusion, and cardiac output [18]. To prevent a rapid drop in circulating blood volume, this mode was developed to slowly remove volume and monitor the patient's response to volume removal. This slow, stable volume removal is particularly helpful in managing patients with cardiorenal syndrome [19]. This modality has a potential application in patients with diuretic-resistant heart failure [20].

Table 28.2 Typical starting prescription for various CRRT modes

Mode of therapy	Blood flow rate ml/min	Replacement fluid rate ml/h	Dialysate flow rate ml/h	Ultrafiltrate (net fluid removal) ml/h
SCUF	50–200	None	None	50–500
CVVH	100–400	2000–4000	None	0–500
CVVHD	100–400	None	2000–4000	0–500
CVVHDF	100–400	2000–4000	1000–2000	0–500

Continuous Venovenous Hemofiltration (CVVH)

Continuous venovenous hemofiltration uses convective clearance to clear solutes from the blood using replacement fluid. Replacement fluid can be circulated into the blood pre-hemofilter and post-hemofilter or split between the two if you are using the Prismaflex®. Delivering replacement fluid pre-hemofilter can lengthen the life of the filter as it dilutes the blood prior to filtration which will reduce clot formation within the filter. However, this prefilter dilution of the blood can reduce the efficiency of solute clearance (see Fig. 28.3). Volume management can be achieved by adding an ultrafiltration rate which can be set independently on top of the replacement fluid rate. CVVH is a relatively simple modality that leverages the advantages of convective clearance to clear middle molecules. These middle molecules include inflammatory cytokines that can worsen a patient's multi-organ failure due to sepsis. In patients with AKI and sepsis, clearance of inflammatory cytokines using CVVH can benefit patients. The authors prefer this mode of therapy for treating critically ill patients with AKI.

Continuous Venovenous Hemodialysis (CVVHD)

Continuous venovenous hemodialysis is a mode that cleanses the blood using diffusion and is applied to the patient continuously. The same premade or premixed solutions which were called "replacement fluid" are called "dialysate" when this mode is utilized. This modality offers the advantage of being able to more easily control electrolyte levels and avoid needing to replace them and is preferred by most nephrologists.

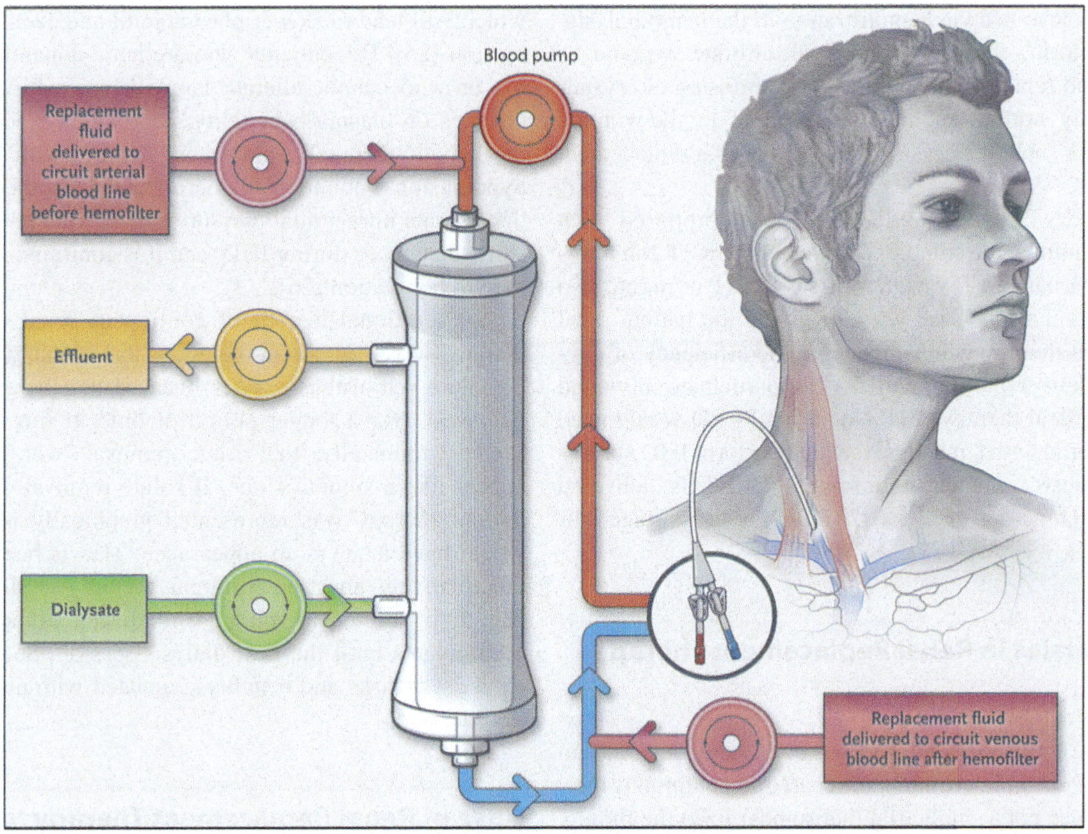

Fig. 28.3 Circuit components in continuous renal replacement therapy. Continuous renal replacement therapy requires a central double-lumen venovenous catheter, an extracorporeal circuit and hemofilter, a blood pump, and an effluent pump. Depending on the type of continuous renal replacement therapy, dialysate, replacement fluid pumps, or both are required. In continuous venovenous hemofiltration, solutes and plasma water are forced across the semipermeable membrane by high ultrafiltration rates (convection). Simultaneously, replacement fluid is infused into the blood with the use of a replacement pump. The replacement fluid replenishes both the volume and electrolytes removed. Replacement fluid can be infused before or after the hemofilter. In continuous venovenous hemodialysis, solutes and plasma move across the semipermeable membrane into the dialysate compartment of the hemofilter by means of diffusion and ultrafiltration. The flow of dialysate is in the opposite direction from the flow of blood. In continuous venovenous hemodiafiltration, solutes and plasma water are removed by diffusion, convection, and ultrafiltration (Used with permission) [50]

Continuous Venovenous Hemodiafiltration (CVVHDF)

This mode of RRT combines solute removal by diffusion using a dialysate and convection via hemofiltration. Combining the two modalities allows the clinician more control over specific electrolytes while taking advantage of the benefits of convective clearance.

Hybrid Modalities

Sustained Low-Efficiency Dialysis (SLED)

SLED is a form of dialysis that uses decreased blood flow rates, allowing therapy to be delivered over a more extended period of time, and is indicated in those who are hemodynamically unstable. This mode is delivered using a conventional dialysis machine and requires less anticoagulation than CRRT. Sessions can be delivered daily or every other day. SLED-f is a hybrid renal replacement therapy that adds convective clearance via hemofiltration to the hemodialysis-based platform. Typically, extra ultrafiltrate volume is removed and replaced by an intravenous infusion of crystalloid (usually normal saline) that is equal to the volume removed. As such, the crystalloid is acting as a replacement fluid.

Other ways of delivering RRT have been proposed in an effort to minimize the complexity of care that RRT can introduce. Nocturnal SLED or intermittent CRRT at night (also called "shift dialysis") are ways of giving the patient renal replacement therapy while enhancing the efficiency of daytime care delivery so that patients can participate in wound care or physical therapy [21]. Nocturnal SLED would need to be delivered with a machine that can perform IHD such as the Fresenius®, whereas intermittent CRRT is delivered using a machine designed for CRRT such as NxStage® or Prismaflex®.

Controversies in Renal Replacement Therapy

Mode

In a review of nine randomized trials comparing outcomes in patients placed on intermittent compared to continuous therapy, there was not a single trial that standardized the timing, criteria for initiation, or dose of renal replacement therapy [22]. This review concluded that there was no statistically significant evidence that the initial RRT modality influenced mortality or recovery of renal function. There was a trend observed that CRRT was associated with less hemodynamic instability and better control of the patient's fluid balance. Another meta-analysis reviewed 23 randomized controlled trials and 16 observational studies to investigate if there was any difference in rates of renal recovery among severe AKI survivors [23]. Pooled analysis of the RCTs did not reveal a statistically significant difference in renal recovery based on RRT modality used. A pooled analysis of the observational studies did demonstrate a higher rate of renal recovery among patients receiving continuous therapy.

The main factor to be considered in deciding to use intermittent or continuous RRT is the patient's hemodynamic stability. Treatment-related hypotension occurs in 10–70% of patients during their dialysis session, depending on the definition of hypotension used [24]. Advanced age, female gender, diabetes, low blood pressure prior to dialysis, hypoalbuminemia, and higher BMI are all associated with increased risk for intradialytic hypotension [24]. If removal of intravascular volume exceeds the patient's ability to refill their plasma volume, then hypotension will occur. The level of sodium in the dialysate, plasma albumin levels, and hydrostatic capillary force all influence plasma refill [25]. The patient's osmolality declines during dialysis due to the rapid removal of urea and shifts in plasma sodium concentrations which will lead to slower plasma refill and eventually hypotension [25]. For patients who are hemodynamically unstable or who cannot tolerate large volume shifts and rapid changes on plasma osmolality, continuous modalities offer the benefit of renal replacement therapy with less risk of hypotension. Patients with neuro-trauma or other conditions that elevate intracranial pressure cannot tolerate the osmotic shifts that occur during IHD, and it is contraindicated in this patient population [26].

An additional benefit of continuous renal replacement therapy over intermittent therapy is that in many cases, mass or solute removal is greater because the therapy is being delivered over a longer period of time. If this were represented graphically, the solute removal over time would appear like a smooth slope. If solute removal during intermittent therapy was represented graphically over time, it would have a sawtooth appearance. This is because during the relatively short intermittent therapy sessions, a high amount of solute and volume is removed and then gradually accumulates until the next dialysis session. See Table 28.3 for a list of risks and benefits associated with using IHD vs. CRRT.

Dose of Renal Replacement Therapy

For continuous modes, the currently recommended dose for renal replacement therapy is 20–25 ml/kg/h [26]. Most patients do not have day after day of uninterrupted CRRT. Therapy can be interrupted by trips to radiology for imaging studies, dysfunction with the circuit caused by clotting, or malfunction of the dialysis access line. In one study, interruptions in RRT ranged from 8% to 28% of the total

Table 28.3 Risks and benefits of different forms of renal replacement therapy

Modality	Benefits	Risks
IHD	Rapid removal of low-molecular-weight substances and toxins Fewer interruptions in other patient care activities Less expensive than CRRT Does not require constant anticoagulation of the circuit	Hypotension due to rapid solute and fluid removal Osmotic shifts that can worsen cerebral edema Requires a specially trained dialysis technician
CRRT	Hemodynamic stability Continuous removal of toxins and volume. Volume removal can be titrated based on patient tolerance Simple machines with user friendly interfaces Safe for patients with elevated ICP	Increased cost Limits participation in physical therapy when on the circuit Circuit must be anticoagulated continuously Slower clearance of toxins

treatment time [27]. Clinicians should target a prescription of 25–30 ml/kg/h and above so as to account for interruptions in therapy and insure that the patient is receiving the minimal delivered dose of 20–25 ml/kg/h. The current recommended dose is based on several clinical trials that compared different doses of renal replacement therapy and their impact on clinical outcomes. The VA/NIH Acute Renal Failure Trial Network randomized 1124 patients with acute kidney injury and failure of at least one non-renal organ or sepsis to intensive therapy (CRRT dose of 35 ml/kg/h) or less intensive therapy (CRRT dose of 20 ml/kg/h). The primary end point was all-cause mortality by day 60. There was no difference in the rate of all-cause mortality or in duration of renal replacement therapy or the rate of renal recovery [28]. The RENAL Replacement Therapy Study Investigators conducted a multicenter, randomized controlled trial to compare the effect of different doses of renal replacement therapy on 90-day mortality. They randomized patients with AKI and critical illness to post-dilution CVVH with a dose of 40 ml/kg/h or 25 ml/kg/h. There was no statistically significant difference in all-cause 90-day mortality or renal recovery or duration of renal replacement therapy [29].

Given the seeming absence of any benefit to higher doses, the KDIGO guideline recommends a dose of 20–25 ml/kg/h for CRRT in AKI [26]. However, this may not be the case for patients with postsurgical AKI. In a recent Cochrane review, postsurgical patients who developed AKI had a statistically significant reduction in mortality if they received a dose greater than 35 ml/kg/h [30]. This was based on two studies that enrolled 531 patients and was deemed by reviewers to be high quality evidence. We therefore recommend the consideration of an initial higher delivered dose of 35 ml/kg/hr. of RRT for patients with postsurgical AKI, especially when dealing with severe metabolic disturbance.

Table 28.4 Complications of acute kidney injury that are traditional indications for initiating renal replacement therapy

Complication	Criteria for initiating renal replacement therapy
Metabolic acidosis	Refractory to sodium bicarbonate infusion
Electrolyte imbalance	Hyperkalemia refractory to medical management
Toxic ingestion	Small molecular size and low level protein binding so as to be cleared by dialysis
Uremia	Uremic encephalopathy, pericarditis, gastropathy, or bleeding due to uremic platelets
Intravascular volume overload	Pulmonary edema refractory to diuretic therapy

Timing

Based on current literature, we believe that early initiation of intensive renal replacement therapy will provide the most benefit [31]. Traditional complications of AKI that would warrant immediate initiation of renal replacement therapy are included in Table 28.4. The literature demonstrates that early and intensive RRT may provide the best benefit for critically ill patients, particularly those with AKI diagnosed early in their clinical course, those in shock, and those with ARDS. Critically ill burn patients who develop AKI have mortality rates that are over 20% higher than the general critical care population [32–34]. Historically, these patients were often not considered candidates for intermittent hemodialysis (IHD) due to their hemodynamic instability by the time they had developed a traditional indication for RRT. The US Army Burn Center remedied this situation by developing an aggressive continuous venovenous hemofiltration (CVVH) program. Patients with greater than 40% total body surface area burn and AKIN stage 3 AKI or AKIN stage 2 AKI with shock were started on CVVH, even if they did not meet traditional criteria for initiating RRT. When these patients were compared to historical controls, they had a 24% lower in-hospital mortality rate, a 33% lower 28-day mortality rate, a dramatic reduction in vasopressor requirement, and an average PaO_2/FiO_2 ratio increase of 153 within 24 h [35].

Two recently published trials attempted to answer the question of when to initiate renal replacement therapy in AKI. The Artificial Kidney Initiation in Kidney Injury (AKIKI) study group performed a multicenter randomized controlled trial on patients with KDIGO stage 3 AKI who required mechanical ventilation, catecholamine infusion. These patients did not have a life-threatening complication directly related to renal failure and were designated to an early or delayed strategy for RRT initiation [36]. Early initiation consisted of starting RRT at the time of randomization. Delayed initiation consisted of starting RRT when the patient developed a potentially life-threatening complication of AKI to include severe hyperkalemia, metabolic acidosis, pulmonary edema, BUN higher than 112 mg/dl, or oliguria for more than 72 h after randomization. The primary outcome was survival at 60 days. The results of the trial demonstrated no difference in mortality but did demonstrate an increased incidence of catheter-related bloodstream infection in the early initiation group, and half of the patients in the delayed initiation arm never needed renal replacement therapy. While the trial did not demonstrate a mortality reduction attributable to early initiation, it may be that waiting to initiate RRT once the patient has KDIGO stage 3 AKI is already too late to see a benefit in "early" initiation.

The Early Versus Late Initiation of Renal Replacement Therapy in Critically Ill Patients with Acute Kidney Injury (ELAIN) randomized clinical trial was a single-center study that randomized 231 patients with KDIGO stage 2 AKI and plasma neutrophil gelatinase-associated lipocalin levels higher than 150 ng/ml to early initiation of RRT (within 8 h of diagnosis of KDIGO stage 2 AKI) or delayed initiation (within 12 h of diagnosis of KDIGO stage 3 AKI) or no initiation [37]. Ninety-day mortality in the early RRT group was 39% and 54% in the delayed group. In the early group, 53% experienced renal recovery, whereas in the delayed group, 38% experienced renal recovery. Duration of renal replacement therapy and hospital length of stay were also shorter in the early initiation group. These results led the authors to call for larger, multicenter trials to be performed using a similar protocol so as to demonstrate whether these results can be generalized to all critical care patients with KDIGO stage 2 AKI.

In the critical care surgery patient population with AKI, early initiation strategies are associated with improved outcomes. One center that used CVVH as their mode of CRRT reported on 73 patients they treated who had AKI in the postoperative period [38]. They initiated CRRT if patients had AKI with hyperkalemia, severe metabolic acidosis, pulmonary edema refractory to diuretics, or oliguria with progressive azotemia in the setting of shock. These patients' AKI were classified using the RIFLE criteria. Patients in the Risk stage who were started on CRRT were considered to be in the early initiation group, and those in the Injury or Failure stages who were initiated on CRRT were considered to be in the late group. The mortality rate in the late-initiation group was 35% higher, and there were no significant differences in demographics, type of surgery, or physiologic scores [38]. The KDIGO guideline for the management of AKI encourages clinicians to "consider the broader clinical context, the presence of conditions that can be modified with RRT, and trends in laboratory tests – rather than single BUN and creatinine thresholds alone – when making the decision to start RRT" (26). Thus, with respect to the controversies in the timing of renal replacement therapy, there is no "one-size-fits-all" approach that applies to every patient scenario. Timing of renal replacement therapy initiation should be individualized to the patient condition with evidence demonstrating that early initiation, in the presence of a metabolic disturbance or fluid overload, is associated with improved outcomes.

Daily Management of the Patient on Renal Replacement Therapy

The daily management of patients on CRRT involves assessment of the adequacy of therapy, serial electrolyte monitoring, ensuring appropriate antibiotic dosing, management of anticoagulation, and management of the vascular access catheter. If there are issues with electrolyte derangement, these can be remedied by either replacing the electrolytes in the case of deficiency or by changing the replacement fluid. Changing replacement fluid may not always be necessary because in some cases the issue may be related to the dose of therapy, and this should be considered and discussed by providers as part of the daily management of the patient's CRRT.

Antibiotics vary in molecular size and protein binding, both of which will affect whether or not they are cleared by renal replacement therapy. Because of its ability to clear middle molecules, continuous modalities that utilize convective clearance can often times clear antibiotics at the same level as fully functioning kidneys. Antibiotics will often times need to be dosed as if renal function is preserved, or sometimes, as is the case with vancomycin, patients will often times need to have an increased dose of the drug because it is so effectively cleared by CRRT. Checking drug levels and coordinating dosing with a clinical pharmacist with experience with dose drugs in patients on CRRT can help ensure patients are getting an appropriate antibiotic dose.

Anticoagulation

Some form of anticoagulation is usually required when patients are on CRRT to prevent the formation of thromboses within the dialysis circuit. The most commonly used agents are heparin and citrate although protocols with other agents exist as do protocols using no anticoagulation for patients at high risk of hemorrhage. Regional heparin anticoagulation consists of infusing 500–1000 units of heparin into the RRT circuit. The dose of heparin is increased until an optimal filter life can be achieved without causing a systemic elevation in PTT. Some protocols utilize protamine for heparin reversal post-filter to insure that the heparin does not have an effect on the patient. Anticoagulation can prevent the filter from clotting which is a common cause of patients having therapy interrupted. If the filter is clotting off frequently, then the filtration fraction should be assessed. This is calculated as follows: replacement fluid(L/h) + ultrafiltrate(L/h) / blood flow rate (L/H) + replacement fluid rate (L/h). The goal to minimize the formation of blood clots in the dialysis circuit is a filtration fraction of less than 25%.

Anticoagulation of the circuit can also be achieved with trisodium citrate or acid-citrate-dextrose. The citrate is usually infused into the arterial or inflow port so that it can bind calcium and anticoagulate the dialysis circuit. Since the citrate provides an alkali load, the pH composition of the replacement fluid may need to be adjusted so that metabolic alkalosis can be prevented. Clinical trials comparing the use of heparin and citrate have demonstrated increased filter patency, decreased rates of bleeding, and decreased mortality when citrate was used [39–41]. This has led to the recommendation that citrate be used for anticoagulation in patients receiving CRRT in the KDIGO guidelines [26]. There is no standard FDA-approved citrate preparation that is universally used. This leads some to view it as a potentially cumbersome medication to use in everyday practice. Its implementation in surgical and trauma ICUs did lead to patients having a higher pH, lower ionized calcium, and higher sodium compared to patients treated with heparin, although this difference was noted to not cause any adverse events among patients treated with citrate [42]. Of note, the use of citrate anticoagulation was noted to lead to an average increase in circuit life of 30 h which can have a clinically significant impact on the patient in terms of them receiving their full dose of therapy and not losing blood in clotted off circuits. When using citrate as an anticoagulant, providers need to remember that it converts to bicarbonate so replacement fluids with a lower bicarbonate level should be used to avoid causing a metabolic alkalosis. The use of citrate for anticoagulation can cause toxicity in patients with liver failure that is manifested by a low serum ionized calcium concentration, elevated total serum calcium level, metabolic alkalosis, and an increased anion gap. The accumulation of citrate causes a fall in ionized calcium levels, while the total serum calcium level will continue to rise. When the ratio of total calcium divided by ionized calcium exceeds 2.5, it is indicative of citrate toxicity. When performing this calculation, it is important to pay attention to the unit of measure as it can vary from lab to lab. One mg/dl of calcium is equal to 0.25 mmol/L and 0.5 meq/L.

Vascular Access

Vascular access with a temporary dialysis catheter for RRT needs to be obtained prior to initiating therapy. These catheters can be placed by the intensivist at the bedside and immediately used for therapy. Placement should be confirmed with a chest x-ray if the internal jugular or subclavian sites are used. There are multiple catheters available that typically utilize two lumens with a septum dividing them. The lumens can be arranged in parallel or spiral around each other with the tip of each lumen staggered to prevent recirculation. Some catheters come with a third lumen that can be used to deliver medications or fluids. The right internal jugular vein is preferred over the left as it is usually a larger vessel and this will allow increased blood flow. A meta-analysis recently demonstrated that the femoral site is not associated with an increased risk of catheter infection when compared to the internal jugular vein [43]. One of the disadvantages of the femoral site is that it can interfere with the patient's ability to participate in physical therapy. The subclavian site can be used; however, if there is concern that the patient may require long-term therapy, this site should be avoided. There are higher rates of subclavian stenosis, compared to other sites, which could prevent the limb on that side of the patient from being used for long-term dialysis access with a fistula.

Signs of Renal Recovery and Discontinuing Therapy

Clinical and laboratory signs that renal recovery has occurred include an increase in urine production, the ability to clear urea and creatinine, and laboratory evidence that the kidney is able to manage the patient's electrolytes at safe levels. Once this is detected by clinicians, they can discontinue renal replacement therapy gradually using progressively longer CRRT holidays each day, or therapy can be discontinued with the plan to resume only if a life-threatening complication of renal dysfunction occurs. For those patients who do not experience renal recovery, it may be appropriate to transition them to intermittent therapy once they become more hemodynamically stable. The KDIGO guidelines do not give any more specific criteria regarding when to stop therapy other than recommending cessation of therapy when it is no longer required or it is not consistent with patient care goals [26].

Long-Term Outcomes

Will my patient with AKI progress to end-stage renal disease (ESRD), or will they recover renal function? In a prospective cohort study of 433 patients with severe ATN requiring RRT, the investigators sought to determine the rates of recovery of renal function at hospital discharge and ESRD status at 1 year follow-up. In-hospital mortality in these patients was 47% at the time of hospital discharge, and 57% of the survivors had normal renal function. Only one of the survivors had ESRD at 1 year follow-up leading investigators to conclude that if the patient survives the initial insult that caused their AKI, the majority of survivors would go on to recover renal function to a degree that they would not require RRT long term [44].

Acute tubular necrosis (ATN) is a common cause of AKI. Researches have categorized the cause of ATN as ischemic, nephrotoxic, or both and looked into whether or not the cause affects the long-term outcome. In a review of 425 critically ill patients with AKI, those who had ATN from mixed causes had the highest mortality rate at 55%, while those with purely ischemic or nephrotoxic were at 39% and 29%, respectively. The patients with a mixed cause of their ATN also had the lowest rates of renal recovery. Proportional differences were seen when these patients were followed up 7 years after the initial recovery, and survival rates were reported [45].

Patients who survive critical illness and AKI have reduced long-term health-related quality of life [46]. When AKI survivors were surveyed using an SF-12 questionnaire, they had lower physical and mental competency scores when matched with control groups [46]. Rates of renal recovery and mortality have been assessed at the time of hospital discharge and 5 years later in a cohort of 226 survivors of AKI requiring RRT. None of these patients had pre-existing kidney disease. At hospital discharge, none of the patients were RRT dependent with 57% demonstrating complete recovery and 43% with partial recovery. At 5 years, only 25% of the cohort was still alive, and 5% of those survivors had become dialysis dependent. AKI not only causes increased in-hospital mortality but also "carries significant implications for long-term survival [47]." The use of continuous modalities instead of IHD is associated with a reduced incidence of long-term dialysis dependence. In a meta-analysis of 23 trials, pooled analysis of observational studies suggested a higher rate of dialysis dependence among survivors of AKI who were initially treated with IHD [48]. While CRRT may appear more expensive when compared to IHD, it is actually far more cost-effective. This is the case because of the decreased risk of dialysis dependence and the increase in quality-adjusted life years that patients experience after treatment with CRRT [49].

Conclusion

In order to provide optimal support and reduce morbidity and mortality in critically ill surgical patients with AKI, the intensivist must understand the principles of RRT. The modes of hemodialysis differ with respect to how the blood is purified, what size molecules can be removed, and in terms of hemodynamic tolerability. Hemodialysis can rapidly and effectively clear small molecular weight molecules. Continuous modalities that utilize hemofiltration can remove middle molecules at a steady rate that is well tolerated by hemodynamically unstable patients. Continuous modes are therefore preferred in the most critically ill patients. With respect to the controversies in the mode, dose, and timing of renal replacement therapy, there is no "one-size-fits-all" approach that applies to all patients. The mode, dose, and timing of renal replacement therapy should be individualized to the patient.

References

1. Ozrazgat-Baslanti T, Thottakkara P, Bihorac A, et al. Acute and chronic kidney disease and cardiovascular mortality after major surgery. Ann Surg. 2016;264(6):987–96.
2. Loftus TJ, Bihorac A, Ozrazgat-Baslanti T, et al. Acute kidney injury following exploratory laparotomy and temporary abdominal closure. Shock. 2016;48(1):5–10. Epub ahead of print.
3. Cerda J, Liu KD, Cruz DN, et al. Promoting kidney function recovery in patients with AKI requiring RRT. Clin J Am Soc Nephrol. 2015;10:1859–67.
4. Dennen P, Douglas IS, Anderson R. Acute kidney injury in the intensive care unit: a primer for the intensivist. Crit Care Med. 2010;38:261–75.
5. Uchino S, Kellum JA, Bellomo R, et al. Acute renal failure in critically ill patients: a multinational, multicenter study. JAMA. 2005;294:813–8.
6. Chung KK, Juncos LA, Wolf SE, et al. Continuous renal replacement therapy improves survival in severely burned military casualties with acute kidney injury. J Trauma. 2008;64:S179–87.
7. Osterman M, Chang RW. Acute kidney injury in the intensive care unit according to RIFLE. Crit Care Med. 2007;35:1837–43. quiz1852
8. Lysak N, Bihorac A, Hobson C. Mortality and cost of acute and chronic kidney disease after cardiac surgery. Curr Opin Anaesthesiol. 2017;30:113–7.
9. Chung KK, Stewart IJ, Gisler C, et al. The Acute Kidney Injury (AKIN) criteria applied in burns. J Burn Care Res. 2012;33(4):483–90.
10. Stewart IJ, Tilley MA, Cotant CL, et al. Association of AKI with adverse outcomes in burned military casualties. Clin J Am Soc Nephrol. 2012;7(2):199–206.
11. Teschan PE, Post RS, Smith LH, et al. Post-traumatic renal insufficiency in military casualties. Am J Med. 1955;19:172–86.
12. Chung KK, Perkins RM, Oliver JD. Renal replacement therapy in support of combat operations. Crit Care Med. 2008;36:S365–9.
13. Himmelfarb J, Ikizler TA. Hemodialysis. N Engl J Med. 2010;363:1833–45.
14. Conger JD. A controlled evaluation of prophylactic dialysis in post traumatic acute renal failure. J Trauma. 1975;15:1056–63.
15. Kramer P, Wigger W, Rieger J, et al. Arteriovenous haemofiltration: a new and simple method for treatment of over-hydrated patients resistant to diuretics. Klin Wochenschr. 1977;55:1121–2.
16. Kellum JA, Bellomo R, Ronco C, et al. Continuous renal replacement therapy. 2nd: Oxford University Press; 2016.
17. Kaplan AA, Longnecker RE, Folkert VW. Continuous arteriovenous hemofiltration: a report of six months experience. Ann Intern Med. 1984;100:358–67.
18. Ronco C, Bellomo R, Ricci Z. Hemodynamic response to fluid withdrawal in overhydrated patients treated with intermittent ultrafiltration and slow continuous ultrafiltration: role of blood volume monitoring. Cardiology. 2001;96(3–4):196–201.
19. Ronco C, Giomarelli P. Current and future role of ultrafiltration in CRS. Heart Fail Rev. 2011;16(6):595–602.

20. Costanzo MR, Negoianu D, Jaski BE, et al. Aquapheresis versus intravenous diuretics and hospitalizations for heart failure. JACC Heart Fail. 2016;4(2):95–105.
21. Fliser D, Kielstein JT. Technology insight: treatment of renal failure in the intensive care unit with extended dialysis. Nat Clin Pract Nephrol. 2006;2(1):32–9.
22. Bagshaw SM, Berthiaume LR, Delaney A, Bellomo R. Continuous versus intermittent renal replacement therapy for critically ill patients with acute kidney injury: a meta-analysis. Crit Care Med. 2008;36:610.
23. Schneider AG, Bellomo R, Bagshaw SM, et al. Choice of renal replacement therapy modality and dialysis dependence after acute kidney injury: a systematic review and meta-analysis. Intensive Care Med. 2013;39:987.
24. Flythe JE, Xue H, Lynch KE, et al. Association of mortality risk with various definitions of intradialytic hypotension. J Am Soc Nephrol. 2015;26:724–34.
25. Assimon MM, Flythe JE. Intradialytic blood pressure abnormalities: the highs, the los and all that lies between. Am J Nephrol. 2015;42:337–50.
26. Kidney Disease Improving Global Outcomes (KDIGO) Acute Kidney Injury Work Group. KDIGO clinical practice guideline for acute kidney injury. Kidney Int. 2012;2(suppl):1–138.
27. Monti G, Herrera M, Kindgen-Milles D, et al. The dose responsive multicenter international collaborative initiative (DO-RE-MI). Contrib Nephrol. 2007;156:434–43.
28. Palevsky PM, Zhang JH, O'Conner TZ, et al. Intensity of renal support in critically ill patients with acute kidney injury. N Engl J Med. 2008;359:1–14.
29. Bellomo R, Cass A, Cole L, et al. Intensity of continuous renal-replacement therapy in critically ill patients. N Engl J Med. 2009;361:1627–38.
30. Fayad AI, Buamscha DG, Ciapponi A, et al. Intensity of continuous renal replacement therapy for acute kidney injury. Cochrane Database Syst Rev. 2016;4(10):CD010613.
31. Li SY, Yang WC, Chuang CL. Effect of early and intensive continuous venovenous hemofiltration on patients with cardiogenic shock and acute kidney injury after cardiac surgery. J Thorac Cardiovasc Surg. 2014;148(4):1628–33.
32. Chrysopoulo MT, Jeschke MG, Dziewulski P, et al. Acute renal dysfunction in severely burned adults. J Trauma. 1999;46:141–4.
33. Coca SG, Bauling P, Schifftner T, et al. Contribution of acute kidney injury toward morbidity and mortality in burns: a contemporary analysis. Am J Kidney Dis. 2007;49:517–23.
34. Leblanc M, Thibeault Y, Querin S. Continuous haemofiltration and heamodiafiltration for acute renal failure in severely burned patients. Burns. 1997;23:160–5.
35. Chung KK, Lundy JB, Matson JR, et al. Continuous venovenous hemofiltration in severely burned patients with acute kidney injury: a cohort study. Crit Care. 2009;13:R62.
36. Gaudry S, Hajage D, Schortgen F, et al. Initiation strategies for renal-replacement therapy in the intensive care unit. N Engl J Med. 2016;375(2):122–33.
37. Zarbock A, Kellum JA, Schmidt C, et al. Effect of early vs delayed initiation of renal replacement therapy on mortality in critically ill patients with acute kidney injury: the ELAIN randomized clinical trial. JAMA. 2016;315(20):2190–9.
38. SC W, CY F, Lin HH, et al. Late initiation of continuous venovenous hemofiltration therapy is associated with a lower survival rate in surgical critically ill patients with postoperative acute kidney injury. Am Surg. 2012;78(2):235–42.
39. Oudemans-van Straaten HM, Bosman RJ, Koopmans M, et al. Citrate anticoagulation for continuous venovenous hemofiltration. Crit Care Med. 2009;37:545.
40. Schilder L, Nurmohamed SA, Bosch FH, et al. Citrate anticoagulation versus systemic heparinisation in continuous venovenous hemofiltration in critically ill patients with acute kidney injury: a multi-center randomized clinical trial. Crit Care. 2014;18:472.
41. Gattas DJ, Rajbhandari D, Bradford C, et al. A randomized controlled trial of regional citrate versus regional heparin anticoagulation for continuous renal replacement therapy in critically ill adults. Crit Care Med. 2015;43:1622.
42. Hafner S, Stahl W, Fels T, et al. Implementation of continuous renal replacement therapy with regional citrate anticoagulation on a surgical and trauma intensive care unit: impact on clinical and economic aspects-an observational study. J Intensive Care. 2015;30(1):35.
43. Marik PE, Flemmer M, Harrison W, et al. The risk of catheter-related bloodstream infection with femoral venous catheters as compared to subclavian and internal jugular venous catheters: a systematic review of the literature and meta-analysis. Crit Care Med. 2012;40(8):2479–85.
44. Schiffl H. Renal recovery from acute tubular necrosis requiring renal replacement therapy: a prospective study in critically ill patients. Nephrol Dial Transplant. 2006;21(5):1248–52.
45. Schiffl H, Fischer R. Clinical cause of presumed acute tubular necrosis requiring renal replacement therapy and outcome of critically ill patients: post hoc analysis of a prospective 7-year cohort study. Int Urol Nephrol. 2012;44(6):1779–89.
46. Wang AY, Bellomo R, Cass A, et al. Health-related quality of life in survivors of acute kidney injury: the prolonged outcomes study of the randomized evaluation of normal versus augmented level replacement therapy study outcomes. Nephrology. 2015;20(7):492–8.
47. Schiffl H, Fischer R. Five-year outcomes of severe acute kidney injury requiring renal replacement therapy. Nephrol Dial Transplant. 2008;23(7):2235–41.
48. Schneider AG, Bellomo R, Bagshaw SM, et al. Choic of renal replacement therapy modality and dialysis dependence after acute kidney injury: a systematic review and meta-analysis. Intensive Care Med. 2013;39(6):987–97.
49. Ethgen O, Schneider AG, Bagshaw SM, et al. Economics of dialysis dependence following renal replacement therapy for critically ill acute kidney injury patients. Nephrol Dial Transplant. 2015;30(1):54–61.
50. Tolwani A. Continuous renal-replacement therapy for acute kidney injury. N Engl J Med. 2012;367:2505–14.

Management of Common Urologic Conditions Among the Critically Ill

29

E. Charles Osterberg

Introduction

Many common urologic problems manifest in the treatment of the critical patient overseen by an intensivist or traumatologist. The changing paradigm of healthcare delivery requires clinicians to have a rudimentary understanding of many surgical subspecialties, including urology. In this chapter, common urologic problems are discussed. A specific focus is paid toward the practical management of these conditions whereby the non-urologist may quickly reference this chapter. It is my hope that this chapter serves as a resource for any non-urologist who participates in the critical care of surgical patients.

Hematuria

Microscopic Hematuria

Microscopic hematuria is defined by three or more red blood cells per high-power field on microscopic analysis of a non-contaminated urine sample without any evidence of urinary infection, pyuria, bacteriuria, and/or contamination [1]. Furthermore, recent instrumentation or manipulation of the urinary tract (e.g., Foley catheter placement) should be determined prior to confirming a positive result. In the setting of the critically ill patient, it is not uncommon to have microscopic hematuria especially in the setting of polytrauma, recent catheterization, renal injury, or other nephrogenic causes.

The most common urologic causes of microscopic hematuria include enlargement of the prostate, infection, and urinary stones [1]. A very small subset of patients with microscopic hematuria will ultimately be diagnosed with a urinary tract malignancy. It is estimated that roughly 4% of patients who undergo screening with a microscopic urinalysis are found to have a urinary tract malignancy [2]. Those individuals with a history of smoking, pelvic radiation, history of exposure to carcinogenic agents, male gender, or history of gross hematuria are at increased risk for urinary tract malignancy in the setting of microscopic hematuria [1].

In the setting of critically ill, a diagnosis of microscopic hematuria is unlikely to be paramount to the patient's clinical course. However, once stabilized and discharged, a repeat microscopic urinalysis should be performed. Once benign causes have been ruled out, the presence of asymptomatic microscopic hematuria should prompt a urologic evaluation. The initial urologic evaluation includes an estimate of renal function with creatinine and blood urea nitrogen levels to protect intrinsic renal disease. Certainly the presence of any cellular casts, dysmorphic red blood cells, or proteinuria would indicate the presence of intrinsic renal disease precipitating microscopic hematuria. After excluding other etiologies, a cystoscopy is warranted on any patient over 35 years of age with asymptomatic microscopic hematuria. In addition, a multi-phase computed tomography scan with and without intravenous contrast including a delayed urography phase is also warranted [1]. In those patients who have contraindications to contrast-enhanced imaging, a magnetic resonance urography scan is an acceptable alternative. In patients who have a history of persistent asymptomatic microhematuria and subsequently have two negative annual urinalyses, further evaluation is no longer necessary [3].

The diagnosis of asymptomatic microscopic hematuria should not be overlooked and warrants repeat evaluation once the critically ill are stabilized and/or discharged. With high-risk individuals, the risk of urinary tract malignancy ranges from 0% to 25%; therefore, follow-up is warranted [2].

E. Charles Osterberg (✉)
University of Texas – Dell Medical School, Austin, TX, USA
e-mail: Charles.Osterberg@austin.utexas.edu

A. Salim et al. (eds.), *Surgical Critical Care Therapy*, https://doi.org/10.1007/978-3-319-71712-8_29

Gross Hematuria and Clot Obstruction

Gross hematuria is defined by urine that is visibly discolored by blood or any blood clots. The degree of gross hematuria is oftentimes categorized on a continuum of light pink, red, brown, or frank blood. Akin to a drop of red food coloring, just the slightest amount (e.g., 1 mL) of blood can impart the appearance of gross hematuria. Alternatively, gross hematuria may be a life-threatening condition.

Gross hematuria is a presenting sign of roughly 60% of patients with urologic cancers [4]. Certainly those individuals that are older, are exposed to carcinogenic agents, and have smoking history, history of pelvic radiation, or chronic urinary tract infections are at increased risk. In men over the age of 60, the positive predictive value of malignancy with gross hematuria is roughly 20%, whereas in women it is roughly 8% [4]. Therefore there are several other etiologies that may contribute to gross hematuria such as enlarged prostate, urinary tract infection, urinary tract stones, cystitis, medications (e.g., aspirin, warfarin, etc.), recent urologic trauma, or instrumentation [5].

Evaluation and management of critically ill patients with gross hematuria are dependent on hemodynamic stability and establishing prompt urinary drainage if the patient is not voiding spontaneously. In the hemodynamically unstable patient with gross hematuria that is not transfusion responsive, prompt urologic evaluation is necessary as operative intervention and/or angioembolization may be imminent [5]. In the case of a hemodynamically stable patient with gross hematuria, this can likely be worked up on an outpatient basis with a cystoscopy and a multi-phase computed tomography scan with and without intravenous contrast including a delayed urography.

Prompt urinary drainage should be achieved in critically ill patients suffering from clot obstruction. During this time it is important to identify risk factors and reversible causes for the gross hematuria and clot retention such as anticoagulation status. Urinary drainage is achieved with a large-bore catheter and bladder irrigation to evacuate obstructing clots. Urinary catheters are size in the French system, whereby 1 French equals 0.33 cm in circumference. In patients with clot retention, a 22 French three-way catheter or larger allows for manual clot irrigation and continuous bladder irrigation (CBI). Via a catheter-tipped syringe and saline irrigant, the bladder may be irrigated via the drainage port of a large-bore three-way catheter to evacuate obstructing clots. This process should be repeated until no further clots are seen. Once the bladder is completely free of clot, CBI can be initiated whereby 3 liter bags of normal saline irrigation will flow into the bladder via the catheter-inflow port and promptly will drain out of the bladder via the catheter-outflow port. The continuous irrigation prevents the formation and propagation of obstructing clots, thereby allowing urinary drainage. Vigilant monitoring of the CBI is necessary to ensure that the outflow continues to drain. There is a risk of bladder rupture should the outflow be obstructed by a clot in the inflow that is running continuously. In addition, accurate measurement of urine output in critically ill patients on CBI is impossible.

Determination of the etiology of gross hematuria may be confirmed once patients are clinically stable or on an outpatient basis if non-obstructing. Despite a multitude of etiologies, gross hematuria should always be considered a red flag for urologic malignancy, and thus urologic consultation is warranted.

Urologic Infections

The genitourinary system is a common source for bacterial and fungal infections. In the critically ill patient, prompt identification and isolation of a genitourinary source are necessary for stabilization. Common urologic infections stem from prostatitis, epididymoorchitis, urethritis, prostate abscesses, and pyelonephritis.

Prostatitis and Prostate Abscess

Acute bacterial prostatitis is a rare entity that is characterized by high fevers, perirectal and perineal pain, lower urinary tract symptoms, and incomplete bladder emptying. Patients may report a prior history of recent urinary tract infections, recent urinary instrumentation, immunocompromised states, and/or diabetes. Physical exam will reveal a tender, boggy prostate that is associated with elevation in white blood cell count, bacteriuria, pyuria, and/or bacteremia [6]. Prompt antibiotic therapy should be initiated, and if patients are septic, hospitalization and fluid resuscitation are necessary. Blood and urine cultures off and reveal common genitourinary pathogens including *Escherichia coli*, *Enterobacter*, *Enterococcus*, and *Staphylococcus* species. Typical oral antibiotics for prostatitis include a quinolone or trimethoprim-sulfamethoxazole for at least 4 weeks following the diagnosis [6]. Common intravenous antibiotics include ampicillin and gentamicin. Following cultural susceptibility testing, antibiotics may be tailored accordingly. If patients are unable to void, urethral catheterization is safe. Prior dogma suggests that the urethra should not be instrumented during episodes of acute bacterial prostatitis, and a suprapubic cystotomy tube placement is mandated. No prospective studies or large series have demonstrated such relationship, and it is my practice to commonly place a 12 French Foley catheter in these patients.

A prostate abscess may also be present at the time of bacterial prostatitis or may present independently [7].

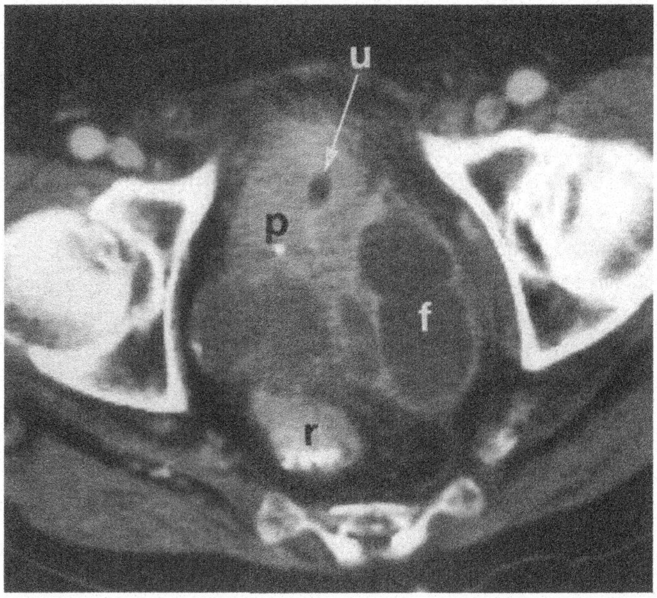

Fig. 29.1 Computed tomography scan demonstrating hypodense areas within the prostate consistent with abscess cavity (Image adapted from Wessels & McAninch "Urologic Emergencies – A Practical Approach" – 2005 Humana Press – Page 138)

Alternatively the prostatic infection may involve a prostate abscess following a prolonged course of oral antibiotics. Typical presentation is similar to that of acute bacterial prostatitis. Often a computed tomography scan or transrectal ultrasound will demonstrate the prostate abscess (see Fig. 29.1) [8]. Surgical management of prostate abscesses is beyond the scope of this chapter; however the urologist may advise prolonged antibiotic therapy, transrectal ultrasound-guided aspiration, or transurethral unroofing of the prostate abscess.

Epididymoorchitis

Epididymoorchitis is the combined infection of the epididymis and the testis [9]. Oftentimes it is a result from bacterial spread from the urethra or bladder. Men will present with an acute-appearing scrotum that is tender and oftentimes erythematous. Associated fever, lower urinary tract symptoms, and testicular induration may also be evident. The clinician should be aware of the possibility of testicular torsion which has an acute onset versus the gradual onset of pain seen in epididymoorchitis. Urinalysis and urine culture may guide antibiotic treatment and should routinely be performed. Common microbes include *Escherichia coli* and *Staphylococcus* [9]. Scrotal sonography will demonstrate a hypervascular epididymis and abnormal echogenicity within the testicle or epididymis. Antimicrobial therapy should last for at least 14 days, and a quinolone or trimethoprim-sulfamethoxazole is recommended [10]. In severe cases that are associated with systemic illness, gentamicin may be added for additional coverage [11]. Scrotal elevation, nonsteroidal anti-inflammatory agents, and scrotal ice pack may all be beneficial to alleviating pain. Surgical exploration is only indicated in cases of severe infection, abscess formation, or testicular infarction.

Urethritis

Urethritis is most often caused by a sexually transmitted infection such as gonorrhea or chlamydia. Often patients will present with a urethral discharge and dysuria; however in some cases, the patient may be entirely asymptomatic. Diagnosis is based upon urine nucleic acid amplification which has improved sensitivity and specificity over the stork urethral swab. Typical treatment for uncomplicated infections includes a single dose of ceftriaxone plus a single dose of azithromycin which will cover both organisms [12].

Pyelonephritis, Renal Abscesses, Emphysematous Pyelonephritis, and Xanthogranulomatous Pyelonephritis (XGP)

Pyelonephritis is a bacterial infection of the kidney that results in inflammation of the renal parenchyma. By definition pyelonephritis is an infection of the renal parenchyma with associated fever and flank pain. The most common organisms causing pyelonephritis are *Escherichia coli*, followed by *Klebsiella*, *Proteus*, *Pseudomonas*, and *Serratia* species [13]. Risk factors for pyelonephritis include underlying anatomic abnormalities of the urinary tract, spinal cord injury, persistent urinary tract infections, pregnancy, and immunocompromised states [14]. Presenting symptoms include lower urinary tract symptoms such as dysuria, frequency, in addition high cyclic fevers, chills, malaise, flank pain, and sepsis. Laboratory evaluation may show a leukocytosis with an elevated creatinine level, blood cultures may be positive for bacteremia, and/or urinalysis usually will show white blood cells and bacteriuria [14]. If patients are clinically stable and there is no anatomic etiology such as ureteral obstruction causing the episode of pyelonephritis, outpatient management may be pursued with 14 days of a fluoroquinolone, amoxicillin-clavulanate, or trimethoprim-sulfamethoxazole [15]. In the critically ill patient, parenteral antibiotics are warranted utilizing broad-spectrum antibiotics and narrowing following culture sensitivities. If blood cultures are positive, parenteral antibiotics should be continued at least for 7 days [14]. Repeat urine culture should be performed if patients fail to improve after 48 h. Furthermore imaging should be obtained if patients fail to improve to identify potential obstruction or perirenal abscesses [14]. In the cases of obstructing pyelonephritis secondary to ureteral stricture or calculi, emergent urinary diversion with nephrostomy tube or indwelling ureteral stent is mandated. Prompt urologic consultation should be performed to decompress the infected system.

Renal abscesses may develop from repeated episodes of pyelonephritis or may result from long-standing, chronic urinary infection. Abscesses present with similar signs and symptoms as acute pyelonephritis and are associated with urinary stasis and calculi [16]. Computed tomography is most accurate way to identify a renal abscess. The mainstay of management revolves around source control and parenteral antibiotics. Those abscesses less than 3 cm in size can usually be treated conservatively with antibiotics; however those abscesses greater than 3 cm in size and those immunocompromised individuals should be managed with image-guided drainage [16]. Follow-up computed tomography scan is important especially if clinical status does not improve.

Emphysematous pyelonephritis is a life-threatening necrotizing infection of the renal parenchyma secondary to gas-forming bacteria commonly among immunocompromised women [17]. The finding of gas within the kidney parenchyma is diagnostic for the condition. Commonly parenteral antibiotics are insufficient, and surgical drainage or nephrectomy is indicated.

Xanthogranulomatous pyelonephritis (XGP) forms after long-standing inflammation of the kidney secondary to chronic urinary obstruction, infections, and stones. The patient often has associated renal insufficiency, and the affected kidney is rendered nonfunctional [18]. Computed tomography shows an enlarged, "bear claw"-like kidney, nephrolithiasis, and little remaining renal parenchyma. (See Fig. 29.2). Antibiotics should be initiated; however XGP is managed with nephrectomy for source control [18].

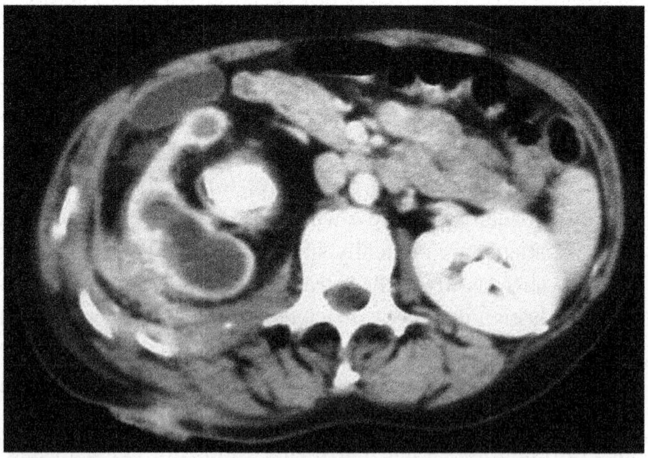

Fig. 29.2 Characteristic appearance of XGP kidney on computed tomography with contrast (Image adapted from Craig et al. Radiographics. Jan 2008)

Fournier's Gangrene

Fournier's gangrene is a necrotizing infection of the skin and subcutaneous tissues overlying the external genitalia and perineum. The disease can involve all images and both genders; however men who are immunocompromised and/or diabetic are most susceptible [19]. The disease is life-threatening and therefore requires a rapid diagnosis as well as immediate surgical management. Mortality has been reported to be as high as 50%, and therefore the astute clinician must recognize the warning signs and symptoms of this necrotizing infection [20].

Pathogenesis

Fournier's gangrene is a result of multiple anaerobic and aerobic bacteria. Common bacteria include *Escherichia coli*, *Staphylococcus*, *Pseudomonas*, *Enterococci*, and *Clostridium perfringens* [21]. Any condition that compromises the immune system puts patients at increased risk of susceptibility and mortality. Conditions such as diabetes, alcoholism, human immunodeficiency virus, malnutrition, and obesity are all such examples of risk factors for Fournier's gangrene [19]. In addition, recent instrumentation and/or surgery to the perineum and scrotum put patients at risk for bacterial penetrance. For example, recent perineal abscess drainage, urethral instrumentation, scrotal abscess drainage, and perirectal abscess drainage all are risk factors for progression to Fournier's gangrene.

Fournier's gangrene carries a high mortality due to the contiguous necrotizing bacterial spread through the fascial anatomy. Bacteria may track along Dartos fascia, into Colles' fascia, along the fascia lata of the thigh, and to Scarpa's fascia along the anterior abdominal wall [21]. As such, surgical control and debridement are necessary to halt any bacterial spread.

Diagnosis

Physical examination is oftentimes the mainstay of Fournier's gangrene diagnosis. Oftentimes genital pain, swelling, and erythema are common findings. Certainly systemic signs of sepsis including fever, malaise, and tachycardia may also be present [20]. Physical exam may demonstrate areas of crepitus and/or purplish discoloration of the perineum and/or scrotum. The skin may be sloughing, and there may be purulent drainage and demarcated necrotic tissue (see Fig. 29.3). These immediate physical exam findings should prompt the clinician to quickly make the diagnosis and proceed forth with surgical intervention [20].

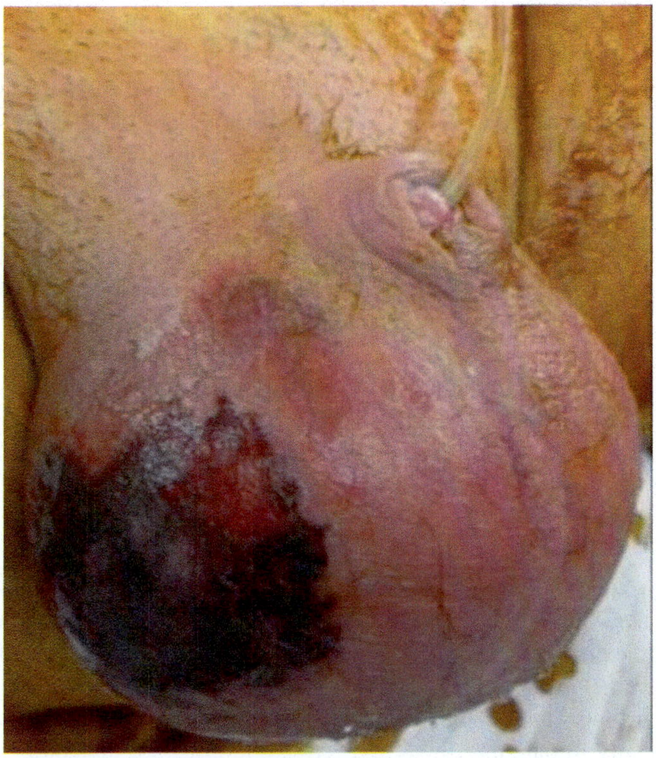

Fig. 29.3 Characteristic appearance of necrotic skin on the scrotum consistent with Fournier's gangrene

Laboratory analysis may demonstrate leukocytosis, hyponatremia, and hypocalcemia; however normal laboratory evaluations should not delay surgical intervention [19]. Radiographic studies may be useful when physical examination is unclear. Such radiographic examinations may include a scrotal ultrasound or computed tomography scan. These imaging studies may reveal gas in the soft tissue and/or an abscess cavity.

Initial Management

Fournier's gangrene is a surgical disease. Initiation of broad-spectrum antibiotics with anaerobic and aerobic coverage, as well as aggressive intravenous fluid resuscitation, is oriented [20]. Those critically ill may require ventilatory and/or pressor support. Surgical debridement requires removal of all devitalized skin and subcutaneous tissue and fascia. Often the penis, corpora spongiosum and cavernosum, and testicles are always preserved because of their rich blood supply [22]. However in the case of epididymoorchitis and/or scrotal abscesses, primary orchiectomy may be performed if the etiology is secondary to these infections [19]. Following debridement, pressure irrigation with antibiotic saline solution is used to reduce bacterial load. A proctoscopy and cystoscopy may be warranted if rectal and/or urethral sources of infection are identified [22].

If the wound has massive contamination, it is possible that a simultaneous fecal diversion is necessary to maintain wound cleanliness. A Foley catheter is also recommended to maintain urinary diversion again for wound cleanliness [21].

Repeat inspection and debridement should be scheduled every 12–24 h for at least two to four consecutive evaluations to ensure that all demarcated and devitalized tissues have been removed [19]. With regard to the testicles should they be totally free, it is my surgical preference to keep them wrapped in moist gauze as opposed to placing them in thigh pouches. In my experience, thigh pouches are difficult to take down as the testicle often scars down, and this creates a more challenging reconstruction in the future. If a testicular thigh pouch is performed, it is important to place the testicles anteriorly so that when the patient abducts his legs, they are not compressed [22].

Postoperative Management

After the wound is clean, the patient has been stabilized, and there are no further plans for debridement, attention should be turned toward reconstruction. The role of hyperbaric oxygen is beyond the scope of this review.

Reconstruction is based on the size of the defect and the presence or absence of the testis and overall skin coverage. Often scrotal skin may be utilized to perform a scrotoplasty, and a split-thickness skin graft is preferred for its ease of use and could take to the penile skin [23]. In general it is my preference to use a mesh to graft over the testicles should there not be sufficient scrotal skin for coverage. For the potent man, it is my preference to use a non-meshed split-thickness skin graft over the phallus for fear that a meshed graft may contract. Tissue expanders may be used to increase the scrotum distensibility, and as a rule of thumb, primary closure is always preferred [23].

The diagnosis and treatment of the patient with Fournier's gangrene is often multidisciplinary involving the critical care team, general surgery team, a urologist, and possibly a plastic surgeon/colorectal surgeon. The team-based approach to care of these complex patients is critical to their success.

Acute Ureteral Obstruction from Calculi

Renal colic secondary to urolithiasis is the most common cause of ureteral obstruction and may manifest as a secondary problem during an inpatient hospitalization. Kidney stones affect anywhere from 1% to 5% of the adult population [24]. The incidence of overlap between a surgical patient and ureteral obstruction secondary to calculi is unknown, and thus the clinician should be aware of the signs and symptoms of ureteral colic.

Evaluation and Diagnosis

It is estimated that up to 50% of patients with a history of stones will have a repeat episode of ureteral colic in the future [24]. A medical history will provide some important clues regarding the etiology of their renal colic. Physical examination may demonstrate evidence of costovertebral angle tenderness and suprapubic tenderness that may radiate to the ipsilateral groin. The pain is often described as intermittent and stabbing. The location of pain often corresponds with stone location with upper ureteral stones oftentimes being felt in the flank versus distal stones oftentimes being reflected in the groin. A stone in the ureterovesical junction may oftentimes present with urinary urgency and frequency [25]. Stones in the mid-ureter may mimic acute appendicitis or peritonitis. Stone size does not correlate with the severity of pain [25].

With clinical suspicion raised, diagnosis can be confirmed with renal imaging. A plain film of the kidney ureter and bladder (KUB) may be used as an initial imaging test as it may help localize stones. However a KUB has limited sensitivity particularly with regard to uric acid stones. A noncontrast computed tomography scan is the mainstay of a renal colic workup [26]. This scan will detect all ureteral calculi except stones produced secondary to long-term antiretroviral, e.g., indinavir. A renal ultrasound may demonstrate pyelo-ureteral dilation; however the etiology secondary to ureteral stone cannot be confirmed with ultrasound. The absence of a urinary ureteral jet from the ureteral orifice may be used as a surrogate for a completely obstructing ureteral stone.

Medical and Surgical Treatment

Data suggest that the likelihood of spontaneous stone passage correlates with stone size and location [27]. In other words, the smaller the stone and the more distal stone, the more likely the stone will pass. Patients who have an uncomplicated ureteral stone less than 1 cm can be offered observation for passage [26], and those with a distal ureteral stone less than 1 cm in size can be offered medical expulsion therapy with an alpha blocker [28]. The routine alpha blocker of choice that I use for medical expulsion therapy is tamsulosin 0.4 mg daily.

While the duration of time for medical expulsion therapy is not clear, conservative therapy should not exceed roughly 6 weeks in time in order to avoid kidney injury [25]. If patients cannot tolerate the trial of passage secondary to recalcitrant pain, nausea, vomiting, a rise in serum creatinine, worsening of hydronephrosis on imaging, or concern for urinary infection, surgical intervention is warranted, and urology consultation should be made [25].

Metabolic testing for stone prevention may be performed as an outpatient. All patients who have a ureteral or renal stone are recommended to increase fluid intake to a voided volume of 2.5 L per day. In general, dietary modification with minimized salt intake, low animal protein intake, and high fluid intake is recommended regardless of the stone etiology.

Surgical intervention for ureteral stone disease is beyond the scope of this chapter. A urologist has an armamentarium of surgical options which include lithotripsy, stenting, nephrostomy tube diversion, and/or open ureterolithotomy. Prompt consultation with a urologist is warranted in the setting of an infected, obstructing ureteral stone [29].

Urinary Diversions

Urinary diversions may be performed for a variety of reasons including extirpative surgery for cancer, strictures in the urinary system, bladder dysfunction, and neurologic and spinal cord issues to name a few. Complications following urinary diversions are frequent and may occur in the critically ill patient.

Types of Urinary Diversions

There are three main types of commonly used urinary diversions. An ileal conduit is an incontinent urostomy and is commonly selected due to its lower complication rate and high patient's satisfaction level. In this diversion, the ureters drained directly into an ileal segment which is matured to the skin [30]. The second most common urinary diversion is an Indiana pouch. This is a continent diversion that requires catheterization to empty urine. Typically a portion of the descending colon and ileum is used to create a pouch with the ileocecal valve functioning as the continence mechanism. A tapered portion of ileum is brought up to the skin and matured to function as a catheterizable continent channel which drains the pouch [31]. Lastly an orthotopic diversion or neobladder utilizes a pouch created by the ileum, ascending colon, or both and is attached following ureteral implantation to the proximal portion of the patient's urethra for an anatomically placed continent urinary diversion (see Fig. 29.4) [32].

Complications with Urinary Diversions

As a result of the complex surgery and urine mixing with a mucosal intestinal surface, these urinary diversions are associated with complications which may occur in the critically ill patient. Several noteworthy complications are highlighted below:

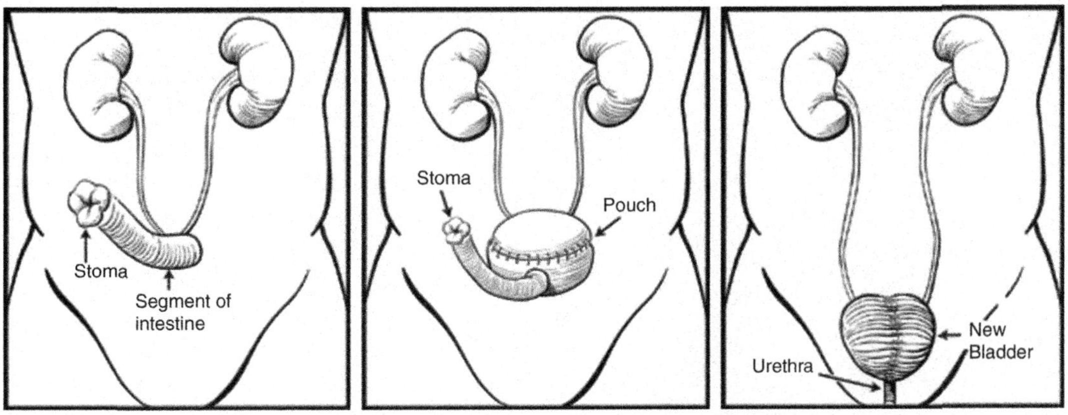

Fig. 29.4 Schematic demonstrating the ileal conduit, Indiana pouch, and neobladder (left to right) (Imaged adapted with permission from – http://bradyurology.blogspot.com/2014/10/quality-of-life-after-surgery-for.html)

Ureteroenteric stricture – Due to the anastomosis of the ureter to the bowel segment, strictures are prone to forming. Causes of stricture formation include tension at the anastomosis, devascularization and ischemia, recurrent infections, and ureteroenteric leakage [33]. The diagnosis of stricture formation can be made with computed tomography scan with delayed contrast. In any patient with a urinary diversion and hydronephrosis, a diagnosis of ureteroenteric stricture is possible [33].

Metabolic complications – The ileum and colon are most commonly used for all urologic urinary diversions. As a result of the intestinal mucosa being exposed to urine, there are associated electrolyte abnormalities. Typically, a hyperchloremic metabolic acidosis is the result of cation and anion exchange [34]. In addition hypokalemia is commonly seen as a result of chronic acidemia [35]. Of note, hypokalemia is less common with ileal diversions versus colonic diversions. Often the kidneys will compensate; however in the critically ill patient, renal function may be impaired, and electrolyte imbalances may occur as a result of the urinary diversion [34].

Malabsorption – The length of bowel utilized is dependent on the type of conduit or continent urinary diversion created. When long segments of bowel are resected, malabsorption may occur, particularly in the case of the terminal ileum [36]. Chronic vitamin B12 deficiency may occur, and level should be monitored periodically [35].

Stone formation – Calculi formation may occur and can predispose patients to infection. As a result of urinary stasis, foreign bodies, and/or repeated infections, stones may form [36]. In patients with urinary diversions and urinary tract infection, a stone may be the nidus, and clearance of the infection necessitates lithotripsy [37].

Pyelonephritis – Patients with urinary diversions are chronically colonized with bacteria and should not undergo treatment with antibiotics if asymptomatic. The most common isolate is *Escherichia coli* [36]. In those patients with asymptomatic bacteriuria and who have *Proteus* or *Pseudomonas* species, treatment is recommended [38]. In those patients who demonstrate systemic signs of infection such as fever or leukocytosis, antibiotics should be initiated, and efforts to maximally drain the urinary system are warranted.

Paraphimosis

Paraphimosis is a medical condition whereby the foreskin of the penis becomes trapped behind the coronal margin of the glans and cannot be reduced to its normal anatomic position secondary to swelling [39]. Oftentimes paraphimosis occurs as a result of improper handling of the foreskin by medical professionals or even the patient. It is imperative during catheter placement, in the circumcised male, that the foreskin, if present, be returned to its normal anatomic position over the coronal margin.

Diagnosis and Treatment

The diagnosis of paraphimosis is exclusively based upon physical examination. Obtaining a history of an uncircumcised phallus in the setting of grossly edematous glans with a concentric ring seen proximally to the coronal margin will include a physician into making the prompt diagnosis of paraphimosis (see Fig. 29.5) [39]. Over time the concentric ring proximal to the glans causes tissue edema and ultimately necrosis.

Manual reduction of the foreskin is the mainstay of treatment for paraphimosis [40]. The provider will place their thumb and index finger at the 3:00 and 9:00 position around the most narrow portion of the concentric phimotic ring. Using slow and steady pressure to reduce the surrounding lymphedema, the provider can slowly begin to pull the

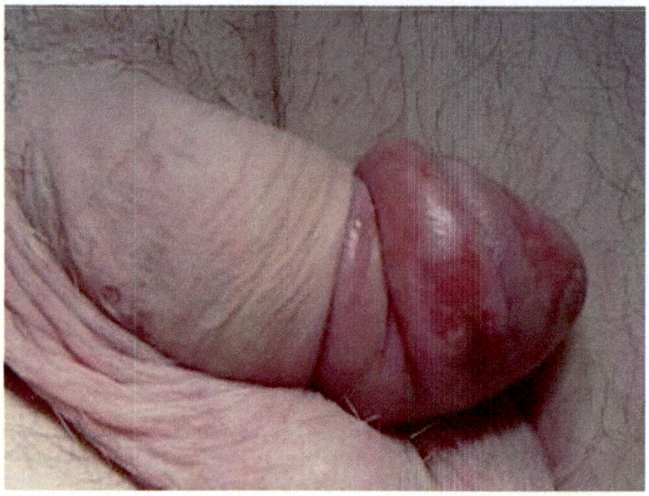

Fig. 29.5 Characteristic appearance of a tight phimotic ring retracted behind the coronal margin consistent with paraphimosis (Image adapted with permission from: http://www.foamem.com/2013/09/07/penile-problems/)

phimotic foreskin back to anatomic position. Typically a penile block with lidocaine can be used for patient comfort during the time of manual reduction [40].

I typically do not recommend the use of cold compression, osmotic diuresis, or other non-reducing interventions. If the phimotic ring is too tight and the edema too great to allow manual reduction of the paraphimosis, a urologic consultation is recommended. A urologist can perform either a dorsal slit across the concentric ring to alleviate the constriction or a circumcision [41].

Acute Urinary Retention

Acute urinary retention is defined by the inability to void and empty the bladder under full additional control. Typically patients present with a distended bladder and suprapubic fullness. In some cases, the patient may void small amounts of urine which is likely overflow incontinence. When acute urinary retention is not diagnosed and left untreated, this may lead to renal compromise, urinary tract infections, hydronephrosis, and/or kidney failure [42].

Urinary retention is most common in men and increases as men age. The etiology of urinary retention is multifactorial. Common etiologies of urinary retention include neurogenic, outlet obstruction, impaired detrusor contractility, medication induced, infection related, and postoperative [43]. Often a detailed history can elucidate whether the etiology is secondary to a neurologic condition versus outlet obstruction versus iatrogenic etiology such as medications.

Diagnosis and Treatment

Regardless of the etiology, urgent bladder decompression is mandated. Diagnosis can quickly be made with suprapubic palpation which may reveal a bladder distended up to the level of the umbilicus. Alternatively a latter ultrasound may be performed to document the amount of residual urine left in the bladder [44]. Laboratory tests are often not useful in the diagnosis of acute urinary retention; however long-standing retention may lead to chronic renal insufficiency.

The mainstay of treatment is urethral catheterization. Foley catheter placement is often low impact and provides an expeditious drainage to a fully distended bladder [42]. In women, urethral catheterization is seldom problematic. In men, however due to the possible outlet obstruction (i.e., and a large prostate, urethral stricture, etc.), urethral catheterization may be challenging [43]. It is my practice to attempt urethral catheterization in a man with suspected enlarged prostate with an 18 French Coudé tip catheter. In a man who I am suspecting a bladder neck contracture or urethral stricture, it is my practice to typically pass a 12 French silicone catheter. If catheterization attempts are not successful, a urologic consultation is warranted. The urologist may need to perform urethroscopy and/or urethral dilation and/or a suprapubic cystotomy.

Urinary Retention Algorithm

My algorithm for urinary retention utilizes a bladder scanner. If the patient has less than 200 mL of urine on bladder scan, an extended trial of void may be considered, i.e., an additional 4 h. If the bladder scanner is not available, my preference is for an in and out catheterization to assess the bladder volume. If the bladder volume is greater than 300 mL after an 8-h trial of void, initial management should utilize an in and out catheterization. This can be done with a Foley catheter with a balloon so that it may be left in place if the residual that is drained is greater than 600 mL. If the catheterization returns less than 600 mL, it is my preference that the catheter should be removed and the patient should be given another trial of void. I would typically wait 2–3 days prior to a repeat trial of void in patients that fail. In the interim, if the patient is an elderly male, I routinely initiate an alpha blocker. Minimizing narcotics, minimizing anticholinergic medications, assisting the patient with ambulation, ensuring there is no constipation, and pulling out infection are all strategies to improve the chances for repeat voiding success [43].

Long-Term Management

Following bladder decompression and failed repeat voiding trial attempts, patients with urinary retention and a catheter require follow-up with a urologist.

Difficult Catheter Insertion and Trauma

Urinary catheters are commonly used in critically ill patients for accurate urine output monitoring and bladder decompression. Despite their benign appearance, urinary catheters may cause urethral or prostatic trauma particularly in the male patient. Men with a large prostate or urethral narrowing (e.g., urethral stricture or bladder neck stenosis) may present extreme difficulty during urinary catheterization attempts. Repeated and unsuccessful attempts at catheterization may lead to catheter-associated trauma, injury to the urethra, pain, urinary tract infection, and potentially urethral stricture formation.

Initial attempt at urinary catheterization may be performed by healthcare providers unless there is a suspicion of urethral injury. If a urethral injury is suspected, a retrograde urethrogram is warranted prior to any attempt at urethral catheterization. Classic presenting symptoms of urethral injury include blood at the urethral meatus, a pelvic fracture with associated urinary retention, or a high riding prostate on digital rectal examination [45]. Assuming no suspicion of urethral injury, the type of urethral catheter chosen is dependent on the desired outcome and patient history.

The main types of urinary catheters include the Foley (self-retaining via inflatable balloon), straight catheters (no balloon), Coudé tip catheters (curved-tip Foley with or without balloon), and irrigation catheters (e.g., three-way catheters with a balloon). In addition, urinary catheters are manufactured with latex or silicone and in a multitude of sizes based on the French scale, whereby 1 French equals to 0.33 mm in circumferential diameter.

If an indwelling catheter is required, patient history can dictate the type of catheter used. For example, an elderly male with no prior urologic procedure history nor pelvic radiation who complains of nocturia and urinary hesitancy may be best served with an 18 French Coudé tip catheter to prevent a false passage due to prostatic enlargement. This is in contrast to a patient with a history of radical prostatectomy or prostatic radiation therapy who would be best served with a 12 French silicone catheter for presumed urethral or bladder neck stenosis.

In addition to determining patient risk factors that will guide catheter choice, here are several tips that I recommend for any routine catheterization: (1) inject 10–15 mL of lubricant or 1% lidocaine jelly via syringe directly into the urethral meatus and allow this to well for 3 min prior to catheterization, (2) place the penis on stretch prior to intubating the urethral meatus with a catheter, (3) always hub the catheter to the port prior to inflating the balloon, (4) ask the patient to breath throughout and not bear down to relax his/her external urinary sphincter during catheterization, and (5), if the first attempt is unsuccessful with a 16 French standard Foley catheter, consider switching to either an 18 French Coudé tip catheter or a 12 French silicone catheter depending on patient history.

The most common injuries related to traumatic urinary catheterization are a false passage created by forceful and repeated catheterization attempts [45]. The location of the false passage usually occurs just distal to the prostatomembranous urethra near the verumontanum. Bleeding is usually the first sign that a urethral injury has occurred secondary to traumatic catheterization. Urologic consultation is warranted after failure of repeated attempts following the catheterization tips provided above. Ironically, the treatment of choice following a traumatic catheterization is urethral rest for at least 7 days with a Foley catheter [46]. This may be achieved with the aid of a cystoscope and/or guide wiring to ensure proper seating of the Foley catheter balloon within the bladder. In the cases of prolonged catheterization attempts, a single dose of oral antibiotics is warranted (i.e., ciprofloxacin 500 mg) [45].

Conclusions

Common urologic problems face many practicing clinicians regardless of surgical subspecialty. The critical care and management of patients in whom a urologic condition is found requires prompt diagnosis and workup. It is my hope that this chapter guides a basic understanding of common urologic problems seen in critically ill patients. The collaborative approach between traumatologist, urologist, and intensivist is necessary for such complex conditions.

References

1. Davis R, et al. Diagnosis, evaluation and follow-up of asymptomatic microhematuria (AMH) in adults: AUA guideline. J Urol. 2012;188(6 Suppl):2473–81.
2. Messing EM, et al. Urinary tract cancers found by homescreening with hematuria dipsticks in healthy men over 50 years of age. Cancer. 1989;64(11):2361–7.
3. Halpern JA, Chughtai B, Ghomrawi H. Cost-effectiveness of common diagnostic approaches for evaluation of asymptomatic microscopic hematuria. JAMA Intern Med. 2017;177(6):800–7.
4. Avellino GJ, Bose S, Wang DS. Diagnosis and management of hematuria. Surg Clin North Am. 2016;96(3):503–15.
5. Patel JV, Chambers CV, Gomella LG. Hematuria: etiology and evaluation for the primary care physician. Can J Urol. 2008;15(Suppl 1):54–61; discussion 62.
6. Brede CM, Shoskes DA. The etiology and management of acute prostatitis. Nat Rev Urol. 2011;8(4):207–12.

7. Susanibar Napuri LF, et al. Prostatic abscess: diagnosis and treatment of an infrequent urological entity. Arch Esp Urol. 2011;64(1):62–6.
8. Vyas JB, et al. Transrectal ultrasound-guided aspiration in the management of prostatic abscess: a single-center experience. Indian J Radiol Imaging. 2013;23(3):253–7.
9. Taylor SN. Epididymitis. Clin Infect Dis. 2015;61(Suppl 8):S770–3.
10. McConaghy JR, Panchal B. Epididymitis: an overview. Am Fam Physician. 2016;94(9):723–6.
11. Redshaw JD, et al. Epididymitis: a 21-year retrospective review of presentations to an outpatient urology clinic. J Urol. 2014;192(4):1203–7.
12. Lancaster JW, et al. Update on treatment options for gonococcal infections. Pharmacotherapy. 2015;35(9):856–68.
13. Matthews SJ, Lancaster JW. Urinary tract infections in the elderly population. Am J Geriatr Pharmacother. 2011;9(5):286–309.
14. Ramakrishnan K, Scheid DC. Diagnosis and management of acute pyelonephritis in adults. Am Fam Physician. 2005;71(5):933–42.
15. Meiland R, Geerlings SE, Hoepelman AI. Management of bacterial urinary tract infections in adult patients with diabetes mellitus. Drugs. 2002;62(13):1859–68.
16. Rubilotta E, et al. Current clinical management of renal and perinephric abscesses: a literature review. Urologia. 2014;81(3):144–7.
17. Ubee SS, McGlynn L, Fordham M. Emphysematous pyelonephritis. BJU Int. 2011;107(9):1474–8.
18. Korkes F, et al. Xanthogranulomatous pyelonephritis: clinical experience with 41 cases. Urology. 2008;71(2):178–80.
19. Hagedorn JC, Wessells H. A contemporary update on Fournier's gangrene. Nat Rev Urol. 2016;14:205–14.
20. Singh A, et al. Fournier's gangrene. A clinical review. Arch Ital Urol Androl. 2016;88(3):157–64.
21. Chennamsetty A, et al. Contemporary diagnosis and management of Fournier's gangrene. Ther Adv Urol. 2015;7(4):203–15.
22. Pernetti R, et al. Fournier's gangrene: clinical case and review of the literature. Arch Ital Urol Androl. 2016;88(3):237–8.
23. Wallner C, et al. Reconstructive methods after Fournier gangrene. Urologe A. 2016;55(4):484–8.
24. Scales CD Jr, et al. Prevalence of kidney stones in the United States. Eur Urol. 2012;62(1):160–5.
25. Kamal BA, et al. Urethral calculi: presentation and management. BJU Int. 2004;93(4):549–52.
26. Pearle MS, et al. Medical management of kidney stones: AUA guideline. J Urol. 2014;192(2):316–24.
27. Segura JW, et al. Ureteral stones clinical guidelines panel summary report on the management of ureteral calculi. The American Urological Association. J Urol. 1997;158(5):1915–21.
28. Loftus C, et al. Medical expulsive therapy is underused for the management of renal colic in the emergency setting. J Urol. 2016;195(4 Pt 1):987–91.
29. Marien T, Miller NL. Treatment of the infected stone. Urol Clin North Am. 2015;42(4):459–72.
30. Liu L, et al. Technique selection of bricker or wallace ureteroileal anastomosis in ileal conduit urinary diversion: a strategy based on patient characteristics. Ann Surg Oncol. 2014;21(8):2808–12.
31. Rowland RG. Present experience with the Indiana pouch. World J Urol. 1996;14(2):92–8.
32. Hollowell CM, Christiano AP, Steinberg GD. Technique of Hautmann ileal neobladder with chimney modification: interim results in 50 patients. J Urol. 2000;163(1):47–50; discussion 50-1.
33. Pantuck AJ, et al. Ureteroenteric anastomosis in continent urinary diversion: long-term results and complications of direct versus nonrefluxing techniques. J Urol. 2000;163(2):450–5.
34. Cruz DN, Huot SJ. Metabolic complications of urinary diversions: an overview. Am J Med. 1997;102(5):477–84.
35. Farnham SB, Cookson MS. Surgical complications of urinary diversion. World J Urol. 2004;22(3):157–67.
36. Madersbacher S, et al. Long-term outcome of ileal conduit diversion. J Urol. 2003;169(3):985–90.
37. Terai A, et al. Urinary calculi as a late complication of the Indiana continent urinary diversion: comparison with the Kock pouch procedure. J Urol. 1996;155(1):66–8.
38. Falagas ME, Vergidis PI. Urinary tract infections in patients with urinary diversion. Am J Kidney Dis. 2005;46(6):1030–7.
39. Williams JC, Morrison PM, Richardson JR. Paraphimosis in elderly men. Am J Emerg Med. 1995;13(3):351–3.
40. Little B, White M. Treatment options for paraphimosis. Int J Clin Pract. 2005;59(5):591–3.
41. Schumacher J, Vaughan JT. Surgery of the penis and prepuce. Vet Clin North Am Equine Pract. 1988;4(3):473–91.
42. Kowalik U, Plante MK. Urinary retention in surgical patients. Surg Clin North Am. 2016;96(3):453–67.
43. Yoon PD, Chalasani V, Woo HH. Systematic review and meta-analysis on management of acute urinary retention. Prostate Cancer Prostatic Dis. 2015;18(4):297–302.
44. Sliwinski A, et al. Acute urinary retention and the difficult catheterization: current emergency management. Eur J Emerg Med. 2016;23(2):80–8.
45. Willette PA, Coffield S. Current trends in the management of difficult urinary catheterizations. West J Emerg Med. 2012;13(6):472–8.
46. Thomas K, Chow K, Kirby RS. Acute urinary retention: a review of the aetiology and management. Prostate Cancer Prostatic Dis. 2004;7(1):32–7.

Venous Thromboembolism, Prophylaxis, and Treatment (Including Fat Embolism Syndrome)

30

Franz S. Yanagawa and Elliott R. Haut

Introduction: Incidence and Impact

In 2008, the Surgeon General issued "a call to action to prevent DVT and PE." March was decreed DVT Awareness Month by the US Congress [1]. These two actions emphasize the importance of this disease that is diagnosed in 600,000 (with reported range of 350,000–900,000) [1] Americans yearly and kills over 100,000. Hence, the AHRQ (Agency for Healthcare Research and Quality) has deemed VTE prophylaxis paramount in the fight against preventable harm in healthcare and as a critically important step toward prevention of in-hospital mortality [2–4].

Now deemed a mostly preventable disease [5], but still not a "never event" [6], VTE prophylaxis protocols, patient risk factors, screening and diagnosing, the scope of the problem, and the impact of the disease need to be addressed and understood.

VTE is encountered more frequently in patients who have undergone surgery, are victims of trauma, harbor malignancy, or are treated in the intensive care unit [7–9]. In trauma patients, VTE is one of the most common complications, reported in up to 50–58% of patients, with potentially deadly outcomes. Patients who have undergone knee and hip replacements have a tenfold risk of developing a VTE [10].

Patients in the ICU (intensive care unit) are also at highly elevated risk for VTE [7], though many of these patients often have other risk factors which may account for this finding. Within this group, those who are mechanically ventilated have an incidence of PE of 10% and DVT of up to 25%, despite being on proper prophylaxis regimens [11, 12]. Some data suggest that despite being on proper prophylaxis, VTE is not preventable in up to 50% of cases [13].

From an economic standpoint, a significant VTE event can add $15,000–20,000 in added cost and can double the length of stay, resulting in yearly national spending as high as $10 billion [5]. Increased hospital readmission rates are also a consequence of VTE. As we move toward a pay-for-performance model, measures to prevent VTE are a significant potential area for advancement.

Definition

DVT (deep venous thrombosis) is either the complete or partial occlusion, typically in the lower extremities, due to the formation of clot within the deep venous system. A proximal DVT is defined as thrombosis involving any deep vein cephalad to the popliteal vein (i.e., iliac vein, common femoral vein). The name "superficial femoral vein" often arouses confusion since it is part of the deep venous system of the leg and a clot there is considered a true DVT. A distal DVT is thrombosis confined to the deep veins of the calf. PE (pulmonary embolism) is an occlusion of the lung vasculature (pulmonary artery system) and traditionally is believed to be an embolic process from a DVT [14]. However, there is literature that also indicates PEs can form primarily in the pulmonary vasculature and are referred to as primary pulmonary thrombosis [14]. PEs can range from small to massive, where a massive PE could occlude enough pulmonary vasculature to cause severe hemodynamic compromise (obstructive shock) and death. Massive PEs require immediate treatment such as thrombolysis, interventional radiology, or surgical intervention to lyse or remove the clot. Submassive PEs may manifest without hemodynamic compromise but can have significant right ventricular dysfunction and subsequent myonecrosis and failure.

F. S. Yanagawa
Department of Surgery, Johns Hopkins University School of Medicine, Baltimore, MD, USA

E. R. Haut (✉)
Department of Surgery, Anesthesiology/Critical Care Medicine (ACCM), and Emergency Medicine, Johns Hopkins University School of Medicine, Baltimore, MD, USA

Johns Hopkins University Bloomberg School of Public Health, Baltimore, MD, USA
e-mail: ehaut1@jhmi.edu

A. Salim et al. (eds.), *Surgical Critical Care Therapy*, https://doi.org/10.1007/978-3-319-71712-8_30

Risk Factors and Pathophysiology

Virchow's triad consists of venous stasis, hypercoagulability, and endothelial damage. A disease that increases any of these factors increases the change of a VTE. In the ICU, many patients have acquired risk factors including immobilization (e.g., secondary to spinal trauma, stroke, pharmacologic paralysis, and critical illness), indwelling venous catheters, and others [12, 15] (see Table 30.1). Patients in the surgical ICU often have preexisting comorbidities such as congestive heart failure or obesity. Many are admitted due to trauma and surgery secondary to neoplastic disease (some of whom are on hormone and chemotherapy) which are known as major or minor VTE risk factors [16] (please see Tables 30.2 and 30.3).

Endothelial damage may occur either through disease process (e.g., trauma) or iatrogenic etiologies (e.g., surgery or venous catheter placement) [17]. Disruption of the vessel causes release of tissue factor, thereby activating the coagulation cascade. Any compression, stretch, or crush of the vessel may cause endothelial injury without disruption of a vein. The body's recognition of vessel integrity and release of cytokines tips the balance to a relative hypercoagulable state. Thrombi can form within minutes of trauma. In the literature, there are cases where VTE in trauma patients manifested as early as the first day [18].

Table 30.2 Major VTE risk factors (In addition to acquired risks in the ICU)

1. Neoplasm/malignancy
2. Family or personal history of VTE
3. Major general surgery or surgical procedure >2 h
4. Multisystem trauma
5. Hip/leg fracture(s)
6. Knee/hip replacement(s)
7. Acute spinal fracture
8. Acute (<1 month) spinal cord injury
9. Acute (<1 month) stroke
10. Pregnancy and post-partum up to 6 weeks
11. Thrombophilias (factor V Leiden, protein C/S deficiency, lupus anticoagulant, Antiocardiolipin antibody, GP 21201A, MTHFR, etc.)
12. Obstructive sleep apnea

Table 30.3 Minor VTE risk factors (In addition to acquired risks in the ICU)

1. Prolonged sitting (e.g. in long automobile or airplane travel)
2. Laparoscopic surgery
3. Inflammatory bowel disease
4. Obesity
5. Infection
6. Varicose veins
7. AV (arteriovenous) malformations
8. Older age
9. Smoking
10. Estrogen and SERMS (selective estrogen receptor modulators)
11. Oral contraceptives

Patient Impact

Patients who develop a VTE, but do not have life-threatening consequences, still remain at risk for long-term sequelae. Patients may develop postphlebitic/post-thrombotic syndrome, chronic pulmonary hypertension, or recurrent VTE. They are also at risk from the necessary anticoagulation, which can cause life-threatening bleeding. In the RIETE (Registry of Patients with Venous Thromboembolism), a computerized registry devoted to elucidating the natural history of VTE started in March of 2001 and, as of 2012, reported 2.4% of patients suffered a major bleeding complication. Of these, 33% of patients died of fatal hemorrhage [19].

Table 30.1 Acquired VTE risk factors in patients in the ICU

1. Mechanical ventilation secondary to respiratory failure
2. New York Heart Association (NYHA) class III-IV heart failure
3. End stage renal disease (ESRD)
4. Sepsis (sepsis, severe sepsis, and septic shock)
5. Use of vasopressors
6. Use of pharmacologic sedation
7. Immobility (secondary to illness or trauma)
8. Central venous catheters
9. Platelet transfusion/factor transfusion
10. HIT (heparin-induced thrombocytopenia)
11. Neuromusclar blockade

Postphlebitic syndrome affects 23–60% of patients with DVT and is the result of venous insufficiency secondary to the destruction of the valves by the clot. Patients will suffer chronic edema, thickening and discoloration of the skin in up to 5–10% of cases, and can progress to ulceration and chronic wounds [20]. Up to 4% of patients following an acute PE will develop chronic pulmonary hypertension with resulting shortness of breath both with exertion and at times with rest, ultimately requiring rehabilitation to retain or improve function [21]. With the right heart in constant strain, many of these patients will die of right heart failure [22, 23]. Finally, the risk of a recurrent thrombosis is highest within the first 6–12 months after the index VTE event; however, it can persist with a 10-year risk of up to 30%.

VTE Prevention

Because the consequences of VTE, both acute and chronic, can be so dire, the cornerstone of managing VTE lies in its primary prevention and is improved the most by evaluating the care system and the component processes [2–4, 21, 24,

25]. Before the movement toward VTE prophylaxis, surgical patients had VTE rates of up to 19.1%, PE of 1.6% with 0.87% being fatal PEs. With the advent of VTE prophylaxis, the rate has fallen considerably to 2–3% after major general and oncologic surgeries. There are several national societies that provide guidelines that are well-researched and evidence-based, e.g., the EAST (Eastern Association for the Surgery of Trauma) [26], AAOS (American Academy of Orthopaedic Surgeons) [27], and ACCP (American College of Chest Physicians). Of these, the one most considered the definitive resource by many is the ACCP guidelines, which are updated every 4 years with the most recent 10th edition update released in February of 2016 [28]. Despite the fact that many guidelines exist, several studies indicate that patients are not routinely given proper prophylaxis [29, 30]. Current reccomendations concentrates on the integration of VTE prophylaxis in the electronic order system rather than the simple distribution of guidelines.

Pharmacologic Prophylaxis: Unfractionated Heparin and LMWH (Low Molecular Weight Heparin)

Because nearly all ICU patients acquire many of the risk factors, unless contraindicated, almost all patients in the ICU should receive pharmacologic prophylaxis. Those who have undergone surgery will likely have received a preoperative dose prior to incision, as this is now noted to be an important part of the preoperative time-out. Most commonly, unfractionated heparin and low molecular weight heparin (LMWH) are used postoperatively, and in many populations, there is no major advantage of one agent over the other. However, in the trauma and orthopedic literature, LMWH has been shown to be more advantageous [31]. For unfractionated heparin, dosing is usually given as 5000 units subcutaneously (SC) every 8 h for majority of patients [9]. For LMWH, the most common dosing for surgical patients is enoxaparin 40 mg SC daily and, in trauma patients, 30 mg two times daily. There is ongoing interest in higher-dose regimens for morbidly obese patients, although there are no definitive recommendations on this topic [32]. Recently, data has shown that missing even a single prophylactic dose is associated with significantly higher risk of developing VTE [33].

Pharmacologic Prophylaxis: Aspirin and Factor Xa Inhibitors

The question of aspirin (ASA) as an effective agent has been explored in the past. Devereaux et al. in 2014 examined 10,010 patients who underwent noncardiac surgery and were randomized to receive a prophylactic aspirin dose of 200 mg (vs. placebo) preoperatively, followed by 100 mg daily (vs. placebo). ASA was not shown to prevent VTE [34]. Though, following this, there have been few studies to suggest the efficacy of VTE prophylaxis [18], in particular in the orthopedic surgery population, making this an area of continued study.

An ongoing study is also evident in the literature for factor Xa inhibitors for VTE prophylaxis as well. Most of these studies are in orthopedic surgery and have been shown to be effective in patients undergoing total hip and knee replacements. In these studies, they suggest effectiveness in preventing VTE while not increasing the risk of bleeding [18]. As this area is still in investigation, there have been no guidelines that suggest the use of Xa inhibitors as primary VTE prophylaxis in other surgical populations or in the ICU.

Newer Approaches to Pharmacologic Prevention

Guidelines currently take a “one-size-fits-all” approach toward VTE prophylaxis. As we enter the age of precision medicine, technology to help tailor prophylaxis according to the risk factors of the individual patient and identification of which patients are at higher risk is in investigation. The rapid thromboelastography (TEG) is gaining attention in the prediction of those who develop DVTs. Van in 2009 explored whether the mA (maximum amplitude) of the TEG, a value which predicts the stability of the clot, could be used to predict patients on enoxaparin that would develop a DVT in critically ill patients [35]. Cotton continued this work in 2012 by examining the admission TEG mA to find those who would be at elevated risk for a PE during admission [36].

The focus on antiplatelet therapy is also changing as in trauma patients, Harr et al. in 2013 found that platelets play a significant role in hypercoagulability and confirmed once again in Allen et al.'s evaluation in 2015, suggesting that antiplatelet therapy could play a role in prophylaxis, adding another class of medications in our armamentarium against VTEs [37, 38].

Inferior Vena Cava (IVC) Filters

In the case where a high-risk patient cannot receive pharmacologic prophylaxis, an IVC filter can be considered for PE prevention, although there remains much disagreement on this recommendation in the literature. This issue has been studied primarily in trauma patients in the ICU who often present with a high risk of bleeding as well as multisystem injury, spinal cord injury, and/or severe traumatic brain injury. The EAST practice management guidelines offers a level III recommendation (based on expert opinion and retrospective studies) that an IVC filter can be placed prophylactically in trauma patients who are not able to be placed on pharmacologic VTE prophylaxis. These filters, when used in high-risk trauma patients, can prevent PE and fatal PE, but the numbers needed to treat are quite high [39]. This remains a controversial topic; other authors and the 2016 ACCP guidelines do not suggest placement of an IVC filter for the primary prevention of VTE [40].

IVC filters carry risk and are shown in certain populations (e.g., bariatric surgery patients) [33, 41] to increase morbidity and mortality and may have a higher risk of DVT thought to be related to the insertion via the femoral vein. Retrievable filters are recommended to be removed as soon as the VTE risk of the patient decreases. If placed in the ICU, planning for follow-up is paramount as in one study of 446 trauma patients who received removable IVC filters, only 22% had them removed after the risk of VTE had decreased [39]. Of newer interest in the ICU, there is now an FDA-approved device for temporary IVC filter placement which is incorporated into an indwelling femoral venous line that assures filter removal [42].

Mechanical Prophylaxis

Thromboembolic deterrent stockings (TEDS) or graduated compression stockings were shown to reduce VTE by nearly 70% compared to placebo, although these data were from the era before pharmacologic prophylaxis [43]. Sequential compression devices (SCDs) are preferred over stockings alone. Interestingly, the length of stockings has been debated in the past and was examined prevention of VTE in patients with stroke. Thigh-length stockings were noted to have a higher VTE prevention rate [44]. Use of SCDs and TEDS is not entirely without risk; they are associated with ulceration and skin breakdown in ICU patients and those with peripheral vascular disease or chronic leg wounds. For patients with acute DVT, a recent change in the ACCP guidelines *does not* recommend usage of compression stockings [45]. Interestingly, although commonly thought to be a risk for in-hospital falls, SCDs have not been shown to increase patient falls [46]. Compliance with these devices is generally poor, even the hospital setting in which they are frequently noted to be in place only about 50% of the time when audited [47]. Ambulation is often emphasized as an effective method of VTE prophylaxis. While ambulation has benefits in ICU patients, there is little evidence to support its use as a replacement for either mechanical or pharmacologic VTE prophylaxis [48].

Diagnosis

For critically ill patients, VTE is often difficult to diagnose as signs and symptoms are non-specific and there is significant variability between patients. Physical examination is unhelpful in the diagnosis as ICU patients rarely manifest signs and symptoms of VTE specifically [49]. DVT can cause generalized fever or local changes including edema, discoloration, or erythema of the leg, but these are common findings in ICU patients. PE may present with tachycardia, tachypnea, hypoxemia, agitation, diaphoresis, or cardiac arrest in the worst of cases. Although PE must be considered in these patients, other diagnoses are also likely and often must be considered simultaneously [50]. In the awake and communicable patient, symptoms may include acute-onset leg or chest pain. Pleuritic chest pain is often the result of smaller emboli which occlude distal branches and cause pleurisy. Larger emboli will manifest with varying degree signs ranging from narrowed pulse pressure, jugular venous distention, pulmonary hypertension, and right heart strain which can lead to overt obstructive shock. An EKG most commonly reveals sinus tachycardia, although classically, the S1-Q3-T3 pattern is suggestive of PE. High suspicion and low threshold for further investigation are required in these patients. PE should be considered in the differential diagnosis for nearly all ICU patients with sudden onset of chest pain, tachycardia, hypoxia, shock, and/or cardiac arrest.

ABG and D-Dimer

The ABG may be used as a screening tool for PE by calculating the pulmonary alveolar-arterial gradient (Aa gradient). An increased Aa gradient suggests a V/Q (ventilation/perfusion) mismatch, therefore increasing the suspicion for PE. However, the specificity of this test is low, given that patients in the ICU may have variable reasons for increased Aa gradient.

The D-dimer is more commonly used in the outpatient and emergency department setting to rule out VTE due to its high sensitivity and high negative predictive value. The D-dimer is a measure of the final degradation product of fibrin, often elevated in patients with VTE. But the D-dimer is non-specific and can be elevated in patients who are post-surgical, victims of trauma, inflammation, or infection [51]. In the ICU, it is likely underused since it is frequently assumed that the level is elevated in all ICU patients. D-dimer can be quite useful if the test is normal, effectively ruling out VTE. However, an elevated D-dimer should not be used in isolation as a confirmatory test for VTE [52].

Duplex Ultrasound

Venography was the historic gold standard for the diagnosis of both DVT and PE [24, 53]. However, in the current era, DVT is almost always diagnosed with a duplex ultrasound. Cheap, non-invasive, and non-contrast, the duplex ultrasound uses the B-mode, color flow Doppler, and pulsed Doppler spectral analysis to identify clot within the venous system. In the era of increasing use of point-of-care ultrasound, the rapid diagnosis of DVT can be within the reach of clinical providers in the ICU [54]. The ultrasound, being inexpensive and noninvasive, can also be used as a surveillance tool but when used to "look for the sake of looking" may detect clinically silent and insignificant DVTs, raising the rate of DVT, and when used as a measure of quality may hurt the reputation of the health system [52].

An acute DVT is diagnosed by a *hypo*echoic thrombus within a non-compressible vein with accompanied "spongy" clot texture and acute venous dilatation secondary to venous hypertension. The possibility for embolization is increased in clots that have flow around the clot, signifying an incomplete adherence to the vessel wall. In contrast, a chronic DVT is *hyper*echoic, adherent to a non-compressible or partially compressible vessel, and accompanied by valvular reflux [55].

CTA (Computed Tomography Angiography)

A multidetector helical CT angiography, though sometimes limited by the patient who cannot receive contrast, has replaced the traditional invasive angiography as the choice modality for diagnosis of PE [56]. The benefits of CTA are the speed and accuracy with which it can be obtained, along with the other diagnoses it can rule in or out [53]. Unfortunately, there remain real risks including those associated with IV contrast and the need for transport of an unstable ICU patient [57, 58]. With the recent advancements in CT resolution, it is able to visualize segmental and subsegmental branches of the pulmonary arteries [53, 56]. However, the clinical significance and the treatment of these smaller emboli are still controversial.

Echocardiogram (Echo)

With the increasing use of bedside point-of-care ultrasound in the ICU, echo can be quite useful for the patient with undifferentiated shock [59]. The benefits of echo include the rapidity of diagnosis and no need for transport, and it may also be used in patients who cannot tolerate IV contrast. Findings such as right ventricular dilation, right atrial dilation, ventricular shift toward the left ventricle, or pulmonary artery dilation are signs suggestive of PE. In a patient with confirmed PE, the degree of right ventricular strain and dilation could prompt a more aggressive treatment than therapeutic anticoagulation.

V/Q Scan

Ventilation/perfusion (V/Q) scan is used in patients who have severe allergy to contrast or with renal insufficiency and cannot undergo contrast-enhanced computed tomography angiography (CTA). It is a two-part study where a patient inhales radioisotopes to evaluate ventilation and receives radioisotopes also to evaluate pulmonary flow. The study determines whether there is a mismatch. Results are presented as low, medium, or high probability of PE. Although still an option, it is rarely used in ICU patients as it is more likely to be indeterminate in patients with an underlying abnormal CXR from other simultaneous underlying pathologies.

Treatment

Therapeutic Anticoagulation

Once VTE is diagnosed, first-line treatment is therapeutic (vs. prophylactic) anticoagulation. Most commonly, patients are placed on an unfractionated heparin drip, ideally with a bolus, with a goal activated partial thromboplastin time (aPTT) of 65–90 s. There is some data to suggest that the use of LMWH at 2 mg/kg SC daily or 1 mg/kg SC twice daily is superior to unfractionated heparin (in selected patients), although this approach may be less useful in the ICU [60]. In patients with high suspicion for VTE, therapy should be immediately initiated while diagnostic tests are underway. Duration of therapy by the most recent ACCP guidelines is 3 months for both DVT and PE, although the exact duration can depend on the underlying condition, whether the event was provoked (i.e., by surgery), response to therapy, and whether it was a first-time or recurrent VTE.

Thrombolysis and Thrombectomy

Clot burden that produces hemodynamic instability should prompt consideration of emergent therapy with thrombolysis (please see Fig. 30.1). The ACCP guidelines delineate a grade 2C recommendation of "systemically administered thrombolytic therapy" for 2 h through a peripheral catheter. In the same guidelines, catheter-directed thrombolysis is recommended in patients with contraindication to systemic thrombolysis or for patients in shock that would result in

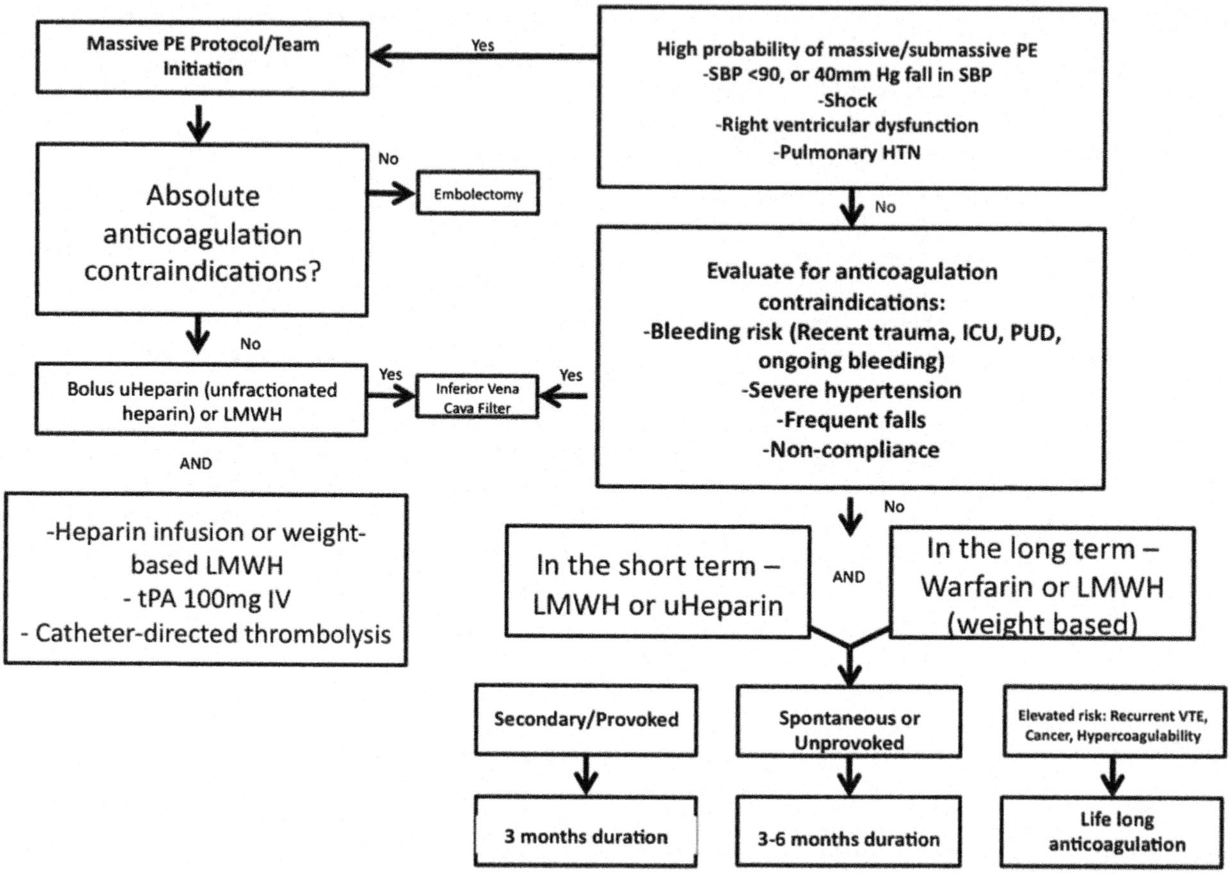

Fig. 30.1 Massive PE protocol

death before systemic thrombolysis can take effect [50]. In the case where patients are refractory to thrombolysis or are moribund secondary to severe shock, a surgical pulmonary embolectomy is recommended. Recently, newer technology such as PAT (percutaneous aspiration thrombectomy) and/or PMT (percutaneous mechanical thrombectomy) balloon maceration of clot has gained some popularity and is shown to have promising results [61]. The ongoing ATTRACT trial is examining the use of percutaneous treatment options for an expanded group of patients with DVT in hopes to lessen the long-term risk and complications of DVT [62].

Pulmonary Embolism Response Team Model

Considering the wide range of therapeutic options for patients with acute PE, there is a surge in the development of rapidly deployable, multidisciplinary teams to consider all therapeutic options for acute PE management. These teams usually consist of combination of critical care intensivists, cardiologists, pulmonologists, cardiac surgeons, vascular surgeons, and/or interventional radiologists. These teams have been proposed as the fastest way to get input from experts who can consider local expertise to devise and execute the optimal treatment in a timely fashion [63–65].

Fat Embolism

Fat embolism is a rare (1–2% incidence in trauma patients) complication, usually after orthopedic surgery or long bone fracture, but described sparsely in the literature secondary to other surgical procedures [61, 65]. A fat embolus is thought to be caused by the presence of droplets of fat in the circulation. The syndrome manifests with a classic triad of pulmonary, skin, and central nervous system changes. It is diagnosed with at least one major and four minor criteria originally described in 1874 by Gurd. Respiratory symptoms dominate with 90% of cases reporting dyspnea (please see Table 30.4). The symptoms, like VTE, are non-specific and may not be easily separated from other cases of respiratory distress [61].

Pathophysiology is poorly understood but consists primarily of two potential mechanisms. Though usually associated with a history of trauma and long bone fracture, there

Table 30.4 Gurd's (1974) criteria: major and minor of FES

Major criteria	Minor criteria
1. Hypoxemia (<60 mmHg O_2)	1. Fever (>39 °C)
2. Confusion	2. Tachycardia (>120 beats/min)
3. Petechial rash	3. Retinal petechiae
	4. Oliguria/anuria
	5. Anemia (Hemoglobin drop of 20%)
	6. Thrombocytopenia (50% drop)
	7. ESR > 71 mm/h
	8. Fat macroglobinemia

have been accounts of fat emboli in patients who did not have any traumatic injury [67]. The mechanical theory was first proposed by Gauss in 1924 [61] and suggests that an acute increase in the intramedullary pressure expels marrow fat into the injured vessels at the site of a fracture. These emboli then obstruct the pulmonary capillaries and cause a V/Q mismatch. Three years later, Moore and Lehmann proposed the biochemical mechanism suggesting that once a fat embolus is trapped in the pulmonary capillary, free fatty acids and glycerol cause an inflammatory cascade that results in what is now known as acute respiratory distress syndrome (ARDS). This latter mechanism may explain the typical subacute presentation of FES about 48–72 h after the initial injury. Unlike VTE, FES has no definitive gold standard diagnostic test or specific treatment other than supportive care. Emphasis is placed on early intramedullary nailing of long bone fractures as there is a fivefold decrease in the incidence of FES when surgery is performed within the first 24 h of injury. Although further investigation is needed, there is some thought that corticosteroids offer a protective measure and decreases the incidence of FES [68].

References

1. US Department of Health and Human Services. Surgeon general's call to action to prevent deep vein thrombosis and pulmonary embolism 2008. Available at: http://www.ncbi.nlm.nih.gov/books/NBK44178/.
2. Maynard G, Stein J. Preventing hospital-acquired venous thromboembolism: a guide for effective quality improvement. Prepared by the Society of Hospital Medicine. AHRQ publication no. 08-0075. Agency for Healthcare Research and Quality: Rockville, MD; 2008.
3. Shekelle PG, Pronovost PJ, Wachter RM, et al. The top patient safety strategies that can be encouraged for adoption now. Ann Intern Med. 2013;158:365–8.
4. Haut ER, Lau BD. Chapter 28: prevention of venous thromboembolism: brief update review. In: Making health care safer II: an updated critical analysis of the evidence for patient safety practices, vol. 211. Rockville, MD: Agency for Healthcare Research and Quality; 2013. p. C-62.
5. Shojania KG, Duncan BW, McDonald KM, Wachter RM, Markowitz AJ. Making health care safer: a critical analysis of patient safety practices. Evid Rep Technol Assess (Summ). 2001;i-x:1–668.
6. Streiff MB, Haut ER. The CMS ruling on venous thromboembolism after Total knee or hip arthroplasty: weighing risks and benefits. JAMA – J Am Med Assoc. 2009;301(10):1063–5.
7. Attia J, Ray JG, Cook DJ, Douketis J, Ginsberg JS, Geerts WH. Deep vein thrombosis and its prevention in critically ill adults. Arch Intern Med. 2001;161(10):1268–79.
8. Minet C, Potton L, Bondadona A, et al. Venous thromboembolism in the ICU: main characteristics, diagnosis and thromboprophylaxis. Crit Care. 2015;19(1):287.
9. McLeod AG, Geerts W. Venous thromboembolism prophylaxis in critically ill patients. Crit Care Clin. 2011;27:765–80.
10. Kabrhel C, Rosovsky R, Channick R, et al. A multidisciplinary pulmonary embolism response team (PERT): initial 30-month experience with a novel approach to delivery of care to patients with sub-massive and massive PE. Chest. 2016;150(2):384–93.
11. Ibrahim EH, Iregui M, Prentice D, Sherman G, Kollef MH, Shannon W. Deep vein thrombosis during prolonged mechanical ventilation despite prophylaxis. Crit Care Med. 2002;30(4):771–4.
12. Cook D, Crowther M, Meade M, et al. Deep venous thrombosis in medical-surgical critically ill patients: prevalence, incidence, and risk factors. Crit Care Med. 2005;33:1565–71.
13. Haut ER, Lau BD, Kraus PS, et al. Preventability of hospital-acquired venous thromboembolism. JAMA Surg. 2015;150(9):912–5.
14. Velmahos GC, Spaniolas K, Tabbara M, et al. Pulmonary embolism and deep venous thrombosis in trauma: are they related? Arch Surg. 2009;144(10):928–32.
15. Merrer J, De Jonghe B, Golliot F, et al. Complications of femoral and subclavian venous catheterization in critically ill patients: a randomized controlled trial. JAMA. 2001;286:700–7.
16. Kaplan D, Casper TC, Elliott CG, et al. VTE incidence and risk factors in patients with severe sepsis and septic shock. Chest. 2015;148(5):1224–30.
17. Caprini JA, Arcelus JI, Hasty JH, et al. Clinical assessment of venous thromboembolic risk in surgical patients. Semin Thromb Hemost. 1991;17(suppl 3):304–12.
18. Kapoor A, et al. Comparative effectiveness of venous thromboembolism prophylaxis options for the patient undergoing total hip and knee replacement: a network meta-analysis. J Thromb Haemost. 2016;14:1–11.
19. Ruíz-Giménez N, Suárez C, González R, et al. Predictive variables for major bleeding events in patients presenting with documented acute venous thromboembolism. Findings from the RIETE registry. Thromb Haemost. 2008;100:26–31.
20. Kearon C. Natural history of venous thromboembolism. Circulation. 2003;107(23 Suppl 1):I22–30.
21. Haut ER, Lau BD, Kraenzlin FS, et al. Improve prophylaxis and decreased rates of preventable harm with the use of a mandatory computerized clinical decision support tool for prophylaxis for venous thromboembolism in trauma. Arch Surg. 2012;147(10):901–7.
22. Ozier Y, Dubourg O, Farcot JC, Bazin M, Jardin F, Margairaz A. Circulatory failure in acute pulmonary embolism. Intensive Care Med. 1984;10(2):91–7.
23. Gazmuri RJ, Patel DJ, Stevens R, Smith S. Circulatory collapse, right ventricular dilation, and alveolar dead space: a triad for the rapid diagnosis of massive pulmonary embolism. Am J Emerg Med. 2016;35:936.e1–4. (online publication).
24. Bilimoria KY. Facilitating quality improvement: pushing the pendulum back toward process measures. JAMA. 2015;314(13):1333–4.
25. Aboagye JK, Lau BD, Schneider EB, Streiff MB, Haut ER. Linking processes and outcomes: a key strategy to prevent and report harm from venous thromboembolism in surgical patients. JAMA Surg. 2013;148(3):299–300.

26. Rogers FB, Cipolle MD, Velmahos G, Rozycki G, Luchette FA. Practice management guidelines for the prevention of venous thromboembolism in trauma patients: the EAST practice management guidelines work group. J Trauma. 2002;53(1):142–64.
27. Johanson NA, Lachiewicz PF, Lierberman JR, et al. American Academy of Orthopaedic Surgeons clinical practice guideline on prevention of symptomatic pulmonary embolism in patients undergoing total hip or knee arthroplasty. J Bone Joint Surg Am. 2009;91(7):1756–7.
28. Guyatt GH, Akl EA, Crowther M, et al. Antithrombotic therapy and prevention of thrombosis, 9th ed: American College of Chest Physicians evidence-based clinical practice guidelines. Chest. 2012;141(2):48–52.
29. Goldhaber SZ, Tapson VF, DVT FREE Steering Committee. A prospective registry of 5,451 patients with ultrasound-confirmed deep vein thrombosis. Am J Cardiol. 2004;93(2):259.
30. Cohen AT, Tapson VF, Bergmann JF, Goldhaber SZ, Kakkar AK, Deslandes B, Huang W, Zayaruzny M, Emery L, Anderson FA Jr, Investigators ENDORSE. Venous thromboembolism risk and prophylaxis in the acute hospital care setting (ENDORSE study): a multinational cross-sectional study. Lancet. 2008;371(9610):387–94.
31. Beitland S, Sandven I, Lill-Kristin K, Sandset PM, Sunde K, Eken T. Thromboprophylaxis with low molecular weight heparin versus unfractionated heparin in intensive care patients: a systematic review with meta-analysis and trial sequential analysis. Intensive Care Med. 2015;4:1209–19.
32. Brotman DJ, Shihab HM, Prakasa KR, et al. Pharmacologic and mechanical strategies for preventing venous thromboembolism after bariatric surgery: a systematic review and meta-analysis. JAMA Surg. 2013;148(7):675–86.
33. Louis SG, Sato M, Geraci T, et al. Correlation of missed doses of enoxaparin with increased incidence of deep vein thrombosis in trauma and general surgery patients. JAMA Surg. 2014;149(4):365–70.
34. Devereaux PJ, et al. Aspirin in patients undergoing non-cardiac surgery. NEJM. 2014;370(16):1494–502.
35. Van P, Cho D, Underwood S, et al. Thromboelastography versus antifactor Xa levels in the assessment of prophylactic dose enoxaparin in critically ill patients. J Trauma. 2009;66(6):1509–15.
36. Cotton BA, Minei KM, Radwan Z, et al. Admission rapid thromboelastography predicts development of pulmonary embolism in trauma patients. J Trauma Acute Care Surg. 2012;72(6):1470–5.
37. Harr J, Moore E, Chin T, et al. Platelets are dominant contributors to hypercoagulability after injury. J Trauma Acute Care Surg. 2013;74(3):756–65.
38. Allen C, Clark M, Meizoso J, et al. Coagulation profile changes due to thromboprophylaxis and platelets in trauma patients at high risk for venous thromboembolism. Am Surg. 2015;81:663–8.
39. Haut ER, Garcia LJ, Shihab HM, et al. The effectiveness of prophylactic inferior vena cava (IVC) filters in trauma patients: a systematic review and meta-analysis. JAMA Surg. 2014;149(2):194–202.
40. Hemmila M, Osborne N, Henke P, Kepros J, Patel S, Cain-Nielsen A, Birkmeyer N. Prophylactic inferior vena cava filter placement does not results in a survival benefit for trauma patients. Ann Surg. 2015;262(4):577–85.
41. Sing RF, Camp SM, Heniford BT, Rutherford EJ, Dix S, Reilly PM, Holmse JH, Haut E, Hayanga A. Timing of pulmonary emboli after trauma: implications for retrievable vena cava filters. J Trauma. 2006;60:732–4; discussion 734–5.
42. Taccone FS, Bunker N, Waldmann C, De Backer D, Brohi K, Jones RG, Vincent JL. A new device for the prevention of pulmonary embolism in critically ill patients: results of the European Angel Catheter Registry. J Trauma Acute Care Surg. 2015;79(3):456–62.
43. Sachdeva A, Dalton M, Amaragiri SV, Lees T. Graduated compression stockings for prevention of deep vein thrombosis. Cochrane Database Syst Rev. 2014;17(12):CD001484.
44. The CLOTS (Clots in Legs Or sTockings after Stroke) Trial Collaboration. Thigh-length versus below-knee stockings for deep venous thrombosis prophylaxis after stroke: a randomized trial. Ann Intern Med. 2010;153(9):553–62.
45. Hobson DB, Chang TY, Aboagye JK, Lau BD, Shihab HM, Fisher B, Young S, Sujeta N, Shaffer DL, Popoola VO, Kraus PS, Knorr G, Farrow NE, Streiff MB, Haut ER. Prevalence of graduated compression stocking associated pressure injuries in surgical intensive care units. J Crit Care. 2017;40:1–6. accepted, in press.
46. Boelig M, Streiff MB, Hobson DB, Kraus PS, Pronovost PJ, Haut ER. Are sequential compression devices commonly associated with in-hospital falls? A myth-busters review using the patient safety net database. J Patient Saf. 2011;7:77–9.
47. Chang D, Velmahos G, Jindal A, Baker D, Phillips J, Bonar J, Campbell K. Compliance with sequential compression device prophylaxis in at-risk trauma patients: a prospective analysis. Am Surg. 2002;68(5):470–3.
48. Lau BD, Streiff MB, Kraus PS, et al. No evidence to support ambulation for reducing postoperative venous thromboembolism. J Am Coll Surg. 2014;219(5):1101–3. Haut ER, Garcia LJ, Shihab HM, et al. The effectiveness of prophylactic inferior vena cava (IVC) filters in trauma patients: a systematic review and meta-analysis. JAMA Surg. 2014;149(2):194–202.
49. Crowther MA, Cook DJ, Griffith LE, et al. Deep venous thrombosis: clinically silent in the intensive care unit. J Crit Care. 2005;20:334–40.
50. Goktay A, Senturk C. Endovascular treatment of thrombosis and embolism. In: Shaidul Islam M, editor. Thrombosis and embolism: from research to clinical practice. 1st ed. Philadelphia, PA: Elsevier; 2016. p. 195–213.
51. Crowther MA, Cook DJ, Griffith LE, et al. Neither baseline tests of molecular hypercoagulability nor d dimer levels predict deep venous thrombosis in critically ill medical surgical patients. Intensive Care Med. 2005;31(1):48–55.
52. Bilimoria KY, Chung J, Ju M, et al. Evaluation of surveillance bias and the validity of the venous thromboembolism quality measure. JAMA. 2013;310(14):1482–9.
53. Quiroz R, Kucher N, Zou KH, et al. Clinical validity of a negative computed tomography scan in patients with suspected pulmonary embolism: a systematic review. JAMA. 2005;293:2012–7.
54. Oks M, Cleven KL, Cardenas-Garcia J, Schaub JA, Koenig S, Cohen RI, Mayo PH, Narasimhan M. The effect of point-of-care ultrasonography on imaging studies in the medical ICU: a comparative study. Chest. 2014;146(6):1574–7.
55. Barleben A, Bandyk D. Interpretation of peripheral venous duplex testing. Semin Vasc Surg. 2013;26(2-3):111–9.
56. Meinel FG, Nance JW Jr, Schoepf UJ, et al. Predictive value of computed tomography in acute pulmonary embolism: systematic review and meta-analysis. Am J Med. 2015;128(7):747–59.
57. Hurst JM, Davis K, Johnson DJ, Branson RD, Campbell RS, Branson PS. Cost and complications during in-hospital transport of critically ill patients: a prospective cohort study. J Trauma. 1992;33(4):582–5.
58. Szem JW, Hydo LJ, Fischer E, Kapur S, Klemperer J, Barie PS. High-risk intrahospital transport of critically ill patients:safety and outcome of the necessary "road trip". Crit Care Med. 1995;23(10):1660–6.
59. Atkinson P, Bowra J, Milne J, Lewis D, Lambert M, Jarman B, Noble EV, Lamprecht H, Harris T, Connolly J. International Federation for Emergency Medicine Consensus Statement: sonography in hypotension and cardiac arrest (SHoC): an international consensus on the use of point of care ultrasound for undifferentiated hypotension and during cardiac arrest. CJEM. 2016;21:1–12.
60. Byrne J, Geerts M, Stephanie A, Gomez D, Hoeft C, Murphy R, Neal M, Nathens A. Effectiveness of low-molecular-weight heparin versus unfractionated heparin to prevent pulmonary embolism

following major trauma: a propensity-matched analysis. J Trauma Acute Care Surg. 2017;82(2):252–62.
61. Gauss H. Pathophysiology of fat embolism, a review. Arch Surg. 1924;9:593–603.
62. Vedantham S, Goldhaber SZ, Kahn SR, Julian J, Magnuson E, Jaff MR, Murphy TP, Cohen DJ, Comerota AJ, Gornik HL, Razavi MK, Lewis L, Kearon C. Rationale and design of the ATTRACT study: a multicenter randomized trial to evaluate pharmacomechanical catheter-directed thrombolysis for the prevention of postthrombotic syndrome in patients with proximal deep vein thrombosis. Am Heart J. 2013;165(4):523–30.
63. Kabrhel C, Jaff MR, Channick RN, Baker JN, Rosenfield K. A multidisciplinary pulmonary embolism response team. Chest. 2013;144(5):1738–9.
64. Provias T, Dudzinski DM, Jaff MR, et al. The Massachusetts general hospital pulmonary embolism response team (MGH PERT): creation of a multidisciplinary program to improve care of patients with massive and submassive pulmonary embolism. Hosp Pract. 2014;42(1):31–7.
65. Deveraux PJ, et al. The perioperative ischemia evaluation-2 trial and a pooled analysis of randomized trials. Anesthesiology. 2016;125:1121–9.
66. Scarpino M, et al. Cerebral fat embolism after video-assisted thoracic surgery. Ann Thorac Surg. 2016;102:409–11.
67. Lehman P, Moore E. Fat embolism including experimental production without trauma. Arch Surg. 1927;14:621–62.
68. Moreau JP. Fat embolism: a review and report of 100 cases. Can J Surg. 1974;17:196–9.

Blood Products and Transfusion Therapy in the ICU

31

Damon Forbes

Introduction

Anemia and coagulopathy are among the most commonly encountered hematologic disorders in critically ill and injured patients [1]. Approximately two-thirds of ICU patients present with a hemoglobin of less than 12 g/dL on admission [2–5]. In addition, greater than one-third of patients develop some form of coagulation abnormality during their ICU stay to include thrombocytopenia, prolonged coagulation times, and abnormal thrombolysis [6–8]. These disorders are particularly prevalent in surgical and trauma ICU populations, where major hemorrhage and coagulopathy are frequently both present and interrelated. The multifactorial nature and multisystem impacts of major hemorrhage and coagulopathy must be taken into consideration and factored in to decisions regarding treatment and interventions, of which transfusion therapy is arguably among the most important (Fig. 31.1).

Given the high incidence of these hematologic disorders, greater than 50% of patients receive blood transfusions during their ICU stay [5, 9]. As with many other critical care interventions, these therapies are not without risks and can result in overall harm, rather than benefit, if used improperly. Most transfusion reactions are benign in nature, although more severe, potentially fatal reactions can occur. The optimal treatment of ICU-related anemia and coagulopathy remains an area of ongoing controversy and research. Like many other areas of critical care, past transfusion paradigms often focused on attempting to "normalize" the physiology and laboratory values of critically ill patients. This approach has not only been shown to have little benefit, but in many cases it can result in net harm to the patient. Consequently, it is of paramount importance that ICU physicians have a firm grasp of these concepts. In this chapter, we will briefly review the etiology and physiological effects of anemia, as well as key aspects of transfusion medicine, focusing on specific types of blood products, indications for transfusion, and potential transfusion-related complications.

D. Forbes (✉)
Pulmonary & Critical Care Service, Womack Army Medical Center, 2817 Reilly Rd, Ft. Bragg, 28310 NC, USA
e-mail: damon.a.forbes.mil@mail.mil

Etiology of Anemia in Critical Illness

In critically ill patients, anemia typically results from two fundamental processes: loss of circulating red blood cells (RBCs) and decreased RBC production [2]. Anemia due to blood loss can be subdivided into disease-specific and secondary factors. Traumatic injuries, gastrointestinal hemorrhage, intrinsic coagulopathy, and hemolysis are examples of disease-specific processes that may contribute to the loss of circulating RBC volume. Other secondary causes are largely iatrogenic and include repetitive blood sampling for diagnostic testing, vascular cannulation, renal replacement therapy, and various surgical procedures [10]. Serial phlebotomy is a near-universal, but often underappreciated, source of blood loss in ICU patients. The average volume of blood drawn for routine laboratory testing is 40–70 milliliters (mL) per day [3, 11]. The cumulative effect of this ongoing blood loss can be substantial and may account for up to 30% of blood transfusions in the ICU setting [12]. Minimizing unnecessary laboratory testing may help to mitigate this problem.

Diminished RBC production is often multifactorial. Nutritional deficiencies (e.g., iron, folate, and vitamin B12) result in decreased metabolic substrates for RBC production. In addition, many critically ill patients develop an "anemia of inflammation" (also referred to as the anemia of chronic disease) during their ICU course. Systemic inflammation can lead to a blunted erythropoietin response, alterations in iron metabolism, and impaired bone marrow cellular signaling [13, 14]. These processes, in total, contribute to the development of anemia in critically ill patients.

A. Salim et al. (eds.), *Surgical Critical Care Therapy*, https://doi.org/10.1007/978-3-319-71712-8_31

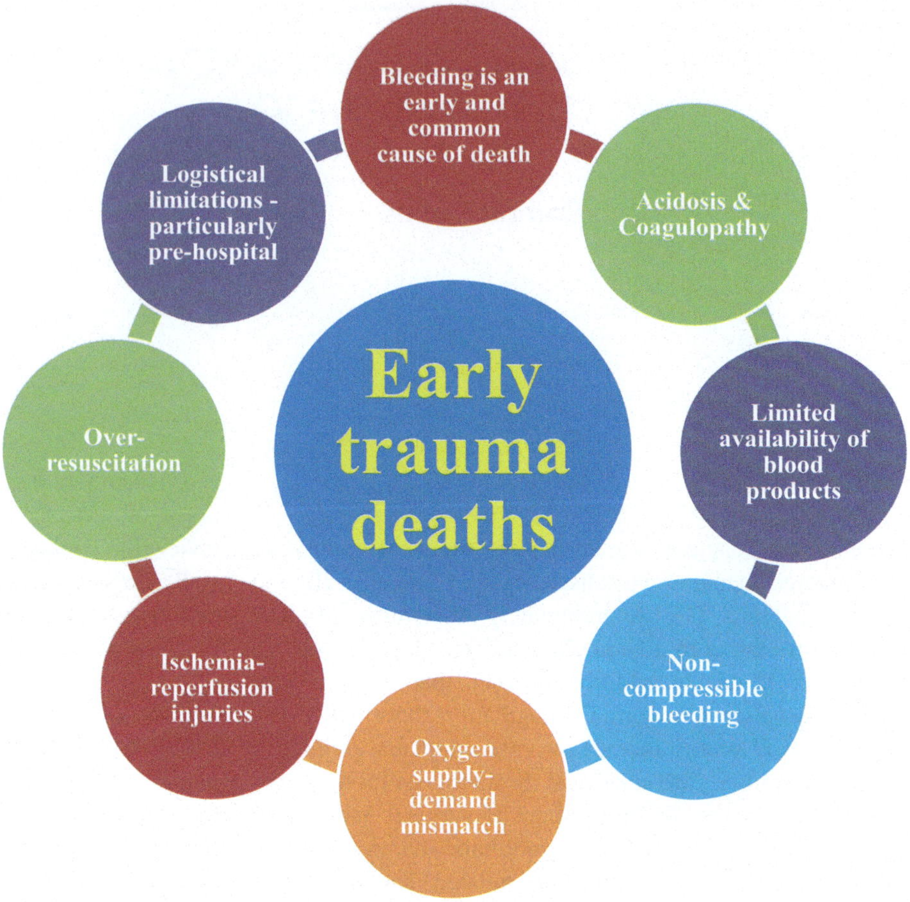
Bleeding is an early and common cause of death
Acidosis & Coagulopathy
Limited availability of blood products
Non-compressible bleeding
Oxygen supply-demand mismatch
Ischemia-reperfusion injuries
Over-resuscitation
Logistical limitations - particularly pre-hospital
Early trauma deaths

Fig. 31.1 Multiple challenges and issues surrounding the central problem of early trauma deaths due to massive bleeding requiring transfusion therapy (Modified with permission from Martin et al. [133])

Physiological Effects of Anemia

Anemia triggers a variety of compensatory physiologic changes. In healthy patients subjected to normovolemic hemodilution, cardiac output *increases* due to decreased blood viscosity and catecholamine-mediated increases in heart rate and myocardial contractility. Other physiologic responses include redistribution of blood flow to critical organs (e.g., heart and brain) and increases in the oxygen extraction ratio [15]. The extent to which these changes occur depends greatly on how quickly the hemoglobin concentration decreases, the physiologic reserve of the patient, and the volume status of the patient.

Patients generally tolerate chronic anemia better due to changes that occur at the cellular level [16]. However, the presence of significant underlying cardiopulmonary disease may impair a patient's ability to compensate for reductions in hemoglobin concentration. The myocardium is particularly at risk in the setting of acute, severe anemia, as the compensatory tachycardia and increased myocardial contractility lead to an increased myocardial oxygen demand. In patients with baseline structural heart disease, acute myocardial infarctions, arrhythmias, and decompensated heart failure may be provoked by severe decreases in hemoglobin concentration [17].

It is often the associated reductions in plasma volume, as opposed to the drop in hemoglobin, that worsen the hemodynamic responses to anemia. In healthy patients, acute, severe isovolemic reductions in hemoglobin concentration to as low as 5 grams per deciliter (g/dL) are generally well tolerated [16, 18]. These individuals experience progressive increases in heart rate, stroke volume, oxygen extraction, and cardiac index without evidence of tissue hypoxia [18]. These compensatory changes are frequently insufficient in the setting of significant volume depletion (e.g., hemorrhage), which can result in decreases in cardiac output and subsequent end-organ hypoperfusion and tissue hypoxia [19, 20]. In these instances, restoration of *both* circulatory volume and oxygen-carrying capacity is necessary to reduce the risk of subsequent organ failure. In acutely bleeding patients, this is best accomplished by transfusion of blood products, either as individual components (e.g., packed red blood cells, plasma, platelets, or cryoprecipitate) or whole blood (Table 31.1).

Table 31.1 Characteristics of blood components [21, 30, 37, 50, 51]

Blood product	Volume (per unit)	Shelf life	Indications	Dosage and response
Red blood cells	250–300 mL	35–42 days	Symptomatic anemia, active bleeding, massive transfusion	1–2 units, depending on hemodynamic stability; 1 unit should increase hemoglobin by 1 g/dL in *non-bleeding* patients
Platelets (single donor or pooled donor)	200–300 mL	3–5 days	Thrombocytopenia, active bleeding, massive transfusion	1–2 units depending on severity of thrombocytopenia; 1 unit should increase platelet count by 20,000–40,000 platelets/μL
Cold-stored platelets	200–300 mL	5–10 days (and potentially longer)	Same as above	Same as above
Frozen plasma	250–300 mL	1 year (24 h after thawing, stored at 1–6 °C)	Multiple clotting factor deficiencies, active bleeding, liver failure, massive transfusion, warfarin reversal, plasma exchange	10–15 mL/kg of body weight; intrinsic INR of 1.3–1.7 in each unit of plasma
"Thawed" plasma	250–300 mL	5 days	Multiple clotting factor deficiencies, active bleeding, liver failure, massive transfusion, warfarin reversal, plasma exchange	10–15 mL/kg of body weight; intrinsic INR of 1.3–1.7 in each unit of plasma
Liquid plasma	250–300 mL	26 days	Active bleeding, massive transfusion	10–15 mL/kg of body weight; intrinsic INR of 1.3–1.7 in each unit of plasma
Cryoprecipitate	10–20 mL	1 year (4–6 h after thawing, stored at 20–24 °C)	Hypofibrinogenemia, DIC, liver failure, von Willebrand disease, massive transfusion	5–10 pooled units; fibrinogen level should increase by 5–10 mg/gL per unit transfused
Fresh warm whole blood	450–500 mL	24–72 h	Massive transfusion, insufficient availability of blood components	Variable dose based on severity of bleeding
Stored whole blood	450–500 mL	35–42 days	Massive transfusion, insufficient availability of blood components	Variable dose based on severity of bleeding

Blood Component Therapy

Red Blood Cell Concentrates

Red blood cell concentrates, commonly referred to as packed red blood cells (pRBCs) or red blood cells (RBCs), are the most commonly administered blood component [21]. They are used to increase hemoglobin levels, thereby theoretically improving the oxygen-carrying capacity of blood [22]. Indications for transfusion of RBCs include hemorrhagic shock, acute anemia with inadequate oxygen delivery (e.g., altered mental status, lactic acidosis, etc.), and symptomatic anemia, regardless of chronicity [23, 24]. RBCs are prepared by centrifugation of 1 unit of whole blood obtained from a single donor (450–500 mL), which provides approximately 200 mL of RBCs. Various anticoagulant-preservative solutions are then added to reduce clotting and prolong shelf life, which increases the volume of each unit by another 50–100 mL [21]. The most commonly used additives are CPDA-1 (citrate, phosphate, dextrose, adenine) and ADSOL (adenine, dextrose, sorbitol, sodium chloride, and mannitol) [21, 25]. Citrate binds calcium and inhibits the clotting cascade. Consequently, the transfusion of large quantities of citrate-containing pRBCs requires administration of supplemental intravenous calcium to prevent significant hypocalcemia [26]. The dextrose and adenine molecules support RBC metabolism. Regardless of which preservative solution is used, RBCs must be stored at 1–6 °C. The average shelf life of each unit is 35–42 days [21, 27]. Additional processing is often performed to RBCs, including leukocyte reduction, washing, and irradiation. These modifications may be indicated in unique patient populations to reduce the risk of specific adverse reactions. However, discussing these variants is beyond the scope of this chapter.

RBC transfusions must be serologically compatible with the patient. The most important blood typing system involves the ABO antigens, which are present on most RBCs [21]. During infancy humans generally develop immunoglobulin M (IgM) antibodies against the antigens that they lack. For example, a person with type A blood will typically have anti-B antibodies and vice versa. Patients with type O blood lack ABO antigens on their RBCs. For this reason, their blood can be transfused to patients with other blood types, making them "universal donors." In contrast, patients with type AB blood have both A and B antigens present on their RBCs and lack both anti-A and anti-B antibodies. As a result, they can receive blood from donors with any blood type, making them "universal recipients." It is critically important to ensure patients receive appropriately typed donor RBCs, as ABO incompatibility can result in a complement-mediated immune response against donor cells, leading to potentially life-threatening intravascular hemolysis [28].

The Rh system is another group of RBC antigens that has important clinical implications. The D antigen is the one used to determine whether a patient is considered "Rh negative" or "Rh positive." Patients who are Rh negative can develop anti-D antibodies, either during pregnancy or from prior transfusion. In contrast to antibodies that develop against A or B antigens, the anti-D antibodies are mostly immunoglobulin G (IgG). This allows anti-D antibodies to cross the placenta and cause hemolytic disease of the newborn, a potentially fatal perinatal condition [29]. For this reason, Rh-negative females of childbearing age should be given Rh-negative RBCs, if possible [21, 22]. Similarly, pregnant female trauma patients who are Rh negative and have proven or suspected exposure to Rh-positive blood (either via maternofetal isoimmunization or administration of Rh-positive blood products) should receive Rho(D) immune globulin to decrease the risk of future Rh disease of the fetus and newborn in future pregnancies.

In most adult patients, transfusion of one unit of RBCs should increase the hemoglobin level by 1 g/dL and the hematocrit by approximately 3% [30]. However, this response may not be seen in patients who are acutely bleeding or actively hemolyzing. In general, each unit should be transfused within 3–4 h. For patients with severe hemorrhagic shock or signs of active bleeding, RBCs can be administered within a matter of minutes via a rapid infuser device, which offer infusion rates up to 30 liters per hour [21, 22]. All blood products should typically be warmed to at least 37 °C. Transfusion guidelines commonly recommend against coadministration of blood products and any calcium-containing intravenous fluid (e.g., lactated Ringer's solution). This recommendation is based on concerns that calcium may bind with citrate in the blood products, thereby promoting clotting and reducing infusion rates [31, 32]. However, studies have demonstrated that blood products can be safely infused with a variety of isotonic crystalloid solutions, including lactated Ringer's and Plasma-Lyte A [33–35].

Platelets

Platelets are prepared by one of two processes: (1) centrifugation of whole blood followed by separation and pooling of the platelet-rich layer from several donors, also known as "random donor platelets," or (2) single-donor apheresis or plateletpheresis. The former involves removal of approximately 50 mL of platelet-rich plasma. Approximately four to six of these units are then combined to give 200–300 mL of platelets. This is commonly referred to as a "six pack" of platelets. Conversely, single-donor apheresis platelets are separated from whole blood at the time of donation, and the remainder of the blood is returned to the patient. One advantage of the apheresis technique is that it can provide 250–500 mL unit of platelets from a single donor. A single apheresis session can yield up to two single-donor units (500–1000 mL). Other advantages of using the apheresis technique over random donor pooling include fewer donor exposures, fewer leukocytes per unit (decreasing risk of some transfusion reactions), and lower risk of bacterial contamination and septic transfusion reactions [36].

Some plasma is retained in each unit of platelets, which increases the risk of some acute transfusion reactions. Unlike RBCs, platelets are stored at room temperature (20–24 °C), increasing the risk of bacterial growth and transmission. These transfusion-related complications are discussed in more detail later in the chapter. Gentle agitation is used to reduce platelet aggregation and to improve the oxygenation of the platelets. The shelf life of a unit of platelets is approximately 5 days [37]. More recently the FDA has approved the use of "cold-stored platelets" that are stored at 1–6 °C, with an extended shelf life of up to 10 days [38]. In addition to extending the longevity of the platelets, there is now evidence that cold storage may have additional benefits including improved platelet function and decreased risk of bacterial contamination compared to standard room temperature storage [39, 40].

ABO incompatibility is less of a concern with platelet transfusions than with packed red blood cells. This is due, in part, to the fact that the concentration of ABO antigens in platelet concentrates is approximately 5% of that of RBC units [21]. Nevertheless, recipient anti-A or anti-B antibodies may affect platelet survival, which can result in a lower platelet count increment following transfusion. In addition, ABO-incompatible transfusions may rarely result in acute hemolytic reactions [41]. For these reasons, many blood bank centers advocate using ABO-compatible platelets.

Indications for platelet transfusion vary depending on the severity of the underlying thrombocytopenia, whether the patient is actively bleeding, and the need for potential invasive procedures. In stable non-bleeding patients, a platelet count as low as 10,000 platelets per microliter (μL) may be acceptable. For patients who are bleeding and/or scheduled to undergo surgery or other invasive procedures, the transfusion threshold is often 40,000–50,000 platelets/μL. Higher cutoffs may be appropriate for patients with intracranial hemorrhage and other serious bleeding disorders [42].

In general, the platelet count is expected to rise by 20,000–40,000 platelets/μL within 1 h following transfusion of one unit. Platelet refractoriness is defined as an inappropriately low rise in the posttransfusion platelet count [43]. This may occur for a variety of reasons. Sepsis and other infectious complications can decrease platelet survival. Splenic sequestration, intravascular platelet consumption (e.g., disseminated intravascular coagulation), and active bleeding can lead to reduced platelet counts. Alloimmunization by human leukocyte antigen (HLA) system, ABO incompatibility, and other antiplatelet antibodies frequently result in platelet destruction, as well [21, 43, 44].

Plasma

Plasma is the protein-rich fraction of whole blood that contains albumin, immunoglobulins, coagulation factors, intrinsic anticoagulants, protease inhibitors, and multiple other important enzymes and cofactors. For these reasons, plasma is an important blood component for the treatment of various coagulopathies and bleeding disorders. Pretransfusion ABO typing is required as anti-A and anti-B antibodies are present in plasma. The Rh status may be an important consideration, as well, particularly if the patient is a female of childbearing age. "AB-negative" plasma is considered the "universal donor" type, as it lacks both anti-A and anti-B antibodies.

Indications for plasma transfusion include multiple clotting factor deficiencies, patients with liver disease, active bleeding, reversal of warfarin therapy, and exchange transfusions. Plasma can be collected via centrifugation of whole blood, during which the supernatant is siphoned off into a separate collection bag, yielding approximately 250–300 mL of plasma fluid [21, 45]. Plasma can also be derived by apheresis collection from a single donor, allowing for collection of 500–600 mL of plasma (e.g., two units) during a single session. Plasma is then processed into several variants: fresh frozen plasma (FFP), plasma frozen within 24 hours after phlebotomy (PF24), Thawed Plasma, liquid plasma, dried or freeze-dried plasma (FDP), plasma cryoprecipitate reduced (also referred to as cryo-poor plasma), and solvent/detergent plasma (S/D plasma). For the purposes of this chapter, we will focus on FFP, PF24, Thawed Plasma, liquid plasma, and FDP.

FFP is the most commonly used plasma formulation, although PF24 is becoming increasingly popular. By definition, FFP is frozen within 8 h of collection and maintained at a temperature of −18 to −30 °C. Conversely, PF24 can be initially stored in a refrigerator (1–6 °C) for up to 8 h after collection, although it must be frozen and maintained at ≤18 °C within 24 h. As noted above, each unit contains approximately 250–300 mL of volume. FFP essentially contains all of the coagulation factors, immunoglobulins, and proteins contained in the original unit of blood, although there is some mild dilution that occurs by the citrate-containing anticoagulant-preservative solution that is added at the time of collection. PF24 maintains similar clotting factor concentrations as FFP, except for a 15–35% reduction in factor VIII levels [46, 47]. For this reason, PF24 cannot be used to make cryoprecipitate. Otherwise, PF24 and FFP are often used interchangeably. When appropriately stored, both FFP and PF24 have a shelf life of 1 year from the date of collection.

Prior to transfusion, each unit of FFP or PF24 must be thawed in water at 37 °C, a process that typically takes 20–30 min. Unless intended for immediate use, the unit(s) must be stored at refrigerator temperature (e.g., 1–6 °C). Technically, the shelf life of *thawed* FFP or PF24 is only 24 h. However, these units can be relabeled as "Thawed Plasma" (note the capital "T" and "P"), which allows them to be stored under the same conditions for a total of 5 days from the time they were thawed. Thawed Plasma has the advantage of being available for immediate use, which is particularly important in the setting of massive hemorrhage. However, when compared to frozen plasma, factors V and VIII levels are typically reduced [48, 49]. The other factor levels are generally unaffected by the thawing process.

Regardless of whether FFP, PF24, or Thawed Plasma is used, each unit of plasma has an intrinsic international normalized ratio (INR) of approximately 1.3–1.7 [50]. Therefore, transfusing these components to achieve an INR less than 1.7 is generally futile. Furthermore, the common practice of transfusing one to two units of plasma is often ineffective. In general, a weight-based dosing protocol is recommended, e.g., 10–15 mL/kg of body weight [51, 52]. For an average 70 kg adult man, this would amount to a plasma dose of 700–1050 mL, or three to four units total (assuming an average unit volume of 250–300 mL). However, the dose can be adjusted based on the clinical scenario and laboratory parameters. In addition, these considerations may not necessarily apply to other forms of plasma such as liquid plasma and FDP.

Unlike FFP and PF24, liquid plasma is never frozen. It is separated from whole blood at any time from collection to 5 days *after* the whole blood has expired. It must be kept at 1–6 °C and has a shelf life of up to 26 days when stored appropriately. Liquid plasma has the advantage of being immediately available, which may be useful in the setting of massive transfusions. The potential drawback of liquid plasma is that it may contain reduced levels of some coagulation factors, namely, factors V and VII, which are a by-product of storing non-frozen blood products for more than 24–48 h. At least one study suggests liquid plasma has a better hemostatic profile compared to thawed FFP [53]. These findings have not yet been confirmed in large, multicenter, randomized studies, and its role has largely been confined to massive transfusion protocols in many US trauma centers.

FDP is a unique form of plasma, which was originally developed in the 1930s and 1940s and used in the treatment of hemorrhage during World War II [54]. Unlike FFP and PF24, FDP is prepared by removal of the liquid component of plasma. The remaining coagulation factors, immunoglobulins, and other proteins are then used to make a powdered formulation that can be reconstituted using sterile water at the time of infusion [55]. FDP can be prepared by one of two processes: lyophilization (removal of liquid via cryodesiccation under vacuum pressure) or spray drying (exposure of plasma to a high-temperature gas to remove liquid without causing protein denaturation). The principal advantage of FDP is that it can be stored at room temperature. Other benefits include a 2-year shelf life, a reconstitution time of less than 6 min, universal ABO compatibility, and reduced risk of transmission of pathogens [56]. French, German, and South African armed forces units have been using FDP since the mid-1990s and have demonstrated an excellent safety record to date [56–58]. Similar products are currently under development in the United States and are of particular interest to US military forces for battlefield use [59].

Cryoprecipitate

Cryoprecipitated antihemophilic factor, commonly abbreviated "cryoprecipitate" or "cryo," consists of cold-insoluble high molecular weight proteins from plasma. Fibrinogen, factor VIII, and von Willebrand factor represent the largest fraction of these cryoglobulins. Cryo is prepared by controlled thawing of frozen plasma to 1–6 °C for 24 h, which results in a residual liquid component and an insoluble *precipitate*. The mixture is then centrifuged allowing separation of the two layers, yielding a 10–20 mL of unit of cryoprecipitate, which must be rapidly refrozen (−18 to −30 °C). If appropriately stored, the shelf life is 1 year.

The principal indication for transfusion of cryoprecipitate is a replacement for fibrinogen, a protein that gets converted to insoluble fibrin strands during the clotting process. Several disorders can lead to hypofibrinogenemia to include disseminated intravascular coagulation, liver failure, and massive transfusion. Cryoprecipitate can be dosed by weight (e.g., 5–10 units per kilogram of body weight). However, the typical dose for an average size adult is ten units. Each unit is expected to increase the fibrinogen level by 5–10 milligrams per deciliter (mg/dL), which corresponds to a total increase of approximately 100–150 mg/dL following an average adult dose. As is the case with plasma, ABO compatibility is recommended to minimize the risk of hemolytic transfusion reactions [21, 51].

Whole Blood Transfusion

History of Whole Blood Use

The first known human whole blood transfusion was performed in France in 1667, prescribed for the treatment of psychosis [60]. However, it was not until the 1820s that the practice of transfusing whole blood for acute hemorrhage became popular. Dr. James Blundell, a British physician, transfused human whole blood into ten women with postpartum hemorrhage [61]. Despite mixed results, the practice of unmatched whole blood transfusion continued in parts of Europe and the United States. Nearly 80 years later, Dr. Karl Landsteiner discovered the ABO antigens. In 1912, Dr. Reuben Ottenberg developed crossmatching techniques [62]. The creation of blood storage solutions soon followed in 1915. These developments represented major breakthroughs in blood transfusion therapy, allowing numerous combat casualties in World War I to receive stored whole blood. This practice was later expanded on a large scale during World War II. In fact, nearly 500,000 units were shipped to US hospitals during a 13-month period spanning 1944 and 1945 [63]. The practice of whole blood transfusion continued through the end of World War II and into the subsequent conflicts in the Korean Peninsula and Vietnam in the 1950 and 1960s, respectively. However, the ongoing need for large amounts of readily available blood products eventually led to the development of whole blood fractionation. The availability of individual blood components allowed for targeted treatment of hematologic abnormalities: RBCs for anemia, platelets for thrombocytopenia, plasma for coagulopathy, etc. In addition, some of these blood components offered substantially longer shelf lives when compared to whole blood. For these reasons, blood component therapy largely replaced whole blood transfusion in most civilian centers beginning in the late 1960s to early 1970s [63, 64]. Nevertheless, whole blood continued to be used during military operations, which were often carried out in challenging environments without access to apheresis and other modern blood banking techniques. The relatively short shelf life of some refrigerated blood products (e.g., platelets and Thawed Plasma) often made blood component therapy impractical in austere environments [65, 66]. Even in the more recent conflicts in Southwest Asia, whole blood has continued to play a critical role in trauma resuscitations, especially in remote locations [67–69].

Stored Versus Fresh Whole Blood

There are two categories of whole blood: (1) stored whole blood and (2) warm fresh whole blood (WFWB). Stored whole blood must be refrigerated immediately after collection. An anticoagulant-preservative fluid is added to each unit, as is the case with other forms of stored blood products. The advantage of stored whole blood versus stored RBCs is that it contains a smaller volume of preservative solution and offers greater conservation of platelet function compared to other stored components [61, 70].

WFWB is defined as whole blood transfused within 24 h of collection. WFWB is not approved by the US Food and

Drug Administration (FDA) and, consequently, is not available for routine use in most civilian centers. For logistical reasons and out of situational necessity, WFWB has continued to be utilized in military settings [71–73]. The most significant safety concerns center around the increased risk for transmission of blood-borne pathogens associated with WFWB, which is largely due to the limited time from WFWB donation to transfusion. Department of Defense guidelines limit the collection and administration of WFWB to situations when blood component therapy is either unavailable or unable to sustain resuscitation efforts [74]. Practices that have been put into place in order to minimize the risk of infectious transmission include routine mandatory screening of all US military service members for HIV and the hepatitides, prescreening of potential whole blood donors, and rapid viral testing of donor blood at the time of collection.

WFWB has several distinct advantages over blood components and stored whole blood. One obvious advantage is that whole blood best mimics the fluid that patients lose in the setting of severe hemorrhage. Regardless of the ratio chosen, blood component therapy cannot perfectly replicate whole blood [62]. WFWB has the additional benefit of avoiding the "storage lesion" associated with blood components and stored whole blood. The "storage lesion" refers to several changes that RBCs undergo when stored in preservative solution, including a significant decline in adenosine triphosphate and 2,3-diphosphoglycerate, as well as cell membrane deformability and increased osmotic fragility [75–77]. These changes result in increased hemolysis, release of microparticles, release of free hemoglobin, and increased extracellular potassium levels [76, 78]. Platelets are also significantly affected by the storage process, resulting in impaired aggregation and function [79, 80]. With 12–18 h of storage at 4 °C, stored whole blood has decreased function of factors V and VIII, both of which have important roles in the clotting cascade [62, 79]. Conversely, WFWB that is stored at room temperature has been shown to maintain normal coagulation function for up to 72 h [62, 81].

"Walking Blood Bank"

Collection of WFWB often requires activation of a "walking blood bank," which is a loosely defined protocol that utilizes a prescreened pool of donors who are immediately available to provide blood [82]. These protocols have been used numerous times during the most recent conflicts in Iraq and Afghanistan. A population of military donors provides a group of individuals who are regularly tested for human immunodeficiency virus (HIV) and whose vaccinations are generally up to date. The donors then undergo standard pretransfusion screening questionnaires. Donors are subsequently screened for anemia and tested for hepatitis B, hepatitis C, and HIV. Blood typing is most commonly determined using a standard EldonCard™ (Fig. 31.2). If all screening measures are passed, the donors are added to a database for future recall [71]. The "walking blood bank" can be activated during mass casualty events or whenever the local blood supply has been exceeded. This latter scenario may occur with only one or two casualties in a deployed setting when there is little availability of stored blood products [83].

Transfusion Thresholds in the ICU

Restrictive Versus Liberal Transfusion Strategies

In 1942 Adams and Lundy published an article proposing several suggestions aimed at improving surgical outcomes in high-risk patients. One such recommendation involved transfusing patients who had a hemoglobin concentration less than 8–10 g/dL [84]. For unclear reasons, this recommendation eventually became the basis for the "10/30 rule," the idea that hemoglobin and hematocrit should be maintained above 10 g/dL and 30%, respectively. This unofficial rule became medical dogma, driving transfusion practices for several decades thereafter [85]. In the early 1980s, the term "transfusion trigger" was introduced, which created the notion that there was a standard hemoglobin threshold at which transfusion should be initiated [86]. Subsequent studies demonstrated an association between anemia and increased mortality in critically ill patients. Hébert et al. published one of the largest studies at the time, a combined retrospective and prospective cohort study of 4470 critically ill patients. The data showed a trend toward increased mortality in the subset of patients with anemia and underlying cardiac disease. This trend was most pronounced when the hemoglobin concentration decreased below 9.5 g/dL [87]. Similar results were demonstrated by Carson et al. in a retrospective cohort study of 1958 patients who underwent surgery and declined blood transfusion for religious reasons [88]. Patients with severe preoperative anemia had a 25-fold increase in risk of death compared to patients with a preoperative hemoglobin concentration greater than 12 g/dL. The risk of death was greatest in patients with underlying cardiovascular disease.

Although these studies served to reinforce common transfusion practices at the time, other authors began questioning the safety of blood product transfusions in the early to mid-1990s [89, 90]. This controversy formed the basis for the Transfusion Requirements in Critical Care (TRICC) trial, a landmark study that has greatly impacted

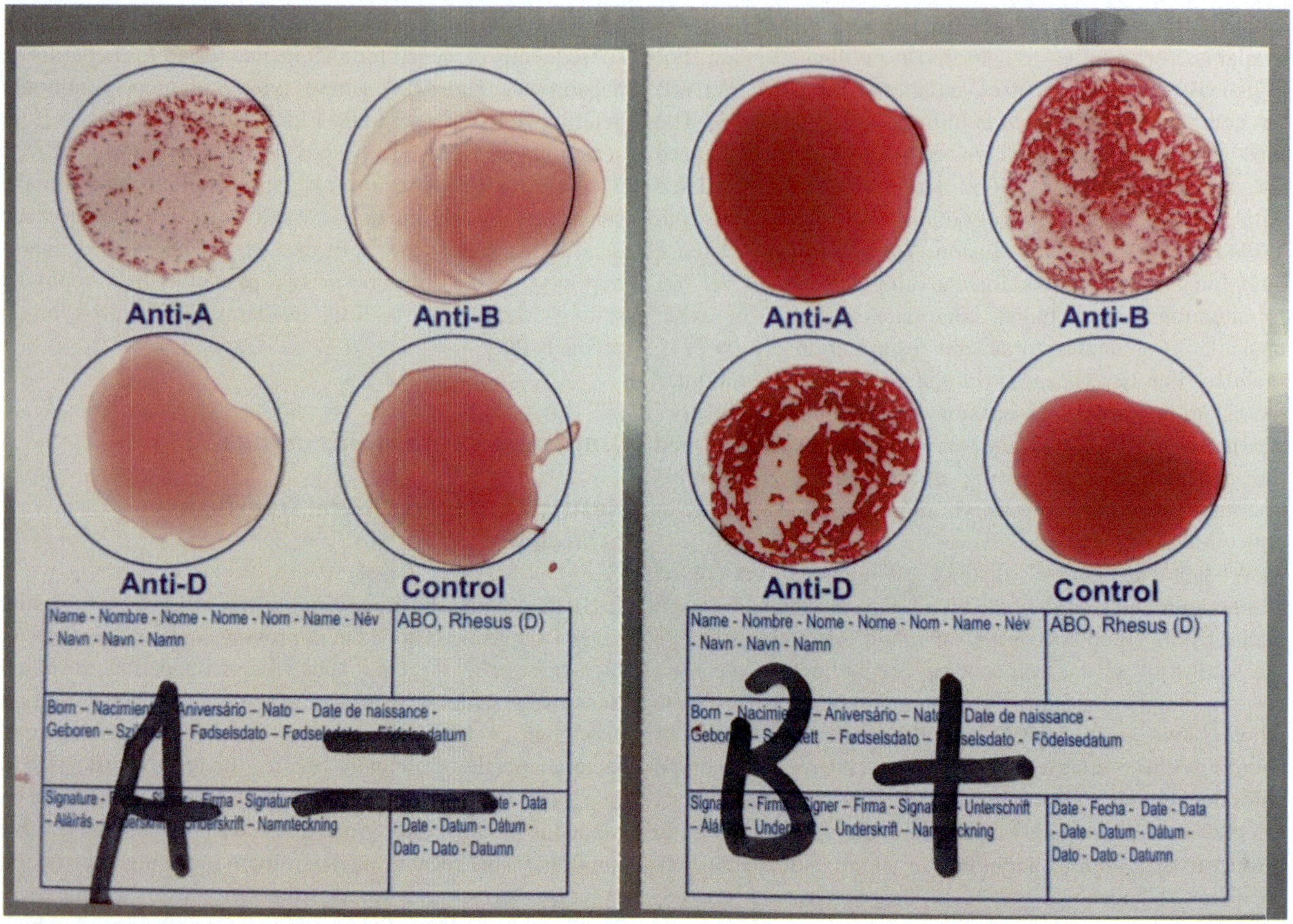

Fig. 31.2 Blood typing is performed using an EldonCard™ (Eldon Biologicals A/S, Gentofte, Denmark). There are four prelabeled circles each containing a reagent. Three of the circles contain antibodies to the A, B, and Rh antigens as noted above. The fourth circle is used for quality control to demonstrate that the test was performed properly. A small drop of water is then added to each circle. A fingertip is then cleaned with a sterile swab, and a lancet is used to make a small puncture. A drop of blood is transferred to each circle. Using an EldonSticks™, the blood is spread over the entire surface of each circle. A new EldonSticks™ is used for each circle to avoid cross contamination. After this step, the card is held upright for 10 s and then turned upside down, right-side up, and then left-side up for 10 s on each side. The circles containing agglutinated blood indicate the presence of an underlying blood antigen. For example, the EldonCard™ on the left contains agglutinated blood only in the anti-A circle, suggesting the presence of A antigen in the blood and no Rh antigens. This patient's blood type is A negative. The EldonCard™ on the right demonstrates agglutinated blood in the anti-B and anti-D circles, suggesting the presence of B and Rh antigens. Therefore, the patient's blood type is B positive

transfusion practices in the ICU over the last 20 years [91]. Hébert and colleagues enrolled 838 critically ill patients from 25 Canadian ICUs over a 3-year period beginning in November 1994. All patients had to be euvolemic and with a hemoglobin concentration below 9.0 g/dL within 72 h of ICU admission. Patients with active bleeding were excluded from enrollment. The patients were then randomized to two groups: *restrictive* or *liberal* transfusion strategies. The restrictive strategy participants received RBC transfusions only if their hemoglobin concentration dropped below 7.0 g/dL. Their hemoglobin concentrations were then maintained at 7.0–9.0 g/dL for the remainder of the trial. The liberal strategy participants received RBC transfusions when their hemoglobin concentrations fell below 10 g/dL, targeting a hemoglobin concentration of 10–12 g/dL. There was no statistical difference in a 30-day mortality between the restrictive and liberal transfusion groups, 18.7% and 23.3%, respectively ($P = 0.11$). However, the mortality rate during hospitalization was significantly lower in the restrictive group (22.2% vs 28.1%, $P = 0.05$). In addition, the restrictive strategy was associated with a lower 30-day mortality rate in less acutely ill patients, as indicated by the Acute Physiologic Assessment and Chronic Health Evaluation (APACHE) II score of less than 20 (8.7% vs 16.1%, $P = 0.03$), and in patients who were less than 55 years old (5.7% vs 13.0%, $P = 0.02$). Overall complication rates (e.g., cardiac events, infectious complications, and multi-organ failure) were comparable between the two groups. The authors concluded that a restrictive RBC transfusion strategy is at least as effective as a liberal transfusion strategy in hemodynamically stable ICU patients with anemia. They cautioned against adopting a restrictive strategy in patients with active myocardial ischemia, although this study did not demonstrate increased complication rates in subgroup analysis.

In 2002 Vincent and colleagues published the ABC (Anemia and Blood Transfusion in Critical Care) trial, a prospective observational study of 3534 critically ill medical and surgical patients from 146 ICUs in Western Europe [3]. Several outcome measures were monitored, including frequency and volume of blood drawn for laboratory testing, hemoglobin levels, transfusion rate, organ dysfunction, and mortality. The transfusion rate during the ICU stay was 37% with a mean number of transfusions per patient of 4.8 +/− 5.2 units per patient. The mean pretransfusion hemoglobin level was 8.4 g/dL. Both ICU and overall mortality rates were significantly higher in patients who had versus had not received a blood transfusion (ICU rates, 18.5 vs 10.1%, respectively [$P < 0.001$]; overall rates, 29.0 vs 14.9%, respectively [$P < 0.001$]). This finding was maintained, even after adjusting for severity of organ dysfunction: 28-day mortality rate of 22.7% among patients who were transfused and 17.1% among those who were not ($P = 0.02$). This study clearly demonstrated an association between blood transfusions and increased risk of death irrespective of severity of illness.

The CRIT study was subsequently performed in the United States [4], which was a multicenter, prospective, observational trial designed to examine the incidence of anemia and RBC transfusion in critically ill patients, as well as the impact of anemia and transfusion on clinical outcomes. A total of 4892 patients were enrolled from 284 ICUs. The patient population consisted of a mixture of medical and surgical patients. A total of 44% of patients received one or more RBC transfusions while in the ICU. The mean pretransfusion hemoglobin level was 8.6 g/dL, nearly identical to the mean value reported in the ABC trial [3]. The number of transfusions a patient received was independently associated with increased ICU and hospital lengths of stay, as well as mortality. A nadir hemoglobin concentration of less than 9 g/dL was also a predictor of increased length of stay and mortality. Baseline hemoglobin, on the other hand, did not predict either of these factors.

Following publication of the CRIT study, three additional randomized, controlled trials were conducted comparing liberal versus restrictive transfusion strategies in different patient populations [92–94]. The FOCUS (Functional Outcomes in Cardiovascular Patients Undergoing Surgical Hip Fracture Repair) trial included a total of 2016 patients enrolled after hip surgery, who were aged 50 years or older with either a history of or risk factors for cardiovascular disease, as well as a hemoglobin concentration of less than 10 g/dL [92]. The patients were then randomly assigned to a liberal (hemoglobin threshold of 10 g/dL) or restrictive (hemoglobin threshold of 8 g/dL). The primary outcome was death or inability to walk across a room without human assistance on a 60-day follow-up. There were no statistically significant differences in outcomes between the two groups, including primary outcome, rates of in-hospital acute coronary syndrome, and rates of death at 60 days. Complication rates were similar between both groups, as well.

In 2013 Villanueva et al. published results of another randomized, controlled study comparing transfusion strategies [93]. However, the study population consisted of adult patients with severe acute upper gastrointestinal bleeding. A total of 921 patients were enrolled from a single tertiary care hospital in Spain over a 6-year period starting in June 2003. Patients were randomized to receive either a restrictive strategy (transfusion when the hemoglobin level fell below 7 g/dL) or a liberal strategy (transfusion when the hemoglobin fell below 9 g/dL). All patients underwent emergent endoscopic evaluation and treatment, performed within 6 h of admission. The etiologies of upper gastrointestinal bleeding were broad and included varying degrees of cirrhosis-related variceal bleeding in both groups. The authors found several improved outcomes favoring the restrictive strategy, including higher probability of survival at 6 weeks ($P = 0.02$), reduced bleeding post-endoscopic intervention ($P = 0.01$), and fewer transfusion reactions and adverse cardiac events ($P = 0.02$). The probability of survival was also significantly higher in the subgroup of patients with Child-Pugh A and B cirrhosis who received a restrictive transfusion strategy.

One year after Villanueva's group published their results, the TRISS (Transfusion Requirements in Septic Shock) trial group published a large, multicenter, randomized study comparing transfusion strategies in critically ill patients with septic shock [94]. A total of 998 patients were enrolled from 32 Scandinavian ICUs. All patients had a primary diagnosis of septic shock and had a baseline hemoglobin concentration of less than 9 g/dL at the time of enrollment. They were randomized to receive either a restrictive or liberal strategy: transfusion for a hemoglobin level below 7 g/dL or 9 g/dL, respectively. Primary outcome was death at 90 days after randomization. The 90-day mortality rate was nearly identical between the two groups, 43% in the lower-threshold group versus 45% in the higher-threshold group ($P = 0.44$). Adverse events (e.g., cardiac ischemia, severe transfusion reaction, need for life support therapies) were similar in both groups, as well. The only statistically significant difference between the two groups was the number of blood transfusions administered with the restrictive strategy group receiving fewer blood products, as expected.

Current Clinical Practice Guidelines

By the time the TRICC trial was published, clinical practice had already begun to change, and an increasing number of ICU clinicians began adopting a more restrictive transfusion strategy. Various clinical practice guidelines began to endorse this approach, as well. The Society of Critical Care Medicine and Eastern Association for the Surgery of Trauma joint clinical practice guidelines were published in 2009, stating a "restrictive" strategy (e.g., transfusing when hemoglobin is less than 7 g/dL) was as effective as a "liberal" transfusion strategy in hemodynamically stable, anemic patients [23]. This recommendation excluded patients with active coronary ischemia, given the lack of high-quality transfusion studies in that patient population. In 2011 the European Society of Cardiology addressed this issue in their updated acute coronary syndrome guidelines. The authors endorsed a "restrictive" strategy in which blood transfusions should be withheld in hemodynamically stable patients with hematocrit above 25% and/or hemoglobin concentration above 7 g/dL [95]. The Society of Thoracic Surgeons/Society of Cardiovascular Anesthesiologists and the British Committee for Standards in Haematology similarly endorsed a "restrictive" transfusion approach [24, 96]. The American Association of Blood Banks red cell transfusion guidelines were updated in 2016, and a hemoglobin concentration of 7 g/dL was the recommended threshold below which transfusion should be considered [97]. This recommendation is for hemodynamically stable adults. Patients with acute coronary syndrome, severe thrombocytopenia, active hematological or solid organ malignancies, and chronic transfusion-dependent anemia were excluded, as the authors felt there was insufficient high-quality evidence to make a recommendation in these patient populations.

These various clinical practice guidelines have reached a consensus that a restrictive transfusion strategy is preferred in most hemodynamically stable, anemic, critically ill adults. Although a hemoglobin concentration of 7 g/dL is most often listed as the "threshold" below which transfusion should be considered, none of these guidelines recommend using a specific hemoglobin value as a transfusion trigger. The decision to transfuse should be based on the overall clinical context of the patient. It is worth emphasizing that these guidelines do not apply to patients who are actively bleeding, hemodynamically unstable, and/or requiring massive transfusion [23, 24, 96, 97]. Additional important considerations for a higher transfusion trigger in surgical and trauma patients include an upcoming surgical procedure with expected significant blood loss, the need for invasive procedures with a significant risk of rapid hemorrhage, and the presence of injuries with a high risk of bleeding in patients with poor functional reserve.

Transfusion-Associated Complications

Overview

Blood product transfusions carry inherent risks, as is the case with any medical intervention. These risks include potential transmission of blood-borne infections and a wide spectrum of transfusion reactions. The severity of these reactions can range from benign to life-threatening (Table 31.2). Nearly 1 out of every 100 patients that receives a blood product transfusion will develop some form of transfusion reaction [98]. In the United States, approximately 40 patients have fatal transfusion-related complications every year [99]. For these reasons, it is of paramount importance that all critical care physicians be familiar with the recognition, diagnosis, and treatment of the various types of adverse reactions and infectious complications.

Urticarial Transfusion Reaction

Mild allergic reactions are the most common type of transfusion reaction with annual incidence of 1–3% in the United States [100]. Symptoms are mediated by histamine release by activation of basophils and mast cells [101]. Mild allergic reactions are generally characterized by urticaria (hives), rash, pruritus, and localized angioedema.

As with other forms of transfusion reactions, the transfusion should be discontinued. Antihistamine therapy, specifically with an H_1-receptor antagonist, should be administered for symptom relief [101, 102]. If symptoms resolve, the transfusion can typically be resumed at the same or reduced rate with close monitoring for symptom recurrence.

Anaphylactic Transfusion Reaction

Anaphylactic transfusion reactions represent the most severe form of allergic transfusion reaction. Anaphylaxis can be triggered in IgA-deficient patients who produce anti-IgA antibodies that react with donor blood products. Other patients may react to the additive solution or other constituents in the transfused product, while many other anaphylactic reactions are idiopathic.

Clinical manifestations can include flushing, urticaria, pruritus, upper airway angioedema, stridor, bronchospasm, and hypotension. Prompt cessation of the blood transfusion and administration of epinephrine, dual H_1-H_2 antihistamine therapy, and systemic corticosteroids are often necessary, depending on the severity of the symptoms. The blood bank should be notified as soon as possible, once the patient has been stabilized.

Table 31.2 Acute transfusion reactions [10]

Complication	Risk (per unit)	Clinical features	Treatment
Urticarial transfusion reaction	1:100	Urticaria, flushing, pruritus, localized angioedema; onset during or up to 4 h after transfusion	Antihistamine, antipyretics
Febrile non-hemolytic transfusion reactions	1:300	Fever, chills, rigors; onset during or up to 6 h after transfusion	Antipyretics; rule out infection and hemolysis
Transfusion-associated circulatory overload	1:700	Dyspnea, tachycardia, hypertension, jugular venous distension, hypoxemic respiratory failure; onset within 2–6 h of transfusion	Discontinue transfusion, supplemental oxygen, loop diuretics, positive pressure ventilation
Transfusion-related acute lung injury	1:5000 [109]	Dyspnea, fever, hypotension, hypoxemic respiratory failure; onset within 2–6 h of transfusion	Discontinue transfusion, supplemental oxygen, vasopressor support, invasive mechanical ventilation with low-tidal-volume ventilation
Anaphylactic transfusion reaction	1:40,000	Bronchospasm, dyspnea, angioedema, hypotension, abdominal cramping; onset during transfusion	Discontinue transfusion, epinephrine, antihistamines, systemic corticosteroids
Acute hemolytic transfusion reaction	1:40,000	Fever, chills, rigors, flank pain, acute kidney injury, pigmenturia; onset during or up to 24 h after transfusion	Discontinue transfusion; hemolysis workup; IV fluid administration +/− urine alkalinization
Septic transfusion reaction	1:60,000 [98]	Fever, chills, hypotension, tachycardia, hypotension, nausea, vomiting; onset during or up to 24 h after transfusion	Discontinue transfusion; rule out hemolysis; culture donor and recipient blood; appropriate broad-spectrum antibiotics; vasopressor support

Febrile Non-hemolytic Transfusion Reaction

Febrile non-hemolytic transfusion reactions are one of the most common of all transfusion reactions, occurring in approximately 1% of all transfusion episodes [103]. As the name implies, these reactions are characterized by fever (temperature ≥38 °C) with or without chills. Other systemic symptoms are generally absent. Because other more serious transfusion reactions may initially present with fever, this is a diagnosis of exclusion. These reactions are typically caused by release of proinflammatory cytokines from donor white blood cells (WBCs) or recipient antibodies targeted against donor antigens. Management is supportive in nature. Although there are few high-quality studies supporting the use of prophylactic antihistamines and antipyretics, it is common practice to pretreat patients with these medications to reduce the occurrence of febrile non-hemolytic transfusion reactions [104].

Transfusion-Associated Circulatory Overload

Transfusion-associated circulatory overload (TACO) is a form of pulmonary edema due to iatrogenic volume overload, which is likely underreported [105]. Some authors suggest that TACO may be the second leading cause of transfusion-associated mortality in the United States [106]. Blood product transfusions represent a source of significant iatrogenic volume administration in ICU patients. Many critically ill patients are particularly susceptible to volume overload due to underlying left or right heart dysfunction, advanced pulmonary disease, and other comorbidities. However, even patients without significant underlying cardiopulmonary disease can develop TACO in the setting of large-volume transfusions delivered over a relatively short time span (minutes to hours).

The clinical manifestations are indistinguishable from acute decompensated heart failure: respiratory distress, hypoxemia, jugular venous distention, etc. The onset of symptoms is generally within 2 h of transfusion onset, although delayed presentations can occur [107]. Chest imaging typically shows evidence of pulmonary edema. Laboratory studies may be normal except for an elevated brain natriuretic peptide (BNP) or N-terminal pro-brain natriuretic peptide (NT-Pro-BNP) level [108].

Avoiding unnecessary transfusions, reducing infusion rates, and minimizing concurrent intravenous fluid therapy may help mitigate the risk of developing volume overload. When TACO develops, the transfusion should be discontinued, and supplemental oxygen should be considered. Diuresis is the cornerstone of medical therapy and should be administered as soon as possible. For patients who develop acute hypoxemic respiratory failure, non-invasive positive pressure ventilation or invasive mechanical ventilation may be necessary.

Transfusion-Related Acute Lung Injury

Transfusion-related acute lung injury (TRALI) is a relatively rare, potentially severe complication associated with blood product transfusions. Based on historical data, the estimated rate of occurrence is 1 in 5000 transfusions, although the true incidence is likely underreported [109, 110]. TRALI is primarily manifested by acute-onset respiratory distress, often progressing to hypoxemic respiratory failure. Fever, tachycardia, and hypotension are other common findings. These changes usually begin with 1–2 h of initiating a blood product transfusion, although they can be delayed as long as 6 h [111]. The diagnosis is largely clinical and should be suspected on a combination of factors: the development of acute hypoxemic respiratory failure, temporal relationship associated with blood product transfusion, chest radiograph demonstrating bilateral pulmonary infiltrates, and the exclusion of alternative causes of acute respiratory distress syndrome.

The exact pathogenesis of the condition is not fully understood, although TRALI likely requires a "two-hit" model. The first event is the presence of an underlying injury to the pulmonary vascular endothelium, which leads to sequestration of neutrophils within the lung [98]. Multiple conditions predispose to pulmonary endothelial injury including hepatic surgery, chronic alcohol abuse, high peak airway pressures during mechanical ventilation, smoking, and positive fluid balance [98, 112]. The second event occurs during blood transfusion with transmission of proinflammatory mediators or donor antibodies targeting HLA or human neutrophil antigens (HNA) on the recipient WBCs. This, in turn, causes activation of the recipient's pulmonary neutrophils and propagation of the immune response and end-organ injury.

Historically, plasma transfusions were associated with a much greater risk of TRALI than platelet or RBC transfusions. In the mid-to-late 2000s, most blood banks in the United States and Europe transitioned to male-only plasma donation following the discovery that most anti-HLA and anti-HNA antibodies were transmitted in plasma from multiparous female donors [113, 114]. These changes, along with improvements in crossmatching and adherence to blood component guidelines, have led to a significant decrease in the risk of TRALI [115]. Even though the overall risk is lower, plasma and platelet transfusions remain more strongly associated with TRALI compared to RBC transfusions due to their higher average volume of plasma per unit.

When suspected, the transfusion should be stopped immediately. Prompt notification of the blood bank is necessary to assist with investigation of the transfusion reaction. Supplemental oxygen should be administered to maintain appropriate oxygenation. If respiratory failure develops, prompt intubation and mechanical ventilation may be necessary. If the patient requires mechanical ventilation, a lung protective ventilator strategy should be employed [116]. Any accompanying hemodynamic instability should be addressed with appropriate vasopressor therapy, as is the case with other forms of distributive shock. Once the patient is initially stabilized, a chest radiograph and laboratory studies (e.g., complete blood count, chemistry panel, bilirubin levels, haptoglobin, direct antiglobulin test, BNP or NT-Pro-BNP) should be obtained. An elevated BNP or NT-Pro-BNP is more suggestive of an acute volume overload state like decompensated heart failure or TACO [108].

Acute Hemolytic Transfusion Reaction

Unlike febrile non-hemolytic transfusion reactions, acute hemolytic transfusion reactions are potentially life-threatening. Fortunately, they are much less common (Table 31.2). These reactions are characterized by acute intravascular hemolysis of transfused RBCs related to immune incompatibility between the donor and the recipient [117]. These reactions can occur at any point within 7 days of receiving a blood transfusion. The more hyperacute variant, often termed "hyperhemolysis," frequently occurs within minutes to hours of initiation of the transfusion [98, 117].

Typical clinical manifestations include fever, chills, flank pain, bleeding from intravenous or surgical incision sites, dyspnea, and hypotension. More severe complications can occur to include disseminated intravascular coagulation, acute renal failure, shock, and even death. Both ABO and non-ABO antigens can be involved. Often these reactions stem from clerical errors in which patients receive RBCs that were intended for someone else, mislabeling of blood products, and other processing errors [118]. The severity of the reaction depends on recipient antibody and titer, as well as the volume of incompatible blood that gets transfused [119].

Given that acute hemolytic transfusions may initially present with only a fever, the ICU clinician must remain vigilant to make a timely diagnosis and avoid progression to more severe manifestations. Other than the clinical signs mentioned above, several laboratory tests are available to aid in the diagnosis. Increased indirect bilirubin and lactate dehydrogenase levels, as well as decreased haptoglobin levels, suggest underlying hemolysis. Other tests that may support the diagnosis include elevated serum potassium, serum creatinine, plasma-free hemoglobin, and urine hemoglobin, as well as abnormal fibrinogen and coagulation panels. A positive direct antiglobulin test for IgG and/or complement may help to confirm the diagnosis, although it is not always positive in the acute phase of the reaction [120].

Once the diagnosis is suspected, the blood transfusion should be discontinued immediately, and the blood bank should be contacted to assist with confirmation of the diagnosis. Additional management of these reactions is largely supportive with intravenous fluids to maintain adequate urine output and urinary alkalinization. Although 0.9% saline is often recommended in the setting of rhabdomyolysis-associated pigmenturia, lactated Ringer's solution may better promote urine alkalinization, favoring excretion of hemoglobin in the urine [121, 122]. Similarly, diuretics may be an adjunctive therapy to augment clearance of urinary hemoglobin [122]. Vasopressor therapy may be necessary to treat associated hemodynamic instability. Management of additional end-organ dysfunction (e.g., renal failure, disseminated intravascular coagulation, etc.) may be necessary, as well.

Infectious Complications

Transfusion-transmitted infections have been a recognized complication of blood product administration since at least the 1940s [123, 124]. As microbiologic testing has advanced over the last several decades, screening programs have greatly reduced the risk of microbial transmission (Table 31.3). Transfusion-transmitted infections can vary in acuity and severity, largely depending on the microorganism involved and the size of the inoculum.

The most common nonbacterial transfusion-transmitted infections in the United States include both viral and parasitic diseases. Hepatitis B virus (HBV), hepatitis C virus (HCV), West Nile virus (WNV), human immunodeficiency virus (HIV), human T-cell lymphotropic virus (HTLV), cytomegalovirus (CMV), and Zika virus are the most common blood-borne viral infections. Babesiosis, Chagas disease, and malaria represent the most commonly transmitted parasitic infections. The average risk of acquiring one of these infections varies from a high of approximately 1 in 150,000 for HBV to a low of 1 in greater than 7,000,000 for HIV [10, 125, 126].

Bacterial infections are much more common and, generally, more severe than other types of transfusion-transmitted infections [127, 128]. Severe septic transfusion reactions occur in approximately 1 out of every 60,000–75,000 transfusions [98, 129]. The risk of bacterial transmission is much higher with platelet transfusions compared to other blood components, because they are stored at room temperature [130]. Healthcare-associated pathogens are the most common culprits in most hospital systems (e.g., *Staphylococcus aureus*, *Pseudomonas aeruginosa*, *Klebsiella pneumoniae*, etc.).

Transfusion-transmitted bacterial infections (TTBI) present with clinical signs and symptoms that are identical to any other acute bloodstream infection. Fevers, chills, and hypotension are the most common manifestations. Patients may progress to septic shock with associated multisystem organ failure. In general, labs do not demonstrate significant hemolysis, which may help to differentiate this condition from other acute transfusion reactions. To confirm a TTBI, blood cultures should be obtained from the donor blood and the patient [131]. Growth of the same organism from both the donor blood and recipient suggests a true TTBI rather than simple contamination [132]. Treatment involves appropriate empiric antibiotic therapy, hemodynamic support, and other supportive therapies as clinically indicated.

Table 31.3 Transfusion-transmitted infections [10]

Infection	Risk (per unit)
HBV	1:150,000
HCV	1:2,000,000
West Nile virus	1:1,000,000
HTLV	1:4,000,000
HIV	1:7,000,000
Bacteria (sepsis)	1:60,000 [98]

Conclusions

Like many other areas of surgical critical care, the science and practice related to blood products and transfusion therapies have significantly advanced over the past several decades and appear to be poised for even more significant advances in the near future. With the large number of currently available blood products to choose from, and the expected continued increase in newer products and formulations, it is imperative that all ICU providers have a solid understanding of these products, their major indications and contraindications, the expected effects and benefits of transfusion, and the potential risks and associated complications. The one overarching concept that directly applies to ICU transfusion strategies, and to most areas of critical care medicine, is to treat the patient and not the numbers. Restrictive transfusion triggers and meaningful transfusion targets should be utilized in order to maximize patient benefit while minimizing the risks of adverse events or other types of patient harm.

References

1. Hunt BJ. Bleeding and coagulopathies in critical care. N Engl J Med. 2014;370(9):847–59.
2. Hayden SJ, et al. Anemia in critical illness: insights into etiology, consequences, and management. Am J Respir Crit Care Med. 2012;185(10):1049–57.
3. Vincent JL, et al. Anemia and blood transfusion in critically ill patients. JAMA. 2002;288(12):1499–507.
4. Corwin HL, et al. The CRIT Study: anemia and blood transfusion in the critically ill--current clinical practice in the United States. Crit Care Med. 2004;32(1):39–52.
5. Thomas J, et al. Anemia and blood transfusion practices in the critically ill: a prospective cohort review. Heart Lung. 2010;39(3):217–25.
6. Levi M, Opal SM. Coagulation abnormalities in critically ill patients. Crit Care. 2006;10(4):222.
7. Baughman RP, et al. Thrombocytopenia in the intensive care unit. Chest. 1993;104(4):1243–7.
8. MacLeod JB, et al. Early coagulopathy predicts mortality in trauma. J Trauma. 2003;55(1):39–44.

9. Rao MP, et al. Blood component use in critically ill patients. Anaesthesia. 2002;57(6):530–4.
10. English SW, McIntyre L. Anemia and RBC transfusion. In: Vincent JL, et al., editors. Textbook of critical care. Philadelphia: Elsevier; 2017. p. 1188–94.
11. Nguyen BV, et al. Time course of hemoglobin concentrations in nonbleeding intensive care unit patients. Crit Care Med. 2003;31(2):406–10.
12. Corwin HL, Parsonnet KC, Gettinger A. RBC transfusion in the ICU. Is there a reason? Chest. 1995;108(3):767–71.
13. Roy CN. Anemia of inflammation. Hematology Am Soc Hematol Educ Program. 2010;2010:276–80.
14. Gangat N, Wolanskyj AP. Anemia of chronic disease. Semin Hematol. 2013;50(3):232–8.
15. Lelubre C, Vincent JL. Red blood cell transfusion in the critically ill patient. Ann Intensive Care. 2011;1:43.
16. Semenza GL. Regulation of oxygen homeostasis by hypoxia-inducible factor 1. Physiology (Bethesda). 2009;24:97–106.
17. Bellotto F, et al. Anemia and ischemia: myocardial injury in patients with gastrointestinal bleeding. Am J Med. 2005;118(5):548–51.
18. Weiskopf RB, et al. Human cardiovascular and metabolic response to acute, severe isovolemic anemia. JAMA. 1998;279(3):217–21.
19. Zollinger A, et al. Extreme hemodilution due to massive blood loss in tumor surgery. Anesthesiology. 1997;87(4):985–7.
20. Leone BJ, Spahn DR. Anemia, hemodilution, and oxygen delivery. Anesth Analg. 1992;75(5):651–3.
21. Gurevitz SA. Update and utilization of component therapy in blood transfusions. Lab Med. 2010;41(12):739–44.
22. Allard S. Blood components and their contents. In: Thachil J, Hill QA, editors. Haematology in critical care: a practical handbook. Chichester: Wiley; 2014. p. 77–84.
23. Napolitano LM, et al. Clinical practice guideline: red blood cell transfusion in adult trauma and critical care. Crit Care Med. 2009;37(12):3124–57.
24. Retter A, et al. Guidelines on the management of anaemia and red cell transfusion in adult critically ill patients. Br J Haematol. 2013;160(4):445–64.
25. Beutler E, West C. The storage of hard-packed red blood cells in citrate-phosphate-dextrose (CPD) and CPD-adenine (CPDA-1). Blood. 1979;54(1):280–4.
26. Dzik WH, Kirkley SA. Citrate toxicity during massive blood transfusion. Transfus Med Rev. 1988;2(2):76–94.
27. Buchholz DH, et al. Comparison of Adsol and CPDA-1 blood preservatives during simulated massive resuscitation after hemorrhage in swine. Transfusion. 1999;39(9):998–1004.
28. Strobel E. Hemolytic transfusion reactions. Transfus Med Hemother. 2008;35(5):346–53.
29. Murray NA, Roberts IA. Haemolytic disease of the newborn. Arch Dis Child Fetal Neonatal Ed. 2007;92(2):F83–8.
30. Wiesen AR, et al. Equilibration of hemoglobin concentration after transfusion in medical inpatients not actively bleeding. Ann Intern Med. 1994;121(4):278–30.
31. Norfolk DR. Safe transfusion – right blood, right patient, right time, and right place. In: Norfolk DR, editor. Handbook of transfusion medicine. Norwich: TSO; 2013. p. 27–40.
32. World Health Organization BTST. The clinical use of blood: handbook; 2001. [cited 2017 08/07/2017]; Available from: http://www.who.int/iris/handle/10665/42396.
33. Cull DL, Lally KP, Murphy KD. Compatibility of packed erythrocytes and Ringer's lactate solution. Surg Gynecol Obstet. 1991;173(1):9–12.
34. Albert K, et al. Ringer's lactate is compatible with the rapid infusion of AS-3 preserved packed red blood cells. Can J Anaesth. 2009;56(5):352–6.
35. Han WY, Wang J. The effect of red blood cells function during autologus blood salvage using by plasmalyte A: 6AP6-4. Eur J Anaesthesiol. 2010;27(47):114–5.
36. van der Meer PF. Apheresis versus whole-blood-derived platelets: pros and cons. ISBT Sci Ser. 2012;7(1):112–6.
37. Green L, Allard S, Cardigan R. Modern banking, collection, compatibility testing and storage of blood and blood components. Anaesthesia. 2015;70(3):373.
38. Reddoch KM, et al. Hemostatic function of apheresis platelets stored at 4 degrees C and 22 degrees C. Shock. 2014;41(Suppl 1):54–61.
39. Berzuini A, Spreafico M, Prati D. One size doesn't fit all: should we reconsider the introduction of cold-stored platelets in blood bank inventories? F1000Res. 2017;6:95.
40. Mondoro TH, Vostal JG. Cold temperatures reduce the sensitivity of stored platelets to disaggregating agents. Platelets. 2002;13(1):11–20.
41. Dunbar NM, Ornstein DL, Dumont LJ. ABO incompatible platelets: risks versus benefit. Curr Opin Hematol. 2012;19(6):475–9.
42. Davenport RD, Mintz PD. Transfusion Medicine. In: McPherson RA, Pincus M, Henry JB, editors. Henry's clinical diagnosis and management by laboratory methods. Philadelphia: Saunders Elsevier; 2007. p. 670.
43. Rebulla P. A mini-review on platelet refractoriness. Haematologica. 2005;90(2):247–53.
44. Hod E, Schwartz J. Platelet transfusion refractoriness. Br J Haematol. 2008;142(3):348–60.
45. Pietersz RNI, Van der Meer PF. Processing and storage of blood components: strategies to improve patient safety. Int J Clin Transfus Med. 2015;3:55–64.
46. Scott E, et al. Evaluation and comparison of coagulation factor activity in fresh-frozen plasma and 24-hour plasma at thaw and after 120 hours of 1 to 6 degrees C storage. Transfusion. 2009;49(8):1584–91.
47. Cardigan R, et al. Coagulation factor content of plasma produced from whole blood stored for 24 hours at ambient temperature: results from an international multicenter BEST Collaborative study. Transfusion. 2011;51(Suppl 1):50s–7s.
48. Yazer MH, Cortese-Hassett A, Triulzi DJ. Coagulation factor levels in plasma frozen within 24 hours of phlebotomy over 5 days of storage at 1 to 6 degrees C. Transfusion. 2008;48(12):2525–30.
49. von Heymann C, et al. Activity of clotting factors in fresh-frozen plasma during storage at 4 degrees C over 6 days. Transfusion. 2009;49(5):913–20.
50. Abdel-Wahab OI, Healy B, Dzik WH. Effect of fresh-frozen plasma transfusion on prothrombin time and bleeding in patients with mild coagulation abnormalities. Transfusion. 2006;46(8):1279–85.
51. O'Shaughnessy DF, et al. Guidelines for the use of fresh-frozen plasma, cryoprecipitate and cryosupernatant. Br J Haematol. 2004;126(1):11–28.
52. Calder L, et al. Review of published recommendations and guidelines for the transfusion of allogeneic red blood cells and plasma. Can Med Assoc J. 1997;156(11 Suppl):S1–8.
53. Matijevic N, et al. Better hemostatic profiles of never-frozen liquid plasma compared with thawed fresh frozen plasma. J Trauma Acute Care Surg. 2013;74(1):84–90; discussion 90–1.
54. Strumia MM, McGraw JJ. Frozen and dried plasma for civil and military use. JAMA. 1941;116(21):2378–82.
55. Pusateri AE, et al. Dried plasma: state of the science and recent developments. Transfusion. 2016;56(Suppl 2):S128–39.
56. Martinaud C, et al. Use of freeze-dried plasma in French intensive care unit in Afghanistan. J Trauma. 2011;71(6):1761–4; discussion 1764–5.

57. Bux J, Dickhorner D, Scheel E. Quality of freeze-dried (lyophilized) quarantined single-donor plasma. Transfusion. 2013;53(12):3203–9.
58. Solheim BG, Chetty R, Flesland O. Indications for use and cost-effectiveness of pathogen-reduced ABO-universal plasma. Curr Opin Hematol. 2008;15(6):612–7.
59. Pusateri AE, et al. Comprehensive US government program for dried plasma development. Transfusion. 2016;56(Suppl 1):S16–23.
60. Starr D. Blood: an epic history of medicine and commerce. 1st ed. New York: Harper Collins; 2000.
61. Zielinski MD, et al. Back to the future: the renaissance of whole-blood transfusions for massively hemorrhaging patients. Surgery. 2014;155(5):883–6.
62. Spinella PC. Warm fresh whole blood transfusion for severe hemorrhage: U.S. military and potential civilian applications. Crit Care Med. 2008;36(7 Suppl):S340–5.
63. Hess JR, Thomas MJ. Blood use in war and disaster: lessons from the past century. Transfusion. 2003;43(11):1622–33.
64. Moss GS, Valeri CR, Brodine CE. Clinical experience with the use of frozen blood in combat casualties. N Engl J Med. 1968;278(14):747–52.
65. Goforth CW, et al. Fresh whole blood transfusion: military and civilian implications. Crit Care Nurse. 2016;36(3):50–7.
66. Kaufman R. A fresh take on whole blood. Transfusion. 2011;51(2):230–3.
67. Kauvar DS, et al. Fresh whole blood transfusion: a controversial military practice. J Trauma. 2006;61(1):181–4.
68. Spinella PC, et al. Warm fresh whole blood is independently associated with improved survival for patients with combat-related traumatic injuries. J Trauma. 2009;66(4 Suppl):S69–76.
69. Murdock AD, et al. Whole blood: the future of traumatic hemorrhagic shock resuscitation. Shock. 2014;41(Suppl 1):62–9.
70. Pidcoke HF, et al. Primary hemostatic capacity of whole blood: a comprehensive analysis of pathogen reduction and refrigeration effects over time. Transfusion. 2013;53(Suppl 1):137S–49S.
71. Repine TB, et al. The use of fresh whole blood in massive transfusion. J Trauma. 2006;60(6 Suppl):S59–69.
72. Grosso SM, Keenan JO. Whole blood transfusion for exsanguinating coagulopathy in a US field surgical hospital in postwar Kosovo. J Trauma. 2000;49(1):145–8.
73. Mabry RL, et al. United States Army rangers in Somalia: an analysis of combat casualties on an urban battlefield. J Trauma. 2000;49(3):515–28; discussion 528–9.
74. Guideline JTTSCP. Fresh whole blood (FWB) transfusion; 2012. 10/24/2012 [cited 2017 08/08/2017]; Available from: http://www.usaisr.amedd.army.mil/cpgs/Fresh_Whole_Blood_Transfusion_24_Oct_12.pdf.
75. Grazzini G, Vaglio S. Red blood cell storage lesion and adverse clinical outcomes: post hoc ergo propter hoc? Blood Transfus. 2012;10(Suppl 2):s4–6.
76. Kim-Shapiro DB, Lee J, Gladwin MT. Storage lesion: role of red blood cell breakdown. Transfusion. 2011;51(4):844–51.
77. Liumbruno GM, Aubuchon JP. Old blood, new blood or better stored blood? Blood Transfus. 2010;8(4):217–9.
78. Latham JT Jr, Bove JR, Weirich FL. Chemical and hematologic changes in stored CPDA-1 blood. Transfusion. 1982;22(2):158–9.
79. Golan M, et al. Transfusion of fresh whole blood stored (4 degrees C) for short period fails to improve platelet aggregation on extracellular matrix and clinical hemostasis after cardiopulmonary bypass. J Thorac Cardiovasc Surg. 1990;99(2):354–60.
80. Lavee J, et al. The effect of transfusion of fresh whole blood versus platelet concentrates after cardiac operations. A scanning electron microscope study of platelet aggregation on extracellular matrix. J Thorac Cardiovasc Surg. 1989;97(2):204–12.
81. Hughes JD, Macdonald VW, Hess JR. Warm storage of whole blood for 72 hours. Transfusion. 2007;47(11):2050–6.
82. Hrezo RJ, Clark J. The walking blood bank: an alternative blood supply in military mass casualties. Disaster Manag Response. 2003;1(1):19–22.
83. Garcia Hejl C, et al. The implementation of a multinational "walking blood bank" in a combat zone: the experience of a health service team deployed to a medical treatment facility in Afghanistan. J Trauma Acute Care Surg. 2015;78(5):949–54.
84. Adams RC, Lundy JS. Anesthesia in cases of poor surgical risk: some suggestions for decreasing the risk. Surg Gynecol Obstet. 1942;74:1011–101.
85. Wang JK, Klein HG. Red blood cell transfusion in the treatment and management of anaemia: the search for the elusive transfusion trigger. Vox Sang. 2010;98(1):2–11.
86. Friedman BA, Burns TL, Schork MA. An analysis of blood transfusion of surgical patients by sex: a question for the transfusion trigger. Transfusion. 1980;20(2):179–88.
87. Hebert PC, et al. Does transfusion practice affect mortality in critically ill patients? Transfusion Requirements in Critical Care (TRICC) Investigators and the Canadian Critical Care Trials Group. Am J Respir Crit Care Med. 1997;155(5):1618–23.
88. Carson JL, et al. Effect of anaemia and cardiovascular disease on surgical mortality and morbidity. Lancet. 1996;348(9034):1055–60.
89. Bordin JO, Heddle NM, Blajchman MA. Biologic effects of leukocytes present in transfused cellular blood products. Blood. 1994;84(6):1703–21.
90. Langenfeld JE, Livingston DH, Machiedo GW. Red cell deformability is an early indicator of infection. Surgery. 1991;110(2):398–403; discussion 403–4.
91. Hebert PC, et al. A multicenter, randomized, controlled clinical trial of transfusion requirements in critical care. Transfusion Requirements in Critical Care Investigators, Canadian Critical Care Trials Group. N Engl J Med. 1999;340(6):409–17.
92. Carson JL, et al. Liberal or restrictive transfusion in high-risk patients after hip surgery. N Engl J Med. 2011;365(26):2453–62.
93. Villanueva C, et al. Transfusion strategies for acute upper gastrointestinal bleeding. N Engl J Med. 2013;368(1):11–21.
94. Holst LB, et al. Lower versus higher hemoglobin threshold for transfusion in septic shock. N Engl J Med. 2014;371(15):1381–91.
95. Hamm CW, et al. ESC Guidelines for the management of acute coronary syndromes in patients presenting without persistent ST-segment elevation: the Task Force for the management of acute coronary syndromes (ACS) in patients presenting without persistent ST-segment elevation of the European Society of Cardiology (ESC). Eur Heart J. 2011;32(23):2999–3054.
96. Ferraris VA, et al. 2011 update to the Society of Thoracic Surgeons and the Society of Cardiovascular Anesthesiologists blood conservation clinical practice guidelines. Ann Thorac Surg. 2011;91(3):944–82.
97. Carson JL, et al. Clinical practice guidelines from the AABB: red blood cell transfusion thresholds and storage. JAMA. 2016;316(19):2025–35.
98. Delaney M, et al. Transfusion reactions: prevention, diagnosis, and treatment. Lancet. 2016;388(10061):2825–36.
99. Savage WJ. Transfusion reactions. Hematol Oncol Clin North Am. 2016;30(3):619–34.
100. Tobian AA, King KE, Ness PM. Transfusion premedications: a growing practice not based on evidence. Transfusion. 2007;47(6):1089–96.
101. Hirayama F. Current understanding of allergic transfusion reactions: incidence, pathogenesis, laboratory tests, prevention and treatment. Br J Haematol. 2013;160(4):434–44.

102. Runge JW, et al. Histamine antagonists in the treatment of acute allergic reactions. Ann Emerg Med. 1992;21(3):237–42.
103. Sanders RP, et al. Premedication with acetaminophen or diphenhydramine for transfusion with leucoreduced blood products in children. Br J Haematol. 2005;130(5):781–7.
104. Marti-Carvajal AJ, et al. Pharmacological interventions for the prevention of allergic and febrile non-haemolytic transfusion reactions. Cochrane Database Syst Rev. 2010:Cd007539.
105. Narick C, Triulzi DJ, Yazer MH. Transfusion-associated circulatory overload after plasma transfusion. Transfusion. 2012;52(1):160–5.
106. Raval JS, et al. Passive reporting greatly underestimates the rate of transfusion-associated circulatory overload after platelet transfusion. Vox Sang. 2015;108(4):387–92.
107. Andrzejewski C Jr, Casey MA, Popovsky MA. How we view and approach transfusion-associated circulatory overload: pathogenesis, diagnosis, management, mitigation, and prevention. Transfusion. 2013;53(12):3037–47.
108. Zhou L, et al. Use of B-natriuretic peptide as a diagnostic marker in the differential diagnosis of transfusion-associated circulatory overload. Transfusion. 2005;45(7):1056–63.
109. Silliman CC, et al. Transfusion-related acute lung injury: epidemiology and a prospective analysis of etiologic factors. Blood. 2003;101(2):454–62.
110. Wallis JP. Transfusion-related acute lung injury (TRALI)--under-diagnosed and under-reported. Br J Anaesth. 2003;90(5):573–6.
111. Silliman CC, Ambruso DR, Boshkov LK. Transfusion-related acute lung injury. Blood. 2005;105(6):2266–73.
112. Toy P, et al. Transfusion-related acute lung injury: incidence and risk factors. Blood. 2012;119(7):1757–67.
113. Gajic O, et al. Transfusion from male-only versus female donors in critically ill recipients of high plasma volume components. Crit Care Med. 2007;35(7):1645–8.
114. Endres RO, et al. Identification of specificities of antibodies against human leukocyte antigens in blood donors. Transfusion. 2010;50(8):1749–60.
115. Chapman CE, et al. Ten years of hemovigilance reports of transfusion-related acute lung injury in the United Kingdom and the impact of preferential use of male donor plasma. Transfusion. 2009;49(3):440–52.
116. Arora S, Singh PM, Trikha A. Ventilatory strategies in trauma patients. J Emerg Trauma Shock. 2014;7(1):25–31.
117. Garratty G. What do we mean by "Hyperhaemolysis" and what is the cause? Transfus Med. 2012;22(2):77–9.
118. Maskens C, et al. Hospital-based transfusion error tracking from 2005 to 2010: identifying the key errors threatening patient transfusion safety. Transfusion. 2014;54(1):66–73; quiz 65.
119. Dasararaju R, Marques MB. Adverse effects of transfusion. Cancer Control. 2015;22(1):16–25.
120. Zantek ND, et al. The direct antiglobulin test: a critical step in the evaluation of hemolysis. Am J Hematol. 2012;87(7):707–9.
121. Cho YS, Lim H, Kim SH. Comparison of lactated Ringer's solution and 0.9% saline in the treatment of rhabdomyolysis induced by doxylamine intoxication. Emerg Med J. 2007;24(4):276–80.
122. Parekh R, Care DA, Tainter CR. Rhabdomyolysis: advances in diagnosis and treatment. Emerg Med Pract. 2012;14(3):1–15; quiz 15.
123. Whitby LEH. The hazards of transfusion. Lancet. 1942;239(6194):581–608.
124. Drummond JR. Dangerous contaminants in stored blood. Lancet. 1956;271(6955):1267–8.
125. Schreiber GB, et al. The risk of transfusion-transmitted viral infections. The Retrovirus Epidemiology Donor Study. N Engl J Med. 1996;334(26):1685–90.
126. Bihl F, et al. Transfusion-transmitted infections. J Transl Med. 2007;5:25.
127. Hillyer CD, et al. Bacterial contamination of blood components: risks, strategies, and regulation: joint ASH and AABB educational session in transfusion medicine. Hematology Am Soc Hematol Educ Program. 2003;1:575–89.
128. Fang CT, et al. Detection of bacterial contamination in apheresis platelet products: American Red Cross experience, 2004. Transfusion. 2005;45(12):1845–52.
129. Funk MB, et al. Transfusion-transmitted bacterial infections – haemovigilance data of German blood establishments (1997–2010). Transfus Med Hemother. 2011;38(4):266–71.
130. Murphy WG, Coakley P. Testing platelet components for bacterial contamination. Transfus Apher Sci. 2011;45(1):69–74.
131. Tinegate H, et al. Guideline on the investigation and management of acute transfusion reactions. Prepared by the BCSH Blood Transfusion Task Force. Br J Haematol. 2012;159(2):143–53.
132. Eder AF, Goldman M. How do I investigate septic transfusion reactions and blood donors with culture-positive platelet donations? Transfusion. 2011;51(8):1662–8.
133. Martin M, et al. Battlefield resuscitation of the future. In: Martin MJ, Beekley AC, Eckert MJ, editors. Front line surgery. 2nd ed. New York: Springer Publishing Inc; 2017.

Damage Control Resuscitation

32

Kyle J. Kalkwarf and John B. Holcomb

Background

Williams Harvey described blood circulation and its function almost 400 years ago [1]. 200 years later, the first recorded human blood transfusion was performed in London, England [2]. In the subsequent century, the frequency and utility of blood transfusion were limited by a lack of technology to inject the blood, an inability to store donated blood, and safety issues because of not understanding blood types [3]. As a result, crystalloid infusions became the standard of care for bleeding patients for most of the nineteenth century [4–6].

With the onset of World War I (WWI) and the subsequent influx of soldiers with profound hemorrhage, allied physicians observed the limitations of crystalloid resuscitation and deemed it "unsatisfactory" for the treatment of hemorrhagic shock because of dilution [7]. For the treatment of severe hemorrhage and shock, they preferred rewarming the patient while providing limited, early blood transfusions to maintain a low blood pressure, noting that this resulted in the "most dramatic improvement" [8, 9]. These transfusions were possible because of recently developed techniques to crossmatch for incompatible blood and store it for several weeks in a cold solution of citrate and dextrose to prevent coagulation [8, 10, 11]. At the end of WWI, the Royal Army Medical Corps determined that developments in blood transfusions were the most important medical advancement resulting from the war [10].

A lack of preservation techniques and storage capacity outside of large institutions prevented the large-scale use of blood transfusions in the decades after WWI, so crystalloid returned as the most common therapy for blood loss [12]. However, physician experience during WWII mirrored that of WWI and resulted in a renewed focus on the principles espoused by Walter Cannon and his colleagues three decades prior, including avoiding saline and using whole blood to replace blood loss in combat casualties who were in hemorrhagic shock [13, 14]. WWII physicians also recommended using the smallest quantities of blood necessary to achieve a systolic blood pressure of 85 mmHg, maintaining good skin color and warmth, and expeditiously stopping blood loss with an operation or tourniquet [14, 15]. The biggest change from previous conflicts was the development of blood fractionation just prior to US entry into the WWII [16]. This allowed for reconstituted dried plasma to be used while whole blood was being prepared for transfusion [17].

At the conclusion of WWII, Dr. Henry Beecher wrote, "It will be tragic if medical historian can look back on the WWII period and write of it as a time when so much was learned and so little remembered" [15]. Unfortunately, most of these lessons were soon forgotten and not employed by civilian trauma surgeons during the second half of the twentieth century. The reasons for disregarding the concepts learned while taking care of huge numbers of combat casualties were many. Surgical leaders in the 1960s were conducting studies (which were subsequently refuted) that were interpreted as demonstrating that isotonic fluid administration was required to replace extracellular fluid lost from fluid shifts and edema at sites of injury [18, 19]. A number of these trials included bleeding dogs to hypotension before stopping the blood loss with a stop-cock and resuscitating the animal with either whole blood or Ringer's lactate (LR) followed by whole blood [12, 20–22]. The outcomes for these dogs were significantly improved when isotonic fluid was administered prior to whole blood resuscitation, but this model did not account for the potential for rebleeding if a normal blood pressure was achieved prior to hemorrhage control, as had been described by Cannon and Beecher based on their respective experiences in WWI and WWII [9, 14]. The protective effect of permissive hypotension was subsequently confirmed in a randomized controlled trial which showed that delaying resuscitation to a normal blood pressure until after operative control of bleeding resulted in improved outcomes and in laboratory models of uncontrolled

K. J. Kalkwarf (✉) · J. B. Holcomb
Department of Surgery, McGovern Medical School,
University of Texas Health Science Center at Houston (UTHealth),
Houston, TX, USA

A. Salim et al. (eds.), *Surgical Critical Care Therapy*, https://doi.org/10.1007/978-3-319-71712-8_32

hemorrhagic shock in animals, including one that demonstrated rebleeding occurs in swine at an average systolic blood pressure of 94 mmHg and a mean arterial pressure of 64 mmHg [23–26].

In addition to reintroducing crystalloid, further changes were made in the resuscitation of injured patients because of improvements in blood fractionation techniques following WWII. These advances caused many in the medical community to call for blood component transfusions to maximize resources by separating whole blood into red blood cells (RBCs), plasma, and platelets so that four to five pediatric or oncology patients could be treated with each unit of whole blood [27–29]. During this time, surgeons continued to emphasize that acute blood loss should be replaced with whole blood and that balanced salt solutions should only be used in circumstances when whole blood was not available [21, 28, 30]. However, by 1970 the American Medical Association pronounced that there was virtually no indication for the use of whole blood and advised that hemorrhagic shock could be treated by packed RBCs and balanced salt solutions or plasma expanders [27]. The result was that large-volume crystalloid resuscitation was regularly employed for casualties during the Vietnam Conflict, and subsequently in civilian trauma centers, despite a lack of rigorous studies to demonstrate the efficacy of component therapy, compared with whole blood, in treating massive hemorrhage [31, 32]. These changes occurred at the same time that hospitals were adopting component therapy to the point where it became the standard practice in the 1970s and patients were often being resuscitated exclusively with RBCs and LR [33, 34]. A subsequent article stated that 1–2 liters of LR could be safely administered to patients in hemorrhagic shock during the time required to crossmatch type-specific blood, and another said that RBCs and LR could be used exclusively in moderate transfusions (average 6.5 units of RBCs) without producing coagulopathy [35, 36]. Additional groups reported that it was not necessary to supplement blood transfusions with plasma or platelets in the absence of clinical or laboratory coagulopathy, further fueling decisions to limit transfusions at the onset of the HIV epidemic in the early 1980s [37–41]. What was often overlooked in these articles was that they were referring to whole blood as the primary resuscitation fluid and not RBCs, as had become the standard therapy throughout most of the country by that time.

Infusing large volumes of crystalloid and RBCs while transfusing plasma and platelets only after alterations were identified in laboratory values probably did not matter in more than 90% of trauma patients who were not in hemorrhagic shock, but the principles were adopted by Advanced Trauma Life Support (ATLS) and subsequently became the standard of care for all trauma patients in the United States and the world for the final two decades of the twentieth century [31, 42]. With the exception of a retrospective review in 1985 that recommended transfusing plasma at an equal ratio with RBCs to avoid dilutional coagulopathy in patients with large wounds, major surgery, and neurologic injuries, little was done to break the trend of limiting plasma and platelet infusion and increasing crystalloid administration until the advent of the twenty-first century [43].

The final step in the transition away from the lessons learned during the World Wars was the adoption of supranormal hemodynamic goals. After observing that patients who survived critical illnesses achieved considerably higher, or "supranormal," cardiodynamic parameters compared with non-survivors, multiple small studies were conducted to monitor and attempt to achieve supranormal levels for cardiac index, oxygen delivery, and oxygen consumption. These studies showed a significant reduction in mortality for patients who achieved supranormal values compared to those who did not achieve these levels [44–49]. Large volumes of intravenous (iv) crystalloid were administered while attempting to achieve these supranormal values. There are published descriptions of infusing an average of 16–21 liters of crystalloid and transfusing 12–19 units of RBCs within the first 24 h in order to achieve these goals and an average of more than twice these volumes (38 liters of crystalloid and 26 units of RBCs) in patients who subsequently developed secondary abdominal compartment syndrome [50, 51]. Large-volume resuscitation continued at many centers despite reports of adverse side effects and studies rebuking the survival benefits of supratherapeutic resuscitation. These studies included a large multicenter, randomized trial published in 1995 that showed no advantage of instituting a protocol to achieve supranormal values in critically ill patients [52]. This study, and other smaller studies in trauma patients, attributed the survival advantage found in previous supratherapeutic studies to comparing the survival of the minority of patients who were able to achieve such supranormal values with those who were not able to achieve such goals [53]. It was later postulated that the inability to achieve supranormal values forecasted a poor outcome relative to those patients who were able to achieve them, rather than a benefit resulting from treatment targeting therapeutic goals [54]. When outcomes for supranormal resuscitation were reviewed, it was shown to result in more isotonic fluid administration, decreased intestinal perfusion, and an increased incidence of abdominal compartment syndrome, organ failure, and death [55].

At the same time studies were recognizing the adverse effects of large-volume crystalloid transfusion, others were rediscovering previous work that showed trauma and shock are associated with hypocoagulable states [56]. This was confirmed by new studies which found that a quarter of patients who arrived in the emergency department after severe trauma were coagulopathic, despite limited prehospital resuscitation or penetrating mechanism [57–59]. This coagulopathy was associated with a mortality rate three to five times greater than patients with normal coagulation laboratory values on admission [58, 60, 61]. Other groups were simultaneously using mathematical modeling and retrospective data to determine that higher ratios of plasma to RBCs were required to limit coagulopathy and improve survival [62–68].

Damage Control Resuscitation

Early in the twenty-first century, military trauma leaders brought together new research on bleeding to change the way that severely injured patients were treated during the conflicts in Southwest Asia. They combined the knowledge that many severely injured patients were coagulopathic on arrival and that low ratios of plasma to RBCs increased coagulopathy with newly implemented changes in military prehospital care. These prehospital recommendations included stopping the bleeding with pressure or tourniquets, only providing enough iv fluids to titrate the patient's mental status to baseline (assuming no head injury) with a normal radial pulse, and rapid evacuation to a facility with surgical capabilities [31, 69, 70]. These prehospital recommendations were based on experience gained from previous wars, permissive hypotension studies, and animal models all of which showed decreased bleeding and mortality with limited resuscitation rather than attempting to achieve normal vital signs [7, 14, 23, 31, 71, 72]. As a result, in time for the conflicts in Iraq and Afghanistan, the military implemented protocols to limit bleeding and resuscitate to a low blood pressure with fluid approximating whole blood, harkening back to care provided during the World Wars.

This care was codified as damage control resuscitation (DCR) and was focused on preventing or reversing coagulopathy by employing permissive hypotension, avoiding hypothermia, limiting crystalloids, rapidly controlling hemorrhage, delivering high ratios of plasma and platelets to approximate whole blood, and applying appropriate adjuncts to limit bleeding [73]. The changes in the standard of care for military physicians treating the severely injured paved the way for investigations into the outcomes of soldiers injured in the Middle East. The first retrospective trial looking at massively transfused patients in US Army combat hospitals who were resuscitated with a 1:1 ratio of plasma/RBC showed that a higher ratio of plasma to RBCs (1:1.4) was associated with significantly lower hemorrhage and a greater than 50% reduction in mortality compared to patients who received lower ratios of plasma to RBCs (1:8) [67]. Multiple subsequent retrospective trials replicated the improved outcomes for those receiving a 1:1 ratio of plasma to RBCs in patients with ruptured abdominal aortic aneurysms as well as trauma patients in military and civilian settings [60, 74–79]. Similar results were also found for patients receiving 4–9 units of blood or more than 10 units of blood in patients who were injured by penetrating or blunt mechanism [80–82]. Other trials showed that including balanced ratios of platelets was also associated with improved survival [83–88]. There were also a few studies that showed no benefit with balanced ratios of plasma to RBCs [34, 89]. When DCR has been implemented for patients in hemorrhagic shock or undergoing damage control laparotomy, retrospective results have demonstrated decreased crystalloid infusion as well as less plasma and platelet utilization despite earlier transfusions with higher initial ratios of plasma and platelets [90, 91]. DCR has also resulted in decreased rates of abdominal compartment syndrome, infection, organ failure, morbidity, and mortality from hemorrhage despite an overall increased rate of trauma deaths in the United States during the same period [90–95].

The limitation of retrospective studies was highlighted by a 2009 study focused on time to transfusion for different blood components. Because of the significantly increased time required to give fresh frozen plasma (FFP) (93 min) compared to RBCs (18 min) when attempting to transfuse at a balanced ratio, those who died early were able to receive RBCs but not the appropriate ratio of FFP and platelets, while those who survived were eventually able to achieve the goal ratios, thus creating a survival bias [96]. As a result, the PROPPR trial was designed as a prospective, randomized, multicenter trial to evaluate the two most common resuscitation ratios [97]. The PROMMTT study observed transfusion practices in ten level 1 trauma centers and found 1:1:1 and 1:1:2 (plasma/platelet/RBCs) were the most common resuscitative ratios [88]. While the PROPPR study showed no improvement in 24-h survival for 1:1:1 v. 1:1:2, it did show a decrease in exsanguination as the cause of death at 24 h for higher ratios of plasma and platelets (9.2% 1:1:1 group v. 14.6% in 1:1:2 group), and there was no difference in complications for the two groups, indicating that plasma and platelets are safe to transfuse in a massive transfusion (MT) protocol. There was also improved mortality at 3 h for the 1:1 group, which is the median time to hemorrhagic death and within the 6-h period when 85% of hemorrhagic deaths occur [94, 97–101].

DCR Concepts

Hypothermia

Hypothermia is common in severely injured patients because of exposure on the scene of the accident, during transport, and while being treated in the emergency department or operating room. It causes a coagulopathy by reducing platelet function and decreasing the reactions of coagulation enzymes and fibrinogen synthesis, thus increasing mortality [34, 102–106]. As a result, rewarming techniques such as heating blankets, body cavity lavage, and warmed iv fluids are important to improve coagulation and correct other physiology [107].

Limit Crystalloid

Large-volume crystalloid infusion worsens the "bloody vicious cycle" of coagulopathy, hypothermia, and acidosis as initially described 35 years ago by causing dilution of the clotting factors in the blood, cooling with unwarmed fluids, and producing a hyperchloremic metabolic acidosis from the isotonic fluid administration [34, 90, 108–110]. Iv fluids have also been shown to disrupt cellular mechanisms, resulting in inflammatory states that cause edema and end organ dysfunction [107, 111, 112]. These processes are associated with a plethora of complications including immune dysfunction, hyperfibrinolysis, acute respiratory distress syndrome, cardiac dysfunction, gastrointestinal delays, decreased wound healing, anastomotic leak, abdominal compartment syndrome, and open abdomens, all of which contribute to multiple organ failure and increased mortality [51, 55, 90, 92, 113–118]. Furthermore, minimizing crystalloid infusions in favor of blood products for those with life-threatening injuries results in fewer transfusions and subsequent complications [119–121].

Whole Blood/Plasma/Platelets

More than a million units of whole blood were transfused by military doctors in WWI, WWII, Korea, Vietnam, Somalia, Kosovo, Afghanistan, and Iraq, and it was successfully used in civilian trauma until it fell out of favor in the 1970s because it was considered to be wasteful and potentially unsafe [10, 11, 122, 123]. A resurgence of whole blood for the treatment of the most severely injured occurred during the recent military conflicts in the Middle East where more than 10,000 units were transfused to 13% of those who received blood products during Operation Iraqi Freedom [41, 122, 124]. Retrospective reviews from recent military conflicts have shown that warm fresh whole blood is superior to component therapy in massively transfused casualties with increased 24-h and 30-day survival [68, 125]. This is consistent with in vitro studies showing whole blood is more hemostatic, a retrospective review which found fresh whole blood (FWB) transfusions resulted in reduced blood loss, and a prospective trial that showed less transfusions of plasma and platelets, when patients with head injuries were excluded [126–128]. The reasons for the superiority of whole blood is that a 500-ml unit of fresh whole blood has a hematocrit of 38–50%, 150,000–400,000 platelets per microliter, and 100% activity of clotting factors. As a comparison, transfusion of one unit of plasma, platelets, and RBCs results in 660 ml of fluid with a hematocrit of 29%, 88,000 platelets per microliter, and 65% coagulation factor activity with reduced flow characteristics and increased additives including anticoagulants [41, 122]. Whole blood also benefits from full platelet activity and aggregation with one unit producing the hemostatic effect of ten units of platelets [122, 129, 130].

When whole blood is not available, balanced component transfusion practices, as adopted by the military in Iraq and Afghanistan, quickly spread to civilian practices throughout the United States and have become the standard of care as more than 85% of major trauma centers currently employ a 1:1:1 ratio for MT protocols, up from just a few institutions a decade ago [131, 132]. The improvement that follows plasma transfusions in massively transfused patients is attributed to its impact on decreasing inflammation, edema, and vascular permeability by repairing the vascular endothelium tight junctions and endothelial glycocalyx as well as by improving platelet function and clot formation [133–135]. At the other end of the spectrum, plasma also decreases hypercoagulability by modulating thrombin generation [136]. One of the limiting factors in FFP administration is the time required to thaw the plasma. Thawed or liquid plasma can therefore be used in the emergency department to decrease the time to initial plasma transfusion, and 69% of Level I and II American College of Surgeons Trauma Quality Improvement Program (ACS TQIP) trauma centers have plasma immediately available for MT protocol activations [137]. This has been shown to allow for earlier transfusions, balanced resuscitation, decreased overall blood product transfusions, and improved mortality [138, 139].

Similar to higher ratios of transfused plasma, higher ratios of platelets have been correlated with improved survival in multiple studies [84, 86, 87]. This is not unexpected as platelet inhibition and decreased function is common in brain and minor trauma, even before administration of extensive fluid or blood [140–142]. Initial platelet dysfunction is thought to result from tissue injury and shock, and it is associated with increased morbidity and mortality [142]. Platelets are also known to improve wound healing, vascular integrity, and immune response [87]. 79% of ACS TQIP trauma centers target balanced ratios of platelets to RBCs in their MT protocols [137].

At the end of WWII, Beecher said, "About 2.5 per cent (sic) of those wounded would fall into the group that is in bad enough condition to require special resuscitative care" [14]. That percentage currently holds true for civilian admissions with 2.6% requiring more than 10 units of blood within the first 6–24 h, while two to three times that percentage of injured military combatants will require a MT [67,84,152]. The mortality rates for those receiving a MT are between 20 and 65%, but balanced ratio MT protocols have been shown to decrease mortality by more than 50%, when employed in these patients [67, 93, 143–146].

The decision to employ DCR is based on hemorrhagic shock or the future need for a MT, so a good way to predict this need is necessary for appropriate initiation. In WWII, Beecher used vital signs and clinical exam with increasing pulse, decreasing blood pressure, and cool skin as prognosticators for a blood transfusion [14]. A decade ago, the military showed that a physical exam could be used to reliably predict the need for a lifesaving intervention and that radial pulse was the best predictor [147]. This method was codified a few years later as the Field Triage Score which gives points for a radial pulse and a normal motor component of Glasgow Coma Scale to allow prehospital personnel to more accurately triage and treat patients in an austere environment [148]. In locations where more resources are available, the ABC Score allows for an accurate assessment of the likelihood for requiring a MT by giving points for penetrating mechanism, positive Focused Assessment Sonography for Trauma (FAST), systolic blood pressure $\leq$ 90 mmHg, and an arrival heart rate >120 beats per minute [149]. This scoring system was verified in a multicenter trial and is currently being used to determine if blood should be given in the prehospital setting on civilian medical transport helicopters [150, 151].

The current practice of resuscitation for hemorrhagic shock differs little from the methods utilized by our surgical forefathers in WWI and WWII. Their concept of limited whole blood transfusions was developed based on treating vast quantities of severely bleeding men during two of the deadliest wars in human history. Migration away from these practices during the second half of the twentieth century was recently rejected based on experiences during more limited conflicts in Southwest Asia. Implementation of damage control resuscitation into civilian trauma care will result some in nuanced changes, but hopefully not to the degree that occurred previously, so we are not forced to relearn the same lessons again.

Acknowledgements Dr. Holcomb reports a conflict of interest as a co-inventor of the Junctional Emergency Treatment Tool.

References

1. Harvey W. Exercitatio anatomica de motu cordis et sanguinis in animalibus. Frankfurt am Main. 1628. pt. 1. Facsimile of the original Latin ed. (1628)-pt. 2. The English translation by Chauncey Depew. Springfield: Thomas; 1928.
2. Blundell J. Some account of a case of obstinate vomiting, in which an attempt was made to prolong life by the injection of blood into the veins. Med Chir Trans. 1819;10(Pt 2):296–311.
3. Schmidt PJ. Transfusion in America in the eighteenth and nineteenth centuries. N Engl J Med. 1968;279(24):1319–20.
4. Jennings CE. The intra-venous injection of fluid for severe haemorrhage. Lancet. 1882;120(3081):436–7.
5. Jennings CE. The intra-venous injection of fluid for severe haemorrhage. Lancet. 1883;121(3102):228–9.
6. Pye-Smith RJ. Sheffield public hospital and dispensary: five cases of intravenous injection of saline fluid for haemorrhage and collapse. Lancet. 1892;139(3582):913–5.
7. Fraser J, Cowell EM. Clinical study of blood pressure in wound conditions. JAMA. 1918;70:520–35.
8. Robertson OH. Transfusion with preserved red blood cells. Br Med J. 1918;1(2999):691.
9. Cannon WB. Traumatic shock. New York: D. Appleton; 1923.
10. Hess JR, Thomas MJ. Blood use in war and disaster: lessons from the past century. Transfusion. 2003;43(11):1622–33.
11. Spinella PC. Warm fresh whole blood transfusion for severe hemorrhage: US military and potential civilian applications. Crit Care Med. 2008;36(7):S340–5.
12. Wolfman EF, Neill SA, Heaps DK, Zuidema GD. Donor blood and isotonic salt solution. Effect on survival after hemorrhagic shock and operation. Arch Surg. 1963;86:869–73.
13. Cannon WB, Fraser J, Cowell EM. The preventive treatment of wound shock. JAMA. 1918;70:618–21.
14. Beecher HK. Preparation of battle casualties for surgery. Ann Surg. 1945;121(6):769–92.
15. Beecher HK. Early care of the seriously wounded man. J Am Med Assoc. 1951;145(4):193–200.
16. Giangrande PL. The history of blood transfusion. Br J Haematol. 2000;100:758–67.
17. Beecher HK. Resuscitation, and anesthesia for wounded men, the management of traumatic shock. Springfield: Charles C. Thomas; 1949.
18. Shires T, Williams J, Brown F. Acute change in extracellular fluids associated with major surgical procedures. Ann Surg. 1961;154:803–10. PMID: 13912109.
19. Shires T, Jackson DE. Postoperative salt tolerance. Arch Surg. 1962;84:703–6. PMID: 13912108.
20. Fogelman MJ, Wilson BJ. A different concept of volume replacement in traumatic hypovolemia observations on injured man and animal. Am J Surg. 1960;99(5):694–701.
21. Shires T, Coln D, Carrico J, Lightfoot S. Fluid therapy in hemorrhagic shock. Arch Surg. 1964;88:688–93.
22. McClelland RN, Shires GT, Baxter CR, Coln CD, Carrico J. Balanced salt solution in the treatment of hemorrhagic shock. JAMA. 1967;199:830–4.
23. Bickell WH, Wall MJ Jr, Pepe PE, Martin RR, Ginger VF, Allen MK, Mattox KL. Immediate versus delayed fluid resuscitation for hypotensive patients with penetrating torso injuries. N Engl J Med. 1994;331(17):1105–9.
24. Kowalenko T, Stern S, Dronen S, Wang X. Improved outcome with hypotensive resuscitation of uncontrolled hemorrhagic shock in a swine model. J Trauma Acute Care Surg. 1992;33(3):349–53.
25. Holmes JF, Sakles JC, Lewis G, Wisner DH. Effects of delaying fluid resuscitation on an injury to the systemic arterial vasculature. Acad Emerg Med. 2002;9:267–74.
26. Sondeen JL, Coppes VG, Holcomb JB. Blood pressure at which rebleeding occurs after resuscitation in swine with aortic injury. J Trauma Injury Infect Crit Care. 2003;54(5 suppl):S110–7.
27. AMA Committee on Transfusion and Transplantation. Something old, something new. JAMA. 1970;212(1):147.
28. Moore FD. Should blood be whole or in parts? N Engl J Med. 1969;280(6):327–8.
29. Westphal RG. Rational alternatives to the use of whole blood. Ann Intern Med. 1972;76(6):987–90.
30. Moore FD, Shires G. Moderation. Ann Surg. 1967;166:300–1.
31. Holcomb JB. Fluid resuscitation in modern combat casualty care: lessons learned from Somalia. J Trauma. 2003;54 (5 Suppl):S46–51. Review.
32. Holcomb JB. Reconstitution: reverse engineering. J Trauma. 2011;70(5 Suppl):S65–7.

33. Sheldon GF, Lim RC, Blaisdell FW. The use of fresh blood in the treatment of critically injured patients. J Trauma. 1975;15:670–7.
34. Kashuk JL, Moore EE, Millikan JS, Moore JB. Major abdominal vascular trauma-a unified approach. J Trauma Acute Care Surg. 1982;22(8):672–9. RJ Lowe in Discussion.
35. Carrico CJ, Canizaro PC, Shires GT. Fluid resuscitation following injury: rationale for the use of balanced salt solutions. Crit Care Med. 1976;4(2):46–54.
36. Shackford SR, Virgilio RW, Peters RM. Whole blood versus packed-cell transfusions: a physiologic comparison. Ann Surg. 1981;193(3):337–40.
37. Counts RB, Haisch C, Simon TL, Maxwell NG, Heimbach DM, Carrico CJ. Hemostasis in massively transfused trauma patients. Ann Surg. 1979;190(1):91–9.
38. Lucas CE, Ledgerwood AM. Clinical significance of altered coagulation tests after massive transfusion for trauma. Am Surg. 1981;47(3):125–30.
39. Reed RL 2nd, Ciavarella D, Heimbach DM, Baron L, Pavlin E, Counts RB, Carrico CJ. Prophylactic platelet administration during massive transfusion. A prospective, randomized, double-blind clinical study. Ann Surg. 1986;203:40–8.
40. Lee L, Moore EE, Hansen KC, Silliman CC, Chandler JG, Banerjee A. It's not your grandfather's field plasma. Surgery. 2013;153(6):857–60.
41. Spinella PC, Pidcoke HF, Strandenes G, Hervig T, Fisher A, Jenkins D, Yazer M, Stubbs J, Murdock A, Sailliol A, Ness PM. Whole blood for hemostatic resuscitation of major bleeding. Transfusion. 2016;56(S2):S190–202.
42. American College of Surgeons Committee on Trauma. Advanced trauma life support (ATLS) student course manual. 9th ed. Chicago: American College of Surgeons; 2012. p. 62–81.
43. Hewson JR, Neame PB, Kumar N, Ayrton A, Gregor P, Davis C, Shragge BW. Coagulopathy related to dilution and hypotension during massive transfusion. Crit Care Med. 1985;13(5):387–91.
44. Bland R, Shoemaker WC, Shabot MM. Physiologic monitoring goals for the critically ill patient. Surg Gynecol Obstet. 1978;147(6):833–41.
45. Shoemaker WC, Appel PL, Kram HB, Waxman K, Lee TS. Prospective trial of supranormal values of survivors as therapeutic goals in high-risk surgical patients. Chest J. 1988;94(6):1176–86.
46. Fleming A, Bishop M, Shoemaker W, Appel P, Sufficool W, Kuvhenguwha A, Kennedy F, Wo CJ. Prospective trial of supranormal values as goals of resuscitation in severe trauma. Arch Surg. 1992;127:1175–9. Discussion 1179–1181.
47. Bishop MH, Wo CCJ, Appel PL, et al. Relationship between supranormal circulatory values, time delays, and outcome in severely traumatized patients. Crit Care Med. 1993;21:56–60.
48. Boyd O, Grounds RM, Bennett ED. A randomized clinical trial of the effect of deliberate perioperative increase of oxygen delivery on mortality in high-risk surgical patients. JAMA. 1993;270(22):2699–707.
49. Bishop MH, Shoemaker WC, Appel PL, Meade P, Ordog GJ, Wasserberger J, Wo CJ, Rimle DA, Kram HB, Umali R. Prospective, randomized trial of survivor values of cardiac index, oxygen delivery, and oxygen consumption as resuscitation endpoints in severe trauma. J Trauma. 1995;38(5):780–7.
50. McKinley BA, Marvin RG, Cocanour CS, Marquez A, Ware DN, Moore FA. Blunt trauma resuscitation: the old can respond. Arch Surg. 2000;135(6):688–95.
51. Balogh Z, McKinley BA, Cocanour CS, Kozar RA, Holcomb JB, Ware DN, Moore FA. Secondary abdominal compartment syndrome is an elusive early complication of traumatic shock resuscitation. Am J Surg. 2002;184(6):538–43; discussion 543–4.
52. Gattinoni L, Brazzi L, Pelosi P, Latini R, Tognoni G, Pesenti A, Fumagalli R. A trial of goal-oriented hemodynamic therapy in critically ill patients. N Engl J Med. 1995;333(16):1025–32.
53. Durham RM, Neunaber K, Mazuski JE, Shapiro MJ, Baue AE. The use of oxygen consumption and delivery as endpoints for resuscitation in critically III patients. J Trauma Acute Care Surg. 1996;41(1):32–40.
54. Velmahos GC, Demetriades D, Shoemaker WC, Chan LS, Tatevossian R, Wo CC, Vassiliu P, Cornwell EE III, Murray JA, Roth B, Belzberg H. Endpoints of resuscitation of critically injured patients: normal or supranormal?: a prospective randomized trial. Ann Surg. 2000;232(3):409–18.
55. Balogh Z, McKinley BA, Cocanour CS, Kozar RA, Valdivia A, Sailors RM, Moore FA. Supranormal trauma resuscitation causes more cases of abdominal compartment syndrome. Arch Surg. 2003;138:637–42.
56. Simmons RL, Collins JA, Heisterkamp CA 3rd, Mills DE, Andren R, Phillips LL. Coagulation disorders in combat casualties, I: acute changes after wounding. Ann Surg. 1969;169(4):455–82.
57. MacLeod JB, Lynn M, McKenney MG, Cohn SM, Murtha M. Early coagulopathy predicts mortality in trauma. J Trauma. 2003;55(1):39–44.
58. Brohi K, Singh J, Heron M, Coats T. Acute traumatic coagulopathy. J Trauma. 2003;54:1127–30.
59. Niles SE, McLaughlin DF, Perkins JG, Wade CE, Li Y, Spinella PC, Holcomb JB. Increased mortality associated with the early coagulopathy of trauma in combat casualties. J Trauma Injury Infect Crit Care. 2008;64(6):1459–63; discussion 1463–5.
60. Gunter OL Jr, Au BK, Isbell JM, Mowery NT, Young PP, Cotton BA. Optimizing outcomes in damage control resuscitation: identifying blood product ratios associated with improved survival. J Trauma Injury Infect Crit Care. 2008;65(3):527–34.
61. Pidcoke HF, Aden JK, Mora AG, Borgman MA, Spinella PC, Dubick MA, Blackbourne LH, Cap AP. Ten-year analysis of transfusion in Operation Iraqi Freedom and Operation Enduring Freedom: increased plasma and platelet use correlates with improved survival. J Trauma Acute Care Surg. 2012;73(6):S445–52.
62. Ho AM, Dion PW, Cheng CA, Karmakar MK, Cheng G, Peng Z, Ng YW. A mathematical model for fresh frozen plasma transfusion strategies during major trauma resuscitation with ongoing hemorrhage. Can J Surg. 2005;48:470–8.
63. Hirshberg A, Dugas M, Banez EI, Scott BG, Wall MJ Jr, Mattox KL. Minimizing dilutional coagulopathy in exsanguinating hemorrhage: a computer simulation. J Trauma Acute Care Surg. 2003;54(3):454–63.
64. Ledgerwood AM, Lucas CE. A review of studies on the effects of hemorrhagic shock and resuscitation on the coagulation profile. J Trauma Acute Care Surg. 2003;54(5):S68–74.
65. Ketchum L, Hess JR, Hiippala S. Indications for early fresh frozen plasma, cryoprecipitate, and platelet transfusion in trauma. J Trauma. 2006;60(Suppl):S51–S8.
66. Gonzalez EA, Moore FA, Holcomb JB, Miller CC, Kozar RA, Todd SR, Cocanour CS, Balldin BC, McKinley BA. Fresh frozen plasma should be given earlier to patients requiring massive transfusion. J Trauma. 2007;62(1):112–9.
67. Borgman MA, Spinella PC, Perkins JG, Grathwohl KW, Repine T, Beekley AC, Sebesta J, Jenkins D, Wade CE, Holcomb JB. The ratio of blood products transfused affects mortality in patients receiving massive transfusions at a combat support hospital. J Trauma. 2007;63(4):805–13.
68. Holcomb JB, Spinella PC. Optimal use of blood in trauma patients. Biologicals. 2010;38(1):72–7.
69. Meredith W, Rutledge R, Hansen AR, Oller DW, Thomason M, Cunningham P, Baker CC. Field triage of trauma patients based upon the ability to follow commands: a study in 29,573 injured patients. J Trauma Acute Care Surg. 1995;38(1):129–35.
70. McManus J, Yershov AL, Ludwig D, Holcomb JB, Salinas J, Dubick MA, Convertino VA, Hinds D, David W, Flanagan T, Duke JH. Radial pulse character relationships to systolic blood pressure and trauma outcomes. Prehosp Emerg Care. 2005;9(4):423–8.

71. Mabry RL, Holcomb JB, Baker AM, Cloonan CC, Uhorchak JM, Perkins DE, Canfield AJ, Hagmann JH. United States Army Rangers in Somalia: an analysis of combat casualties on an urban battlefield. J Trauma Acute Care Surg. 2000;49(3):515–29.
72. Burris D, Rhee P, Kaufmann C, Pikoulis E, Austin B, Eror A, DeBraux S, Guzzi L, Leppäniemi A. Controlled resuscitation for uncontrolled hemorrhagic shock. J Trauma. 1999;46:216–23.
73. Holcomb JB, Jenkins D, Rhee P, Johannigman J, Mahoney P, Mehta S, Cox ED, Gehrke MJ, Beilman GJ, Schreiber M, Flaherty SF. Damage control resuscitation: directly addressing the early coagulopathy of trauma. J Trauma Acute Care Surg. 2007;62(2):307–10.
74. Johansson PI, Stensballe J, Rosenberg I, Hilsløv TL, Jørgensen L, Secher NH. Proactive administration of platelets and plasma for patients with a ruptured abdominal aortic aneurysm: evaluating a change in transfusion practice. Transfusion. 2007;47(4):593–8.
75. Spinella PC, Perkins JG, Grathwohl KW, Beekley AC, Niles SE, McLaughlin DF, Wade CE, Holcomb JB. Effect of plasma and red blood cell transfusions on survival in patients with combat related traumatic injuries. J Trauma. 2008;64(2 Suppl):S69–77; discussion S77–8.
76. Duchesne JC, Hunt JP, Wahl G, Marr AB, Wang YZ, Weintraub SE, Wright MJ, McSwain NE Jr. Review of current blood transfusions strategies in a mature level I trauma center: were we wrong for the last 60 years. J Trauma. 2008;65:272–6. Discussion 276–278.
77. Maegele M, Lefering R, Paffrath T, Tjardes T, Simanski C, Bouillon B. Working Group on Polytrauma of the German Society of Trauma Surgery (DGU). Red-blood-cell to plasma ratios transfused during massive transfusion are associated with mortality in severe multiple injury: a retrospective analysis from the Trauma Registry of the Deutsche Gesellschaft für Unfallchirurgie. Vox Sang. 2008;95(2):112–9.
78. Teixeira PG, Inaba K, Shulman I, Salim A, Demetriades D, Brown C, Browder T, Green D, Rhee P. Impact of plasma transfusion in massively transfused trauma patients. J Trauma Injury Infect Crit Care. 2009;66(3):693–7.
79. Brown LM, Aro SO, Cohen MJ, Trauma Outcomes Group, Holcomb JB, Wade CE, Brasel KJ, Vercruysse G, MacLeod J, Dutton RP, Hess JR, Duchesne JC, McSwain NE, Muskat P, Johannigamn J, Cryer HM, Tillou A, Pittet JF, Knudson P, De Moya MA, Schreiber MA, Tieu B, Brundage S, Napolitano LM, Brunsvold M, Sihler KC, Beilman G, Peitzman AB, Zenait MS, Sperry J, Alarcon L, Croce MA, Minei JP, Kozar R, Gonzalez EA, Stewart RM, Cohn SM, Mickalek JE, Bulger EM, Cotton BA, Nunez TC, Ivatury R, Meredith JW, Miller P, Pomper GJ, Marin B. A high fresh frozen plasma: packed red blood cell transfusion ratio decreases mortality in all massively transfused trauma patients regardless of admission international normalized ratio. J Trauma. 2011;71(2 Suppl 3):S358–63.
80. Wafaisade A, Maegele M, Lefering R, Braun M, Peiniger S, Neugebauer E, Bouillon B, Trauma Registry of DGU. High plasma to red blood cell ratios are associated with lower mortality rates in patients receiving multiple transfusion (4≤ red blood cell units< 10) during acute trauma resuscitation. J Trauma Acute Care Surg. 2011;70(1):81–9.
81. Rowell SE, Barbosa RR, Diggs BS, Schreiber MA, Trauma Outcomes Group, Holcomb JB, Wade CE, Brasel KJ, Vercruysse G, MacLeod J, Dutton RP, Hess JR, Duchesne JC, McSwain NE, Muskat P, Johannigamn J, Cryer HM, Tillou A, Cohen MJ, Pittet JF, Knudson P, De Moya MA, Schreiber MA, Tieu B, Brundage S, Napolitano LM, Brunsvold M, Sihler KC, Beilman G, Peitzman AB, Zenait MS, Sperry J, Alarcon L, Croce MA, Minei JP, Kozar R, Gonzalez EA, Stewart RM, Cohn SM, Mickalek JE, Bulger EM, Cotton BA, Nunez TC, Ivatury R, Meredith JW, Miller P, Pomper GJ, Marin B. Effect of high product ratio massive transfusion on mortality in blunt and penetrating trauma patients. J Trauma. 2011;71(2 Suppl 3):S353–7.
82. Sperry JL, Ochoa JB, Gunn SR, Alarcon LH, Minei JP, Cuschieri J, Rosengart MR, Maier RV, Billiar TR, Peitzman AB, Moore EE, Inflammation the Host Response to Injury Investigators. An FFP:PRBC transfusion ratio >/=1:1.5 is associated with a lower risk of mortality after massive transfusion. J Trauma. 2008;65:986.
83. Holcomb JB, Wade CE, Michalek JE, Chisholm GB, Zarzabal LA, Schreiber MA, Gonzalez EA, Pomper GJ, Perkins JG, Spinella PC, Williams KL, Park MS. Increased plasma and platelet to red blood cell ratios improves outcome in 466 massively transfused civilian trauma patients. Ann Surg. 2008;248(3):447–58.
84. Perkins JG, Cap AP, Spinella PC, Blackbourne LH, Grathwohl KW, Repine TB, Ketchum L, Waterman P, Lee RE, Beekley AC, Sebesta JA, Shorr AF, Wade CE, Holcomb JB. An evaluation of the impact of apheresis platelets used in the setting of massively transfused trauma patients. J Trauma. 2009;66:S77–85.
85. Zink KA, Sambasivan CN, Holcomb JB, Chisholm G, Schreiber MA. A high ratio of plasma and platelets to packed red blood cells in the first 6 hours of massive transfusion improves outcomes in a large multicenter study. Am J Surg. 2009;197(5):565–70; discussion 570.
86. Inaba K, Lustenberger T, Rhee P, Holcomb JB, Blackbourne LH, Shulman I, Nelson J, Talving P, Demetriades D. The impact of platelet transfusion in massively transfused trauma patients. J Am Coll Surg. 2010;211:573–9.
87. Holcomb JB, Zarzabal LA, Michalek JE, Kozar RA, Spinella PC, Perkins JG, Matijevic N, Dong JF, Pati S, Wade CE, Trauma Outcomes Group, Holcomb JB, Wade CE, Cotton BA, Kozar RA, Brasel KJ, Vercruysse GA, MacLeod JB, Dutton RP, Hess JR, Duchesne JC, McSwain NE, Muskat PC, Johannigamn JA, Cryer HM, Tillou A, Cohen MJ, Pittet JF, Knudson P, DeMoya MA, Schreiber MA, Tieu BH, Brundage SI, Napolitano LM, Brunsvold ME, Sihler KC, Beilman GJ, Peitzman AB, Zenati MS, Sperry JL, Alarcon LH, Croce MA, Minei JP, Steward RM, Cohn SM, Michalek JE, Bulger EM, Nunez TC, Ivatury RR, Meredith JW, Miller PR, Pomper GJ, Marin B. Increased platelet:RBC ratios are associated with improved survival after massive transfusion. J Trauma. 2011;71(2 Suppl 3):S318–28.
88. Holcomb JB, del Junco DJ, Fox EE, Wade CE, Cohen MJ, Schreiber MA, Alarcon LH, Bai Y, Brasel KJ, Bulger EM, Cotton BA, Matijevic N, Muskat P, Myers JG, Phelan HA, White CE, Zhang J, Rahbar MH, PROMMTT Study Group. The prospective, observational, multicenter, major trauma transfusion (PROMMTT) study: comparative effectiveness of a time-varying treatment with competing risks. JAMA Surg. 2013;148(2):127–36.
89. Scalea TM, Bochicchio KM, Lumpkins K, Hess JR, Dutton R, Pyle A, Bochicchio GV. Early aggressive use of fresh frozen plasma does not improve outcome in critically injured trauma patients. Ann Surg. 2008;248:578.
90. Cotton BA, Reddy N, Hatch QM, LeFebvre E, Wade CE, Kozar RA, Gill BS, Albarado R, McNutt MK, Holcomb JB. Damage control resuscitation is associated with a reduction in resuscitation volumes and improvement in survival in 390 damage control laparotomy patients. Ann Surg. 2011;254(4):598–605.
91. Joseph B, Azim A, Zangbar B, Bauman ZM, O'Keeffe T, Ibraheem K, Kulvatunyou N, Tang A, Latifi R, Rhee P. Improving mortality in trauma laparotomy through the evolution of damage control resuscitation: analysis of 1,030 consecutive trauma laparotomies. J Trauma Acute Care Surg. 2016;82:328–33.

92. Hatch QM, Osterhout LM, Podbielski J, Kozar RA, Wade CE, Holcomb JB, Cotton BA. Impact of closure at the first take back: complication burden and potential overutilization of damage control laparotomy. J Trauma. 2011;71(6):1503–11.
93. Cotton BA, Au BK, Nunez TC, Gunter OL, Robertson AM, Young PP. Predefined massive transfusion protocols are associated with a reduction in organ failure and postinjury complications. J Trauma. 2009;66:41–8; discussion 48–49.
94. Oyeniyi BT, Fox EE, Scerbo M, Tomasek JS, Wade CE, Holcomb JB. Trends in 1029 trauma deaths at a level 1 trauma center: impact of a bleeding control bundle of care. Injury. 2016;48:5–12.
95. Rhee P, Joseph B, Pandit V, Aziz H, Vercruysse G, Kulvatunyou N, Friese RS. Increasing trauma deaths in the United States. Ann Surg. 2014;260(1):13–21.
96. Snyder CW, Weinberg JA, McGwin G Jr, Melton SM, George RL, Reiff DA, Cross JM, Hubbard-Brown J, Rue LW 3rd, Kerby JD. The relationship of blood product ratio to mortality: survival benefit or survival bias. J Trauma Injury Infect Crit Care. 2009;66(2):358–62.
97. Holcomb JB, Tilley BC, Baraniuk S, Fox EE, Wade CE, Podbielski JM, del Junco DJ, Brasel KJ, Bulger EM, Callcut RA, Cohen MJ, Cotton BA, Fabian TC, Inaba K, Kerby JD, Muskat P, O'Keeffe T, Rizoli S, Robinson BR, Scalea TM, Schreiber MA, Stein DM, Weinberg JA, Callum JL, Hess JR, Matijevic N, Miller CN, Pittet JF, Hoyt DB, Pearson GD, Leroux B, van Belle G, PROPPR Study Group. Transfusion of plasma, platelets, and red blood cells in a 1:1:1 vs a 1:1:2 ratio and mortality in patients with severe trauma: the PROPPR randomized clinical trial. JAMA. 2015;313(5):471–82.
98. Demetriades D, Murray J, Charalambides K, Alo K, Velmahos G, Rhee P, Chan L. Trauma fatalities: time and location of hospital deaths. J Am Coll Surg. 2004;198(1):20–6.
99. Demetriades D, Kimbrell B, Salim A, Velmahos G, Rhee P, Preston C, Gruzinski G, Chan L. Trauma deaths in a mature urban trauma system: is "trimodal" distribution a valid concept? J Am Coll Surg. 2005;201(3):343–8.
100. Tisherman SA, Schmicker RH, Brasel KJ, Bulger EM, Kerby JD, Minei JP, Powell JL, Reiff DA, Rizoli SB, Schreiber MA. Detailed description of all deaths in both the shock and traumatic brain injury hypertonic saline trials of the Resuscitation Outcomes Consortium. Ann Surg. 2015;261(3):586–90.
101. Fox EE, Holcomb JB, Wade CE, Bulger EM, Tilley BC. PROPPR Study Group. Earlier endpoints are required for hemorrhagic shock trials among severely injured patients. Shock. 2017;47(5):567–73.
102. Hess JR, Holcomb JB. Transfusion practice in military trauma. Transfus Med. 2008;18(3):143–50.
103. Martini WZ, Holcomb JB. Acidosis and coagulopathy: the differential effects on fibrinogen synthesis and breakdown in pigs. Ann Surg. 2007;246(5):831–5.
104. Jurkovich GJ, Greiser WB, Luterman A, Curreri PW. Hypothermia in trauma victims: an ominous predictor of survival. J Trauma. 1987;27(9):1019–24.
105. Ferrara A, MacArthur JD, Wright HK, Modlin IM, McMillen MA. Hypothermia and acidosis worsen coagulopathy in the patient requiring massive transfusion. Am J Surg. 1990;160:515–8.
106. Cosgriff NM, Ernest E, Sauaia A, Kenny-Moynihan M, Burch JM, Galloway B. Predicting life-threatening coagulopathy in the massively transfused patient: hypothermia and acidosis revisited. J Trauma Injury Infect Crit Care. 1997;42(5):857–62.
107. Duchesne JC, Kimonis K, Marr AB, Rennie KV, Wahl G, Wells JE, Islam TM, Meade P, Stuke L, Barbeau JM, Hunt JP, Baker CC, McSwain NE Jr. Damage control resuscitation in combination with damage control laparotomy: a survival advantage. J Trauma. 2010;69:46–52.
108. Maegele M, Lefering R, Yucel N, Tjardes T, Rixen D, Paffrath T, Simanski C, Neugebauer E, Bouillon B. AG Polytrauma of the German Trauma Society (DGU). Early coagulopathy in multiple injury: an analysis from the German Trauma Registry on 8724 patients. Injury. 2007;38:298.
109. Tieu BH, Holcomb JB, Schreiber MA. Coagulopathy: its pathophysiology and treatment in the injured patient. World J Surg. 2007;31:1055–64.
110. Myburgh JA, Mythen MG. Resuscitation fluids. N Engl J Med. 2013;369:1243–51.
111. Feinman M, Cotton BA, Haut ER. Optimal fluid resuscitation in trauma: type, timing, and total. Curr Opin Crit Care. 2014;20(4):366–72.
112. Shah SK, Uray KS, Stewart RH, Laine GA, Cox CS. Resuscitation-induced intestinal edema and related dysfunction: state of the science. J Surg Res. 2011;166(1):120–30.
113. Cotton BA, Guy JS, Morris JA Jr, Abumrad NA. The cellular, metabolic, and systemic consequences of aggressive fluid resuscitation strategies. Shock. 2006;26:115–21.
114. Cotton BA, Harvin JA, Kostousouv V, Minei KM, Radwan ZA, Schöchl H, Wade CE, Holcomb JB, Matijevic N. Hyperfibrinolysis at admission is an uncommon but highly lethal event associated with shock and prehospital fluid administration. J Trauma Acute Care Surg. 2012;73(2):365–70; discussion 370.
115. Brandstrup B, Tønnesen H, Beier-Holgersen R, Hjortsø E, Ørding H, Lindorff-Larsen K, Rasmussen MS, Lanng C, Wallin L, Iversen LH, Gramkow CS. Effects of intravenous fluid restriction on postoperative complications: comparison of two perioperative fluid regimens: a randomized assessor-blinded multicenter trial. Ann Surg. 2003;238(5):641.
116. Lobo DN, Bostock KA, Neal KR, Perkins AC, Rowlands BJ, Allison SP. Effect of salt and water balance on recovery of gastrointestinal function after elective colonic resection: a randomized control trial. Lancet. 2002;359:1812–8.
117. Schnüriger B, Inaba K, Wu T, Eberle BM, Belzberg H, Demetriades D. Crystalloids after primary colon resection and anastomosis at initial trauma laparotomy: excessive volumes are associated with anastomotic leakage. J Trauma Acute Care Surg. 2011;70(3):603–10.
118. Ley EJ, Clond MA, Srour MK, Barnajian M, Mirocha J, Margulies DR, Salim A. Emergency department crystalloid resuscitation of 1.5 L or more is associated with increased mortality in elderly and nonelderly trauma patients. J Trauma. 2011;70:398–400.
119. Spinella PC, Perkins JG, Grathwohl KW, Repine T, Beekley AC, Sebesta J, Jenkins D, Azarow K, Holcomb JB, 31st CSH Research Working Group. Fresh whole blood transfusions in coalition military, foreign national, and enemy combatant patients during Operation Iraqi Freedom at a US combat support hospital. World J Surg. 2008;32(1):2–6.
120. Duchesne JC, Heaney J, Guidry C, McSwain N Jr, Meade P, Cohen M, Schreiber M, Inaba K, Skiada D, Demetriades D, Holcomb J. Diluting the benefits of hemostatic resuscitation: a multi-institutional analysis. J Trauma Acute Care Surg. 2013;75(1):76–82.
121. Shrestha B, Holcomb JB, Camp EA, Del Junco DJ, Cotton BA, Albarado R, Gill BS, Kozar RA, Kao LS, McNutt MK, Moore LJ, Love JD, Tyson GH 3rd, Adams PR, Khan S, Wade CE. Damage-control resuscitation increases successful nonoperative management rates and survival after severe blunt liver injury. J Trauma Acute Care Surg. 2015;78(2):336–41.
122. Kauvar DS, Holcomb JB, Norris GC, Hess JR. Fresh whole blood transfusion: a controversial military practice. J Trauma. 2006;61(1):181–4.
123. Murdock AD, BersÈus O, Hervig T, Strandenes G, Lunde TH. Whole blood: the future of traumatic hemorrhagic shock resuscitation. Shock. 2014;41:62–9.

124. Holcomb JB. Damage control resuscitation. J Trauma. 2007;62 (6 Suppl):S36–7. Review.
125. Spinella PC, Perkins JG, Grathwohl KW, Beekley AC, Holcomb JB. Warm fresh whole blood is independently associated with improved survival for patients with combat-related traumatic injuries. J Trauma Injury Infect Crit Care. 2009;66 (4 Suppl):S69–76.
126. Golan M, Modan M, Lavee J, Martinowitz U, Savion N, Goor DA, Mohr R. Transfusion of fresh whole blood stored (4 degrees C) for short period fails to improve platelet aggregation on extracellular matrix and clinical hemostasis after cardiopulmonary bypass. J Thorac Cardiovasc Surg. 1990;99(2):354–60.
127. Erber WN, Tan J, Grey D, Lown JA. Use of unrefrigerated fresh whole blood in massive transfusion. Med J Aust. 1996;165:11–3.
128. Cotton BA, Podbielski J, Camp E, Welch T, del Junco D, Bai Y, Hobbs R, Scroggins J, Hartwell B, Kozar RA, Wade CE, Holcomb JB, Early Whole Blood Investigators. A randomized controlled pilot trial of modified whole blood versus component therapy in severely injured patients requiring large volume transfusions. Ann Surg. 2013;258(4):527–32; discussion 532–3.
129. Repine TB, Perkins JG, Kauvar DS, Blackborne L. The use of fresh whole blood in massive transfusion. J Trauma Injury Infect Crit Care. 2006;60(6 suppl):S59–69.
130. Nepstad I, Reikvam H, Strandenes G, Hess JR, Apelseth TO, Hervig TA. Comparison of in vitro responses to fresh whole blood and reconstituted whole blood after collagen stimulation. Blood Transfus. 2014;12(1):50.
131. Hess JR, Holcomb JB. Resuscitating PROPPRly. Transfusion. 2015;55(6):1362–4.
132. Malone DL, Hess JR, Fingerhut A. Massive transfusion practices around the globe and a suggestion for a common massive transfusion protocol. J Trauma. 2006;60(6 Suppl):S91–6.
133. Pati S, Matijevic N, Doursout MF, Ko T, Cao Y, Deng X, Kozar RA, Hartwell E, Conyers J, Holcomb JB. Protective effects of fresh frozen plasma on vascular endothelial permeability, coagulation, and resuscitation after hemorrhagic shock are time dependent and diminish between days 0 and 5 after thaw. J Trauma. 2010;69(Suppl 1):S55–63.
134. Watson JJ, Pati S, Schreiber MA. Plasma transfusion: history, current realities, and novel improvements. Shock. 2016;46(5):468–79.
135. Sillesen M, Johansson PI, Rasmussen LS, Jin G, Jepsen CH, Imam A, Hwabejire JO, Deperalta D, Duggan M, Velmahos GC, Alam HB. Fresh frozen plasma resuscitation attenuates platelet dysfunction compared with normal saline in a large animal model of multisystem trauma. J Trauma Acute Care Surg. 2014;76(4):998–1007.
136. Cardenas JC, Cap AP, Swartz MD, Huby Mdel P, Baer LA, Matijevic N, Cotton BA, Holcomb JB, Wade CE. Plasma resuscitation promotes coagulation homeostasis following shock-induced hypercoagulability. Shock. 2016;45(2):166–73.
137. Camazine MN, Hemmila MR, Leonard JC, Jacobs RA, Horst JA, Kozar RA, Bochicchio GV, Nathens AB, Cryer HM, Spinella PC. Massive transfusion policies at trauma centers participating in the American College of Surgeons Trauma Quality Improvement Program. J Trauma Acute Care Surg. 2015;78(6):S48–53.
138. Radwan ZA, Bai Y, Matijevic N, del Junco DJ, McCarthy JJ, Wade CE, Holcomb JB, Cotton BA. An emergency department thawed plasma protocol for severely injured patients. JAMA Surg. 2013;148(2):170–5.
139. Holcomb JB, Pati S. Optimal trauma resuscitation with plasma as the primary resuscitative fluid: the surgeon's perspective. Hematology Am Soc Hematol Educ Program. 2013;2013:656–9.
140. Jacoby RC, Owings JT, Holmes J, Battistella FD, Gosselin RC, Paglieroni TG. Platelet activation and function after trauma. J Trauma. 2001;51:639–47.
141. Sirajuddin S, Valdez C, DePalma L, Maluso P, Singhal R, Schroeder M, Sarani B. Inhibition of platelet function is common following even minor injury. J Trauma Acute Care Surg. 2016;81(2):328–32.
142. Wohlauer MV, Moore EE, Thomas S, Sauaia A, Evans E, Harr J, Silliman CC, Ploplis V, Castellino FJ, Walsh M. Early platelet dysfunction: an unrecognized role in the acute coagulopathy of trauma. J Am Coll Surg. 2012;214(5):739–46.
143. Como JJ, Dutton RP, Scalea TM, Edelman BB, Hess JR. Blood transfusion rates in the care of acute trauma. Transfusion. 2004;44(6):809–13.
144. Perkins JG, Schreiber MA, Wade CE, Holcomb JB. Early versus late recombinant factor VIIa in combat trauma patients requiring massive transfusion. J Trauma. 2007;62(5):1095–9.
145. Biffl WL, Smith WR, Moore EE, Gonzalez RJ, Morgan SJ, Hennessey T, Offner PJ, Ray CE Jr, Franciose RJ, Burch JM. Evolution of a multidisciplinary clinical pathway for the management of unstable patients with pelvic fractures. Ann Surg. 2001;233(6):843–50.
146. Riskin DJ, Tsai TC, Riskin L, Hernandez-Boussard T, Purtill M, Maggio PM, Spain DA, Brundage SI. Massive transfusion protocols: the role of aggressive resuscitation versus product ratio in mortality reduction. J Am Coll Surg. 2009;209:198–205.
147. Holcomb JB. Manual vital signs reliably predict need for lifesaving interventions in trauma patients. J Trauma. 2005;59:821–9.
148. Eastridge BJ, Butler F, Wade CE, Holcomb JB, Salinas J, Champion HR, Blackbourne LH. Field triage score (FTS) in battlefield casualties: validation of a novel triage technique in a combat environment. Am J Surg. 2010;200(6):724–7; discussion 727.
149. Nunez TC, Voskresensky IV, Dossett LA, Shinall R, Dutton WD, Cotton BA. Early prediction of massive transfusion in trauma: simple as ABC (assessment of blood consumption). J Trauma. 2009;66:346.
150. Cotton BA, Dosseett LA, Haut EH, Shafi S, Nunez TC, Au BK, Zaydfudim V, Johnston M, Arbogast P, Young PP. Multicenter validation of a simplified score to predict massive transfusion in trauma. J Trauma. 2010;69:S33–9.
151. Holcomb JB, Donathan DP, Cotton BA, Del Junco DJ, Brown G, Wenckstern TV, Podbielski JM, Camp EA, Hobbs R, Bai Y, Brito M, Hartwell E, Duke JR, Wade CE. Prehospital transfusion of plasma and red blood cells in trauma patients. Prehosp Emerg Care. 2015;19(1):1–9. Epub 2014 Jun 16.

Anticoagulants and Antiplatelet Agents

33

Dave D. Paskar and Sandro B. Rizoli

Diagnosis of Active Anticoagulation/Antiplatelet Therapy

Detection of active anticoagulation or antiplatelet therapy in the awake and oriented patient is, ideally, straightforward: asking the patient if they are on any such agent and, if so, when it was last taken and what the indication for the therapy is. Recall may be prompted by naming common agents for the patient. In the obtund patient, the detection of these agents can be more difficult. Possible confirmation strategies include family inquisition, review of medical records, medical condition/medication notification jewelry (i.e., *MedicAlert* © bracelets), and inquiry into drug insurance and commercial pharmacy databases.

If direct confirmation is not possible, certain patient and clinical factors may suggest that antiplatelet or anticoagulant agents may be present. For example, elderly patients are more likely to be on these agents than younger individuals. Patients in atrial fibrillation in the trauma bay and/or those with seemingly inappropriate bradycardia (suggesting beta blockade) also have a higher likelihood of being anticoagulated for stroke prevention (in light of atrial fibrillation).

Finally, depending on the specific agent, laboratory investigations ordered in the acute trauma setting may help in suggesting the presence of anticoagulant or antiplatelet medications. However, confirmatory drug detection assays are not typically available in trauma care environments. Laboratory investigations are only reliable for suggesting the presence of these medications early in the immediate post-injury period, before hemorrhagic consumption and/or acute traumatic coagulopathy result in abnormal values, independent of anticoagulant medications.

D. D. Paskar
Divisions of General Surgery Trauma & Critical Care Medicine, University of Toronto, Toronto, ON, Canada

S. B. Rizoli (✉)
Department of Trauma & Acute Care Surgery, St. Michael's Hospital, University of Toronto, Toronto, ON, Canada
e-mail: RizoliS@smh.ca

Prothrombin time (PT) (measured by INR – *international normalized ratio*), which assesses the vitamin K-dependent extrinsic clotting pathway, is elevated (2.0 or higher; normal 0.9–1.2) in a calibrated fashion in patients undergoing warfarin therapy. PT is also often elevated in patients receiving direct oral anticoagulants (DOACs) such as dabigatran (*Pradaxa* ©), albeit in a non-calibrated ("qualitatively elevated"), and thus unreliable, manner [1]. PT is also elevated in patients with liver disease with synthetic dysfunction and other medical conditions. Partial thromboplastin time (PTT), which measures the intrinsic clotting pathway, is usually elevated in patients undergoing most forms of anticoagulation, including DOACs, and unfractionated and low-molecular-weight heparin. Furthermore, PT and PTT may be of limited clinical utility as they represent measurements of only portions of the overall coagulation process.

Antiplatelet agents such as clopidogrel (*Plavix* ©) and acetylsalicylic acid (ASA; *Aspirin* ©) inhibit platelet function rather than synthesis, and as such, platelet counts as part of a complete blood count (CBC) are not helpful in the detection of these agents as total platelet counts are typically normal in these patients. Specific assays of platelet function exist, but are not rapidly available in the trauma setting, but may be employed as the resuscitation enters the operative and critical care environments.

Finally, "traditional" lab tests such as INR/PTT and CBC are often slow to return results, further contributing to their limited utility in detecting the presence of anticoagulant or antiplatelet medications. Point-of-care tests of whole blood clotting activity are being increasingly employed in acute care environments due to their rapidity and perceived external validity.

Activated clotting time (ACT) testing simply measures time to whole blood clotting. While simple to interpret, ACT provides one value that may be lengthened by any of a host of sources of coagulopathy (i.e., thrombocytopenia, hemophilia) and thus does not provide insight into the specific cause of coagulopathy, only confirming that it is present. On the other hand, viscoelastic tests, such as rotational thromboelastometry (*ROTEM* ©), are dynamic whole blood

A. Salim et al. (eds.), *Surgical Critical Care Therapy*, https://doi.org/10.1007/978-3-319-71712-8_33

assays which distinguish and characterize different phases of the clotting process by measuring different parameters: clot initiation (*clotting time*), propagation (*alpha angle*), maintenance (*amplitude*), and destruction (*lysis*) [14] (Fig. 33.1a).

As such, these tests are able to provide additional insight into the cause(s) of coagulopathy, including the possible activity of pro-bleeding medications, information which is not available from traditional hematological tests, or ACT. An isolated delay in clot initiation (lengthened clotting time) is a product of inhibited or depleted clotting factors, and in the appropriate clinical context, is suggestive of the presence of anticoagulant therapy (Fig. 33.1b). Impaired clot propagation (reduced alpha angle) and reduced amplitude suggests a deficiency of the raw materials that make up physical clot, which include fibrin (fibrinogen) and activated platelets (Fig. 33.1c). In the setting of a patient with such ROTEM © characteristics but normal fibrinogen and platelet counts, the possibility of inhibited platelet function should be considered. Our institution routinely performs ROTEM © on all trauma patients as part of their initial bloodwork panel.

Management of Anticoagulant/Antiplatelet Agents in the Setting of Acute Trauma

The management of acute trauma patients with known or possible anticoagulant or antiplatelet therapy starts with adherence to good trauma care principles (i.e. ATLS), the aforementioned efforts to diagnose or suspect the presence of these agents, preventing exacerbation of coagulopathy by other sources such as hypothermia, and, where possible, expedited surgical control of anatomical bleeding. In regard to the latter, we have a lower injury severity (grade) threshold for triggering operative management of solid organ injuries (i.e., liver and spleen) in initially hemodynamically stable patients on nonreversible anticoagulant or antiplatelet agents.

It is our routine practice to administer tranexamic acid (TXA) to all patients with suspected bleeding, especially those with active nonreversible anticoagulant and antiplatelet therapy (two 1 gram boluses, with additional amounts in patients with suspected hyperfibrinolysis) [5]. Discussion of the management of specific agents follows.

Antiplatelet Agents

The common antiplatelet agents, ASA and clopidogrel, irreversibly inhibit the function of platelets, and as such, effects of these medications persists for the life span of individual platelets (up to 9 days). Moreover, these medications will also similarly inhibit any transfused platelets that are administered in response to bleeding while these agents are still active (up to 30 h for both agents). Since these agents do not currently have reversal agents, their presence potentially represents a significant problem for affected patients with traumatic bleeding and their care providers [13].

Historically, platelet transfusion was advised for these patients as this results in temporary increases in circulating activated platelets [16]. However, recent RCT evidence regarding the use of platelet transfusion in the setting of clopidogrel-treated patients with spontaneous (nontraumatic) intracerebral hemorrhage demonstrated increased harm relative to standard care alone [3], further casting doubt on the role of platelet transfusion in the trauma patient on clopidogrel, although this, overall, remains an unanswered question. Our practice is to urgently consult with our transfusion medicine (hematology) colleagues and consider transfusion depending on the severity of bleeding and time since the last ingestion of the antiplatelet agent.

Another described maneuver is the administration of synthetic vasopressin (desmopressin [ddAVP]) which stimulates the release of von Willebrand factor, hypothetically improving the aggregation of any non-inhibited platelets [7]. However, the clinical data supporting this intervention is lacking [16].

Warfarin

Warfarin remains the most commonly prescribed anticoagulant agent, although it is losing ground to the DOACs [10]. One of its persisting appeals has been the drug's ability to be rapidly reversed with prothrombin complex concentrates (PCCs) (i.e., *Octaplex* ©). However, a growing number of the DOACs now have reversal agents, and furthermore, there is increasing evidence in trauma that warfarin results in equivalent or even poorer outcomes relative to the DOACs despite its potentially more robust reversibility profile (awareness and availability of its reversal agent) [6, 9, 12].

Warfarin works via inhibition of vitamin K reactivation that is required for the clotting function of numerous clotting factors. As such, the foundation of its reversal is the administration of supplemental vitamin K (phytomenadione), which when appropriately dosed according to the patient's INR, will reverse the effect of warfarin within 6–12 h as the liver generates vitamin K-dependent clotting factors. Obviously, this time frame is inadequate for acute trauma management, and direct replacement of vitamin K-dependent clotting factors is also needed. Historically, this was via the administration of fresh frozen plasma (FFP). However, this has been replaced in the recent era by the PCCs which have been shown to reverse warfarin faster, more cost-effectively, completely, and safely than the administration of FFP [11] and, thus, are the standard of care for this purpose. We administer PCC to potentially bleeding trauma patients with known or suspected warfarin use at a dose of 50 U/kg intravenously (IV) in conjunction with a 5–10 mg dose of

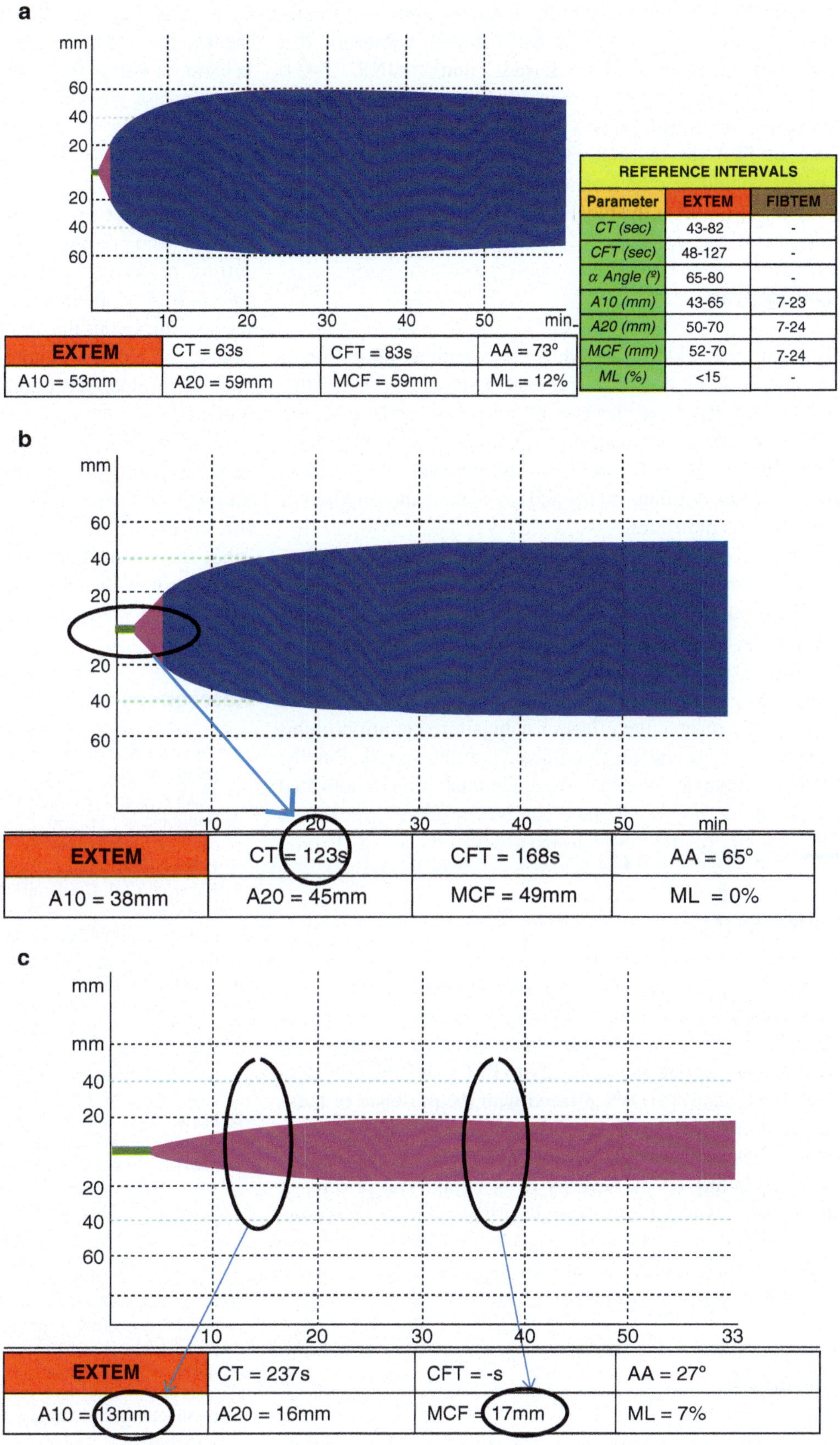

Fig. 33.1 (**a**) Normal ROTEM© (EXTEM) example results and reference parameters. (**b**) Example ROTEM © data in the setting of active anticoagulant therapy. (**c**) Example ROTEM © data in setting of inhibited platelet function

vitamin K. (The latter is still required as some of the elements of PCC have a shorter half-life than warfarin). If a PCC is not available, FFP is advised: 2 units for INR 1.6–2.0 and 4 units for INR greater than 2.0. The predominant acute complication of FFP (versus PCC) is volume overload. (The role of FFP for reversal of pre-existing coagulopathy in trauma should now be isolated to the sole indication to that resulting from liver dysfunction.)

Dabigatran

Dabigatran is a DOAC and thus acts via direct inhibition of thrombin. A monoclonal antibody reversal agent for this medication has been developed and has recently achieved full approval for use in most jurisdictions. This agent, idarucizumab (*Praxbind* ©), achieves full reversal of dabigatran in the matter of minutes [15] and, as such, is the standard of care for this indication.

If not available, other less optimal reversal strategies include hemodialysis, which is typically impractical for use in acute trauma, and PCCs, which do not reverse as rapidly or as fully, and are not as readily available at the point of care as idarucizumab which can be stored in the trauma bay or emergency department [7]. Activated PCCs (aPCCs) more profoundly reverse the effect of dabigatran, but are prohibitively expensive and have significant thrombosis risk. Finally, for dabigatran, as for all DOACs, administration of activated charcoal via nasogastric tube can be considered to exclude any recently (under 2 h) ingested doses of the agent [15].

Other DOACs

Other DOAC agents such as rivaroxaban (*Xarelto* ©) and apixaban (*Eliquis* ©) do not have as robust reversal strategies as dabigatran, as they lack available specific reversal agents and do not respond as vigorously to PCCs and aPCCs (especially apixaban) [2]. When faced with the presence of these medications, we consult urgently with our transfusion medicine colleagues and will consider PCC or aPCC administration depending on the severity of bleeding. The priority in these patients is definitive bleeding control, where possible, and prevention of additional sources of coagulopathy. There are currently reversal agents in development for these agents, albeit none currently available in the clinical setting.

Heparins

The heparin family of injectable anticoagulants includes unfractionated heparin (UFH) and more modern low-molecular-weight heparins (LMWH) (i.e., dalteparin [*Fragmin* ©] and enoxaparin [*Lovenox* ©]). Protamine is the IV reversal agent for the heparins and its dosing depends on the type and dose of the heparin, as well as the time since last administration.

Summary

Trauma care providers are increasingly faced with injured patients who present with possible significant bleeding in the setting of active anticoagulant and/or antiplatelet therapy. The upfront challenge is first identifying these patients and the specific agents that are on board, which can be difficult in obtund or elderly trauma patients. Modern investigations such as thromboelastography may help in identifying these patients.

Some agents, such as warfarin and dabigatran, have robust reversal agents and strategies, whereas others, such as the antiplatelet agents and the other DOACs, do not. In the setting of the latter, the priorities are preventing and treating other sources of coagulopathy, increased emphasis on surgical control of bleeding, and the consideration of aforementioned incomplete reversal strategies.

References

1. Adcock DM, Gosselin RC. The danger of relying on the APTT and PT in patients on DOAC therapy, a potential patient safety issue. Int J Lab Hematol. 2017;39(s1):37–40.
2. Babilonia K, Trujillo T. The role of prothrombin complex concentrates in reversal of target specific anticoagulants. Thromb J. 2014;12:8.
3. Baharoglu MI, Cordonnier C, Salman RAS, et al. Platelet transfusion versus standard care after acute stroke due to spontaneous cerebral haemorrhage associated with antiplatelet theraphy (PATCH): a randomised, open-label, phase 3 trial. Lancet. 2016;387:2605–13.
4. Coleman J, Baldawi M, Heidt D. The effect of anticoagulation status on geriatric fall trauma patients. Am J Surg. 2016;212:1237–42.
5. CRASH-2 Trial Collaborators. Effects of tranexamic acid on death, vascular occlusive events, and blood transfusion in trauma patients with significant hemorrhage (CRASH-2): a randomised, placebo-controlled trial. Lancet. 2010;376:23–32.
6. Feeney JM, Santone E, DiFiori M, et al. Compared to warfarin, direct oral anticoagulants are associated with lower mortality in patients with blunt traumatic intracranial hemorrhage: a TQIP study. J Trauma Acute Care Surg. 2016;81(5):843–8.
7. Gordon JL, Fabian TC, Lee MD. Anticoagulant and antiplatelet medications encountered in emergency surgery patients: a review of reversal strategies. J Trauma Acute Care Surg. 2013;75:475–86.
8. Kannel KB, Wolf PA, Benjamin EJ, Levy D. Prevalence, incidence, prognosis and predisposing conditions for atrial fibrillation: population-based estimates. Am J Cardiol. 1998;82(7):2N–9N.
9. Kobayashi L, Barmparas G, Bosarge P, et al. Novel oral anticoagulants and trauma: the results of a prospective American Association for the Surgery of Trauma Multi-Institutional Trial. J Trauma Acute Care Surg. 2017;82(5):827–35.
10. Levi M. Epidemiology and management of bleeding in patients using vitamin K antagonists. J Thromb Haemost. 2009;7(s1):103–6.

11. McBeth PB, Weinberg JA, Sarani B, Yeung LY, May AK. Surgeon's guide to anticoagulant and antiplatelet medications part one: warfarin and new direct oral anticoagulant medications. Trauma Surg Acute Care Open. 2016;1:1–5.
12. Myers SP, Dadashzadeh ER, Cheung J, et al. Management of anticoagulation with rivaroxaban in trauma and acute care surgery: complications and reversal strategies as compared to warfarin therapy. J Trauma Acute Care Surg. 2017;82(3):542–9.
13. Nishijima DK, Offerman SR, Ballard DW, Vinson DR, Chettipally UK, Rauchwager AS, Reed ME, Holmes JF. Immediate and delayed traumatic hemorrhage in patients with head trauma and preinjury warfarin or clopidogrel use. Ann Emerg Med. 2012;59(6):460–8.
14. Veigas PV, Callum J, Rizoli S, Nascimento B, da Luz LT. A systematic review on the rotational thrombelastometry (ROTEM) values for the diagnosis of coagulopathy, prediction and guidance of blood transfusion and prediction of mortality in trauma patients. Scand J Trauma Resusc Emerg Med. 2016;24(1):114.
15. von Heymann C, Rosenthal C, Kaufner L, Sander M. Management of direct oral anticoagulants-associated bleeding in the trauma patient. Curr Opin Anesthesiol. 2016;29(2):222–8.
16. Yeung LY, Sarani B, Weinberg JA, McBeth PB, May AK. Surgeon's guide to anticoagulant and antiplatelet medications part two: antiplatelet agents and perioperative management of long-term anticoagulation. Trauma Surg Acute Care Open. 2016;1:1–7.

Laboratory Assessment of Coagulation

34

Hunter B. Moore, Eduardo Gonzalez, and Ernest E. Moore

Cell-Based Model of Hemostasis

Enzymatic protease pathways taught during medical school do not accurately assess the living coagulation system. While assays used to measure therapeutic anticoagulation such as an international normalized ratio of prothrombin time (INR) or partial thromboplastin time (PTT) are based on the proteases of the intrinsic and extrinsic pathway, they artificially partition coagulation. The importance of assessing coagulation with its cellular constituents has been highlighted by the work of Hoffman and Monroe [1], in which cell-based interactions coordinate hemostasis. While the INR was the gold standard for identifying trauma-induced coagulopathy (TIC) [2], this laboratory assay is limited to the first 5% of clot formation [3]. It has been argued that whole blood viscoelastic assays can replace all plasma-based assays for the initial assessment of both adult [4] and pediatric [5] trauma patients. Because these viscoelastic assays measure whole blood coagulation, they not only detect coagulation abnormalities but can be used for goal-directed resuscitation as a single test [6, 7]. Viscoelastic assays use warm whole blood to assess coagulation. Therefore, platelets, coagulation proteases, and fibrinogen are tested as a whole. The two additional actors in cell-based hemostasis that are not taken into consideration with viscoelastic assays are tissue factor (TF) bearing cells and endothelial cells.

TF is considered the key protein in initiation of cell-based coagulation. While viscoelastic assays do not include TF cells, the soluble protein is used as an ex vivo agonist to initiate coagulation in viscoelastic assays. TF in vivo provides a constitutively active hemostatic envelope around blood vessels in the body that is prebound to factor VII [8]. This TF-FVII (coagulation factor seven) complex produces activated FX (coagulation factor ten) around the vascular system [9]. Essentially the entire perivascular space is already primed for coagulation, but large proteins and platelets confined to the intravascular space prevent propagation. This is a key technical point for drawing blood samples. When collecting a fresh venous or arterial sample, the initial 1 ml of blood should be discarded, as it will contain a core of TF rich cells, which will cause artifact in the viscoelastic readout.

Amplification of coagulation after TF initiation is predominantly through the release of FV (coagulation factor five) from platelets [10]. There are numerous additional protease interactions including FIX and tissue factor pathway inhibitor (TFPI) that regulate this process, but ultimately when platelets bind to an area of injury, coagulation begins to rapidly proceed. This process is thought to be mediated by platelets that have dual activation of both collagen (binding site of injury) and thrombin (local initiation of coagulation). These COAT (collagen- and thrombin-stimulated) platelets are highly procoagulant [11]. This leads to platelet aggregation and assembly of coagulation factors to promote clot propagation. Platelets orchestrate the thrombin burst resulting in clot propagation by localization of FV and FVIII to their phospholipid surface [12]. This results in high levels of thrombin cleaving fibrinogen and strengthening the forming hemostatic plug, which is further strengthened by fibrin cross-linking from factor XIII.

Coagulation in vivo is a continuous process with circulating factors and endothelial surface receptors limiting clot to the site of injury and preventing clot formation in distant uninjured intravascular sites. Ultimately all clot will begin to degrade through a process termed fibrinolysis. Furthermore, endothelial glycocalyx [13] and receptors such a thrombomodulin [14] are believed to be endogenous anticoagulants. Viscoelastic assays lack an endothelial component and are an inherent limitation of the test. However, the complexity of the endothelial response to coagulation is beyond the capacity of a single test. The endothelium

H. B. Moore (✉) · E. Gonzalez
Department of Surgery, University of Colorado, Denver, CO, USA
e-mail: mjdaley@seton.org

E. E. Moore
Department of Surgery, University of Colorado Denver, Denver, CO, USA

Department of Surgery, Denver Health, Denver, CO, USA

A. Salim et al. (eds.), *Surgical Critical Care Therapy*, https://doi.org/10.1007/978-3-319-71712-8_34

depending on the vascular type (arterial, venous, capillary) and organ-specific location has diverse functions and compositions. This is important to consider when assessing viscoelastic assays. A readout of these coagulation tests is coagulation of the systemic circulation and not the local environment of injury.

While viscoelastic assays do not completely replicate the living coagulation system, they offer superior results to conventional plasma-based assays. The clear importance of including platelets and coagulation factors when assessing coagulation is not of debate. The major limitations of these assays are their relatively limited clinical use in trauma. While manufactures have recommended guidelines for normal ranges, the indices of these assays directing patient care remain to be clearly defined in specific patient populations. Certain specialties such as cardiothoracic and transplant surgery have been using these devices to guide intra-operative resuscitation for decades, but these patients may harbor coagulation dysfunction that is dissimilar from trauma. The fact that the only randomized controlled trauma trial assessing the impact of viscoelastic assays over conventional laboratory tests [15] was not published until 2016, it is clear we are in our infancy in utilizing viscoelastic assays to understand coagulation in trauma.

Viscoelastic Assays

Blood transitions through different states of viscoelasticity during coagulation and fibrinolysis. Viscoelasticity is the property of a material that exhibits both viscous and elastic characteristics during deformity. Viscoelastic devices employ variable techniques for causing deformity. The most common methodology is with a pin and cup. Thrombelastography (TEG) uses a rotating cup to deform blood, while ROTEM uses a rotating pin in a stationary cup. Additional methodologies can be used, but are beyond the scope of this chapter. As blood transitions from a liquid to solid state, the shear strain created by cross-linking fibrin and platelet aggregation is transmitted to the device. Resistance is then quantified by the machine, which is visualized on a display as a single line splitting into two. The distance between the two lines is proportional to resistance transmitted from the clot. This resistance is measured over time until the clot forms its maximum strength, represented by the two lines reaching their maximum amplitude. This concludes the clot formation aspect of the device. After this point, the clot begins to lose strength through fibrinolysis, via cleavage of cross-linked fibrin. The two lines of amplitude decreases and are quantified over time. The end result of a viscoelastic assay is an hourglass-shaped tracing, which has numerous properties that can be calculated to approximate abnormalities of the different components of coagulation.

Anticoagulant and Blood Sampling

Blood samples run on viscoelastic assays can be stored in citrate (light blue top), heparin (green top), and no anticoagulant (white top) vacuum-sealed containers. Manufactures have specific recommendations on the timing between blood sample draw and time to run assay. In the setting of trauma for whole blood analysis, a citrated sample or non-anticoagulant tube can be used. The argument for using a non-anticoagulated blood sample is that these samples can be run within 5 min of blood draw and represent an unaltered blood sample, which in one small retrospective study had reported superiority to predicting FFP administration compared to a citrated sample [16]. Citrated samples must also be filled to the appropriate level as under and over fills can alter results [17]. However, non-citrated blood samples are at risk of clotting before they reach the viscoelastic device in the clinic setting due to delay in delivery of blood sample to the lab and the potential of expedited onset to coagulation from injury. Despite the limitations of running a citrated sample, our institution switched from non-anticoagulant blood collection to citrated samples because premature clotting in the non-anticoagulant blood sample was problematic, particularly during emergency department evaluation.

Functional fibrinogen assays are also typically run using citrated blood samples. Heparin anticoagulation is the typical manufacture recommendation for assessing platelet function due to concerns of citrate chelation of calcium causing artificial platelet impairment. Heparin is also known to cause platelet dysfunction, and there is an argument for using a direct thrombin inhibitor tube, although these inhibitors are significantly more expensive and likely confined to a non-clinical setting. Platelet mapping can be performed in both heparin and citrated samples, but if repeat measures are performed, the same anticoagulant should be used. As these assays are not currently used to guide trauma resuscitation, they will be discussed in brevity in the following section.

The location of the blood draw is also relevant when interpreting TEG results. Arterial blood samples in both animal [18] and human [19] samples tend to have slightly more hypercoagulable readouts than venous sample. As early arterial blood draws may be challenging on hypotensive trauma patients, it is the authors' recommendations to attempt venous blood draws when possible. In the more stable patients, while a fresh venous stick would be ideal, existing arterial and central venous catheters can be used for blood sampling. When trending the effects of blood products during resuscitation, it would be optimal to not alternate between blood sampling sites. There is also animal data to support that smaller-diameter catheters are more prone to underestimate coagulation than larger-diameter catheters [20]. Therefore, we would recommend central venous sample over arterial in patients undergoing serial blood draws. In the end, the differences between sampling sites may be more of an academic argument, as those patients who are profoundly hypocoagulable will likely demonstrate abnormalities regardless of blood draw source. Interestingly the fibrinolytic readout does not appear to be affected by the location of blood draw.

Activation of TEG-/ROTEM-Based Assay

Whole blood generation of clot can be initiated through various mechanisms. The two classic pathways of coagulation are the intrinsic and extrinsic activators. As we have previously discussed, hemostasis is a cell-mediated process, and both of these pathways do not act in isolation of each other. However, activation of blood with different agonist can produce different results, which need to be taken into clinical consideration. Extrinsic pathway activation is typically via tissue factor, while intrinsic, also known as contact pathway, is activated through kaolin. ROTEM has simplified the naming of their assays as EXTEM for tissue factor-based activation and In-TEM for kaolin-based activation. TEG uses both tissue factor and kaolin in the rapid TEG (rTEG) to expedite clotting and uses a kaolin TEG (kTEG) for intrinsic activation. Both ROTEM and TEG can be run as native assays (nTEG or nat-TEM), which are presumably activated through contact of the whole blood with an artificial surface (predominantly intrinsic).

The decision for running the optimal assay is dependent on the clinical scenario. For example, the time to obtain clotting indices in an rTEG to guide resuscitation is >10 min quicker than kTEG due to rapid activation of the clotting. Therefore, an rTEG is optimal for use in hemodynamically unstable patients in both the emergency department and operating room. Detection of hypercoagulability may be better assessed with a native or kaolin-activated assay. Native TEG [21] and kTEG [22] demonstrate that the majority of trauma patients are hypercoagulable on presentation to the hospital, which is not appreciated with rTEG. This could be attributable to saturating the activation of the coagulation system with supraphysiologic levels of tissue factors. An important caveat of differences between ROTEM and TEG parameters is that despite assays targeted toward specific coagulation pathways, the composition of the reagents in these assays is not the same between companies, and indices are not interchangeable. The authors routinely use rTEG to guide blood product transfusions and kTEG to guide antiplatelet therapy in the intensive care unit for post-injury deep venous thrombosis prophylaxis. The nTEG, which appears to be the most sensitive for detecting hypercoagulability, is currently not used clinically in the United States because it has not been approved for use by the Federal Drug Administration.

Specialized TEG assays to evaluate platelet function employ specific sets of agonists to assess if specific receptors are inhibited. The two most common agonists are adenosine diphosphate (ADP) and arachidonic acid (AA). Additional activators include thrombin receptor activator protein (TRAP) and collagen. Assessment of platelet function is dependent on blocking fibrinogen contribution to clot propagation and strength. This is accomplished by blocking different methods in both TEG and ROTEM.

The converse is true for assessment of fibrinogen function, in which the goal of the assay is to inhibit platelet contribution to clot. Their clinical application for trauma of these assays is limited in the United States, but in Europe, the ROTEM FIBTEM heavily relied on in specialized trauma centers.

Viscoelastic Index Correlation to Coagulation Abnormality

Viscoelastic indices are correlated to specific abnormalities of the coagulation system. However, assumptions are made that these processes are independent of each other to help guide resuscitation, but the reality is that these variables are representative of multiple processes occurring at the same time. In both TEG [21] and ROTEM [23], regression analysis of specific indices correlates with platelet versus fibrinogen contribution to clot. However, at times a dysfunction of platelets or fibrinogen can be compensated by over activity of another. For example, patients in renal failure tend to have an increased maximum amplitude on TEG [24], which is the variable commonly attributed to platelet function. These patients tend to have platelet dysfunction, and that is overcompensated by hyperfibrinogen function causing a strong clot, which is likely attributable to poor long-term patency of fistulas. The goal of the future generation of viscoelastic assays will have simultaneous readouts of whole blood coagulation paired to platelet and fibrinogen function to help guide resuscitation. However, despite the existing limitation of these assays, reproducible results can be determined in both TEG and ROTEM to predict patients at risk of massive transfusion and guide resuscitation of specific blood products. Abnormalities of the manufactured reported normal limits of TEG and ROTEM can be used as crude indications for blood product transfusion. However, the optimal threshold for transfusions based on readout of these assays in trauma is yet to be defined. The following sections describe the anatomy of these viscoelastic assays and association with blood product use.

Transition from Liquid to Solid State (Initiation)

As previously described blood transitions from a liquid to solid phase and indices measured by the viscoelastic assays correlate to particular components of coagulation. The initial transition from liquid to start of solid phase is in theory representative of the patient's coagulation factor status. Patients on systemic anticoagulation with heparin for bypass surgery will form a flat line and no evidence of clot, unless their blood is run in a specialized heparinase assay (heparinase cup TEG or ROTEM hepTEM), reversing the effects of this anticoagulant. Prolongation of this initial time is indicative of a patient benefitting from a plasma transfusion to replete their coagulation factors. The name of this indices varies by company and type of activator used.

The R time is the measurement of this initial phase of coagulation in both kaolin and native TEG. R time represents the time required from the baseline tracing to split and achieve an amplitude of >2 mm. While TEG will also record the actual split time (time when line splits into 2), the R time tends to be more reliable as small air bubbles can artificially shorten the split time, but the sample can retain a normal R time. The R time in rapid TEG is described as an activated clotting time (ACT). Since the ACT is available in minutes before these other assays, the utility of using a kaolin or native TEG in emergent situations is of limited value. However, these slower assays may be useful for the detection of hypercoagulability early after injury. But their significance remains to be defined.

ACT is the first actionable data for rTEG. The time to obtain ACT is short and in an attempt to normalize the distribution of data, the actual time is converted to an artificial number called the ACT. ACT in TEG is not the same as point of care Hemochron® ACT tests and should not be used interchangeably. TEG ACT has been demonstrated to predict massive transfusion and mortality [4]. The optimal threshold for plasma transfusion based on ACT remains to be validated by prospective data but appears to be 128 s [16, 25]. A markedly prolonged ACT (>140) is also indicative of dysfunction of both platelets and fibrinogen and can be an indication for transfusing cryoprecipitate and platelets before obtaining additional TEG indices in a hemodynamically unstable patient [6]. It is important to take into context that the rapid TEG uses supraphysiologic levels of tissue factor. This should evoke rapid clot formation in a patient with a functional coagulation system, and the delayed onset of activation of a clot in severely injured trauma patient in this setting should generate immediate concerns (especially if it is beyond 200 s based on authors personal experience).

The ROTEM comparable variable is called the coagulation time (CT). An EXTEM greater than 79 s has been associated with an elevated INR and FFP transfusion [26]. CT is not commonly used as a transfusion threshold. This may be attributable to transfusion practice differences between the United States and Europe. The Eurocentric approach to trauma resuscitation tends to favor fibrinogen replacement over plasma. However, the use of prothrombin complex or plasma for a prolonged CT (>80 s) has been advocated [27]. European trauma centers more often use ROTEM and often employ the A5 and A10 (amplitude of clot after 5 and 10 min after CT) as the first indices to guide resuscitation. The rationale for using these variables is that they serve as surrogates for predicting maximum clot firmness in an expedited fashion in trauma patients. Low amplitude A5 and A10 (<30 mm and <40 mm in EXTEM) predicted coagulopathy and increased transfusion requirements with high specificity and sensitivity [28]. These assays were used with the presumption of empiric blood product ratio resuscitation and have not been validated to guide specific blood product transfusions. The TEG A5 and A10 compared to ROTEM variables also suggest that these indices can be used to predict coagulopathy and massive transfusion [29].

Kinetics of Clot Strengthening (Propagation and Amplification)

After the clot has transitioned to its solid state, the rate at which it strengthens can be quantified by the rate required to reach maximum clot strength. To expedite the time to achieve this result without waiting for the clot to reach its maximum strength, a tangential line to the curve generated by the growing clot that passes through the 2 mm deflection point creates an angle to the baseline tracing. The resulting angle between the two lines is called alpha or angle in both TEG and ROTEM. An angle of less than 65 degrees has been proposed to be the threshold for cryoprecipitate transfusions in trauma patients using TEG [30]. ROTEM angle has also been correlated to fibrinogen dysfunction following trauma, but its utilization to guide fibrinogen repletion remains controversial [31]. The preferred methodology of guiding fibrinogen replacement with ROTEM is using the FIBTEM assay. This assay can have gradated transfusion triggers based on the A10 level of the FIBTEM which starts at a cutoff of <7 mm or in patients at risk of severe coagulopathy with an EXTEM A10 < 30 mm [27]. TEG also has a function fibrinogen assay which performs similarly to FIBTEM. Both of these specialized assays have been reported fibrinogen function with the same specificity of the gold stand Claus assay [32]. Additional kinetic parameters exist for TEG and ROTEM called the K time and clot formation time (CFT), but are rarely used clinically to guide resuscitation, although they are correlated with coagulopathy and massive transfusion.

Maximum Clot Strength

The maximum clot strength called the maximum amplitude (MA) in TEG and maximum clot firmness (MCF) in ROTEM represents the ultimate clot contribution to hemostasis. An MA of less than 55 mm in a rTEG is associated with massive transfusion [25], while a cutoff of 52 mm has been used as a transfusion threshold for platelets in trauma [16]. An MCF of less than 45 mm has been identified as an indicator of early mortality following trauma [33]. The European thresholds for ROTEM-based platelet transfusions are much more stringent and dependent on a low platelet count (<50,000) and a FIBTEM suggestive of normal fibrinogen levels (A5 > 12) and a A 10 of <40 mm in EXTEM [27]. But retrospective review of this protocol failed to mention the number of platelet transfusion in 157 patients who were receiving blood product resuscitation [33]. Most of the transfusions in ROTEM-based hospitals use platelet count to guide platelet transfusions. These trans-Atlantic differences in transfusion practice represent the confusion associated with the use of viscoelastic assays during resuscitation. To some extent the fact that neither resuscitation strategy id proven superior may be reflective that both platelets and fibrinogen contribute to clot strength and deficiency in one can be compensated in another. The decision to use maximum clot strength to guide platelet resuscitation therefore is hospital dependent. Of note, platelet function assays have not been validated for transfusion triggers in trauma patients and to date remain confined to the research setting.

Fibrinolysis

Both ROTEM- and TEG-based assays have been used to detect increased fibrinolysis in trauma patients, which has been associated with massive transfusion and mortality [7, 34, 35]. TEG quantifies the amount the lysis at 30 min after MA (LY30). ROTEM quantifies fibrinolysis as the percent decrease in clot strength after MA at 30 min (l130), which is comparable to the TEG CL30 variable (not commonly reported clinically). These indices can also be measured at 60 min. While it was originally believed that the goal-directed antifibrinolytics could be used in patients with excessive fibrinolysis, recent retrospective data has failed to identify a survival advantage [36]. Furthermore, research of fibrinolysis following acute injury has identified that the majority of patients already have impaired fibrinolysis (fibrinolysis shutdown) within an hour of injury which is associated with increased mortality [37]. These data suggest that antifibrinolytics should be used selectively, but the optimal patient population is yet to be defined.

Rationale for Goal-Directed Resuscitation

Trauma-induced coagulopathy is not a single etiology. Unique phenotypes of coagulation abnormalities after injury have been identified by principal component analysis using plasma-based assays [38], viscoelastic assays [39], and combinations of both modalities [40]. While a high injury severity and hypotension drive coagulopathy identified by an increased INR [14], the reason that these patients continue to bleed is multifactorial. Coagulation-based assessment of bleeding has been predominantly descriptive and associated with massive transfusion or mortality, and previous research has failed to delineate if patients were actually bleeding to death from their coagulopathy or if they were bleeding to death from their injury [41]. While there is enthusiasm for empiric high ratios of plasma to red blood cells in bleeding patients based on the military experience in Iraq [42], the most recent randomized control trial in the United States did not demonstrate an overall survival advantage when using empiric high ratios of plasma and platelets to red blood cells [43]. Retrospective evidence supporting individualized resuscitation with TEG was superior to ratios in massively bleeding patients that preexisted in this trial [44].

The evidence for TEG-guided resuscitation have been validated prospectively in a randomized control trial of patients at risk of massive transfusion [15]. Mortality was reduced to 19% in the TEG-based resuscitation group compared to the standard of care group (36%) based on intention to treat. Of note, by the end of the trial, the treating surgeons preferentially unblinded the study to obtain TEG results to guide resuscitation, and the survival benefit based was even greater with TEG (18% vs. 40% mortality). TEG-guided resuscitation did not result in less red blood cell transfusions compared to the standard of care group but resulted in patients receiving less platelets and plasma. While the mechanism remains unclear why this resulted in a survival advantage, it supports the importance of a goal-directed resuscitation, as blindly transfusing patients with blood products does not provide a survival advantage. Since the publication of this study, the authors have adopted an initial empiric 2:1 ratio of red blood cells to plasma in patients meeting activation of our massive transfusion protocol, followed by rTEG-guided resuscitation for additional blood products. Multicenter validation of these findings is warranted before global adoption of this protocol, but due to the large survival advantage appreciated at our trauma center, rTEG-guided resuscitation is the standard of care.

ROTEM-directed resuscitation algorithms also exist. As previously mentioned due to differences in transfusion practices, there are different strategies utilized to achieve hemostasis based on ROTEM indices, which put an emphasis on fibrinogen replacement, PCC, and tranexamic acid. Using ROTEM vs TEG is based on hospital/surgeon/anesthesia preference and local transfusion practices. While results between TEG and ROTEM are not interchangeable, they are in agreement with each other in identifying coagulopathy and transfusion requirements [45].

There are currently no standardized transfusion thresholds that have been agreed upon for TEG and ROTEM following significant injury. This is of significant clinical importance as implementation of goal-directed therapy resuscitation is likely to be a major logistic challenge. In a recent survey of 125 level I and II trauma centers, 98% reported having a massive transfusion protocol, yet the indications for activating this protocol were only based on a validated score system 7% of the time [46]. In this survey a coagulation test was only routinely measured a third of the time, and a viscoelastic assay was only available in 9% of centers, yet over a quarter continued to use activated factor VII and more than half of these center used tranexamic acid. In Europe similar concerns about a lack of consensus for guiding resuscitation in bleeding trauma patients also exist [47]. The American-based Trans-Agency Consortium for Trauma-Induced Coagulopathy and European-based Targeted Action for Curing Trauma Induced Coagulopathy are working on standardizing and validating goal-directed transfusion triggers with viscoelastic and other assays. While these collaborative efforts may not provide the definitive answer to treating coagulopathy, the need for a starting point on a consensus of how to perform goal-directed resuscitation is essential, as the continued publication of descriptive changes of trauma induced coagulopathy will not improve survival.

References

1. Hoffman M, Monroe DM 3rd. A cell-based model of hemostasis. Thromb Haemost. 2001;85(6):958–65.
2. Brohi K, Singh J, Heron M, Coats T. Acute traumatic coagulopathy. J Trauma. 2003;54(6):1127–30.
3. Peltan ID, Vande Vusse LK, Maier RV, Watkins TR. An international normalized ratio-based definition of acute traumatic coagulopathy is associated with mortality, venous thromboembolism, and multiple organ failure after injury. Crit Care Med. 2015;43(7):1429–38.
4. Cotton BA, Faz G, Hatch QM, Radwan ZA, Podbielski J, Wade C, et al. Rapid thrombelastography delivers real-time results that predict transfusion within 1 hour of admission. J Trauma. 2011;71(2):407–14; discussion 14-7.
5. Vogel AM, Radwan ZA, Cox CS Jr, Cotton BA. Admission rapid thrombelastography delivers real-time "actionable" data in pediatric trauma. J Pediatr Surg. 2013;48(6):1371–6.
6. Moore HB, Moore EE, Chin TL, Gonzalez E, Chapman MP, Walker CB, et al. Activated clotting time of thrombelastography (T-ACT) predicts early postinjury blood component transfusion beyond plasma. Surgery. 2014;156(3):564–9.
7. Schochl H, Frietsch T, Pavelka M, Jambor C. Hyperfibrinolysis after major trauma: differential diagnosis of lysis patterns and prognostic value of thrombelastometry. J Trauma. 2009;67(1):125–31.
8. Hoffman M, Colina CM, McDonald AG, Arepally GM, Pedersen L, Monroe DM. Tissue factor around dermal vessels has bound factor VII in the absence of injury. J Thromb Haemost JTH. 2007;5(7):1403–8.
9. Rao LV, Rapaport SI. Activation of factor VII bound to tissue factor: a key early step in the tissue factor pathway of blood coagulation. Proc Natl Acad Sci U S A. 1988;85(18):6687–91.
10. Tracy PB, Giles AR, Mann KG, Eide LL, Hoogendoorn H, Rivard GE, Factor V. (Quebec): a bleeding diathesis associated with a qualitative platelet factor V deficiency. J Clin Invest. 1984;74(4):1221–8.
11. Mazepa M, Hoffman M, Monroe D. Superactivated platelets: thrombus regulators, thrombin generators, and potential clinical targets. Arterioscler Thromb Vasc Biol. 2013;33(8):1747–52.
12. Monroe DM, Roberts HR, Hoffman M. Platelet procoagulant complex assembly in a tissue factor-initiated system. Br J Haematol. 1994;88(2):364–71.
13. Ostrowski SR, Johansson PI. Endothelial glycocalyx degradation induces endogenous heparinization in patients with severe injury and early traumatic coagulopathy. J Trauma Acute Care Surg. 2012;73(1):60–6.
14. Brohi K, Cohen MJ, Ganter MT, Matthay MA, Mackersie RC, Pittet JF. Acute traumatic coagulopathy: initiated by hypoperfusion: modulated through the protein C pathway? Ann Surg. 2007;245(5):812–8.
15. Gonzalez E, Moore EE, Moore HB, Chapman MP, Chin TL, Ghasabyan A, et al. Goal-directed hemostatic resuscitation of trauma-induced coagulopathy: a pragmatic randomized clinical trial comparing a viscoelastic assay to conventional coagulation assays. Ann Surg. 2016;263(6):1051–9.
16. Kashuk JL, Moore EE, Le T, Lawrence J, Pezold M, Johnson JL, et al. Noncitrated whole blood is optimal for evaluation of postinjury coagulopathy with point-of-care rapid thrombelastography. J Surg Res. 2009;156(1):133–8.
17. Haas T, Spielmann N, Cushing M. Impact of incorrect filling of citrate blood sampling tubes on thromboelastometry. Scand J Clin Lab Invest. 2015;75(8):717–9.
18. Doering CJ, Wagg CR, Caulkett NA, McAllister RK, Brookfield CE, Paterson JM, et al. Comparison of arterial and venous whole blood clot initiation, formation, and strength by thromboelastography in anesthetized swine. Blood Coagul Fibrinolysis: Int J Haemost Thromb. 2014;25(1):20–4.
19. Manspeizer HE, Imai M, Frumento RJ, Parides MK, Mets B, Bennett-Guerrero E. Arterial and venous Thrombelastograph variables differ during cardiac surgery. Anesth Analg. 2001;93(2):277–81. 1st contents page.
20. Neate SL, Boysen SR, Wagg CR, Radics SL, Caulkett NA. Comparison of thromboelastography parameters between different catheter lumen diameters in an uncontrolled haemorrhagic shock model in swine. Blood Coagul Fibrinolysis: Int J Haemost Thromb. 2013;24(6):581–6.
21. Moore HB, Moore EE, Chapman MP, Gonzalez E, Slaughter AL, Morton AP, et al. Viscoelastic measurements of platelet function, not fibrinogen function, predicts sensitivity to tissue-type plasminogen activator in trauma patients. J Thromb Haemost JTH. 2015;13(10):1878–87.
22. Schreiber MA, Differding J, Thorborg P, Mayberry JC, Mullins RJ. Hypercoagulability is most prevalent early after injury and in female patients. J Trauma. 2005;58(3):475–80; discussion 80-1.
23. Schlimp CJ, Solomon C, Ranucci M, Hochleitner G, Redl H, Schochl H. The effectiveness of different functional fibrinogen polymerization assays in eliminating platelet contribution to clot strength in thromboelastometry. Anesth Analg. 2014;118(2):269–76.
24. Chapman MP, Moore EE, Burneikis D, Moore HB, Gonzalez E, Anderson KC, et al. Thrombelastographic pattern recognition in renal disease and trauma. J Surg Res. 2015;194(1):1–7.
25. Holcomb JB, Minei KM, Scerbo ML, Radwan ZA, Wade CE, Kozar RA, et al. Admission rapid thrombelastography can replace conventional coagulation tests in the emergency department: experience with 1974 consecutive trauma patients. Ann Surg. 2012;256(3):476–86.
26. David JS, Durand M, Levrat A, Lefevre M, Rugeri L, Geay-Baillat MO, et al. Correlation between laboratory coagulation testing and thromboelastometry is modified during management of trauma patients. J Trauma Acute Care Surg. 2016;81(2):319–27.

27. Schochl H, Schlimp CJ, Voelckel W. Potential value of pharmacological protocols in trauma. Curr Opin Anaesthesiol. 2013;26(2):221–9.
28. Woolley T, Midwinter M, Spencer P, Watts S, Doran C, Kirkman E. Utility of interim ROTEM((R)) values of clot strength, A5 and A10, in predicting final assessment of coagulation status in severely injured battle patients. Injury. 2013;44(5):593–9.
29. Meyer AS, Meyer MA, Sorensen AM, Rasmussen LS, Hansen MB, Holcomb JB, et al. Thrombelastography and rotational thromboelastometry early amplitudes in 182 trauma patients with clinical suspicion of severe injury. J Trauma Acute Care Surg. 2014;76(3):682–90.
30. Kashuk JL, Moore EE, Pinski S, Johnson JL, Moore JB, Morgan S, et al. Lower extremity compartment syndrome in the acute care surgery paradigm: safety lessons learned. Patient Saf Surg. 2009;3(1):11.
31. Solomon C, Schochl H, Ranucci M, Schlimp CJ. Can the viscoelastic parameter alpha-angle distinguish fibrinogen from platelet deficiency and guide fibrinogen supplementation? Anesth Analg. 2015;121(2):289–301.
32. Harr JN, Moore EE, Chin TL, Chapman MP, Ghasabyan A, Stringham JR, et al. Viscoelastic hemostatic fibrinogen assays detect fibrinolysis early. Eur J Trauma Emerg Surg. 2015;41(1):49–56.
33. Tauber H, Innerhofer P, Breitkopf R, Westermann I, Beer R, El Attal R, et al. Prevalence and impact of abnormal ROTEM(R) assays in severe blunt trauma: results of the 'Diagnosis and treatment of trauma-induced coagulopathy (DIA-TRE-TIC) study'. Br J Anaesth. 2011;107(3):378–87.
34. Chapman MP, Moore EE, Ramos CR, Ghasabyan A, Harr JN, Chin TL, et al. Fibrinolysis greater than 3% is the critical value for initiation of antifibrinolytic therapy. J Trauma Acute Care Surg. 2013;75(6):961–7.
35. Cotton BA, Harvin JA, Kostousouv V, Minei KM, Radwan ZA, Schochl H, et al. Hyperfibrinolysis at admission is an uncommon but highly lethal event associated with shock and prehospital fluid administration. J Trauma Acute Care Surg. 2012;73(2):365–70; discussion 70.
36. Harvin JA, Peirce CA, Mims MM, Hudson JA, Podbielski JM, Wade CE, et al. The impact of tranexamic acid on mortality in injured patients with hyperfibrinolysis. J Trauma Acute Care Surg. 2015;78(5):905–11.
37. Moore HB, Moore EE, Liras IN, Gonzalez E, Harvin JA, Holcomb JB, et al. Acute fibrinolysis shutdown after injury occurs frequently and increases mortality: a multicenter evaluation of 2,540 severely injured patients. J Am Coll Surg. 2016;222(4):347–55.
38. Kutcher ME, Ferguson AR, Cohen MJ. A principal component analysis of coagulation after trauma. J Trauma Acute Care Surg. 2013;74(5):1223–9; discussion 9-30.
39. Chin TL, Moore EE, Moore HB, Gonzalez E, Chapman MP, Stringham JR, et al. A principal component analysis of postinjury viscoelastic assays: clotting factor depletion versus fibrinolysis. Surgery. 2014;156(3):570–7.
40. White NJ, Contaifer D Jr, Martin EJ, Newton JC, Mohammed BM, Bostic JL, et al. Early hemostatic responses to trauma identified with hierarchical clustering analysis. J Thromb Haemost JTH. 2015;13(6):978–88.
41. Morton AP, Moore EE, Wohlauer MV, Lo K, Silliman CC, Burlew CC, et al. Revisiting early postinjury mortality: are they bleeding because they are dying or dying because they are bleeding? J Surg Res. 2013;179(1):5–9.
42. Borgman MA, Spinella PC, Perkins JG, Grathwohl KW, Repine T, Beekley AC, et al. The ratio of blood products transfused affects mortality in patients receiving massive transfusions at a combat support hospital. J Trauma. 2007;63(4):805–13.
43. Holcomb JB, Tilley BC, Baraniuk S, Fox EE, Wade CE, Podbielski JM, et al. Transfusion of plasma, platelets, and red blood cells in a 1:1:1 vs a 1:1:2 ratio and mortality in patients with severe trauma: the PROPPR randomized clinical trial. JAMA. 2015;313(5):471–82.
44. Tapia NM, Chang A, Norman M, Welsh F, Scott B, Wall MJ Jr, et al. TEG-guided resuscitation is superior to standardized MTP resuscitation in massively transfused penetrating trauma patients. J Trauma Acute Care Surg. 2013;74(2):378–85; discussion 85-6.
45. Hagemo JS, Naess PA, Johansson P, Windelov NA, Cohen MJ, Roislien J, et al. Evaluation of TEG((R)) and RoTEM((R)) interchangeability in trauma patients. Injury. 2013;44(5):600–5.
46. Etchill E, Sperry J, Zuckerbraun B, Alarcon L, Brown J, Schuster K, et al. The confusion continues: results from an American Association for the Surgery of Trauma survey on massive transfusion practices among United States trauma centers. Transfusion. 2016;56:2478–86.
47. Schafer N, Driessen A, Frohlich M, Sturmer EK, Maegele M, Partners T. Diversity in clinical management and protocols for the treatment of major bleeding trauma patients across European level I Trauma Centres. Scand J Trauma Resusc Emerg Med. 2015;23:74.

Coagulopathies and Hypercoagulable States

35

Aaron Strumwasser and Erin Palm

Introduction

Coagulopathies in the intensive care unit (ICU) are present in as many as 50% of critically ill patients. A prolongation of prothrombin time (PT) or activated partial thromboplastin time (aPTT) occurs in 14–28% of the critically ill, with thrombocytopenia evident in 35–50% [1, 2]. Clinical outcomes are dependent on rapid identification and treatment of hemostatic disturbances [3, 4]. Traditional measures of clotting factors via PT, aPTT, thrombin (bleeding) time (TT), and activated clotting time (ACT) are being replaced by more modern, timely, cost-effective, blood conserving point-of-care viscoelastic testing that assesses the exact prothrombotic/antithrombotic state of the patient [5]. The modern intensivist familiar with coagulopathies in the ICU must be facile with these diagnostic modalities (Fig. 35.1). In post-surgical ICUs, coagulopathies often arise as a result of trauma, sepsis, or recent surgery [6]. With heparin-derived products commonplace for venous thromboembolism prophylaxis and treatment, the ubiquitous use of renal replacement therapy, and the mechanical and pharmacologic disturbances induced by cardiovascular surgery, heparin-induced thrombocytopenia (HIT) is an increasing cause of thrombophilia and bleeding in the ICU. Intensivists must also possess a thorough knowledge of common inherited clotting disorders, such as hemophilia, factor deficiencies, and von Willebrand disease as these syndromes can complicate the clinical picture. The following discussion will highlight important features of coagulopathies and hypercoagulable states in the surgical ICU.

A. Strumwasser · E. Palm (✉)
Los Angeles County, University of Southern California Medical Center, Los Angeles, CA, USA
e-mail: aaron.strumwasser@med.usc.edu

Heparin-Induced Thrombocytopenia (HIT)

HIT Epidemiology

Heparin-induced thrombocytopenia maximal risk estimates of 5% are observed in patients exposed to heparin-containing products [7]. Higher incidence in women is observed (two to three times estimated risk compared to men of comparable age) [8] and higher incidence in surgical ICUs compared to medical ICUs (three times higher) due to prevalence of trauma and cardiovascular disease in postsurgical patients. The syndrome is more observed with unfractionated as opposed to low molecular weight heparin (Lovenox) [8]. Heparin-induced thrombocytopenia may be associated with older age, is rare in patients less than the age of 40, and pregnancy may confer protection [9].

HIT Pathophysiology

Autoantibodies form to platelet factor 4 (in platelet alpha granules) complex with heparin causing further platelet aggregation and downstream thrombosis in propagating fashion. The reaction is IgG-mediated as the heparin-PF4 complex depends on the Fc receptor on the platelet surface [10–14]. Antibody formation usually takes more than 4 days to promulgate [15, 16]. There are thought to be five different etiologies of thrombocytopenia with heparin exposure. Type I HIT causes a small, insignificant clinical drop in platelets, not related to an immune reaction and can usually be managed expectantly by stopping heparin. Type II HIT is due to IgG-PF4-heparin complex antibody formation, where platelets are scavenged by macrophages in the spleen, liver, and bone marrow, causing clinically significant thrombosis. HIT type II requires anticoagulation with non-heparin formulations. Subclinical HIT occurs in patients that have prior HIT IgG antibodies in their system due to initial adverse exposure to heparin. Spontaneous HIT (3–8% incidence) includes the syndrome of HIT type II with positive laboratory findings for

A. Salim et al. (eds.), *Surgical Critical Care Therapy*, https://doi.org/10.1007/978-3-319-71712-8_35

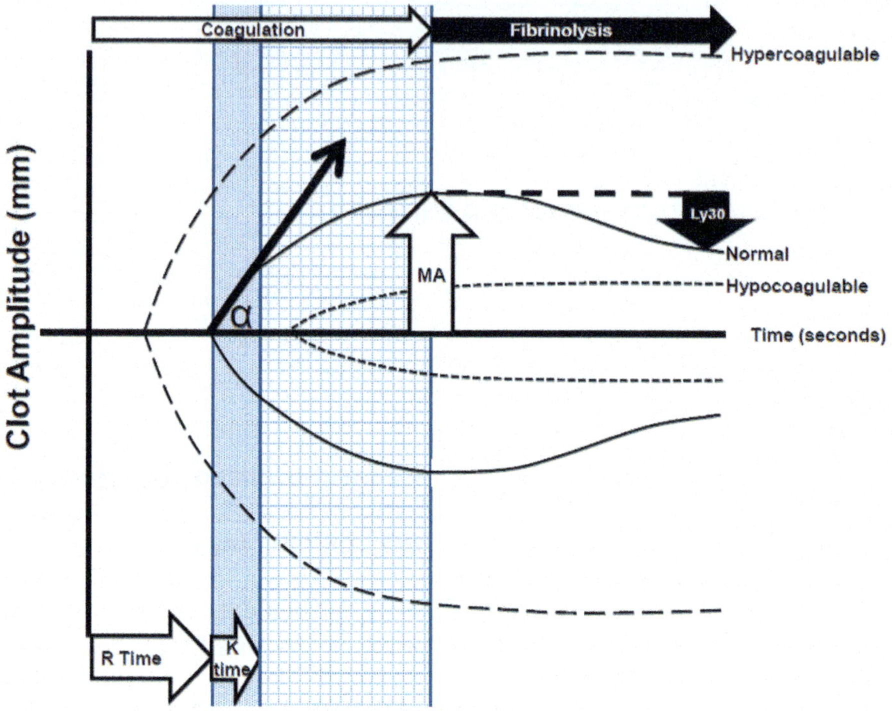

Fig. 35.1 Thromboelastography Thromboelastography reveals clinically relevant information regarding real-time coagulation status. In this figure, three different curves are depicted for each coagulation state. For reference, R time refers from time of injury to the time to start forming clot (2 mm amplitude – usually 5–10 min). K time refers to the time it takes for the clot to propagate from 2 to 20 mm or the time it takes for the clot to reach a fixed strength (normal 1–3 min). The line that is drawn from clot initiation to the maximum rate of clot formation constitutes an angle (α) reflecting the rapidity of clot formation or speed of fibrin accumulation (normal 53–72°). The maximum amplitude (MA) refers to the maximal height of clot formation (fixed strength) (normal 50–70 mm). During the fibrinolysis phase, Ly30 refers to the percentage of maximum amplitude reduction after 30 min. During the hypocoagulable state, prolongations of R and K times and decreased α and MA are observed. During the hypercoagulable state, shortened R and K and increased α and MA are observed. In the terminal stages of coagulopathy (fibrinolysis), Ly30 is increased. The morphology of each coagulopathic state dictates therapy. Derangements of R, K, or α are usually corrected with FFP or cryoprecipitate (reflective of a factor or fibrinogen problem). Derangements of MA are corrected with platelet transfusions, and derangements of Ly30 are usually corrected with antifibrinolytics (tranexamic acid, e-aminocaproic acid)

HIT without recent evidence of heparin exposure. Finally, heparin-induced antibodies form with recent exposure to heparin and cross-react with HIT assays but do not develop the syndrome of HIT [17–20]. Heparin-induced antibodies are more frequently found with the use of unfractionated heparin (UFH) due to the ability to form ultralarge complexes. Patients undergoing cardiopulmonary bypass, while having 50% positivity with HIT assays, do not develop the clinical syndrome as they do not form ultracomplexes as easily [15, 21]. In cardiac and orthopedic surgery, the estimates of developing HIT syndrome with UFH as opposed to LMWH range from 5% (UFH) to less than 1% (LMWH) [22]. Prior exposure to UFH or LMW heparin more than quintuples the risk of developing HIT (0.3% vs. 1.7%) [23].

HIT Clinical Manifestations

Type I HIT has no clinical sequelae if heparin is discontinued. Type II HIT sees a platelet drop of approximately 50% (usually counts hover around 100,000 to 150,000 platelets/μL), a finding seen in 85–90% of patients [21, 24]. Rarely do platelet counts drop below 20,000 platelets/μL in type II HIT, and 5% demonstrate reduced platelet counts but remain in the normal range [21, 25]. Type II HIT usually appears on days 5–10 post-heparin administration. Antibody-associated HIT, on the other hand, may appear within 24 h if exposure was recent (within 3 months) [26, 27]. Type II HIT is associated with significant arterial and venous thrombosis that may manifest as petechiae, gangrene, and limb threat. Thrombosis presents as the initial finding in 25–50% (usually venous); arterial thrombosis is less common (3–10%). Sites of thrombosis are usually seen in the extremities, skin, and cardiac vasculature, but platelet complexes can occur in any organ, causing ischemia and infarction. Thrombosis may be also catheter-associated. On pathologic analysis thrombi form a characteristic "white clot" due to their platelet-rich nature. Anaphylactic reactions with respiratory failure and severe immune responses with catastrophic life-threatening thrombosis have been described [21, 28–30]. Bleeding is a rare complication of type II HIT, due to the fact that thrombocytopenia associated with spontaneous bleeding rarely results in platelet counts less than 10,000 platelets/μL. Case studies of bleeding in HIT have been limited to adrenal and orthopedic surgery [31–33].

HIT Diagnosis

Clinical scoring systems exist for the diagnosis of HIT, and HIT requires both clinical and laboratory criteria to properly diagnose. The 4 Ts clinicopathologic scoring system interprets (1) tally, degree of thrombocytopenia (>50% reduction in platelets); (2) timing, onset of thrombocytopenia, expected within 5–10 days of administration of heparin; (3) thrombosis (presence of); and (4) thrombosis (alternative causes). Each T gets a point, and pretest probability is assessed (<3 low probability, three to five intermediate probability and six or more high probability) [34]. If the T-score confers low probability, do not perform laboratory testing. For intermediate probability, seek laboratory testing. For high probability, treat for HIT presumptively. The most common assays are the ELISA immunoassay that screens for IgG to PF4 (sensitivity 98%, specificity 83%) and the C^{14}-serotonin release assay which tests the ability for patient serum to activate test platelets (sensitivity and specificity greater than 95%). If the ELISA is positive, the patient has HIT and should be treated presumptively. If the ELISA yields an indeterminate result, then proceed to C^{14}-serotonin release assay [35, 36]. In patients on heparin-bonded circuits (renal replacement therapy) despite one in five patients developing HIT antibodies, only 1% produce the clinical syndrome (within 90 days usually), and heparin therapy does not need to be stopped [37]. The prothrombotic/antithrombotic features of HIT make it difficult to assess by viscoelastic testing. While the clinical syndrome is usually prothrombotic (R and K decreased and maximum amplitude increased), thrombocytopenia may manifest as diminished maximum amplitude on viscoelastic testing and severe thrombocytopenia with bleeding manifesting as decreased (or absent) R, K, and alpha angle and increased Ly30 in terminal stages. In situations where conventional testing is not sufficient, viscoelastic testing demonstrates utility. In patients with negative HIT antibodies, TEG may be used to predict complications of HIT type II [38]. Rotational thromboelastometry (ROTEM) has been used to titrate anticoagulation in the setting of HIT in cardiac patients with ventricular assist devices, particularly in cases where ACT levels were not able to reach goal levels [39]. In patients with HIT and posttransfusion purpura, ROTEM helped differentiate causes of hypofibrinogenemia for appropriate titration of anticoagulation with argatroban and lepirudin [40].

HIT Treatment

Prompt therapy is crucial in HIT because between 10% and 25% of cases are associated with arterial or venous thromboembolic complications [41]. The cardinal treatment for HIT includes discontinuation of all forms of heparin, initiation of alternative anticoagulation, and avoidance of vitamin K antagonists (VKA), such as warfarin [42]. With cessation of heparin therapy, platelet counts rebound in approximately 1 week. Platelet normalization should occur in the first 4 days, and if not observed to be significantly increasing, other etiologies of thrombocytopenia should be sought. Anticoagulation is paramount; without treatment, HIT confers an additional risk of 34–53% of subsequent thrombosis [43, 44]. Alternative anticoagulant agents include the direct thrombin inhibitor class – argatroban (for patients with normal hepatic and renal function), fondaparinux (for patients with abnormal liver function), and bivalirudin (for patients with abnormal liver and kidney function). Reduced dosages of argatroban may be considered to prevent further toxicity; otherwise, full therapeutic anticoagulation is the standard [45–47]. The duration of anticoagulation is controversial, but most authors recommend transition to Coumadin with outpatient anticoagulation for 1 week to 1 month [41]. Treatment specifics are shown in Table 35.1.

HIT Outcomes

With arterial and venous thrombosis, mortality approaches 20%. Current therapy rates have significantly dropped (less than 2% due to early recognition and cessation of heparin therapy). Because HIT antibodies can persist 1–3 months after exposure to heparin, patients must be counseled on being HIT reactive, and these findings should be conveyed to future treating physicians [26].

Von Willebrand Disease

Von Willebrand Disease Epidemiology

Von Willebrand disease (VWD) is the most common bleeding disorder, present in up to 1% of the population [48, 49]. It encompasses a group of related disorders with clinical manifestations ranging from mild to severe.

Von Willebrand Disease Pathophysiology

Von Willebrand disease is an inherited defect in von Willebrand factor (VWF). It has an autosomal inheritance pattern, in contrast to the most common forms of hemophilia

Table 35.1 Selected anticoagulants for HIT

Drug agent	Dose	Steady state achieved	Potential contraindications, adverse effect considerations	Monitoring
Argatroban	Initial dose 2 mcg/kg/min; maintenance dosage not to exceed 10 mcg/kg/min	2 h	Dose adjustment is necessary for patients with hepatic dysfunction (if total bilirubin ≥1.5 mg/dL, adjust initial dose to 0.5–1.2 mcg/kg/mi) Also consider dose adjustment (0.2 mcg/kg/min) for patients with MOF	Titrate to aPTT 1.5–3 times baseline
Fondaparinux	5–10 mg/day	68–85 h (half-life of 17 h)	Patients should have periodic monitoring of renal function; no antidote	No monitoring necessary
Bivalirudin	0.15 mg/kg/h	2 h	Caution if patient has demonstrated anti-lepirudin antibodies; need to overlap with warfarin therapy; FDA has not officially approved this for use for HIT	Titrate to aPTT 1.5–2.5 times baseline

(A and B), which are X-linked. Von Willebrand factor is a protein present in both the endothelium of blood vessels and within platelets, circulating in complex with factor VIII. When injury occurs to the vascular endothelium, VWF is activated and released locally, where it binds to the vessel wall and triggers platelet adherence, aggregation, and formation of a hemostatic plug. Von Willebrand factor also protects factor VIII from clearance, thereby increasing circulating levels of factor VIII, which facilitates clot formation [50]. Von Willebrand disease occurs when VWF is either low in supply or deficient in function. Patients with type I VWF have decreased levels of circulating VWF, whereas type II encompasses various qualitative defects in VWF. The most severe type III, which describes a complete deficiency of VWF, is also the rarest form [51].

Von Willebrand Disease Clinical Presentation

Symptoms of VWD often manifest on mucosal surfaces because of the specifics of hemostasis in these tissues. The most common presenting symptom of VWD is bleeding from skin or mucous membranes, usually not requiring medical intervention [48]. Patients may have a history of epistaxis, profuse bleeding from small wounds, or after tonsillectomy or tooth extraction. Women with VWD often complain of menorrhagia [52]. Uncommonly, patients with severe VWF deficiency can experience spontaneous joint bleeding and life-threatening bleeding in the central nervous system or GI tract [53].

Von Willebrand Disease Diagnosis

A careful history and physical examination should be performed to evaluate for bleeding symptoms and bleeding risk prior to laboratory testing. A family history of bleeding disorder can be helpful in making a diagnosis but does not exclude VWD. Once a positive bleeding history is established, initial hemostasis tests should include a complete blood count with platelets, PT, and PTT. If bleeding history is strong or if an isolated PTT elevation is identified, VWD assays should be performed. In the past, VWD was diagnosed by prolonged PTT and thrombin (bleeding) time (TT). However, in milder forms of VWD, these tests may be normal. Therefore in patients with symptomatic bleeding that lacks another explanation, specific VWF assays should be performed. The most common initial assays for VWD include (1) VWF:Ag, an assay measuring the concentration of VWF; (2) VWF:RCo, which measures the binding activity of VWF to platelets; and (3) a factor VIII level, which estimates the ability of VWF to act as a carrier. If an abnormality is identified, genetic testing is performed [48, 54]. In the absence of a personal or family history of abnormal bleeding, a VWF:Ag assay will identify moderately low levels of VWF (approximately 2.5% of the population). The clinical significance of this finding in otherwise normal individuals has not been established [55]. Thromboelastography (demonstrating prolonged R time corresponding to diminished factor VIII activity) has been used successfully in patients with VWD in the setting of cardiac bypass surgery [56], and TEG as opposed to ROTEM appears to be superior in diagnosing VWD [57].

Von Willebrand Disease Treatment

Desmopressin (DDAVP) is a synthetic derivative of vasopressin that increases plasma concentration of VWF and FVIII. The mechanism is thought to be cAMP-mediated release of VWF from endothelial cells. Desmopressin is effective as surgical prophylaxis and treatment of bleeding episodes in most patients with VWD. Standard dosing is 0.3 mcg/kg given subcutaneously or intravenously, alternatively intranasally [58]. There is variation in VWD response to DDAVP and tachyphylaxis may occur [59, 60]. For those reasons, guidelines recommend monitoring VWF:RCo and factor VIII levels to achieve minimum targets (~approximately 50%). If target levels are not achieved, plasma-derived VWF concentrate can be administered [61]. Patients with severe forms of the disease can be managed effectively with concentrated VWF infusions [62]. For anticipated major surgery (cardiac surgery, orthopedic surgery, trauma) and childbirth, patients with VWD should be treated at specialized hemophilia centers [48]. Compared to patients with hemophilia, in which approximately half of patients require prophylactic clotting factor infusions to prevent spontaneous bleeding, only about 10–13% of patients with severe VWD require prophylactic VWF infusions [63].

Von Willebrand Disease Outcomes

Even in patients with mild forms of VWD, bleeding complications from surgical procedures and mild trauma are anticipated. In women with VWD, childbirth-related hemorrhage and need for blood transfusion are significantly more common [52]. With appropriate monitoring and prophylactic factor administration, bleeding episodes can be mitigated.

Hemophilia and Factor Deficiencies

Hemophilia/Factor Deficiency Epidemiology

Approximately 95% of hemophilia is accounted by deficiencies of factor VIII, IX, and XI. The remainder, "rare hemophilias," is seen in 5% of the world's population, localized mainly to Turkey, Asia, and Japan. Of the common hemophilias, factor VIII deficiency occurs in 1/5000 live male births. Of those, two-thirds have severe disease (X-linked pattern of inheritance). Factor IX deficiency (Christmas disease) occurs in 1/30,000 male births, of which half have severe disease (X-linked pattern of inheritance). Factor XI deficiency (Rosenthal syndrome) is rare (1/1,000,000 births), with disproportionate incidence in Ashkenazi Jews [64]. Of the rare hemophilias, in order, the most common are factor XI deficiency, followed by V, VII, X, fibrinogen, and XIII [65, 66]. Compared to common hemophilia, the age of bleeding onset in rare coagulopathies varies (median age 7 years, range birth to 73 years) [66, 67].

Hemophilia/Factor Deficiency Pathophysiology

Pathophysiology differs for the type of hemophilia and/or factor deficiency. Dysfibrinogenemias result from mutations in the coding region of the fibrinogen gene (over 100 mutations exist) and can result in quantitative reduction of fibrinogen, qualitative alterations of fibrinogen, or deficiencies of both [68]. The disease in most severe form is autosomal recessive, as are the majority of the rare factor deficiencies (V, VII, X, XIII). Factor V deficiency is usually involved with genetic mutation associated with severe reduction in factor V levels. The majority of mutations associated with factor VII deficiency are mild-to-moderate expressors of phenotype. The minority (33%) have severe mutations that cause significant bleeding tendency. Factor X deficiency involves a mutation that results in low but detectable levels of factor X activity. Factor XIII deficiency depends on the appropriate manufacturing of two subunits of factor XIII, which usually results in marked reduction of factor XIII levels and bleeding with a mutation of the gene coding for either the A or B subunit of the factor XIII protein [66]. The common hemophilia mutations (A and B) are sex-linked, expressed in males (or lyonized females undergoing dual inactivation of the factor VIII and IX genes).

Hemophilia/Factor Deficiency Clinical Presentation

Hemophilia is usually classified by severity (related to factor level deficit) – mild bleeding occurs at factor levels 5–40% of normal ($\geq$0.05 to <0.40 IU/mL), moderate at factor levels 1–5% of normal ($\geq$0.01 to <0.05 IU/mL), and severe bleeding less than 1% of normal (<0.01 IU/mL). Severe hemophilia is characterized by spontaneous bleeding and severe bleeding at a younger age at first bleeding episode. Spontaneous bleeds usually occur when factor levels are less than 20% [67]. It is not uncommon for severe hemophilia to present at the time of birth, with umbilical cord separation as the presenting finding. Delayed bleeding can present as massive hemorrhage or slower ooze occurring over longer periods of time, inducing chronic anemia [67]. Intracranial hemorrhage may occur, particularly after trauma. Excessive bleeding with minor surgical procedures such as tooth extraction or circumcision may be the presenting finding. In contrast to platelet disorders, mucosal (epistaxis), muscle, and joint bleeding (joint contractures) may occur in chronic form and are characteristic of hemophilia and factor deficiencies. Although patients have bleeding tendency, this feature is not protective against acute coronary syndrome or stroke. In patients that are heterozygous for disease, the normal allele compensates for deficient factor level which usually does not present with clinical disease. Classification systems address the severity of bleeding in order to guide therapy and appropriately prognosticate [69]. Grade I bleeding occurs after trauma or antithrombotic therapy. Grade II bleeding is minor mucosal-associated or menorrhagic bleeding that occurs spontaneously. Grade III bleeding is major bleeding into organs and tissue spaces (muscles/joints) and may be immediately life-threatening (intracranial hemorrhage). Pregnancy loss has been associated with deficiencies of factor XIII, factor X, and fibrinogen. Thrombosis is rare in the hemophilias/factor deficiencies and may be attributable to iatrogenesis (thrombophilic medications, central venous catheters, inherited or acquired prothrombotic conditions (factor V Leiden, trauma, vascular disease) and appears to be reported most frequently with factors V, VII, and XI [70, 71]. Late complications of disease include joint contractures from repeated hemarthroses and neurologic dysfunction from intracranial hemorrhage [64].

Hemophilia/Factor Deficiency Diagnosis

Proper evaluation includes family history-taking and clinical assessment (obstetric details for infants/kids and bleeding/bruising patterns in adults). Attention in the record to bleeding during minor trauma and dental procedures should be noted. Patients with family history significant for bleeding disorders or coagulopathies should be sought (approximately one-third of patients with hemophilia have a negative family history). Standard laboratory testing for prothrombin time (PT) and activated partial thromboplastin time (aPTT) should be performed [64]. Thromboelastography may better estimate the degree of deficiency in patients with hemophilia. Whereas patients with mild-to-moderate hemophilia may demonstrate prolonged R and K times with preserved alpha and maximum amplitude, severe disease has no formation of clot with absence of a visualizable TEG waveform [72] These values correlate with aPTT measurements early in the disease process. However, at 24 h, aPTT levels (normal) are discordant with TEG findings (abnormal), which may suggest sub-therapeutic factor replacement in patients having undergone therapy [73].

Hemophilia/Factor Deficiency Treatment

Cornerstones of therapy include raising factor activity levels to arrest hemorrhage and achieve definitive hemostasis (target factor level above 50% usually). The distinction between mild and serious/life-threatening bleeding guides management. For patients with intracranial hemorrhage, severe organ system dysfunction, or life-threatening bleeding, therapy should be initiated immediately (pre-hospital phase) prior to complete diagnostic assessment (do not delay greater than 30 min, and if diagnosis is in question, treat) [74, 75]. Specific pharmacotherapy dosing is based on the severity and the location of the bleed [66, 70, 76–79]. For hemarthrosis, specific concern should be placed regarding intra-articular bleeds at the femoral head and hip (increased risk of osteonecrosis) [80]. Avoidance of weight bearing, ice packs, immobilization/splinting, and analgesic therapy is indicated. Avoid medications with anticoagulant effects. Arthrocentesis is not necessary and may exacerbate the problem. If aspiration is planned, make sure factor replacement has been performed (100% repletion). For repeated aspirations, prednisone (3–5 day short-course therapy) should be used to minimize inflammation and permanent joint contracture [81]. Factor replacement is dictated by location of the hemarthrosis. Hemarthrosis in the hip, iliopsoas target factor levels should reach 80–100%. For hemarthrosis in the knees, elbows, or ankles, activity level should be raised to 40–50%. These levels should be maintained for a minimum of 3 days [82]. After resolution of the hemarthrosis, rehabilitation is crucial to maintain healthy joint function. For muscle and soft tissue bleeding, replacement to maintain 50% peak factor levels is sufficient [83]. For patients planning surgery, DDAVP test-dosing should be performed 1 week before planned surgery, and inhibitor screening should be performed. For at-risk patients with positive screens, perioperative factor administration should be given 30–60 min before the procedure, with repeat dosing based on the half-life of each factor and the total duration of surgery. Most recommendations suggest a preoperative factor for major surgery (orthopedic surgery, cardiac surgery) to be 80–100% for hemophilia A and 60–80% for hemophilia B, with factors tapering to 50% for 2 weeks post-op [84, 85]. In those patients receiving substantial amounts of perioperative and intraoperative factor, screening for inhibitors should be performed at the completion of surgery and as an outpatient [86]. Antifibrinolytic agents (tranexamic acid, aminocaproic acid) can be used as an adjunct with factor replacement in individuals with less severe bleeding (mucosal bleeding) but should be avoided in severe cases [87, 88].

Management of patients with factor inhibitors (usually the patient is affected with hemophilia A) depends on the severity of bleeding and the type and titer of the inhibitor [89]. High responding inhibitor titers by Bethesda assay (>5 Bethesda units) are resistant to factor infusions whereas those with lower inhibitor titers (<5 Bethesda units) may benefit from factor infusion. Bypassing products (recombinant factor VIIa, 90–120 mcg/kg, and FEIBA, 50–100 units/kg every 6–12 h) are used in patients with high inhibitor titers [90]. If patients are nonresponders to one type of bypassing product, they may respond to the alternative. Comparable efficacy has been demonstrated for rFVIIa and FEIBA [89, 91–94]. Plasmapheresis is reserved for patients that fail bypassing therapy. Surgical or interventional techniques are last resort options for uncontrollable hemorrhage [95]. At the completion of treatment, eradication of the inhibitor and immunotolerance should be addressed.

A summary of the epidemiology, clinical presentation, diagnosis, and management of major hemophilias and factor deficiencies are shown in Table 35.2.

Table 35.2 Factor deficiencies, hemophilias, and inhibitors

Factor deficiency	Epidemiology	Clinical presentation	Laboratory profile	Treatment
Factor II deficiency (prothrombin)	Rare, 1 in 2,000,000	Usually mild. Rarely presents with clinically severe bleeding. Severe factor II (prothrombin) deficiency is characterized by excessive bleeding after invasive procedures, and umbilical cord, joint, muscle, and mucosal bleeding. Life-threatening bleeding may also occur	Increased PT/INR and PTT	Maintain coagulation factors between 20 and 30% (higher threshold compared to other deficiencies). Can treat bleeding with either 3 or 4 factor PCC, only in severe cases due to thrombogenicity of PCC. If PCC is not available FFP should be used.
		Rarely thrombosis is observed (procoagulant state with thrombosis rather than bleeding has been reported in factor V deficiency)		
Factor V deficiency (parahemophilia)	Rare, 1 in 1,000,000, individuals from Turkey have a higher than average incidence of factor VII deficiency (one-third to one-quarter of RICDs)	Usually mild. Rarely presents with clinically severe bleeding (factors <1%). The most common clinical symptoms are excessive bleeding after invasive procedures and mucosal tract bleeding. Intracranial hemorrhage has been reported	Increased PT/INR and PTT	Fresh frozen plasma should be used as specific recombinant products, or coagulation factor V concentrates are not available
Factor VII deficiency (Alexander's disease)	Rare, 1 in 500,000, usually acquired. Most commonly seen following VKA therapy, early liver disease, vitamin K deficiency, and in early DIC (rare)	Factor VII levels do not correlate with clinical severity of bleeding. Bleeding is unlikely with factor VII activity levels >10% and usually patients are asymptomatic. If bleeding occurs, the most common symptoms are excessive bleeding with invasive procedures, menorrhagia, and mucosal tract, joint, and muscle bleeding. Intracranial bleeding may occur (20%). Thrombosis (3–4%) may occur	Increased PT, normal PTT	Recombinant-activated factor VII (rfVIIa) is first-line treatment. If not available, PCC or FFP
Factor VIII deficiency (hemophilia A)	Factor VIII deficiency occurs in 1/5000 live male births	Severe bleeding when factor levels are below 1%. Factor activity levels above approximately 15–20% are often sufficient to prevent spontaneous bleeding and to produce a normal PT and aPTT	Normal PT/INR, increased PTT	Recombinant factor VIII first line. Goal is to maintain levels above 50% at all times. In the setting of an acute bleed, an immediate dose of factor VIII should be given to raise the peak factor level to 80–100%, re-dosing when factor levels drop below 50%. Check factor VIII trough every 4–6 h and re-dose accordingly
		Patients with mild deficiency bleed with hemostatic challenge (surgery, trauma, pregnancy)		In mild bleeding settings, antifibrinolytics may be used. Tranexamic acid (TXA – 25 mg/kg per dose every 6 to 8 h) or aminocaproic acid (EACA – 75 to 100 mg/kg every 6 h, not to exceed a single dose of 3–4 g with administration)
				DDAVP can be used in mild-to-moderate disease, not an emergency (30–60 min window), adult patient (not kids because of increased risk of SIADH). Moreover, DDAVP will not work with severe disease (< 1% factor activity). Typical dosing for DDAVP is 0.3 mcg/kg (maximum dose, 20 mcg), administered intravenously or subcutaneously or as a nasal spray (Stimate), one puff (150 mcg) in one nostril in patients weighing <50 kg and two puffs (150 mcg in both nostrils) in patients weighing ≥50 kg. A repeat dose may be given at 12 h, and subsequent doses are often administered once daily

(continued)

Table 35.2 (continued)

Factor deficiency	Epidemiology	Clinical presentation	Laboratory profile	Treatment
Factor IX deficiency (hemophilia B, Christmas disease)	Factor IX deficiency (Christmas disease) occurs in 1/30,000 male births	Severe bleeding when factor levels are below 1%. Factor activity levels above approximately 15 to 20% are often sufficient to prevent spontaneous bleeding and to produce a normal PT and aPTT, although this varies by specific factor level. However, patients with mild deficiency of a coagulation factor may have increased bleeding with hemostatic challenges (e.g., excessive surgical bleeding, menorrhagia)	Normal PT/INR, increased PTT	Recombinant factor IX first line. Administer initial dose of 100–120 units/kg and maintain peak factor levels at >50%. The peak factor activity level should be checked approximately 5 to 15 min after the first dose. Check trough at 8–12 h, re-dose accordingly
				In mild bleeding settings, antifibrinolytics may be used. Tranexamic acid (TXA – 25 mg/kg per dose every 6 to 8 h) or aminocaproic acid (EACA – 75 to 100 mg/kg every 6 h, not to exceed a single dose of 3–4 g with administration)
				DDAVP ineffective (not stored or released)
Factor X deficiency (Stuart-Prower disease)	Rare, 1 in 1,000,000	Factor X deficiency is associated with bleeding in individuals who have a factor X activity level < 10%, manifesting as bleeding after invasive procedures, intracranial, umbilical cord, joint, and muscle bleeding. As opposed to factor VII, the risk of bleeding correlates well with factor X levels	Increased PT/INR and PTT	Can treat bleeding with either 3 or 4 factor PCC, only in severe cases due to thrombogenicity of PCC. If PCC is not available FFP should be used
Factor XI deficiency (hemophilia C)	Rare, Ashkenazi Jews (8–9% heterozygous); sporadic form 1/1,000,000	Associated with thrombosis more than bleeding; bleeding occurs when factor levels are less than 15%	Normal PT/INR, increased PTT	Multiple options:FFP or factor XI concentrate (15 units/kg) to maintain factor levels at 30–40%
				Hormone therapy (OCPs) – Dosing varies
				DDAVP (0.3 mcg/kg SQ or IV)
				Antifibrinolytic therapy – TXA 25 mg/kg PO or 10 mg/kg IV every 6 h
				Low dose rFVIIa (20 mcg/kg bolus, followed by continuous infusion at 1.8–3.6 mcg/kg per hour)
Factor XII deficiency	Rare, Asians have a higher than average prevalence of factor XII deficiency (which is not associated with bleeding)	NOT associated with clinical bleeding; relatively benign	Normal PT/INR, increased PTT	Treatment is usually unnecessary
Factor XIII deficiency	Rare, 1 in 2,000,000 (higher in southeastern Iran)	Usually severe bleeding is observed. Most patients with factor XIII activity level < 5% are symptomatic from bleeding, and the severity of bleeding correlates relatively well with plasma factor XIII levels	Normal PT/INR and normal PTT	Bleeding can be treated with recombinant factor XIII A subunit or factor XIII concentrate. If one of these is not available, FFP or cryoprecipitate may be used
		Severe bleeding manifests as umbilical cord, surgical, joint, intracranial hemorrhage, and menorrhagia.		
		Patients may also have recurrent pregnancy loss and impaired wound healing		
		Factor XIII deficiency may present with delayed bleeding, usually 24 to 36 h after surgery or trauma; spontaneous bleeding also occurs		

Combined factor deficiency	Rare; less than 100 people in 60 families have been identified in the world to date; in high-risk populations (Mediterranean) may be as high as 1/100,000	Patients with combined factor V and VIII deficiency generally have higher baseline factor levels than those with isolated factor V or VIII deficiencies and bleeding is mild to moderate (does not correlate with factor levels).	Increased PT/INR and PTT	Treat only for trauma, perioperative, or obstetrical bleeding. FFP is the agent of choice (repletes factors V and VIII). The recommended starting dosage of FFP is 15 to 20 mL/kg IV, repeated daily to keep factor V at hemostatic levels (>20%). Due to high volumes transfused, consider diuretics for volume overload
		Typical stigmata include surgical, traumatic, and mucocutaneous bleeding (epistaxis, menorrhagia)		
		Rarely spontaneous bleeding, hemarthrosis, or intracranial hemorrhage		
Fibrinogen deficiency (factor I)	Rare; 1/1,000,000	Usually mild. Overall, dysfibrinogenemias can be silent (55%) or lead to a hemorrhagic (25%) or thrombotic diathesis (10–30%); patients with fibrinogen levels less than 50 to 100 mg/dL have a higher frequency of bleeding complications	Increased PT/INR and PTT	Prophylactic fibrinogen replacement (cryoprecipitate, FFP, or fibrinogen concentrates) indicated before delivery and before major surgery. Goal is fibrinogen 50–100 mg/dL in nonsurgical settings, 100–200 mg/dL for surgical and obstetric prophylaxis. Keep levels above 50 mg/dL until complete wound healing post-op (~ 2 weeks)
		Most bleeding manifestations are mild, but some can be severe. Spontaneous life-threatening bleeds are rare		
		The clinical presentation is diverse – Mucosal, surgical, traumatic, obstetric, and intracranial have all been described		
Factor inhibitor	Varies, depends on etiology – Myeloproliferative disease, inflammatory disorders, rheumatologic disorders (antiphospholipid syndrome), malignancy	Varies, depends on etiology but thrombosis associated (rarely bleeding)	Normal PT/INR, increased PTT (abnormal, does not correct with mixing)	Treatment is based on Bethesda assay; for low titer (< 5 BU), factor replacement may be sufficient. For high titer response, bypassing products (rFVIIa, FEIBA) are used. Plasmapheresis can be used in select cases of patients failing bypassing therapy
			Inhibitors are diagnosed and classified by titer using the Bethesda assay, in which serial dilution of patient plasma is used to determine an inhibitor titer in Bethesda units (BU). Inhibitors with a titer of <5 BU despite repeated factor infusions are referred to as low responding inhibitors. Any inhibitor >5 BU/mL at any time is considered high responding, even if the titer subsequently becomes undetectable due to lack of re-exposure	

PT prothrombin time, *INR* international normalized ratio, *PTT* partial thromboplastin time (activated), *FFP* fresh frozen plasma, *DDAVP* desmopressin acetate

Hemophilia/Factor Deficiency Outcomes

As treatment for hemophilia has improved, chronicity has led to long-term complications. In addition to late intracranial hemorrhage and joint contractures from repeated hemarthrosis, infections from repeated product infusions (HIV, hepatitis), an increased risk of bleeding from cancer, increased incidence of chronic kidney disease, and challenges in managing heart disease have all been described in hemophiliacs. The most common cause of death in non-HIV individuals affected by hemophilia is liver disease (related mainly to factor depletion and not coinfection with the Hepatitis virus). Liver transplantation is curative for hemophilia. Overall awareness and treatment options have estimated life expectancy statistics among hemophiliacs to be similar to those of the general population [96–98].

References

1. Levi M, Opal SM. Coagulation abnormalities in critically ill patients. Crit Care. 2006;10:222.
2. Vanderschueren S, De Weerdt A, Malbrain M. Thrombocytopenia and prognosis in intensive care. Crit Care Med. 2000;28:1871–6.
3. Ahmed A, Kojicic M, Herasevich V, Gajic O. Early identification of patients with or at risk of acute lung injury. Neth J Med. 2009;67:268–71.
4. Schultz MJ. Early recognition of critically ill patients. Neth J Med. 2009;67:266–7.
5. Whiting P, Al M, Westwood M, Ramos IC, Ryder S, Armstrong N, Misso K, Ross J, Severens J, Kleijnen J. Viscoelastic point-of-care testing to assist with the diagnosis, management and monitoring of haemostasis: a systematic review and cost-effectiveness analysis. Health Technol Assess. 2015;19(58):1–228.
6. Levy JH, Faraoni D, Sniecinski RM. Perioperative coagulation management in the intensive care unit. Curr Opin Anaesthesiol. 2013;26(1):65–70.
7. Coutre S, Leung L, Tirnauer JS. Clinical presentation and diagnosis of heparin-induced thrombocytopenia. UpToDate Online. Nov 02, 2016.
8. Warkentin TE, Sheppard JA, Sigouin CS, Kohlmann T, Eichler P, Greinacher A. Gender imbalance and risk factor interactions in heparin-induced thrombocytopenia. Blood. 2006;108(9):2937.
9. Stein PD, Hull RD, Matta F, Yaekoub AY, Liang J. Incidence of thrombocytopenia in hospitalized patients with venous thromboembolism. Am J Med. 2009;122(10):919.
10. Visentin GP, Ford SE, Scott JP, Aster RH. Antibodies from patients with heparin-induced thrombocytopenia and thrombosis are specific for platelet factor 4 complexed with heparin or bound to endothelial cells. J Clin Invest. 1994;93(1):81.
11. Rauova L, Zhai L, Kowalska MA, Arepally GM, Cines DB, Poncz M. Role of platelet surface PF4 antigenic complexes in heparin-induced thrombocytopenia pathogenesis: diagnostic and therapeutic implications. Blood. 2006;107(6):2346.
12. Kelton JG, Smith JW, Warkentin TE, Hayward CP, Denomme GA, Horsewood P. Immunoglobulin G from patients with heparin-induced thrombocytopenia binds to a complex of heparin and platelet factor 4. Blood. 1994;83(11):3232.
13. Rauova L, Poncz M, McKenzie SE, Reilly MP, Arepally G, Weisel JW, Nagaswami C, Cines DB, Sachais BS. Ultralarge complexes of PF4 and heparin are central to the pathogenesis of heparin-induced thrombocytopenia. Blood. 2005;105(1):131.
14. Khandelwal S, Arepally GM. Immune pathogenesis of heparin-induced thrombocytopenia. Thromb Haemost. 2016;116(5):792–8.
15. Martel N, Lee J, Wells PS. Risk for heparin-induced thrombocytopenia with unfractionated and low-molecular-weight heparin thromboprophylaxis: a meta-analysis. Blood. 2005;106(8):2710.
16. Girolami B, Prandoni P, Stefani PM, Tanduo C, Sabbion P, Eichler P, Ramon R, Baggio G, Fabris F, Girolami A. The incidence of heparin-induced thrombocytopenia in hospitalized medical patients treated with subcutaneous unfractionated heparin: a prospective cohort study. Blood. 2003;101(8):2955.
17. Warkentin TE, Makris M, Jay RM, Kelton JG. A spontaneous prothrombotic disorder resembling heparin-induced thrombocytopenia. Am J Med. 2008;121(7):632.
18. Krauel K, Pötschke C, Weber C, Kessler W, Fürll B, Ittermann T, Maier S, Hammerschmidt S, Bröker BM, Greinacher A. Platelet factor 4 binds to bacteria, [corrected]inducing antibodies cross-reacting with the major antigen in heparin-induced thrombocytopenia. Blood. 2011;117(4):1370.
19. Greinacher A, Holtfreter B, Krauel K, Gätke D, Weber C, Ittermann T, Hammerschmidt S, Kocher T. Association of natural anti-platelet factor 4/heparin antibodies with periodontal disease. Blood. 2011;118(5):1395.
20. Warkentin TE, Basciano PA, Knopman J, Bernstein RA. Spontaneous heparin-induced thrombocytopenia syndrome: 2 new cases and a proposal for defining this disorder. Blood. 2014;123(23):3651.
21. Linkins LA, Dans AL, Moores LK, Bona R, Davidson BL, Schulman S, Crowther M. American College of Chest Physicians. Treatment and prevention of heparin-induced thrombocytopenia: antithrombotic therapy and prevention of thrombosis, 9th ed: American College of Chest Physicians Evidence-Based Clinical Practice Guidelines. Chest. 2012;141(2 Suppl):e495S.
22. Warkentin TE, Sheppard JA, Horsewood P, et al. Impact of the patient population on the risk for heparin-induced thrombocytopenia. Blood. 2000;96:1703.
23. Prandoni P, Siragusa S, Girolami B, Fabris F, BELZONI Investigators Group. The incidence of heparin-induced thrombocytopenia in medical patients treated with low-molecular-weight heparin: a prospective cohort study. Blood. 2005;106(9):3049.
24. Warkentin TE. Heparin-induced thrombocytopenia: a clinicopathologic syndrome. Thromb Haemost. 1999;82(2):439.
25. Warkentin TE. Clinical presentation of heparin-induced thrombocytopenia. Semin Hematol. 1998;35(4 Suppl 5):9.
26. Warkentin TE, Kelton JG. Temporal aspects of heparin-induced thrombocytopenia. N Engl J Med. 2001;344(17):1286.
27. Lubenow N, Kempf R, Eichner A, Eichler P, Carlsson LE, Greinacher A. Heparin-induced thrombocytopenia: temporal pattern of thrombocytopenia in relation to initial use or reexposure to heparin. Chest. 2002;122(1):37.
28. Hong AP, Cook DJ, Sigouin CS, Warkentin TE. Central venous catheters and upper-extremity deep-vein thrombosis complicating immune heparin-induced thrombocytopenia. Blood. 2003;101(8):3049.
29. LaMonte MP, Brown PM, Hursting MJ. Stroke in patients with heparin-induced thrombocytopenia and the effect of argatroban therapy. Crit Care Med. 2004;32(4):976.
30. Giossi A, Del Zotto E, Volonghi I, Costa P, Bertuetti R, Remida P, Magoni M, Gasparotti R, Padovani A, Pezzini A. Thromboembolic complications of heparin-induced thrombocytopenia. Blood Coagul Fibrinolysis. 2012;23(6):559.
31. Rosenberger LH, Smith PW, Sawyer RG, Hanks JB, Adams RB, Hedrick TL. Bilateral adrenal hemorrhage: the unrecognized cause of hemodynamic collapse associated with heparin-induced thrombocytopenia. Crit Care Med. 2011;39(4):833.

32. Thota R, Porter J, Ganti AK, Peters E. Hemodynamic collapse following bilateral knee arthroplasty: a mysterious case. J Thromb Thrombolysis. 2012;33(1):3–5.
33. Goel R, Ness PM, Takemoto CM, Krishnamurti L, King KE, Tobian AA. Platelet transfusions in platelet consumptive disorders are associated with arterial thrombosis and in-hospital mortality. Blood. 2015;125(9):1470.
34. www.hematology.org/Practice/Guidelines/11747.aspx. Accessed on 07 Jan 2014.
35. Nagler M, Bachmann LM, ten Cate H, ten Cate-Hoek A. Diagnostic value of immunoassays for heparin-induced thrombocytopenia: a systematic review and meta-analysis. Blood. 2016;127(5):546.
36. Nagler M, Bakchoul T. Clinical and laboratory tests for the diagnosis of heparin-induced thrombocytopenia. Thromb Haemost. 2016;116(5):823–34.
37. Asmis LM, Segal JB, Plantinga LC, Fink NE, Kerman JS, Kickler TS, Coresh J, Gardner LB. Heparin-induced antibodies and cardiovascular risk in patients on dialysis. Thromb Haemost. 2008;100(3):498.
38. Kouerinis IA, El-Ali M, Theakos N, Dedeilias P. Can thromboelastography predict which patients with heparin-induced thrombocytopenia may suffer thrombotic complications of type II? Eur J Cardiothorac Surg. 2007;32(3):544–6.
39. Iwanski J, Kazui T, Le Tran P, Basken R, Wong RK, Khalpey Z. Novel method using rotational thromboelastography analysis for intraoperative management of device patient with heparin-induced thrombocytopenia. Blood Coagul Fibrinolysis. 2016;27(8):943–7.
40. Haeberle HA, Menzel D, Unertl K, Nohé B. Management of complex thrombocytopenia with thrombelastometry : a case of simultaneous posttransfusion purpura and heparin-induced thrombocytopenia. Anaesthesist. 2011;60(12):1135–40.
41. Marks PW. Coagulation disorders in the ICU. Clin Chest Med. 2009;30(1):123–9.
42. Coutre S, Leung L, Tirnauer JS. Management of heparin-induced thrombocytopenia. UpToDate Online. Nov 02, 2016.
43. Warkentin TE, Kelton JG. A 14-year study of heparin-induced thrombocytopenia. Am J Med. 1996;101(5):502.
44. Wallis DE, Workman DL, Lewis BE, Steen L, Pifarre R, Moran JF. Failure of early heparin cessation as treatment for heparin-induced thrombocytopenia. Am J Med. 1999;106(6):629.
45. Lewis BE, Wallis DE, Leya F, Hursting MJ, Kelton JG, Argatroban-915 Investigators. Argatroban anticoagulation in patients with heparin-induced thrombocytopenia. Arch Intern Med. 2003;163(15):1849.
46. Lewis BE, Wallis DE, Berkowitz SD, Matthai WH, Fareed J, Walenga JM, Bartholomew J, Sham R, Lerner RG, Zeigler ZR, Rustagi PK, Jang IK, Rifkin SD, Moran J, Hursting MJ, Kelton JG, ARG-911 Study Investigators. Argatroban anticoagulant therapy in patients with heparin-induced thrombocytopenia. Circulation. 2001;103(14):1838.
47. Lewis BE, Wallis DE, Hursting MJ, Levine RL, Leya F. Effects of argatroban therapy, demographic variables, and platelet count on thrombotic risks in heparin-induced thrombocytopenia. Chest. 2006;129(6):1407.
48. Nichols W, Hultin M, James A, et al. von Willebrand disease (VWD): evidence-based diagnosis and management guidelines, the national heart, lung, and blood institute (NHLBI) expert panel report (USA). Haemophilia. 2008;14:171–232.
49. Rodeghiero F, Castaman G, Dini E. Epidemiological investigation of the prevalence of von Willebrand's disease. Blood. 1987;69:454–9.
50. Lillicrap D. von Willebrand disease: advances in pathogenetic understanding, diagnosis, and therapy. Hematol Am Soc Hematol Educ Program. 2013;2013:254–60.
51. Sadler JE, Budde U, Eikenboom JC, et al. Working party on von Willebrand disease classification. Update on the pathophysiology and classification of von Willebrand disease: a report of the Subcommittee on von Willebrand factor. J Thromb Haemost. 2006;4:2103–14.
52. Kouides PA, Phatak PD, Burkart P, et al. Gynaecological and obstetrical morbidity in women with type I von Willebrand disease: results of a patient survey. Haemophilia. 2000;6:643–8.
53. Federici A, Bucciarelli P, Castaman G, et al. The bleeding score predicts clinical outcomes and replacement therapy in adults with von Willebrand disease: a prospective cohort study of 796 cases. Blood. 2014;123:4037–44.
54. Neff AT. Current controversies in the diagnosis and management of von Willebrand disease. Ther Adv Hematol. 2015;6(4):209–16.
55. Bucciarelli P, Siboni S, Stufano F, et al. Predictors of von Willebrand disease diagnosis in individuals with borderline von Willebrand factor plasma levels. J Thromb Haemost. 2015;13:228–36.
56. Stolla M, Chang S, Schulman S, Bauer K, Haspel R, Lerner AB. Use of thromboelastography in the management of a patient with acquired von Willebrand disease undergoing cardiac bypass surgery. Br J Haematol. 2017.
57. Schmidt DE, Majeed A, Bruzelius M, Odeberg J, Holmström M, Ågren A. A prospective diagnostic accuracy study evaluating rotational thromboelastometry and thromboelastography in 100 patients with von Willebrand disease. Haemophilia. 2016;23(2):309–18.
58. Svensson P, Bergqvist P, Juul K, Berntorp E. Desmopressin in treatment of haematological disorders and in prevention of surgical bleeding. Blood Rev. 2014;28:95–102.
59. Federici A, Mazurier C, Berntorp E, et al. Biologic response to desmopressin in patients with severe type 1 and type 2 von Willebrand disease: results of a multicenter European study. Blood. 2004;103:2032–8.
60. Rodeghiero F, Castaman G, Di Bona E, et al. Consistency of responses to repeated DDAVP infusions in patients with von Willebrand's disease and hemophilia A. Blood. 1989;74:199–200.
61. Mannucci PM, Chediak J, Hanna W, et al. Treatment of von Willebrand disease with a high-purity factor VIII/von Willebrand factor concentrate: a prospective, multicenter study. Blood. 2002;99:450–6.
62. Abshire T, Federici A, Alvarez M, et al. Prophylaxis in severe forms of von Willebrand's disease: results from the von Willebrand disease prophylaxis network (VWD PN). Haemophilia. 2013;19:76–81.
63. Sumner M, Williams J. Type 3 von Willebrand disease: assessment of complications and approaches to treatment – results of a patient and hemophilia treatment center survey in the United States. Haemophilia. 2004;10:360–6.
64. Hoots KW, Shapiro AD. Clinical manifestations and diagnosis of hemophilia. UpToDate Nov 11, 2014.
65. Ruiz-Saez A. Occurrence of thrombosis in rare bleeding disorders. Semin Thromb Hemost. 2013;39(6):684–92. Epub 2013 Aug 8. [Giansily-Blaizot M, Biron-Andreani C, Aguilar-Martinez P, de Moeloose P, Briquel ME, Goudemand J, Stieltjes N, Barrot C, Chambost H, Durin A, Gay V, Peynet J, Pouymayou K, Schved JF. Inherited factor VII deficiency and surgery: clinical data are the best criteria to predict the risk of bleeding. Br J Haematol. 2002;117(1):172].
66. Mannucci PM, Duga S, Peyvandi F. Recessively inherited coagulation disorders. Blood. 2004;104(5):1243.
67. Acharya SS, Coughlin A, Dimichele DM, North American Rare Bleeding Disorder Study Group. Rare Bleeding Disorder Registry: deficiencies of factors II, V, VII, X, XIII, fibrinogen and dysfibrinogenemias. J Thromb Haemost. 2004;2(2):248.
68. Hanss M, Biot F. A database for human fibrinogen variants. Ann N Y Acad Sci. 2001;936:89.
69. Peyvandi F, Palla R, Menegatti M, Siboni SM, Halimeh S, Faeser B, Pergantou H, Platokouki H, Giangrande P, Peerlinck K, Celkan T, Ozdemir N, Bidlingmaier C, Ingerslev J, Giansily-Blaizot M, Schved JF, Gilmore R, Gadisseur A, Benedik-Dolničar M, Kitanovski L, Mikovic D, Musallam KM, Rosendaal FR, European

Network of Rare Bleeding Disorders Group. Coagulation factor activity and clinical bleeding severity in rare bleeding disorders: results from the European Network of Rare Bleeding Disorders. J Thromb Haemost. 2012;10(4):615–21.

70. Giansily-Blaizot M, Biron-Andreani C, Aguilar-Martinez P, de Moeloose P, Briquel ME, Goudemand J, Stieltjes N, Barrot C, Chambost H, Durin A, Gay V, Peynet J, Pouymayou K, Schved JF. Inherited factor VII deficiency and surgery: clinical data are the best criteria to predict the risk of bleeding. Br J Haematol. 2002;117(1):172. [Mannucci PM, Duga S, Peyvandi F. Recessively inherited coagulation disorders. Blood. 2004;104(5):1243].
71. Girolami A, Sartori MT, Simioni P. An updated classification of factor XIII defect. Br J Haematol. 1991;77(4):565.
72. Nogami K. The utility of thromboelastography in inherited and acquired bleeding disorders. Br J Haematol. 2016;174(4):503–14.
73. Al Hawaj MA, Martin EJ, Venitz J, Barrett JC, Kuhn JG, Nolte ME, Brophy DF. Monitoring rFVIII prophylaxis dosing using global haemostasis assays. Haemophilia. 2013;19(3):409–14.
74. Fowler H, Lacey R, Keaney J, Kay-Jones C, Martlew V, Thachil J. Emergency and out of hours care of patients with inherited bleeding disorders. Haemophilia. 2012;18(3):e126–31.
75. Hoots WK. Emergency management in hemophilia. In: Lee CA, Berntorp EE, Hoots WK, editors. Textbook of hemophilia. 2nd ed. Oxford, UK: Wiley-Blackwell; 2010. p. 394.
76. Schulman S, Varon D, Keller N, Gitel S, Martinowitz U. Monoclonal purified F VIII for continuous infusion: stability, microbiological safety and clinical experience. Thromb Haemost. 1994;72(3):403.
77. Martinowitz UP, Schulman S. Continuous infusion of factor concentrates: review of use in hemophilia A and demonstration of safety and efficacy in hemophilia B. Acta Haematol. 1995;94(Suppl 1):35.
78. Hay CR, Doughty HI, Savidge GF. Continuous infusion of factor VIII for surgery and major bleeding. Blood Coagul Fibrinolysis. 1996;7(Suppl 1):S15.
79. Schulman S, Wallensten R, White B, Smith OP. Efficacy of a high purity, chemically treated and nanofiltered factor IX concentrate for continuous infusion in haemophilia patients undergoing surgery. Haemophilia. 1999;5(2):96.
80. Paton RW, Evans DI. Silent avascular necrosis of the femoral head in haemophilia. J Bone Joint Surg Br. 1988;70(5):737.
81. Kisker CT, Burke C. Double-blind studies on the use of steroids in the treatment of acute hemarthrosis in patients with hemophilia. N Engl J Med. 1970;282(12):639.
82. Manco-Johnson MJ, Abshire TC, Shapiro AD, Riske B, Hacker MR, Kilcoyne R, Ingram JD, Manco-Johnson ML, Funk S, Jacobson L, Valentino LA, Hoots WK, Buchanan GR, DiMichele D, Recht M, Brown D, Leissinger C, Bleak S, Cohen A, Mathew P, Matsunaga A, Medeiros D, Nugent D, Thomas GA, Thompson AA, McRedmond K, Soucie JM, Austin H, Evatt BL. Prophylaxis versus episodic treatment to prevent joint disease in boys with severe hemophilia. N Engl J Med. 2007;357(6):535.
83. Franchini M, Favaloro EJ, Lippi G. Mild hemophilia A. J Thromb Haemost. 2010;8(3):421.
84. Poon MC, Aledort LM, Anderle K, Kunschak M, Morfini M. Comparison of the recovery and half-life of a high-purity factor IX concentrate with those of a factor IX complex concentrate. Factor IX Study Group. Transfusion. 1995;35(4):319.
85. Powell JS, Pasi KJ, Ragni MV, Ozelo MC, Valentino LA, Mahlangu JN, Josephson NC, Perry D, Manco-Johnson MJ, Apte S, Baker RI, Chan GC, Novitzky N, Wong RS, Krassova S, Allen G, Jiang H, Innes A, Li S, Cristiano LM, Goyal J, Sommer JM, Dumont JA, Nugent K, Vigliani G, Brennan A, Luk A, Pierce GF, B-LONG Investigators. Phase 3 study of recombinant factor IX Fc fusion protein in hemophilia B. N Engl J Med. 2013;369(24):2313.
86. Srivastava A, Brewer AK, Mauser-Bunschoten EP, Key NS, Kitchen S, Llinas A, Ludlam CA, Mahlangu JN, Mulder K, Poon MC, Street A, Treatment Guidelines Working Group on Behalf of The World Federation Of Hemophilia. Guidelines for the management of hemophilia. Haemophilia. 2013;19(1):e1–47.
87. Djulbegovic B, Marasa M, Pesto A, Kushner GM, Hadley T, Joseph G, Goldsmith G. Safety and efficacy of purified factor IX concentrate and antifibrinolytic agents for dental extractions in hemophilia B. Am J Hematol. 1996;51(2):168.
88. StajcićZ. The combined local/systemic use of antifibrinolytics in hemophiliacs undergoing dental extractions. Int J Oral Surg. 1985;14(4):339.
89. Berntorp E, Shapiro AD. Modern haemophilia care. Lancet. 2012;379(9824):1447–56. Epub 2012 Mar 27.
90. Kempton CL, White GC. How we treat a hemophilia A patient with a factor VIII inhibitor. Blood. 2009;113(1):11.
91. Astermark J, Donfield SM, DiMichele DM, Gringeri A, Gilbert SA, Waters J, Berntorp E, FENOC Study Group. A randomized comparison of bypassing agents in hemophilia complicated by an inhibitor: the FEIBA NovoSeven Comparative (FENOC) Study. Blood. 2007;109(2):546.
92. Young G, Shafer FE, Rojas P, Seremetis S. Single 270 microg kg(−1)-dose rFVIIa vs. standard 90 microg kg(−1)-dose rFVIIa and APCC for home treatment of joint bleeds in haemophilia patients with inhibitors: a randomized comparison. Haemophilia. 2008;14(2):287.
93. Santagostino E, Mancuso ME, Rocino A, Mancuso G, Scaraggi F, Mannucci PM. A prospective randomized trial of high and standard dosages of recombinant factor VIIa for treatment of hemarthroses in hemophiliacs with inhibitors. J Thromb Haemost. 2006;4(2):367.
94. Kavakli K, Makris M, Zulfikar B, Erhardtsen E, Abrams ZS, Kenet G. NovoSeven trial (F7HAEM-1510) investigators. Home treatment of haemarthroses using a single dose regimen of recombinant activated factor VII in patients with haemophilia and inhibitors. A multi-centre, randomised, double-blind, cross-over trial. Thromb Haemost. 2006;95(4):600.
95. Mauser-Bunschoten EP, Zijl JA, Mali W, van Rinsum AC, van den Berg HM, Roosendaal G. Successful treatment of severe bleeding in hemophilic target joints by selective angiographic embolization. Blood. 2005;105(7):2654.
96. Mazepa MA, Monahan PE, Baker JR, Riske BK, Soucie JM, US Hemophilia Treatment Center Network. Men with severe hemophilia in the United States: birth cohort analysis of a large national database. Blood. 2016;127(24):3073–81.
97. Kulkarni R, Soucie JM, Evatt BL, Hemophilia Surveillance System Project Investigators. Prevalence and risk factors for heart disease among males with hemophilia. Am J Hematol. 2005;79(1):36–42.
98. Chronic complications and age-related comorbidities in patients with hemophilia. UpToDate Online. Nov 17, 2016.

36 Antibiotic and Antifungal Therapy in the ICU

Mitchell J. Daley, Emily K. Hodge, and Dusten T. Rose

Abbreviations

5-FC	Flucytosine
ABLC	Amphotericin B lipid complex
ADR	Adverse drug reaction
AMB-d	Amphotericin B deoxycholate
AMG	Aminoglycoside
ARC	Augmented renal clearance
AUC	Area under the curve
Cmax	Peak drug concentration
CNS	Central nervous system
CPK	Creatinine phosphokinase
CrCl	Creatinine clearance
CRE	Carbapenem-resistant *Enterobacteriaceae*
CRRT	Continuous renal replacement therapy
CSF	Cerebrospinal fluid
ESBL	Extended-spectrum β-lactamase
FDA	Food and Drug Administration
FLQ	Fluoroquinolones
hVISA	Heterogeneous vancomycin-intermediate *Staphylococcus aureus*
ICU	Intensive care unit
IHD	Intermittent hemodialysis
INR	International normalized ratio
L-AMB	Liposomal amphotericin B
MAOI	Monoamine oxidase inhibitor
MDR	Multidrug resistant
MIC	Minimum inhibitory concentration
MRSA	Methicillin resistant *Staphylococcus aureus*
MSSA	Methicillin susceptible *Staphylococcus aureus*
NS	Nonsusceptible
PAE	Post-antibiotic effect
PBP	Penicillin binding protein
PCN	Penicillin
PD	Pharmacodynamics
PK	Pharmacokinetics
SMX	Sulfamethoxazole
SSTI	Skin and soft tissue infection
TMP	Trimethoprim
Vd	Volume of distribution
VISA	Vancomycin-intermediate *Staphylococcus aureus*
VRE	Vancomycin-resistant enterococcus
VRSA	Vancomycin-resistant *Staphylococcus aureus*

M. J. Daley · E. K. Hodge (✉) · D. T. Rose
Department of Pharmacy, Dell Seton Medical Center at the University of Texas, Austin, TX, USA
e-mail: mjdaley@ascension.org

Introduction

Few diseases challenge the critical care provider as frequent as the prevention or treatment of infection. In non-cardiac intensive care units (ICU), infection and related sepsis are the leading cause of death with reported mortality rates as high as 60%, accounting for approximately 40% of total ICU expenditures [1]. In a 1-day point-prevalence study in 1265 ICUs from 75 countries, 71% of critically ill patients were receiving an anti-infective agent for either prophylaxis (20%) or treatment (51%), most commonly for respiratory (64%), intra-abdominal (20%), and bloodstream (15%) infections [2]. The success of preventing or eradicating an infection is determined based on the interaction of an anti-infective drug, host, and pathogen. Although a complete discussion of each of these components is outside of the scope of this chapter, knowledge of antimicrobial pharmacology (e.g., mechanism of action, spectrum of activity, toxicity) and strategies to optimize pharmacokinetics (PK) and pharmacodynamics (PD) are key tools for the intensivist to improve the probability of eradicating infection in critically ill patients while preventing the emergence of antimicrobial resistance [3].

General PK-PD Concepts

PK describes the action of the patient toward a drug, including absorption, distribution, metabolism, and excretion, ultimately determining systemic exposure [4]. Contrarily, PD is

A. Salim et al. (eds.), *Surgical Critical Care Therapy*, https://doi.org/10.1007/978-3-319-71712-8_36

the physiologic and biochemical response to a drug, typically stated "what the drug does to the body." The PK-PD properties are integrated to describe the exposure-response relationship and determine the ability for an anti-infective to kill (bactericidal) or inhibit (bacteriostatic) the growth of a pathogen [5].

To apply PK-PD principles of anti-infectives (Fig. 36.1), it is important to first understand a pathogen factor known as the minimum inhibitory concentration (MIC). The MIC is the lowest serum concentration of an antimicrobial required to inhibit the visible growth of the microorganism. Antibiotics considered to have "time-dependent" pathogen kill activity, such as β-lactams, are entirely dependent on the time the free drug concentration remains above the MIC during the dosing interval ($T_{>MIC}$) [6]. To optimize the dose of "time-dependent" antibiotics, more frequent administration or extended infusions are preferred to prolong the time the antibiotic concentration remains above the MIC, as compared to simply giving larger doses. In this scenario, PK-PD studies suggest you can actually give a smaller total daily dose of an antimicrobial while achieving similar or greater probability of achieving the PK-PD target and associated outcome. Using cefepime as an example, the probability of achieving at least 67% of the $T_{>MIC}$, a standard PK-PD goal, when the pathogen MIC is 8 μg/mL is similar for a dose of 1 g q6h as compared to 2 g q8h, despite the fact that the patient is receiving one third the total daily dose [7].

Alternatively, concentration-dependent antibiotics, such as aminoglycosides (AMG), elicit kill characteristics that are exclusively influenced by the degree of free drug concentration above the MIC for a specific pathogen (Cmax/MIC). The optimal dosing strategy of concentration-dependent antibiotics is to give larger doses that achieve a higher maximum concentration with less frequent administration. Finally, certain antibiotics, such as vancomycin and fluoroquinolones (FLQ), have a hybrid approach where bactericidal or static activity can be described as concentration-dependent with time dependence. Known as the ratio of area under the curve (AUC) to MIC (AUC/MIC), optimal dosing of these antibiotics includes a combination of larger doses with either more frequent administration or prolonged infusions. Goal PK-PD targets are specific to individual classes of antimicrobial agents, and strategies to optimize PK-PD properties will be discussed with each antimicrobial class subsequently in this chapter. Some antibiotics, such as AMGs, demonstrate a post-antibiotic effect (PAE), where bacterial regrowth is suppressed after the free drug concentration falls below the MIC. When applying these concepts, only unbound or "free" drug should be considered as the microbiologically active drug that can pass through capillary endothelium.

(*AMG* aminoglycoside, *AUC* area under the concentration-time curve, *Cmax* peak concentration, *FLQ* fluoroquinolones, *MIC* minimum inhibitory concentration, *T* time, *PAE* post-antibiotic effect).

The last general concept relates to the influence of the physiochemical properties of a drug on PK, ultimately impacting the achievement of adequate concentrations at the site of infection. Generally, drugs that are hydrophilic or have "water loving" properties tend to achieve low intracellular penetration, have limited distribution, and are predominantly excreted through the kidneys [8]. Hydrophilic antibiotics include β-lactams, AMGs, glycopeptides (e.g., vancomycin), and colistin. Alternatively, lipophilic antimicrobials or drugs with "fat loving" properties are extensively distributed, achieve high intracellular penetration, and undergo predominantly hepatic metabolism and excretion. Lipophilic antibiotics include FLQs,

Fig. 36.1 PK-PD parameters of antibiotics on a concentration vs. time curve [6]

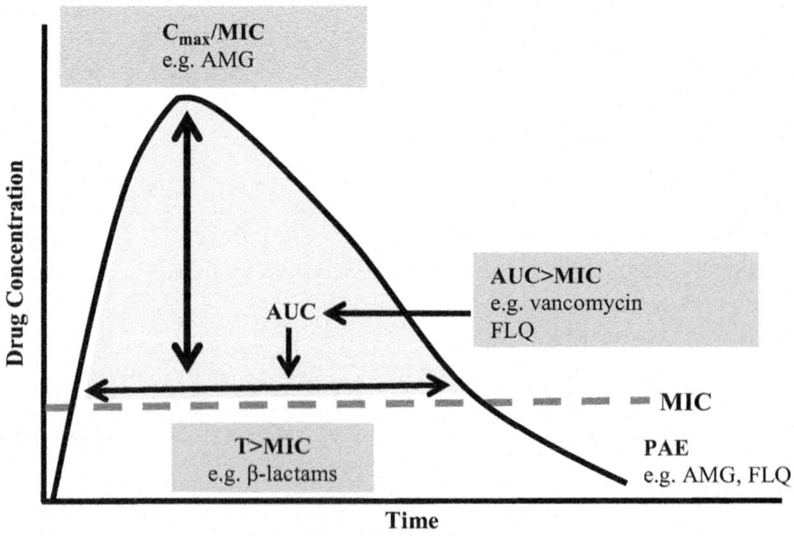

macrolides, linezolid, tigecycline, and lincosamides (e.g., clindamycin).

Altered PK-PD in Critically Ill

Unfortunately, critically ill patients experience deranged physiology with numerous medical interventions that can have a tremendous impact on achieving PK-PD targets and desired patient outcomes. Generally, these alterations tend to affect volume of distribution (Vd) and clearance.

In critical illness, fluid resuscitation, hypoalbuminemia, and capillary leak syndrome result in fluid shift from the intravascular compartment into the interstitial space [6]. For hydrophilic drugs, this generally results in "dilution" where the Vd can be substantially increased with resultant reductions in plasma concentrations. On the contrary, Vd of lipophilic drugs is largely unchanged due to more extensive adipose tissue penetration [8]. The risk with standard antibiotic doses is clearly suboptimal antibiotic exposure and associated worse outcomes. For example, in early septic shock, only one third of patients who received an initial standard dose of cefepime or piperacillin-tazobactam achieved target PK-PD goals [10]. To overcome expanded Vd and ensure therapeutic concentration, consider giving a loading dose of hydrophilic drugs to fully "load the tank," regardless of clearance irregularities [8].

Following an assessment of volume status, one must next consider the impact of clearance abnormalities, and historically "end organ dysfunction" has received the greatest attention. Generally, acute or chronic renal impairment will reduce clearance and increase concentrations of hydrophilic anti-infectives whereas hepatic insufficiency may increase concentrations of lipophilic antimicrobials. Given the increased risk for toxicities with standard doses, maintenance dose reductions are typically recommended in the setting of impaired organ function, respectively. However, over the past decade, a greater understanding of augmented renal clearance (ARC) has been identified effecting 50–85% of patients managed in a surgical ICU [11]. ARC results from enhanced renal elimination of solutes from baseline, including glomerular filtration, secondary to increased renal blood flow from augmented cardiac output. Given that serum creatinine appears "normal," the risk is enhanced elimination of antimicrobial agents leading to treatment failure, resistance, or possibly worse outcomes [12]. In fact, ARC has been shown to be an independent predictor of subtherapeutic antibiotic concentrations in critically ill patients, where only 58% of patients with ARC achieved standard PK-PD targets [13]. Therefore, routine screening for ARC with an 8–24 h continuous urine creatinine clearance (CrCl) is recommended for patients at risk, including less than 55 years, male, trauma, surgery, burns, or neurologic insult. When starting hydrophilic antibiotics for patients identified to have ARC with a CrCl greater than 130 mL/min from direct measure, consider more aggressive doses that maximize PK-PD properties (e.g., cefepime 2 g q6–8 h infused over 3 h) [12].

Antibacterial Agents

Ideally, antibiotic selection for the prevention or treatment of specific infections should be based on rigorous clinical trials. In reality, with a few exceptions, such data rarely exists [14]. Therefore, appropriate selection of antimicrobial agents is determined by pharmacologic properties (e.g., spectrum of activity, penetration into source of infection), host factors, suspected organisms given a specific infection, and local susceptibilities (e.g., your institutions antibiogram). Relevant discussions of anti-infectives for specific disease properties are discussed in other sections of this book. The purpose of this chapter is to understand the pharmacologic properties of commonly used antibiotics and antifungals prescribed in the ICU, with an emphasis on mechanism of action, spectrum of activity, and clinical pearls as organized by drug classes.

β-Lactams

β-lactam antibiotics, including penicillins, cephalosporins, carbapenems, and monobactams, are collectively the most commonly prescribed antibiotics in the ICU, accounting for more than 40% of all antibiotic orders [15]. As a drug class, these antibiotics share a common β-lactam ring within the chemical structure, critical for inhibiting bacterial cell wall and the associated bactericidal activity. Generally, bacterial killing from exposure to β-lactam antibiotics is determined by ideally 100% $T_{>MIC}$, with minimal impact of C_{max} or PAE, particularly for gram-negative organisms [16]. Given the hydrophilic nature of these antibiotics, no β-lactam covers intracellular pathogens, such as the atypical organisms *Legionella pneumophilia or Chlamydia pneumoniae* [9].

Penicillins and β-Lactamase Inhibitors

Mechanism of action Penicillins (PCN) are natural or semi-synthetic compounds that generally display bactericidal activity by binding to PCN binding proteins (PBP) within the cell wall of susceptible bacteria. PCN binding to PBPs inhibits peptidoglycan cross-linking, a key structure within the cell wall, resulting in bacterial cell lysis and cell death during cellular division [16].

Classification/spectrum of activity Spectrum of activity, in part, is related to the affinity of PBP for β-lactam antibiotics and chemical modifications, such as stability against β-lactamase production or improved penetration through lipopolysaccharide within gram-negative organisms. PCN can be divided into four clinically relevant classes based on spectrum (Table 36.1). Of note, natural PCN, such as penicillin G, has largely fallen out of favor for treatment of *Staphylococcus aureus* and gram-negative rods secondary to production of β-lactamase, an enzyme which hydrolyzes the β-lactam ring rendering the antibiotic ineffective. Considering β-lactamase production is the most common mechanism of resistance for bacteria, aminopenicillins can be given with β-lactamase inhibitors (e.g., ampicillin/sulbactam) to extend the spectrum of activity, including anaerobes. Specific to the ICU, ampicillin/sulbactam is the drug of choice for *Acinetobacter baumannii* infections, a common ventilator-associated pneumonia pathogen, if susceptible [18]. However, the same drug is often avoided as empiric therapy for common infections (e.g., intra-abdominal) due to increasing resistance among *Escherichia coli* [19]. Although methicillin is no longer available secondary to high rates of interstitial nephritis, penicillinase-resistant PCN (e.g., nafcillin, oxacillin) is the drug of choice for methicillin susceptible *Staphylococcus aureus* (MSSA) [14]. Extended-spectrum PCN in combination with β-lactamase inhibitors (e.g., piperacillin/tazobactam) provides the broadest antibacterial spectrum of this class, including *Pseudomonas aeruginosa*.

Cephalosporins

Mechanism of action The mechanism of action of cephalosporins is identical to penicillins, ultimately disrupting bacterial cell wall [14].

Classification/spectrum of activity Cephalosporins are arbitrarily classified into five generations based solely but loosely on microbial spectrum of activity (Table 36.1). A common generalization as you advance through the classes is diminishing gram-positive activity with enhanced gram-negative coverage. *First-generation* cephalosporins, such as cefazolin, are potent inhibitors of gram-positive cocci with moderate activity against gram-negative bacilli and some anaerobic oropharyngeal organisms. In many situations, cefazolin is an alternative to nafcillin or oxacillin for the treatment of MSSA, other than central nervous system (CNS) infections where penetration is poor. As a whole, *second-generation* cephalosporins generally provide enhanced activity against *E. Coli*, *K. pneumonia*, and some *Proteus* species while individual agents have enhanced β-lactamase activity (e.g., cefuroxime) or anaerobic coverage (e.g., cefoxitin, a cephamycin). However, there is a growing prevalence of cefoxitin-resistant *Bacteroides fragilis* indicating the need to validate cefoxitin appropriateness for intra-abdominal infections to your local antibiogram [20]. *Third-generation* cephalosporins, such as ceftriaxone, have markedly increased potency against gram-negative bacilli which are often resistant to extended-spectrum penicillins or early generation cephalosporins yet may lack adequate empiric coverage of *S. aureus*. Ceftriaxone is particularly unique in that it is primarily hepatically metabolized and excreted. Within this generation, ceftazidime is considered to have activity against most gram-negative bacilli, including *P. aeruginosa* [21]. Cefepime, a *fourth-generation* cephalosporin, has the widest spectrum of activity, including *P. aeruginosa* while maintaining activity against gram-positive cocci. The "new" fifth-generation cephalosporin, known as ceftaroline, represents the first β-lactam antibiotics to have activity against MRSA with similar gram-negative coverage as ceftriaxone. Finally, ceftolozane/tazobactam and ceftazidime/avibactam are cephalosporins and β-lactamase inhibitor combinations indicated for multidrug-resistant *Pseudomonas* spp.

Carbapenems

Mechanism of action Similar to other β-lactams, carbapenems inhibit cell wall synthesis by binding PBP [22]. The broad spectrum of activity of these agents is related to "compact" chemical structures that readily diffuse through porin channels of gram-negative bacilli and are particularly resistant to β-lactamases [14].

Classification/spectrum of activity As a class, the carbapenems provide the broadest spectrum of activity of all β-lactams (Table 36.1) [23]. Imipenem was the first available carbapenem. It is co-administered with cilastatin to prevent deactivation by dehydropeptidase within the renal brush boarder cells. Imipenem inhibits most gram-positive cocci, *Enterobacteriaceae*, and gram-negative rods, including *P. aeruginosa* and anaerobes. Meropenem and doripenem differ from imipenem in that they have enhanced activity against gram-negative rods due to rapid penetration through the cell wall yet may have reduced *Enterococcus* activity. Ertapenem is unique within the carbapenems, in that its long half-life and extensive protein binding allow for once daily administration, yet it has no appreciable activity against *P. aeruginosa* or *Acinetobacter* spp. Given its limited spectrum of activity against prominent ICU pathogens, it should be limited to step-down therapy for targeted treatment (e.g., extended-spectrum β-lactamase (ESBL) producing organisms) [24].

Table 36.1 General spectrum of activity for common intravenous β-lactams for common ICU pathogens [17]

	Penicillin G	Ampicillin	Oxacillin Nafcillin	Ampicillin/ sulbactam	Piperacillin/ tazobactam	Cefazolin	Cefoxitin	Ceftriaxone	Cefepime	Imipenem Doripenem Meropenem	Ertapenem	Aztreonam
Gram-positive												
MSSA	–	–	+	+	+	+	±	±	+	+	+	–
MRSA	–	–	–	–	–	–	–	–	–	–	–	–
Coag – Staph	–	–	±	–	–	–	–	–	+	–	–	–
Strep viridans	±	±	±	±	±	+	±	+	+	+	+	–
B-hemolytic strep	+	+	±	+	±	+	+	+	+	+	+	–
S. pneumoniae	+	+	±	+	±	±	±	+	+	+	+	–
E. faecalis	+	+	–	+	+	–	–	–	–	±	±	–
E. faecium	±	±	–	±	±	–	–	–	–	±	±	–
Gram-negative												
H. influenza	–	±	–	+	+	–	+	+	+	+	+	+
E. coli	–	±	–	±	+	+	+	+	+	+	+	+
Klebsiella sp.	–	±	–	+	+	+	+	+	+	+	+	+
Enterobacter sp.	–	–	–	–	±	–	–	–	+	+	+	+
Serratia sp.	–	–	–	–	±	–	–	–	+	+	+	±
Proteus sp.	–	±	–	±	+	±	±	±	+	+	+	±
Citrobacter sp.	–	–	–	–	±	–	–	–	+	+	+	±
Aeromonas sp.	–	–	–	–	±	–	–	+	+	+	+	±
Acinetobacter sp.	–	–	–	±	±	–	–	–	±	±	–	–
Pseudomonas sp.	–	–	–	–	+	–	–	–	+	+	–	+
ESBL positive	–	–	–	–	±	–	–	–	–	+	+	–
Anaerobes												
B. Fragilis	–	–	–	+	+	–	±	–	–	+	+	–
Oral anaerobes*	+	+	+	+	+	–	+	+	+	+	+	–

(+) = active; (–) = not active; (±) = less active to potential resistance; sp. = species

Monobactams

Mechanism of action Aztreonam, the only monobactam currently available, has high affinity for PBP3, causing bacterial cell wall lysis [22].

Spectrum of activity Aztreonam has no clinical utility against any gram-positive or anaerobic organisms, but has moderate activity against *Enterobacteriaceae* and gram-negative rods (Table 36.1). Aztreonam is completely synthetic and lacks the allergenic chemical structure common among all other β-lactams, meaning aztreonam can be safely used in patients with significant penicillin or cephalosporin allergies [14]. If indicated, consideration should be given for double coverage of gram-negative organisms with an AMG or FLQ if resistance from your local antibiogram exceeds 10–20% [25].

β-Lactam Mechanism of Resistance

The mechanism of antimicrobial resistance is complex and dependent on pathogen and drug characteristics. Although some resistance is mediated through efflux pumps or porin channel modifications, the vast majority of resistance for β-lactam antibiotics is enzymatic hydrolysis by β-lactamases produced by the pathogen [26]. The "new" β-lactamase enzymes of most relevance in the ICU include AmpC enzymes, ESBL, and carbapenem-hydrolyzing β-lactamase (carbapenemases).

Although most *Enterobacteriaceae* have AmpC-encoding genes within their chromosomes, these are considered clinically problematic among the SPACE (*Serratia*, *Pseudomonas aeruginosa*, *Acinetobacter*, *Citrobacter*, and *Enterobacter*) organisms [14]. Among these pathogens, production of AmpC β-lactamase occurs either "all the time" or following induction from specific antibiotics, such as imipenem, leading to the concept of "inducible resistance." Once produced, AmpC β-lactamase confer resistance of most penicillins (potentially including piperacillin/tazobactam), through third-generation cephalosporins and monobactams, necessitating treatment with cefepime or carbapenems. ESBLs, although originally common among *E. coli* and *K. pneumoniae*, are plasmid-mediated genes that can be easily transferred from one organism to the next. ESBLs hydrolyze broad and extended-spectrum cephalosporins, PCN, and monobactams, necessitating treatment with carbapenems. Recently, carbapenemases have gained more attention, especially *K. pneumoniae* carbapenemase, which confers resistance to nearly all β-lactams. Given a lack of novel antibiotics in development, optimization of current antibiotics by applying antimicrobial stewardship principles with good infection control practices is key to combat antibiotic resistance [27].

β-Lactam Adverse Drug Reactions

Although β-lactam antibiotics are considered to have a wide therapeutic window and are generally well tolerated, there are some common adverse drug reactions (ADR) that warrant consideration. First and foremost is the concern for hypersensitivity reactions. Although most common with the PCN class, where up to 15% of patients "self-report" an allergy, hypersensitivity reactions have also been reported with cephalosporins and carbapenems [28]. Yet, hypersensitivity reactions are likely overestimated, where 95% of patients with a history of a PCN allergy had a negative confirmatory skin test [29]. In addition, IgE-mediated reactions wane over time, effecting less than 20% of patients 10 years after an initial event [30]. Given the "work horse" nature of β-lactams, labeling someone with any type of a β-lactam allergy is not without risk, potentially leading to suboptimal antibiotic prescriptions and antimicrobial resistance [28]. In these situations, it is critical for the healthcare team to critically evaluate "self-reported" allergies to distinguish non-immunogenic adverse effects (e.g., rash) from IgE-medicated hypersensitivity reactions (e.g., hives, airway swelling, anaphylaxis). In the modern era, it is also recognized that the cross-reactivity among β-lactams is much lower than previously reported. If a patient has a proven PCN allergy, approximately 2% of patients may react to a cephalosporin and 10% to a carbapenem [31, 32]. Risk is higher among β-lactams with similar side chains (e.g., amoxicillin and piperacillin). Of note, cefazolin, a drug commonly implicated for hypersensitivity reactions in the ICU or operating room, has sufficiently different side chains from all other agents leading to decreased risk of cross-reactivity. Management of patients with β-lactam allergies includes challenge with an alternative β-lactam class (preferably with a different side chain); choose a different antimicrobial class (if antibiogram suggests sufficient empiric coverage of intended organisms) or β-lactam desensitization.

There are numerous other ADRs relevant for the β-lactam class, including drug fever, serum sickness, rash, encephalopathy, *Clostridium difficile* colitis, interstitial nephritis, neutropenia, and thrombocytopenia. Some ADRs are more specific to individual β-lactams. For example, seizures, although rare, may occur most frequently following exposure to penicillin G, imipenem, and even cefepime (e.g., nonconvulsive status epilepticus) [14]. Generally, risk of seizures is related to preexisting CNS disease, advanced age, and renal insufficiency which can usually be avoided by reducing the dose.

Drugs for Gram-Positive Organisms

Vancomycin

Mechanism of action Vancomycin is a glycopeptide that binds to peptidoglycan precursors of the cell wall, D-alanyl-D-alanine, which inhibits cell wall synthesis by PBP [33].

Spectrum of activity Vancomycin has broad activity against gram-positive bacteria. Traditionally, it has been the drug of choice for empiric/targeted therapy for MRSA with susceptible MICs of ≤2 μg/mL. However, due to reported treatment failures with elevated, yet susceptible, MICs ≥ 1.5–2 μg/mL, it is debated when alternative agents should be used [35, 36]. Although vancomycin has activity against MSSA, it should not be used, as nafcillin and cefazolin have superior clinical outcomes [37, 38]. Several *Streptococcus* species are routinely susceptible including *S. pneumoniae*, *S. pyogenes*, *S. agalactiae*, and group C and G streptococci. Vancomycin is active against *Enterococcus faecalis* and *E. faecium*, although resistance is increasing. Combination therapy with an AMG is often recommended for severe infections. Gram-positive anaerobes are usually susceptible such as *Peptostreptococcus* spp., *Propionibacterium* spp., and most *Clostridium* spp., including *C. difficile* [33].

Clinical pharmacology and dosing The best PK-PD parameter to predict treatment success with vancomycin is an AUC/MIC ratio ≥ 400. An initial loading dose of 25–30 mg/kg is recommended to "fill the tank," especially during early stages of sepsis when Vd is increased [39, 40]. Maintenance doses and frequencies should be determined by several factors but none more important than renal function (e.g., CrCl) and body weight. The usual dose in adults with normal renal function is 15–20 mg/kg every 12 h. This dose may be inadequate to produce desired trough concentrations of 15–20 μg/mL, and most institutions use a nomogram for more accurate initial dosing (Table 36.2). Dosing in obesity and critically ill patients remains a challenge secondary to interpatient variability and unpredictable PK due to ARC or acute kidney injury [41]. Research is ongoing in these patient populations for optimal dosing regimens. Oral, not intravenous, vancomycin should be reserved for *C. difficile* colitis at doses of 500 mg every 6 h for disease complicated by hypotension, shock, ileus, or toxic megacolon [42].

Therapeutic drug monitoring The most reliable surrogate for AUC/MIC ratio is trough concentrations. Trough concentrations can be obtained prior to the fourth or fifth dose with targets of 15–20 μg/mL for more severe infections, despite limited evidence supporting higher troughs with improved outcomes [43, 44]. Routine trough concentrations are unnecessary, but should be strongly considered for worsening clinical status, documented MRSA infections, changing renal function, or in populations with unreliable pharmacokinetics (i.e., burn, trauma, obese, febrile neutropenia).

Table 36.2 Vancomycin dosing nomogram

Target troughs 15–20 mcg/mL			
Dose based on weight		Frequency based on CrCl	
Weight (kg)	Maintenance dose (mg)	CrCl (mL/min)	Dose frequency (hours)
>90	1500–1750	≥80	Q8[a]
76–90	1250–1500	50–79 (CRRT ≥ 3 L/HR)	Q12
55–75	1000–1250	25–49 (CRRT ≥ 1.5 L/HR)	Q24
<55	750–1000	< 25, IHD, CRRT < 1.5 L/HR	~Q48; based on levels

[a]Maximum empiric dose, 1.5 g q8h if < 40 years old, *CRRT* continuous renal replacement therapy, *IHD* intermittent hemodialysis

Resistance *Staphylococcus aureus* resistance to vancomycin can be categorized into three groups: vancomycin-resistant *Staphylococcus aureus* (VRSA), vancomycin-intermediate *Staphylococcus aureus* (VISA), and heterogeneous VISA (hVISA) [47]. VISA and hVISA are both caused by a thickened cell wall. VISA, defined as "intermediate" with MICs of 4–8 μg/mL, requires alternative anti-MRSA treatment. Alternatively, hVISA is interpreted as susceptible, and controversy persists as to whether it is associated with failure. VRSA possesses the *VanA* gene, a common mechanism of resistance for *Enterococcus faecalis* and *E. faecium*, causing high-level resistance by substituting D-ala-D-ala to D-ala-D-lactate of the peptidoglycan precursors [47].

Adverse events The most common adverse reactions include red man syndrome and nephrotoxicity. Red man syndrome is associated with a rash and pruritus affecting the head, neck, and face often during the infusion. This can be mitigated by prolonging the infusion time or administering antihistamines prior to subsequent doses. Potential risk factors for nephrotoxicity include troughs ≥15 μg/mL, critically ill, obesity, and concomitant use of piperacillin-tazobactam [33, 45, 46]. Anaphylaxis and ototoxicity are uncommon.

Daptomycin

Mechanism of action Daptomycin inserts a lipophilic tail into the cell membrane of gram-positive organisms, causing membrane depolarization [33].

Spectrum of activity Daptomycin has similar activity of aerobic and anaerobic gram-positive organisms typically covered by vancomycin (see 36.4.2.1). It is often reserved for MRSA infections failing vancomycin therapy, VISA, and vancomycin-resistant *Enterococcus* (VRE).

Clinical pharmacology and dosing Daptomycin exerts concentration-dependent bactericidal activity. FDA dosing recommends 4–6 mg/kg every 24 h; however, higher doses (8–12 mg/kg) may be more effective for deep-seated MRSA infections and elevated enterococcal MICs of 3–4 μg/mL [48–51]. The drug is primarily renally eliminated and requires increasing dosing interval to every 48 h for CrCl ≤30 mL/min or administered after IHD [52]. Daptomycin is inactivated by lung surfactant and should not be used for pneumonia [33].

Resistance Nonsusceptible (NS) daptomycin *Staphylococcus aureus* (MIC > 1 μg/mL) may develop on therapy when the source of the infection is uncontrolled or the drug is underdosed. Resistance is more common with *E. faecium* compared to *E. faecalis.* In vitro data and case reports demonstrate synergy for resistant organisms when daptomycin is combined with some β-lactams [53, 54].

Adverse events Muscle toxicity presenting with upper extremity myopathy and increases in creatinine phosphokinase (CPK) levels is the most common toxicity (6.7%). The drug should be discontinued for unexplained myopathy with CPK > 1000 units/L or for CPK > 2000 units/L without muscle pain. Daptomycin may cause a falsely elevated prothrombin time depending on reagents used [33].

Oxazolidinones: Linezolid/Tedizolid

Mechanism of action Linezolid and tedizolid act by inhibiting protein synthesis through inhibition of the 50S ribosome [55].

Spectrum of activity The spectrum of activity of the oxazolidinones is similar to daptomycin (see 36.4.2.2) and is often reserved for MRSA infections failing vancomycin, VRE, and NS-daptomycin isolates. Unlike daptomycin, these drugs are bacteriostatic. Tedizolid exhibits a four- to eightfold increase in potency compared to linezolid [56]. Both agents display activity to *Mycobacterium* spp. [57].

Clinical pharmacology Both agents are available in IV and PO formulations and are dosed in a 1:1 ratio, attributing to 100% bioavailability. Due to its longer half-life, tedizolid is dosed at 200 mg daily versus 600 mg twice daily for linezolid. Neither agent requires dosing adjustment for renal or hepatic dysfunction. These agents are used for several infection types as they penetrate into many body sites; however, they should be used with caution for endovascular infections as outcomes are mixed [58, 59].

Resistance Resistance is expressed via binding site modifications and is associated with prolonged use. Tedizolid may retain activity against linezolid resistant isolates [56, 62].

Adverse events These agents are well tolerated with GI symptoms predominating. Hematologic (e.g., anemia, thrombocytopenia, neutropenia) and mitochondrial toxicities (e.g., lactic acidosis, neuropathies) limit prolonged use and have been seen as early as 10 days after initiation [60, 61]. Linezolid is a reversible monoamine oxidase inhibitor (MAOI) and has been associated with serotonin syndrome. Although rare, caution should be exercised when used with concurrent serotonergic agents. Tedizolid, a weaker MAOI, may have less risk [56].

Other Drugs for Gram-Positive Organisms

Telavancin Telavancin, a once-daily lipoglycopeptide approved for skin and soft tissue infections (SSTI) and pneumonia, has activity against gram-positive organisms, including resistant isolates [33]. It should be used with caution in patients with a baseline CrCl ≤ 50 mL/min as mortality rates were higher compared to vancomycin for MRSA-associated hospital-acquired pneumonia [63, 64]. Common adverse events include infusion-related reactions similar to vancomycin. It interferes with coagulation assays, but testing can be performed just prior to telavancin doses to mitigate this interaction [33].

Quinupristin/dalfopristin Quinupristin/dalfopristin, a combination of two streptogramins, is bactericidal against most gram-positive organisms, with the exception of *E. faecalis.* It is often reserved for salvage therapy against multidrug-resistant VRE due to the availability of newer, better-tolerated alternatives. Common side effects leading to drug cession include infusion site irritation, arthralgia, and myalgia [33].

Clindamycin Clindamycin inhibits ribosomal subunits with activity against *S. aureus*, including MRSA, most Streptococcal spp., and anaerobic gram-positives including *Peptostreptococcus* spp., *Peptococcus* spp., and *Clostridium perfringens.* It has some activity against gram-negative anaerobes; however, due to increased resistance to *B. fragilis,* it should be avoided for intra-abdominal infections. Streptococcus milleri group resistance continues to rise; therefore, it should be reserved for β-lactam allergic patients for odontogenic infections [65–67]. With the exception of the CNS, clindamycin achieves excellent concentrations into most tissues and can be used to reduce toxin production (e.g., streptococci). The most concerning adverse event is *Clostridium difficile*-associated colitis.

Fluoroquinolones

Mechanism of action FLQs achieve bactericidal activity by interfering with the activity of DNA gyrase and topoisomerase which ultimately impedes bacterial DNA synthesis [68].

Clinical pharmacology The FLQs are concentration-dependent antibiotics that are well absorbed from the GI tract and have excellent bioavailability (~70–100%). However it should be noted that co-administration with cations, which are often found in enteral tube feeds, can have a significant impact and administration and should ideally be separated by at least 2 h. Due to a large Vd, concentrations of FLQs in tissues can exceed that of the serum, particularly in the kidneys and urine. Some exceptions to this include the bones, prostatic fluid, and cerebrospinal fluid (CSF) where tissue concentrations are typically lower. Both levofloxacin and ciprofloxacin require dose adjustment in patients with renal dysfunction due to primarily renal elimination and mixed renal and nonrenal elimination, respectively. In contrast, moxifloxacin requires no renal dose adjustment since hepatic metabolism and biliary excretion are the primary routes of elimination.

Spectrum of activity FLQs have a broad spectrum of activity including many aerobic gram-negatives, including *Enterobacteriaceae*, *Haemophilus* spp., *Neisseria* spp., and *Moraxella catarrhalis* [68]. Ciprofloxacin and levofloxacin are unique in that they have additional activity against *P. aeruginosa*, with ciprofloxacin being more potent. Respiratory pathogens such as *Streptococcus* spp. are best covered by levofloxacin and moxifloxacin. FLQ also has activity against atypical organisms and most mycobacteria.

Adverse drug reactions QT interval prolongation is the most significant adverse effect associated with FLQ therapy. Risk is highest in patients receiving concomitant medications which can prolong the QT interval and in older patients or those with underlying risk factors for arrhythmias [68]. Other side effects include GI upset, CNS effects (headaches and dizziness), and the risk of potential arthropathy and tendinitis. In July of 2016, the Food and Drug Administration (FDA) administered a black box warning regarding the use of FLQ to treat uncomplicated infections such as acute sinusitis, bronchitis, and uncomplicated urinary tract infections since the risks of therapy likely outweigh the benefits [69]. FLQ use is also a risk factor for *C. difficile* diarrhea.

Resistance For serious infections with a high bacterial burden, it is important to be aware that resistance to FLQs can develop while on therapy [68]. This is particularly true when treating pathogens like *P. aeruginosa* and *S. aureus* where resistance is more likely. In practice, increasing resistance to nosocomial pathogens has limited empiric FLQ use. Strategies for minimizing FLQ resistance include judicious FLQ use, optimizing selection of FLQ, dose, and duration of treatment as well as infection control procedures to prevent spread of resistant organisms.

Aminoglycosides

AMGs are a class of antibiotics that have been in use since the 1940s to treat serious gram-negative infections [70]. The most commonly used AMGs in clinical practice today include amikacin, gentamicin, and tobramycin, which have similar physical, chemical, and pharmacologic properties.

Mechanism of action AMGs exert their activity by inhibiting protein synthesis [70]. Unlike most other antibiotics that exert their activity via this mechanism, AMGs are unique in that they are bactericidal, rather than bacteriostatic [70]. The exact mechanism for achieving cell death is unknown. AMGs are concentration-dependent antibiotics; therefore, the Cmax/MIC ratio must be maximized for efficacy, where concentrations are ideally ten times higher than the MIC. Antibacterial activity of AMGs is also due to a prolonged PAE which allows suppression of bacterial growth after short antibiotic exposure.

Spectrum of activity Due to toxicities and complicated dosing, AMGs are primarily used for their activity against resistant gram-negative bacilli, including *Enterobacteriaceae*, *Pseudomonas aeruginosa*, and *Acinetobacter* spp., but may also be used synergistically with cell wall active agents for certain gram-positive infections [70]. When comparing antimicrobial spectrum across the AMG class, it should be noted that tobramycin is more potent against *Pseudomonas*. AMGs require aerobic metabolism to exert their antibacterial effect and thus do not have activity against anaerobic organisms.

Clinical pharmacology Since AMGs are highly water soluble and have a low level of protein binding, they distribute widely throughout the extracellular space [70]. Low lipid solubility contributes to the limited ability of AMGs to cross cellular membranes and thus potential sites of infection, with the exception of the synovial fluid. AMGs are largely excreted unchanged in the urine, and thus therapeutic concentrations after one systemic dose can remain therapeutic for days.

Dosing and monitoring Traditionally, AMG was dosed two to three times per day requiring the measurement of peak and trough concentrations to determine efficacy and safety. This dosing scheme has largely fallen out of favor due to the optimization of PAE and peak concentrations (efficacy) and decreased rates of toxicity with once-daily dosing [70]. In a study of more than 2000 patients, only 1.2% developed nephrotoxicity with once-daily dosing [71]. For most patient populations and infections, 5–7 mg/kg/day of gentamicin/tobramycin and 15 mg/kg/day for amikacin will be efficacious. In patients with renal impairment, this dosing interval may need to be prolonged. Once-daily AMG dosing generally eliminates the need for peak serum level monitoring with the exception of some critically ill patients and cystic fibrosis patients where significant alterations in pharmacokinetics may be seen. Therapeutic drug monitoring for once-daily dosing may be achieved by using a nomogram or obtaining trough concentrations. When a nomogram is used (Fig. 36.2), AMG serum levels are obtained 6–14 h post-infusion and plotted on a graph to determine the appropriate dosing interval [71]. Conversely, true trough concentrations (18–24 h post-dose) may be obtained to document AMG clearance. If undetectable troughs are not achieved (<0.5–1 mcg/mL for gentamicin/tobramycin; <3–5 mcg/mL for amikacin), dosing interval should be adjusted to minimize toxicity [70].

Adverse drug reactions AMGs share the potential for causing nephrotoxicity, ototoxicity, and rarely, neuromuscular blockade [70]. AMG-induced injury to renal proximal tubular cells is the primary mechanism of nephrotoxicity. Fortunately, tubular injury is generally reversible, and once-daily dosing can be used to minimize renal insult due to saturable uptake of AMG into tubular cells. In contrast, AMG-induced ototoxicity caused by cochlear damage, vestibular damage, or both is irreversible. Risk of ototoxicity increases with age, renal impairment, concomitant vancomycin therapy, and prolonged AMG duration (≥3 weeks). Rarely, neuromuscular blockade, which can be fatal, can occur. To avoid, AMGs should be infused over at least 30 min, but preferably longer, and minimize use with other neuromuscular blocking drugs (e.g. neuromuscular blocking agents).

Sulfamethoxazole/Trimethoprim

Mechanism of action Sulfamethoxazole (SMX) is a bacteriostatic antibiotic that exerts its activity via interfering with bacterial folic acid synthesis. When used together with trimethoprim (TMP), a dihydrofolate reductase inhibitor, these two agents display synergistic antimicrobial activity [72]. Therefore, the fixed ratio combination product, available in both oral and parenteral forms, is most commonly used today. It should be noted that when dosing these products, dosing is based on the TMP component.

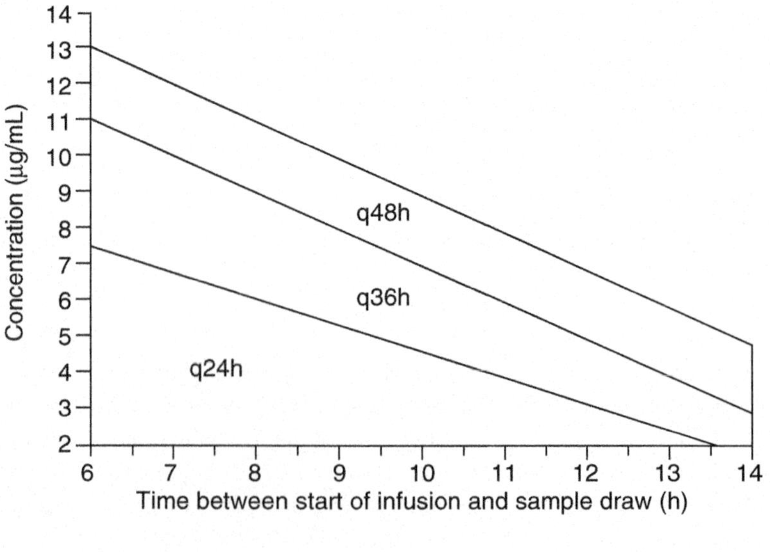

Fig. 36.2 Adapted Hartford nomogram for aminoglycoside dose adjustment [71]

Spectrum of activity The gram-positive activity of TMP-SMX includes MSSA, MRSA, *S. pneumoniae*, and *S. pyogenes*. TMP-SMX can be effective against a wide range of *Enterobacteriaceae* as well as *Acinetobacter* spp.; however, susceptibilities vary widely, so empiric therapy with TMP-SMX is not generally recommended when other more effective agents are available [72]. TMP-SMX also plays an important role in therapy for the treatment of *Stenotrophomonas maltophilia* and *Pneumocystis jirovecii* pneumonia. Most enterococci and *P. aeruginosa* display resistance.

Clinical pharmacology TMP-SMX has excellent oral bioavailability, with peaks similar to that of intravenous administration [72]. In general, TMP-SMX is well distributed throughout the body, including the kidney, lung, and sputum where higher concentrations than serum may be achieved. TMP-SMX also penetrates the CSF with concentrations of about 25–50% of that measured in the serum. TMP-SMX is hepatically metabolized and excreted in the urine as metabolites and unchanged drug; therefore, dosing must be adjusted in patients with renal dysfunction to prevent accumulation. Several clinically relevant drug-drug interactions exist. TMP-SMX can increase the risk of bleeding in patients on warfarin; empiric warfarin dose reductions are warranted with concomitant therapy. Drug interactions also exist with phenytoin, digoxin, and certain antiretroviral medications. Toxicity of these medications should be monitored along with drug levels where possible.

Adverse drug reactions GI upset and hypersensitivity reactions are the most common adverse effects observed with TMP-SMX. In rare cases, Stevens-Johnson syndrome and toxic epidermal necrolysis can occur [72]. Renal dysfunction due to TMP-SMX is also possible, particularly in patients with preexisting renal disease. Patients should be monitored for sodium disorders and hyperkalemia, especially in elderly patients and those on concomitant medications known to increase serum potassium.

Metronidazole

Mechanism of action Metronidazole is considered a prodrug since it must be activated by the target pathogen prior to exerting its concentration-dependent bactericidal or parasiticidal activity [73]. Once activated, metronidazole induces cell death by inhibiting DNA synthesis and causing oxidative DNA structural damage leading to DNA degradation.

Spectrum of activity Metronidazole is well known for its use in treating anaerobic infections, including those caused by *Bacteroides* and *Clostridium* [73]. However, some anaerobes possess intrinsic resistance to metronidazole, including non-spore-forming gram-positive anaerobic bacteria (*Actinomyces*, *Bifidobacterium*, *Lactobacillus*, and *Propionibacterium*), and therefore metronidazole should not be used to empirically treat these pathogens. Facultative anaerobes are not reliably treated with metronidazole due to variable susceptibility, with the exception of the use of metronidazole to treat bacterial vaginosis where *Gardnerella* may be implicated [74]. Metronidazole also remains an important member of many *Helicobacter pylori* treatment regimens despite increasing resistance. Of note, metronidazole has activity against several protozoa: *Giardia*, *Entamoeba histolytica*, and *Trichomonas vaginalis* [75].

Clinical pharmacology Metronidazole has excellent bioavailability and is widely distributed throughout the body due to its lipophilicity, low protein binding, and relatively large Vd. Thanks to these properties, metronidazole achieves great penetration into the CSF, peritoneal fluid, pancreatic and appendix tissue, and abscesses. Metronidazole has several clinically significant drug interactions that clinicians should be aware of prior to prescribing. First, patients should avoid consuming alcohol within 3 days of metronidazole therapy due to disulfiram-like reactions, producing severe nausea and vomiting that can occur with any route of administration. Also, warfarin and metronidazole should be used with caution due to the inhibition of warfarin metabolism and increased risk of bleeding. Preemptive warfarin dose reduction with close monitoring of international normalized ratio (INR) is warranted in most patients. Although rare, it is possible that metronidazole can prolong the QT interval and lead to risk of torsades de pointes, particularly in combination with other QT interval prolonging drugs.

Adverse drug reactions Metronidazole should be avoided in pregnant women, particularly in the first trimester where its use is contraindicated due to the risk of fetal malformation [73].

Tetracyclines

Mechanism of action Tetracyclines induce their bacteriostatic activity by reversibly binding to the 30S ribosomal subunit which inhibits bacterial protein synthesis [75]. Uniquely, doxycycline can also bind to the 70S subunit which inhibits protein synthesis in mitochondria allowing anti-protozoal activity.

Spectrum of activity The gram-positive spectrum of tetracyclines is very broad and includes community-acquired MSSA and MRSA, *Streptococcus pneumoniae*, and gram-positive anaerobes [75]. Tetracyclines are also highly active against atypical bacteria and play a pivotal role in the treatment of spirochetes and the rickettsial family which include pathogens that cause Lyme disease and Rocky Mountain spotted fever. The gram-negative coverage of tetracyclines is much narrower but typically includes *Neisseria*, *Moraxella*, *Haemophilus*, and *Campylobacter*.

Clinical pharmacology Tetracyclines are most commonly used as their oral preparations due to high bioavailability; however, doxycycline may be administered parenterally when needed [75]. Administration should be separated from multivalent cations and enteral tube feeds containing these elements by about 3 h due to chelation and subsequent decrease in drug absorption of up to 90%. Overall, tetracyclines achieve good tissue and body fluid penetration with the exception of the CSF. Each tetracycline antibiotic is eliminated slightly differently, and all, except doxycycline, require dose adjustment in the setting of renal dysfunction.

Adverse drug reactions The most common side effect is GI upset leading to nausea, vomiting, diarrhea, and epigastric pain. Tetracyclines are pregnancy category D and should be avoided during pregnancy primarily due to their potential to stain teeth and cause enamel hypoplasia in the fetus [75].

Polymyxins

Due to high rates of nephrotoxicity, the polymyxin class of antibiotics is primarily reserved for oral and topical use. Unfortunately, because of emerging resistance among some gram-negative pathogens, their parenteral use, as polymyxin B and polymyxin E (colistin), is again finding a niche. Parenteral polymyxins have bactericidal activity against many gram-negative bacilli, but their use is primarily reserved for multidrug-resistant (MDR) *P. aeruginosa*, *Acinetobacter baumannii*, and carbapenem-resistant *Enterobacteriaceae* (CRE) when no other less toxic or more effective drug is available [76]. Inhalation therapy may also be used to treat colonization or infection of the pulmonary system, particularly in the CF population. To complicate matters, there is debate upon optimal dosing strategies as well as defined breakpoints for susceptibility. When used to treat serious infections, it is preferred that polymyxins are used as combination therapy whenever possible.

Rifamycins

The rifamycins are a class of antibiotics that inhibit bacterial RNA synthesis and are most commonly used to treat tuberculosis and *Mycobacterium avium* complex infections [77]. However, two of the more commonly used antibiotics of the class, rifampin and rifaximin, may be used more frequently in the standard critical care population.

Rifampin In addition to the abovementioned activity, rifampin is effective against many gram-positive bacteria including *Staphylococcus* and *Streptococcus* spp. However, rifampin should not be used as monotherapy for these pathogens due to rapid emergence of resistance [77]. Rifampin is highly lipophilic, has a large Vd, and has the ability to penetrate metabolically dormant bacteria that are commonly seen in biofilms. Due to these properties, rifampin has been studied for use in combination with β-lactams, vancomycin, and other antimicrobials to improve clinical outcomes or provide synergistic effects in certain infections [78, 51]. Ultimately, the role of rifampin as adjunctive therapy is still under debate but may be considered when treating prosthetic valve endocarditis, foreign-body or prosthetic joint infections, and chronic osteomyelitis [77, 78, 51]. Many drug interactions are possible with rifampin due to multiple different mechanisms including modulation of cytochrome P450 enzymes [77]. It is essential that providers evaluate for drug interactions and adjust therapy appropriately.

Rifaximin Rifaximin is a bactericidal oral rifamycin with low systemic absorption and high fecal concentrations that is effective against many enteric pathogens [77]. In the ICU, rifaximin is primarily used for hepatic encephalopathy or for *C. difficile* infections refractory to first-line therapies. However, rifaximin should be used with caution for treating *C. difficile* due to resistance development while on therapy. Compared with systemic rifamycins, rifaximin is associated with minimal side effects and drug interactions.

Macrolides

The macrolide class of antibiotics consists of erythromycin, azithromycin, and clarithromycin. This section will focus primarily on azithromycin since the other two members are rarely used in the critical care setting.

Erythromycin Erythromycin exerts its antibiotic activity by inhibiting RNA-dependent protein synthesis during chain elongation [79]. Today, there are few indications where erythromycin would be the antimicrobial of choice. Additionally, there are significant toxicities associated with its use including QT interval prolongation, GI toxicity, drug interactions, and the induction of bacterial resistance. Therefore, in the critical care setting, erythromycin is more commonly used for its motilin receptor agonist properties which promote GI motility in patients with gastroparesis or acute colonic pseudo-obstruction, although evidence use in this setting is limited [79, 80].

Azithromycin

Mechanism of action Similar to erythromycin, azithromycin produces its bacteriostatic antimicrobial properties by binding to the bacterial 50S ribosomal subunit to inhibit protein synthesis [65]. Because of structural changes from erythromycin, azithromycin has improved oral absorption, longer half-life, fewer GI adverse effects, and a greater antimicrobial spectrum.

Spectrum of activity The spectrum of azithromycin includes *Streptococcus* spp., MSSA, *Haemophilus influenzae*, *Moraxella catarrhalis*, and atypical organisms making this agent useful for treating community-acquired upper and lower respiratory tract infections. However, clinicians should be aware that there has been increasing macrolide resistance among *S. pneumoniae* and MSSA isolates [65]. Azithromycin plays an important role in the treatment of sexually transmitted diseases including *Chlamydia trachomatis* and dual therapy for *Neisseria gonorrhoeae* [74]. Azithromycin also has activity against *Mycobacterium avium* complex. In addition to their antimicrobial properties, there have been proposed benefits for the use of macrolides due to their anti-inflammatory and immunomodulatory effects in patients with inflammatory lung diseases and severe pneumonia [65, 81, 82].

Clinical pharmacology Azithromycin is available in both oral and parenteral forms; however, the bioavailability after a single oral dose is only about 35%, and this is further decreased when taken with food or cations [65]. Due to relatively low protein binding, azithromycin achieves concentrations in most tissue equal to or greater than that of the serum, especially in the lungs, and effective concentrations can remain present for days after therapy discontinuation. Azithromycin is primarily hepatically metabolized; no data exists regarding dose adjustment in patients with organ failure.

Adverse drug reactions Azithromycin is generally well tolerated with the most common adverse effect being GI upset. In 2013, the FDA released a warning regarding the risk of QT prolongation and torsades de pointes with azithromycin use [83]. In one study, there was a 2.88 increased risk of death in patients taking a 5-day course of azithromycin as compared to no antibiotic therapy, and this risk was increased in patients with underlying cardiac disease [84]. When azithromycin must be used, it is prudent to monitor electrolyte levels and limit other medications that can prolong the QT interval.

Antifungal Agents

Amphotericin B

Mechanism of action Amphotericin B is fungicidal by disrupting membrane function by binding to ergosterol [84].

Spectrum of activity and resistance Amphotericin B has activity against most fungi (Table 36.3). Acquired resistance on therapy for susceptible organisms is relatively uncommon [85, 86].

Clinical pharmacology Amphotericin B is available as deoxycholate formulation (AmB-d) and two lipid-based formulations – liposomal amphotericin B (L-AmB) and amphotericin B lipid complex (ABLC). Amphotericin B colloidal dispersion is no longer available. The three available agents are compared below (Table 36.4) [85–88].

Table 36.3 General spectrum of activity for common intravenous antifungals for ICU pathogens [17]

	AMB	5-FC	FLU	ITR	VOR	POS	ISA	ECH
C. albicans	+	+	+	+	+	+	+	+
C. glabrata	+	+	±	±	+	+	+	±
C. parapsilosis	+	+	+	+	+	+	+	±
C. tropicalis	+	+	+	+	+	+	+	+
C. krusei	+	±	–	±	+	+	+	+
C. lusitaniae	–	+	+	+	+	+	+	+
A. fumigatus	+	–	–	±	+	+	+	±
C. neoformans	+	+	+	+	+	+	+	–
Mucormycosis	+	–	–	–	–	+	+	–
Fusarium spp.	±	–	–	±	+	+	+	–
Scedosporium spp.	±	–	–	±	±	±	±	–
Histo/blasto	+	–	±	+	+	+	+	–
C. Immitis	+	–	±	+	+	+	+	–

5-FC flucytosine, *AMB* amphotericin, *ECH* echinocandins, *FLU* fluconazole, *ISA* isavuconazole, *ITR* itraconazole, *POS* posaconazole, *VOR* voriconazole

Table 36.4 Clinical pharmacology and adverse events of amphotericin formulations

Drug	Dose (IV)	Comments
AmB-d	0.7–1 mg/kg/d	No dose adjustments for renal/hepatic dysfunction, HD Half-life: 15 days Continuous infusion nephrotoxicity rates ~L-AmB ADE: Nephrotoxicity (25%), electrolyte wasting, infusion reactions (chills, fevers, tachypnea) Cost: $
L-AmB	3–6 mg/kg/d	No dose adjustment for organ dysfunction Minimal concentrations in urine ADE: Similar to AmB-d - lower rates Cost: $$$$
ABLC	5 mg/kg/d	↑ lung concentrations; clinical significance unknown ADE: Similar to AmB-d – Lower rates Cost: $$$

ABLC amphotericin B lipid complex, *ADE* adverse drug events, *AmB-d* amphotericin B deoxycholate, *HD* hemodialysis, *L-AmB* liposomal amphotericin B

Imidazoles and Triazoles

Mechanism of action "Azoles" inhibit C-14α demethylation of lanosterol by binding to a cytochrome P450 enzyme, which ultimately leads to impairment of ergosterol synthesis and cell membrane integrity [85, 86]. All agents are CYP450 inhibitors and/or substrates, and drug interactions must be assessed upon initiation.

Spectrum of activity and resistance See Table 36.2 for detailed spectrum of activity. Intrinsic azole resistance has increased among *C. glabrata* isolates to fluconazole from 9% to 14% [86]. Resistance is mediated by mutations on the drug target, 14α-demethylase, and upregulation of efflux pumps (Table 36.5).

Table 36.5 Clinical pharmacology and adverse events of azoles [86–90]

Drug	Dose	Comments
Fluconazole (IV/PO)	ICI: 12 mg/kg LD; 400 mg/d (~6 mg/kg) Mucosal candidiasis: 100–200 mg/d	Excellent bioavailability (> 90%) CrCl < 50: ↓ dose 50% Distributes into brain, CSF, eye ADR: Tolerated well, ↑LFTs
Itraconazole (PO)	200 mg TID × 3d, 200 mg BID Capsule/solution available	Bioavailability: Solution > capsule Dose adjust: ↓ dose 50% (severe hepatic impairment; CrCl < 50 (caution IV form) ADR: GI, ↑LFTs Concentrations: 2–10 μg/mL
Voriconazole (IV/PO)	6 mg/kg Q12h × 2 doses, 4 mg/kg Q12h (~200 mg Q12h)	Excellent bioavailability (> 90%) Distributes into brain, CSF, eye Caution with severe hepatic impairment ADR: Visual impairment, QTc prolongation Concentrations: 1–5.5 μg/mL
Posaconazole (IV/PO)	IV: 300 mg/d PO: 400 mg BID (susp), 300 mg BID × 2 doses; 300 mg/d (DR)	Bioavailability: DR > susp Dose adjust: CrCl < 50 (caution IV form) ADR: GI, ↑LFTs, QTc prolongation Ideal concentrations undetermined
Isavuconazole (IV/PO)	372 mg Q8h × 6 doses, 372 mg/d	Excellent bioavailability (> 90%) Caution with severe hepatic impairment ADR: GI, ↑LFTs, QTc shortening Concentrations not currently recommended

ADR adverse drug reactions, *BID* twice daily, *CSF* cerebrospinal fluid, *CrCl* creatinine clearance, *DDI* drug-drug interactions, *DR* delayed-release tablet, *GI* gastrointestinal, *ICI* invasive candidiasis, *LFT* liver function tests, susp suspension, *TID* three times daily

Echinocandins: Caspofungin, Micafungin, and Anidulafungin

Mechanism of action The echinocandins are generally fungicidal by disrupting the synthesis of the cell wall by inhibiting 1,3-β-glucan synthase [86].

Spectrum of activity and resistance All three agents demonstrate a similar spectrum of activity (Table 36.6). These agents are fungicidal for all *Candida* spp. Although *C. parapsilosis* and *C. guilliermondii* demonstrate elevated MICs, outcomes are rarely affected. *C. glabrata*, once thought routinely susceptible, now has reported rates of resistance up to 3–15% [86]. Echinocandins are fungistatic against *Aspergillus* spp. and do not have activity against *Cryptococcus* spp., endemic dimorphic fungi, mucormycosis, *Fusarium* spp., or *Scedosporium* spp. Resistance to echinocandins by candida is mediated by adaptive stress responses or target site *FKS* mutations on glucan synthase. Resistance is still relatively uncommon with prevalence rates ranging between 2.9% and 3.1% [89].

Table 36.6 Clinical pharmacology and adverse events of echinocandins [85–87]

Drug	Dose (IV)	Comments
Caspofungin	70 mg LD; 50 mg/d	Moderate hepatic impairment: 35 mg/d Minimal concentrations in urine, CNS DDI: Cyclosporine (avoid), rifampin (↓ levels)
Micafungin	100–150 mg/d	No dose adjustment for organ dysfunction Minimal concentrations in urine, CNS No DDI
Anidulafungin	200 mg LD; 100 mg/d	See micafungin

CNS central nervous system, *DDI* drug-drug interactions, *IV* intravenous, *LD* loading dose

Adverse events Mild histamine-mediated reactions (e.g., rash urticaria, flushing, pruritus, hypotension), GI upset, and transaminitis are relatively uncommon [86].

References

1. Angus DC, Linde-Zwirble WT, Lidicker J, et al. Epidemiology of severe sepsis in the United States: analysis of incidence, outcome, and associated costs of care. Crit Care Med. 2001;29:1303–10.
2. Vincent JL, Rellow J, Marshall J, et al. International study of the prevalence and outcomes of infection in intensive care units. JAMA. 2009;302:2323–9.
3. Pai MP, Cottrell ML, Kashuba ADM, et al. Pharmacokinetics and pharmacodynamics of anti-infective agents. In: Bennett JE, editor. Mandell, Douglas, and Bennett's principles and practice of infectious diseases. 8th ed. Philadelphia: Saunders; 2015. p. 252–62.
4. Blumenthal DK, Garrison JC. Pharmacodynamics: molecular mechanisms of drug action. In: Brunton LL, Chabner BA, Knollman BC, editors. Goodman and Gilman's the pharmacological basis of therapeutics. 12th ed. New York: McGraw-Hill; 2011. p. 97–146.
5. Craig WA. Basic pharmacodynamics of antibacterials with clinical applications to the use of β-lactams, glycopeptides, and linezolid. Infect Dis Clin N Am. 2003;17:479–501.
6. Roberts JA, Lipman J. Pharmacokinetic issues for antibiotics in the critically ill. Crit Care Med. 2009;37:840–51.
7. Lodise TP, Lomaestro BM, Drusano GL. Application of antimicrobial pharmacodynamic concepts into clinical practice: a focus on β-lactam antibiotics. Pharmacotherapy. 2006;26:1320–32.
8. Tsai D, Lipman J, Roberts JA. Pharmacokinetic/pharmacodynamics considerations for the optimization of antimicrobial delivery in the critically ill. Curr Opin Crit Care. 2015;21:412–20.
9. Pea F, Viale P, Furlanut M. Antimicrobial therapy in critically ill patients. Clin Pharmacokinet. 2005;44:1009–34.
10. Taccone FS, Laterre PF, Dugernier T, et al. Insufficient β-lactam concentrations in the early phase of severe sepsis and septic shock. Crit Care. 2010;14:R126.
11. Udy AA, Roberts JA, Boots RJ, et al. Augmented renal clearance: implications for antibacterial dosing in the critically ill. Clin Pharm. 2010;49:1–16.
12. Hobbs ALV, Shea KM, Roberts KM, et al. Implications of augmented renal clearance on drug dosing in critically ill patients: a focus on antibiotics. Pharmacotherapy. 2015;35:1063–75.
13. Udy AA, Varghese JM, Altukroni M, et al. Subtherapeutic initial β-lactam concentrations in select critically ill: association between ARC and low trough drug concentrations. Chest. 2012;142:30–9.
14. Oki FY. Principles of critical care. 3rd ed. New York: The McGraw-Hill Companies; 2005. p. 641–97.
15. Thomas Z, Bandali F, Sankaranarayanan J, et al. A multicenter evaluation of prolonged empiric antibiotic therapy in adult ICUs in the United States. Crit Care Med. 2015;43:2527–34.
16. Doi Y, Chambers HF. Penicillin and beta-lactamase inhibitors. In: Bennett JE, editor. Mandell, Douglas, and Bennett's principles and practice of infectious diseases. 8th ed. Philadelphia: Saunders; 2015. p. 263–77.
17. Cosgrove SE, Avdic E, Dzintars K, et al. Johns Hopkins Antibiotic Guideline 2015–2016. Available at: https://www.hopkinsmedicine.org/amp/guidelines/antibiotic_guidelines.pdf. (2015). Accessed 10 Jan 2017.
18. Munoz-Price LS, Weinstein RA. Acinetobacter infection. N Engl J Med. 2008;358:1271–81.
19. Solomkin JS, Mazuski JE, Bradley JS, et al. Diagnosis and management of complicated intra-abdominal infections in adults and children. Clin Infect Dis. 2010;50:133–64.
20. Bieluch VM, Cuchural GJ, Snydman DR, et al. Clinical importance of cefoxitin-resistant *Bacteroides fragilis* isolates. Diagn Microbial Infect Dis. 1987;7:119–26.
21. Craig WA, Andes DR. Cephalosporins. In: Bennett JE, editor. Mandell, Douglas, and Bennett's principles and practice of infectious diseases. 8th ed. Philadelphia: Saunders; 2015. p. 278–92.
22. Doi Y, Chambers HF. Other β-lactams. In: Bennett JE, editor. Mandell, Douglas, and Bennett's principles and practice of infectious diseases. 8th ed. Philadelphia: Saunders; 2015. p. 293–7.
23. Bhalodi AA, Nicolau. Principles of critical care. 4th ed. New York: The McGraw-Hill Companies; 2015. Available at: http://accessmedicine.mhmedical.com.ezproxy.lib.utexas.edu/content.aspx?bookid=1340&Sectionid=80033680. Accessed 12 Jan 2017.
24. Collins VL, Marchaim D, Pogue JM, et al. Efficacy of ertapenem for treatment of bloodstream infections caused by extended spectrum β-lactamase producing enterobacteriaceae. Antimicrob Agents Chemother. 2012;56:2173–7.
25. Kalil AC, Metersky ML, Klompas M, et al. Management of adults with hospital-acquired and ventilator-associated pneumonia. Clin Infect Dis. 2016;63:1–51.
26. Jacoby GA, Munoz-Price LS. The new β-lactamases. N Engl J Med. 2005;352:380–91.
27. Barlam TF, Cosgrove SE, Abbo LM, et al. Implementing an antibiotic stewardship program: guidelines by the IDSA and SHEA. Clin Infect Dis. 2016;62:51–77.
28. Kuruvilla ME, Khan DA. Antibiotic allergy. In: Bennett JE, editor. Mandell, Douglas, and Bennett's principles and practice of infectious diseases. 8th ed. Philadelphia: Saunders; 2015. p. 298–303.
29. Salkind AR, Cuddy PG, Foxworth JW. The rational clinical examination; is this patient allergic to penicillin? JAMA. 2001;285:2498–505.
30. Sullivan T, Wedner HJ, Shatz GS, et al. Skin testing to detect penicillin allergy. J Allergy Clin Immunol. 1981;68:171–80.
31. Frumin J, Gallagher JC. Allergic cross-sensitivity between penicillin, carbapenem and monobactam antibiotics: what are the chances? Ann Pharmacother. 2009;43:304–15.
32. Solensky R, Khan DA. Drug allergy: an updated practice parameter. Ann Allergy Asthma Immunol. 2010;105:e1–78.
33. Murray BE, Arias CA, Nannini EC. Glycopeptides (vancomycin and teicoplanin), streptogramins (Quinupristin-dalfopristin), lipopeptides (daptomycin), and lipoglycopeptides (telavancin). In: Bennett JE, editor. Mandell, Douglas, and Bennett's principles

and practice of infectious diseases. 8th ed. Philadelphia: Saunders; 2015. p. 377–400.
34. Alvarez R, Lopez Cortes LE, Molina J, et al. Optimizing the clinical use of vancomycin. Antimicrob Agents Chemother. 2016;60:2601–9.
35. van Hal SJ, Lodise TP, Paterson DL. The clinical significance of vancomycin minimum inhibitory concentration in Staphylococcus aureus infections: a systemic review and meta-analysis. Clin Infect Dis. 2012;56:755–71.
36. Wunderink RG, Niederman MS, Kollef MH, et al. Linezolid in methicillin-resistance Staphylococcus aureus nosocomial pneumonia: a randomized, controlled study. Clin Infect Dis. 2012;54:621–9.
37. Stryjewski ME, Szczech LA, Benjamin DK, et al. Use of vancomycin or first-generation cephalosporins for the treatment of hemodialysis-dependent patients with methicillin-susceptible Staphylococcus aureus bacteremia. Clin Infect Dis. 2007;44:190–6.
38. Schwizer ML, Furuno JP, Harris AD, et al. Comparable effectiveness of nafcillin of cefazolin versus vancomycin in methicillin-susceptible Staphylococcus aureus bacteremia. BMC Infect Dis. 2011;11:279–86.
39. Rosini JM, Laughner J, Levine BJ, et al. A randomized trial of loading vancomycin in the emergency department. Ann Pharmacother. 2015;49:6–13.
40. Rybak M, Lomaestro B, Rotschafer JC, et al. Therapeutic monitoring of vancomycin in adult patients: a consensus review of the American society of health-system pharmacists, the infectious diseases society of America, and the society of infectious diseases pharmacists. Am J Health-Syst Pharm. 2009;66:82–98.
41. Aubron C, Corallo CE, Nunn MO, et al. Evaluation of the accuracy of a pharmacokinetic dosing program in predicting serum vancomycin concentrations in critically ill patients. Ann Pharmacother. 2011;45:1193–8.
42. Cohen SH, Gerding DN, Johnson S, et al. Clinical practice guidelines for Clostridium difficile infection in adults: 2010 update by the society for healthcare epidemiology of America (SHEA) and the infectious diseases society of America (IDSA). Infect Control Hosp Epidemiol. 2010;31:431–55.
43. Kullar R, Davis SL, Levine DP, et al. Impact of vancomycin exposure on outcomes in patients with methicillin-resistant Staphylococcus Aureus bacteremia: support for consensus guidelines suggested targets. Clin Infect Dis. 2011;52:975–81.
44. van Hal SJ, Paterson DL, Lodise TP. Systematic review and meta-analysis of vancomycin-induced nephrotoxicity associated with dosing schedules that maintain troughs between 15 and 20 milligrams per liter. Antimicrob Agents Chemother. 2013;57:734–44.
45. Giuliano CA, Patel CR, Kale-Pradhan PB. Is the combination of piperacillin-tazobactam and vancomycin associated with development of acute kidney injury? A meta-analysis. Pharmacotherapy. 2016;36:1217–28.
46. Lodise TP, Lomaestro B, Graves J, et al. Larger vancomycin doses (at least four grams per day) are associated with an increased incidence of nephrotoxicity. Antimicrob Agents Chemother. 2008;52:1330–6.
47. Fraimow HS, Tsigrelis C. Antimicrobial resistance in the intensive care unit: mechanisms, epidemiology, and management of specific resistant pathogens. Crit Care Clin. 2011;27:163–205.
48. Steenbergen JN, Alder J, Thorne GM, et al. Daptomycin: a lipopeptide antibiotic for the treatment of serious gram-positive infections. J Antimicrob Chemother. 2005;55:283–8.
49. Kullar R, Davis SL, Levine DP, et al. High-dose daptomycin for treatment of complicated gram-positive infections: a large, multicenter, retrospective study. Pharmacotherapy. 2011;31:527–36.
50. Britt NS, Potter EM, Patel N, et al. Comparative effectiveness and safety of standard-, medium-, and high-dose daptomycin strategies for the treatment of vancomycin-resistant Enterococcal bacteremia among veterans affairs patients. Clin Infect Dis. 2016;64(5):605–13. [Epub ahead of print].
51. Liu C, Bayer A, Cosgrove SE, et al. Clinical practice guidelines by the infectious diseases society of America for the treatment of methicillin-resistant Staphylococcus aureus infections in adults and children. Clin Infect Dis. 2011;52:e18–55.
52. Haselden M, Leach M, Bohm N. Daptomycin dosing strategies in patients receiving thrice-weekly intermittent dialysis. Ann Pharmacother. 2013;47:1342–7.
53. Humphries RM, Pollett S, Sakoulas G. A current perspective on daptomycin for the clinical microbiologist. Clin Microbiol Rev. 2013;26:759–80.
54. Mehta S, Singh C, Plata KB, et al. β-Lactams increase the antibacterial activity of daptomycin against clinical methicillin-resistant Staphylococcus aureus strains and prevent selection of daptomycin-resistant derivatives. Antimicrob Agents Chemother. 2012;56:192–200.
55. Cox HL, Donowitz GR. Linezolid and other oxazolidinones. In: Bennett JE, editor. Mandell, Douglas, and Bennett's principles and practice of infectious diseases. 8th ed. Philadelphia: Saunders; 2015. p. 406–9.
56. Zhanel GG, Love R, Adam H, et al. Tedizolid: a novel oxazolidinone with potent activity against multidrug-resistant gram-positive pathogens. Drugs. 2015;75:253–70.
57. Ashtekar DR, Costa-Periera R, Shrinivasan T, et al. Oxazolidinones, a new class of synthetic antituberculosis agent. In vitro and in vivo activities of DuP-721 against Mycobacterium tuberculosis. Diagn Microbiol Infect Dis. 1991;14:465–71.
58. Kullar R, Sakoulas G, Deresinski S, et al. When sepsis persists: a review of MRSA bacteraemia salvage therapy. J Antimicrob Chemother. 2016;7:576–86.
59. Sperber SJ, Levine JF, Gross PA. Persistent MRSA bacteremia in a patient with low linezolid levels. Clin Infect Dis. 2003;36:675–6.
60. Nambiar S, Rellosa N, Wassel RT, et al. Linezolid-associated peripheral and optic neuropathy in children. Pediatrics. 2011;127:1528–32.
61. Gerson SL, Kaplan SL, Bruss JB, et al. Hematologic effects of linezolid: summary of clinical experience. Antimicrob Agents Chemother. 2002;46:2723–6.
62. Sanchez-Garcia M, De la Torre MA, Morales G, et al. Clinical outbreak of linezolid-resistant Staphylococcus aureus in an intensive care unit. JAMA. 2010;303:2260–4.
63. Corey GR, Kollef MH, Shorr AF, et al. Telavancin for hospital-acquired pneumonia: clinical response and 28-day survival. Antimicrob Agents Chemother. 2014;58:2030–7.
64. Rubinstein E, Lalani T, Corey GR, et al. Telavancin versus vancomycin for hospital-acquired pneumonia due to gram-positive pathogens. Clin Infect Dis. 2011;52:31–40.
65. Sivapalasingam S, Steigbigel NH. Macrolides, clindamycin, and ketolides. In: Bennett JE, editor. Mandell, Douglas, and Bennett's principles and practice of infectious diseases. 8th ed. Philadelphia: Saunders; 2015. p. 358–75.
66. Rams TE, Degener JE, van Winkelhoff AJ. Antibiotic resistance in human chronic periodontitis microbiota. J Periodontol. 2014;85:160–9.
67. Plum AW, Mortelliti AJ, Walsh RE. Microbial flora and antibiotic resistance in peritonsillar abscesses in upstate New York. Ann Otol Rhinol Laryngol. 2015;124:875–80.
68. Hooper DC, Strahilevitz J. Quinolones. In: Bennett JE, editor. Mandell, Douglas, and Bennett's principles and practice of infectious diseases. 8th ed. Philadelphia: Saunders; 2015. p. 419–39.
69. FDA Drug Safety Communication: FDA advises restricting fluoroquinolone antibiotic use for certain uncomplicated infections; wars about disabling side effects that can occur together. Available at: http://www.fda.gov/Drugs/DrugSafety/ucm500143.htm (2017). Accessed 10 Jan 2017.

70. Leggett JE. Aminoglycosides. In: Bennett JE, editor. Mandell, Douglas, and Bennett's principles and practice of infectious diseases. 8th ed. Philadelphia: Saunders; 2015. p. 310–21.
71. Nicolau DP, Freeman CD, Belliveau PP, et al. Experience with a once-daily aminoglycoside program administered to 2,184 adults patients. Antimicrob Agents Chemother. 1995;39:650–5.
72. Zinner SH, Mayer KH. Sulfonamides and trimethoprim. In: Bennett JE, editor. Mandell, Douglas, and Bennett's principles and practice of infectious diseases. 8th ed. Philadelphia: Saunders; 2015. p. 410–8.
73. Nagel JL, Aronoff DM. Metronidazole. In: Bennett JE, editor. Mandell, Douglas, and Bennett's principles and practice of infectious diseases. 8th ed. Philadelphia: Saunders; 2015. p. 350–7.
74. Workowski KA, Bolan GA. Sexually transmitted diseases treatment guidelines 2015. MMWR. 2015;64:1–138.
75. Moffa M, Brook I. Tetracyclines, glycylcyclines, and chloramphenicol. In: Bennett JE, editor. Mandell, Douglas, and Bennett's principles and practice of infectious diseases. 8th ed. Philadelphia: Saunders; 2015. p. 322–38.
76. Kaye KS, Pogue JM, Kaye D. Polymyxins (Polymyxin B and colistin). In: Bennett JE, editor. Mandell, Douglas, and Bennett's principles and practice of infectious diseases. 8th ed. Philadelphia: Saunders; 2015. p. 401–5.
77. Maslow MJ, Portal-Celhay C. Rifamycins. In: Bennett JE, editor. Mandell, Douglas, and Bennett's principles and practice of infectious diseases. 8th ed. Philadelphia: Saunders; 2015. p. 339–49.
78. Baddour LM, Wilson WR, Bayer AS, et al. Infective endocarditis in adults: diagnosis, antimicrobial therapy, and management of complications. Circulation. 2015;132:1–52.
79. Dive A, Miesse C, Galanti L, et al. Effect of erythromycin on gastric motility in mechanically ventilated critically ill patients a double-blinded, randomized, placebo-controlled study. Crit Care Med. 1995;23:1356–62.
80. Bonacini M, Smith OJ, Pritchard T. Erythromycin as therapy for acute colonic pseudo-obstruction (Ogilvie's syndrome). J Clin Gastroenterol. 1991;13:475.
81. Restrepo MI, Mortensen EM, Waterer GW, et al. Impact of macrolide therapy on mortality for patients with severe sepsis due to pneumonia. Eur Respir J. 2009;33:153–9.
82. Martin-Loeches I, Lisboa T, Rodriguez A, et al. Combination antibiotic therapy with macrolides improves survival in intubated patients with community-acquired pneumonia. Intensive Care Med. 2010;36:612–20.
83. FDA Drug Safety Communication: azithromycin (Zithromax or Zmax) and the risk of potentially fatal heart rhythms. Available at: http://www.fda.gov/drugs/drugsafety/ucm341822.htm (2017). Accessed 10 Jan 2017
84. Ray WA, Murray KT, Hall K, et al. Azithromycin and the risk of cardiovascular death. N Engl J Med. 2012;366:1881–90.
85. Rex JH, Stevens DA. Drugs active against fungi, Pneumocystis, and Microsporida. In: Bennett JE, editor. Mandell, Douglas, and Bennett's principles and practice of infectious diseases. 8th ed. Philadelphia: Saunders; 2015. p. 479–94.
86. Nett JE, Andes DR. Antifungal agents spectrum of activity, pharmacology, and clinical indications. Infect Dis Clin N Am. 2016;30:51–83.
87. Felton T, Troke PF, Hope WM. Tissue penetration of antifungal agents. Clin Microbiol Rev. 2014;27:66–88.
88. Falci DR, dos Santos RP, Wirth F, et al. Continuous infusion of amphotericin B deoxycholate: an innovative, low-cost strategy in antifungal treatment. Mycoses. 2011;54:91–8.
89. Beyda ND, Lewis RE, Garey KW. Echinocandin resistance in Candida species: mechanisms of reduced susceptibility and therapeutic approaches. Ann Pharmacother. 2012;46:1086–96.
90. Dodds-Ashley E. Management of drug and food interactions with azole antifungal agents in transplant recipients. Pharmacotherapy. 2010;30:842–54.

SIRS/Sepsis/Septic Shock/MOSF

37

Thomas J. Herron and David J. Ciesla

Introduction

The systemic inflammatory response syndrome (SIRS), multiple organ dysfunction syndrome (MODS), and multiple organ failure (MOF) refer to a spectrum of physiologic changes resulting from a dysfunctional immune response to infection or tissue injury. Sepsis and septic shock refer to conditions due specifically to the host's response to infection. In the mildest form, this dysfunctional immune response manifests as SIRS (Table 37.1). More severe states progress to end organ dysfunction and failure which have been characterized by numerous definitions and scoring systems, each with particular advantages and disadvantages [1]. The purpose of such scoring systems is to provide a common definition for comparative study and outcome prediction. An ideal scoring system would consist of readily available clinical information and have the ability to accurately and reproducibly predict the outcome of interest. The most commonly used in contemporary studies are the Denver MOF score, the SOFA score, and the qSOFA score [2, 3] (Figs. 37.1 and 37.2).

Sepsis and septic shock are currently defined by the Society of Critical Care Medicine (SCCM) and European Society of Intensive Care Medicine (ESICM) consensus [4]. Sepsis is defined as a life-threatening organ dysfunction caused by a deregulated host response to injury and a SOFA score greater than 1. Sepsis is associated with an in-hospital mortality rate in excess of 10%. Septic shock is defined as a euvolemic patient who meets sepsis criteria, has evidence of tissue dysoxia (acidosis), and requires vasopressors to maintain a mean arterial pressure greater than 65 mmHg. Septic shock is associated with an in-hospital mortality rate in excess of 40% (Fig. 37.3).

Although post-injury MODS and sepsis have different etiologies and several unique features, they share a common pathway of unbridled host hyper-inflammation that leads to a self-sustaining cycle of indiscriminate tissue destruction and organ dysfunction. Scientific research on one has regularly complimented the other, and treatment strategies are often similar. In this chapter we focus on the common pathophysiology, inflammatory syndromes, and treatment of these conditions.

T. J. Herron · D. J. Ciesla (✉)
Department of Surgery, University of South Florida
College of Medicine, Tampa, FL, USA
e-mail: therron2@health.usf.edu; dciesla@health.usf.edu

Historical Perspective

Much of our understanding of post-injury shock, inflammation, and death was advanced during times of major military conflicts. Deaths during World War I were thought to be a result of toxins released from wounds that lead to cardiovascular collapse. Recognition that deaths were due to exsanguination and the ability to store and transfuse blood improved survival in World War II and Korea, but death came to many as a result of oliguric renal failure. The importance of replacing the extracellular fluid losses in addition to circulating blood volume was demonstrated in the work of Shires and associates in 1964. The addition of balanced salt solutions to resuscitation strategies during the Vietnam Era decreased deaths from renal failure, but a new pattern of refractory hypoxic respiratory failure leading to death emerged in some patients. Originally referred to as shock lung or Da Nang lung, it was further characterized by Ashbaugh in 1967 and termed adult respiratory distress syndrome. Development of mechanical ventilators improved survival, but again a new syndrome of progressive multiple organ failure became the leading cause of late post-injury deaths. Eiseman and associates introduced the term multiple organ failure (MOF) in a series of patients with progressive organ dysfunction at Denver General Hospital in 1977 [5].

Originally thought to be due to uncontrolled abdominal sepsis, MOF was also observed in patients with no evidence of infection [6]. Subsequent studies identified a pattern to the onset of MOF. Faist and colleagues identified two distinct patterns: early MOF, which was associated with massive tissue injury, shock, and no infection, and late MOF, which followed moderate tissue injury, shock, and delayed sepsis

A. Salim et al. (eds.), *Surgical Critical Care Therapy*, https://doi.org/10.1007/978-3-319-71712-8_37

[7]. From this work came the inflammatory model of multiple organ failure manifesting in several patterns [8]. In mild cases, patients are resuscitated into an early SIRS state, which is beneficial and resolves as the patient recovers. In massive injury associated with severe shock, patients can develop overwhelming post-injury hyper-inflammation that leads to organ failure and death. Alternatively, serial sublethal insults lead to either hyper-inflammation and organ failure or delayed immunosuppression and susceptibility to sepsis (Fig. 37.4).

As the pathophysiology underlying the systemic inflammatory response became better understood, resuscitation strategies, operative approaches, and ICU care improved such that in the 1990s and 2000s, the incidence of MOF and its associated mortality diminished substantially [9, 10]. Far fewer patients developed MOF despite having higher risk factors and fewer patients with MOF died early deaths [11]. Yet hyper-inflammatory states are common after severe injury; its victims continue to suffer high morbidity and consume substantial medical resources.

Table 37.1 Criteria for SIRS

Parameter	Value
Temperature	>38 or <36 °C
Heart rate	>90 beats/min
Respiratory rate	>20 breaths/min or $PaCO_2 < 32$ mmHg
White blood cell count	>12,000/mm³ or <4000/mm³ or >10% immature bands

Pathophysiology

The cascade of events that lead to MOF begins with tissue injury or infection mediated primarily through the innate immune system which is composed of mediators and cells with invariant receptors that respond to conditions which threaten the functional integrity of the host [12]. Direct tissue injury results in localized cellular disruption, microvascular thrombosis, and tissue ischemia. The degree of the inflammatory response is dependent on the amount of tissue injury, the severity of shock, the resultant the ischemia/reperfusion injury, infection, and host factors.

Both mechanical injury and ischemia reperfusion cause cellular disruption and release of noxious intracellular contents. Ischemia-reperfusion elicits a localized and systemic inflammatory response by a number or mechanisms. Cells depleted of oxygen shift to anaerobic intracellular metabolism and eventually exhaust the intracellular supply of adenosine

Sequential [Sepsis-Related] Organ Failure Assessment Score[a]

	Score				
System	**0**	**1**	**2**	**3**	**4**
Respiration					
PaO_2/FIO_2, mm Hg (kPa)	≥400 (53.3)	<400 (53.3)	<300 (40)	<200 (26.7) with respiratory support	<100 (13.3) with respiratory support
Coagulation					
Platelets, ×10³/μL	≥150	<150	<100	<50	<20
Liver					
Bilirubin, mg/dL (μmol/L)	<1.2 (20)	1.2–1.9 (20–32)	2.0–5.9 (33–101)	6.0–11.9 (102–204)	>12.0 (204)
Cardiovascular	MAP ≥70 mm Hg	MAP <70 mm Hg	Dopamine <5 or dobutamine (any dose)[b]	Dopamine 5.1–15 or epinephrine ≤0.1 or norepinephrine ≤0.1[b]	Dopamine >15 or epinephrine >0.1 or norepinephrine >0.1[b]
Central nervous system					
Glasgow Coma Scale score[c]	15	13–14	10–12	6–9	<6
Renal					
Creatinine, mg/dL (μmol/L)	<1.2 (110)	1.2–1.9 (110–170)	2.0–3.4 (171–299)	3.5–4.9 (300–440)	>5.0 (440)
Urine output, mL/d				<500	<200

Abbreviations: FIO_2, fraction of inspired oxygen; MAP, mean arterial pressure; PaO_2, partial pressure of oxygen.

Fig. 37.1 Sequential [sepsis-related] Organ Failure Assessment score

Parameter	Value
Respiratory Rate	≥22/min
Mentation	Altered
Systolic Blood Pressure	≥ 100 mmHg

Fig. 37.2 Quick SOFA

triphosphate. Under these conditions, xanthine dehydrogenase converts to xanthine oxidase and catalyzes the production of the superoxide (O_2^-) anion upon reperfusion. This triggers a peroxidation chain reaction which generates more toxic oxygen species which act on local cell membranes leading to rupture. Local vasoconstriction also occurs as a result Nitric Oxide scavenging by the now abundant oxygen free radicals leading to further local tissue ischemia, decreased platelet aggregation, and PMN adherence to endothelium [13].

Among the intracellular contents released following non-apoptotic cell death are damage-associated molecular patterns (DAMPS), endogenous molecules (ATP, mitochondrial DNA and proteins, high mobility group box 1) which promote the production of inflammatory cytokines (e.g., tumor necrosis factor alpha, interleukin-1 [IL-1], IL-6). These inflammatory mediators have local (paracrine) as well as systemic (endocrine) effects. Specifically, inflammatory cytokines act locally as chemoattractants that activate endothelial cells and further recruit PMNs and monocytes to the injury site and act systemically to signal to circulating immune cells and end organs [14–17] .

In addition to DAMPS, activated immune and endothelial cells recognize exogenous (bacterial, fungal, and viral) pathogen-associated molecular patterns (PAMPs) [18]. Bacterial lipopolysaccharide (LPS), a glycolipid component of the bacterial outer membrane, is the prototypical class of PAMPs. Lipopolysaccharides and bacterial-derived formylated peptides (fMLP) synergistically induce pro-inflammatory gene expression in circulating neutrophils and monocytes similar to DAMPS.

Polymorphonuclear (PMN) leukocytes are responsible for majority of indiscriminate tissue destruction as well as the production of inflammatory mediators [19, 20]. Circulating PMNs reside primarily in the pulmonary venules until acted upon by circulating inflammatory mediators at which time they demarginate and enter the blood stream. Upon arrival to injured tissue, PMNs adhere to activated endothelium, transmigrate to the interstitial space, and then degranulate releasing proteolytic enzymes and reactive oxygen species through the respiratory burst. Together, these agents are responsible for the bulk of inflammatory-mediated tissue damage which mostly occurs in the lung. Simultaneously, activated PMNs produce additional cytokines which in turn recruit more PMNs to the area.

Phenotypically, PMNs express cytotoxicity via two principal modes: a standard response triggered by a single stimulus and an enhanced response where a "priming" stimulus precedes an activating stimulus [21]. Primed PMNs express more adhesion molecules, release greater amounts of proteolytic enzymes, and have an enhanced respiratory burst to an activating stimulus than unprimed PMNs. Priming also is observed in endothelial cells via upregulating the expression of adhesion molecules.

The responses at the cellular level in individual tissues are triggered by system wide changes in physiology. Local inflammation begins in mechanically damaged tissue while shock redistributes blood flow to vital organs at the expense of other. Visceral blood flow is greatly reduced causing in visceral ischemia and breakdown of the gut mucosal barrier [22, 23]. This results in bacterial translocation into the gut interstitium, a consequent local inflammatory response to gut pathogens and production inflammatory mediators, primarily lipids, which are delivered to the pulmonary vasculature via mesenteric lymph and the thoracic duct as it empties into the subclavian vein [24]. Pulmonary endothelial cells and sequestered PMNs exposed to these inflammatory lipids become primed. Both increase the expression of adhesion molecules, and the PMNs demarginate and enter the circulation. This is observed clinically as an increase in the peripheral white blood cell count shortly after injury. If exposed to activating stimuli in the periphery, circulating PMNs firmly adhere to pulmonary endothelium, transmigrate to the pulmonary interstitium via diapedesis, and degranulate releasing their cytotoxic contents. This is observed clinically as a precipitous drop in the white blood cell count, a harbinger of impending MOF. At the same time, activated PMNs produce inflammatory cytokines that attract additional immuno-inflammatory cells creating a self-sustaining cycle of indiscriminate tissue destruction. Pro-inflammatory cytokines released into the circulation act on remote organs leading to brain dysfunction (delirium), acute renal failure, liver failure, and cardiac failure.

Systemic Inflammatory Modulation: SIRS, CARS, and PICS

The host post-injury immune environment is influenced by inflammatory and anti-inflammatory signaling that both begin immediately following injury [25] (Fig. 37.5). In this conceptual model early MOF can follow a massive traumatic insult that overwhelms the patient's ability to respond to resuscitation ("one" hit model). Alternatively, a sublethal traumatic event provokes a mild pro-inflammatory primed state (SIRS), presumed to be beneficial, which lasts up to 72 h and resolves as the patient recovers. A second sublethal event in this primed state can provoke enhanced destructive immune response ("two hit" model) precipitating MOF. Secondary insults that can precipitate

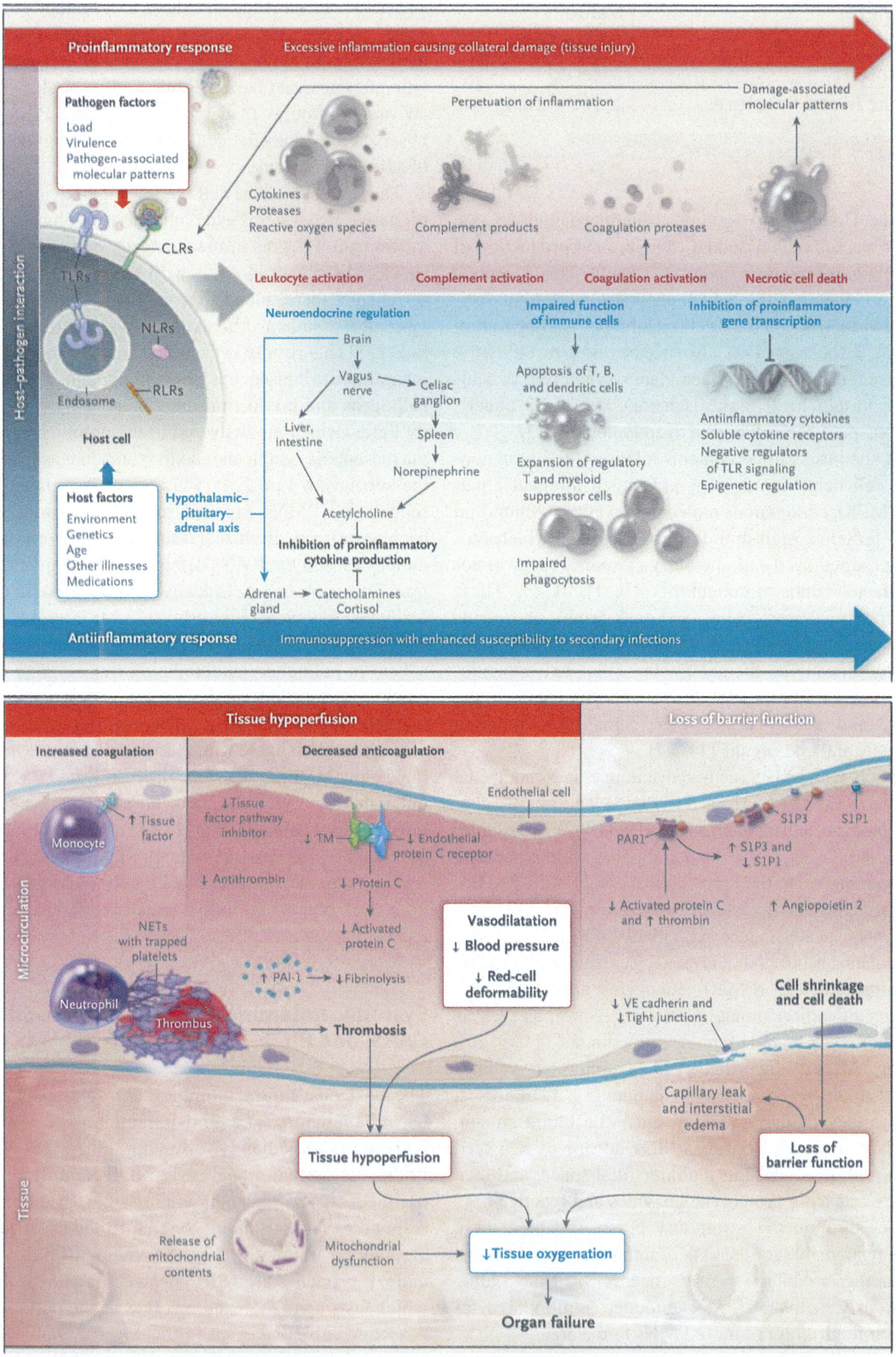

Fig. 37.3 Sepsis diagram

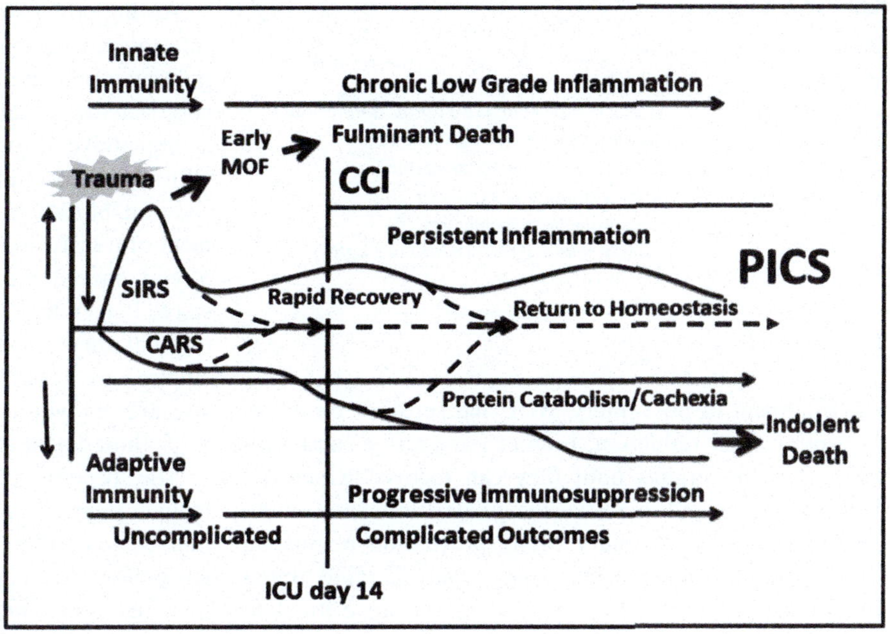

Fig. 37.4 MOF diagram

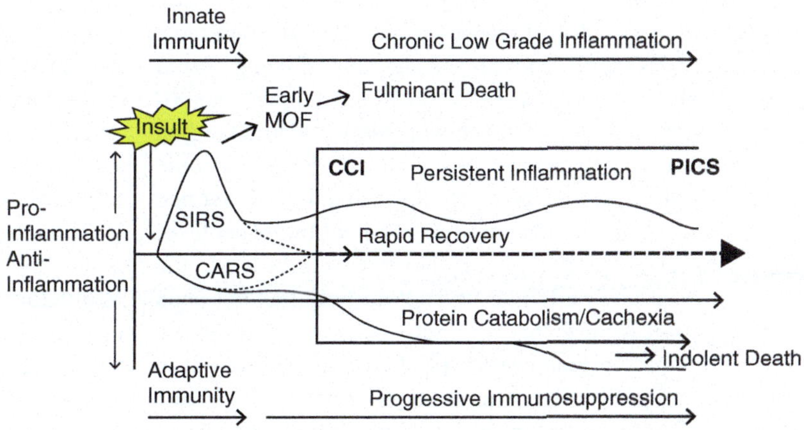

Fig. 37.5 Inflammatory regulation

dysfunctional hyper-inflammation include recurrent shock, ischemia/reperfusion, blood transfusions, ventilator-induced lung injury, long bone fixation, fat embolus, and infection.

In addition to SIRS and hyper-inflammation mediated by the innate immune system, the compensatory anti-inflammatory response syndrome (CARS) mediated by the adaptive immune system also begins immediately after injury. As with SIRS, mild CARS is thought to be beneficial and protect the host from excessive early hyper-inflammation. However, CARS persists after the early pro-inflammatory state subsides, and the patient enters a state of relative immunosuppression. This phase is characterized by poor wound healing and susceptibility to recurrent infections. If infected during this window, patients are at risk of developing systemic sepsis, late MOF, and death.

As more severely injured patients survive the initial hospitalization in the ICU, death from late MOF is decreasing, and delayed effects of dysfunctional immunomodulation after trauma have been observed. While some patients recover quickly and return to normal immunologic homeostasis, most demonstrate abnormal regulation of both the innate and adaptive immune systems for weeks following ICU discharge. Many enter into a state of chronic critical illness (CCI) with prolonged ICU lengths of stay and mild organ dysfunction. These patients are too ill to progress to the rehabilitation phase of recovery and are referred to subacute and long-term care facilities where they often suffer late deaths [26]. This persistent inflammation-immunosuppression catabolism syndrome (PICS) is characterized by ongoing protein catabolism, poor nutritional status, poor wound healing, immunosuppression, and recurrent infections. Criteria for PICS are listed in Table 37.2.

Table 37.2 Criteria for PICS

Parameter	Value
ICU stay	≥14 days
Persistent inflammation	C-reactive protein >150 μg/dL *and* retinol binding protein <10 μg/dL
Immunosuppression	Total lymphocyte count <800/mm^3
Catabolic state	Serum albumin < 3.0 mg/dL Creatinine height index <80% Weight loss > 10% of BMI < 18 kg/m^2

Treatment

The treatment of post-injury MOF and sepsis is based on prevention, risk reduction, prompt recognition, and support of failing organs until they can recover. Since the degree of injury and shock has the greatest influence on the development of post-injury MOF, prevention begins on initial patient contact. Hemorrhage control, rapid transport, and initiation of volume restoration are critical to minimize the time in shock. In septic patients, prompt recognition, initiation of antibiotics, source control, and volume resuscitation play analogous roles. For bleeding patients, damage control resuscitation employing massive transfusion protocols that replace shed blood using stored components that approximate whole blood achieves hemostasis faster and consumes fewer blood products than resuscitation in the absence of such protocols. Isotonic balanced salt solutions, typically normal saline or lactated Ringer's solution, are also used to augment blood replacement and restore volume in septic patients, and while the superiority of any particular crystalloid fluid has not been established, it is clear that care must be taken to avoid too much fluid and volume overload [27, 28]. Once thought to augment oxygen delivery to tissues, crystalloid volume loading to supra-normal levels was later found to be associated with higher incidences of abdominal compartment syndrome, ARDS, and MOF.

Concurrent with restoration of intravascular volume in the trauma patient is the operative care of major injuries. Initial efforts are targeted at achieving hemorrhage control, controlling enteric spillage, reestablishing organ and limb perfusion, reconstruction of the GI tract, stabilization or fixation of long bone fractures, and wound closure. Ideally, all patients should undergo definitive operative care as expeditiously as practical. However, extreme physiologic derangements can prohibit the safe completion of all repairs. Under such conditions, a damage control strategy is recommended where only essential maneuvers to stop surgical bleeding, control spillage, temporarily stabilize fractures and cover wounds are done [29]. A period of resuscitation aimed at correcting acidosis, hypothermia, and coagulopathy is taken in the ICU before returning to the operating room for definitive reconstruction and wound closure.

An important strategy to prevent MOF is to limit exposure to secondary activating events in a primed host. Since priming can be established within 3 h of injury, a thoughtful approach toward interventions during the resuscitative phase is imperative. Blood transfusions independently correlate with major infections, multi-organ failure, and mortality. In addition, blood transfusions are associated with the development of transfusion-related acute lung injury (TRALI) [30]. Stored packed red blood cells (PRBC), especially those stored longer than 2 weeks, contain pro inflammatory mediators that can prime or activate circulating PMNs for enhanced cytotoxicity. Once hemorrhage control is achieved, permissive anemia with a lower transfusion threshold of 7 mg/dL helps limit potentially unnecessary transfusions.

The benefits of early definitive facture stabilization include improvements in pulmonary toilet, early mobilization, decreased thromboembolic events, and decreased mortality. However, major operations in primed patients have the potential to precipitate MOF. Early temporary external fixation of major long bone fractures with delayed definitive care timed to a more favorable inflammatory state may be indicated in patients at high risk for post-injury MOF [31].

Often described as "the motor that drives MOF," [32, 33] the lung plays a central role in progression of SIRS to overt organ failure. Lung-protective ventilation with lower tidal volumes (6 cc/kg ideal body weight) reduces the risk of progression from acute lung injury to ARDS. The purpose is to minimize ventilator-induced lung injury and the resultant systemic release of inflammatory mediators. Also important is the prevention of ventilator-associated pneumonia (VAP). Ventilator bundles consisting of selective oral or gut decontamination, elevating the head of bed, and judicious pulmonary toilet decrease the incidence of VAP.

Infection prevention is paramount in the immunosuppressed phase of CARS. Eliminating known infection risk factors (central venous catheters, Foley catheters) as early as possible helps to minimize the stress on the weakened immune capacity. History and physical examination of the postoperative surgical patient should direct the radiographic and laboratory work-up. Close attention should be paid to the pulmonary exam, prosthetic catheters, all surgical wounds, and the extremities. The clinical diagnosis of pneumonia in critically ill patients is often inaccurate [14]. A quantitative culture should be obtained, and empiric antibiotics based on the ICU antibiogram should be started while awaiting culture results depending on the overall clinical suspicion. Urinalysis should be obtained prior to a urine culture. When negative it is a strong predictor of a negative urine culture, excluding a urinary tract infection.

Once MOF is established, treatment consists of continuing to minimize additional insults and support failing organs. Acute brain dysfunction is common in patients in the intensive care unit. Patients are evaluated clinically by various scoring systems such as the Richmond Agitation Sedation Scale (RASS), the Glasgow Coma Scale (GCS), and Confusion Assessment Method for the ICU (CAM-ICU). Delirium in patients on the mechanical ventilator is associated with higher mortality at 6 months. Targeted pain and sedation plans, daily awakening and breathing trials, early mobilization, and non-pharmacologic sleep protocols decrease the risk of delirium. Antipsychotics (haloperidol/olanzapine) are effective in the acutely agitated patient.

Support of the cardiovascular system must balance the need for adequate perfusion pressure with the increase in peripheral vascular resistance that comes with most vasopressors. The goal is to deliver enough oxygen to the tissues to meet metabolic demands, which depends on the blood's oxygen content and cardiac output. A strategy of ensuring sufficient hemoglobin levels and optimal hemoglobin oxygen saturation followed by optimizing cardiac preload, afterload, and contractility optimizes oxygen delivery. Interventions to augment each factor come with potentially harmful effects. Equivocation of blood pressure with blood flow is a common pitfall that must be recognized. Specifically, augmenting blood pressure with peripheral vasoconstrictors increases cardiac workload and, since their locus of action is the precapillary arterioles, can decrease perfusion of capillary beds. At particular risk is mesenteric blood flow where excessive use of peripheral vasoconstrictors can cause visceral ischemia and threaten bowel anastomoses. Moreover, since dysoxia associated with sepsis and septic shock is more a function of oxygen utilization than oxygen delivery, the use of peripheral vasoconstrictors to drive blood pressure is of unclear value.

Renal replacement therapy is often indicated in critically ill patients with acute renal failure to correct volume overload, metabolic acidosis, uremic encephalopathy, and electrolyte abnormalities. Continuous hemofiltration (CAVH, CVVH) uses convection for solute transport, which decreases the risk of hypotension compared to intermittent hemodialysis. Hyperglycemia is common in critically ill patients due to insulin resistance.

Patients in the ICU should have a nutritional assessment within 24 h of their admission. Early enteral nutrition support should be started as soon as fluid resuscitation is complete and the patient is hemodynamically stable, ideally within the first 24–72 h. Enteral nutrition support decreases gut permeability and diminishes release of inflammatory cytokines. Multiple studies have shown a reduction in infections and decreased length of stay.

Hyperglycemia is common in critically ill patients due to insulin resistance. The NICE-SUGAR investigators showed that intensive glucose control (81– 108 mg/dL) increased mortality in adults in the ICU and saw a reduction in mortality with a target blood glucose of <180 mg/dL.

Targeted pharmacological interventions to modulate inflammatory signaling pathways have not been effective. The onset of post-injury inflammation and activation of the innate immune system occur immediately upon injury or sepsis usually before symptoms manifest thus denying an opportunity to interrupt signaling. Additionally, the redundancy signaling pathways limit the effectiveness of inhibiting any one pathway.

Conclusion

Although the development of SIRS following injury and sepsis remains relatively common, progression to MODS, MOF, and death has diminished as our understanding of the pathophysiology and our treatment strategies improved. The most effective approach has been to minimize the risks of further immune-mediated injury through careful application of validated resuscitation and intensive care principals. Our understanding of this disease and its treatments is a culmination of continuous integrated clinical, translational, and basic science research [34]. At each stage, recognition of underlying pathophysiology prompted scientific study, targeted treatment, and improved outcome only to witness the emergence of new syndromes in some patients that would have otherwise died. Also at each stage, the time frame of clinical focus has expanded from the survival immediately following injury to chronic conditions and deaths occurring months or years later. The resultant advances in clinical care and improvements in outcome are extraordinary achievements comparable to any in human disease.

References

1. Sauaia A, Moore EE, Johnson JL, Ciesla DJ, Biffl WL, Banerjee A. Validation of postinjury multiple organ failure scores. Shock. 2009;31(5):438–47.
2. Raith EP, Udy AA, Bailey M, McGloughlin S, MacIsaac C, Bellomo R, Pilcher DV, Australian, New Zealand Intensive Care Society Centre for, O, Resource, E. Prognostic accuracy of the SOFA score, SIRS criteria, and qSOFA score for in-hospital mortality among adults with suspected infection admitted to the intensive care unit. JAMA. 2017;317(3):290–300.
3. Williams JM, Greenslade JH, McKenzie JV, Chu K, Brown AF, Lipman J. Systemic inflammatory response syndrome, quick sequential organ function assessment, and organ dysfunction: insights from a prospective database of ED patients with infection. Chest. 2017;151(3):586–96.
4. Singer M, Deutschman CS, Seymour CW, Shankar-Hari M, Annane D, Bauer M, Bellomo R, Bernard GR, Chiche JD, Coopersmith CM, Hotchkiss RS, Levy MM, Marshall JC, Martin GS, Opal SM, Rubenfeld GD, van der Poll T, Vincent JL, Angus DC. The third international consensus definitions for sepsis and septic shock (Sepsis-3). JAMA. 2016;315(8):801–10.
5. Eiseman B, Beart R, Norton L. Multiple organ failure. Surg Gynecol Obstet. 1977;144(3):323–6.
6. Eiseman B, Sloan R, Hansbrough J, McIntosh R. Multiple organ failure: clinical and experimental. Am Surg. 1980;46(1):14–9.
7. Faist E, Baue AE, Dittmer H, Heberer G. Multiple organ failure in polytrauma patients. J Trauma. 1983;23(9):775–87.

8. Moore FA, Moore EE. Evolving concepts in the pathogenesis of postinjury multiple organ failure. Surg Clin North Am. 1995;75(2):257–77.
9. Ciesla DJ, Moore EE, Johnson JL, Burch JM, Cothren CC, Sauaia A. A 12-year prospective study of postinjury multiple organ failure: has anything changed? Arch Surg. 2005;140(5):432–8; discussion 438-440.
10. Sauaia A, Moore EE, Johnson JL, Chin TL, Banerjee A, Sperry JL, Maier RV, Burlew CC. Temporal trends of postinjury multiple-organ failure: still resource intensive, morbid, and lethal. J Trauma Acute Care Surg. 2014;76(3):582–92, discussion 592-583.
11. Nast-Kolb D, Aufmkolk M, Rucholtz S, Obertacke U, Waydhas C. Multiple organ failure still a major cause of morbidity but not mortality in blunt multiple trauma. J Trauma. 2001;51(5):835–41; discussion 841-832.
12. Moore EE, Moore FA, Harken AH, Johnson JL, Ciesla D, Banerjee A. The two-event construct of postinjury multiple organ failure. Shock. 2005;24(Suppl 1):71–4.
13. Meneshian A, Bulkley GB. The physiology of endothelial xanthine oxidase: from urate catabolism to reperfusion injury to inflammatory signal transduction. Microcirculation. 2002;9(3):161–75.
14. Raoof M, Zhang Q, Itagaki K, Hauser CJ. Mitochondrial peptides are potent immune activators that activate human neutrophils via FPR-1. J Trauma. 2010;68(6):1328–32; discussion 1332-1324.
15. Hauser CJ, Sursal T, Rodriguez EK, Appleton PT, Zhang Q, Itagaki K. Mitochondrial damage associated molecular patterns from femoral reamings activate neutrophils through formyl peptide receptors and P44/42 MAP kinase. J Orthop Trauma. 2010;24(9):534–8.
16. Krysko DV, Agostinis P, Krysko O, Garg AD, Bachert C, Lambrecht BN, Vandenabeele P. Emerging role of damage-associated molecular patterns derived from mitochondria in inflammation. Trends Immunol. 2011;32(4):157–64.
17. Kuipers MT, van der Poll T, Schultz MJ, Wieland CW. Bench-to-bedside review: damage-associated molecular patterns in the onset of ventilator-induced lung injury. Crit Care. 2011;15(6):235.
18. Raymond SL, Holden DC, Mira JC, Stortz JA, Loftus TJ, Mohr AM, Moldawer LL, Moore FA, Larson SD, Efron PA. Microbial recognition and danger signals in sepsis and trauma. Biochim Biophys Acta. 2017;1863(10 Pt B):2564–73.
19. Windsor AC, Mullen PG, Fowler AA, Sugerman HJ. Role of the neutrophil in adult respiratory distress syndrome. Br J Surg. 1993;80(1):10–7.
20. Borregaard N, Cowland JB. Granules of the human neutrophilic polymorphonuclear leukocyte. Blood. 1997;89(10):3503–21.
21. Botha AJ, Moore FA, Moore EE, Kim FJ, Banerjee A, Peterson VM. Postinjury neutrophil priming and activation: an early vulnerable window. Surgery. 1995;118(2):358–64; discussion 364-355.
22. Moore EE, Moore FA, Franciose RJ, Kim FJ, Biffl WL, Banerjee A. The postischemic gut serves as a priming bed for circulating neutrophils that provoke multiple organ failure. J Trauma. 1994;37(6):881–7.
23. Hassoun HT, Kone BC, Mercer DW, Moody FG, Weisbrodt NW, Moore FA. Post-injury multiple organ failure: the role of the gut. Shock. 2001;15(1):1–10.
24. Moore EE. Mesenteric lymph: the critical bridge between dysfunctional gut and multiple organ failure. Shock. 1998;10(6):415–6.
25. Sauaia A, Moore FA, Moore EE. Postinjury inflammation and organ dysfunction. Crit Care Clin. 2017;33(1):167–91.
26. Mira JC, Brakenridge SC, Moldawer LL, Moore FA. Persistent inflammation, immunosuppression and catabolism syndrome. Crit Care Clin. 2017;33(2):245–58.
27. Balogh Z, McKinley BA, Cocanour CS, Kozar RA, Valdivia A, Sailors RM, Moore FA. Supranormal trauma resuscitation causes more cases of abdominal compartment syndrome. Arch Surg. 2003;138(6):637–42; discussion 642-633.
28. Joseph B, Zangbar B, Pandit V, Vercruysse G, Aziz H, Kulvatunyou N, Wynne J, O'Keeffe T, Tang A, Friese RS, Rhee P. The conjoint effect of reduced crystalloid administration and decreased damage-control laparotomy use in the development of abdominal compartment syndrome. J Trauma Acute Care Surg. 2014;76(2):457–61.
29. Joseph B, Azim A, Zangbar B, Bauman Z, O'Keeffe T, Ibraheem K, Kulvatunyou N, Tang A, Latifi R, Rhee P. Improving mortality in trauma laparotomy through the evolution of damage control resuscitation: analysis of 1,030 consecutive trauma laparotomies. J Trauma Acute Care Surg. 2017;82(2):328–33.
30. Silliman CC. The two-event model of transfusion-related acute lung injury. Crit Care Med. 2006;34(5 Suppl):S124–31.
31. Taeger G, Ruchholtz S, Waydhas C, Lewan U, Schmidt B, Nast-Kolb D. Damage control orthopedics in patients with multiple injuries is effective, time saving, and safe. J Trauma. 2005;59(2):409–16; discussion 417.
32. Ciesla DJ, Moore EE, Johnson JL, Burch JM, Cothren CC, Sauaia A. The role of the lung in postinjury multiple organ failure. Surgery. 2005;138(4):749–57; discussion 757-748.
33. dos Santos CC, Slutsky AS. The contribution of biophysical lung injury to the development of biotrauma. Annu Rev Physiol. 2006;68:585–618.
34. Nathens AB, Johnson JL, Minei JP, Moore EE, Shapiro M, Bankey P, Freeman B, Harbrecht BG, Lowry SF, McKinley B, Moore F, West M, Maier RV. Inflammation and the host response to injury, a large-scale collaborative project: patient-oriented research Core – standard operating procedures for clinical care. I. Guidelines for mechanical ventilation of the trauma patient. J Trauma. 2005;59(3):764–9.

CLABSI

38

Tarek Madni and Alexander L. Eastman

Introduction

According to the Centers for Disease Control and Prevention (CDC), central line-associated bloodstream infections (CLABSIs) result in thousands of deaths and add billions of dollars of burden to the United States (US) healthcare system each year [1]. CLABSIs have an estimated mortality rate of 12–25% and are thought to be one of the deadliest types of healthcare-associated infections (HAIs) [2]. Following catheter-associated urinary tract infections, CLABSIs are estimated to be the second most preventable HAI [3] and have been estimated to be as high as the eighth leading cause of death in the United States [4]. In recent years, the Centers for Medicare and Medicaid Services developed a policy to both deny hospital payments for treatment of hospital acquired preventable events and potentially impose financially penalties [5]. Through a number of preventative measures, the rate of CLABSI has significantly declined over the past decade, with roughly 18,000 reported occurrences among patients hospitalized in intensive care units (ICUs) in the United States in 2009 [2].

According to the CDC, CLABSI is defined as a pathogen from a blood culture (a single blood culture for organisms not commonly present on the skin and two or more blood cultures for organisms commonly present on the skin) in a patient who had a central line at the time of infection or within 48 h before development of the infection [2, 4]. In addition, the infection cannot be related to any other infection the patient might have and may not have been present or incubating when the patient was admitted to the hospital [2].

T. Madni · A. L. Eastman (✉)
Department of Surgery, Division of Burns, Trauma, and Critical Care, University of Texas Southwestern, Dallas, TX, USA
e-mail: alexander.eastman@utsouthwestern.edu

Prevention

A number of preventative measures have been recommended by both the CDC and the Joint Commission to significantly reduce preventable CLABSI in the ICU setting [1, 6]. Specifically, the 2011 CDC guidelines for the prevention of CLABSI include [1, 7]:

- Removal of unwarranted central lines through daily audit
- Proper insertion practices
  - Hand hygiene prior to insertion.
    - Conventional soap and water or alcohol-based rubs
  - Maximum sterile barrier precaution.
    - Mask, cap, gown, sterile gloves, sterile body drape
  - Prepare skin via aseptic technique.
    - Preferably >0.5% chlorhexidine with alcohol solution
  - Choose best site to minimize infection.
    - Current recommendations include avoidance of femoral site in adult patients.
    - Preference for subclavian site if mechanical complications can be avoided [8].
  - Cover site with sterile gauze or sterile, transparent, semipermeable dressing.
- Appropriate maintenance practices
  - Hand hygiene prior to access/use.
  - Access port or hub must be scrubbed with antiseptic immediately prior to each use.
  - Access catheters only with sterile devices.
  - Replace wet/soiled/dislodged dressings.
  - Perform dressing changes under aseptic technique using sterile gloves.

The aforementioned practices have been demonstrated in the literature to significantly decrease a facility's overall CLABSI rate. Specifically, the practice of a central line insertion bundle (i.e., maximum barrier precautions, hand washing, skin preparation, use of a central line cart, and avoidance of femoral lines) has demonstrated to significantly decrease

A. Salim et al. (eds.), *Surgical Critical Care Therapy*, https://doi.org/10.1007/978-3-319-71712-8_38

CLABSI after bundle initiation [9, 10]. In addition, adherence to maintenance practices such as daily line audits, replacing wet/soiled dressings, and hand hygiene prior to handling has been shown to even further decrease the risk of CLABSI in healthcare facilities [11]. Further topics of insertion and maintenance practices not mentioned in the checklist have been explored by multiple Cochrane and systemic reviews:

- Skin cleansing with chlorhexidine solution may reduce CLABSI rates greater than povidone iodine [12].
- No clear evidence demonstrating longer intervals between central line dressing changes are associated with more CLABSI [13].
- While impregnation of catheters with antimicrobials demonstrated a significant decrease in CLABSI in the ICU, there was no change in all-cause mortality or clinically diagnosed sepsis [14].
- Medication impregnated dressing, such as Biopatch use, reduces the incidence of CLABSI [15].
- Daily bathing with 2% chlorhexidine solution significantly decreased rates of CLABSIs in adult ICUs (RR = 0.46) [16, 17].

Pathology

A review of the recent literature has verified a number of organisms responsible for CLABSI. A review of HAIs reported to the National Healthcare Safety Network (NHSN) between 2006 and 2007 noted the following selected pathogen percentages [18]:

- Coagulase-negative staphylococci (34%)
- *Staphylococcus aureus* (10%)
- *Enterococcus species* (16%)
- *Candida species* (12%)
- Gram-negative rods (18%)
  - *Escherichia coli* (3%)
  - *Pseudomonas aeruginosa* (3%)
  - *Klebsiella pneumoniae* (5%)
  - *Enterobacter species* (4%)
  - *Acinetobacter baumannii* (2%)
  - *Klebsiella oxytoca* (1%)
- Other (10%)

This same review by Hidron et al. (2008) explored several antimicrobial resistance percentages within each of the aforementioned subgroups [18]. Specific highlights include:

- Methicillin-resistant *Staphylococcus aureus* (MRSA): 56.8%
- Vancomycin-resistant *Enterococcus*: 36.4%

Another review of over 1700 ICUs reporting to the National Healthcare Safety network in 2011 demonstrated the following resistance updates [19]:

- 48.9% of *S. aureus* CLABSI were due to MRSA.
- 27.7% of *Klebsiella* CLABSI demonstrated non-susceptibility to extended spectrum cephalosporins.
- 10.6% of *Klebsiella* CLABSI demonstrated non-susceptibility to carbapenems.

The results of these studies are based on the contribution of a large number of facilities; however, specific facility resistance may vary due to a number of variables such as location, patient demographics, ICU versus non-ICU, medical versus surgical, oncology related, etc. [20, 21] In addition, while the overall incidence of CLABSI appears to be declining annually over the last decade [22], increases in antimicrobial resistances, such as MRSA, may continue to increase [23]. These results further suggest the need for facility-specific data when considering the appropriate treatment for a verified CLABSI.

Diagnosis

Two important distinctions should be made, specifically between CLABSI and a catheter-related bloodstream infection (CRBSI). According to the CDC, CLABSI is defined as a pathogen from a blood culture (a single blood culture for organisms not commonly present on the skin and two or more blood cultures for organisms commonly present on the skin) in a patient who had a central line at the time of infection or within 48 h before development of the infection. In addition, the infection cannot be related to any other infection the patient might have and may not have been present or incubating when the patient was admitted to the hospital [2]. The CDC recognizes this definition may overestimate the true incidence of CLABSI, as some bloodstream infections may be secondary to sources other than the central line but are not easily diagnosed or known [1]. Thus, the clinical diagnosis of CRBSI requires the clinical manifestation of an infection, such as a fever, in addition to:

- Two blood cultures drawn through the central venous catheter and a peripheral vein positive for the same microorgansims [24, 25].
- Positive culture from removed catheter of the same microorganism isolated from the blood [24].

It is imperative to draw a venipuncture blood sample in addition to a catheter-drawn blood culture to avoid diagnosing an infection based on a contaminant. Previous research has demonstrated almost a double the chance of contamination from a catheter-drawn culture versus a direct venipuncture [26].

In 2009, the Infectious Diseases Society of America (IDSA) published updated clinical practice guidelines for the diagnosis of CRBSI [25]. While fairly extensive, key points for diagnosis include:

- Catheter cultures should be performed when a catheter is removed for suspected CRBSI.
- Obtain blood cultures prior to antibiotic initiation.

Treatment

While removing a central venous catheter can aid in establishing the diagnosis of a CRBSI, the risks of additional iatrogenic injury or healthcare costs cannot be negated [27]. The IDSA has recommended immediate removal based on the following circumstances [25]:

- Severe sepsis
- Hemodynamic instability
- Endocarditis
- Suppurative thrombophlebitis
- If susceptible organisms are present, but persistent bacteremia after 72 h of antimicrobial therapy

Attempts at catheter salvage may be considered if a long-term catheter is present and the isolated pathogens are not: *Staphylococcus aureus*, *Pseudomonas aeruginosa*, fungi, or mycobacteria [25].

Basic antimicrobial guidelines published by the IDSA in 2009 include but are not limited to [25]:

- Day 1 of antimicrobial therapy is the first day negative cultures are obtained.
- Empirical therapy in the healthcare setting with an elevated prevalence of MRSA should be vancomycin.
- Empirical coverage for gram-negative bacteria should be based on local susceptibility data.
- Empirical coverage for *Candida* should begin with either echinocandin or fluconazole.
- Empirical coverage for suspected CRBSI involving femoral catheters should include coverage for gram-negative pathogen and *Candida* in addition to gram-positive pathogens.
- Consider *Candida* coverage in septic patients with TPN use, prolonged antibiotic use, femoral catheters, hematologic malignancy, or other colonization with *Candida* and who are prior transplant recipients.

Treatment length will vary depending on the clinical situation and pathogens isolated from the cultures.

References

1. Center for Disease Control and Prevention. Central Line-associated Bloodstream Infection (CLABSI) 2016 updated 3/1/2016. Available from: https://www.cdc.gov/hai/bsi/bsi.html.
2. Center for Disease Control and Prevention. Vital signs: central line-associated blood stream infections--United States, 2001, 2008, and 2009. MMWR Morb Mortal Wkly Rep. 2011;60(8):243–8.
3. Umscheid CA, Mitchell MD, Doshi JA, Agarwal R, Williams K, Brennan PJ. Estimating the proportion of healthcare-associated infections that are reasonably preventable and the related mortality and costs. Infect Control Hosp Epidemiol. 2011;32(2):101–14.
4. Miller SE, Maragakis LL. Central line-associated bloodstream infection prevention. Curr Opin Infect Dis. 2012;25(4):412–22.
5. Clancy CM. CMS's hospital-acquired condition lists link hospital payment, patient safety. Am J Med Qual. 2009;24(2):166–8.
6. The Joint Commission. CLABSI Toolkit – Preventing Central-Line Associated Bloodstream Infections: Useful Tools, An International Perspective 2017 updated 2017. Available from: https://www.jointcommission.org/topics/clabsi_toolkit.aspx.
7. O'Grady NP, Alexander M, Burns LA, Dellinger EP, Garland J, Heard SO, Lipsett PA, Masur H, Mermel LA, Pearson ML, et al. Guidelines for the prevention of intravascular catheter-related infections. Am J Infect Control. 2011;39(4 Suppl 1):S1–34.
8. Ramritu P, Halton K, Cook D, Whitby M, Graves N. Catheter-related bloodstream infections in intensive care units: a systematic review with meta-analysis. J Adv Nurs. 2008;62(1):3–21.
9. Galpern D, Guerrero A, Tu A, Fahoum B, Wise L. Effectiveness of a central line bundle campaign on line-associated infections in the intensive care unit. Surgery. 2008;144(4):492–5; discussion 5.
10. Pronovost P, Needham D, Berenholtz S, Sinopoli D, Chu H, Cosgrove S, Sexton B, Hyzy R, Welsh R, Roth G, et al. An intervention to decrease catheter-related bloodstream infections in the ICU. N Engl J Med. 2006;355(26):2725–32.
11. Guerin K, Wagner J, Rains K, Bessesen M. Reduction in central line-associated bloodstream infections by implementation of a postinsertion care bundle. Am J Infect Control. 2010;38(6):430–3.
12. Lai NM, Lai NA, O'Riordan E, Chaiyakunapruk N, Taylor JE, Tan K. Skin antisepsis for reducing central venous catheter-related infections. Cochrane Database Syst Rev. 2016;(7):Cd010140.
13. Gavin NC, Webster J, Chan RJ, Rickard CM. Frequency of dressing changes for central venous access devices on catheter-related infections. Cochrane Database Syst Rev. 2016;(2):Cd009213.
14. Lai NM, Chaiyakunapruk N, Lai NA, O'Riordan E, Pau WS, Saint S. Catheter impregnation, coating or bonding for reducing central venous catheter-related infections in adults. Cochrane Database Syst Rev. 2016;(3):Cd007878.
15. Ullman AJ, Cooke ML, Mitchell M, Lin F, New K, Long DA, Mihala G, Rickard CM. Dressings and securement devices for central venous catheters (CVC). Cochrane Database Syst Rev. 2015;(9):Cd010367.
16. Shah HN, Schwartz JL, Luna G, Cullen DL. Bathing with 2% chlorhexidine gluconate: evidence and costs associated with central line-associated bloodstream infections. Crit Care Nurs Q. 2016;39(1):42–50.
17. O'Horo JC, Silva GL, Munoz-Price LS, Safdar N. The efficacy of daily bathing with chlorhexidine for reducing healthcare-associated bloodstream infections: a meta-analysis. Infect Control Hosp Epidemiol. 2012;33(3):257–67.

18. Hidron AI, Edwards JR, Patel J, Horan TC, Sievert DM, Pollock DA, Fridkin SK. NHSN annual update: antimicrobial-resistant pathogens associated with healthcare-associated infections: annual summary of data reported to the National Healthcare Safety Network at the Centers for Disease Control and Prevention, 2006-2007. Infect Control Hosp Epidemiol. 2008;29(11):996–1011.
19. Soe MM, Edwards JR, Sievert DM, Ricks PM, Magill SS, Fridkin SK. Evaluating state-specific antibiotic resistance measures derived from central line-associated bloodstream infections, national healthcare safety network, 2011. Infect Control Hosp Epidemiol. 2015;36(1):54–64.
20. Duane TM, Kikhia RM, Wolfe LG, Ober J, Tessier JM. Understanding gram-negative central line-associated blood stream infection in a surgical trauma ICU. Am Surg. 2015;81(8):816–9.
21. See I, Freifeld AG, Magill SS. Causative organisms and associated antimicrobial resistance in healthcare-associated, central line-associated bloodstream infections from oncology settings, 2009–2012. Clin Infect Dis. 2016;62(10):1203–9.
22. Fagan RP, Edwards JR, Park BJ, Fridkin SK, Magill SS. Incidence trends in pathogen-specific central line-associated bloodstream infections in US intensive care units, 1990–2010. Infect Control Hosp Epidemiol. 2013;34(9):893–9.
23. Burton DC, Edwards JR, Horan TC, Jernigan JA, Fridkin SK. Methicillin-resistant Staphylococcus aureus central line-associated bloodstream infections in US intensive care units, 1997–2007. JAMA. 2009;301(7):727–36.
24. Chatzinikolaou I, Hanna H, Hachem R, Alakech B, Tarrand J, Raad I. Differential quantitative blood cultures for the diagnosis of catheter-related bloodstream infections associated with short- and long-term catheters: a prospective study. Diagn Microbiol Infect Dis. 2004;50(3):167–72.
25. Mermel LA, Allon M, Bouza E, Craven DE, Flynn P, O'Grady NP, Raad II, Rijnders BJ, Sherertz RJ, Warren DK. Clinical practice guidelines for the diagnosis and management of intravascular catheter-related infection: 2009 update by the Infectious Diseases Society of America. Clin Infect Dis. 2009;49(1):1–45.
26. Everts RJ, Vinson EN, Adholla PO, Reller LB. Contamination of catheter-drawn blood cultures. J Clin Microbiol. 2001;39(9):3393–4.
27. Rijnders BJ, Peetermans WE, Verwaest C, Wilmer A, Van Wijngaerden E. Watchful waiting versus immediate catheter removal in ICU patients with suspected catheter-related infection: a randomized trial. Intensive Care Med. 2004;30(6):1073–80.

Catheter-Associated Urinary Tract Infections

39

Stephanie Nitzschke

Introduction

Urinary tract infections are the most common health-care-acquired infections and a significant source of patient morbidity, increased length of stay, as well as increased hospital costs. The placement or prolonged use of an indwelling urinary catheter is the most common risk factor. The overall rate of infection in the intensive care unit are 1–4 per 1000 catheter days and are, infrequently, a source of bloodstream infection as well at approximately 1.4 bloodstream infections per 10,000 patient days.

Complications

CAUTIs (Catheter Associated Urinary Tract Infections) are associated with an incidence of bacteremia but are less likely (around 3%) to be the primary cause of bacteremia in critically ill ICU patients. Clinically significant complications can occur to patients secondary to trauma that occurs during foley catheter placement with some literature showing complication rates as high as one third of patients who undergo catheterization. This may lead to other necessary interventions, such as cystoscopy, if there is an injury to the urinary tract or any clinically significant bleeding [1]. It is imperative for a hospital system to try to avoid these more severe complications, as well as CAUTIs, as they increase hospital costs, and hospital length of stay, and most importantly, increase patient discomfort.

S. Nitzschke (✉)
Department of Trauma, Burn, Surgical Critical Care & Emergency General Surgery, Brigham and Women's Hospital, Boston, MA, USA
e-mail: snitzschke@partners.org

Risk Factors

The main risk factor for development of a CAUTI is the duration of catheterization, as the incidence of bacteriuria increases the longer a catheter is in place and is present in 25% of patients who have their catheter in place for greater than 2 days. This is very telling as similar data shows that for patients who have a catheter in place for more than 24 hours: 25% will develop a CAUTI and 3.4% of patients will then go on to develop bacteremia (which is a rare complication of CAUTIs) [2]. There are other risk factors for CAUTIs such as female gender, chronic health conditions such as diabetes mellitus, patients that require chronic indwelling catheters, and at risk populations such as elderly patients or patients who are immunocompromised. Certainly, another important risk factor would be improper placement with a breach in sterile technique during placement or manipulation from the patient or caregiver as well as any defect in the catheter system.

The majority of infections are acquired from bacteria that are present at the urethra and then are able to ascend along the catheter into the bladder. The catheter allows the bacteria a direct pathway to access the bladder and occurs more frequently in women (due to a short urethra). The bacteria cultured in CAUTIs are most commonly the same bacteria found on the patient's own skin or in their stool. The catheter can cause mucosal injury that facilitates bacterial translocation as it is a foreign body that can become contaminated/colonized with bacteria that now have access into a sterile space. Patients can still have a CAUTI after catheter removal as bacteria can still be present on the patient's meatus.

Diagnosis

The diagnosis of a catheter-associated urinary tract infection (CAUTI) can be challenging as there may not be any clinical symptoms especially in the critically ill patient. Frequently it

A. Salim et al. (eds.), *Surgical Critical Care Therapy*, https://doi.org/10.1007/978-3-319-71712-8_39

Table 39.1 Definitions of CAUTI and CA-ASB

CA-ASB	1. Presence of indwelling catheter or recent removal within 48 h 2. Presence of $\geq 10^5$ of at least one bacterial species 3. **No** symptoms compatible with UTI
CAUTI	1. Presence of an indwelling catheter or removed within 48 h 2. Signs and symptoms of a UTI 3. $\geq 10^3$ colony-forming units (CFU)/ml of bacteria

Table 39.2 Recommendations for empiric antibiotic choices for catheter-associated urinary tract infections (CAUTI)

Microbe	Antibiotic	Alternative antibiotic	Duration
Gram-negative bacteria	Ceftriaxone 1 g IV daily or cefotaxime 1 g IV Q 8 h	Cefepime 1 g IV Q 12 h or ceftazidime 1 g IV Q 8 h. Decision for MRSA or VRE should be driven by prior culture data	10–14 days
Candida	Fluconazole 200–400 mg daily		14 days

Specific therapy should be based on an individual hospital's antibiogram for empiric therapy

is diagnosed in the setting of a fever and a positive urine culture. However, patients may have other symptoms of pelvic pain, mental status changes, costovertebral tenderness, or hematuria. Pyuria alone is not enough for the diagnosis, and for those patients with an indwelling catheter, the diagnosis is made when the clean catch urine sample grows $>10^5$ colony-forming units (CFU) of a single species (Table 39.1). For patients who have had their catheter removed in the past 48 h and the clean catch specimen grows $>10^3$ CFU of a single species, this would also meet criteria for the diagnosis of a CAUTI if the patient is clinically symptomatic (such as a complaint of dysuria). Table 39.1 compares CAUTI and Catheter associated asymptomatic bacteria (CA-ASB). The most important difference between the CAUTI and the CA-ASB is that the patient with CA-ASB has no clinical symptoms of a urinary tract infection as previously described above. Currently there is no evidence that CA-ASB requires treatment with antibiotics but there are specific patient populations that warrant special considerations and are out of the scope of this chapter.

Microbiology

For patients with short term catheterization the organism is typically a single isolate, usually an aerobic gram negative bacteria, and is most frequently E.Coli. In patients with long-term catheterization the isolates are usually polymicrobial. Fungal isolates are rare and are not typically associated with an infection. For patients that have long-term catheterization, the isolates are typically polymicrobial.

Treatment

The treatment of CAUTIs is also a source of controversy, and the optimal duration of antimicrobial therapy is not known. Current recommendations published by the Infectious Diseases Society of America recommend treatment for 7 days for those who respond to treatment and a longer 10–14-day course for patients in whom response to treatment is delayed. For young healthy women who no longer have a catheter, a short 3-day course can be considered, and there is some evidence a 5-day course of levofloxacin could be sufficient treatment in a non-critically ill patient.

The initial empiric therapy in a patient who does not require broad-spectrum therapy for other reasons, is ceftriaxone 1 g IV daily or cefotaxime 1 g IV every 8 h until culture results are back and the antibiotics can be tailored to a specific isolate with sensitivities (Table 39.2). If the patient has specific resistance patterns that require broader empiric coverage or is critically ill, then appropriate empiric coverage should be determined by the clinical team.

The removal and re-insertion of a foley catheter as part of the treatment regimen is another area of controversy and is not necessarily backed by strong evidence. However, if a patient has a chronic indwelling catheter, then the catheter should/could be changed at the time of treatment due to poor penetration of antibiotics into the biofilm. Though this last recommendation lacks sufficient evidence.

Candidal infections of the urinary tract are rare, and determining colonization from a true urinary tract infection is difficult. Patients at highest risk for a candidal infection are patients with a chronic indwelling catheter, diabetes mellitus, anatomic abnormalities, or those with chronic antibiotic use. Typically, isolated candiduria does not require treatment without evidence of clinical symptoms such as flank pain or costovertebral pain.

Patients with an isolated growth of candiduria should not be treated unless there is clinical concern for disseminated candidiasis. A patient with persistent candiduria should have imaging of their kidneys to rule out renal or upper urinary tract involvement. Those patients who are at high risk for disseminated candidiasis can be treated with fluconazole 200–400 mg daily for 14 days. However, antifungal therapy should be tailored to resistance patterns and if there is concern for fluconazole resistance then amphotericin B (0.3 mg to 0.6 mg/kg daily) (the non-lipid formula as the lipid formula is not excreted in the urine) should be used.

The routine removal and replacement of catheters as part of the treatment regimen is not supported by the IDSA or the CDC in the setting of a diagnosis of a CAUTI or a patient with candiduria; however, if a catheter has been in place for greater than 2 weeks and cannot be removed, then the catheter should/could be replaced to decrease the risk of future CAUTIs. Again, this last recommendation lacks sufficient evidence.

Prevention

The CDC publishes guidelines to help prevent CAUTIs with an emphasis on decreasing catheter use as the primary target for prevention. There have been studies that have used silver impregnated catheters or nitrofurazone impregnated catheters that have shown a small decrease in CAUTI rates, but more research is needed to assess the cost:benefit ratios. However, the most effective strategies for reducing CAUTIs focus on early catheter removal and education regarding the indication for catheter placement [3].

Cho et al.'s recently published work demonstrates an intervention to reduce CAUTIs by educating nursing and physician staff about the indications for a urinary catheter and a daily prompt regarding removal. Their paper shows a reduction in CAUTIs as well as a decrease in hospital costs [4].

Once a catheter is inserted, it is important to maintain the integrity of the system to decrease contamination. However, once the catheter is in place there are little or no evidence based prevention strategies that can be utilized to decrease CAUTI rates outside of early removal. For example, there is no evidence to suggest that meatal care provides any protection from CAUTI or CA-ASB. This is also true for bladder irrigation or antimicrobials added to the drainage bag as these techniques do not provide any protection against CAUTIs or CA-ASB and at the same time increase hospital costs. Empiric catheter exchange protocols have not shown a benefit in decreasing CAUTIs in patients with chronic or long-term indwelling catheters.

Prevention, which is an important and effective strategy that has the strongest evidence for its effectiveness, also involves teaching the appropriate techniques for catheter placement so that breaches in sterile technique are minimized. Standardized education of all staff who place catheters (nurses, residents, as well as medical students) could minimize errors in placement technique which could put the patient at risk for a future CAUTI. This could be done through simulation curriculums or observed training that ensures appropriate placement techniques before catheters can be placed independently.

Conclusion

CAUTIs are a significant burden to the patient and the health-care system and can be difficult to diagnose or separate from CA-ASB. Patient's with CAUTIs require empiric treatment that is subsequently tailored to specific culture data once it is available. There are many strategies that help to prevent CAUTIs which include education around placement and protocols for early removal.

References

1. Leuk AM, Wright D, Ellingson L, Kraemer L, Kuskowski MA, Johnson JR. Complications of Foley catheters—is infection the greatest risk? J Urol. 2012;187(5):1662–6.
2. Saint S. Clinical and economic consequences of nosocomial catheter-related bacteriuria. Am J Infect Control. 2000;28(1):68.
3. CDC Catheter-associated Urinary Tract Infections (CAUTI). Centers for Disease Control and Prevention 2015. Retrieved from https://www.cdc.gov/hai/ca_uti/uti.htmlDecember 2017.
4. Cho HJ, Khalil S, Poeran J, Mazumdar M, Bravo N, Wallach F, Markoff B, Lee N, Dunn AS. "Lose the Tube": a choosing wisely initiative to reduce catheter-associated urinary tract infections in hospitalist-led inpatient units. Am J Infect Control. 2017;45:333–5.

Ventilator-Associated Pneumonia

40

Dina M. Filiberto and Martin A. Croce

Introduction

Ventilator-associated pneumonia is a surgical disease. It is responsible for significant morbidity, mortality, resource utilization, and increased hospital costs in our surgical patients. In this chapter, we will focus on risk factors, diagnosis, treatment, and prevention of this scourge in our surgical and trauma intensive care units.

Epidemiology

Ventilator-associated pneumonia (VAP) is a common cause of infection in the intensive care unit (ICU) and is a significant cause of morbidity and mortality in critically ill patients. Patients with VAP have prolonged lengths of stay in the ICU and hospital [1], and reported mortality rates range from 15% to 25% [2–4]. The incidence of VAP ranges from 4% to 87% in the literature [3, 5, 6]. Such wide variability can be attributed to the different methods of diagnosis, the population studied, and the lack of a uniform definition of VAP. However, it is clear that the incidence of VAP increases with duration of mechanical ventilation. Cook et al. investigated 1014 mechanically ventilated patients to determine risk factors in VAP during their hospital course. They found the cumulative risk of VAP increased over time, but the daily risk decreased after day 5, suggesting a high risk of early VAP [7]. Furthermore, in a study evaluating trauma patients, the authors noted a linear relationship between duration of mechanical ventilation and the incidence of VAP [8].

Risk Factors

Risk factors for the development of VAP in medical patients include chronic disease, lung disease, age, aspiration, supine positioning, and use of paralytic agents. As expected, patients with comorbidities, patients with immunosuppressive disease, and patients that are elderly have decreased physiologic reserve are at an increased risk of VAP. A randomized controlled trial identified aspiration and use of paralytic agents as risk factors for VAP. Decreasing the cough reflex and impairing endotracheal secretion clearance may put patients at higher risk of VAP [7]. Drakulovic et al. found a higher frequency of pneumonia in patients positioned supine compared to patients in a semirecumbent position. The risk of VAP was even more apparent in patients positioned supine that received enteral feeding, alluding to aspiration as a risk factor [9].

The trauma and surgical populations have been analyzed in various studies, and predictors of VAP were identified as increased injury severity score (ISS), increased Glasgow Coma Scale (GCS) score, blunt injury, emergent intubation, shock, age, increased transfusion requirement, and specific injury patterns such as spinal cord injury, chest injury, and need for emergent craniotomy, femur fixation, or laparotomy. The relationship between increasing severity of traumatic brain injury and development of VAP is striking (Fig. 40.1). The incidence of pneumonia in patients with a GCS score of 3–8 is 40% [1]. The trauma literature suggests that more critically injured patients, evidenced by ISS and GCS, are more likely to develop VAP [1, 3].

Diagnosis

Despite its relative frequency, there is no universally accepted definition of VAP. Clinical features such as purulent sputum, fever, leukocytosis, worsening oxygenation, difficulty to wean from the ventilator, and new or worsening infiltrate on chest radiograph are often used as criteria in patients with suspected VAP.

D. M. Filiberto · M. A. Croce (✉)
University of Tennessee Health Science Center, Memphis, TN, USA
e-mail: mcroce@uthsc.edu

A. Salim et al. (eds.), *Surgical Critical Care Therapy*, https://doi.org/10.1007/978-3-319-71712-8_40

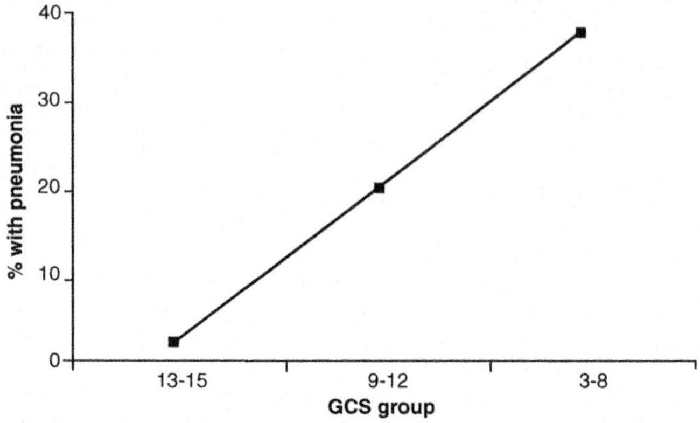

Fig. 40.1 Demonstrates the relationship between GCS score and incidence of VAP

The Clinical Pulmonary Infection Score (CPIS) is constructed from multiple clinical parameters and was developed by Pugin to assist in pneumonia diagnosis. The parameters selected to comprise the score are patient's temperature, blood leukocytes, trachea secretions, PaO_2/FiO_2, chest radiograph, and tracheal aspirate culture. CPIS >6 correlated to a diagnosis of pneumonia when compared to quantitative culture data. The study only used 28 patients who underwent BAL; however, this score has subsequently become a popular method for diagnosis of pneumonia [10]. Others have even described a strategy that utilizes the CPIS to guide antibiotic duration in medical patients [11]. However, its utility in guiding treatment duration and diagnosis of VAP in surgical patients is limited. Croce et al. evaluated 285 patients that underwent quantitative BAL with clinical evidence of VAP. The CPIS was calculated in each patient, and the average score in patients without VAP and with VAP (organism with 10^5 CFU/mL) was 6.8 and 6.9, respectively. The sensitivity and specificity was 61% and 43% utilizing a CPIS of >6 as a threshold for VAP, demonstrating that CPIS is not a good tool in trauma patients [12]. Parks et al. investigated the potential use of CPIS in determining duration of antimicrobial therapy in VAP. There was no correlation between VAP resolution and CPIS score. In fact, the mean CPIS score was greater than 6 when VAP had resolved on quantitative culture. Antibiotics would have been unnecessarily continued in 59% of patients [13]. The CPIS attempts to measure the inflammatory response in pneumonia; however, it is not successful in distinguishing inflammation from infection. Surgical patients frequently demonstrate systemic inflammatory response syndrome (SIRS) from operations, trauma, burns, atelectasis, transfusions, and wounds. Fever and leukocytosis are common findings. Additionally, pulmonary contusions and acute respiratory distress syndrome (ARDS) can make radiograph interpretation difficult [8].

A more invasive diagnostic technique can be utilized to differentiate SIRS from infection in surgical patients. Using bronchoscopy to sample the distal airways, quantitative bronchoalveolar lavage (BAL) culture improves diagnostic accuracy with the ability to distinguish between SIRS and VAP [4, 14–17]. Quantitative BAL is more specific than a combination of clinical findings and sputum culture. In fact, less than 50% of patients with clinical signs and symptoms of VAP will have an infection based on quantitative BAL. A bronchoscope is advanced into the involved lung segment without using suction, and with the tip of the bronchoscope in the lower airway, a BAL is performed with 100 mL of sterile nonbacteriostatic saline in 20 mL aliquots. The effluent is aspirated and sent to the microbiology laboratory for gram stain, culture, and sensitivity, which generally finalizes in 72 h [4].

Other methods for obtaining cultures include tracheal aspiration, protected specimen brush, or mini-BAL. Tracheal aspirates can identify causative organisms; however, upper airways and endotracheal tubes are frequently colonized, which may yield false-positive sputum cultures [18]. Protected brush specimen (PBS) is obtained by inserting a brush-tipped catheter into a bronchoscope and then brushing the tip along the lining of the bronchiole. Mini-BAL is performed by placing a catheter into the endotracheal tube, injecting 20 mL of sterile nonbacteriostatic saline through the catheter, and re-aspirating the saline.

Comparison between tracheal aspirate, PBS, and BAL was performed in 107 patients with clinical evidence of pneumonia. The incidence of pneumonia according to each method was tracheal aspirate 73%, PSB 34%, and BAL 25%. Even in patients with classic clinical pneumonia, tracheal aspirate demonstrated a pathogen only 73% of the time. As previously stated, tracheal aspirates are often inaccurate, but the presence of a pathogen on tracheal aspirate in combination with clinical parameters is frequently an indication for antibiotics at many institutions. This study highlights the large difference in incidence of pneumonia between diagnostic modalities. In addition to bronchoscopically obtained quantitative cultures being more accurate, their use is more cost-effective. Because the incidence of pneumonia is lower with PSB and BAL, costly unnecessary antibiotics are discontinued [19].

The diagnostic threshold of quantitative BAL has been debated in the literature with values of 10^4 [20, 21] and 10^5 [22, 23] colony-forming units/mL (CFU/mL) used. A value of 10^3 CFU/mL is considered diagnostic with protective specimen brush [24]. A higher threshold for quantitative BAL is expected because a larger area of lung tissue is exposed to the effluent. With approximately one million alveoli sampled, more organisms are recovered [4, 25]. At our institution, a threshold of 10^5 CFU/mL demonstrated few false-negative quantitative BAL cultures and a pneumonia-related mortality comparable to what is described in the literature. In a prospective study, 232 mechanically ventilated patients underwent 443 bronchoscopies with quantitative BAL. Incidence of pneumonia was 39% and was not different regardless of the number of BALs a patient received during their hospitalization. The false-negative rate of quantitative BAL was low at 7%. This demonstrates SIRS may occur at any time during a patient's ICU course and the use of BAL with a threshold of 10^5 CFU/mL can effectively diagnose VAP. In most studies using quantitative BAL as a method of diagnosis, antibiotics were continued in patients who still had clinical signs and symptoms of pneumonia. However, in this study antibiotics were discontinued with insignificant colony counts as determined by BAL, irrespective of the patients' clinical parameters [4]. When the threshold was reduced to 10^4 CFU/mL, the sensitivity was similar, and the specificity and positive predictive values were much lower [21].

Treatment

The causative pathogens of VAP are widely variable in bacterial etiology. Effective treatment of VAP depends on early administration of empiric antibiotics with broad coverage after cultures have been obtained. The antibiotic selection should then be narrowed based on the speciation and sensitivity of the culture. Antibiotics should be discontinued if the bacterial diagnostic threshold is not achieved. The goal of treatment is to adequately eradicate the infection while limiting exposure to unnecessary antibiotics to prevent overuse and development of multidrug-resistant organisms [26].

Empiric antibiotic selection should be based on the most likely causative pathogens. Resistant or unexpected organisms can limit the success of antibiotic regimens resulting in inadequate empiric antibiotic therapy [19, 27, 28]. In a study that evaluated 82 patients with multiple VAP episodes, there were 39% with inadequate empiric antibiotic therapy. Inadequate empiric antibiotic therapy means there was no antibiotic with activity again the causative pathogen. Most of the episodes were attributed to *Acinetobacter* sp. and *Stenotrophomonas* sp. The mortality rate for patients with no episodes of inadequate therapy was 3.6% and for multiple episodes of inadequate therapy was 45%. In addition, inadequate therapy was associated with prolonged ICU length of stay and prolonged length of mechanical ventilation [29]. A meta-analysis on 32 VAP studies found the odds of death were 2.34 times greater for patients with inappropriate empiric therapy compared to those receiving adequate antibiotic therapy [30]. These risks support the notion that broad therapy is important to decrease the risk of missing a drug-resistant organism. Factors to consider in empiric antibiotic selection are time from admission, previous antibiotic use, and the antibiogram of the ICU [20, 31]. The gram stain from the quantitative BAL does not help in identifying causative organisms and should not be used to select empiric antibiotic therapy [4].

The timing of VAP development is associated with distribution patterns of organisms. BAL cultures performed within the first week of admission primarily identified *Haemophilus influenza*, *Streptococcus pneumonia*, methicillin-sensitive *Staphylococcus aureus* (MSSA), enteric gram-negative bacilli, *Escherichia coli*, *Klebsiella pneumonia*, *Enterobacter* sp., *Proteus* sp., and *Serratia marcescens*. Many of these early pathogens are community acquired with a low likelihood of antibiotic resistance. After 1 week of admission, *Pseudomonas aeruginosa*, extended-spectrum beta-lactamase-producing bacteria, *Acinetobacter* sp., methicillin-resistant *Staphylococcus aureus* (MRSA), *Stenotrophomonas* sp., and *Legionella pneumophila* become more common [4, 32]. A clinical algorithm for diagnosis and empiric management of VAP was developed and validated at our institution (Fig. 40.2). The antibiotic selection is based on time from admission and our antibiogram. Empiric therapy is continued when BAL culture has "no growth to date" on the preliminary report. This is because the reports are done everyday at the same time in the microbiology laboratory, regardless of when the specimen is received. A specimen can be incubated up to 23 h longer than a different one, yet both will have a report at 24 h.

The Infectious Diseases Society of America and the American Thoracic Society (IFDSA/ATS) released updated clinical practice guidelines in 2016. Initial antibiotic therapy options should cover *S. aureus*, *P. aeruginosa*, and other gram-negative bacilli. Suggested antibiotics include piperacillin-tazobactam, cefepime, ceftazidime, levofloxacin, imipenem, or meropenem.

Concern for MRSA or *P. aeruginosa* justifies the use of more aggressive empiric therapy. In patients with increased risk of antimicrobial resistance or if >10–20% of the local ICU's *S. aureus* isolates are MRSA, then vancomycin or linezolid should be used empirically.

IFDSA/ATS recommends monotherapy for treatment of *P. aeruginosa* in low-risk patients; however, in patients with high risk of antimicrobial resistance or if >10% of the local ICU's gram-negative organisms resistant to the monotherapy, dual therapy is suggested [33].

The recommendations emphasize antibiotic regimens should be based on an institutional antibiogram, where the most common pathogens and their susceptibilities are tracked. For example, our institution found monotherapy with cefepime was successful in treating trauma patients with *Pseudomonas* VAP; therefore, dual therapy is not routinely administered [34]. If the ICU has a high rate of multidrug-resistant organisms, uncommon organisms, or an immunosuppressed patient population (i.e., transplant patients or oncology patients), standard antibiotic selection may not be appropriate [35].

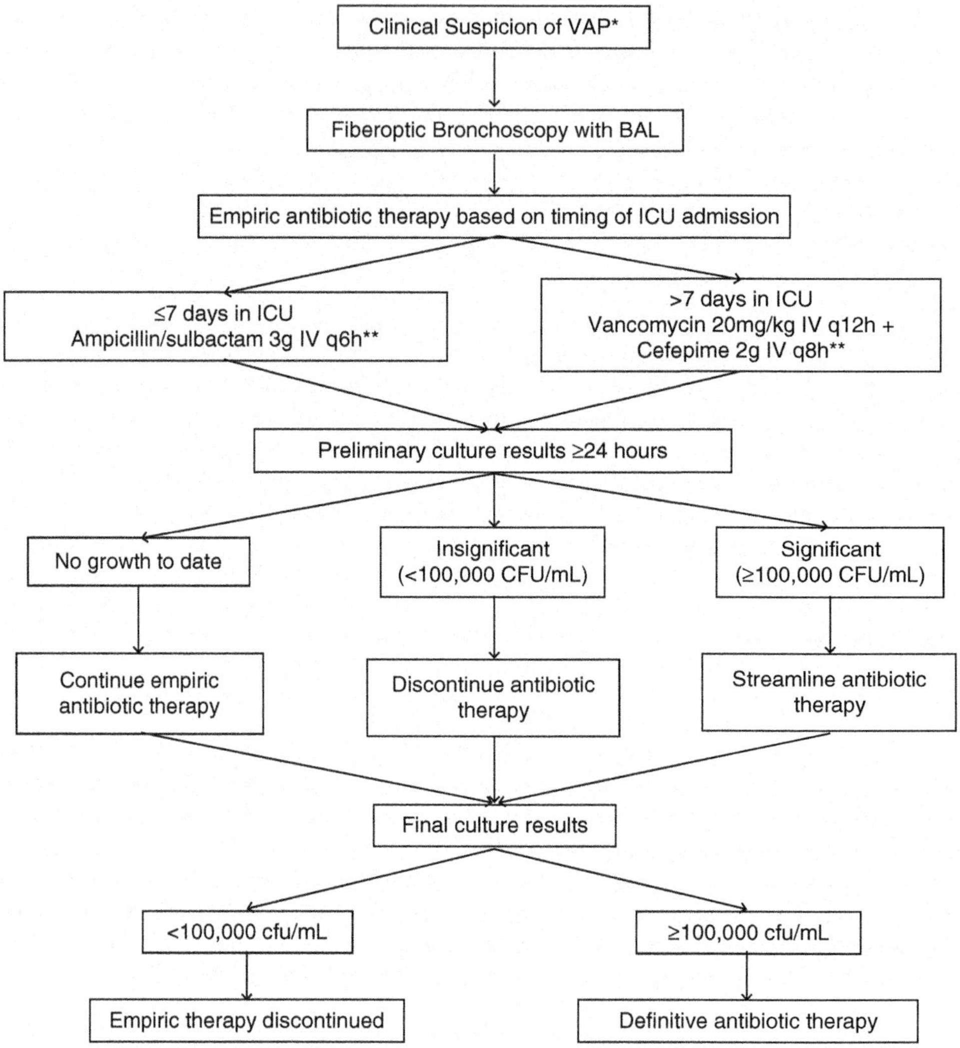

Fig. 40.2 Clinical algorithm for diagnosis and empiric management of ventilator-associated pneumonia. *Defined as any three of the following: appearance of a new or changing infiltrate on chest x-ray; abnormal temperature (>38.3 or <35.6 °C); abnormal white blood cell count (>10,000 cells/mm^3 or >10% immature bands); macroscopically purulent sputum. **If severe β-lactam allergy, change ampicillin/sulbactam to moxifloxacin 400 mg IV q24h and cefepime to ciprofloxacin 400 mg IV q8h

The duration of antibiotic treatment of VAP historically ranged from 14 to 21 days. However, modern data supports shorter duration depending on the causative pathogen. Ibrahim et al. evaluated 102 medical patients with VAP and found a limited 7-day course of antibiotic therapy decreased VAP recurrence without increasing morbidity and mortality [26].

Chastre et al. performed a randomized controlled trial comparing 8 days versus 15 days of antibiotic therapy in patients with VAP. The clinical outcomes were similar in both groups. The long-course antibiotic group grew more multidrug-resistant organisms when there was a VAP recurrence. Lastly, the study found patients with VAP caused by nonfermenting gram-negative bacilli, such as *P. aeruginosa,* had a higher recurrence rate in the short-course antibiotic group and suggested a longer treatment course may be necessary [36].

Using an arbitrary duration of time for treatment may result in VAP recurrence or antibiotic resistance. Determining the optimal duration of definitive antibiotic therapy for VAP limits unnecessary antibiotic exposure. Mueller et al. used serial quantitative BAL to determine if antibiotic duration can be abbreviated. Repeat BAL was performed at day 4 of appropriate antibiotic therapy, and antibiotics were discontinued if quantitative BAL was <10^4 CFU/mL; otherwise, they were continued. This group was compared to a control group of patients that were not treated with repeat BAL. Antibiotic duration was shorter in the repeat BAL group compared to the control group (9.8 vs 16.7 days), and there were no differences in VAP recurrence or mortality. 82.7% of VAP isolates in the repeat BAL group were either community-acquired pathogens or early pathogens such as MSSA, *H. influenza*, and *S. pneumoniae*. These organisms were treated with 7–8 days of antibiotics. Late pathogens such as *P. aeruginosa*, *Acinetobacter* sp., and *Stenotrophomonas* sp. commonly required a longer duration of therapy [37].

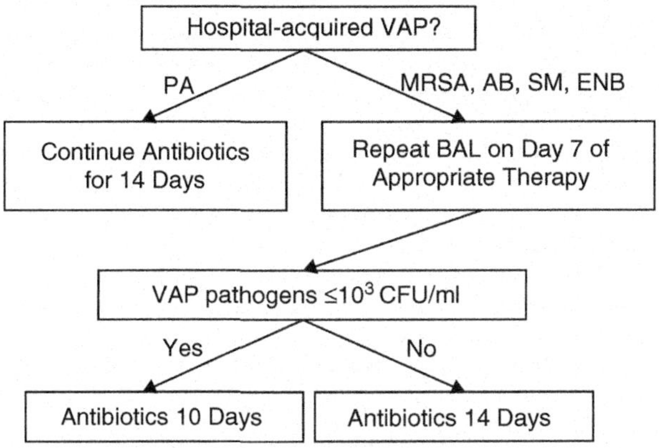

Fig. 40.3 Clinical pathway for definitive management of hospital-acquired VAP. AB *Acinetobacter baumannii*, ENB *Enterobacteriaceae*, PA *Pseudomonas aeruginosa*, SM *Stenotrophomonas maltophilia*

To evaluate the optimal duration of antibiotics for patients with hospital-acquired pathogens, Magnotti et al. performed repeat BAL on days 4, 7, and 10 (if necessary) of appropriate antibiotic therapy. Antibiotics were continued until there was microbiological resolution of VAP based on quantitative BAL. This study demonstrated MRSA and *P. aeruginosa* mostly resolved after 14 days of therapy. Sixty percent of *Acinetobacter* sp., *Stenotrophomonas* sp., and *Enterobacter* sp. resolved after 10 days of therapy; however, an additional 30% of the patients required prolonged antibiotic therapy (14 days). By performing a repeat BAL on day 7, the subset of patients requiring prolonged therapy is identified. The recurrence rate in this study was 2% [32]. The clinical practice algorithm for definitive VAP management at our institution has subsequently incorporated repeat BAL into the schema (Fig. 40.3). The use of repeat BAL provides an objective measure to determine the resolution of VAP in hospital-acquired pathogens and therefore avoids arbitrary endpoints. Antibiotic selection and duration of therapy are tailored to the causative organism.

There is increased emphasis on antibiotic stewardship in most hospital systems. Overuse can result in increased costs, antibiotic-related complications, and increased resistant organisms. When the diagnostic threshold is not achieved, antibiotics should be discontinued. When the speciation and sensitivity is determined, antibiotics should be de-escalated and tailored to the organism [33]. Using our clinical algorithm, the pathogen sensitivities have not significantly changed. It must be emphasized, however, that the colonization patterns of other ICUs may be different from our institution. It is important to track the prevalence of organisms and their antimicrobial susceptibilities to guide and refine empiric therapy.

Prevention

Every effort should be made to decrease the occurrence of VAP in critically ill patients. The Institute for Healthcare Improvement introduced the concept of a VAP bundle, an assortment of prophylactic interventions, to prevent VAP development in the ICU. The original bundle consists of head of bed elevation and semirecumbent positioning to decrease the risk of aspiration, daily sedation holidays, daily spontaneous breathing trials and assessment for weaning and extubation, stress gastritis prophylaxis, and mechanical and chemical venous thromboembolism prophylaxis. The bundle was later modified to add use of chlorhexidine and oral hygiene to decrease oropharyngeal colonization. Multiple studies claim success with implementation of the VAP bundle or various other protocols, which include components of the bundle [38–40]. However, there are methodologic issues with these studies, and any conclusive statement about the effectiveness of the VAP bundle should be tempered. It is not known which interventions or factors contribute to its success [41, 42]. A multi-institutional, prospective study of trauma patients demonstrated that the original ventilator bundle (excluding the oral hygiene component) had no impact on the development of ventilator-associated pneumonia [42]. However, since the bundle is not detrimental to patient care, it is still typically used in intensive care units.

Other preventative measures to decrease VAP are to maintain the endotracheal cuff pressures at 20 cm H_2O, to prevent tracking of bacterial pathogens around the cuff, and to change the ventilator circuit when it's contaminated from secretions and condensation. It has been demonstrated that routine change of the ventilator circuit does not decrease risk for VAP [43].

Aerosolized antibiotics have been introduced as a potential prophylactic measure. A randomized controlled trial was performed to evaluate aerosolized ceftazidime in the prevention of VAP. Forty patients were enrolled, and there were significant reductions in VAP in the antibiotic group compared to the placebo group at ICU day 14 and for the entire ICU stay. Additionally, aerosolized ceftazidime did not change the sensitivity patterns of gram-negative bacilli in the ICU. The study was limited by its small patient population [44]. With this promising preliminary data, another randomized controlled trial was performed that compared aerosolized ceftazidime with placebo in 105 patients. There was no significant difference between the groups in VAP incidence at 2 weeks or at 30 days, and therefore, routine use of prophylactic aerosolized antibiotic cannot be recommended [45].

Conclusion

VAP is a common disease process in the ICU, resulting in significant morbidity, mortality, and hospital expenditure. Without a uniform definition of VAP, interpretation of data and management remain a challenge. The utilization of quantitative diagnostic modalities in surgical patients appears superior to clinical strategies due to the prevalence of SIRS in this patient population. Treatment of VAP relies on early, appropriate empiric antibiotic therapy that covers the most probable pathogens. Regimens should be guided by local antibiograms and likelihood of antibiotic resistance. Therapy should be narrowed when the causative organism is determined. It is important to find a balance between adequate empiric coverage and overuse of antibiotics. Prolonged exposure to unnecessary antibiotics can develop resistance; however, inadequate treatment can result in increased morbidity and mortality. Short-course antibiotic duration is favored in community-acquired pathogens, while optimal duration of hospital-acquired pathogens ranges from 10 to 14 days. Prevention measures should be undertaken to decrease the incidence of VAP in the ICU population.

References

1. Croce MA, Fabian TC, Waddle-Smith L, Maxwell RA. Identification of early predictors for post-traumatic pneumonia. Am Surg. 2001;67(2):105–10.
2. Croce MA, Fabian TC, Schurr MJ, et al. Using bronchoalveolar lavage to distinguish nosocomial pneumonia from systemic inflammatory response syndrome: a prospective analysis. J Trauma. 1995;39:1134–40.
3. Rodriguez JL, Gibbons KJ, Bitzer LG, et al. Pneumonia: incidence, risk factors, and outcome in injured patients. J Trauma. 1991;31:907–14.
4. Croce MA, Fabian TC, Waddle-Smith L, et al. Utility of Gram's stain and efficacy of quantitative cultures for posttraumatic pneumonia. Ann Surg. 1998;227:743–55.
5. Miller EH, Caplan ES. Noscocomial hemophilus pneumonia in patients with severe trauma. Surg Gynecol Obstet. 1984;159:153–6.
6. Trinkle JK, Richardson JD, Frank JL, Grover FL, Arom KV, Holmstrom FM. Management of flail chest without mechanical ventilation. Ann Thorac Surg. 1975;19:355–63.
7. Cook DJ, Walter SD, Cook RJ, et al. Incidence of and risk factors for ventilator-associated pneumonia in critically ill patients. Ann Intern Med. 1998;129:433–40.
8. Croce MA, Tolley EA, Fabian TC. A formula for prediction of posttraumatic pneumonia based on early anatomic and physiologic parameters. J Trauma. 2003;54:724–30.
9. Drakulovic MB, Torres A, Bauer TT, Nicolas JM, Nogue S, Ferrer M. Supine body position as a risk factor for nosocomial pneumonia in mechanically ventilated patients: a randomized trial. Lancet. 1999;354:1851–8.
10. Pugin J, Auckenthaler R, Mili N, Janssens JP, Lew PD, Suter PM. Diagnosis of ventilator-associated pneumonia by bacteriologic analysis of bronchoscopic and nonbronchoscopic "blind" bronchoalveolar lavage fluid. Am Rev Respir Dis. 1991;143:1121–9.
11. Singh N, Rogers P, Atwood CW, Wagener MM, Yu VL. Short-course empiric antibiotic therapy for patients with pulmonary infiltrates in the intensive care unit. A proposed solution for indiscriminate antibiotic prescription. Am J Respir Crit Care Med. 2000;162:505–11.
12. Croce MA, Swanson JM, Magnotti LJ, Claridge JA, Weinberg JA, Wood GC, Boucher BA, Fabian TC. The futility of the clinical pulmonary infection score in trauma patients. J Trauma. 2006;60:523–8.
13. Parks NA, Magnotti LJ, Weinberg JA, Zarzaur BL, Schreoppel TJ, Swanson JM, Fabian TC, Croce MA. Use of the clinical pulmonary infection score to guide therapy for ventilator-associated pneumonia risks antibiotic overexposure in patients with trauma. J Trauma Acute Care Surg. 2012;73:52–9.
14. Wimberly N, Faling LJ, Barrlett JG. A fiberoptic bronchoscopy technique to obtain uncontaminated lower airway secretions for bacterial culture. Am Rev Respir Dis. 1979;119:337–43.
15. Stover DE, Zaman MB, Hajdu SI, et al. Bronchoalveolar lavage in the diagnosis of diffuse pulmonary infiltrates in the immunosuppressed host. Ann Intern Med. 1984;101:1–7.
16. Meduri GU, Wunderink RG, Leeper KV, et al. Management of bacterial pneumonia in ventilated patients: protected bronchoalveolar lavage as a diagnostic tool. Chest. 1992;101:500–8.
17. Polk HC Jr. Quantitative tracheal cultures in surgical patients requiring mechanical ventilator assistance. Surgery. 1975;78:485–91.
18. Meduri GU. Ventilator-associated pneumonia in patients with respiratory failure: a diagnostic approach. Chest. 1990;97:1208.
19. Croce MA, Fabian TC, Shaw B, et al. Analysis of charges associated with diagnosis of nosocomial pneumonia: can routine bronchoscopy be justified? J Trauma. 1994;37(5):721–7.
20. Luna CM, Vujacich P, Niederman MS, et al. Impact of BAL data on the therapy and outcome of ventilator-associated pneumonia. Chest. 1997;111:676–85.
21. Chastre J, Fagon JY. Ventilator-associated pneumonia. Am J Respir Crit Care Med. 2002;165:867–903.
22. Croce MA, Fabian TC, Mueller EW, et al. The appropriate diagnostic threshold for ventilator-associated pneumonia using quantitative cultures. J Trauma. 2004;56:931–6.
23. Miller PR, Meredith JW, Chang MC. Optimal threshold for diagnosis of ventilator associated pneumonia using bronchoalveolar lavage. J Trauma. 2003;55:263–8.
24. Fagon JY, Chastre J, Hance AJ, et al. Detection of nosocomial lung infection in ventilated patients: use of a protected specimen brush and quantitative culture techniques in 147 patients. Am Rev Respir Dis. 1988;138:110.
25. Baselski V. Microbiologic diagnosis of ventilator-associated pneumonia. Infect Dis Clin N Am. 1993;7:331.
26. File TM. Recommendations for treatment of hospital-acquired and ventilator-acquired pneumonia: review of recent international guidelines. Clin Infect Dis. 2010;51:S42–7.
27. Ibrahim EH, Ward S, Sherman G, et al. Experience with a clinical guideline for the treatment of ventilator-associated pneumonia. Crit Care Med. 2001;29:1109–15.
28. Magnotti LJ, Schroeppel TJ, Fabian TC, Clement LP, Swanson JM, Fischer PE, Bee TK, Maish GO 3rd, Minard G, Zarzaur BL, Croce MA. Reduction in inadequate empiric antibiotic therapy for ventilator-associated pneumonia: impact of a unit-specific treatment pathway. Am Surg. 2008;74(6):516–22.
29. Mueller EW, Hanes SD, Croce MA, et al. Effect from multiple episodes of inadequate empiric antibiotic therapy for ventilator-associated pneumonia on morbidity and mortality among critically ill trauma patients. J Trauma. 2005;58:94–101.
30. Kuti EL, Patel AA, Coleman CI. Impact of inappropriate antibiotic therapy on mortality in patients with ventilator-associated pneumonia and blood stream infection: a meta-analysis. J Crit Care. 2008;23:91–100.

31. Kollef MH. Inadequate antimicrobial treatment: an important determinant of outcome for hospitalized patients. Clin Infect Dis. 2000;31(suppl 4):S131–8.
32. American Thoracic Society; Infectious Diseases Society of America. Guidelines for the management of adults with hospital-acquired, ventilator-associated, and healthcare-associated pneumonia. Am J Respir Crit Care Med. 2005;171:388–416.
33. Kalil AC, Metersky ML, et al. Management of adults with hospital-acquired and ventilator-associated pneumonia: 2016 clinical practice guidelines by the Infectious Diseases Society of American and the American Thoracic Society. Clin Infect Dis. 2016;63(5):61–111.
34. Magnotti LJ, Schroeppel TJ, et al. Efficacy of monotherapy in the treatment of *Pseudomonas* ventilator-associated pneumonia in patients with trauma. J Trauma. 2009;66:1052–9.
35. Rello J, Sa-Borges M, Correa H, Leal SR, Baraibar J. Variations in etiology of ventilator-associated pneumonia across four treatment sites: implications for antimicrobial prescribing practices. Am J Respir Crit Care Med. 1999;160:608–13.
36. Chastre J, Wolff M, Fagon JY, Chevret S, Thomas F, Wermert D, Clementi E, Gonzalez J, Jusserand D, Asfar P, Perrin D, Fieux F, Aubas S. Comparison of 8 vs 15 days of antibiotic therapy for ventilator-associated pneumonia in adults: a randomized trial. JAMA. 2003;290:2588–98.
37. Mueller EW, Croce MA, Boucher BA, Hanes SD, Wood C, Swanson JM, Chennault SK, Fabian TC. Repeat bronchoalveolar lavage to guide antibiotic duration for ventilator-associated pneumonia. J Trauma. 2007;63:1329–37.
38. Bird D, Zambuto A, et al. Adhereance to ventilator-associated pneumonia bundle and incidence of ventilator-associated pneumonia in the surgical intenseive care unit. Arch Surg. 2010;145:465–70.
39. Cachecho R, Dobkin E. The application of human engineering inteventions reduces ventilator-associated pneumonia in trauma patients. J Trauma. 2012;73:939–43.
40. Sinuff T, Muscedere J, et al. Implementation of clinical practice guidelines for ventilator-associated pneumonia: a multicenter prospective study. Crit Care Med. 2013;41:15–23.
41. Croce MA, Brasel KJ, et al. National Trauma Institute prospective evaluation of the ventilator bundle in trauma patients. Does it really work? J Trauma. 2013;74(2):354–62.
42. Wip C, Napolitano L. Bundles to prevent ventilator-associated pneumonia: how valuable are they? Curr Opin Infect Dis. 2009;22:159–66.
43. Han J, Liu Y. Effect of ventilator circuit changes on ventilator-associated pneumonia: a systematic review and meta-analysis. Respir Care. 2010;55:467–74.
44. Wood CG, Boucher BA, et al. Aerosolized ceftazidime for prevention of ventilator-associated pneumonia and drug effects on the proinflammatory response in critically ill trauma patients. Pharmacotherapy. 2002;22(8):972–82.
45. Claridge JA, Edwards NM, et al. Aerosolized ceftazidime prophylaxis against ventilator-associated pneumonia in high-risk trauma patients: results of a double-blind randomized study. Surg Infect. 2007;8(1):83–90.

Fungal, Viral, and Other Oddball Infections and the Immunosuppressed Patient

41

Sameer A. Hirji, Sharven Taghavi, and Reza Askari

Introduction

Infections with fungal and viral pathogens in the surgical intensive critical unit (ICU) are not uncommon. Often, however, diagnosis tends to be either delayed or superimposed on bacterial infections. In some scenarios, definitive diagnosis can be challenging and a high index of suspicion is warranted to promptly manage critically ill patients. This approach is critical especially in immunosuppressed patients given their relative vulnerability to a multitude of infectious processes. Although rare, oddball infections with rare viruses and fungi can significantly affect the clinical course and recovery of patients if timely diagnosis is delayed. This chapter highlights important fungal, viral, and rare infections in the context of critically ill and high-risk patients, including the immunosuppressed patients, in the surgical ICU.

Common Fungal Infections

Fungal infections in the critical setting are associated with increasing morbidity and mortality when undiagnosed promptly. These pathogens can place a huge burden on the existing health-care system. Isolated cases of fungal infections are possible, but often these infections occur concurrently with bacterial or viral infections. More than 50% of all fungal infections tend to occur in surgical patients, and a significant portion are prevalent in the surgical ICU [1]. Common infectious fungal species include *Candida*, aspergillosis, and mucormycosis. Fungal infections can affect any organ but most likely affect the brain, lungs, abdomen, and soft tissues [2].

S. A. Hirji · S. Taghavi
Department of Surgery, Brigham and Women's Hospital, Harvard Medical School, Boston, MA, USA

R. Askari (✉)
Department of Surgery, Brigham and Women's Hospital, Harvard Medical School, Boston, MA, USA

Trauma, Burn, and Surgical Critical Care, Brigham and Women's Hospital, Boston, MA, USA
e-mail: RASKARI@PARTNERS.ORG

Candidiasis

Epidemiology: Incidence, Mortality

Candida is prevalent in the surgical patients with reported mortality between 30 and 40%, depending on the patient and associated infection site. Most often, the major cause of mortality is patient acuity at the time of diagnosis and the delay in treatment initiation. *Candida* infections typically arise from intravascular catheters, bladder catheters, or the gastrointestinal tract. It is for this reason that sterile precautions should be maintained in the ICU setting at all times [1].

Risk Factors

Several populations of surgical patients are more susceptible to *Candida* infections. These include patients on immunosuppression such as those who have had solid organ transplants (i.e., kidney, pancreas) and those with various rheumatologic and endocrine disorders. Other at risk populations include patients with prior history of *Candida* colonization, those receiving parenteral nutrition, those with poor hygiene, those who have undergone multiple abdominal operations, neutropenic patients in the setting of chemotherapy, and those with a prolonged ICU stay, defined as greater than 7 days [1, 2].

The presence of indwelling catheters in moist areas as well as failure to adhere to sterile techniques during catheter care can predispose these patients to *Candida* colonization. The GI tract also serves as a reservoir for candida organisms, and overgrowth can be precipitated in critically ill patients through changes in GI flora due to prolonged ileus, as well as prolonged antiacid and antibiotic use [1].

Subtypes

There are hundreds of different species of *Candida* but only nine that are clinically significant and pathogenic to humans. Some of these species include *C. albicans*, *C. glabrata,* and *C. krusei*,

A. Salim et al. (eds.), *Surgical Critical Care Therapy*, https://doi.org/10.1007/978-3-319-71712-8_41

although the majority of the diseases are caused by *C. albicans*. However, with increasing resistance to antifungal therapies, these rare species of *Candida* are becoming increasingly prevalent.

C. glabrata infections are more commonly seen in older patients and transplant recipients. *C. krusei* infections, on the other hand, are seen in the setting of prior antifungal use, hematologic malignancies, neutropenic patients, and patients with ongoing corticosteroid use. Patients affected with *C. krusei* also tend to be much younger and less likely to have concomitant bacterial infections. *C. parapsilosis* are seen in patients with recent surgery while *C. tropicalis*, although less common, are most virulent and indicative of concurrent invasive infection. *Candida* infections can occur in the bloodstream, respiratory mucosa, and urine with or without endophthalmitis, with varying severity [1, 2].

Aspergillosis

Epidemiology: Incidence, Mortality

Aspergillosis infection can be devastating and associated with significant morbidity and mortality. In the ICU setting, *Aspergillus* may harbor in the ICU ventilation and water systems that have been poorly maintained and various other equipment. The lowest incidence for invasive aspergillosis is reported in HIV patients and in patients with hematologic malignancy, which is 0.4%. The incidence in solid organ transplant recipients is more variable, 0.1– 2.4%. Overall mortality rates are about 17% and can rise to more than 50% in transplant recipients [2, 3].

Risk Factors

Populations at risk for infections with aspergillosis are similar to the ones affected by *Candida* species. Notably neutropenic patients and transplant patients receiving corticosteroid therapy or antirejection medications are increasingly vulnerable. Specifically, patients receiving steroids are at increased risk for having cavitating lesions and aspergillomas, and neutropenic patients develop angioinvasive aspergillosis, as neutrophils play a pivotal role in disease clearance [2].

Subtypes

Aspergillosis can be caused by hundreds of molds, but the pertinent species affecting critically ill patients include *A. fumigatus*, *A. flavus,* and *A. terreus*. These species have a wide environmental distribution and can be found in the soil, water, and air as well as may colonize immunosuppressed patients.

Mucormycosis

Epidemiology: Incidence, Mortality

Mucorales are saprophytes with mortality ranging from 35% up to 70% in patients with existing malignancy [2].

Risk Factors

Populations at risk for infections include neutropenic patients, patients with diabetes mellitus, and patients with co-existing malignancy. Renal failure patients and those with penetrating trauma are also vulnerable.

Subtypes

Mucormycosis can be caused by hundreds of species but the pertinent species affecting critically ill patients include *Rhizopus, Mucor, and Rhizomucor.*

Common Diagnostics Tests

Despite the advent of newer technologies and diagnostics tests, blood cultures remain the gold standard to identify candidemia. Negative blood cultures do no entirely exclude an infection because the sensitivity is only about 50%, and cultures can take as long as 4 days to become positive. Thus, prompt treatment should be initiated based on clinical evaluation. Common serologic tests include galactomannan and1,3 B-D-glucan that can be obtained while awaiting blood cultures. Galactomannan is detected in body fluids and a galactomannan index is calculated based on the concentration. When a certain minimum threshold is surpassed, the diagnosis of invasive aspergillosis is made. B-D glucan is a cell wall component found in body fluid and indicates the probability of infection although it fails to discriminate between colonization and infection. Moreover, these tests are specific but they lack sensitivity [2]. Additionally, depending on the location of suspected infection, thoracentesis, interventional radiology guided drainage or aspiration, diagnostic paracentesis, or bronchoalveolar lavages can be obtained to help guide treatment decisions although these techniques are invasive. In cases of aspergillosis infection of the lung, radiographic signs such as the halo sign can be suggestive but not necessarily diagnostic. Moreover, histopathology can be useful in identifying certain species, e.g., periodic acid-Schiff stains for *Mucor*, and Grocott-methenamine-silver for yeastlike fungus *Pneumocystis jiroveci*.

Current Treatment Options

Optimization of treatment strategies in the context of fungal infections is extremely essential in order to avoid excessive medication use, which could ultimately lead to disease resistance. In recent years, several risk scores have been developed to help guide treatment strategies. While many have not been validated clinically, the Candida Score (CS) or the Candida Colonization Index (CCI) is one that is often utilized clinically. This is defined as the ratio of the number of culture-positive surveillance sites for *Candida* spp. over the number of sites cultured. If the ratio of CCI is greater than 0.4, preemptive antifungal therapy should be initiated [2, 4].

Candidiasis

Candidemia and invasive candidiasis are associated with varying degrees of mortality if untreated promptly. There are many treatment options for *Candida* infections including polyenes, triazoles, echinocandins, and flucytosine (oral). Triazoles include fluconazole, itraconazole, and voriconazole, and they inhibit fungal cytochrome P450. For this reason, they can be used as first-line treatment or empiric treatment although drug interactions are common. Of note, fluconazole has the greatest penetration into the cerebrospinal fluid. Echinocandins include caspofungin and micafungin, and these fungicidals inhibit the synthesis of beta-1,3-D-glucan, which results in fungal cell wall disruption. Polyenes include amphotericin B, which inhibits ergosterol, an essential component of fungal cell wall. *C. glabrata* and *C. krusei* species are most commonly treated with echinocandins listed above [1].

Candida in Blood

All patients with candidemia or invasive candidiasis should be treated with a loading dose of either fluconazole (triazoles) or caspofungin (echinocandins). In critically ill patients, patients with severe sepsis, and those with recent triazole exposure, echinocandins are preferred. This must be followed by repeat blood cultures, and treatment is continued for 10–14 days after the last positive blood culture or if clinical symptoms improve.

Candida in Urine

Candida is a common pathogen found in many ICU patients with urinary tract infections. Moreover, colonization of the urine by *Candida* is also seen in patients that have diabetes or those that routinely require catheterization. Treatment is not indicated unless the patient is immunosuppressed, in which case oral fluconazole is effective. Removal and replacement of the catheter is the most important treatment strategy.

Candida in Respiratory Mucosa

Oral candidiasis (thrush) is also common in ICU patients, especially those on the ventilator. Effective treatment involves nystatin suspensions, oral ketoconazole, fluconazole, or itraconazole. Oropharyngeal candidiasis should be treated with fluconazole for 7 days and perhaps beyond for immunocompromised patients. Treatment should be altered as needed if there is no interval improvement in symptoms, so as to avoid disease progression to esophageal candidiasis. Pneumonia due to *Candida* is very rare and growth of candida on respiratory cultures often represents contamination or colonization. No treatment is indicated in this case.

Candida in the GI Tract

While candida can be isolated in intraabdominal cultures, they are rarely the etiology of the infection especially when there are concurrent bacterial pathogens. In these circumstances, antifungal therapy should not be typically used. The only exceptions are when there is failed treatment of previous intraabdominal infection or when there is spillage of GI contents due to anastomotic leak. As previously mentioned, fluconazole is the preferred empiric treatment choice unless there is prior evidence of resistance. Intraabdominal abscesses due to fungi are associated with high failure rate when managed via percutaneous drainage, so most often operative drainage is utilized with antifungal therapy for definitive treatment. Renal patients with peritoneal dialysis catheters can develop candida infections as well. Treatment in this case involves fluconazole therapy and timely removal of catheter, which can be replaced once the infection clears [1].

Aspergillosis

Timely diagnosis and treatment of invasive aspergillosis is essential particularly because the infection is transmitted airborne and can lead to detrimental sequela if left untreated. Invasive pulmonary aspergillosis is the most common form of infection, which manifests initially as a pneumonia but can lead to thrombotic, hemorrhagic events or complicated necrotizing bronchopneumonia that eventually necessitates surgical treatment. In most cases, the first line of treatment is voriconazole, but it is associated with high treatment failures. The dose is initially administered intravenously as a loading dose of 6 mg/kg twice a day and then lowered to 4 mg/kg twice daily. Amphotericin B is another alternative antifungal that can be utilized with varying success. It is administered intravenously as liposomal amphotericin B in a dosage of 3–5 mg/kg/day usually. The duration of treatment is often variable, but patients should be treated for at least 6–12 weeks and perhaps longer in immunosuppressed patients. In cases of medically refractory infection or recurrent infection despite optimal treatment, surgical treatment with Clagett window is often performed [1, 2].

Mucormycosis

Like other fungal infections, infections with mucor warrant timely intervention. Amphotericin B is the preferred antifungal in most cases. Recommended doses include 1–1.5 mg/kg/day for the deoxycholate formulary. The duration for treatment is not established and so should be individualized for each patient depending on clinical response.

Role of Antifungal Prophylaxis

Routine use of antifungal prophylaxis is effective in reducing the incidence of fungal infections in selected high-risk patients, although its effect on overall mortality remains unclear. Widespread use of antifungal prophylaxis should be limited to carefully selected patients based on their clinical condition, in order to prevent the development of disease resistance and avoid unnecessary toxic exposure. Fluconazole can be used empirically for invasive candidiasis in patients recently undergoing abdominal surgery and/or those with recurrent GI perforations or leakages. In the ICU setting, empiric treatment for aspergillosis in patients with neutropenia is not common and not recommended [1, 2].

Common Viral Infections

While viral infections are common in the community and outpatient setting, they are less common in the ICU. However, viral infections can present in the ICU setting. These viral infections have a broad spectrum of presentation, from fulminant organ failure and shock, to chronic latent disease in immunosuppressed patients.

Respiratory Infections

Most viral respiratory infections seen in the ICU are community-acquired cases that evolve into lower respiratory disease that progresses into respiratory failure. In their most severe form, they can cause acute respiratory distress syndrome (ARDS) requiring prolonged mechanical ventilator dependence. Viral respiratory infections in some patients can be part of a larger community outbreak. Some of the more common viral pathogens causing respiratory infection in the ICU include influenza, respiratory syncytial virus (RSV), SARS, varicella-zoster virus (VZV), herpes simplex virus (HSV), adenovirus, and cytomegalovirus (CMV) [5, 6].

While most community-acquired pneumonia requiring ICU admission is bacterial, 3 to 10% of cases can be caused by viruses. The most common viral infection causing viral pneumonia is influenza A and B. Patients that are immunocompromised are more likely to have viral pneumonia caused by RSV, CMV, VZV, or adenovirus. In general, clinical presentation and radiographic findings for patients with viral pneumonia are not specific to viral infection and resemble bacterial respiratory infection. Respiratory viruses can also cause hospital- or ventilator-associated pneumonias [5, 6].

Central Nervous System

Viral infections of the central nervous system can cause inflammation of the meninges and brain parenchyma. In the ICU setting, these can present as meningitis, encephalitis, seizure, coma, or neuromuscular weakness. In most cases of viral infection of the central nervous system, a specific cause is not found. In cases, where the specific pathogen is determined, the most common causes are HSV and VZV. Other less common pathogens associated with central nervous system infection include enteroviruses, arboroviruses, influenza, CMV, mumps, measles, rubella, and rabies [7, 8].

Cardiac Infections

Viral myocarditis can be the cause of cardiogenic shock in the ICU setting. These patients will present with clinical findings consistent with heart failure. More severe cases can require mechanical assist device support. Coxsackievirus groups A and B can cause viral myocarditis, but several other pathogens are also known to cause myocarditis such as influenza, adenovirus, parvovirus, RSV, CMV, HIV, and echovirus [8, 9].

Abdomen

The vast majority of abdominal infections seen in the ICU are caused by bacterial pathogens. CMV colitis can occur in immunocompromised hosts such as transplant recipients or patients with HIV/AIDS with low CD4 counts. CMV colitis can present with fever, weight loss, abdominal pain, and diarrhea. More severe forms of the disease may present with colon ulceration or toxic megacolon with perforation. Typical findings on endoscopic exam include patchy erythema of the colon with ulcerations. Inclusion bodies are seen on histopathological examination [10].

Viral hepatitis in the ICU setting is most commonly seen in chronic hepatitis C patients at end stages of liver disease. Acute viral hepatitis outbreaks in the ICU caused by hepatitis A or B infection, while still possible, have become more rare with more modern infection control practices [11].

Common Diagnostic Tests

Diagnostic testing for viral infection is organ specific and centered around obtaining culture and molecular detection data. Patients with respiratory infections will often show evidence of an infiltrate on X-ray or CT scan. Viral infection can be a diagnosis of exclusion, with clinical findings of infection with negative bacterial or fungal cultures. CMV colitis has typical findings on endoscopy and histopathology that are discussed above. Viral serologies in viral hepatitis infection can make a diagnosis of viral hepatitis [8].

Current Treatment Options

Treatment of viral infections in the ICU is centered around early diagnosis, supportive care, and antiviral agents. Treatment of herpesvirus infection can be treated with acyclovir, ganciclovir, or valacyclovir and valganciclovir. Acyclovir and valacyclovir can be also used against HSV, VZV, and EBV. CMV can be treated with acyclovir, ganciclovir, and foscarnet. Amantadine can be used against influenza A, and ribavirin can be used against RSV.

Role of Antiviral Prophylaxis

Patients who are immunocompromised due to solid organ transplant are often on prophylactic antiviral medications to prevent viral infection. Antiviral medications can be used to suppress latent and/or chronic viral infections in organ transplant recipients. In addition, they can be used to prevent transmission of viral infections to seronegative transplant recipients. Viruses that are common and that can warrant prophylactic antiviral therapy include CMV, VZV, HSV, and EBV. Solid organ transplant recipients should also receive Influenza vaccination prophylaxis [12].

Oddball Infections

Oddball infections in the context of critically ill patients are rare but can present with significant diagnostic and management challenges. They represent a spectrum of rare pathogens, including parasites, viruses, fungus, and bacteria. Some of these infections include cryptococcosis, blastomycosis, histoplasmosis, and coccidioidosis. Often, diagnosis is delayed because symptoms tend to be atypical in most patients. These infections are diagnosed by a variety of means including blood, urine, and respiratory cultures, as well as radiography, similar to fungal and viral infections. In certain circumstances, coinfection with bacteria, virus, or fungus is also possible, so treatment decisions are made on a case-by-case basis, usually with the assistance of infectious disease specialists.

Immunosuppressed Patients

As previously discussed, these patients are increasingly susceptible to bacterial, fungal, and viral infections. These patients include those on corticosteroid therapy, neutropenic patients, and transplant patients on antirejection therapy. Neutropenia can be a result of blood disorders such as leukemia, aplastic anemia, and ongoing or recent chemotherapy. In these patients, enteric gram-negative bacilli, *Pseudomonas aeruginosa*, *Staphylococcus aureus,* and *Aspergillus* commonly cause infections.

Likewise, patients who lack the ability to mount a cell-mediated response to infection, such as those with lymphoma, on chronic corticosteroid use and chemotherapy, are also vulnerable. Infection in this unique cohort is often due to *Pneumocystis jiroveci*, *Legionella*, herpes, coccidioidomycosis, and *Cryptococcus*. In patients with lack of humoral response to infection, such as those with multiple myeloma, chemotherapy, and post-splenectomy, *Streptococcus pneumonia*, *Haemophilus influenza*e, and enteric gram-negative bacilli infections are common. Treatment decisions should be carefully weighed in these patients because most often, these patients lack the immune reserve to mount a response to ongoing infection. Thus, empiric treatment, as previously described, should be initiated when a particular infection is suspected as delay in treatment could have adverse consequences on the patient. Adjunctive therapy with GCSF (granulocyte colony-stimulating factor) or interferon gamma can be utilized and recommended.

Conclusions

Timely diagnosis and treatment of fungal and viral infections in the ICU setting is essential to improve patient morbidity and mortality. Sometimes, diagnosis can be challenging or difficult to establish for multiple reasons. This chapter highlights the common infections affecting critically ill patients and pertinent treatment strategies to utilize when viral and fungal infections are suspected.

References

1. Cameron JL, Cameron AM. Current surgical therapy. 10th ed. Philadelphia: Elseiver Saunders; 2011. ISBN: 978-1-4377-0823-3.
2. Matthaiou DK, Christodoulopoulou T, Dimopoulos G. How to treat fungal infections in ICU patients. BMC Infect Dis. 2015;15:205.
3. Tong KB, Lau CJ, Murtagh K, et al. The economic impact of aspergillosis: analysis of hospital expenditures across patient subgroups. Int J Infect Dis IJID Off Publ Int Soc Infect Dis. 2009;13(1):24–36.
4. Pittet D, Monod M, Suter PM, et al. Candida colonization and subsequent infections in critically ill surgical patients. Ann Surg. 1994;220(6):751–8.
5. Stollenwerk N, Harper RW, Sandrock CE. Bench-to-bedside review: rare and common viral infections in the intensive care unit--linking pathophysiology to clinical presentation. Crit Care. 2008;12(4):219.
6. Mandell LA, Wunderink RG, Anzueto A, et al. Infectious Diseases Society of America/American Thoracic Society consensus guidelines on the management of community-acquired pneumonia in adults. Clin Infect Dis. 2007;44(Suppl 2):S27–72.
7. Kramer AH. Viral encephalitis in the ICU. Crit Care Clin. 2013;29(3):621–49.
8. Kelesidis T, Mastoris I, Metsini A, et al. How to approach and treat viral infections in ICU patients. BMC Infect Dis. 2014;14:321.
9. Liu P, Martino T, Opavsky MA, et al. Viral myocarditis: balance between viral infection and immune response. Can J Cardiol. 1996;12(10):935–43.
10. Rafailidis PI, Mourtzoukou EG, Varbobitis IC, et al. Severe cytomegalovirus infection in apparently immunocompetent patients: a systematic review. Virol J. 2008;5:47.
11. Soultati A, Dourakis S. Liver dysfunction in the intensive care unit. Ann Gastroenterol. 2005;18(1):35–45.
12. Slifkin M, Doron S, Snydman DR. Viral prophylaxis in organ transplant patients. Drugs. 2004;64(24):2763–92.

Postoperative Intra-abdominal Infection

42

Paul B. McBeth and Andrew W. Kirkpatrick

Introduction

Abdominal surgery is by definition invasive and thus carries the risk of postoperative intra-abdominal infection (PIAI) necessitating difficult therapeutic management. Infectious complications are the main cause of postoperative morbidity in abdominal surgery. Mortality from intra-abdominal sepsis depends on severity and ranges from 7.5% to 43% [1]. Despite many advances, postoperative intra-abdominal infections are common after both elective and emergency surgery. The assessment and evaluation of patients suspected of having postoperative infections are often challenging. A high index of suspicion is required. The use of prophylactic antibiotics has decreased the incidence of abdominal infections; however, there exists a growing challenge in managing multiresistant organisms. Thus the corollary to the importance in administering appropriate antibiotics early is not to needlessly administer or prolong inappropriate antibody therapy. Thus, knowledge of common postoperative complications and having a specific management approach is essential for all physicians caring for postoperative patients. In this chapter, we will discuss the evaluation of patients with suspected postoperative abdominal infections. A review of likely etiologies, common diagnoses, and therapeutic approaches is provided. These principles will provide the foundations for management of patients with PIAI. The fundamental principles of management of intra-abdominal infections are predicated on early clinical recognition and diagnosis followed by goal-directed resuscitation, broad-spectrum antimicrobial therapy, and early source control.

P. B. McBeth (✉)
Departments of Surgery and Critical Care Medicine, Foothills Medical Centre, Calgary, AB, Canada

A. W. Kirkpatrick
Regional Trauma Services, Departments of Surgery, Critical Care Medicine, University of Calgary, Calgary, AB, Canada

Risk Factors for Postoperative Intra-abdominal Infections

Certain characteristics make one more vigilant at the bedside. Factors that raise concerns for and may influence the severity of an event can be considered as either patient-specific or procedural-specific factors. Patient factors contributing to increased risk of intra-abdominal infections include diabetes, immune deficiency (long-term steroids, immunosuppressive therapy), smoking, elderly, functional status, frailty, obesity, and malnutrition. Procedural factors contributing to increased risk of intra-abdominal infections include poor blood supply, excess suture tension, degree of contamination, hypotension, hypothermia, use of vasopressors, and emergency surgeries lasting more than 2 h.

Strategies to Avoid Postoperative Infections

Any infection is easier to treat if it never occurs in the first place. The prevention of PIAI is thus an area of expanding research. The basic principles of infection prevention are as follows:

- Preoperative weight control
- Optimal nutritional status including the early administration of feeding postoperatively if possible
- Bowel preparation in selected cases (recognizing some controversies that exist)
- Correction of anemia
- Prophylactic use of antibiotics
- Minimizing tissue handling
- Minimizing operative time while maintaining attention to detail
- Reduced blood loss
- Smoking cessation

A. Salim et al. (eds.), *Surgical Critical Care Therapy*, https://doi.org/10.1007/978-3-319-71712-8_42

Characterization of Postoperative Infections

When a PIAI occurs or is suspected, it is important to understand the clinical and technical details of the original surgery are important as these will relate to the risk of occurrence and often dictate the subsequent clinical course. A relative advantage that surgical intensivists have is being familiar with the actual surgical procedures conducted on the patients who subsequently develop PIAI requiring critical care. A useful classification tool developed by the American College of Surgeons and based on the pioneering efforts of Simmons forms the basis of surgical wound classification and the evaluation of surgical site infections [2]. The classification system is based on four classes outlined in Table 42.1.

Evaluation of the Postoperative Abdomen Infection

Recognizing and making the diagnosis of PIAI are essential to minimize patient morbidity and mortality. However, the diagnosis of an intra-abdominal infection in the postoperative period may be difficult. Delays in source control may make the difference between a minor setback in recovery and spiraling multisystem organ dysfunction (MSOD). A detailed evaluation of a patient's history of presenting illness, a thorough knowledge of the procedure performed, a comprehensive physical exam, and a review of laboratory investigations and diagnostic imaging are needed to evaluate patients with suspected PIAI. When the anticipated progress of a postoperative patient deviates from that expected, a high index of suspicion is important to potentially permit rapid diagnosis and treatment.

PIAI should be considered in patients with a deteriorating clinical condition following abdominal surgery. Such postoperative intra-abdominal infections can arise from a variety of sources including perforated viscous, ischemic bowel, anastomotic failure, or biliary leakage. Generalized or local peritonitis developing postoperatively is always concerning. Infected fluid collections will typically form an abscess after 5–7 days, again. Therefore, even despite the most vigilant bedside care, the diagnosis may be unclear. We believe that liberal use of cross-sectional imaging such as CT scan should be made, as many abscesses are only detected this way.

Table 42.1 Surgical wound classification

Class I: Clean
Uninfected operative wound where no inflammation is encountered.
The respiratory, GI, genital, and urinary tracts are not entered.
Wounds are primarily closed. Drains are connected to a closed system.
Risk of infection: 2% or lower.
Class II: Clean/contaminated
Operative wound that enters the respiratory, GI, genital, or urinary tract under controlled conditions
No contamination or major break in surgical technique
Risk of infection: 5–15%
Class III: Contaminated
Open wound from surgery with a major break in sterile technique or gross spillage from GI tract
Acute nonpurulent inflammation of operative site
Risk of infection: > 15%
Class IV: Dirty/infected
Old traumatic wounds with retained devitalized tissue
Procedures with existing clinical infection or perforated viscera
Risk of infection: > 30%

History

Patients with suspected PIAI require a careful review of the presenting illness and the index surgical procedure and a review of the intra- and postoperative course. A detailed review of medications, allergies, and immunosuppressive treatments is required. Patient complaints should be identified in detail such as nausea, vomiting, fever/chills, bloating, dysuria or urinary retention, unexplained pleural effusion, and change in bowel function (diarrhea). A full characterization of abdominal pain is also required. Persistent abdominal pain and focal tenderness combined with spiking fevers, tachycardia, and a prolonged ileus suggest an intra-abdominal infection in patients with recent abdominal surgery. Patients under sedation in critical care units are more difficult to elicit complaints and therefore require a careful review of their course in ICU including hemodynamic status, and medications and tolerance to enteral feeds are required. Conversely, the uncomplicated tolerance of enteral feeds in any critically ill patient is very reassuring and generally directs attention away from the abdomen. These details are helpful to focus diagnostic and therapeutic interventions. Clinical factors predicting failure of source control for intra-abdominal infections are outlined in Table 42.2 [3].

Table 42.2 Clinical factors predicting failure of source control for intra-abdominal infection [4]

Delay in the initial intervention (>24 h)
High severity of illness (APACHE II score > 5)
Advanced age
Comorbidity and degree of organ dysfunction
Low albumin level
Poor nutritional status
Degree of peritoneal involvement or diffuse peritonitis
Inability to achieve adequate debridement or control of drainage
Presence of malignancy

Physical Examination

The physical examination begins with reviewing the vital signs. Unexplained tachycardia especially if new may represent infection, as do high-spiking fevers. Hypotension is extremely concerning, carries a high risk of death, and demands both urgent interventions and an explanation as to the presumed cause. Similarly, a new spontaneous onset of intra-abdominal hypertension (IAH) must be explained in any postoperative patient as this may be a hard sign of PIAI. Physical examination of patients with a suspected PIAI can be a challenge, particularly those patients who are critically ill who maybe sedated, paralyzed, and intubated. Further, it has been shown that physical examination has poor performance in determining the IAP. Thus, we believe routinely measuring IAP is required in all critically ill patients. A thorough review of current and recorded vital signs will help determine the clinical course of a patient. A detailed examination of the patient is required to determine volume status and sources of nonsurgical site infections and surgical site infection. Assessment of intravascular volume status and hemodynamics of a patient will help guide appropriate fluid resuscitation. The abdominal exam should include a careful inspection of the incision site for increased pain and redness, cellulitis, delayed healing, foul smell or wound drainage, and viability of the facial closure. This examination will help confirm a suspected diagnosis or guide appropriate diagnostic investigations. A focused examination of the abdomen can also illicit important underlying pathology. The presence of bowel sounds does not always correlate with normal bowel function. Abdominal wall guarding or rigidity may indicate peritoneal irritation. We also consider surgeon-performed bedside ultrasound as a simple extension of the physical examination which will be elaborated upon.

Laboratory Investigations

The diagnostic work-up of a patient with suspected PIAI requires a selection of laboratory investigations. A complete blood count (CBC) including hematocrit, hemoglobin, platelets, and white blood cell count with differential is routine. Infectious work-up should include cultures of all sources of fluid (blood, urine, abdominal drains). Serum amylase may be increased in patient with pancreatitis, ischemic bowel disease, and a perforated ulcer. Serum lipase is a specific marker of acute pancreatitis. An elevated serum bilirubin level is associated with sepsis, resolving hematoma, hemolysis, and hepatobiliary disease. During resuscitation of a septic patient, laboratory data will help guide management and correction of fluids, electrolytes, and acid-base derangements. Although a number of biomediators have been investigated, for their utility at diagnosing infection earlier, prognosticating infection, or distinguishing sterile from septic inflammation, none are clearly superior to more traditional laboratory tests [4].

Diagnostic Imaging

Modern diagnostic imaging techniques are essential in the evaluation and management of patients with PIAI. The most common modalities used are plain X-ray, CT scan, and ultrasound, with abdominal CT being the mainstay of diagnosis.

Standard abdominal X-rays can be used for the evaluation of free air, postoperative ileus, bowel obstruction, and fecal loading. They have the benefit of being portable and available at the patient's bedside. Abdominal X-rays are most commonly used to determine the position of intra-abdominal tubes, excluding retained foreign objects, and to evaluate abnormal intra-abdominal gas patterns.

Cross-sectional imaging involving CT scan is the mainstay for evaluation of PIAI, however, as it provides greater detail of intra-abdominal organs and pathology than standard abdominal X-rays or ultrasound [5–9]. Contrast enhancement with intravenous, oral, and rectal contrast can help characterize vascular structures and enhance intra-abdominal anatomy. Oral and rectal contrast can further help detect the presence of anastomotic leak, as differentiation of fluid-filled extra-luminal structure from a normal intestine is enhanced with oral contrast. Caution with oral contrast must be taken in patients with ileus to avoid aspiration. Intra-abdominal free fluid can be characterized as ascites or blood based on Hounsfield units. Postoperative tissue edema is reduced along with reabsorption of nonsuppurative fluid by postoperative day 7. In most postoperative patients, signs of intra-abdominal abscesses will develop after 4–5 days. Suspicious features on CT suggestive of an intra-abdominal abscess are contrast enhancement of the cavity wall, the presence of debris, loculations, and extra-luminal gas. Inflammatory edema and stranding in the adjacent tissues are features which help support the diagnosis of an intra-abdominal abscess. Once the diagnosis of an abscess has been established, then CT- or US-guided percutaneous drainage is routinely performed unless there is an anatomic or physical contraindication to proceeding.

Point-of-care ultrasonography is an essential adjunct for diagnostic and interventional procedures in the ED, ICU, and OR. It has the advantage of being portable with capabilities of providing diagnostic evaluation of intra-abdominal organ pathology. This technology is less expensive than CT but relies on an experienced and trained user for image acquisition and interpretation. Ultrasound is highly sensitive for detection of intra-abdominal fluid. In the postoperative period, however, bowel distention is common and often limits the interpretability and diagnostic capabilities of ultrasonography. Even in the presence of a "gaseous" abdomen, sonographic windows may be located in gravitationally dependent locations, and there is no contraindication to attempting visualization except for emergent time-critical situations.

Treatment of Postoperative Abdomen Infection

Management of PIAI currently requires concurrent resuscitation for any hemodynamic compromise, early administration of broad-spectrum antibiotics, and source control. Mortality rates in patients with intra-abdominal infections have improved with advances in critical care, availability of broad-spectrum antibiotics, improved nutrition, and earlier recognition and diagnosis. Initial management is outlined in Fig. 42.1 [3].

Resuscitation

Early goal-directed therapies should be initiated in patients with suspected intra-abdominal infection or sepsis [10]. It is critical, however, not to over-resuscitate, especially with crystalloid fluids, any patient with postoperative IAS, as they are physiologically "leaky" with global endothelial dysfunction and tend to be immunologically "primed" to undergo physiological tertiary, quaternary "hits" with massive edema generation if over-resuscitated. Cases of abdominal compartment syndrome, formally epidemic in critical care units, are now much less common but are still seen if resuscitation fluids are not carefully titrated to effect as any medication should be [11–13].

Antibiotics

Pharmacologic therapy involves the empiric administration of antibiotics and at least a consideration of immunoglobulins if there is a suspicion of a potential toxigenic infective organism [14, 15]. At present, despite decades and billions of dollars in research and development, pharmacologic or biologic approaches do not have utility in improving outcomes in cases of PIAS. Attempting to derive pharmacologic therapies for combating post-infective inflammation has proved to be an incredibly expensive and frustrating process so far. There have been literally 100 s of failed anti-mediator trials and even the one potential promising drug APC, being taken

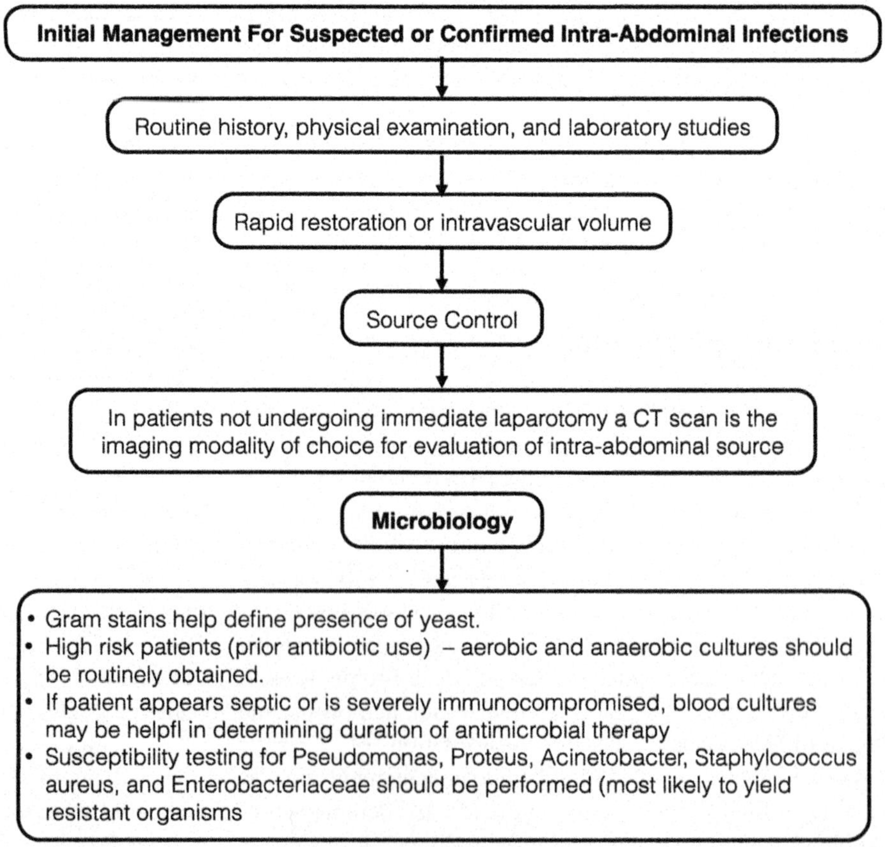

Fig. 42.1 Early management of intra-abdominal infections (Adapted from IDSA – Complicated Intra abdominal Infection – In Adults, http://www.idsociety.org)

off the market [16]. Over 100 attempts at blocking single biological response mediators have failed examining the early cytokine storm of sepsis [17]. Thus, in 2017 it is readily apparent that attempt to neutralize, block, or promote a single biomediator(s) after they have been generated is not currently helpful, and more integrated approaches to understanding and hopefully addressing the complex mediator interactions will be required to fundamentally improve outcomes in PIAS [18].

In patients with suspected PIAI, the initial empiric therapy must be directed against a mixture of aerobic (Gram-positive and Gram-negative bacteria) and anaerobic organisms. The microbiology of abscesses is dependent on the organ involved and duration of critical illness. Figure 42.2 outlines the antibiotic management guidelines of patients with community acquired intra-abdominal infections [3]. Antimicrobial therapy is accomplished with antibiotic combination therapy or with broad-spectrum single-agent therapy. The results of cultures retrieved by source control should be used to target therapy for the patient. Review of local resistance patterns is also required when selecting appropriate antibiotic coverage.

Antibiotics: Special Circumstances

Intra-abdominal Candidiasis

Abdominal candidiasis is rare and most commonly seen in patients following major abdominal surgery or trauma. The incidence depends on the presence of immunodeficiency or prolonged exposure to antibiotics. Routine treatment for *Candida* spp. isolated in uncomplicated repair of an intra-abdominal perforation is not recommended in healthy patients. Surgical source control with elimination of contaminated peritoneal fluid is essential in the treatment of intra-abdominal candidiasis. Pharmacologic therapy using fluconazole or amphotericin B is recommended [19–21]. However, when PIAS is unexplained, unusually severe, or not responsive, *Candida* should be considered as being possibly causative or at least complicating.

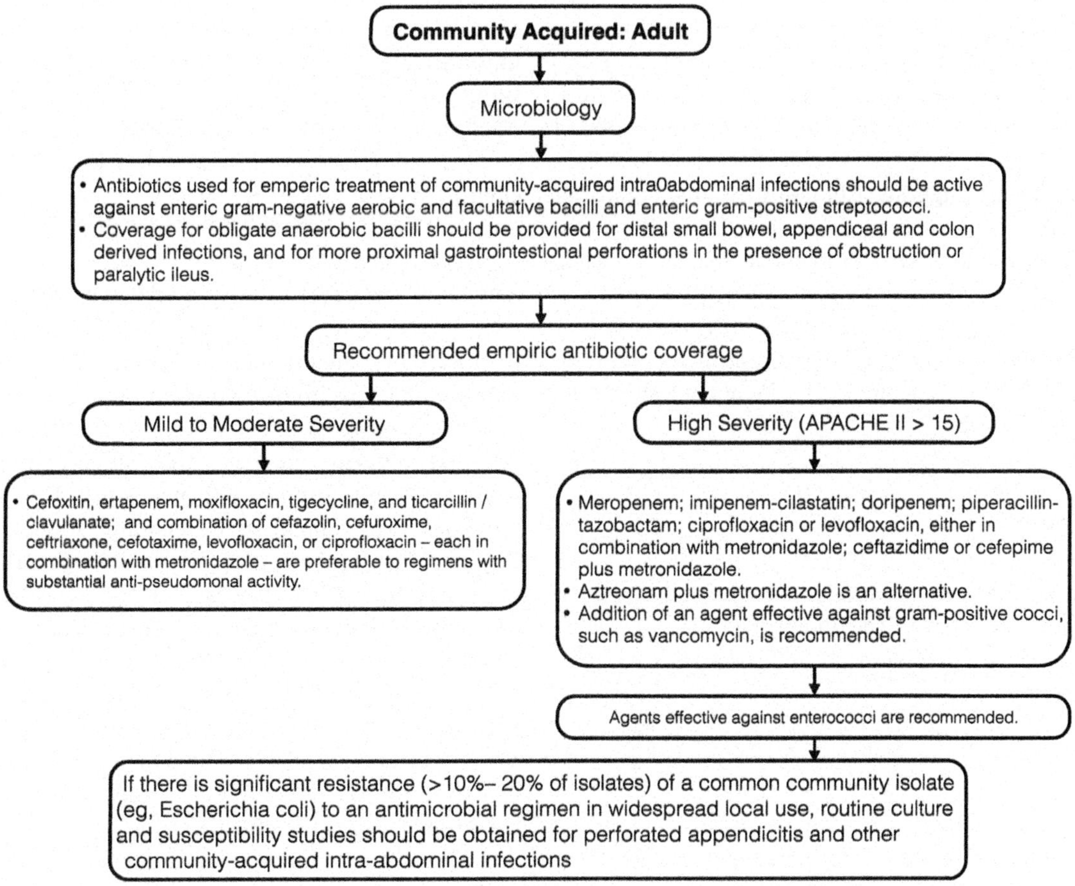

Fig. 42.2 Microbiology and management of intra-abdominal infections (Adapted from IDSA – Complicated Intra-abdominal Infection – In Adults, http://www.idsociety.org)

Antimicrobial Resistance in Intra-abdominal Infections

The empirical use of antibiotics for PIAI must consider risk factors for the likelihood of resistant pathogens, resistant microorganism colonization, prolonged hospitalization, and previous use of antibiotics. The emergence of resistant microorganisms often limits the choice of antibiotic coverage. This challenge is generally limited to patients with complicated intra-abdominal infections [22–24]. Knowledge of local resistance patterns is important since they may differ substantially between hospitals. In patients with prolonged hospitalization or prior antibiotic exposure, antibiotic treatment should include antipseudomonal coverage. Routine coverage against enterococcal is not required in patients with uncomplicated intra-abdominal infections. However, indications for enterococcal coverage include (1) patients in septic shock with previous treatment using cephalosporins, (2) immunosuppressed patients, (3) presence of prosthetic heart valves, and (4) recurrent intra-abdominal infection with severe sepsis [25, 26].

Duration of Antimicrobial Therapy

The duration of antimicrobial therapy is dependent on a patient's clinical course. In patients with established intra-abdominal infections managed with early source control, antibacterial therapy can be safely stopped after resolution of clinical signs of infection [27]. Persistent sepsis after 7 days of antibiotic therapy suggests a failure of source control or another focus of hospital-acquired infection. Recurrent infections are less likely when symptoms such as fever and leukocytosis have resolved and bowel function has returned. Patients with *Candida* spp. and *Staphylococcus aureus* intra-abdominal infections required close monitoring for recurrent infection and bloodstream infections. Treatment should be continued for 2–3 weeks.

Source Control

Early source control of intra-abdominal infections is essential for improved survival. The three principles of source control are drainage, debridement, and restoration of anatomy and function.

Drainage

The primary goal is to drain all infected material from the abdomen. If not completely drained, source control will fail. Abscess drainage can be done surgically or percutaneously depending on the clinical severity of a patient's septic state or distribution of infected fluid and presence of anastomotic leak requiring surgical intervention. Patients with generalized peritonitis or hemodynamic instability with suspected intra-abdominal infection require emergent surgical exploration to identify the cause. The primary source of the infection is controlled by repair or resection followed by a thorough washout of the abdominal cavity. In patients with severe contamination and hemodynamically unstable, the abdominal cavity may be temporarily left open for additional washout in 24–48 h. This is our preferred approach but remains controversial. Management of the open abdomen is discussed below. In stable patients with localized collections, percutaneous abscess drainage is the preferred method in most situations provided adequate drainage is possible. Surgical drainage is indicated when percutaneous drainage fails or cannot be performed. Surgical drainage must be approached with caution as re-exploration of the abdomen maybe fraught with difficulty.

Debridement

Surgical debridement consists of removing dead tissue and foreign material from the abdominal cavity accomplished surgically. The extent of debridement is controversial. "Defibrination" with mechanical debridement of the bowel at laparotomy is not helpful and may lead to a catastrophic enterotomy that results in a fistula.

Restoration of Anatomy and Function

Restoration of anatomy and function is the final step in the management of intra-abdominal infections. This is the goal of the surgical intervention. In most patients it can be established during the first operation, but in some patients a damage control approach is necessary. The choice of the procedure will depend on the anatomic source of infection, degree of peritoneal inflammation and generalized septic response, patient's physiological reserve, and comorbidities. These factors must be considered when deciding whether to provide a bowel anastomosis, exteriorization of bowel, or temporary closure. Operative characteristics may serve as a guide to the surgeon on the decision to construct a protective stoma. The construction of a protective stoma relies on the surgeon's experience. Anastomotic leak risk factors for consideration are diabetes, tobacco and alcohol use, duration of surgery, intraoperative fecal spillage, duration of operation, blood transfusion, or rectal anastomoses.

The Gut Microbiome and Human Health

Clinicians should be aware, however, that in reality any human being is not living in isolation but is in reality a complex commensal organism in conjunction with trillions of microbiological organisms. Thus, clinicians should start to consider the microbiome of their patients, which is defined as all of the microbial consortia (both commensal and pathogenic bacteria, viruses, and fungi), their genes, their gene products (proteins, metabolites), their community structure (distribution, diversity, evenness), and the particulars of the environment in which they reside when they consider microbiological infection and treatment in their patients [28]. It is not only possible but likely that many of the current approaches to intestinal antisepsis prior to an IAS complication and the medical responses to these complications will radically alter with a great understanding of human physiology health in health and disease. As an example, antiseptic preparations for gastrointestinal surgery run counter to emerging concepts of intestinal microbiota health contributing to immune function and recovery from injury [28, 29]. In the future in addition to a beside presence diagnosing and resuscitation as surgeons have best done for generations, they may also need to consider a molecular, genetic, and functional understanding of the implications of IAS and both the contribution of the flora within and the heath of gastrointestinal tract to course of systemic sepsis and the homeostasis of the critically ill host in all aspects of treatment [28, 29].

The Open Abdomen: A Complication or an Adjunct to Severe Complicated Intra-abdominal Sepsis (SCIAS)

Outcomes are particularly poor in PIAS, when patients present with septic shock and outcomes are compounded by medical comorbidities and frailty. However, even young previously healthy patients can tragically die from postoperative IAS despite the best efforts of their caregivers when IAS is severe and complicated. The World Society of Emergency Surgery has defined severe IAS as being denoted by the presence of any organ dysfunction or positive qSOFA score (systolic blood pressure < 100 mmHg, respiratory rate > 22/min, altered mentation) and complicated with the presence of purulent, feculent, or enteric spillage over at least two intraperitoneal quadrants [30–32]. In such cases, despite the appeal of a single curative operation, re-laparotomy has been considered necessary to eliminate persistent peritonitis or new infectious foci [31, 33]. Until recently, two debated surgical approaches to ensuring source control in the peritoneal cavity consisted of "laparotomy on demand (LOD)" versus "planned re-laparotomy" (PRL). In a planned re-laparotomy strategy, re-laparotomy was routinely performed every 36–48 h in order to inspect, drain, and lavage the abdominal cavity until the intraoperative findings were negative for peritonitis. Re-laparotomy on demand offers repeat laparotomy only in those patients in whom the lack of clinical improvement or even clinical deterioration has suggested that ongoing peritonitis has resulted from either persistent peritonitis or a new infectious focus. The relative merits of either approach have been widely debated for many years but were best addressed by the large RCT conducted by van Ruler [34], which noted no difference in mortality between the two approaches, although the ROL strategy reduced direct medical costs by 23%. The equivalence in outcomes, coupled with an apparent cost savings, has generated consensus guidelines that recommended that LOD after laparotomy for peritonitis be adopted as the standard of care [35]. Upon critical review the mortality in this RCT of severe secondary peritonitis well illustrates the devastating nature of this disease with the resultant mortality of approximately 1/3 of all afflicted patients. No matter which cohort is considered, such a dismal outcome demands alternate approaches to attempt to save more lives. It should be clearly stated that in neither of these strategies was an open abdomen approach to intra-abdominal sepsis considered.

Secondary (and tertiary) IAS with severe complicated peritonitis ultimately remains a surgical disease. Thus, if reoperation is required for postoperative IAS, the morbid but potentially lifesaving technique of adopting an open abdomen may be a valuable adjunct to management. The focused aim is to arrest the physiologic insult of severe trauma which most often includes hemorrhage and resultant progressive ischemia. Although not typically due to hemorrhage, SCIAS also induces progressive ischemia and tissue damage that must be reversed as soon as possible for patient survival. Ultimately this organ dysfunction is associated with a progressive oxygen deficit, ongoing organ failure, and massive biomediator generation, in a progressive downward spiral. Nontrauma damage control surgery thus attempts to break this downward spiral, through emergent surgical intervention, aimed at controlling enteric leakage and removal of ischemic tissue, without regard to completing the formal laparotomy. It is increasingly being reported in uncontrolled series, as another potentially desirable option for the sickest SCIAS patients [30, 36–39]. Integration of OA in severe sepsis may allow early identification and increased drainage of any residual infection, control any persistent source of infection, more effectively remove biomediator-rich peritoneal fluid, enable prophylaxis against the abdominal compartment syndrome, and allow for the safe deferral of gastrointestinal reanastomosis. Compared to trauma patients, however, patients undergoing OA management for intra-abdominal sepsis have greater risks subsequent to OA utilization, including entero-atmospheric fistula (EAF), intra-abdominal abscesses, and lower rates of definitive fascial closure. Besides the practical need to avoid inducing IAH, a more fundamental attribute to consider offering an OA is the fact that OA with newer active negative peritoneal pressure therapy (ANPPT) may facilitate the delivery of a new novel therapy to the peritoneal cavity that of ANPPT [11, 35, 40]. Although unexplained, significantly improved survival with ANPPT does warrant further exploration as a means of breaking the progression toward MSOF and death in cases of severe SCIAS. Thus the lifesaving potential of ANNPT after laparotomy for SCIAS coupled with global clinical equipoise warrants a carefully conducted randomized prospective study.

Summary

Postoperative abdominal infections are common in trauma and acute care surgical patients. Therefore, in a patient with a deteriorating clinical presentation, physicians must have a high level of suspicion of an intra-abdominal source of infection. History and physical examination will guide further laboratory and diagnostic imaging investigations. Early fluid resuscitation, antibiotic administration, and source control are the foundations of treatment.

References

1. Dellinger EP, Wertz MJ, Meakins JL, et al. Surgical infection stratification system for intra-abdominal infection: multicenter trial. Arch Surg. 1985;120:21.
2. Simmons BP. Guideline for prevention of surgical wound infections. Infect Control. 1982;3:185–96.
3. Solomkin JS, Mazuski JE, Bradley JS, Rodvold KA, Goldstein EJ, Baron EJ, O'Neill PJ, Chow AW, Dellinger EP, Eachempati SR, Gorbach S, Hilfiker M, May AK, Nathens AB, Sawyer RG, Bartlett JG. Diagnosis and management of complicated intra-abdominal infection in adults and children: guidelines by the Surgical Infection Society and the Infectious Diseases Society of America. Clin Infect Dis. 2010;50(2):133–64.
4. Xiao Z, Wilson C, Robertson HL, Roberts DJ, Ball CG, Jenne CN, et al. Inflammatory mediators in intra-abdominal sepsis or injury - a scoping review. Crit Care. 2015;19(1):373.
5. Ogilvie H. Large intestine colic due to sympathetic deprivation: a new clinical syndrome. Br J Med. 1948;2:671.
6. Ponec RJ, Saunders MD, Kimmey MB. Neostigmine for the treatment of acute colonic pseudo-obstruction. N Engl J Med. 1999;341:137.
7. Edwards MS, Cherr GS, Craven TE, et al. Acute occlusive mesenteric ischemia: surgical management and outcomes. Ann Vasc Surg. 2003;17:72.
8. Birnabaum W, Rudy L, Wylie EJ. Colonic and rectal ischemia following abdominal aneurysmectomy. Dis Colon Rectum. 1964;7:293.
9. Stoney RJ, Cunningham CG. Acute mesenteric ischemia. Surgery. 1993;114:489.
10. Rivers E, Nguyen B, Havstad S, Ressler J, Muzzin A, Knoblich B, et al. Early goal-directed therapy in the treatment of severe sepsis and septic shock. N Engl J Med. 2001;345:1368–77.
11. Roberts DJ, Ball CG, Kirkpatrick AW. Increased pressure within the abdominal compartment: intra-abdominal hypertension and the abdominal compartment syndrome. Curr Opin Crit Care. 2016;22(2):174–85.
12. Malbrain ML, De Laet I. AIDS is coming to your ICU: be prepared for acute bowel injury and acute intestinal distress syndrome. Intensive Care Med. 2008;34(9):1565–9.
13. Malbrain ML, De Laet I. It's all in the gut: introducing the concept of acute bowel injury and acute intestinal distress syndrome. Crit Care Med. 2009;37(1):365–6.
14. Alejandria MM, Lansang MA, Dans LF, Mantaring JB. Intravenous immunoglobulin for treating sepsis, severe sepsis and septic shock. Cochrane Database Syst Rev. 2013;9:CD001090.
15. Laupland KB, Kirkpatrick AW, Delaney A. Polyclonal intravenous immunoglobulin for the treatment of severe sepsis and septic shock in critically ill adults: a systematic review and meta-analysis. Crit Care Med. 2007;35(12):2686–92.
16. Opal SM, Dellinger RP, Vincent JL, Masur H, Angus DC. The next generation of sepsis clinical trial designs: what is next after the demise of recombinant human activated protein C?*. Crit Care Med. 2014;42(7):1714–21.
17. Gentile LF, Moldawer LL. HMGB1 as a therapeutic target for sepsis: it's all in the timing! Expert Opin Ther Targets. 2014;18(3):243–5.
18. Malig MS, Jenne CN, Ball CG, Roberts DJ, Xiao Z, Kirkpatrick AW. High mobility group Box-1 protein and outcomes in critically ill surgical patients requiring open abdominal management. Mediat Inflamm. 2017;2017:1-8.
19. Pappas PG, Rex JH, Sobel JD, et al. Guidelines for treatment of candidiasis. Clin Infect Dis. 2004;38:161–89.
20. Holzheimer RG, Dralle H. Management of mycoses in surgical patients: review of the literature. Eur J Med Res. 2002;7:200–26.
21. Blot S, Vandewoude K. Management of invasive candidiasis in critically ill patients. Drugs. 2004;64:2159–75.
22. De Waele JJ, Vogelaers D, Hoste E, et al. Emergence of antibiotic resistance in infected pancreatic necrosis. Arch Surg. 2004;139:1371–5.
23. Blot S, Vandewoude K. Early detection of systemic infection. Acta Clin Belg. 2004;59:20–3.
24. Blot S, Depuydt P, Vogelaers D, et al. Colonization status and appropriate antibiotic therapy in nosocomial bacteremia caused by antibiotic-resistant gram- negative bacteria in an ICU. Infect Control Hosp Epidemiol. 2005;26:575–9.
25. Harbarth S, Cosgrove S, Carmeli Y. Effects of antibiotics on nosocomial epidemiology of vancomycin-resistant enterococci. Antimicrob Agents Chemother. 2002;46:1619–28.
26. Fernandez-Guerrero ML, Herrero L, Bellver M, et al. Nosocomial enterococcal endocarditis: a serious hazard for hospitalized patients with enterococcal bacteraemia. J Intern Med. 2002;252:510–5.
27. Solomkin JS, Mazuski JE, Baron EJ, et al. Guidelines for the selection of anti-infective agents for complicated intra-abdominal infections. Clin Infect Dis. 2003;37:997–1005.
28. Alverdy JC, Hyoju SK, Weigerinck M, Gilbert JA. The gut microbiome and the mechanism of surgical infection. Br J Surg. 2017;104(2):e14–23.
29. Guyton K, Alverdy JC. The gut microbiota and gastrointestinal surgery. Nat Rev Gastroenterol Hepatol. 2017;14(1):43–54.
30. Sartelli M, Catena F, Ansaloni L, Coccolini F, Corbella D, Moore EE, et al. Complicated intra-abdominal infections worldwide: the definitive data of the CIAOW Study. World J Emerg Surg. 2014;9:37.
31. Sartelli M, Abu-Zidan FM, Ansaloni L, Bala M, Beltran MA, Biffl WL, et al. The role of the open abdomen procedure in managing severe abdominal sepsis: WSES position paper. World J Emerg Surg. 2015;10:35.

32. Singer M, Deutschman CS, Seymour CW, Shankar-Hari M, Annane D, Bauer M, et al. The third international consensus definitions for sepsis and septic shock (Sepsis-3). JAMA. 2016;315(8):801–10.
33. Dellinger RP, Levy MM, Carlet JM, Bion J, Parker MM, Jaeschke R, et al. Surviving sepsis campaign: international guidelines for management of severe sepsis and septic shock: 2008. Crit Care Med. 2008;36(1):296–327.
34. van Ruler O, Mahler CW, Boer KR, Reuland EA, Gooszen HG, Opmeer BC, et al. Comparison of on-demand vs planned relaparotomy strategy in patients with severe peritonitis: a randomized trial. JAMA. 2007;298(8):865–72.
35. Kirkpatrick AW, Roberts DJ, De Waele J, Jaeschke R, Malbrain ML, De Keulenaer B, et al. Intra-abdominal hypertension and the abdominal compartment syndrome: updated consensus definitions and clinical practice guidelines from the World Society of the Abdominal Compartment Syndrome. Intensive Care Med. 2013;39(7):1190–206.
36. Khan A, Hsee L, Mathur S, Civil I. Damage-control laparotomy in nontrauma patients: review of indications and outcomes. J Trauma Acute Care Surg. 2013;75(3):365–8.
37. Leppaniemi A, Kimball EJ, De Laet I, Malbrain ML, Balogh ZJ, De Waele JJ. Management of abdominal sepsis--a paradigm shift? Anaesthesiol Intensive Ther. 2015;47(4):400–8.
38. Bruns BR, Ahmad SA, O'Meara L, Tesoriero R, Lauerman M, Klyushnenkova E, et al. Nontrauma open abdomens: a prospective observational study. J Trauma Acute Care Surg. 2016;80(4):631–6.
39. Goussous N, Jenkins DH, Zielinski MD. Primary fascial closure after damage control laparotomy: sepsis vs haemorrhage. Injury. 2014;45(1):151–5.
40. Roberts DJ, Zygun DA, Grendar J, Ball CG, Robertson HL, Ouellet JF, et al. Negative-pressure wound therapy for critically ill adults with open abdominal wounds: a systematic review. J Trauma Acute Care Surg. 2012;73(3):629–39.

New Fever in the Surgical Intensive Care Unit Patient

43

Evan Ross, Deidra Allison, Athena Hobbs, and Ben Coopwood

Introduction

Fever is defined as an increase in core body temperature above 38.3 °C (101 °F). It can be considered part of the body's adaptive and regulated response to infection, trauma, and tissue injury, or it can be considered maladaptive and dysregulated, as when caused by a drug side effect, venous thrombosis, thyroid storm, or a neurological injury [1]. Fever has been shown to enhance the immune response to invading pathogens, while on the other hand, fever increases cardiac output, oxygen consumption, carbon dioxide production, and energy expenditure, which can have untoward effects in those with poor cardiopulmonary reserve, those suffering from neurologic insult, and pregnant patients [2]. Determining the etiology of fever and the appropriate clinical treatment is therefore an important element in improving outcomes for critically ill patients.

Etiology

Fever is the result of an elevation in the body's thermal homeostatic set point that is maintained by the hypothalamus. This process is driven by receptors in the ventromedial preoptic area (VMPOA) of the hypothalamus in response to elevated levels of the prostaglandin E2 (PGE2) [3]. Pyrogens, a catch-all term for the broad set of small molecules that stimulate fever, cause circulating leukocytes to release cytokines IL-1, IL-6, and TNF-α into circulation [4]. These pyrogenic cytokines in turn drive the synthesis of phospholipase A2, which releases arachidonic acid from cell membranes, and cyclooxygenase-2, which converts the arachidonic acid into PGE2 [5]. These actions are inhibited by steroids and nonsteroidal anti-inflammatory drugs, respectively [6].

The PGE2 receptor family is highly conserved from mice to humans and includes four different subtypes, EP1–EP4 [7]. EP3, the PGE2 receptor in the VMPOA thought to be responsible for the induction of fever, is a G-protein-coupled receptor with up to eight possible isoforms that mediates a decrease in cyclic AMP [8]. In rats, the EP3-positive neurons in the VMPOA are GABAergic and project to both the rostral raphe pallidus nucleus (rRPN) as well as the dorsomedial hypothalamus (DMH) where they constitutively inhibit the function of excitatory neurons that drive brown adipose tissue thermogenesis and cutaneous vasoconstriction [9, 10]. The PGE2 signal releases the rRPN and the DMH from baseline inhibition, thus promoting thermogenesis [11].

Epidemiology of Fever

Depending upon the definition, elevated core body temperature will complicate the intensive care course of approximately 25% of all patients in the surgical ICU and approximately 40% of patients in the trauma ICU; of those patients who become febrile, approximately half will be found to have an infectious etiology and bacteremia will be present in approximately one quarter [12, 13]. Fever is more common in younger patients than older patients, and severe fever is a herald of poorer outcomes in surgical ICU patients [12].

E. Ross
Department of Surgery, The University of Texas Medical Branch, Galveston, TX, USA

D. Allison
Dell Seton Medical Center at University of Texas, Surgical Intensive Care Unit, Austin, TX, USA

A. Hobbs
Department of Clinical Pharmacy, Baptist Memorial Health Care & The University of Tennessee Health Science Center – Memphis, Memphis, TN, USA

B. Coopwood (✉)
Department of Surgery, Dell Medical School, University of Texas at Austin, Austin, TX, USA
e-mail: tbcoopwoodjr@seton.org

A. Salim et al. (eds.), *Surgical Critical Care Therapy*, https://doi.org/10.1007/978-3-319-71712-8_43

Definition

ACCCM and IDSA guidelines suggest the use of 38.3 °C (101 °F) as the threshold for triggering a clinical evaluation for a source of fever [14]. It is important to remember that infection can present with euthermia or low-grade temperatures in immunocompromised patients such as the elderly, patients receiving steroids and anti-inflammatory drugs, neutropenic patients, patients with an open abdominal wound, those with extensive burns, patients on ECMO, and patients receiving CRRT. As this population may have an impaired ability to increase their thermostatic set point, a temperature of 37.0 °C (100.4 °F) for more than 1 h should trigger further clinical evaluation.

In practical terms, it is useful to divide fever into early (first 48 h of hospitalization) versus late since, in the absence of pre-existing infection, early fevers are likely inflammatory unless a breach in sterile technique, aspiration pneumonia, or anastomotic leak are suspected. Fevers may also be classified as moderate (between 38.3 °C and 39.5 °C – 101 °F and 103.1 °F) versus severe (>39.5 °C - > 103.1 °F). While moderate fevers likely signal an appropriate immune response, severe fevers exceed the physiological range and should be considered maladaptive. Sever fevers should always be managed aggressively.

Finally we can divide fevers into infectious and noninfectious causes; while a fever of 38.3–38.9 °C may represent either infectious or noninfectious causes, fevers of 38.9–39.4 °C are rarely secondary to noninfectious causes with the exception of drug fever and posttransfusion fevers. Evaluation of fever in the surgical intensive care unit must take into consideration many factors such as onset relative to hospitalization, timing in relation to operative procedures, immune status, age, medications, indwelling line and catheters, therapeutic procedures, as well as previous infections and antibiotics usage. Therefore evaluation of fever requires a thorough review of the hospital course to include a review of injuries, operative procedures, pre-existing illnesses, temperature trend, previous cultures, radiologic studies, invasive lines/catheter insertion dates, and medication administrations throughout the hospital stay.

Monitoring

The bladder temperature represents the best combination of convenience and accuracy of all options for central temperature measurement and is our preferred method; other options include rectal and esophageal probes. In awake, non-intubated patients, oral or tympanic membrane measurements are acceptable alternatives.

Treatment

Whether or not to treat elevated body temperature remains controversial and depends upon the clinical circumstances; on the one hand, the pharmacologic control of fever in suspected infection has been assessed and found to offer no clear benefits, while on the other hand, external cooling has been shown to be beneficial in select circumstances [15]. When the fever is within the physiological range and is in response to infection, fever can be thought of as an adaptive response that facilitates clearance of the infection through various mechanisms. For instance, fever promotes leukocyte trafficking through the high endothelial venules of the lymphatic system [16], increases their phagocytic activity [17], enhances their motility [18], and increases their responsiveness to mitogens [19].

However, when the elevated temperature is supraphysiologic, as it often is in response to neurological injury, endocrine derangement, or adverse drug reaction, the fever should be considered maladaptive and attempts should be made to control it, whether via pharmacologic means or external cooling.

The pharmacologic treatment of fever revolves around the usage of antipyretic drugs, so-called because of their ability to interfere with the cascade of events leading to thermogenesis. The most efficacious medicine is acetaminophen, which is thought to exert its antipyretic effect via the semi-selective inhibition of COX-2-mediated PGE2 synthesis [20]. However, the capacity of acetaminophen to suppress PGE2 synthesis can be overwhelmed, obviating the antipyretic effect at therapeutic doses in certain cases – as in isolated neurotrauma.

Infectious Causes of Fever

Sepsis

New onset fever in the ICU should always raise the possibility of sepsis, though fever is not required for the diagnosis; nearly 10% of septic patients will be hypothermic at diagnosis [21]. Sepsis is defined as "life-threatening organ dysfunction caused by a dysregulated host response to infection [22]." It was the single most expensive condition to treat in hospitals in 2013, accounting for $23.7 billion (6.2% of total) in costs and requiring 1.3 million hospital stays [23]. Recent data estimates mortality from sepsis to be 29% across all settings [24].

The three fundamental principles of sepsis management in the surgical ICU are the early initiation of appropriate antibiotic therapy, infectious source control, and adequate hemodynamic support. Because the critically ill surgical patient has numerous potential sites of infection that could cause sepsis, initial antibiotic selection should be empiric, broad-spectrum therapy with antimicrobial activity against MRSA, pseudomonal species, and other gram-negative organisms. Our combination of choice is vancomycin and cefepime. Consideration should be given to covering for fungal infections as well, especially if the intestines have been violated by trauma or the threat of anastomotic leak is present.

A source of the sepsis should be determined and treated aggressively. While the most common cause of sepsis across all ICUs is pneumonia, a high index of suspicion for intra-abdominal catastrophe should be maintained for both postoperative and trauma patients as intra-abdominal processes are the second most common cause of sepsis and require intervention beyond the initiation of antibiotic therapy.

Aggressive fluid resuscitation is often required to maintain a mean arterial pressure $\geq$ 65 mmHg and a urine output of $\geq$0.5 ml/kg/hour. Administration of 5% albumin in saline should be considered as an adjunct to crystalloid for fluid resuscitation [25, 26]. We begin vasopressor support in patients who have been adequately volume resuscitated, as measured by a stroke volume variability of $\leq$10%, yet still show signs of shock [27]. Central venous pressure should not be used as a measure of volume status or as a predictor of fluid responsiveness [28, 29]. We begin vasopressor support with norepinephrine, titrated to a maximum dose of *** mcg/kg/min. If the patient remains in shock, we add vasopressin at a dose of 0.4 mcg/kg/min. As opposed to norepinephrine, we do not titrate the dose of vasopressin. If a third vasoactive medication is required, we add epinephrine and titrate to a maximum dose of *** mcg/kg/min.

Ventilator-Associated Pneumonia

Ventilator-associated pneumonia may develop in up to 20% of ventilated patients, cost between $10,000 and $40,000 extra per episode, and increase mortality rates from 10 to 50% [30, 31]. While various surveillance definitions exist for ventilator-associated pneumonia, the diagnosis and decision to treat are largely based on clinical characteristics.

When we suspect a respiratory infection to be the source of the fever, we begin by obtaining plain films of the chest. The presence of a new infiltrate is highly suspicious in the ventilated patient and prompts a microbiological analysis. We obtain qualitative cultures of the airway secretions by aspirating the endotracheal tube, an approach which has been shown to have equivalent outcomes to the quantitative culture of bronchoalveolar lavage fluid [32]. We also simultaneously obtain blood cultures, given the approximately 18% incidence of concomitant bacteremia, which requires a longer duration of antibiotic therapy [33, 34].

We empirically begin broad-spectrum antibiotics to cover MRSA and pseudomonal species – making use of the antibiogram to guide initial selection of medications; a usual combination for our center based upon local patterns of organism prevalence and resistance is vancomycin and cefepime. We continue broad-spectrum antibiotics until culture results are available, and we narrow or expand the antibiotic coverage to the narrowest possible spectrum of antimicrobial activity. If the culture results do not show any apparent pathogen (but rather show normal respiratory organisms), we discontinue antibiotic therapy. We treat ventilator-associated pneumonia with a total of 7 days of antibiotics [31].

Central Venous Catheter Management

In patients with a CVC or arterial catheter, a febrile episode should immediately prompt an assessment of the insertion site for signs of infection and consideration of obtaining blood cultures. If no other source for the fever is identified, we recommend drawing two blood cultures; one culture sample should be drawn through the catheter, while the other should be obtained via a peripheral stick. If the insertion site is purulent, a swab for culture and gram stain is also obtained. If the fever is moderate (below 39.5 °C or 103.1 °F) and there are no signs of organ dysfunction, the catheter can be left in place during the workup, while cultures are growing. If the catheter is thought to be infected, it should be replaced and the tip sent for culture. Alternatively, if the patient is in extremis, there are signs of organ dysfunction, or the fever is severe (above 39.5 °C or 103.1 °F), the catheter should be removed immediately after cultures are drawn and replaced, either in a new position or over a guidewire, and the tip should be collected in a sterile cup and sent for culture [35].

Urinary Catheter Management

While urinary tract infections (UTI) are the most common nosocomial infections in healthcare worldwide, they are an uncommon source of symptoms, fever, and septicemia in the ICU patient [36]. UTI should not be considered the infectious source of fever until all other possibilities are excluded.

In our center, the diagnostic workup for urinary tract infection begins by obtaining a urinalysis with microscopic analysis. If the UA shows >10 WBC per high-powered field, then the sample is reflexively sent for culture and gram stain, and antibiotics are started empirically. This is based on the fact that a WBC count below 10 per high-powered field has a 98.6% negative predictive value for a positive urinary culture result [37]. This rule should not be applied to neutropenic patients or patients who are otherwise immunosuppressed and incapable of mounting a leukocyte response to infection. An epithelial cell count serves as quality control, and if there are more than two per high-powered field, the sample is considered to have been contaminated and is re-collected.

Urinary tract infection is often suspected in catheterized patients. Complicating this diagnosis is the fact that catheterized patients have a high rate of asymptomatic bacteriuria. When we suspect UTI in a catheterized patient, we first assess the age of the catheter; catheters that have been in place for longer than 24 h are replaced prior to collection of the specimen. In patients with a culture-confirmed UTI and no other source of fever, we treat with 7 days of antibiotics beginning with an empiric selection based upon our antibiogram that we then narrow based on culture results [36].

C. difficile Infection and C. difficile Colitis

Diarrhea can be a common occurrence in hospitalized patient and occurs due to both infectious and noninfectious causes. According to the Centers for Disease Control, the most common cause of infectious diarrhea in the critically ill patient is *Clostridium difficile* infection. C. difficile, a spore forming gram-positive anaerobic bacillus, is transmitted via the fecal-oral route by spore ingestion. The spores are heat, acid, and antibiotic resistant and can survive on hospital surfaces for months. Infection with C. difficile most commonly occurs as a result of depletion of normal intestinal flora by antimicrobial drug therapy. This disruption of the intestinal microbiome allows C. difficile to grow unencumbered and inflame the gastrointestinal tract causing mucosal injury and fluid secretion. The exotoxins produced by the C. difficile bacteria, Toxin A and Toxin B, induce colonocyte death, loss of intestinal barrier, and neutrophilic colitis. The most prominent risk factor for C. difficile infection is antibiotic or chemotherapy administration within 60 day of the onset of symptoms. While any antibiotic can lead to C. difficile infection, the usual culprits are clindamycin, cephalosporins, and fluoroquinolones. Other risk factors for C. difficile infection include prolonged hospitalization, advanced age, and the usage of H2 blockers and proton-pump inhibitors.

C. difficile infection is usually characterized by loose stools, with or without blood or mucous, abdominal pain, leukocytosis, and fever. While diarrhea and fever are usually the hallmark signs of C. difficile infection, in the postoperative patient, C. difficile infection may instead present as a leukemoid reaction, ileus, or toxic megacolon.

The gold standard for diagnosing C. difficile infection is a tissue culture assay because it is highly sensitive and specific. However, due to long turnaround time, limited availability, and cost, it is not often employed. We utilize the GDH antigen (glutamate dehydrogenase), a metabolic enzyme expressed at high levels in all strains of C. difficile, and toxin A/B with reflex PCR to diagnose C. difficile. This test simultaneously detects the presence of GDH and toxins A and B in a single reaction. The nucleic acid amplification test is only utilized if the GDH antigen and A/B toxin test are discordant. Direct visualization of pseudomembranes via the use of sigmoidoscopy or colonoscopy is pathognomonic for C. difficile colitis but is only used in cases of severe illness in need of rapid diagnosis.

Oral metronidazole and vancomycin are the mainstays for treatment of C. difficile infection. In the case of complete ileus, rectal vancomycin can be considered. For severely ill patients, empiric antibiotic treatment should be initiated before laboratory confirmation. Care should be taken to avoid antiperistaltic agents as these may increase the risk of toxic megacolon and may mask worsening symptoms. Any unnecessary antibiotic should be discontinued immediately; if antibiotics are necessary to treat a confirmed infection, they should be discontinued as soon as clinically able.

In our institution, we continue C. difficile therapy for 10–14 days after other antibiotics are stopped. Recurrence is treated with the same antibiotic regimen initially used unless the severity has increased. For any subsequent reoccurrence, therapy is escalated to vancomycin if metronidazole has been used twice due to concerns for neurotoxicity; if vancomycin was used for prior treatment, then therapy is escalated to taper and/or pulse regimen. Operative management of C. difficile infection is reserved for severely ill patients with serum lactate >5 and WBC > 50,000.

Acute Acalculous Cholecystitis

Acute acalculous cholecystitis (AAC) is defined as acute cholecystitis in the absence of gallstones [38]. It is an increasingly recognized and fulminant complication of critical illness. Though it is rare, occurring in approximately 0.2–0.4% of all admissions to the ICU, it is highly lethal, with a mortality rate of approximately 30% [39]. The most common precipitating events (in descending order) are trauma, recent surgery, shock, burns, and sepsis [39].

AAC is likely due to a combination of bile stasis and ischemia of the gallbladder and presents with nonspecific findings, including fever, right upper quadrant pain, and jaundice [40]. There may be an associated transaminitis and leukocytosis, though diagnosis relies more on ultrasound imaging than on laboratory findings [39]. AAC is managed with percutaneous gallbladder drainage by the interventional radiologist.

Noninfectious Causes of Fever

SIRS/Postoperative Fever

The systemic inflammatory response syndrome (SIRS) is group of clinical signs exhibited in response to physiological stress. SIRS may be incited by both infectious and noninfectious causes. Noninfectious SIRS can be secondary to ischemia, acute trauma, burns, surgical procedures, endocrine derangements, immune system activation, critical illness, and various other types of cellular injury. These and other cytokines stimulate the production of a pro-inflammatory cytokine cascade that induces both a local and a systemic reaction. The local reaction involves the cardinal signs of inflammation: redness, swelling, pain, warmth, and loss of function, while the systemic response is manifested as fever, hypotension, procoagulant activity, muscle breakdown, catabolism, anorexia, heat conservation, and the release of stress hormones. Systemic activation also stimulates the production growth factor, activation of macrophages, and platelet activation. A counter-inflammatory response typically limits the SIRS response by producing IL-4 and IL-10, the antagonists to TNFα and IL-1. The SIRS response is propagated when this negative feedback mechanism fails, and continued inflammation leads to tissue destruction, humoral cascade activation, activation of the reticular endothelial system, tissue hypoxia, and subsequent end-organ dysfunction.

SIRS is clinically defined as the presence of two or more of the following symptoms: temperature > 38.5 °C or <36 °C, heart rate > 90 BPM, respiratory rate > 20 breaths per minute or pCO_2 < 32 mmHg, or WBC count >12,000 cells/ml or <4000 cells/ml or 10% bands (bone). Patients who undergo surgical procedures will often meet SIRS criteria solely due to activation of the inflammatory cascade due to tissue injury. Short of a break in sterile technique or suspected aspiration, fever in the first 48 h post-op is rarely secondary to infection; infection secondary to indwelling urinary catheters, surgical site infections, and pneumonia will typically take 48–72 h to incubate unless the condition existed prior to the operative procedure.

Treatment of fever in the immediate postoperative period is largely supportive unless there are obvious signs of infection present. The use of antipyretics such as acetaminophen and ibuprofen is typically effective. Medication review to rule out drug fever as well as review of transfusion records to rule out transfusion reaction should be done in cases of fever >38.9. Additional environment cooling may also be helpful but care must be taken to avoid shivering. Continued assessment for infection and other noninfectious etiologies is pertinent for fever lasting longer than 96 h.

Blood Transfusion

We will focus on the two adverse reactions to blood transfusion that result in fever, the febrile non-hemolytic transfusion reaction (FNHTR) and the hemolytic transfusion reaction. While the FNHTR is a benign, self-limited fever caused by the cytokines present in the donor blood, the hemolytic transfusion reaction is a life-threatening, antibody-mediated immune response to ABO-incompatible donor blood.

In a multicenter, prospective, observational study of nearly 5000 ICU patients in the United States, blood transfusion caused a fever in 1.9% of recipients [41]. Leukocytes in the stored donor blood have been known to be responsible for the febrile transfusion reaction since the 1950s, but it wasn't until the 1990s that pyrogenic cytokines elaborated by the stored leukocytes were found to be the direct cause [42–44]. Prestorage leukoreduction, a process by which the number of leukocytes in the blood is reduced prior to storage so as to decrease the amount of cytokines present in the stored blood, has been shown to decrease the incidence of febrile transfusion reactions [45–47].

The use of premedication with acetaminophen to prevent febrile hemolytic reactions is controversial [48]. The consensus from several reviews of the literature is that there is no evidence to support the practice of premedication to prevent the febrile transfusion reaction [49]. We do not routinely administer prophylaxis, and we do not recommend it. We do, however, immediately stop transfusion and discard the donor blood in case the fever heralds a hemolytic transfusion reaction.

Hemolytic transfusion reactions present with fever and are thought to be caused by the presence of pre-existing antibodies to the donor blood's AB antigens. Hemolytic transfusion reactions can be fatal, causing between 10 and 37% of all transfusion-related deaths, but only 2% of patients who receive ABO incompatible blood will die from it [50–52]. Treatment for the hemolytic transfusion reaction is supportive, with special attention paid to preserving renal function [53].

Drug Fever

As the name implies, drug fever is a fever that coincides with administration of a drug and that resolves after discontinuation of the inciting agent. The diagnosis is often one of exclusion in patients with fever of unknown origin. It poses a unique challenge to physicians in that some of the most common provoking agents can be antimicrobials, yet these are initiated for suspected infection in febrile patients [54]. Disease processes other than infection that can cause fever and should be ruled out in fever of unknown origin include malignancy, thromboembolic disease, cerebrovascular accident, and acute gout [55]. Clinicians should also consider drug fever in patients with fever of unknown origin, not only because drug fever leads to excessive cost reflected by unnecessary laboratory and radiologic studies, treatment, and length of stay but because it can also precede more serious adverse drug reactions including hypersensitivity reactions and cutaneous manifestations, which occur in 18–29% of patients [55–59].

Numerous agents can cause drug fever, though the most common implicated agents include antimicrobials, anticonvulsants, antiarrhythmic agents, and other cardiac agents [57, 59]. The true incidence of drug fever is unknown due to misdiagnosis and underreporting, but it is estimated to occur in 3–5% of reported adverse effects [60]. There are primarily five mechanisms by which drugs can cause fever including altered thermoregulation (e.g., anticholinergic agents, levothyroxine, monoamine oxidase inhibitors, sympathomimetic agents), administration related (e.g., amphotericin B, cephalosporins, vancomycin, vaccines, bleomycin), pharmacologic action of the drug (e.g., antineoplastic agents, heparin, penicillin, warfarin), idiosyncratic reactions (e.g., anesthetic agents, methyldopa, nitrofurantoin, sulfonamides, chloramphenicol), and hypersensitivity reactions (e.g., allopurinol, antimicrobial agents, carbamazepine, heparin, phenytoin, sulfonamides) [54, 61].

The median time to initiation of the causative agent and onset of fever is 7–10 days, though drug fever can occur at any point during a course of drug therapy, and some agents can provoke a faster response [55]. Fever can be characterized as continuous, intermittent, or a combination of both, and the degree of pyrexia can range from 99 °F to 109 °F, though elevations from 102 to 104 °F are most common [55, 57–59]. Though laboratory values are not always elevated in those with drug fever, leukocytosis occurs in approximately 22%, eosinophilia in 22%, and skin rash in 18% of cases [57].

Treatment of drug fever involves discontinuing the offending agent if possible. If the reaction is severe and involves a hypersensitivity reaction, it may be most appropriate to stop all nonessential drugs [54]. Defervescence typically occurs 48–72 h after discontinuation, though factors such as a more severe reaction like those involving maculopapular rash or delayed elimination may delay resolution of fever by days or weeks [54, 60]. In some instances where fever is the primary culprit, the benefit of continuing therapy may outweigh the risk of drug fever, in which case clinicians can consider switching to a chemically unrelated substitute. Alternative agents may not be available in some situations like chemotherapy for a particular type of cancer or infection with a multidrug-resistant organism. In these cases, it might be possible to continue therapy by using pretreatment with corticosteroids, antihistamines, and/or prostaglandin inhibitors while monitoring for signs of hypersensitivity [62]. Rechallenge is not typically recommended, especially when the initial drug fever was accompanied by severe adverse effects [14, 54].

Isolated Neurotrauma

Prevention of secondary brain injury is paramount in the recovery of the neurotrauma patient. Processes such as neurotransmitter-mediated excitotoxicity, electrolyte imbalances, mitochondrial dysfunction, the inflammatory response, and secondary ischemia have all been shown to cause neuronal death, worsen cerebral edema, and increase intracranial pressure causing further exacerbation of the primary brain injury. Fever in brain-injured patients is known to increase metabolic demands, increase intracranial pressure, worsen the local inflammatory response in brain tissue, and increase mortality [63]. Therefore, efforts must be made to rapidly identify the cause, promptly control fevers, and maintain euthermia in brain-injured patients. Unfortunately, brain-injured patients are uniquely susceptible to a maladaptive fever termed neurogenic fever, a diagnosis of exclusion.

The proposed etiology of neurogenic fever is prostaglandin-induced elevation in the hypothalamic set point trigger by both local and systemic inflammatory responses. Blood in the ventricles, DAI, and frontal lobe damage are known risk factors for the development of fever in neurotrauma. Timing of fever onset may help to differentiate infectious and noninfectious causes of fever as development of fever prior to 72 h of admission is strong predictor of noninfectious etiology. Otherwise, if the patient is >72 h since hospital admission, it is prudent to pursue both infectious and common noninfectious cases for fever. A new onset fever in patients who have an invasive monitoring line in place should prompt CSF cultures along with gram stain and cell counts.

Because a large portion of patients with TBI can be expected to be refractory to antipyretic medication (one study found that only 7% of patients with traumatic brain injury defervesced with pharmacological means alone), external cooling devices should be considered to maintain euthermia [64]. Adverse reactions of concern with external cooling devices include shivering and skin breakdown. Shivering increases metabolic demands and may thwart the cooling effort and can be managed via established protocols like the Columbia Anti-Shivering Protocol that ranges from acetaminophen administration through neuromuscular blockade with vecuronium [65]. These patients may also benefit from counter-warming techniques such as application of warm blanket to extremities. Infusion of cold IV fluids and esophageal cooling has also been shown to decrease fever burden without increased adverse events [66].

Thyroid Storm

Thyroid storm is a rare but life-threatening "augmentation of the manifestations of hyperthyroidism" that occurs in the setting of stress, as seen after severe infection, surgery, or trauma [67]. An objective scale has been developed to assist in the diagnosis of thyroid storm, though no uniform definition yet exists [68]. Thyroid storm is characterized by a pronounced, severe fever (above 39.5 °C or 103.1 °F) with diaphoresis, tachyarrhythmia due to sympathetic hyperactivity, CNS dysfunction, and gastrointestinal disturbances [69].

There are four major principles of managing thyroid storm: source control, reducing circulating thyroid hormone levels, sympathetic blockade, and supportive measures [69, 70]. As the source of the storm is usually exposure to stress, source control generally takes the form of supportive measures. When the inciting stress is suspected infection, empiric antibiotics should be initiated immediately. Propylthiouracil is the drug of choice for reducing both the intrathyroid organification of iodine as well as the peripheral conversion of T4 to T3 while iodine, administered as either Lugol's solution or saturated solution of potassium iodide, will block the release of already synthesized T4 [69, 70]. For sympathetic blockade, propranolol is the drug of choice. Supportive measures include maintenance of normothermia using external cooling devices and considering the use of corticosteroids to manage the possible relative adrenal insufficiency [69, 70].

Deep Venous Thrombosis

Depending upon many clinical factors as well as the frequency of ultrasound surveillance, the reported incidence of deep venous thrombosis (DVT) ranges widely, from 0.35% of general surgical patients up to 65% of trauma patients [71]. In a prospective, multicenter study of nearly 14,500 ICU patients with DVT, a fever was present at the time of diagnosis for approximately 5% [72].

Alcohol Withdrawal Syndrome and Delirium Tremens

The prevalence of chronic alcohol abuse ranges from 10 to 33% in all ICU patients and can be as high as 50% in the trauma ICU [73, 74]. Alcohol withdrawal causes fever due to reflex sympathetic hyperactivity, itself thought to be a consequence of releasing pyrogenic neurons from the chronic suppression of GABAergic neuronal activity caused by alcohol consumption [73]. AWS and DT are both managed with symptom-triggered benzodiazepine therapy using the CIWA scoring system developed by the Clinical Institute [75, 76].

References

1. Kluger MJ, Kozak W, Conn CA, Leon LR, Soszynski D. Role of fever in disease. Ann N Y Acad Sci. 1998;856(1):224–33.
2. Manthous CA, Hall JB, Olson D, et al. Effect of cooling on oxygen consumption in febrile critically ill patients. Am J Respir Crit Care Med. 1995;151(1):10–4.
3. Scammell TE, Elmquist JK, Griffin JD, Saper CB. Ventromedial preoptic prostaglandin E2 activates fever-producing autonomic pathways. J Neurosci. 1996;16(19):6246–54.
4. Netea MG, Kullberg BJ, Van der Meer JW. Circulating cytokines as mediators of fever. Clin Infect Dis. 2000;31(Supplement 5):S178–84.
5. Dinarello CA. Proinflammatory cytokines*. Chest. 2000;118(2):503.
6. Kalinski P. Regulation of immune responses by prostaglandin E2. J Immunol. 2012;188(1):21–8.
7. Narumiya S, FitzGerald GA. Genetic and pharmacological analysis of prostanoid receptor function. J Clin Invest. 2001;108(1):25–30.
8. An S, Yang J, So SW, Zeng L, Goetzl EJ. Isoforms of the EP3 subtype of human prostaglandin E2 receptor transduce both intracellular calcium and cAMP signals. Biochemistry. 1994;33(48):14496–502.
9. Nakamura K, Matsumura K, Kaneko T, Kobayashi S, Katoh H, Negishi M. The rostral raphe pallidus nucleus mediates pyrogenic transmission from the preoptic area. J Neurosci. 2002;22(11):4600–10.
10. Nakamura Y, Nakamura K, Matsumura K, Kobayashi S, Kaneko T, Morrison SF. Direct pyrogenic input from prostaglandin EP3 receptor-expressing preoptic neurons to the dorsomedial hypothalamus. Eur J Neurosci. 2005;22(12):3137–46.
11. Saper CB, Romanovsky AA, Scammell TE. Neural circuitry engaged by prostaglandins during the sickness syndrome. Nat Neurosci. 2012;15(8):1088–95.
12. Laupland KB, Shahpori R, Kirkpatrick AW, Ross T, Gregson DB, Stelfox HT. Occurrence and outcome of fever in critically ill adults. Crit Care Med. 2008;36(5):1531–5.
13. Barie PS, Hydo LJ, Eachempati SR. Causes and consequences of fever complicating critical surgical illness. Surg Infect. 2004;5(2):145–59.
14. O'Grady NP, Barie PS, Bartlett JG, et al. Guidelines for evaluation of new fever in critically ill adult patients: 2008 update from the American College of Critical Care Medicine and the Infectious Diseases Society of America. Crit Care Med. 2008;36(4):1330–49.
15. Young P, Saxena M, Bellomo R, et al. Acetaminophen for fever in critically ill patients with suspected infection. N Engl J Med. 2015;373(23):2215–24.
16. Chen Q, Fisher DT, Clancy KA, et al. Fever-range thermal stress promotes lymphocyte trafficking across high endothelial venules via an interleukin 6 trans-signaling mechanism. Nat Immunol. 2006;7(12):1299–308.
17. Van Oss C, Absolom D, Moore L, Park B, Humbert J. Effect of temperature on the chemotaxis, phagocytic engulfment, digestion and O2 consumption of human polymorphonuclear leukocytes. J Reticuloendothel Soc. 1980;27(6):561.
18. Nahas G, Tannieres M, Lennon J. Direct measurement of leukocyte motility: effects of pH and temperature. Exp Biol Med. 1971;138(1):350–2.
19. Roberts N, Steigbigel R. Hyperthermia and human leukocyte functions: effects on response of lymphocytes to mitogen and antigen and bactericidal capacity of monocytes and neutrophils. Infect Immun. 1977;18(3):673–9.
20. Graham GG, Davies MJ, Day RO, Mohamudally A, Scott KF. The modern pharmacology of paracetamol: therapeutic actions, mechanism of action, metabolism, toxicity and recent pharmacological findings. Inflammopharmacology. 2013;21(3):201–32.
21. Clemmer TP, Fisher CJ Jr, Bone RC, Slotman GJ, Metz CA, Thomas FO. Hypothermia in the sepsis syndrome and clinical outcome. Crit Care Med. 1992;20(10):1395–401.
22. Singer M, Deutschman CS, Seymour CW, et al. The third international consensus definitions for sepsis and septic shock (sepsis-3). JAMA. 2016;315(8):801–10.
23. Torio CM, Moore BJ. National inpatient hospital costs: the most expensive conditions by payer, 2013. Agency for Healthcare Research and Quality; 2016.

24. Stevenson EK, Rubenstein AR, Radin GT, Wiener RS, Walkey AJ. Two decades of mortality trends among patients with severe sepsis: a comparative meta-analysis. Crit Care Med. 2014;42(3):625.
25. Caironi P, Tognoni G, Masson S, et al. Albumin replacement in patients with severe sepsis or septic shock. N Engl J Med. 2014;370(15):1412–21.
26. Investigators SS. Impact of albumin compared to saline on organ function and mortality of patients with severe sepsis. Intensive Care Med. 2011;37(1):86–96.
27. Khwannimit B, Bhurayanontachai R. Prediction of fluid responsiveness in septic shock patients: comparing stroke volume variation by FloTrac/Vigileo and automated pulse pressure variation. Eur J Anaesthesiol (EJA). 2012;29(2):64–9.
28. Marik PE, Cavallazzi R. Does the central venous pressure predict fluid responsiveness? An updated meta-analysis and a plea for some common sense. Crit Care Med. 2013;41(7):1774–81.
29. Marik PE, Baram M, Vahid B. Does central venous pressure predict fluid responsiveness?: a systematic review of the literature and the tale of seven mares. Chest J. 2008;134(1):172–8.
30. Safdar N, Dezfulian C, Collard HR, Saint S. Clinical and economic consequences of ventilator-associated pneumonia: a systematic review. Crit Care Med. 2005;33(10):2184–93.
31. Kalil AC, Metersky ML, Klompas M, et al. Management of adults with hospital-acquired and ventilator-associated pneumonia: 2016 clinical practice guidelines by the Infectious Diseases Society of America and the American Thoracic Society. Clin Infect Dis. 2016;63(5):e61–e111. ciw353.
32. Group CCCT. A randomized trial of diagnostic techniques for ventilator-associated pneumonia. N Engl J Med. 2006;2006(355):2619–30.
33. Morata L, Cobos-Trigueros N, Martínez JA, et al. Influence of multidrug resistance and appropriate empirical therapy on Pseudomonas Aeruginosa bacteremia 30-days mortality. Antimicrob Agents Chemother. 2012;56(9):4833–7. AAC. 00750-00712.
34. Agbaht K, Diaz E, Muñoz E, et al. Bacteremia in patients with ventilator-associated pneumonia is associated with increased mortality: a study comparing bacteremic vs. nonbacteremic ventilator-associated pneumonia. Crit Care Med. 2007;35(9):2064–70.
35. Mermel LA, Allon M, Bouza E, et al. Clinical practice guidelines for the diagnosis and management of intravascular catheter-related infection: 2009 update by the Infectious Diseases Society of America. Clin Infect Dis. 2009;49(1):1–45.
36. Hooton TM, Bradley SF, Cardenas DD, et al. Diagnosis, prevention, and treatment of catheter-associated urinary tract infection in adults: 2009 International Clinical Practice Guidelines from the Infectious Diseases Society of America. Clin Infect Dis. 2010;50(5):625–63.
37. Stovall RT, Haenal JB, Jenkins TC, et al. A negative urinalysis rules out catheter-associated urinary tract infection in trauma patients in the intensive care unit. J Am Coll Surg. 2013;217(1):162–6.
38. Owen CC, Jain R. Acute acalculous cholecystitis. Curr Treat Options Gastroenterol. 2005;8(2):99–104.
39. Huffman JL, Schenker S. Acute acalculous cholecystitis: a review. Clin Gastroenterol Hepatol. 2010;8(1):15–22.
40. Barie PS, Eachempati SR. Acute acalculous cholecystitis. In:Acute cholecystitis: Springer; 2015. p. 187–96.
41. Corwin HL, Gettinger A, Pearl RG, et al. The CRIT Study: anemia and blood transfusion in the critically ill-current clinical practice in the United States. Crit Care Med. 2004;32(1):39–52.
42. Brittingham TE, Chaplin H. Febrile transfusion reactions caused by sensitivity to donor leukocytes and platelets. J Am Med Assoc. 1957;165(7):819–25.
43. Muylle L, Joos M, Wouters E, Bock R, Peetermans M. Increased tumor necrosis factor alpha (TNF alpha), interleukin 1, and interleukin 6 (IL-6) levels in the plasma of stored platelet concentrates: relationship between TNF alpha and IL-6 levels and febrile transfusion reactions. Transfusion. 1993;33(3):195–9.
44. Muylle L. The role of cytokines in blood transfusion reactions. Blood Rev. 1995;9(2):77–83.
45. King KE, Shirey RS, Thoman SK, Bensen-Kennedy D, Tanz WS, Ness PM. Universal leukoreduction decreases the incidence of febrile nonhemolytic transfusion reactions to RBCs. Transfusion. 2004;44(1):25–9.
46. Yazer MH, Podlosky L, Clarke G, Nahirniak SM. The effect of prestorage WBC reduction on the rates of febrile nonhemolytic transfusion reactions to platelet concentrates and RBC. Transfusion. 2004;44(1):10–5.
47. Paglino JC, Pomper GJ, Fisch GS, Champion MH, Snyder EL. Reduction of febrile but not allergic reactions to RBCs and platelets after conversion to universal prestorage leukoreduction. Transfusion. 2004;44(1):16–24.
48. Geiger TL, Howard SC. Acetaminophen and diphenhydramine premedication for allergic and febrile nonhemolytic transfusion reactions: good prophylaxis or bad practice? Transfus Med Rev. 2007;21(1):1–12.
49. Tobian AA, King KE, Ness PM. Transfusion premedications: a growing practice not based on evidence. Transfusion. 2007;47(6):1089–96.
50. Sazama K. Reports of 355 transfusion-associated deaths: 1976 through 1985. Transfusion. 1990;30(7):583–90.
51. Linden JV, Wagner K, Voytovich AE, Sheehan J. Transfusion errors in New York State: an analysis of 10 years' experience. Transfusion. 2000;40(10):1207–13.
52. Gilliss BM, Looney MR, Gropper MA. Reducing noninfectious risks of blood transfusion. J Am Soc Anesthesiologists. 2011;115(3):635–49.
53. Eder AF, Chambers LA. Noninfectious complications of blood transfusion. Arch Pathol Lab Med. 2007;131(5):708–18.
54. Patel RA, Gallagher JC. Drug fever. Pharmacotherapy. 2010;30(1):57–69.
55. Tabor PA. Drug-induced fever. Drug Intell Clin Pharm. 1986;20(6):413–20.
56. Harris L, Holdsambeck H. Drug fever--surprisingly common and costly. *Alabama medicine*. J Med Assoc State Ala. 1986;56(3):19.
57. Mackowiak PA, LeMAISTRE CF. Drug fever: a critical appraisal of conventional concepts. An analysis of 51 episodes in two Dallas hospitals and 97 episodes reported in the English literature. Ann Intern Med. 1987;106(5):728–33.
58. Johnson DH, Cunha BA. Drug fever. Infect Dis Clin N Am. 1996;10(1):85–91.
59. Tisdale JE, Miller DA. Drug-induced diseases: prevention, detection, and management. Bethesda: ASHP; 2010.
60. Roush MK, Nelson KM. Understanding drug-induced febrile reactions: when a fever of unknown etiology develops it is important to consider drug fever to avoid delays additional costs of treatment. Am Pharm. 1993;33(10):39–42.
61. Tierney L. Drug fever. West J Med. 1978;129(4):321.
62. Oizumi K, Onuma K, Watanabe A, Motomiya M. Clinical study of drug fever induced by parenteral administration of antibiotics. Tohoku J Exp Med. 1989;159(1):45–56.
63. Meier K, Lee K. Neurogenic fever review of pathophysiology, evaluation, and management. J Intensive Care Med. 2016;32(2):124–9. https://doi.org/10.1177/0885066615625194.
64. Albrecht RF, Wass CT, Lanier WL. Occurrence of potentially detrimental temperature alterations in hospitalized patients at risk for brain injury. Paper presented at: Mayo Clinic Proceedings 1998.
65. Choi HA, Ko S-B, Presciutti M, et al. Prevention of shivering during therapeutic temperature modulation: the Columbia anti-shivering protocol. Neurocrit Care. 2011;14(3):389–94.

66. Broessner G, Beer R, Lackner P, et al. Prophylactic, endovascularly based, long-term normothermia in ICU patients with severe cerebrovascular disease. Stroke. 2009;40(12):e657–65.
67. Bajwa SJS, Jindal R. Endocrine emergencies in critically ill patients: challenges in diagnosis and management. Indian J Endocrinol Metab. 2012;16(5):722.
68. Burch HB, Wartofsky L. Life-threatening thyrotoxicosis. Thyroid storm. Endocrinol Metab Clin N Am. 1993;22(2):263–77.
69. Sarlis NJ, Gourgiotis L. Thyroid emergencies. Rev Endocr Metab Disord. 2003;4(2):129–36.
70. Bahn RS, Burch HB, Cooper DS, et al. Hyperthyroidism and other causes of thyrotoxicosis: management guidelines of the American Thyroid Association and American Association of Clinical Endocrinologists. Thyroid. 2011;21(6):593–646.
71. Haut ER, Chang DC, Pierce CA, et al. Predictors of posttraumatic deep vein thrombosis (DVT): hospital practice versus patient factors—an analysis of the National Trauma Data Bank (NTDB). J Trauma Acute Care Surg. 2009;66(4):994–1001.
72. Barba R, Di Micco P, Blanco-Molina Á, et al. Fever and deep venous thrombosis. Findings from the RIETE registry. J Thromb Thrombolysis. 2011;32(3):288–92.
73. de Wit M, Jones DG, Sessler CN, Zilberberg MD, Weaver MF. Alcohol-use disorders in the critically ill patient. Chest J. 2010;138(4):994–1003.
74. Awissi D-K, Lebrun G, Coursin DB, Riker RR, Skrobik Y. Alcohol withdrawal and delirium tremens in the critically ill: a systematic review and commentary. Intensive Care Med. 2013;39(1):16–30.
75. Daeppen J-B, Gache P, Landry U, et al. Symptom-triggered vs fixed-schedule doses of benzodiazepine for alcohol withdrawal: a randomized treatment trial. Arch Intern Med. 2002;162(10):1117–21.
76. Sullivan JT, Sykora K, Schneiderman J, Naranjo CA, Sellers EM. Assessment of alcohol withdrawal: the revised clinical institute withdrawal assessment for alcohol scale (CIWA-Ar). Br J Addict. 1989;84(11):1353–7.

Glycemic Control in Critically Ill Surgical Patients

44

Brian C. Beldowicz, Jeremiah J. Duby, Danielle Pigneri, and Christine S. Cocanour

Introduction

Acute dysglycemia is a collective term for hyperglycemia, hypoglycemia, and glycemic variability that result from short-term, dynamic changes in glucose production, distribution, and utilization. Approximately half (47.7%) of adults that present to the ICU have acute dysglycemia on admission, and roughly one-third (33.2%) of the remaining patients subsequently develop the disorder [1]. Severe hyperglycemia (> 180 mg/dL), severe hypoglycemia (< 40 mg/dL), and wide glycemic variability are independently associated with substantial increases in mortality (50–80%) [1]. However, it is difficult to distinguish whether acute dysglycemia represents a cause or consequence of critical illness. Further, the optimal target levels of and methods for achieving glycemic control remain open questions.

The goals of glycemic control in the ICU are to safely treat hyperglycemia and effectively mitigate hypoglycemia and glycemic variability. Clinical practice guidelines for insulin infusion suggest thresholds for initiating therapy, describe the effects of hypoglycemia, and outline appropriate methods for blood glucose monitoring, among other critical considerations for *what* measures constitute best practice [2]. The purpose of this chapter is to provide a systematic approach for *how* to apply these evidence-based principles. No system or strategy can possibly account for every patient- and disease-specific variable. Therefore, the objective is to assemble the tools and structure to facilitate individualized glycemic control based on the patient's baseline health and clinical course. The background will review landmark trials and emerging research. The discussion will then trace the typical trajectory of critically ill patients through a practical examination of medication reconciliation, insulin infusion, transition to subcutaneous insulin, and prevention and treatment of hypoglycemia. Finally, the unique challenges of diabetic ketoacidosis (DKA) and hyperosmolar hyperglycemic state (HHS) will also be reviewed.

Background

Following the publication of the Leuven Intensive Insulin Therapy Trial in 2001, which demonstrated a 3.4% absolute reduction in ICU mortality, tight glycemic control was rapidly accepted as an indicator of overall quality of institutional healthcare delivery [3]. By 2008, the American Diabetes Association considered maintaining blood glucose levels "as close to 110 mg/dL as possible" a standard of care for critically ill patients [4]. The publication of the NICE-SUGAR trial 1 year later, however, indicated a 2.6% absolute increase in 90-day mortality for patients subjected to Leuven study targets compared to those patients subject to less intensive glycemic control [5], calling into question our entire understanding of the role of hyperglycemia in illness and recovery.

It is well established that critically ill and injured patients can develop stress-related hyperglycemia as part of the response to their systemic insult. Physiologically, these patients typically secrete higher levels of cortisol, glucagon, and growth hormone and have higher circulating levels of catecholamines and cytokines. This neuroendocrine cascade stimulates glycogenolysis, gluconeogenesis, and insulin resistance, elevating blood glucose levels [6].

B. C. Beldowicz
Department of Surgery, Division of Trauma, UC Davis Health, Acute Care Surgery and Surgical Critical Care, Sacramento, CA, USA

J. J. Duby
Department of Pharmacy Services, UC Davis Health, Sacramento, CA, USA

Touro University, College of Pharmacy, Vallejo, CA, USA

UCSF School of Pharmacy, San Francisco, CA, USA

D. Pigneri · C. S. Cocanour (✉)
Department of Surgery, Division of Trauma, UC Davis Health, Sacramento, CA, USA
e-mail: cscocanour@ucdavis.edu

A. Salim et al. (eds.), *Surgical Critical Care Therapy*, https://doi.org/10.1007/978-3-319-71712-8_44

What is not yet understood is what role this hyperglycemia plays in the course of critical illness. Some extrapolate that the pro-inflammatory, pro-thrombotic, and pro-oxidant effects observed in chronic hyperglycemia potentiate a similarly detrimental systemic inflammatory response in acute illness that results in higher mortality. Others, however, suggest stress-related hyperglycemia is an adaptive response that increases the glycemic diffusion gradient, facilitating glucose distribution to cells suffering insufficient perfusion [7].

Multiple investigations have examined the outcome discrepancy between the Leuven and NICE-SUGAR trials. The original Leuven study had a substantially higher proportion of surgical patients than the NICE-SUGAR trial, suggesting surgical patients may benefit from tighter glycemic control. In fact, a follow-up study at Leuven isolating medical ICU patients failed to demonstrate the same degree of mortality benefit as previously observed in their surgical ICU [8]. A 2009 meta-analysis examining the effects of glycemic control in different settings confirmed a greater benefit in surgical ICUs compared to nonsurgical ICUs [9]. Additionally, two-thirds of the original Leuven study population consisted of cardiac surgery patients. Subsequent studies have confirmed a disproportional mortality benefit of insulin infusions [10] and tight glycemic control [11] specific to cardiac surgery patients.

The Leuven study population also included a high proportion of patients receiving parenteral nutrition compared to the NICE-SUGAR population. A 2010 meta-analysis of randomized trials concluded that patients whose blood glucose levels are artificially elevated through the infusion of parenteral nutrition benefit from tighter glycemic control, whereas those taking enteral nutrition fared better with less strict control of blood glucose [12]. It appears that iatrogenic hyperglycemia caused by intravenous carbohydrate loads may be detrimental, and in such instances, blood glucose should be tightly controlled. Mild-to-moderate hyperglycemia unrelated to parenteral nutrition, however, may be part of a natural physiologic response to illness or injury, and its effects may be beneficial. Strict glycemic control in this scenario is not warranted and may, in fact, be harmful.

As the medical community continues its struggle to understand conflicting research regarding the implications of acute hyperglycemia in critical illness, the deleterious effects of abnormally low blood glucose levels have remained consistently apparent. Attempts to regulate glycemic control in critically ill and injured patients results in higher rates of hypoglycemia (blood glucose <70 mg/dL) and severe hypoglycemia (blood glucose <40 mg/dL), though, interestingly, the incidence of this iatrogenic complication is not directly related to the size or level of target glucose windows [2]. Instead, it appears that patient factors such as illness severity and underlying disease as well as the details of glycemic control protocols and their required level of attentiveness portend greater influence on the risk of hypoglycemia.

Studies have consistently demonstrated a direct correlation between the number, severity, and duration of hypoglycemic episodes with increased risk of mortality. Patients subject to acute glycemic control interventions are five times more likely to suffer one or more episodes of severe hypoglycemia resulting in a fivefold greater risk of mortality with even a single episode [1].

To confound the issue, a 2008 study demonstrated the relative inaccuracy of point-of-care (POC) glucometers commonly used in critical care glycemic management protocols. POC glucose monitors prescribed a different protocol intervention than laboratory measurements performed on the same blood sample on up to 13.3% of measurements. Most often, POC monitors overstated the blood glucose levels, which would lead to higher doses of prescribed insulin than would be necessary based on laboratory values. The inaccuracies were spread throughout the entire range of blood glucose measurements, meaning episodes of hypoglycemia would be under-detected and undertreated based on POC monitor findings. Inaccuracy appeared to be exacerbated by states of shock and vasopressor requirements but appeared throughout the spectrum of illness severity [13]. According to the updated standards published by the FDA in 2016, glucometer measurements used in a clinical setting must be within +/− 12% of lab-measured results for >95% of tests and within +/− 15% on 98% [14]. Due to both the ramifications of POC glucometers unique to ICUs and concerns of the concentration of confounding variables that can affect accuracy, there is only a single blood glucose monitoring system that has been approved specifically for POC use in critical care by the FDA [15].

Minimizing the detrimental effects of both hyper- and hypoglycemia requires a systematic approach to glycemic control that incorporates informed decisions on the initiation, titration, and transition of insulin therapy. This chapter will provide an evidence-based, systematic approach for *how* to manage acute dysglycemia.

Medication Reconciliation

Medication reconciliation is the process of creating and reviewing the patient medication profile upon admission to, transfer within, and discharge from the hospital. Patients with diabetes are admitted and discharged with approximately twice as many medications and are subject to four times the rate of severe medication errors as patients without diabetes [16]. Insulin is consistently ranked among high-alert medications in the acute care setting due to the frequency and severity of associated adverse drug events [17]. Transitions to and from the ICU likely amplify the risk of medication error and adverse drug reactions. Changes in clinical status – such as surgery or shock – dynamically affect both insulin sensitivity and nutritional support in critically ill patients, thereby exacerbating acute dysglycemia and precluding long-term diabetic therapy. However, creating and reviewing the "Best Possible Medication History" (BPMH) are critical to providing safe and effective glycemic management and to facilitating efficient transfer and disposition from the ICU. The process for transitioning to long-term, diabetic therapy is discussed separately below. Moreover, medication reconciliation may be used in combination with hemoglobin A1c (A1c) to assess the role of diabetes mellitus (DM) in the patient's acute dysglycemia and to evaluate the effectiveness of chronic glycemic management. An elevated A1c or a medication history indicating prior diabetic therapy may explain persistent insulin insensitivity and expedite transition to basal and nutritional insulin therapy. Further, a high A1c in patients with previously diagnosed DM suggests poor medication compliance, which may indicate the need for outpatient referral or transitions of care services such as patients admitted for DKA. In contrast, a normal A1c in the absence of diabetic medications signals that hyperglycemia likely represents acute dysglycemia. This common scenario demands close glucose monitoring and forewarns against the use of long-acting insulins, especially during clinically dynamic intervals such as the postoperative period. Finally, allogeneic red blood cell transfusion effectively dilutes the level of glycosylated hemoglobin, thereby rendering the laboratory value meaningless. Therefore, a review of the patient's recent transfusion history and early monitoring are prerequisites to ordering and assessing A1c in critically ill patients.

Insulin Therapy in the ICU

The intensity and flexibility needed for glycemic control and the mode of nutritional support determine the method and type(s) of insulin therapy. Table 44.1 illustrates the general advantages, disadvantages, and traps of various methods of insulin support. Figure 44.1 provides a basic algorithm for initiating and directing insulin therapy based on clinical and glycemic status. Table 44.2 outlines the selection and management of insulin therapies based on nutritional support.

The dynamic interplay of insulin sensitivity, nutrition, and insulin tends to parallel the patient's clinical course; the natural starting point for application is ICU admission. One of the presenting characteristics and challenges for critically ill patients is severe hyperglycemia and wide glycemic variability. In the acute phase of critical illness, basal insulin requirements are often obscured or eclipsed by severe and dynamic insulin insensitivity. Chasing hyperglycemia with basal insulin is limited by titration of long- or intermediate-acting insulin, which tends to lag changes in clinical course. The result is ineffective glycemic control as insulin insensitivity worsens and subsequent hypoglycemia as acute dysglycemia resolves. By design then, basal insulin is best initiated as the patient's insulin requirements stabilize (Fig. 44.1). Correctional insulin (i.e., sliding scale) also fails at the goals of treating hyperglycemia and mitigating glycemic variability, because it is merely reactive to hyperglycemia and magnifies glycemic variability. Insulin infusion is the only strategy with the intensity and flexibility to match the demands of hyperdynamic, critically ill patients.

Insulin Infusion

Insulin infusion is the preferred method of initial glycemic control in critically ill patients (Fig. 44.1 and Table 44.2). Moreover, there is some suggestion that the benefits of insulin infusion may extend beyond hyperglycemia and include anti-inflammatory effects and improved endothelial cell function [18]. However, insulin infusion is associated with tremendous workflow demands on nursing staff and with a high risk of medication error and hypoglycemia. These costs

Table 44.1 Overview of insulin support strategies. Complete refers to the combination of basal, nutritional, and correctional insulin therapy

Strategies	Advantages/role	Disadvantages	Traps
Insulin infusion	Preferred for wide glycemic variability (blood glucose ±40 mg/dL) Provides "complete" insulin support Effective for severe hyperglycemia Reduces glycemic variability	Very labor intensive Risk for medication errors High risk for hypoglycemia	Using in combination with diet or bolus feeding Using without continuous carbohydrate source
Correctional insulin (sliding scale)	Effective for monitoring dysglycemia Short-term, dose-finding strategy Least labor-intensive option	Ineffective for severe hyperglycemia Increases glycemic variability	Using as "default" strategy from admission order sets Using for nutritional needs
Complete: Basal + nutritional + correctional	Effective for persistent hyperglycemia Provides complete coverage of insulin needs	Requires daily assessment and titration May be difficult to match nutritional insulin with variable carbohydrate intake	Using basal insulin to cover nutritional insulin needs Overfeeding No hold parameters for nutritional insulin Sudden changes in carbohydrate intake

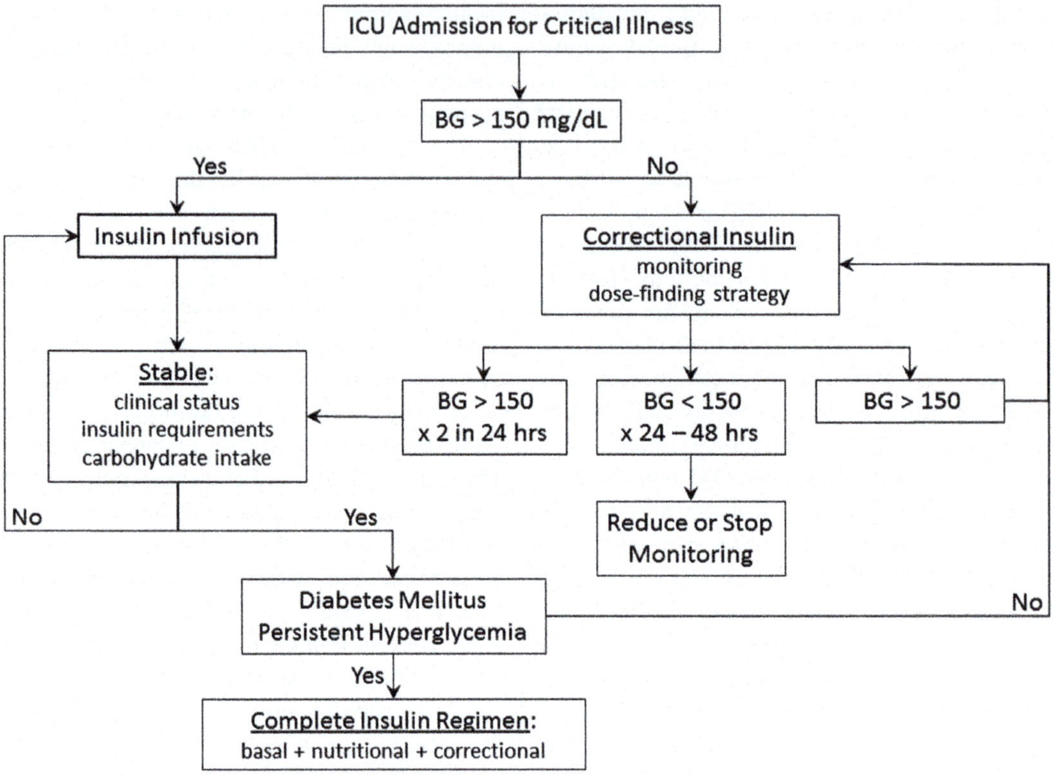

Fig. 44.1 ICU algorithm for glucose control

Table 44.2 Strategies for insulin support based on nutritional source. In reading the table, begin with the nutritional source, and select insulin support based on degree and variability of dysglycemia

Insulin Support	Nutritional Source			
	NPO	TPN	Continuous Enteral Nutrition	Intermittent Enteral Nutrition
Insulin Infusion	• use for severe hyperglycemia and wide glycemic variability • provides basal, nutritional, and correctional insulin • discontinue other sources of insulin (with possible exception of basal insulin such as in TPN)			CONTRAINDICATED
Basal	• Insulin requirements must be stable • titrate to ½ of TDD of insulin every 48 – 72 hours • do NOT adjust dose based on nutritional source or support • decrease dose if "fasting" or lowest BG value is less than 120 mg/dL • do not HOLD or adjust dose for surgery or interruptions in nutrition			
Nutritional	HOLD	• titrate to ½ TDD of insulin every 48 – 72 hours • HOLD for planned interruption of nutrition • unplanned interruption of nutrition: start dextrose-containing fluid at same rate as continuous nutrition • hold parameters: example: hold for pre-meal BG value less than 120 mg/dL • adjust dose based on "carbohydrate counting" method for variable nutritional intake • wide glycemic variability may signal need for carbohydrate restriction		
Correctional (sliding scale)	• dose-finding: include requirements in calculation of TDD insulin • select and titrate range based on insulin insensitivity • do NOT use to cover nutritional or basal support			

TPN **total parenteral nutrition,** *TDD* **total daily dose,** *BG* **blood glucose**

stipulate that the order for insulin infusion is regularly reviewed and justified based on the patient's needs.

Insulin infusion is indicated for initial management of severe hyperglycemia (blood glucose >150 mg/dL) and for wide glycemic variability (blood glucose ±40 mg/dL). It effectively provides for basal, nutritional, and correctional insulin; all other sources of insulin and diabetic therapy must be held or otherwise stopped (Table 44.2). Intermittent enteral nutrition is a relative contraindication to insulin infusion as the resultant, peri-prandial glycemic variability increases the risk of hypoglycemia. The risk for hypoglycemia is compounded by short-term deprivation of nutritional support. Severe and refractory hypoglycemia may then result if there is any disruption in gluconeogenesis, such as surgery, shock, or liver dysfunction, as the patient's glycogen stores may be depleted. The simple but paradoxical strategy to mitigate this complication is to provide a continuous source of dextrose, which may reduce the drive for gluconeogenesis and the risk of hypoglycemia. After the initial resuscitation period, consider using an intravenous (IV) crystalloid that contains dextrose (e.g., D_5-LR, D_{10}-NS) if enteral or parenteral nutrition is not feasible. This risk mitigation strategy is especially important for patients with head injury because of the profound impact of relative hypoglycemia (BG < 100 mg/dL) in this population. Conversely, intermittent doses of medications such as antibiotics may worsen glycemic variability if prepared in dextrose bases.

In initiating an insulin infusion, it is important to recognize that insulin adheres to the wall of the polyvinyl tubing typically used for intravenous infusions. All IV lines must therefore be primed with insulin in order to ensure reliable delivery of the prescribed insulin dose.

The initial rate of insulin infusion ranges from 1 to 5 units/hour based on the patient's blood glucose level at the time of initiation. Dosing adjustments are commonly calculated using a multiple of the current infusion rate rather than titration in an absolute number of units of insulin. Table 44.3 describes an insulin titration regimen that incorporates an adjustment factor that is based on both the absolute blood glucose measurement and its change since the previous measurement.

Blood glucose is measured, and the insulin infusion is titrated every hour until no titration is required for 4 h. Measurements can then be spaced to every 2 h unless there is

Table 44.3 Adjustment factor for insulin infusion. Plot the current BG (left column) and change in BG (top row) to determine the adjustment factor. The NEW RATE = current rate × adjustment factor. Do NOT increase insulin rate by more than 10 units/hour. Monitor the BG 30 min after rate change if insulin infusion is doubled and/or increased by 10 units/hour

CURRENT Blood Glucose (mg/dL)	CHANGE in blood glucose since the prior reading					
	Decreased more than 50	Decreased 31-50	Decreased 11-30	No change (± 10)	Increased 11-30	Increased more than 30
70-110	Stop for 30min restart at x 0.25 if BBG >110	current rate X 0.25 ↓	current rate X 0.5 ↓	current rate X 0.75 ↓	Continue current rate	↑ current rate X 1.5 *Max increase NOT to exceed 10 units
111-150	current rate X 0.25 ↓	current rate X 0.5 ↓	current rate X 0.75 ↓	Continue current rate	↑ current rate X 1.25 *Max increase NOT to exceed 10 units	↑ current rate X 1.5 *Max increase NOT to exceed 10 units
151-180	current rate X 0.5 ↓	current rate X 0.75 ↓	Continue current rate	↑ current rate X 1.25 *Max increase NOT to exceed 10 units	↑ current rate X 1.5 *Max increase NOT to exceed 10 units	↑ current rate X 2 *Max increase NOT to exceed 10 units
181-210	current rate X 0.75 ↓	Continue current rate	Continue current rate	↑ current rate X 1.5 *Max increase NOT to exceed 10 units		↑ current rate X 2 *Max increase NOT to exceed 10 units
Over 210	Continue current rate	Continue current rate	↑ current rate X 1.5 *Max increase NOT to exceed 10 units		↑ current rate X 2 *Max increase NOT to exceed 10 units	

BG **blood glucose**

an alteration in carbohydrate intake such as titration or interruption of enteral or parenteral nutrition. Glucose is checked more frequently (every 30 min) if the dosing adjustment calculation calls for an increase of 10 units/hour or a doubling of the previous infusion rate. Do not increase insulin rate by more than 10 units/hour.

Basal, Nutritional, and Correctional Components of Insulin Therapy

Relative clinical stability and resolution of glycemic variability are reasonable prerequisites to transitioning from insulin infusion to less intensive forms of glycemic control (Table 44.1). Acute dysglycemia may rapidly and completely resolve along with sources of inflammation and stress associated with the acute phase of critical illness. Frequently, however, patients enter an intermediate phase of persistent but dynamic hyperglycemia that requires a more complete regimen. It is useful to divide insulin requirements into basal, nutritional, and correctional components which can be met by a combination of long- and short-acting insulins. Figure 44.2 illustrates approximate onset, peak, and duration of activity for the major types of insulin used in the ICU.

Basal insulin reduces gluconeogenesis and represents the amount of insulin a patient requires regardless of nutritional support. Therefore, changes or interruptions in nutritional support should have minimal risk of causing hypoglycemia. Basal insulin is typically comprised of longer-acting insulins such as glargine or NPH provided once every 12–24 h.

Table 44.4 indicates how to calculate initial basal and nutritional insulin dosing using information gleaned from IV infusions in patients receiving no nutrition or continuous enteral or parenteral nutrition. Basal insulin requirements should only be calculated after the patient is fully resuscitated with a relatively stable insulin requirement over 2–3 days, signifying that the patient has progressed beyond the most physiologically stressful part of their illness and the neuroendocrine cascade that accompanies it. Glargine can be provided as a single bedtime dose of up to 50 units; however daily requirements above 50 units should be divided into two equal doses given 12 h apart. NPH may be more suitable in patients demonstrating varying insulin requirements at different times of day. NPH is initially provided twice daily in equal doses. Patients that demonstrate wide glycemic variability with consistent day and night variation in blood glucose levels may benefit from independent titration of daytime and nighttime NPH dosing. Basal insulin should not be titrated to nutritional support.

Insulin requirements are expected to gradually decline as the patient's acute dysglycemia resolves over days to weeks. Therefore, it is essential to carefully monitor and taper basal insulin based on early morning or "fasting" blood glucose levels (less than 120 mg/dL). Basal insulin requirements should be recalculated no more often than every 48–72 h, using the guidance provided in Table 44.2.

Nutritional insulin is the recurring requirement reliably associated with the timing, quantity, and composition of nutritional intake. Nutritional insulin takes the form of

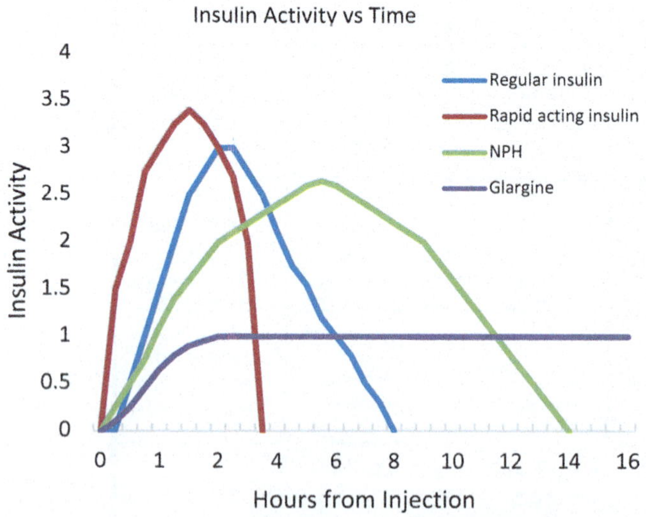

Fig. 44.2 Insulin activity. The graph illustrates the approximate onset, peak, and duration of activity for the major types of insulin

Table 44.4 Calculation of initial basal and nutritional insulin requirements

Step 1	Confirm stable insulin infusion requirements Continue insulin infusion if insulin requirements are dynamic
Step 2	Calculate TDD of IV insulin TDD IV insulin = (average units/hour over last 4 h) × (24 h)
Step 3	Calculate TDD of SC insulin DM: TDD SC insulin = TDD IV insulin × 0.8 Non-DM: TDD SC insulin = TDD IV insulin × 0.7
Step 4	Divide dose between basal and nutritional insulin Basal insulin = TDD SC insulin × 0.5 Glargine dose = basal insulin dose, given once daily OR NPH dose = basal insulin dose × 0.5, given q 12 h Nutritional insulin = TDD SC insulin × 0.5 Divided dose = nutritional insulin dose × 0.25 Continuous enteral nutrition: Administer as regular insulin q 6 h (HOLD for BG < 150 mg/dL) Eating or bolus feeding: Administer as insulin aspart qAC and qHS (HOLD for BG < 150 mg/dL) Parenteral nutrition: TDD IV insulin added to TPN (Stop TPN for BG ≤ 70 mg/dL)

TDD total daily dose, *DM* diabetes mellitus, *IV* intravenous, *SC* subcutaneous, *qAC* before meals, *qHS* at bedtime, *TPN* total parenteral nutrition

short-acting, subcutaneous insulins, such as insulin aspart, in patients taking regular meals or bolus tube feedings. Because the effect of insulin aspart is limited to 1–2 h, its role is most useful with intermittent nutrition. Regular subcutaneous insulin is preferred as nutritional insulin in patients on continuous nutrition. Correctional insulin is given in addition to nutritional insulin; therefore, the same type of insulin should be used for both.

When the route, quantity, or composition of nutrition changes, intentionally or unintentionally, nutritional insulin may require adjustment. In patients receiving intermittent nutrition, subcutaneous correctional insulin can be used as a dose-finding strategy for titrating nutritional insulin requirements. Because such a strategy is reactive, correctional insulin will result in wider variability during the period of dose-seeking. In general, patients on intermittent nutrition are less critically ill, and glycemic variability may be less likely to influence acute outcomes. Table 44.2 illustrates the titration of nutritional insulin requirements. These requirements should be recalculated every 48–72 h. The risk of hypoglycemia may be further mitigated with order parameters on nutritional insulin that stipulate holding for preprandial glucose levels less than 150 mg/dL.

Correctional insulin should be reserved for short-term monitoring and dose-finding purposes (Fig. 44.1). The use for persistent hyperglycemia is of no benefit and only increases glycemic variability. Frequent administration of correctional insulin signals the requirement for basal and/or nutritional insulin. The varying nutritional intake and insulin insensitivity observed in critical illness require the addition of short-acting *correctional insulin*. This component of the inpatient insulin regimen helps fine-tune basal and nutritional insulin requirements. By maintaining a more flexible and responsive component to glycemic management, correctional insulin allows an acceptable degree of glycemic variability in order to minimize the risk of hypoglycemic events. Correctional insulin may be discontinued when blood glucose levels are consistently less than 150 mg/dL and both basal and nutritional insulin are no longer required.

Parenteral Nutrition (TPN)

Parenteral nutrition represents a unique situation as basal and nutritional insulin may be directly coupled with nutrition. The potential advantage is that interruptions or cycles in carbohydrate infusion rates automatically follow parallel profiles. Disadvantages include a limited flexibility in insulin dosing. For example, dose adjustments for the next day's TPN are typically based on data from the previous day. This limitation naturally directs a more conservative dosing approach that may result in poor glycemic control. There is also a danger that dose titration includes correctional insulin, which results in using parenteral nutrition as a de facto insulin infusion. Obvious dangers include the inability to titrate the infusion and unawareness that the parenteral nutrition is a source of insulin during hypoglycemic episodes. The keys, then, are recognizing the limitations of insulin therapy via parenteral nutrition, judiciously titrating to basal and nutritional insulin, and strictly separating correctional insulin requirements by concurrent use of insulin infusion or sliding-scale insulin. Any episode of hypoglycemia should prompt immediate cessation of the insulin-containing TPN. Such interruption can be costly, both financially and nutritionally.

The half-life of regular insulin provided intravenously is only 9 min compared to 1.5 h when that same insulin is administered subcutaneously, so risks of hypoglycemia with the abrupt cessation of TPN are related more to the patient's own insulin response rather than the insulin within the TPN, itself. The risk of hypoglycemia upon abrupt cessation of TPN can be mitigated by the immediate infusion of a $D_{10}W$ at the same rate at which the TPN had been running in order to compensate for the patient's own innate insulin response to the previously flowing TPN. This dextrose infusion can be reduced by 50% every hour for 2 h and then discontinued. Blood glucose should be checked every 30 min until at least 1 h after the dextrose has been discontinued.

Transition to Outpatient Diabetic Regimens

Clinical stability is the first consideration in transitioning back to a patient's home diabetic regimen, because it is typically associated with improvements in glycemic variability and nutritional support. Restarting each diabetic medication requires reconciling current insulin requirements and carbohydrate intake with use and diet prior to admission. Basal and nutritional insulin requirements will gradually approach chronic insulin requirements as acute dysglycemia resolves, necessitating dose titration every 2–3 days. Even for patients that are metabolically stable, it may be prudent to reduce doses of basal and nutritional insulin to 25–50% of what patients reportedly received prior to admission. Oral diabetic agents generally work to improve insulin sensitivity; simply adding or layering these therapies on top of short-term glycemic management strategies may result in hypoglycemia. Therefore, oral agents should be reintroduced in coordination with concurrent de-escalation of basal and nutritional insulin.

Sulfonylureas (e.g., glipizide, glimepiride) generally and glyburide especially are associated with substantially higher rates of hypoglycemia compared to other oral diabetic agents, likely due their insulin-secretagogue activity. These agents should not be restarted until oral nutritional intake is consistent and adequate.

Metformin, in contrast, is associated with low relative risk of hypoglycemia [19]. The risk of metformin-associated lactic acidosis appears to have been grossly exaggerated, occurring with an incidence of 4.3 cases per 100,000 person-years, compared to 4.8 cases per 100,000 person-years with sulfonylureas, respectively [19, 20]. Temporarily holding or reducing the dose is indicated for both metformin and the sulfonylureas in patients with hemodynamic instability, acute kidney injury, or clearance creatinine less than 60 ml/min [21].

The thiazolidinediones (e.g., pioglitazone, rosiglitazone) are associated with prolonged antihyperglycemic effects; therefore, these agents should not be continued in the acute care setting. Emerging agents such as dipeptidyl peptidase inhibitors, glucagon-like peptide-1 agonists, and sodium-glucose cotransporter 2 inhibitors should not be continued as the safety and role have not yet been established in the critical care population.

Insulin pumps in hospitalized patients are associated with significant risks of medication errors and adverse events due to underrecognition that they are present. The identification of a patient with an insulin pump should automatically prompt an endocrine consult as well as hospital pharmacy and nursing safety measures.

Diabetic Ketoacidosis and the Hyperosmotic Hyperosmolar State

DKA and HHS are more often associated with critically ill medical patients; however, it is not uncommon for patients with these conditions to require surgical management. The fundamentals of management for both of these life-threatening, acid-base disorders include resuscitation, electrolyte repletion, blood glucose normalization, and treatment of an inciting cause, when present. Aggressive therapy is prone to overcompensation resulting in wide glycemic variability, hypokalemia, and dangerously low serum osmolarity, which can generate cerebral edema, particularly in younger patients.

Management begins with resuscitation. Hypotensive patients receive boluses of isotonic crystalloid until blood pressure improves; and it is critical to continue resuscitation until anion gap closure occurs. It is important to recognize that these patients demonstrate an osmotic diuresis from their hyperglycemia, so urine output does not correlate with volume status. A corrected serum sodium is then calculated using the formula:

$$\text{Corrected Na+} = \text{measured Na}^{+} + \left[1.6 \text{ x} \left(\text{blood glucose} - 100\right) / 100\right]$$

Patients with elevated corrected serum sodium receive 0.45% NS maintenance fluid. Those with low corrected serum sodium receive 0.9% NS.

The traditional insulin infusion protocol is also modified for patients with DKA and HHS to better mitigate the risks associated specifically with these acid-base disturbances. An IV insulin bolus is not given at the inception of the insulin infusion. DKA and HHS patients already suffer from total body potassium depletion. Bolus doses of IV insulin could cause rapid migration of serum potassium into cells, putting patients at risk for cardiac arrhythmias in a hypokalemic situation where potassium repletion could prove challenging and prolonged.

The insulin infusion protocol is targeted to the rate of blood glucose correction rather than directly to blood glucose normalization. The dosing adjustment calculation guides glycemic correction by no more than 50 mg/dL per hour until blood glucose is less than 300 mg/dL. In patients who are correcting at a rate greater than 50 mg/dL per hour, the insulin infusion is reduced by 25% even if their blood glucose remains above 300 mg/dL. To facilitate a smooth, safe, gradual glycemic correction, oral, enteral, and parenteral nutrition are held for the 12–24 h period required to resolve the acute metabolic disturbance.

To avoid rebound hypoglycemia, 5% dextrose is added to maintenance fluids once blood glucose is reduced to less than 300 mg/dL. Blood glucose is then maintained between 200 and 300 mg/dL until fluid resuscitation has restored the anion gap to less than 12 in DKA patients or plasma osmolality is less than 315 in HHS patients. At that point, critically ill patients are transitioned to a standard insulin infusion protocol (Table 44.3), targeting a stable blood glucose between 110 and 150 mg/dL. Stable patients may be transitioned to subcutaneous insulin (Table 44.4).

A substantial reduction in the prevalence of hypoglycemia and glycemic variability has been observed by targeting a conservative rate of glycemic correction [22]. Though mean blood glucose levels are higher under this protocol, this strategy resulted in consistently shorter hospital and ICU lengths of stay in both DKA and HHS populations.

Hypoglycemia

The largest clinical trials of glycemic control have demonstrated an incidence of severe hypoglycemia ranging from 5 to 18% [2]. Some of the risk factors for severe hypoglycemia are patient-specific, such as severity of illness, pressor requirement, female gender, renal failure, and dialysis. But other risks can be mitigated, particularly those associated with disruption of caloric intake. Interruption of oral intake, tube feeding, or parenteral nutrition requires alternative carbohydrate supplementation, reduced insulin administration, or both. It is important to understand the onset of action and duration of effect for all types of insulin and antihyperglycemic medications prescribed in the ICU setting where nutritional disruption cannot always be anticipated. Even brief deprivation of nutritional support can rapidly deplete glycogen stores in the context of the hypermetabolic demand often present in critical illness. Severe and refractory hypoglycemia may then result from any disruption in gluconeogenesis (e.g., shock, liver injury) or bioaccumulation of insulin (e.g., renal compromise). The simple but counterintuitive strategy to mitigate this complication is to provide a continuous source of dextrose, which may reduce the drive for gluconeogenesis and the risk for hypoglycemia. When enteral or parenteral nutrition is not feasible, then add dextrose to maintenance infusions.

Treatment of hypoglycemia should seek to rapidly resolve patient symptoms and restore euglycemia while avoiding rebound hyperglycemia. Wide ranges of glucose variance have been associated with poor outcomes [23]; though as with many aspects of acute glycemic control, it is unclear if this observation is more of a correlation with severity of illness or if it has a contributory role.

Blood glucose will increase by approximately 4 mg/dL for each gram of dextrose administered acutely for hypoglycemia [24]. Each milliliter of $D_{50}W$ has 0.5 g of dextrose, so each mL of $D_{50}W$ will increase blood glucose by a median of 2 mg/dL. Use these estimates to calculate doses of $D_{50}W$ to be administered to rescue patients from hypoglycemia.

$$(100\ \text{mg/dL} - \text{blood glucose in mg/dL})/2 = \text{volume in mL of } D_{50}W \text{ to be administered}$$

Burn patients, as well as those with diabetes, tend to have a higher blood glucose response to bolus dextrose, while patients with a history of recurrent hypoglycemic episodes typically have responses less than 4 mg/dL per gram of dextrose [24]. The generalized response of giving "one amp" of $D_{50}W$ provides 25 g of dextrose which is capable of raising blood glucose by as much as 100 mg/dL, resulting in hyperglycemia.

Blood glucose is monitored every 15 min until symptoms have resolved in responsive patients and every 30 min until it has remained >70 mg/dL for two consecutive measurements without further intervention. Basal, nutritional, and correctional insulin orders are discontinued, while the strategy for glycemic control is reassessed.

Conclusion

Glycemic control in the ICU continues to evolve, making it essential that critical care providers consistently incorporate updated research into their management strategies. There is already evidence emerging that absolute blood glucose values do not correlate with benefit and harm when a generalized population of critically ill patients are broken into more specific subgroups based on pre-morbid glycemic control. Peak glucose concentrations during critical illness correlate with mortality risk in patients with admission A1C levels <7% but not in those with levels ≥7%. This suggests that patients with hyperglycemia at baseline benefit from higher levels of stress hyperglycemia than nondiabetics or those with good baseline glucose control [25]. Some emerging research also suggests that baseline blood glucose levels may account for inter-study variability and that greater personalization of blood glucose targets relative to this patient-specific baseline may prove beneficial. One expert proposes a modified target glucose of 160–220 mg/dL (8.8–12.2 mmol/L) for patients with admission HbA1C greater than 7 [26]. Another proposes 180–260 mg/dL [27], and still a third proposes a target of 30–40 mg/dL greater than the estimated average glucose, calculated by the formula 28.7 × HbA1C − 46.7 [28]. None of these proposals are currently widely accepted.

Conflicting results in authoritative studies and rescinded recommendations from professional societies indicate that more research is required for glycemic control in the ICU. It appears that its future will likely focus on patient-specific targets that balance individual risks and benefits of observation versus intervention in a variety of clinical scenarios.

References

1. Badawi O, Waite MD, Fuhrman SA, Zuckerman IH. Association between intensive care unit-acquired dysglycemia and in-hospital mortality. Crit Care Med. 2012;40(12):3180–8. https://doi.org/10.1097/CCM.0b013e3182656ae5.
2. Jacobi J, Bircher N, Krinsley J, Agus M, Braithwaite SS, Deutschman C, et al. Guidelines for the use of an insulin infusion for the management of hyperglycemia in critically ill patients. Crit Care Med. 2012;40(12):3251–76. https://doi.org/10.1097/CCM.0b013e3182653269.
3. van den Berghe G, Wouters P, Weekers F, Verwaest C, Bruyninckx F, Schetz M, et al. Intensive insulin therapy in critically ill patients. N Engl J Med. 2001;345(19):1359–67. https://doi.org/10.1056/NEJMoa011300.
4. American Diabetes Association. Standards of medical care in diabetes--2008. Diabetes Care. 2008;31(Suppl 1):S12–54. https://doi.org/10.2337/dc08-S012.
5. Investigators N-SS, Finfer S, Chittock DR, Su SY, Blair D, Foster D, et al. Intensive versus conventional glucose control in critically ill patients. N Engl J Med. 2009;360(13):1283–97. https://doi.org/10.1056/NEJMoa0810625.
6. Dungan KM, Braithwaite SS, Preiser JC. Stress hyperglycaemia. Lancet. 2009;373(9677):1798–807. https://doi.org/10.1016/S0140-6736(09)60553-5.
7. Marik PE, Bellomo R. Stress hyperglycemia: an essential survival response! Crit Care Med. 2013;41(6):e93–4. https://doi.org/10.1097/CCM.0b013e318283d124.
8. Van den Berghe G, Wilmer A, Hermans G, Meersseman W, Wouters PJ, Milants I, et al. Intensive insulin therapy in the medical ICU. N Engl J Med. 2006;354(5):449–61. https://doi.org/10.1056/NEJMoa052521.
9. Griesdale DE, de Souza RJ, van Dam RM, Heyland DK, Cook DJ, Malhotra A, et al. Intensive insulin therapy and mortality among critically ill patients: a meta-analysis including NICE-SUGAR study data. CMAJ. 2009;180(8):821–7. https://doi.org/10.1503/cmaj.090206.

10. Furnary AP, Gao G, Grunkemeier GL, Wu Y, Zerr KJ, Bookin SO, et al. Continuous insulin infusion reduces mortality in patients with diabetes undergoing coronary artery bypass grafting. J Thorac Cardiovasc Surg. 2003;125(5):1007–21. https://doi.org/10.1067/mtc.2003.181.
11. Ouattara A, Lecomte P, Le Manach Y, Landi M, Jacqueminet S, Platonov I, et al. Poor intraoperative blood glucose control is associated with a worsened hospital outcome after cardiac surgery in diabetic patients. Anesthesiology. 2005;103(4):687–94.
12. Marik PE, Preiser JC. Toward understanding tight glycemic control in the ICU: a systematic review and metaanalysis. Chest. 2010;137(3):544–51. https://doi.org/10.1378/chest.09-1737.
13. Hoedemaekers CW, Klein Gunnewiek JM, Prinsen MA, Willems JL, Van der Hoeven JG. Accuracy of bedside glucose measurement from three glucometers in critically ill patients. Crit Care Med. 2008;36(11):3062–6. https://doi.org/10.1097/CCM.0b013e318186ffe6.
14. Food and Drug Aministration U.S. Department of health and human services, blood glucose monitoring test systems for presciption point-of-care use, Guidance for Industry and Food and Drug Administration Staff. Rockville; 2016.
15. Food and Drug Administration. FDA clears glucose monitoring system for use in hospital critical care units. 2014. https://wayback.archive-it.org/7993/20160221101309/fda.gov/NewsEvents/Newsroom/PressAnnouncements/ucm416144.htm . Accessed 04 Nov 2017.
16. Breuker C, Abraham O, di Trapanie L, Mura T, Macioce V, Boegner C, Jalabert A, Villiet M, Castet-Nicolas A, Avignon A, Sultan A. Patients with diabetes are at high risk of serious medication errors at hospital: interest of clinical pharmacist intervention to improve healthcare. Eur J Intern Med. 2016. doi:https://doi.org/10.1016/j.ejim.2016.12.003.
17. (ISMP). IfSMP (Accessed January 13, 2017.) ISMP list of high-alert medications in acute care settings. Available at http://www.ismporg/Tools/highalertmedicationspdf.
18. Clement S, Braithwaite SS, Magee MF, Ahmann A, Smith EP, Schafer RG, et al. Management of diabetes and hyperglycemia in hospitals. Diabetes Care. 2004;27(2):553–91.
19. Bodmer M, Meier C, Krahenbuhl S, Jick SS, Meier CR. Metformin, sulfonylureas, or other antidiabetes drugs and the risk of lactic acidosis or hypoglycemia: a nested case-control analysis. Diabetes Care. 2008;31(11):2086–91. https://doi.org/10.2337/dc08-1171.
20. Salpeter SR, Greyber E, Pasternak GA, Salpeter EE. Risk of fatal and nonfatal lactic acidosis with metformin use in type 2 diabetes mellitus. Cochrane Database Syst Rev. 2010;4:CD002967. https://doi.org/10.1002/14651858.CD002967.pub4.
21. Eppenga WL, Lalmohamed A, Geerts AF, Derijks HJ, Wensing M, Egberts A, et al. Risk of lactic acidosis or elevated lactate concentrations in metformin users with renal impairment: a population-based cohort study. Diabetes Care. 2014;37(8):2218–24. https://doi.org/10.2337/dc13-3023.
22. Firestone RL, Pandya PK, Parker PL, Duby JJ. Effect of a conservative correction DKA protocol on clinical outcomes in hospitalized patients. Crit Care Med. 2013;41(12):A16.
23. Krinsley JS. Glycemic variability: a strong independent predictor of mortality in critically ill patients. Crit Care Med. 2008;36(11):3008–13. https://doi.org/10.1097/CCM.0b013e31818b38d2.
24. Murthy MS, Duby JJ, Parker PL, Durbin-Johnson BP, Roach DM, Louie EL. Blood glucose response to rescue dextrose in hypoglycemic, critically ill patients receiving an insulin infusion. Ann Pharmacother. 2015;49(8):892–6. https://doi.org/10.1177/1060028015585574.
25. Plummer MP, Bellomo R, Cousins CE, Annink CE, Sundararajan K, Reddi BA, et al. Dysglycaemia in the critically ill and the interaction of chronic and acute glycaemia with mortality. Intensive Care Med. 2014;40(7):973–80. https://doi.org/10.1007/s00134-014-3287-7.
26. Marik PE, Egi M. Treatment thresholds for hyperglycemia in critically ill patients with and without diabetes. Intensive Care Med. 2014;40(7):1049–51. https://doi.org/10.1007/s00134-014-3344-2.
27. Krinsley JS, Schultz MJ, Spronk PE, Harmsen RE, van Braam Houckgeest F, van der Sluijs JP, et al. Mild hypoglycemia is independently associated with increased mortality in the critically ill. Crit Care. 2011;15(4):R173. https://doi.org/10.1186/cc10322.
28. Nathan DM, Kuenen J, Borg R, Zheng H, Schoenfeld D, Heine RJ, et al. Translating the A1C assay into estimated average glucose values. Diabetes Care. 2008;31(8):1473–8. https://doi.org/10.2337/dc08-0545.

45 Adrenal Insufficiency

Ellie Cohen and Walter L. Biffl

Introduction

Adrenal insufficiency during critical illness was first described by Hans Selye in 1949, in which he described a stress response that occurs when an event threatens an organism's well-being [1]. Since that time, adrenal insufficiency has been well recognized outside of the critical care setting and is defined as a failing in cortisol production resulting in low baseline cortisol levels, with no response to the ACTH stimulation test. More recently it has been recognized that a transient state of relative adrenal insufficiency occurs in patients within the critical care setting. The reported evidence of this critical illness corticosteroid insufficiency (CIRC) in critically ill patients varies widely (0–77%), depending on the population of patients studied and the diagnostic criteria. In addition, the underlying mechanism surrounding the disorder remains poorly understood.

What Is Adrenal Insufficiency?

The hypothalamic-pituitary-adrenal (HPA) axis and sympathoadrenal system are functionally related, with both playing an important role during times of stress.

The sympathoadrenal system is a physiological connection between the sympathetic nervous system and the adrenal medulla. It activates the secretion of epinephrine and norepinephrine from the adrenal medulla and increases the production of inflammatory cytokines, such as interleukin (IL)-6.

Activation of the HPA axis results in increased secretion from the paraventricular nucleus of the hypothalamus, releasing corticotropin-releasing hormone (CRH). CRH stimulates the release of ACTH by the anterior pituitary, causing the adrenal cortex to produce glucocorticoids.

E. Cohen
Hennepin County Medical Center, Minneapolis, MN, USA

W. L. Biffl (✉)
Scripps Memorial Hosptial La Jolla, San Diego, CA, USA
e-mail: walt@biffl.com

In humans cortisol is the major endogenous glucocorticoid secreted by the adrenal cortex. More than 90% of cortisol is bound to corticosteroid-binding globulin, and to a lesser extent albumin, with <10% free in the biologically active form. It exerts its effects after uptake from circulation by binding to intracellular glucocorticoid receptors (GR), which then causes the activation of a steroid-receptor complex that moves intracellularly to the nucleus and binds to homodimer DNA sequences called glucocorticoid response elements. These response elements are found located in the promoter region of thousands of genes, causing a broad range of effects on transcription, which results in multiple effects aimed at restoring homeostasis during times of stress. It has been estimated that 20% of the genome of mononuclear blood cells is affected by the activation of glucocorticoid.

Metabolically, cortisol increases the blood glucose concentrations through the activation of key enzymes involved in hepatic gluconeogenesis as well as inhibits the uptake of glucose into peripheral tissues, such as skeletal muscle. Lipolysis is also activated in adipose tissue, resulting in a release of free fatty acids into the circulation. It also displays a permissive effect on other hormones, such as catecholamines and glucagon.

It increases blood pressure through several mechanisms involving the kidney and vasculature. By acting directly on vascular smooth muscle, it increases sensitivity to vasopressor agents like catecholamine and angiotensin II. It does this by increasing transcription and expression of receptors for these hormones. It also acts on nitric oxide synthase, an enzyme that increases production of nitric oxide (NO), which helps modulate vascular tone.

Cortisol has multiple anti-inflammatory effects, such as a decreased production of cytokines, chemokines, and eicosanoids. It also enhances the function of various immune cells at sites of inflammation by increasing production of macrophage migratory inhibitory function.

Because of these effects and others, cortisol is essential for our adaption during times of stress, with a pronounced and sustained activation of the HPA axis being vital. It has

A. Salim et al. (eds.), *Surgical Critical Care Therapy*, https://doi.org/10.1007/978-3-319-71712-8_45

been demonstrated in animal models that those that have their adrenal glands removed succumb rapidly to hemorrhagic or septic shock. Likewise, patients with a prior history of adrenal insufficiency are also at increased risk of developing an Addisonian crisis—a life-threatening condition that causes a constellation of symptoms such as severe back pain, abdominal pain, vomiting/diarrhea leading to dehydration, and low blood pressure.

A transient or relative adrenal insufficiency, characterized by an inappropriate cortisol response during times of stress, is recognized in the critical care setting and may relate to morbidity and mortality, particularly in sepsis.

Clinical Scenarios

Overall prevalence of CIRC in critically ill patients remains controversial, with studies citing a prevalence of 10–20% in the general population, with a rate as high as 60% for those diagnosed with septic shock.

Some patients develop this insufficiency through structural damage to the adrenal gland, such as from hemorrhage or infarction, with hemorrhage being seen in cases of blunt trauma, resulting, after major surgery, in disseminated intravascular coagulopathy, associated with sepsis, major burns, HIT syndrome, antiphospholipid syndrome, HIV infection, disseminated fungal infections, or TB.

Medications can also affect adrenal function, with etomidate being a well-known suppressor of cortisol production, even following a single dose. Other common drugs seen in the ICU include anticoagulants, phenobarbital, phenytoin, rifampin, opioids, chlorpromazine, and imipramine. Exogenous glucocorticoid administration is well known to cause a long-term adrenal suppression, creating a secondary adrenal insufficiency.

Tissue cortisol resistance is also well known to manifest in chronic inflammatory diseases, such as COPD, severe asthma, lupus, ulcerative colitis, and rheumatoid arthritis.

Finally it is something that one should suspect in all patients with unexplained hypovolemia or catecholamine-resistant hypotension.

How Is the Diagnosis Made?

Although the mechanisms leading to CIRC are poorly understood, it is generally well accepted that it involves an impaired production of CRH, ACTH, or cortisol. Individuals with this impaired production often become critically ill with illnesses that would otherwise be minor and are unlikely to improve without administration of steroids. It can be very difficult to diagnose, since its clinical features are similar to those of severe illness, and there are variable changes that can occur in the HPA axis during the course of an illness. If unrecognized, corticosteroid insufficiency can be life-threatening. Even with the early diagnosis and institution of therapy, patients have a higher mortality, decreased quality of life, and increased risk of developing an adrenal crisis [2–5].

The gold standard stimulation test is the insulin tolerance test (ITT), which assesses the integrity of the HPA axis. However it is limited in its use in the ICU and is not recommended for use on patients with ischemic heart disease, epilepsy, or severe cortisol deficiency. In normal subjects, peak plasma cortisol exceeds 18 μg/dL. However, the cortisol response to hypoglycemia can be reliably predicted by the ACTH stimulation test—a safer, quicker, and less-expensive study.

Diagnosis is generally made on either a random serum cortisol level or through a short ACTH challenge or (in the specific case of septic shock) the incremental change seen in cortisol levels in response to an ACTH test. This latter test evaluates the cortisol response to acute ACTH stimulation with either a 250-μg dose (high or standard dose) or a 1-μg dose (low dose) [6, 7], with both tests having similar diagnostic accuracy for primary or secondary adrenal insufficiency [8]. Both tests are adequate to rule in, but not rule out secondary adrenal insufficiency. The IV administration of ACTH is used in the initial assessment of adrenal insufficiency, with the short synacthen test, making it easy to assess adrenal reserves. Baseline cortisol function tests are obtained before and 30 or 60 min after administration of 250-μg synacthen is administered, with the highest value being utilized to calculate the delta. As the poststimulation value is used for diagnostic purposes in this test, the effects of the circadian rhythm are negated, and this test may be performed at any time throughout the day [9].

Synthetic glucocorticoids such as prednisolone and methylprednisolone cross-react significantly in most cortisol assays, while prednisone cross-reacts to a smaller extent, but is converted to prednisolone in vivo [10]. Cortisol precursors and cortisol metabolites cross-react in some assays, but do not generally present a problem in clinical use.

Increased cortisol-binding globulin and total cortisol concentrations are associated with estrogen use, and low serum albumin concentrations, such as those commonly found in the ICU setting or with hepatic or renal failure, which may lead to misleading reduced total serum cortisol concentrations despite normal biologically active free cortisol concentrations [9], with the dissociation between free and protein-bound states being the most significant in patients with hypoalbuminemia <2.5.

In addition, random basal serum cortisol levels are of limited value of assessment of HPA axis reserve, and they follow diurnal variation, with higher concentrations seen in the early morning.

The interpretation of these tests is difficult, and the final decision regarding treatment is based on clinical context. There are no current tests in place to measure tissue glucocorticoid resistance or determine the circulating cortisol level needed to overcome tissue resistance. Where there is uncertainty, empiric glucocorticoid replacement is usually indicated.

The biochemical diagnosis is another approach to consider. Although it can be straightforward in an outpatient setting, it often becomes much more difficult in the critical care unit. In established primary hypoadrenalism, hyponatremia is present in 90% of cases and hyperkalemia in 65%. Hyperkalemia occurs due to an aldosterone deficiency and is therefore usually absent in secondary hypoadrenalism. Hyponatremia may be depletional in Addisonian crisis, but elevated vasopressin levels can cause dilutional hyponatremia in secondary adrenal insufficiency as well. Usually, free thyroxine concentrations are low or normal, but TSH values are frequently elevated. This is a direct effect of glucocorticoid deficiency and reverses with glucocorticoid replacement. Thyroxine levels may also be low in secondary hypoadrenalism. Thyroid hormone administration without glucocorticoids in these situations can precipitate adrenal insufficiency and should be avoided. Eosinophilia may be seen and can occasionally alert a clinician to the diagnosis.

Treatment

The benefit of moderate-dose steroids (200–300 mg/day) in divided doses has been evaluated for patients in septic shock in randomized control studies [1]. These have shown a more rapid reversal of shock but no decrease in mortality. It is currently recommended that in states of shock with suspected CIRC, IV doses should be given as 50 mg every 6 h or 100 mg every 8 h. Clinical improvement, especially in blood pressure, should be evident within 6 h if the diagnosis is correct. Mineralocorticoid replacement is generally not required during high-dose hydrocortisone therapy, but should be considered in patients with adrenal disease, when daily hydrocortisone doses drop below 50 mg per day.

In patients with ARDS, the dosing regimen may be either 1 mg/kg/day methylprednisolone as a continuous infusion or a low-dose regimen as described above. Low-dose steroids utilized in the early stages of ARDS may improve hypoxemia and reduce the period of mechanical ventilation and number of ICU days, but it has not been shown to reduce mortality [11]. On the other hand, there are studies that show improvement on short-term mortality if a low-dose steroid administration has started within 14 days of diagnosis [12, 13].

Some complications that can occur with the utilization of steroids during treatment should be kept in mind. These include GI bleeding, hyperglycemia, other major organ failures (kidney, heart, and liver), arrhythmia, pneumothorax, and psychiatric disorders.

Summary

Adrenal insufficiency occurs in critical illness and is associated with morbidity and mortality. Diagnosis is made on either a random serum cortisol level or through a ACTH stimulation test. Early diagnosis and treatment with corticosteroids are keys to optimizing outcomes.

References

1. Gabrelli A, Layon AJ, Yu M. Endocrine disease and dysfunction. In: Gabrelli A, Layon AJ, Yu M. editors. Civetta, Taylor & Kirby's: critical care. 4th ed. Philadelphia: Lippincott, Williams & Wilkins; 2014.
2. Park YJ, Park KS, Kim JH, et al. Reproducibility of the cortisol response to stimulation with the low dose (1 microg) of ACTH. Clin Endocrinol. 1999;51:153–8.
3. Burman D, Morrison GD. Too many infant deaths. Be Med J. 1963;2:1419–20.
4. Benson S, Neumann P, Unger N, et al. Effects of standard glucocorticoid replacement therapies on subjective well being: a randomized, double blind, crossover study in patients with secondary adrenal insufficiency. Eur J Endocrinol. 2012;167:679–85.
5. Hahner S, Loeffler M, Fassnacht M, et al. Impaired subjective health status in 256 patients with adrenal insufficiency or standard therapy based on cross-sectional analysis. J Clin Endocrinol Metab. 2007;92:3912–22.
6. Bancos I, Hahner S, Tommlinson J, Arlt W. 2014 diagnosis and management of adrenal insufficiency. Lancet Diabetes Endocrinol. 2015;3:216–26.
7. de Miguel Novoa P, Vela ET, Garcia NP, et al. Guidelines for the diagnosis and treatment of adrenal insufficiency in the adult. Endocrinol Nutr. 2014;1(61 Suppl):1–35.
8. Ospina NS, Nofal A, Murad H, et al. ACTH stimulation tests for diagnosis of adrenal insufficiency: systematic review and meta-analysis. J Clin Endocrinol Metab. 2016;101(2):427–34.
9. Brennan A, O'Connor KA, Plant WD, O'Halloran DJ. Nephrotic syndrome: cause of an abnormal response to the rapid ACTH stimulation test. Nephrol Dial Transplant. 2004;19:477.
10. Wallace I, Cunningham S, Lindsay J. The diagnosis and investigation of adrenal insufficiency in adults. Ann Clin Biochem. 2009;46:351–67.
11. Cho YJ, Mono JY, Shin ES, Won C, et al. Clinical practice guideline of acute respiratory distress syndrome. Tuber Respir Dis. 2016;79:241–33.
12. Peter JV, John P, Graham PL, Moran JL, George IA, Bersten A. Corticosteroids in the prevention and treatment of ARDS in adults; meta-analysis. Crit Care Med. 2009;37:1594–603.
13. Meduri GU, Marik PE, Chorousos GP, Pastores SM, Arlt W, et al. Steroid treatment in ARDS: a critical appraisal of the ARDS network trial and the recent literature. Intensive Care Med. 2008;34:61–9.

Thyroid Hormone Abnormalities

46

James M. Bardes and Elizabeth Benjamin

Thyroid Hormone

Function

Thyroid hormone is a permissive hormone with action through the body. Secreted primarily as T4, thyroid hormone is bound to thyroid-binding globulin (TBG) while in circulation. T4 is converted to its active form of T3 in the liver and in the peripheral tissues. When T3 enters a cell it binds to chromatin-bound nuclear receptors called thyroid hormone response elements. Active T3 has many effects on metabolism, including influence on the basal metabolic rate and metabolism of proteins and carbohydrates.

Regulation

Thyroid hormone synthesis and secretion is regulated by a negative feedback system. Decreased thyroid hormone stimulates the hypothalamus to secrete thyroid-releasing hormone (TRH). This stimulates the release of thyroid-stimulating hormone (TSH) by the anterior pituitary. Once secreted, TSH acts on the thyroid gland to induce synthesis of thyroid hormone. The thyroid gland then secretes thyroid hormone into circulation in the form of T4, or thyroxine. Once in circulation T4 is converted to T3, which provides negative feedback to the hypothalamus.

Measurement

In a non-critically ill patient, the preferred initial thyroid test is to measure serum TSH levels. High TSH levels indicate the thyroid gland is not producing enough thyroid hormone and represents hypothyroidism. A low TSH level indicates the thyroid gland is producing too much thyroid hormone and the patient is hyperthyroid. Most laboratories will perform reflex T4 or free T4 testing after an abnormal TSH level has been determined. Elevated TSH levels with low T4 point to the thyroid gland as the cause of hypothyroidism. A low TSH with low T4 indicates hypothyroidism due to the pituitary gland. A low TSH with high T4 indicates hyperthyroidism originating at the thyroid gland itself.

Additional testing for thyroid antibodies can be performed for patients with evidence of hyperthyroidism. Antibody tests for antithyroid peroxidases or anti-thyroglobulin in a hypothyroid patient are diagnostic for Hashimoto's thyroiditis. Antibodies to the TSH receptor result in Graves's disease and are often referred to as thyroid-stimulating immunoglobulin (TSI).

Pharmacology

Replacement

Thyroid hormone replacement is indicated to replace the function of a nonfunctioning gland and as suppression therapy to prevent further progression of disease in the setting of thyroid cancer. Hypothyroidism is the most common cause for hormone replacement. Replacement is started based on weight, at a dose of 1.7 μg/kg/day. Older adults can be started safely at 1 μg/kg/day due to changes in their metabolism. Rarely are doses greater than 200 mcg/day required. Patients are advised to take thyroid replacement at the same time each morning, an hour before meals. If patients prefer to take replacement dosing in the evening, it should be more than 3 h after the evening meal. Providers should consider this timing when ordering replacement in an ICU where continuous tube feeds are common. Additionally thyroid hormone should not be administered within 4 h of certain medications and supplements, as they can have effects on serum levels (Fig. 46.1).

J. M. Bardes · E. Benjamin (✉)
Division of Trauma, Emergency Surgery and Surgical Critical Care, Los Angeles County and Univeristy of Southern California Medical Center, Los Angeles, CA, USA
e-mail: elizabeth.benjamin@med.usc.edu

A. Salim et al. (eds.), *Surgical Critical Care Therapy*, https://doi.org/10.1007/978-3-319-71712-8_46

Fig. 46.1 Medications affecting thyroid replacement dosing

<u>Increased Serum Concentration</u>
Androgens
Anabolic Steroids

<u>Decreased Serum Concentration</u>

Calcium Carbonate	Phenobarbitol
Proton Pump Inhibitors	Phenytoin
Aluminum Based Antacids	Carbamazepine
Coleselvalam	Sertraline
Cholestyramine	Rifampin
Selavamer	Tyrosine Kinase Inhibitors
Clofibrate	Tamoxifen and Raloxifene
Orlistat	Estrogens
Ferrous Sulfate	Capecitabine
Mitotane	Fluorourarcil
Opioids	

The most common replacement is levothyroxine or T4. This will be converted peripherally into the active form T3; this conversion is not normally effected by thyroid disease. Additionally T4 has a much longer half-life, making it the preferred replacement hormone. There are synthetic T3 replacements available. This form of replacement must be taken several times daily to maintain adequate thyroid hormone levels due to its short half-life. This form of replacement is not well tolerated; patients frequently complain of hyperthyroid-type symptoms immediately after ingestion due to spikes in this active form of the hormone. Lastly a combined T3 and T4 replacement is available. This is given once daily due to the presence of T4. The T3 in this combination drug will still cause some patients symptoms of hyperthyroidism immediately after ingestion. However, some patients report an overall decrease in hypothyroid symptoms when on either T3 replacement or combination regimens.

Treatment of Hyperthyroidism

Medical treatment of hyperthyroidism can be directed at decreasing available thyroid hormone or against the thyroid gland itself. Two medications are primarily used to decrease the available thyroid hormone. Propylthiouracil (PTU) inhibits enzymes within the thyroid gland to decrease the production of T4. This is done by inhibiting thyroperoxidase, which normally is responsible for adding iodine to tyrosine residues during the formation of T4. PTU additionally inhibits peripheral conversion of T4 to its active T3 form. In this manner PTU acts both centrally and peripherally to decrease available thyroid hormone. Side effects of PTU include agranulocytosis. This can present as infections of the skin or respiratory tract. Thrombocytopenia has also been reported with severe bleeding. Lastly and the most concerning is the rare case of fulminant hepatic failure. While these serious side effects are reported, they are rare; the majority of patients will tolerate PTU well.

Methimazole is another antithyroid medication. Similar to PTU, methimazole works centrally within the thyroid by inhibiting thyroperoxidase, decreasing available thyroid hormone for secretion. Unlike PTU, there is no effect on peripheral thyroid hormone conversion by methimazole. Agranulocytosis is a serious side effect of methimazole as well. Patients and clinicians should be informed that it is also a potent inhibitor of the CY450 system. Plasma concentration of many other medications will be increased substantially while taking methimazole, and dosing should be done with caution.

For patients that require long-term ablation of the thyroid gland itself, radioactive iodide (RAI), I-131, is used. The American Thyroid Association (ATA) recommends pretreating patients with antithyroid hormone medications and β-blockade prior, as the administration of RAI is known to increase serum thyroid hormone levels and could precipitate thyroid storm. Generally RAI is administered based on the size of the patient's thyroid gland. Thyroid hormone levels are then checked 1–2 months after treatment and then serially until the patient becomes hypothyroid. At this time thyroid replacement therapy is initiated.

Acute Infectious Thyroiditis

Normal thyroid gland is resistant to infection due to its high vascularity and high iodine concentrations. In rare cases the thyroid gland can become infected; in these cases acute infectious thyroiditis or suppurative thyroiditis can be a medical emergency. This condition is responsible for less than 1% of thyroiditis but can carry a mortality rate of up to 12%. Common bacteria include *Staphylococcus aureus* and *Streptococcus* species. Other aerobic organisms including *Klebsiella* and *H. influenza* have also been reported and rarely a fungal infection. Most patients will also report a recent upper respiratory tract infection prior to developing thyroiditis.

Patients will present with acute onset fever, pain, erythema, and swelling in the anterior neck. Dysphagia and voice changes are common. A leukocytosis will be present. Ultrasound examination will demonstrate swelling and edema of the thyroid and can assist with diagnosis. Treatment is primarily antimicrobials. Fine needle aspirate can be performed to tailor antibiotic choices. Broad-spectrum antibiotics should be selected to cover common organisms. Coverage for MRSA would rarely be indicated. Penicillins with beta-lactamase inhibitors are excellent first-choice antibiotics. Clindamycin or a macrolide can be considered in the case of penicillin allergy. If antibiotic therapy does not lead to improvements in symptoms, surgical drainage may be required. When performing surgical drainage, a lobectomy is performed.

Hashimoto's Thyroiditis

Also known as chronic lymphocytic thyroiditis, Hashimoto's thyroiditis is an autoimmune destruction of the thyroid gland. With time this leads to symptoms of hypothyroidism and is a leading cause of hypothyroidism in the United States. It primarily affects women age 30–50. A family history of thyroid disease is common, and there appears to be a genetic component. The HLA-DR5 gene and CTLA-4 gene polymorphisms are associated with an increased risk of Hashimoto's thyroiditis development. Pathology will demonstrate a lymphocytic infiltration into the thyroid gland.

Patients may present with goiter as an initial symptom or may present with chronic complaints related to decreased thyroid hormone levels. Laboratory analysis will show an elevated TSH, low thyroid hormone and free hormone levels, and antithyroid antibodies. Treatment is primarily based on symptoms of hypothyroidism. If patients are found to have elevated antibody levels but thyroid hormone levels are still normal, no treatment is indicated. When hormone levels decrease and patients become symptomatic, then levothyroxine should be started. Doses are adjusted every 6–8 weeks by following TSH levels. Once patients reach a steady state, then yearly TSH monitoring is sufficient.

Graves' Disease

Graves' disease is an autoimmune disorder of the thyroid gland, commonly resulting in symptoms of hyperthyroidism. These signs and symptoms include irritability, tachycardia, heat intolerance, weight loss, and diarrhea. Graves' ophthalmopathy is seen in more than 25% of patients and results in an exophthalmos or a bulging of the eyes. Pretibial myxedema is another sign of Graves' disease and usually a late finding. It presents as a waxy discoloration of the skin overlying the shin.

The disorder results from antibodies to the TSH receptor present on the thyroid gland. These TSI antibodies cause the thyroid gland to overproduce thyroid hormone. Laboratory analysis shows elevated T3 and T4 levels and low TSH levels. Testing for TSI will confirm the diagnosis.

Treatment for Graves' disease is multifaceted. Initial treatment includes medications to reduce thyroid hormone synthesis and release. Methimazole and PTU are common treatments. Radioactive iodine-131 (I-131) is an additional treatment modality. As the thyroid gland is hyperstimulated to uptake iodine, it will absorb the majority of the radioactive I-131. Radioactive ablation is less commonly used due to its high rate of hypothyroidism requiring thyroid replacement after therapy. Ablation must be avoided in select patient populations such as pregnant females and patients with prior radiation exposure. Lastly, surgical therapy can be applied to Graves' disease. It is commonly used for young patients who are at prolonged risk of disease progression or recurrence. Additionally, it may be used in the setting of pregnancy to avoid antithyroid medication effects on the fetus. Lastly, surgery is considered for compressive symptoms from a large goiter or glands with suspicious nodules.

Sick Euthyroid Syndrome

Thyroid hormone levels remain challenging to assess among the hospitalized, particularly in those with critical non-thyroidal illness. Many of these patients will present with low levels of both T3 and T4 and TSH. This syndrome has classically been called the sick euthyroid syndrome or acquired transient central hypothyroidism. It is commonly associated with decrease in serum gonadotropin and sex hormone levels and increased cortisol levels.

Patients can present with a variety of thyroid hormone level abnormalities. These abnormalities are often found incidentally during testing for other endocrinopathies or frequently in the evaluation of cardiac arrhythmias. Low T3 is the most common finding and occurs within 24 h of critical illness. This decrease in T3 levels is a result of decreased conversion of T4 in the periphery. Thyroid hormone receptors are also decreased. T4 levels can be elevated during the acute phase of severe illness but will become low as the duration or severity of illness increases. This decrease in T3 and T4 is partially due to a decrease in serum TSH leading to decreased production of thyroid hormone. Additionally, a decrease in thyroid hormone binding to serum proteins also occurs. This decrease in protein binding allows free levels of thyroid hormone to remain close to normal, and patients will appear clinically euthyroid despite decreased hormone production.

Management

Thyroid hormone replacement is not indicated or effective in patients with severe non-thyroidal illness and low T3 or T4 levels. It has been suggested the decrease in thyroid hormone is protective as it prevents excess tissue catabolism in an already stressed patient. Studies of replacement in both burn patients and the critically ill have shown no improvements in mortality, metabolism, or outcomes. These findings were similar in studies of patients undergoing coronary artery bypass surgery who also had lower levels of T3. Recovery is variable post-critical illness. The vast majority of patients will return to normal thyroid function, although recovery may take several weeks, in some cases up to 6 months.

Thyroid Storm

Thyroid storm is an acute and life-threatening clinical entity. It is a severe expression of hyperthyroidism. Its frequency in the surgical literature has varied from as low as 2% to as high as 10% of patients. Classically it was seen postoperatively in patients undergoing thyroid surgery, or after administration of RAI, but can also be seen in the critically ill. Better recognition of the disease has led to a decreased incidence, due to preoperative preventative measures. By giving preoperative thyroid treatment to deplete the thyroid of available hormone, and an increased prevalence of perioperative beta-blockers, the incidence of thyroid storm has declined significantly. Thyroid storm remains a rarely seen event in the modern intensive care unit. However, intensivists must maintain a high index of suspicion in patients with sudden decompensation and a history of thyroid disease. Currently it is most frequently seen in the setting of an infection, pneumonia and upper respiratory being the most common. Other ICU-related stressors such as trauma, diabetic ketoacidosis, and severe cardiac disease could all be precipitators. Providers should also be mindful when stopping antithyroidal medications as this can precipitate thyroid storm as well. Rarely, it has been reported in patients receiving iodinated contrast when they have unrecognized or untreated thyroid disease.

Clinical Presentation

The clinical presentation of thyroid storm is varied. The most common features are fever, tachycardia, and mental status changes. Fever can often range from 104° to 106 °F. Additional symptoms can affect multiple organ systems. Neurologically these patients can exhibit a wide range of symptoms, from psychosis, to delirium and agitation, or even stupor or coma. These patients will often exhibit tremors as well. The gastrointestinal system commonly exhibits nausea and vomiting, diarrhea, and even organomegaly. Some series have also shown jaundice and hepatic failure. Cardiac complications can be the most dangerous and are the most prevalent; more than 60% of patients will have cardiac complications. Patients with thyroid storm will exhibit tachyarrhythmias with heart rates exceeding 140 beats per minute, atrial fibrillation, and congestive heart failure. Complete cardiovascular collapse has been reported with a high mortality rate.

Physical exam can be nonspecific. Clinicians may identify typical findings of hyperthyroidism such as goiter, lid lag, exophthalmos in the settings of Graves' disease, tremor, and skin that is warm and diaphoretic.

Diagnosis

Diagnosis of thyroid storm remains primarily clinical. Lab abnormalities are common, but none are specific for thyroid storm. Patients will demonstrate elevated thyroid hormone levels, with serum T3 levels being greater than T4. TSH is typically low to undetectable.

Physicians should be cognizant of the possible multisystem organ failure that can follow a thyroid storm. Additional laboratory measures to consider are liver function tests, calcium levels, checking of hematocrit, and white blood cell count. As the condition is managed, consider ordering blood cultures and lactate levels to evaluate for a septic source as the precipitating agent. Brain natriuretic peptide and cardiac evaluation with EKG and echo may assist with ruling out cardiac disease as the inciting event or a complication of thyroid storm.

Management

Management of this acute life-threatening condition is directed at supportive measures and treatment for the thyroid itself. Any patient with clinical concern for thyroid storm should be transferred to an ICU for appropriate management. Clinicians must identify the precipitating factor and provide treatment.

To treat the thyroid itself, antithyroid drugs are first-line treatment in the management of thyroid storm. PTU and methimazole are both used in its treatment. PTU is preferred due to its better efficacy at large doses and effects on peripheral conversion of T4 to T3, but either may suffice. PTU can be started at 200 mg every 4 h, or if using methimazole, start at 20 mg every 6 h. One hour after patients are loaded with antithyroid medications, they should be given iodide medication to block the release of already formed thyroid hormone. Lugol's solution is given 10 drops every 8 h until symptoms subside. Steroid administration, dexamethasone 2 mg intravenous (IV) every 6 h or hydrocortisone 100 mg every 8 h, is used as both a supportive and antithyroid treatment. Steroids prevent conversion of T4 to T3 in the periphery and manage any concomitant adrenal insufficiency. Lastly, consider the administration of cholestyramine, 4 g orally four times daily, to reduce enterohepatic circulation of thyroid hormone.

Supportive therapy is aimed at each patient's symptoms. Many will require IV fluid resuscitation secondary to fluid losses from the hyperthermia. IV fluid resuscitation should be titrated to achieve a urine output of greater than 0.5 cc/kg/h. Acetaminophen, other antipyretics, and cooling blankets may also be needed to treat severe hyperthermia. Temperatures greater than 102.2 °F can be treated with cooling blankets and ice packs to the axilla and groin. Hemodynamic support is commonly provided via β-blockade. Propranolol is an ideal choice to manage tachyarrhythmias in the setting of thyroid storm. Its β-blocking ability is augmented by an inhibitory action on T4 to T3 conversion as well. Patients will often require 60–80 mg of oral propranolol every 6 h for control of heart rate. Some patients may require IV esmolol for careful titration in the setting of acute heart failure. Esmolol is given with a loading dose of 250–500 mcg/kg followed by an infusion starting at 50 mcg/kg/min. Esmolol can be increased until a maximum of 300 mcg/kg/min is achieved. If arrhythmias are present, consider the use of calcium channel blockers.

There are small reports using plasmapheresis to remove thyroid hormone during thyroid storm. Lithium has also been given to prevent the release of more thyroid hormone during acute thyroid storm. However, it cannot be recommended for routine use, because the renal and neurotoxicity that accompany its administration limit its effectiveness.

Treatment is continued until there is clinical resolution of symptoms. Central nervous system symptoms will resolve, the patient will become normothermic without antipyretics, and cardiac manifestations will be resolved. At this time iodine therapy, Lugol's solution, can be discontinued. Beta-blockers should continue until the patient's thyroid function tests return to normal. PTU or methimazole can be titrated to maintain a euthyroid state with the assistance of endocrinology.

Myxedema Coma

Myxedema coma is a complication of severe chronic hypothyroidism. There is usually a precipitating stressor that induces this condition. Myxedema coma can be precipitated by cold exposure, infections such as pneumonia or UTI, trauma or surgery, and several common medications. Mortality rates are reported up to 60% for this rare condition.

Clinical Presentation

Myxedema coma presents with hypothermia with cardiovascular depression and altered mental status. Patients will report lethargy and weight gain over the preceding months as a consequence of their severe hypothyroidism. The patients experience cardiac effects due to the severe hypothermia; these include bradycardia and profound hypotension. This cardiac depression can be exacerbated by pleural or pericardial effusions. The gastrointestinal tract will also become atonic presenting with an ileus. Lastly clinicians will note the effects of chronic hypothyroidism, including delayed reflexes, dry and rough skin, periorbital edema, and patchy hair loss.

Diagnosis

Myxedema coma is a clinical diagnosis. Commonly these patients are unable to provide a detailed history; collateral history should be obtained from family and caregivers to demonstrate symptoms of chronic hypothyroidism.

Laboratory testing will reveal an elevated TSH and a low or undetectable T4 level. These labs may be indistinguishable from routine hypothyroidism. Additional laboratory abnormalities are common but not specific to myxedema coma. Providers should still evaluate for laboratory abnormalities to maximize supportive therapy; these include anemia, hyponatremia, acidosis, and elevations in creatine kinase and lactate dehydrogenase. Up to 10% will demonstrate adrenal insufficiency if cortisol levels are evaluated.

Management

Severe thyroid disease resulting in myxedema coma requires admission to an ICU. Therapy for this condition is based on support for symptoms and supplemental thyroid hormone. Thyroid hormone replacement should begin with an IV loading dose of 200–300 μg of T4. IV replacement is mandatory as many of these patients will present with an ileus. Daily dosing of 50–100 μg follows this. If no improvement is seen within 12 h of the initial loading dose, a second load may be given. This rapid rise in thyroid hormone levels can precipitate cardiac arrhythmias, so all of these patients should be on continuous telemetry monitoring. If arrhythmias do develop, they should be managed symptomatically.

Supportive therapy is initially targeted to hypothermia correction. Core temperatures have been reported as low as 23 °C. For severe hypothermia, active warming of 0.5 °C per hour should be performed until the patient's core temperature is above 31 °C. Above this, the patient should receive passive heating; do this by placing them in a warm room and minimizing heat loss with blankets. Hypothermia may cause cardiac arrhythmias requiring antiarrhythmic therapy. Severe hypotension is also common. Initial management should be with crystalloid resuscitation; fluid choice should consider the common hyponatremia seen in this condition. Patients that do not respond to IV fluids will require vasopressor support until T4 replacement begins to take effect. Due to the severe neurologic and cardiac dysfunction, many of these patients will require intubation and ventilator support during their treatment. Laboratory values may demonstrate hypoglycemia, which should be treated with dextrose infusion. Lastly consider treatment with hydrocortisone, 100 mg IV every 8 h for treatment of adrenal insufficiency.

Treatment continues until symptoms clinically resolve. They are then transitioned to oral thyroid replacement. This replacement can be titrated with the assistance of endocrinology as an outpatient after the patient's recovery.

Thyroid Replacement in Potential Organ Donors

Thousands of Americans are currently awaiting life-saving organ donation. The majority will receive these organs from brain-dead donors. Unfortunately the process of brain death often causes a state of malperfusion to develop, severely damaging organs prior to transplantation. This process is a complex system affecting all organ systems with subsequent hemodynamic collapse. The cardiovascular collapse is caused by a shift toward anaerobic metabolism within the myocardium itself. Even with intensive vasopressor support, up to 25% of all available organ donors are lost. When evaluated, these potential organ donors will demonstrate low levels of circulating thyroid hormone, cortisol, and insulin. These hormone deficiencies have been targeted for intervention to stabilize potential donors. Thyroid hormone replacement to improve hemodynamics in the brain-dead donor has been trialed extensively. Finding an optimal regimen would potentially increase the available organ pool and potentially save lives.

1 ampule of 50% dextrose
2 g of methylprednisolone
20 U of insulin
20 μg of levothyroxine bolus
IV continuous infusion of levothyroxine at 10 μg/h

Fig. 46.2 Thyroid replacement protocol after brain death for potential donors

Several studies and protocols have been presented in the literature. One reported regimen is the administration of 1 ampule of 50% dextrose, 2 g of methylprednisolone, 20 U of insulin, and 20 μg of levothyroxine as a bolus followed by a continuous infusion of levothyroxine at 10 μg/h (Fig. 46.2) [5]. This protocol has been reported to decrease the total vasopressor requirement and improve hemodynamics for the brain-dead donor. As a result of thyroid hormone replacement, some centers have shown increased organs donated. Unfortunately, some centers have not shown this same increase in organs. The literature is confounded by a wide variety of thyroid dosing with differences in steroid administration and as a result a wide range of efficacy. This wide range of published effect has tempered enthusiasm for thyroid replacement in all potential donors. Additional work will need to be done to find the optimal regimen and demonstrate its true efficacy. For now, the use of a thyroid hormone replacement protocol should be considered for stabilization of brain-dead donors with high vasopressor requirements.

Suggested Readings

1. Brent GA, Hershman JM. Thyroxine therapy in patients with severe nonthyroidal illnesses and low serum thyroxine concentration. J Clin Endocrinol Metab. 1986;63(1):1.
2. Kapstein EM, Sanchez A, Beale E, et al. Clinical review: thyroid hormone therapy for postoperative nonthyroidal illnesses: a systematic review and synthesis. J Clin Enocrinol Metab. 2010;95(10):4526.
3. Ross DS, Burch HB, Cooper DS, et al. 2016 American Thyroid Association guidelines for diagnosis and management of hyperthyroidism and other causes of thyrotoxicosis. Thyroid. 2016;26(10):1343–421.
4. Chiha M, Samarasinghe S, Kabaker AS. Thyroid storm: an updated review. J Intesive Care Med. 2015;30(3):131–40.
5. Salim A, Vassiliu P, Velmahos GC, et al. The role of thyroid hormone administration in potential organ donors. Arch Surg. 2001;136:1377–80.

Intravenous Fluids

47

Peter Rhee and Paul M. Evans

Introduction

Surgical patients who are critically ill suffer all varieties of physiological insults, such as hemorrhagic, septic, cardiogenic, and neurogenic shock. They often are in renal failure with the resulting fluid and electrolyte imbalance and often cannot tolerate enteral nutrition which also significantly impairs their ability to manage salts and fluids autogenously. Thus, it is the surgeon's responsibility to control the patients' fluids precisely. Thoughtful management of the intravenous fluids is a critical skill in the ICU, and it is incumbent on surgeons to know this topic thoroughly. We will briefly discuss the different fluid compartments within the human body, as well as their major constituents. Then, we will discuss the most common types of fluids encountered in the ICU, as well as briefly covering their historical origin. Finally, we will discuss their use in specific situations and the evidence for their use. Due to the complexity of blood transfusions, this topic will not be addressed in this chapter.

Body Compartments and Constituents

In order to properly understand the effect of administration of intravenous fluids, it is important to have a solid understanding of water and electrolytes. Only for historic interest, the classic two-compartment model of the human body was first proposed by Adolf Magnus-Levy in 1906, who divided the body into the fat and lean tissue compartments [1]. More recently, a four-compartment model has been proposed, dividing the body into water, protein, bone ash, and fat [2] . Of these four compartments, water makes up the greatest proportion of the total body mass. However, the exact percentage varies based on an individual's age, gender, and BMI. Total body water (TBW) is approximately 60% of the total weight of an average male, and 50% for females or those who are obese, given their relatively greater amount of adipose tissue.

TBW is then divided into intracellular fluid (ICF) and extracellular fluid (ECF). ICF is 66% of TBW and consists of all water found within cell membranes. ICF cations are predominantly potassium and magnesium, whereas the major anions are proteins, phosphate, bicarbonate, and sulfate. ECF, on the other hand, is 33% of TBW and consists of all water outside of a cell membrane. This includes both interstitial fluid (75% of ECF) and intravascular fluid (25% of ECF). With some minor differences in the absolute concentrations, both sub-compartments of the ECF have sodium as the predominant cation and chloride and bicarbonate as the major anions (Table 47.1).

Although body water is divided into the intravascular, intracellular, and interstitial spaces, as surgical intensivists we only have access to, and the ability to directly control, the intravascular space, and thus we only indirectly affect the other spaces. Although the intravascular space contains only 8% of the total body water, it is the most important to understand as it is directly related to perfusion of nutrients to tissues.

Types of Intravenous Fluids

Intravenous fluids are drugs and should be given the same level of respect and understanding as any other intravenous medications. There is an optimal dose and it has toxicities associated with it and has a dose effect. Too frequently, fluids are given to a patient without much thought in regard to its pharmacology or any potential side effects. Current intravenous fluids are by no means benign as it is not a naturally found substance in our blood. Because blood is so complex, the recognition that the current fluids are in no way representative of blood and its contents is vital. Excessive fluids have

P. Rhee (✉) · P. M. Evans
Division of Acute Care Surgery, Department of Surgery, Grady Memorial Hospital, Atlanta, GA, USA
e-mail: prhee@gmh.edu

A. Salim et al. (eds.), *Surgical Critical Care Therapy*, https://doi.org/10.1007/978-3-319-71712-8_47

Table 47.1 Body compartments and constituents

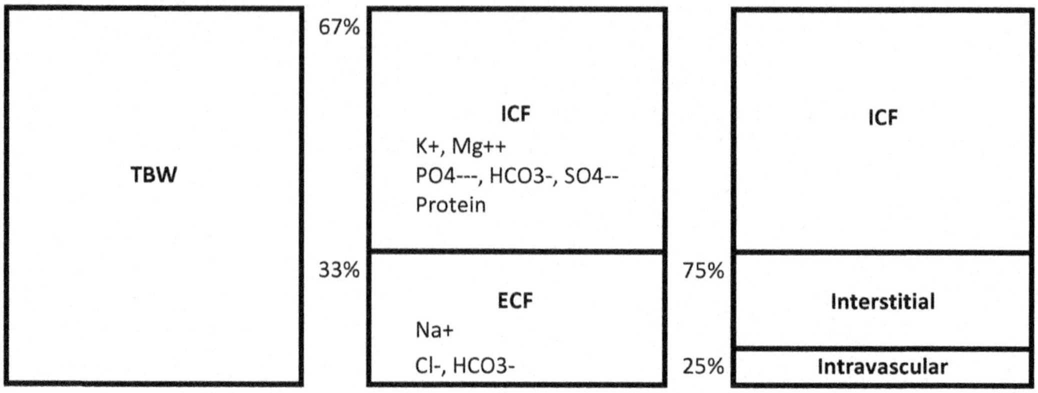

Table 47.2 Composition of common intravenous fluids

Fluid	Na+	Cl-	K+	Ca2+	Mg2+	HCO3- source	Other components	mOsm
NS	154	154						308
LR	130	109	4	3		28 lactate		273
Plasma-Lyte Normosol	140	98	5		3	27 acetate 23 gluconate		296
7.5% HTS	1283	1283						2567
5% albumin	145	145					50 g/L albumin	290
Hespan	154	154					60 g/L hetastarch	308
Hextend	130	109	4	3		28 lactate	60 g/L hetastarch	273
Voluven	154	154					60 g/L tetrastarch	308
D5½ NS + 20KCl	77	97	20				50 g/L dextrose	444

been associated with dysfunction of almost every organ system, including drowsiness and difficulty concentrating [3], worsening heart failure, precipitating myocardial infarction, pulmonary edema, ARDS [4–7], prolonged ileus [8–11], renal vasoconstriction and AKI [12], excessive bleeding from delusional coagulopathy as well as increased risk of DVT from hypercoagulability [13–16], neutrophil activation [17], and wound complications [11].

Currently intravenous fluids are broadly separated into crystalloids and colloids. Crystalloid fluids include normal saline (NS), lactated Ringer's (LR), Ringer's acetate (RA), Plasma-Lyte, Normosol, and hypertonic saline (HTS). Colloids are subdivided into human-derived and synthetic colloids. Human-derived colloids include albumin, which comes in 4%, 5%, 20%, and 25% formulations, and plasma protein fraction (PPF). Synthetic colloids come in essentially three varieties: hydroxyethyl starch (HES), gelatin, and dextran. We will now discuss each of these fluids in greater detail and their relative advantages and disadvantages.

Crystalloids

Normal saline is one of the first crystalloids to come into existence and is still widely used in the ICU. However, its origins are somewhat obscure. In 1831, Irish physician William Brooke O'Shaughnessy first described his idea of giving patients suffering from cholera, salt-containing fluids. High volumes were required to treat the massive dehydration which resulted from cholera. Because of such severe total body water deficit, the high volumes of replacement were required which was often up to 10 liters of fluid. Later, when studying the concentration of salt water that did not cause erythrocytes to burst, Dutch chemist Hartog Jakob Hamburger erroneously concluded that 0.9% saline was the concentration of sodium chloride in the blood. Because this estimation was in error, the currently available and used normal saline (also known as physiologic saline) is by no means normal nor physiologic, with a concentration of 154 mEq/L of Na + and Cl- (Table 47.2), both well above their corresponding normal values in the blood [18]. Excessive use of NS can lead to a non-anion gap acidosis, renal arteriolar vasoconstriction and impaired ability to excrete salt loads, reduction in gastric blood flow, impairment of cardiac contractility, pulmonary inflammation, and activation of neutrophils [3]. Again, while large volumes of normal saline can be useful when there is a large deficit of water and salt, when in excess there are physiologic consequences.

Lactated Ringer's (LR) has also been widely used in the critical care setting for a long time. LR was originally developed by Sydney Ringer (Fig. 47.1) in 1885 while devising a fluid that would allow an isolated frog heart to continue beat-

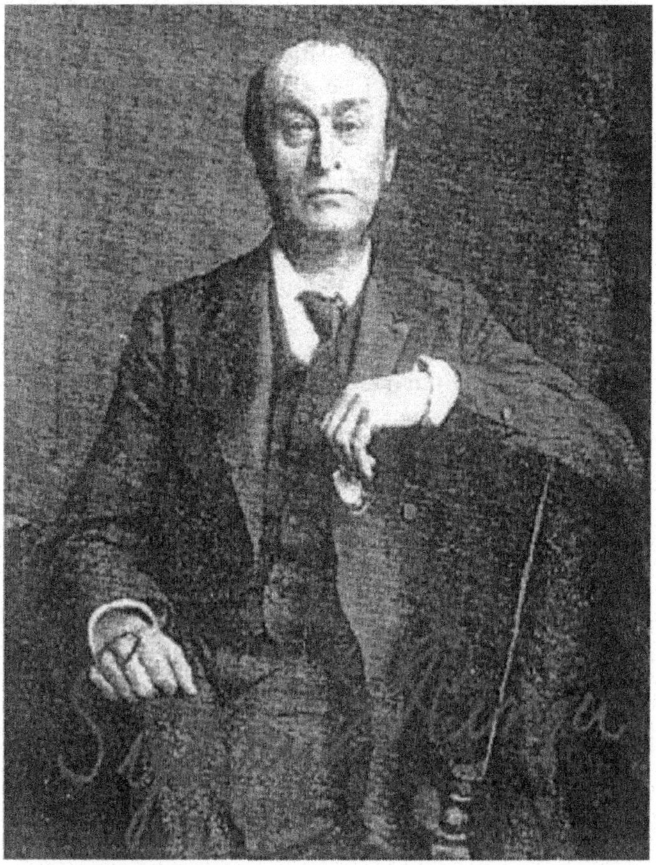

Fig. 47.1 Sidney Ringer

ing longer in vitro. He found that few additional electrolytes and a buffering agent were useful. Then, in 1932, pediatrician Alexis Hartmann modified this solution to include lactate to assist in his treatment of infantile diarrhea. He chose lactate instead of bicarbonate as bicarbonate was thought to cause alkalosis too rapidly, while it took longer for lactate to be converted to bicarbonate by the liver. Thus, just like normal saline, LR was originally created for purposes well out of the scope of the surgical ICU. The difference between the surgical ICU and nonsurgical ICU is that due to trauma or surgery, the patients often have blood loss, and using crystalloids to replace blood loss is now recognized as being the source of iatrogenic injury. It has only been recently recognized that large volumes of crystalloids will cause inflammation and injury as crystalloids do not resemble blood. Of note, the original LR formulation contained a racemic mixture of the L(+) and D(−) lactate; however, only the L(+) enantiomer is produced by humans. This difference is clinically significant as subsequent experiments determined that the D(−) enantiomer is more inflammatory than the L(+) enantiomer [19, 20]. Unfortunately, most LR formulations still contain the racemic mixture, and only one manufacturer (Baxter) makes LR with the L(+) enantiomer of lactate. Both NS and LR quickly leave the intravascular space. Studies have shown that less than 200 mL of a 1 L bolus remains in the intravascular compartment after a couple of hours [21].

Plasma-Lyte is a newer "balanced" crystalloid solutions sold by Baxter International and it has been heavily studied in various patient populations over the past 40 years. Normosol-R is a similar, cheaper alternative to Plasma-Lyte sold by Hospira. In comparison with LR, Plasma-Lyte has a lower chloride level, contains magnesium but no calcium, and uses acetate and gluconate as a buffer and bicarbonate source rather than lactate. Lactate is metabolized mostly by the liver, whereas acetate is rapidly metabolized by most cells in the human body, giving it at least a theoretical advantage [22]. Unlike LR, Plasma-Lyte contains no calcium so it can be used for blood transfusions. Magnesium deficiency is common in the ICU, so Plasma-Lyte may be useful in decreasing its incidence although it should be used carefully in the setting of renal failure. Although there are no studies demonstrating a survival benefit with the use of Plasma-Lyte compared to other crystalloids, Plasma-Lyte does appear to have a lower rate of respiratory failure, cardiac complications, GI bleeding, infection, electrolyte abnormalities, and renal failure when compared to normal saline [23, 24]. When used in trauma resuscitations, use of Plasma-Lyte rather than NS results in a more rapid base deficit clearance, lower chloride levels, and slightly better overall urine output [25].

Hypertonic saline (HTS) is a general term that describes any formulation of salt water that contains sodium chloride at a concentration greater than 0.9%. The most commonly used formulations include 3%, 5%, 7.5%, and 23.4%. Although 7.5% has been the most heavily studied in resuscitation following hemorrhagic shock, this concentration is not FDA-approved and thus not commercially available in the USA. There are no manufacturers that are interested in incurring the costs of getting 7.5% solution through the FDA as the profit margin from a non-patentable product is thought to be none. Unlike NS or other isotonic crystalloids, HTS tends to draw additional fluid from the extravascular compartment into the intravascular space, requiring less overall volume to be given to achieve the same hemodynamic effect [26, 27]. In fact, HTS has been extensively studied in animal models of hemorrhagic shock. In such models, 1 L of NS was required to return to a BP of 120 mmHg, whereas only 182 mL of 5% HTS or 120 mL 7.5% to achieve the same result [28]. This showed how important sodium was in the treatment of acute hemorrhagic shock and not the volume. In acute blood loss setting, there is enough extravascular water in reserve to be drawn into the intravascular compartment by the sodium.

These results attracted the interest of the military, who were interested in fluids that could be easily carried by medics and used for battlefield resuscitation of wounded bleeding soldiers. HTS was particularly attractive as it is stable at room temperature for many years, resistant to a wide range of temperatures, and comes in much smaller volumes than isotonic crystalloids. Due to the high sodium concentration, it is also relatively sterile. This enthusiasm ultimately culminated in the Resuscitation Outcomes Consortium (ROC) trial, which was a randomized multicenter trial in both the USA and Canada, comparing the prehospital use of HTS, HTS with dextran, and NS in patients in hemorrhagic shock trauma or those who suffered traumatic brain injury. Unfortunately, this trial was stopped early for futility, as an interim analysis showed that the likelihood of achieving a statistically significant difference was low [29]. Interestingly, the hypertonic nature of these fluids also causes arterial vasodilation, cutaneous hyperemia, and a sensation of warmth soon after infusion [30]. Moreover, depending on the concentration, HTS can be irritating to peripheral veins sometimes causing discomfort to the infusion site. The numerous prospective randomized studies have always shown that in regard to complications from HTS, there was no higher rate of complications [31, 32].

Human-Derived Colloids

Albumin is the mostly commonly used human-derived colloid in the ICU. Albumin is a 66.5kD protein that consists of 50% of the total protein content found in human plasma but contributes 80% of the intravascular oncotic pressure. As a commercially available fluid, albumin is fractionated from blood and is then dissolved in salt water. It is available in concentrations of 4%, 5%, 20%, and 25%. Plasma protein fraction (PPF) is similar to albumin but simply has fewer purification steps than albumin and thus is of lower purity (>95% vs 88%). The main advantages of albumin over isotonic crystalloids include a smaller volume of fluid needed to achieve the same hemodynamic effect and a longer duration of effect, given that the oncotic pressure generated by albumin may help keep water in the intravascular space and is less inflammatory [33]. In earlier studies in primates, albumin has been shown to eventually lead out of the intravascular space and is thought to possibly be responsible for retaining water in the extravascular and intracellular space. However, there is a small risk of transmission of prion disease with albumin, and it is approximately 30 times more expensive than isotonic crystalloids [34].

A heated debate between camps supporting the use of albumin or crystalloids for resuscitation has been raging on for decades, unfortunately without any definitive conclusions. The SAFE (saline versus albumin fluid evaluation) trial, published in 2004, is frequently cited by both groups. The SAFE trial was a multicenter randomized trial carried out in Australia and New Zealand, looking at 7000 patients admitted to the ICU for a broad variety of reasons. It was designed to demonstrate the safety of albumin. These patients were randomized to either NS or 4% albumin for resuscitation, and no differences were seen between these two groups [35]. Subsequent meta-analyses of all published RCTs studying the use of albumin in critically ill patients reached the same conclusion [36–38]. The SAFE trial excluded cardiac surgery patients, where albumin is widely used. However, notably there is no evidence of benefit in using albumin in this patient population either [12]. Thus, one can conclude either that there is no benefit to albumin compared with crystalloids and therefore given its expense it should be avoided or that there is no evidence of harm in using albumin instead of crystalloid and the choice of fluid should be left up to the individual practitioner.

Synthetic Colloids

Synthetic colloids are not derived from human blood, so they are much cheaper to produce and are much more widely available. They are stable at room temperature for long periods of time, and at least theoretically, synthetic colloids remain in the vascular space longer than crystalloids as they are unable to cross the capillary barrier [39, 40]. These putative benefits originally generated much enthusiasm for their use as a plasma expander, particularly in austere and military settings. Synthetic colloids available can be divided into three subgroups: gelatins, dextrans, and hydroxyethyl starches (HES).

Gelatin is derived from animal collagen and is chemically modified either via urea linkage (polygeline), succinylation (gelofusine, plasmagel, plasmion), or glyoxal and hydrogen peroxide (oxypolyn, gelifundol). Although the US government heavily funded research in the use of gelatins as a plasma expander during World War II, the wide availability of donated blood after the WWII quickly dampened enthusiasm for its use, and more recently its use has been shown to be associated with increased mortality [38].

Dextran is a glucose polymer produced by bacteria grown on sucrose media and is commercially available in either 40 kDa or 70 kDa average molecular weight varieties. Dextrans are effective volume expanders, lower blood viscosity, and prolong bleeding times, making them particularly attractive in protecting vascular suture lines after macro- and microvascular surgery [41, 42]. However, use of dextran is associated with many complications, including anaphylaxis, pulmonary edema, CHF, coagulopathy, and renal failure [43, 44], so any decision for its use should be carefully considered.

HES is a synthetic colloid derived from plant-based amylopectin. Amylopectin is chemically modified via hydrolyzation to varying degrees in order to increase its solubility in water and slow its degradation by enzymes. There are three HESs available in the USA: Hespan (Braun),

Hextend (Biotime), and Voluven (Fresenius Kabi). Both Hespan and Voluven are dissolved in NS, whereas Hextend is dissolved in LR. Unfortunately, no studies have demonstrated any benefit of synthetic colloid use compared to other fluids, and in fact they have been found to have many disadvantages, including severe allergic reactions, long-term deposition in the skin causing pruritis, coagulopathy, renal failure, and even an increased risk of death [45–47]. Thus, it is hard to find a setting where HES should be used. It too in large of concentrations has been shown to increase coagulopathy and thus increase bleeding time.

The artificial colloids are also not naturally found in the body and thus have dose effects just like all intravenous solutions. There are optimal doses that can be used for a variety of purposes. However, it should again be emphasized that in the setting of acute blood loss, the replacement of blood with artificial solutions has consequences. In the right dose, it can be used to benefit the patient. For example, the synthetic colloids interfere with the coagulation and inflammatory cascade as they are interrelated. Thus, in larger doses, it can be used to create coagulopathy which sometimes can be useful in vascular surgery when there are circumstances of wanting a controllable coagulopathic state. In high doses, it is well known that they cause coagulopathy, and that is typically undesirable in acute hemorrhagic shock.

Summary

Thus, in the majority of situations, despite years of effort and thousands of papers published on the subject, there is no clear evidence of benefit between using crystalloids and human-derived colloids for fluid resuscitation in the ICU, whereas the currently available synthetic colloids have clear evidence of harm and should generally be avoided.

Fluid Management in the Intensive Care Unit

Maintenance Fluids

Just as important as choosing the correct fluid in a given situation, if not more so, it is crucial to be able to determine the appropriate volume of fluid to give to a patient at any particular point in time. Although it may sound simple, this is a surprisingly difficult task. Critically ill patients can have significant blood loss from trauma, elective or emergent surgery, or water and electrolyte losses from fevers, vomiting, diarrhea, fistulas, burns, inflammation, sepsis, or intestinal obstruction. Thus, an ongoing challenge facing the intensivist while assessing a patient is to determine their volume status. Patients can be hypervolemic, normovolemic, or hypovolemic. To be on the safe side, if assumed that the normovolemic window is small, then the clinician will be more attuned to the patient's fluid requirements. Acute blood loss or sepsis causes hypovolemia, and replacement with appropriate fluids is needed. If the patient is hypervolemic after surgery, then average maintenance fluid should be avoided. It is nearly impossible to keep a patient precisely normovolemic: more commonly a patient is hypo- or hypervolemic. Clinically, too much volume can result in pulmonary edema and increase time on the ventilator, whereas too little volume could precipitate renal failure and its associated increased mortality, which can be as high as 30%. While it is preferred to not be infused with excess fluids causing longer ventilatory requirements, it is more preferred to avoid acute kidney injury with inadequate fluid infusion.

When a patient is unable to receive enteral nutrition for whatever the reason, they are often started on "maintenance" fluids. Typically, this means D5 ½ NS + 20 KCl at a maintenance rate of (weight in kg + 40) mL/hour in adults. This methodology is probably adequate for normal postoperative patients, but in the critical care setting, this approach is archaic. Despite their wide use, maintenance fluids have not been subjected to rigorous study, and the rationale for using this fluid at this rate is based on the estimated daily salt and water needs of a normal, healthy patient. Obviously, this is not the same patient population as is found in a typical ICU. Moreover, the rationale for adding dextrose to fluids is based on data from the 1920s showing that less urinary nitrogen was lost in fasting medical students if they were given IV dextrose. Thus, the choice of fluid and rate must be made carefully, taking into account the patient's overall volume status, electrolytes, renal function, pulmonary status, age, and nutritional needs. In order to determine how much fluids a person needs, the intravascular volume status needs to be first determined.

Traditional Means of Volume Assessment

Determination of volume status should be part of the overall daily assessment, and although newer technology is helpful in determining the minute-to-minute volume status, addressing any medical problem should always first involve a physical exam of the patient. Clues pointing toward extravascular hypervolemia include pitting extremity or sacral edema, anasarca, and distended neck veins, whereas signs of hypovolemia include poor skin turgor, sunken eyes, dry mucous membranes, flat neck veins, and weak peripheral pulses. A review of the patient's net fluid balance over the previous several days, as well as the total fluid balance since admission are also sometimes helpful and often misleading. Keep in mind that the insensible losses of fluids in a critically ill patient that may have undergone acute blood loss and is now febrile and septic is nearly impossible to assess. Next, review the patient's vitals and urine output. Oliguria, increased heart rate, narrowed pulse pressure due to a rising diastolic blood pressure, and of course overt hypotension are all signs suggestive of hypovolemia. Tachycardia in particular is difficult to use as a guide to a patient's volume status, as it is so easily affected by other variables, such as pain, anxiety, and SIRS. Next, review the patient's laboratory values. BUN/Creatinine ratio > 20, a rising creatinine, BUN, hemoglobin (due to hemoconcentration), lactate, base deficit, or a low HCO3- or ScvO2 are all suggestive of hypovolemia. Low urinary sodium (less than 20 mEq) and a FeNa <1% are also suggestive of hypovolemia, at least as perceived by the kidneys. Currently, the FeNa is still considered to be the most accurate in a patient without acute kidney injury and if not given diuretics. In most surgical critical care setting, the history of chronic renal failure is uncommon. For the average person who is assumed to have normal renal function, close attention to the hourly urine output can be extremely helpful in determining what the kidneys are doing in response to the intravascular renal blood flow. If the urine output is high, it can be assumed that the patient has adequate intravascular volume. If the urine output is low, it should be assumed that the normal functioning kidneys feel that the renal blood flow is lower than desired, and this should be confirmed if possible and maintenance fluids adjusted or increased if needed.

In regard to hypervolemia, in the absence of any acute pulmonary abnormality such as pneumonia, ARDS, or pulmonary contusion, the P/F ratio (PaO2 / FiO2) is quite helpful to determine the amount of interstitial lung water. A high P/F ratio in this setting is suggestive of low interstitial volume which could indicate low intravascular volume. If a patient has been determined to by hypervolemic, then it is imperative that all fluids be minimized and stopped before considering any forced diuresis which has not been shown to be beneficial but is associated with renal failure. Concurrent diuresis while infusing intravenous fluids subjects the patients to harm from the drugs forcing the diuresis. Forced diuresis also eliminates the use of urine output which is typically a reflection of renal blood flow. Thus it is difficult to know if the high urine output is due to the hypervolemia or the scenario of forced diuresis while hypovolemic. Drugs causing forced diuresis can also contribute to acute renal injury if given in the hypovolemic stage. Intravascular volume needs to be critically determined constantly but at the minimum three times a day in the ICU setting. Maintenance fluids should be constantly adjusted in the critical care setting, and a patient being blindly placed on 125 cc per hour of crystalloids irregardless of volume status, age, gender, and size shows lack of expertise in the management of intravenous maintenance fluids. The determination of the rate of fluids again is determined by the clinical assessment of the patient's intravascular and extravascular fluid status.

Invasive Monitoring

The values of any available invasive or advanced monitoring devices could be helpful. Invasive monitoring with a central line can measure a patient's central venous pressure (CVP) and is widely used as a means to infer a patient's volume status, based on the (often rather large) assumption that CVP ultimately correlates with the LVEDV. This has been thoroughly studied, and in fact, there is level 1 evidence that CVP as it is customarily used does not correlate in any way to volume status, and neither its absolute value nor any changes in its value in response to fluid are predictive. Therefore, it is suggested by some that CVP should not be used for this purpose of determining fluid status [48]. The pulmonary artery catheter (PAC) is an even more invasive catheter that can simultaneously measure CVP, pulmonary artery pressure (PAP), SvO2, and cardiac output (CO) via intermittent thermodilution and estimate LVEDV via intermittent measurement of the pulmonary artery occlusion pressure (PAOP or "wedge pressure"). Since its first introduction in 1970 [49], enthusiasm initially surged and then subsequently waned as reports of the many complications associated with its use came to light, including arrhythmias, knotting of catheter, infection, thrombosis, valvular damage, and even perforation of the pulmonary artery. Moreover, use of the PA catheter to guide resuscitation has not been shown to clearly have any benefit, and there may even be some harm [50, 51]. The problem with the PA catheter is the lack of expertise in interpreting the data and the concept that increasing oxygen delivery with a variety of fluids and drugs may not be valid.

Transesophageal echocardiography has been used for decades and can estimate a patient's volume status and CO via several measures in real time. CO is estimated by obtaining a window of the left ventricular outflow tract (LVOT), whereas the cross-sectional area is roughly cylindrical, and then measuring the total rate of flow at this point over systole (the velocity time integral). These two values multiplied together can estimate the CO. The degree of variation of the diameter of the SVC over the respiratory cycle, or the collapsibility index, is also predictive of fluid responsiveness. TEE also has the distinct advantage of being able to assess both LV and RV function and gather an overall assessment of cardiac function rather quickly. Its main disadvantages are its invasiveness, high cost, and need for specific training to be able to perform TEE competently. In the appropriate setting, it takes on average 31 exams to become competent with good interobserver reliability [52]. Another problem is that when looking at the heart in a variety of cross-sectional views, what the heart should look like for a particular individual is not known. There are certain circumstances that infer severe hypovolemia, but otherwise in the absence of these classic findings, the interpretation and action are highly variable. Traditional TEE probes are rather large, whereas a newer probe, the hTEE (ImaCor, USA), is only 6 mm in diameter and can be left in place for up to 72 h, allowing for ongoing, serial assessments with the TEE probe during resuscitation.

CardioQ™ (Deltex Medical, UK) is another device place in the esophagus, but rather than looking at the heart with ultrasound, it instead analyzes blood flow waveforms in the descending aorta to calculate fluid responsiveness, SV, contractility, and CO. The corrected duration of forward flow in the descending aorta, or FTc (flow time corrected), if less than 350 msec, is predictive of hypovolemia. There is good evidence for its use in the perioperative setting after major GI surgery, with the CardioQ™ being associated with a shorter hospital stay, fewer complications, and a quicker return of bowel function [53].

Minimally Invasive and Noninvasive Monitoring

More recently, the trend has been toward creating minimally invasive and even completely noninvasive devices that can measure variables traditionally obtained with a PA catheter. Even more importantly, there has been a trend toward attempting to use these devices in the perioperative or ICU setting in a goal-directed manner with the goal of improving outcomes. There is some evidence this strategy does reduce hospital length of stay and incidence of postoperative complications [54]. Strategies used to help achieve these goals include arterial waveform analysis, gastric tonometry, transesophageal echocardiography (TEE), esophageal Doppler, partial carbon dioxide rebreathing, transthoracic electrical bioimpedance, and electrical bioreactance cardiography.

Arterial waveform analysis, in its most simple form, calculates the degree of variation of the amplitude of the pulse pressure (PP) over the whole of the respiratory cycle. The resultant value, pulse pressure variation (PPV), if greater than 12%, is highly predictive of fluid responsiveness to a fluid challenge [55]. However, it must be kept in mind that fluid responsiveness doesn't necessarily mean that the patient needs fluids, just that the patient's cardiac function is still in the upward-sloping portion of the Frank-Starling curve. More advanced systems such as the FloTrac/Vigileo™ system (Edwards Lifesciences, USA) are based on the assumption that pulse pressure (PP) correlates with stroke volume (SV) and that therefore SV can be used to estimate stroke volume variation (SVV) and CO. These monitors use a large database of historical patients to create an adjustment factor to appropriate calculate the CO based on a given variability in PP. However, the calculated SVV is only accurate if several rather restrictive criteria are met. The patient must be on the ventilator with complete respiratory support, not have any significant arrhythmias (and thus is not useful in the setting of atrial fibrillation), and no RV failure. Moreover, its accuracy is worse if the patient is on a beta blocker or vasoactive agents. With the FloTrac/Vigileo™ system, the calculated CO is not calibrated. Other systems, such as the PiCCO™ (Maquet, France), VolumeView™ (Edwards Lifesciences, USA), and LiDCOplus™ (LiDCO, UK) use various means to externally calibrate CO and thus may be more accurate. The best evidence for their use to date, the OPTIMIZE trial [54], demonstrated that use of the LiDCOplus in the perioperative setting for 6 h after major gastrointestinal surgery resulted in a shorter length of stay and fewer complications, with no effect on mortality. The data for these new devices in the ICU setting, however, is much weaker and consists of mostly small retrospective studies.

More recently, a technology known as electrical bioreactance cardiography has been developed in an attempt to completely noninvasively evaluate fluid responsiveness. Currently, there is only one device on the market that uses this technology, the Cheetah NICOM/Starling SV (Cheetah Medical, USA). This device measures the phase shift of high-frequency alternating current signals transmitted across the thorax caused by pulsatile blood flow to estimate SV. The change in SV with a passive leg raise or 250 mL fluid bolus can be then used to predict fluid responsiveness. Although very attractive given its complete noninvasiveness, it has been minimally studied at this time, and its role remains to be defined.

Summary

Accurate and thoughtful management of a patient's hemodynamic status is a critical skill in the daily work of the modern intensivist. Intravenous fluids, like any other foreign substance injected into the patient's bloodstream, are drugs, and it is crucial that the intensivist has a complete understanding of the fluids being administered. Just as important as the type of fluid chosen are the rate and volume of fluids given, as these have a direct impact on the patient's likelihood of survival, and there are many invasive and noninvasive ways to estimate a given patient's volume status and to estimate the need for further resuscitation.

References

1. Magnus-Levy A. Physiologie des Stoffwechesels: Handbuch der Pathologie des Stoffwechesels. Noorden CV, editor. Berlin: 1906.
2. Baumgartner RN, et al. Body composition in elderly people: effect of criterion estimates on predictive equations. Am J Clin Nutr. 1991;53(6):1345–53.

3. Williams EL, et al. The effect of intravenous lactated Ringer's solution versus 0.9% sodium chloride solution on serum osmolality in human volunteers. Anesth Analg. 1999;88(5):999–1003.
4. Arieff AI. Fatal postoperative pulmonary edema: pathogenesis and literature review. Chest. 1999;115(5):1371–7.
5. Bishop MH, et al. The relationship between ARDS, pulmonary infiltration, fluid balance, and hemodynamics in critically ill surgical patients. Am Surg. 1991;57(12):785–92.
6. Plurad D, et al. The decreasing incidence of late posttraumatic acute respiratory distress syndrome: the potential role of lung protective ventilation and conservative transfusion practice. J Trauma. 2007;63(1):1–7; discussion 8.
7. Martin M, et al. The decreasing incidence and mortality of acute respiratory distress syndrome after injury: a 5-year observational study. J Trauma. 2005;59(5):1107–13.
8. Tambyraja AL, et al. Patterns and clinical outcomes associated with routine intravenous sodium and fluid administration after colorectal resection. World J Surg. 2004;28(10):1046–51; discussion 1051-2.
9. Lobo DN, et al. Effect of salt and water balance on recovery of gastrointestinal function after elective colonic resection: a randomised controlled trial. Lancet. 2002;359(9320):1812–8.
10. Brandstrup B, et al. Effects of intravenous fluid restriction on postoperative complications: comparison of two perioperative fluid regimens: a randomized assessor-blinded multicenter trial. Ann Surg. 2003;238(5):641–8.
11. Nisanevich V, et al. Effect of intraoperative fluid management on outcome after intraabdominal surgery. Anesthesiology. 2005;103(1):25–32.
12. Shaw A, Raghunathan K. Fluid management in cardiac surgery: colloid or crystalloid? Anesthesiol Clin. 2013;31(2):269–80.
13. Tocantins LM, Carroll RT, Holburn RH. The clot accelerating effect of dilution on blood and plasma. Relation to the mechanism of coagulation of normal and hemophilic blood. Blood. 1951;6(8):720–39.
14. Ng KF, Lam CC, Chan LC. In vivo effect of haemodilution with saline on coagulation: a randomized controlled trial. Br J Anaesth. 2002;88(4):475–80.
15. Janvrin SB, Davies G, Greenhalgh RM. Postoperative deep vein thrombosis caused by intravenous fluids during surgery. Br J Surg. 1980;67(10):690–3.
16. Ruttmann TG, Jamest MF, Lombard EH. Haemodilution-induced enhancement of coagulation is attenuated in vitro by restoring antithrombin III to pre-dilution concentrations. Anaesth Intensive Care. 2001;29(5):489–93.
17. Rhee P, et al. Human neutrophil activation and increased adhesion by various resuscitation fluids. Crit Care Med. 2000;28(1):74–8.
18. Awad S, Allison SP, Lobo DN. The history of 0.9% saline. Clin Nutr. 2008;27(2):179–88.
19. Rhee P, et al. Lactated Ringer's solution resuscitation causes neutrophil activation after hemorrhagic shock. J Trauma. 1998;44(2):313–9.
20. Koustova E, et al. Effects of lactated Ringer's solutions on human leukocytes. J Trauma. 2002;52(5):872–8.
21. Nees JE, et al. Comparison of cardiorespiratory effects of crystalline hemoglobin, whole blood, albumin, and Ringer's lactate in the resuscitation of hemorrhagic shock in dogs. Surgery. 1978;83(6):639–47.
22. Rizoli S. PlasmaLyte. J Trauma. 2011;70(5 Suppl):S17–8.
23. Shaw AD, et al. Major complications, mortality, and resource utilization after open abdominal surgery: 0.9% saline compared to Plasma-Lyte. Ann Surg. 2012;255(5):821–9.
24. McFarlane C, Lee A. A comparison of Plasmalyte 148 and 0.9% saline for intra-operative fluid replacement. Anaesthesia. 1994;49(9):779–81.
25. Young JB, et al. Saline versus Plasma-Lyte A in initial resuscitation of trauma patients: a randomized trial. Ann Surg. 2014;259(2):255–62.
26. Younes RN, et al. Hypertonic solutions in the treatment of hypovolemic shock: a prospective, randomized study in patients admitted to the emergency room. Surgery. 1992;111(4):380–5.
27. Dubick MA, Shek P, Wade CE. ROC trials update on prehospital hypertonic saline resuscitation in the aftermath of the US-Canadian trials. Clinics (Sao Paulo). 2013;68(6):883–6.
28. Velasco IT, et al. Hyperosmotic NaCl and severe hemorrhagic shock. Am J Phys. 1980;239(5):H664–73.
29. Bulger EM, et al. Out-of-hospital hypertonic resuscitation after traumatic hypovolemic shock: a randomized, placebo controlled trial. Ann Surg. 2011;253(3):431–41.
30. Holcroft JW. The hypertonic saline trial: a possible downside to the gold standard of double blinding. Ann Surg. 2011;253(3):442–3.
31. Joseph B, et al. The physiological effects of hyperosmolar resuscitation: 5% vs 3% hypertonic saline. Am J Surg. 2014;208(5):697–702.
32. DuBose JJ, et al. Clinical experience using 5% hypertonic saline as a safe alternative fluid for use in trauma. J Trauma. 2010;68(5):1172–7.
33. Powers KA, et al. Twenty-five percent albumin prevents lung injury following shock/resuscitation. Crit Care Med. 2003;31(9):2355–63.
34. Caironi P, Gattinoni L. The clinical use of albumin: the point of view of a specialist in intensive care. Blood Transfus. 2009;7(4):259–67.
35. Finfer S, et al. A comparison of albumin and saline for fluid resuscitation in the intensive care unit. N Engl J Med. 2004;350(22):2247–56.
36. Perel P, Roberts I, Ker K. Colloids versus crystalloids for fluid resuscitation in critically ill patients. Cochrane Database Syst Rev. 2013;(2):CD000567.
37. Delaney AP, et al. The role of albumin as a resuscitation fluid for patients with sepsis: a systematic review and meta-analysis. Crit Care Med. 2011;39(2):386–91.
38. Rochwerg B, et al. Fluid resuscitation in sepsis: a systematic review and network meta-analysis. Ann Intern Med. 2014;161(5):347–55.
39. Conhaim RL, et al. Pulmonary capillary sieving of hetastarch is not altered by LPS-induced sepsis. J Trauma. 1999;46(5):800–8; discussion 808-10.
40. Rosengren S, Ley K, Arfors KE. Dextran sulfate prevents LTB4-induced permeability increase, but not neutrophil emigration, in the hamster cheek pouch. Microvasc Res. 1989;38(3):243–54.
41. Hayes PD, et al. Transcranial Doppler-directed Dextran-40 therapy is a cost-effective method of preventing carotid thrombosis after carotid endarterectomy. Eur J Vasc Endovasc Surg. 2000;19(1):56–61.
42. Cigna E, et al. Postoperative care in finger replantation: our caseload and review of the literature. Eur Rev Med Pharmacol Sci. 2015;19(14):2552–61.
43. Feest TG. Low molecular weight dextran: a continuing cause of acute renal failure. Br Med J. 1976;2(6047):1300.
44. Farber A, et al. Intraoperative use of dextran is associated with cardiac complications after carotid endarterectomy. J Vasc Surg. 2013;57(3):635–41.
45. Brunkhorst FM, et al. Intensive insulin therapy and pentastarch resuscitation in severe sepsis. N Engl J Med. 2008;358(2):125–39.
46. Perner A, et al. Hydroxyethyl starch 130/0.42 versus Ringer's acetate in severe sepsis. N Engl J Med. 2012;367(2):124–34.
47. Bartels K, Thiele RH, Gan TJ. Rational fluid management in today's ICU practice. Crit Care. 2013;17(Suppl 1):S6.
48. Marik PE, Baram M, Vahid B. Does central venous pressure predict fluid responsiveness? A systematic review of the literature and the tale of seven mares. Chest. 2008;134(1):172–8.
49. Swan HJ, et al. Catheterization of the heart in man with use of a flow-directed balloon-tipped catheter. N Engl J Med. 1970;283(9):447–51.

50. Harvey S, et al. Assessment of the clinical effectiveness of pulmonary artery catheters in management of patients in intensive care (PAC-Man): a randomised controlled trial. Lancet. 2005;366(9484):472–7.
51. Barmparas G, et al. Swan-Ganz catheter use in trauma patients can be reduced without negatively affecting outcomes. World J Surg. 2011;35(8):1809–17.
52. Cioccari L, et al. Hemodynamic assessment of critically ill patients using a miniaturized transesophageal echocardiography probe. Crit Care. 2013;17(3):R121.
53. Abbas SM, Hill AG. Systematic review of the literature for the use of oesophageal Doppler monitor for fluid replacement in major abdominal surgery. Anaesthesia. 2008;63(1):44–51.
54. Pearse RM, et al. Effect of a perioperative, cardiac output-guided hemodynamic therapy algorithm on outcomes following major gastrointestinal surgery: a randomized clinical trial and systematic review. JAMA. 2014;311(21):2181–90.
55. Khwannimit B, Bhurayanontachai R. Prediction of fluid responsiveness in septic shock patients: comparing stroke volume variation by FloTrac/Vigileo and automated pulse pressure variation. Eur J Anaesthesiol. 2012;29(2):64–9.

48 Sodium and Potassium Abnormalities

Caroline Park and Daniel Grabo

Introduction

Surgical and trauma patients in the intensive care unit (ICU) often have electrolyte (particularly sodium and potassium) abnormalities due to postoperative or post-injury fluid shifts, intravenous fluid (IVF) therapy, blood transfusions, stress hormones, nutritional support (including re-feeding syndrome), fluid loss (hemorrhage), and trauma (tissue injury). Frequent measurements of plasma electrolytes are indicated in situations of electrolyte excess or deficiency. Monitoring and correcting of electrolytes to normal levels can help avoid common surgical complications such as ileus and more importantly avoid devastating consequences of cardiac arrhythmias and neurologic sequelae.

Fluids and Compartments

Total body water (TBW) is distributed between two major compartments in the body, intracellular and extracellular. The intracellular compartment holds 2/3 of the TBW, with the extracellular compartment holding the remaining 1/3. The extracellular space, or remaining 1/3 of TBW, can be further divided into the interstitial space and intravascular space. The intravascular space comprises the essential 5–10% of TBW that represents the circulating plasma volume. Refer to Table 48.1 for a description of the intracellular and extracellular fluid compartments.

It is important to understand TBW as a percentage of body weight, which can vary in females, children, the obese, and the malnourished. The standard reference for total body water as a percentage of body weight in males is 60%. TBW is slightly less in females at an average of 50–55% and is attributed generally by a decrease in muscle mass percentage. In children, this number can vary widely but generally decreases with age; almost 90% of a fetus' body weight is in water and falls to 60–65% in children. Depending on the severity of obesity, TBW as a percent of body weight may be up to 10-20% lower in the obese patient. In the malnourished, and depending on the severity of chronic malnutrition, TBW may be adjusted up to 10%.

Chemical Composition of Body Fluid Compartments

Understanding the chemical composition of the intracellular and extracellular spaces is paramount in calculating osmolality as well as identifying and treating electrolyte abnormalities, which are oftentimes a result of volume shifts. This relates to shifts in water and not salts, which remain fairly compartmentalized by gradients in the otherwise functioning, dynamic cell membrane. There is significant clinical relevance of the distribution of cations and anions to the regulation of water movement, which is a mostly active, energy-driven phenomenon.

The intracellular fluid compartment, which constitutes 2/3 of TBW, contains mostly potassium and magnesium as its main solutes. The major anions include phosphate, sulfate, and proteins. Within the extracellular space, plasma contains a higher concentration of sodium cations; anions include mostly chloride with some bicarbonate, sulfate, and proteins. Likewise, the interstitial fluid also contains a higher amount of sodium cations with a smaller portion of potassium, calcium, and magnesium. Chloride constitutes the majority of anions in interstitial fluid, followed by bicarbonate, sulfate, phosphate, organic acids, and proteins. See Table 48.2 for the representative cations and anions found within the different body fluid compartments.

C. Park
Department of Acute Care Surgery, LAC-USC Medical Center, Los Angeles, CA, USA

D. Grabo (✉)
Department of Trauma, Acute Care Surgery and Surgical Critical Care, West Virginia University, Morgantown, WV, USA
e-mail: daniel.grabo@hsc.wvu.edu

A. Salim et al. (eds.), *Surgical Critical Care Therapy*, https://doi.org/10.1007/978-3-319-71712-8_48

Table 48.1 Body fluid compartments in relation to TBW

Intravascular space Or Plasma (¼ of ECF)	Extracellular fluid (ECF) 1/3 of TBW
Interstitial space (¾ of ECF)	
Intracellular space	Intracellular fluid (ICF) 2/3 of TBW

TBW = total body water

Table 48.2 Body fluid compartments and respective concentration of cations and anions

Compartment	Cations (mEq/L)	Anions (mEq/L)
Intracellular fluid	Potassium 150 Sodium 10 Magnesium 40	Sulfate/phosphate 150 Protein 40 Bicarbonate 10
Interstitial fluid	Sodium 144 Potassium 4 Calcium 3 Magnesium 2	Chloride 114 Bicarbonate 30 Organic acids/other: 8 Protein 1
Plasma	Sodium 142 Potassium 4 Calcium 5 Magnesium 3	Chloride 103 Bicarbonate 27 Protein 16 Organic acids/other: 8

The ratio of plasma solutes and water determines *plasma osmolality* (P_{osm}). The normal range for plasma osmolality is 275–290 mOsm/kg. Sodium (Na^+) is the principal osmotically active particle in the extracellular space (plasma and interstitial fluid). It follows that the regulation of P_{osm} is mostly driven by Na^+, with minor contributions from glucose and BUN.

Calculating Plasma Osmolality

$$P_{osm} = 2\times\left(\left[\mathrm{Na}^+\right]_p\right) + \frac{\mathrm{BUN}}{2.8} + \frac{\mathrm{glucose}}{18}$$

$$\text{Plasma sodium} = \left[\mathrm{Na}^+\right]_p$$

Osmoregulation is the movement of water between intracellular and extracellular spaces across cell membranes. It is principally directed by the exchange of Na^+ and potassium (K^+) via a transmembrane Na^+/K^+ ATPase pump. Alterations in water balance and sodium homeostasis are intimately associated with and help mediate osmoregulation; with otherwise intact renal function, water intake then must equal output with an overall goal to maintain plasma volume rather than $[Na^+]_p$. Antidiuretic hormone (ADH) is released in response to an increase in P_{osm} or a decrease in effective circulating volume. This fine control of P_{osm} helps maintain plasma sodium ($[Na^+]_p$) within the tight range of 135–145 mEq/L, a range which may vary slightly between institutions.

While P_{osm} is controlled within a relatively tight range, the range for urine is much wider. Accepting a preserved countercurrent concentrating mechanism with overall intact renal function, urine osmolality (U_{osm}) can range from as low as 40m0sm/kg up to1400mOsm/kg. Therefore, in the patient with syndrome of inappropriate ADH (SIADH) or diabetes insipidus (DI), it is important to compare the P_{osm} to the U_{osm} to determine intrinsic renal disease versus other processes, including alterations in the hypothalamic-pituitary axis. Derangements can be encountered in patients with DI, diabetes mellitus, and acute renal dysfunction (refer to subsequent section in "Sodium" for specific examples).

Sodium

As the major cation in the extracellular space, sodium plays a multitude of essential roles in cell physiology, including nerve impulse potentiation, active transport, and osmotic equilibrium. The normal range for plasma sodium is 135–145 mEq/L, which is highly related to volume status. Hyponatremia in general is due to water intake that cannot be excreted, and hypernatremia is a result of water loss without replacement. Loss of sodium and water results in hypovolemia, and retention of sodium and water leads to the development of edema. As such, most derangements in sodium level can be treated with adjustments of volume with fluid restriction, diuretics, or volume administration. There are, in some cases, instances of intrinsic renal dysfunction (acute tubular necrosis from nonsteroidal anti-inflammatories, chemotherapy) or cerebral pathology that require consideration (intracranial hemorrhage with inappropriate antidiuretic hormone release).

Hyponatremia

The classifications are as listed below and based on degree of derivation of plasma sodium from its lower limit of the normal range (135–145 mEq/L):

- Mild hyponatremia, 130–135 mEq/L
- Moderate hyponatremia, 125–129 mEq/L
- Severe hyponatremia, <125 mEq/L

The signs and symptoms are directly related to the rate and degree of hyponatremia. Patients with mild hyponatremia are largely asymptomatic. As moderate hyponatremia develops, nausea, vomiting, and weakness may manifest and progress to headache, lethargy, and altered mental status. With severe hyponatremia, particularly with plasma sodium <120 mEq/L, neurologic symptoms such as seizure and coma can develop.

The diagnosis of hyponatremia can be made with a simple laboratory test, the serum chemistry panel. Understanding the cause, however, relies on detailed history and physical examination with the additional tests of urine and plasma osmolality (U_{osm}, P_{osm}) and plasma and urine [Na^+], [K^+], [Cl^-], [$HCO3^-$], [urea], and [glucose]. After determining the presence and severity of hyponatremia, it is important to evaluate the patient's plasma osmolality ($P_{osm} = 2 \times Na^+ + BUN/2.8 + glucose/18$). Most commonly, hyponatremia is indicative of a hypoosmotic state ($P_{osm} < 275$). Evaluation of urine osmolality is helpful to determine whether water excretion is impaired; a U_{osm} of < 100 mosmol/kg or specific gravity of < 1.003 is suggestive of ADH suppression, which can be found in reset osmostat or polydipsia. Functional management of hypoosmotic hyponatremia is largely based on volume status with three main categories: hypovolemic, euvolemic, and hypervolemic. See Fig. 48.1 for a simple algorithm in approaching the patient with hyponatremia. The specific management concepts for hyponatremic patients with respect to volume status are discussed in the following sections.

Hypovolemic Hyponatremia

Hypovolemic hyponatremia is the most frequent situation encountered and occurs in patients with processes that stimulate ADH secretion and water loss. Excessive renal (diuretics) or gastrointestinal losses (nasogastric suctioning, emesis, or diarrhea) are typically the cause. Additionally, patients with pancreatitis, large surface area burns, and hypoaldosteronism can exhibit hypovolemic hyponatremia.

Treatment of hypovolemic hyponatremia is directly related to addressing the underlying cause and replacing any initial fluid losses in the volume-depleted patient with isotonic normal saline. In addition to the serum chemistry panel, laboratory investigations should also include a urinalysis to check for ketones (diabetes mellitus) and hyaline or tubular casts (renal dysfunction). Specifically, check the urine creatinine and sodium in relation to plasma counterparts, noting that urine sodium of < 15–20 mmol/L is suggestive of preserved renal function with a "prerenal" state secondary to hypovolemia (i.e., gastrointestinal losses, bleeding, or third-spacing). Urine sodium of > 15–20 mmol/L suggests intrinsic renal dysfunction and should warrant additional investigations to identify any offending agents.

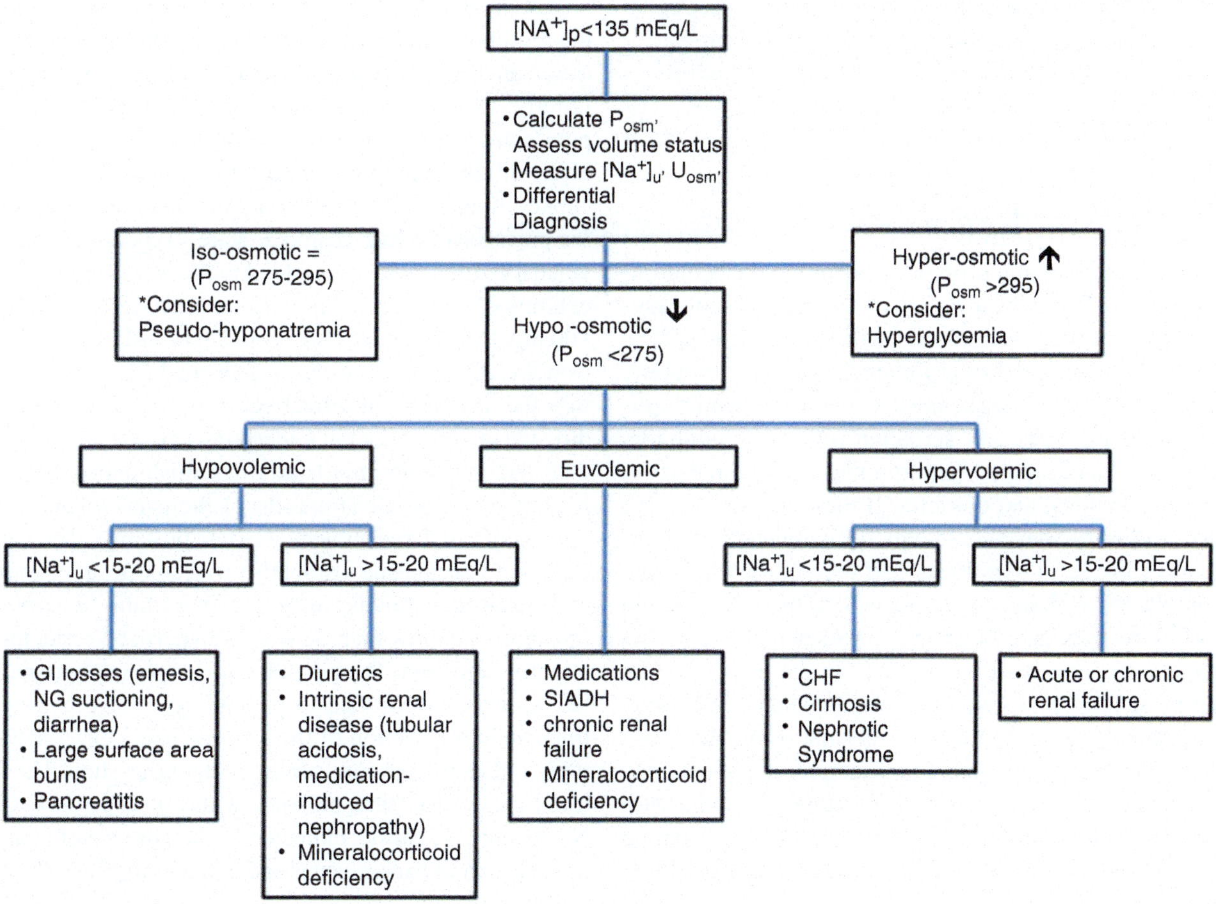

Fig. 48.1 Algorithm for approaching the patient with hyponatremia. $[Na^+]_p$ plasma sodium, P_{osm} plasma osmolality, $[Na^+]_u$ urine sodium, U_{osm} urine osmolality, SIADH syndrome of inappropriate antidiuretic hormone, CHF congestive heart failure

Calculating Sodium Deficit

$$\text{Na}^{+}\text{deficit} = \left(140 - \left[\text{Na}^{+}\right]_{\text{p}}\right) \times 0.6 \times \text{weight in kg}$$

For acute hyponatremia (often associated with neurologic symptoms when severe and $[Na^+] < 120$ mEq/L), the maximal rate of correction is 1–2 mEq/L/h for 3–4 h, more than 10–12 mEq/L in the first 24 h or until plasma Na^+ is >120 mEq/L or symptoms subside. Three percent normal saline or hypertonic saline (HTS) can be administered at a rate of 50 cc/h to achieve this goal. Central intravenous infusion is recommended, as HTS can be caustic to peripheral veins. For chronic hyponatremia, correct the serum sodium level even more slowly at 0.5–1 mEq/L/hr. or no faster than 10–12 mEq/L in the first 24 h. Serial monitoring of $[Na^+]_p$ is important to track the efficacy of treatment as well as prevent too rapid correction, which is more common in chronic hyponatremia. Note that the correction of sodium deficit does not take into account ongoing isosmotic losses, which need to be additionally replaced.

**Pitfall: Caution must be used when correcting hyponatremia as rapid over-correction of sodium can lead to a demyelinating lesion, central pontine myelinolysis.

Euvolemic Hyponatremia

Euvolemic hyponatremia is often diagnosed in the acute-on-chronic setting. There are a variety of causes, including psychogenic polydipsia, tuberculosis, malnutrition, side effects from medications, and inappropriate levels of antidiuretic hormone (or SIADH). Many medications have been implicated, including selective serotonin reuptake inhibitors (SSRIs), carbamazepine, chlorpromazine, amiodarone, vasopressin analogs, and diuretics. If these medications are deemed necessary, they should only be continued with judicious surveillance of symptoms and laboratory follow-up. Also associated with hyponatremia is SIADH (often seen in the early post-traumatic brain injury patient), although this phenomenon is not clearly understood in the acute state. A variant of SIADH, reset osmostat, occurs when ADH secretion and thirst are reset at a lower plasma osmolality with otherwise normal regulation. For example, a patient may have a plasma concentration of 125 mEq/L but otherwise remains euvolemic and asymptomatic. Much less common causes of SIADH include multiple sclerosis and Guillain-Barre syndrome.

Treatment of euvolemic hyponatremia is similarly directed at identifying and correcting the cause, i.e., offending medications, paraneoplastic syndromes, etc. Fluid restriction is often the first line of treatment as water retention and Na^+ loss do not occur if water is restricted. Consider loop diuretics should fluid restriction prove ineffective. In patients with traumatic brain injury, HTS (3% normal saline) can also be administered via central vein access with frequent monitoring of urine and serum osmolality and chemistries.

Hypervolemic Hyponatremia

Hypervolemic hyponatremia is a disorder of sodium balance, specifically, an excess of sodium with an expanded extracellular volume given an impairment in maintaining fluid in the intravascular space and out of the interstitium. There are several causes of hypervolemic hyponatremia, including congestive heart failure, cirrhosis, and mineralocorticoid excess (Cushing's and Conn's syndromes). Renal failure also disturbs the maintenance of these hydrostatic and oncotic pressures at the level of the capillary bed. Nephrotic syndrome similarly may lead to sodium retention with subsequent excess water retention.

The treatment of hypervolemic hyponatremia is directed toward optimization of the underlying decompensated state (i.e., salt restriction and diuretics with cirrhosis and heart failure). Diuretics are often used, including spironolactone, potassium-sparing diuretics, and steroids that block the effect of aldosterone and testosterone.

Additional causes of hyponatremia can be considered in the presence of a hyperosmolar state. Hyperglycemia occurs when a solute (glucose) is added to the extracellular fluid and exhibits effective osmolality. Each increase of $[\text{glucose}]_p$ of 100 mg/dL will reduce $[Na^+]_p$ by 1.6 mEq/L. Calculating the osmolal gap (calculated P_{osm} – measured P_{osm}) will help identify the presence of effective osmoles. Therapy is then directed at correcting the underlying causes.

Pseudohyponatremia is an often misbranded category of hyponatremia that illustrates the phenomenon of an increased percentage of large molecules (fat, proteins) that may not contribute to plasma osmolality (isosmotic hyponatremia) and result in a relative decrease in sodium concentration. Specific examples include severe hypertriglyceridemia and hyperproteinemia. The phenomenon of pseudohyponatremia has also been described in patients who have undergone a transurethral resection of the prostate using excessive hypotonic bladder irrigation; serum chemistries should be monitored closely in these patients in the postoperative setting. No specific therapy is indicated in the absence of symptoms as excretion of excess water and solute will generally correct the abnormality.

Hypernatremia

Hypernatremia is also associated with changes in volume status and is defined as plasma sodium >145 mEq/L. Similar to hyponatremia, hypernatremia can be simplified into three main categories based on evaluation of the patient's volume status:

- Hypovolemic
- Euvolemic
- Hypervolemic

The clinical signs and symptoms of hypernatremia are caused by cellular dehydration and can include irritability, muscle twitching or spasm, excessive thirst, and, in more severe cases, seizures or coma. Patients with altered mental status or those who are debilitated, bedbound, or at the extremes of age are at high risk given their inability to regulate water intake. Measurement of urine [Na^+] will further help elucidate the cause of the hypernatremia. See Fig. 48.2 for an approach to patients with hypernatremia.

Hypovolemic Hypernatremia

Hypovolemic hypernatremia is most often diagnosed with a thorough history and physical exam. Patients at the extremes of age (infants, elderly) or those with altered mental status may present with clinical symptoms and signs of dehydration (thirst, dry mucus membranes, decreased skin turgor). Oftentimes the postoperative patient with high nasogastric output and/or frequent high volume emesis may present with hypernatremia as well as tachycardia and hypotension concerning for hypovolemia. Other causes include diarrhea, osmotic diuretics, prolonged diaphoresis, renal tubular disease, and diabetes insipidus (DI).

The treatment of hypovolemic hypernatremia is to first establish euvolemia and correct any metabolic abnormalities that can lead to or exacerbate cardiac arrhythmias. It is prudent to administer isotonic fluids first to reestablish euvolemia while measuring urine and serum electrolytes, BUN, glucose, and creatinine to identify and correct the source of loss. For example, a patient with a prolonged small intestinal obstruction with relative hypotension and hypernatremia may also have hypokalemia and contraction alkalosis.

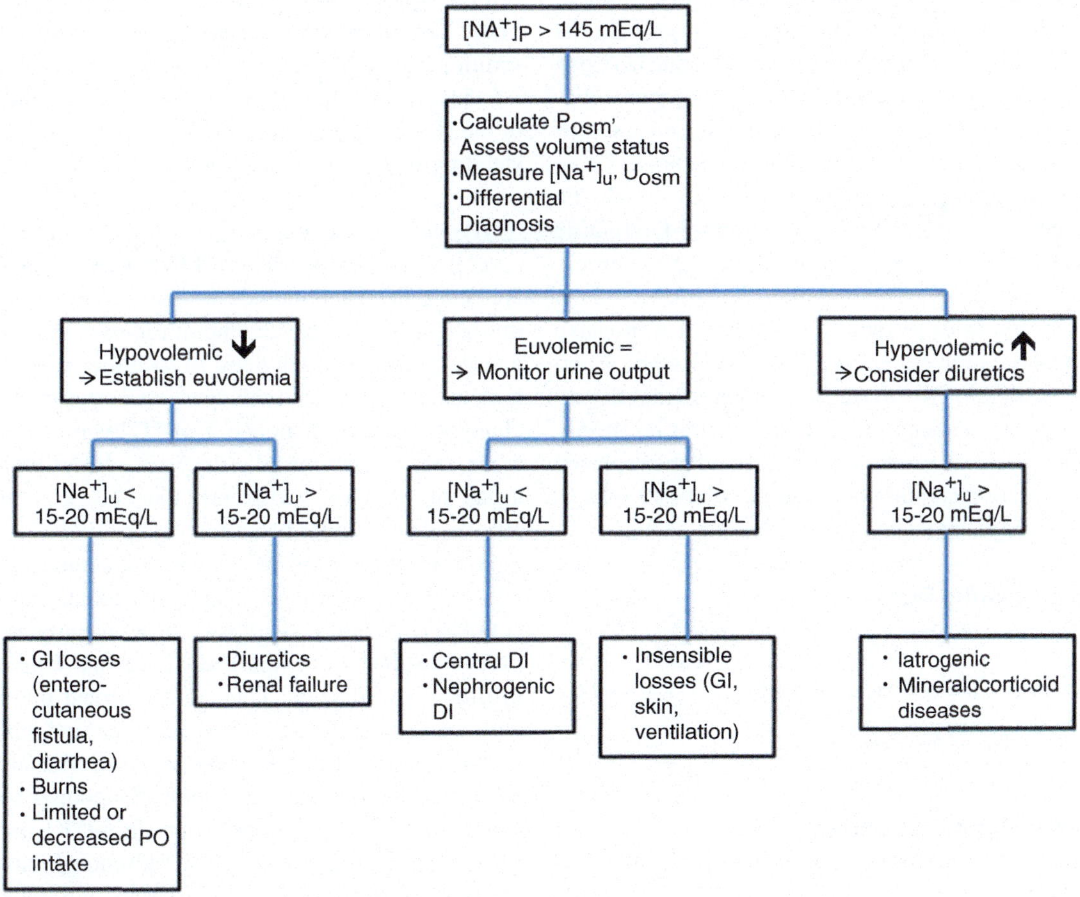

Fig. 48.2 Algorithm for approaching the patient with hypernatremia. $[Na^+]_p$ plasma sodium, P_{osm} plasma osmolality, $[Na^+]_u$ urine sodium, U_{osm} urine osmolality, DI diabetes insipidus

There is a role for diuretics (both loop and non-loop) in addition to mannitol in the treatment of hypernatremia. These medical therapies are usually spared in the initial resuscitative setting, keeping in mind that mannitol, as an osmotic diuretic, can precipitate transient hypotension.

Euvolemic Hypernatremia

Euvolemic hypernatremia is often diagnosed late and remains a difficult entity to capture. It is essential to identify the cause (in most causes either neurogenic or nephrogenic diabetes insipidus) as the treatment algorithm is widely different. In neurogenic diabetes insipidus (DI), there are insufficient levels of antidiuretic hormone (ADH) or a quantitative deficiency. This may be secondary to head trauma with associated cerebral edema, overall acute traumatic state, and surgery or from tumor. Nephrogenic DI is characterized by a decreased sensitivity to ADH, with a subsequent decrease in ability to concentrate urine. There are several causes, including chronic renal disease, interstitial renal disease, and exposure to nephrotoxic medications (most commonly amphotericin and lithium).

The initial treatment of hypernatremia consists of appropriate initial fluid resuscitation if the patient is hypovolemic and monitoring of both serum and urine osmolality, glucose, creatinine, and electrolytes (specifically sodium). Once the patient has achieved euvolemia, proceed to delineate between neurogenic or nephrogenic DI. Patients with neurogenic diabetes insipidus may often develop urine output in excess of 200–400 cc/hr. with high risk for hypovolemic shock. Urine output as well as urine and serum electrolytes should be monitored closely every 4–6 h, and 1-deamino-8-D-arginine vasopressin (DDAVP), IV or intranasal, ought to be administered based on increasing urine output.

Nephrogenic diabetes insipidus is largely not responsive to DDAVP. The initial treatment consists of resuscitation and laboratory investigation as above in addition to identifying the offending agent. Patient intake/output should be strictly monitored and their free water deficit measured and replaced as needed. Correction should not exceed a rate of 12 mEq/L over 24 h (0.5 mEq/L/h) so as to avoid cerebral edema.

Calculating Free Water Deficit

$$\text{Free water deficit} = 0.6 \times \text{weight}(\text{kg}) \times \left(\frac{[\text{Na}^+]_p}{140} - 1 \right)$$

Hypervolemic Hypernatremia

Hypervolemic hypernatremia is often diagnosed in the outpatient setting in the adult population classically as a patient with primary aldosteronism presenting with headaches, weakness, and, less commonly, excessive urination. Besides mineralocorticoid excess states, iatrogenic administration of hypertonic saline can also lead to hypernatremia and should be carefully monitored. The mineralocorticoid excess states include Conn's syndrome, Cushing's syndrome, secondary aldosteronism, and congenital adrenal hyperplasia.

Treatment of hypervolemic hypernatremia is largely directed toward the primary deficiency with loss of negative feedback in the hypothalamic-pituitary axis and/or eliminating the excess state (i.e., tumor). These patients will initially require frequent electrolyte monitoring or replacements and may need steroid supplementation depending on severity and the deficiency. Minimize any excess salt administration and judiciously correct with free water (both PO and IV), and in the inpatient setting, avoid rapid overcorrection, which may result in cerebral edema.

Potassium

As one of the major intracellular cations, potassium plays an essential role in nerve impulse potentiation in addition to maintenance of an ATPase transmembrane pump and cardiac myocyte excitability. Subtle shifts in potassium in the extracellular space can lead to life-threatening consequences. There are numerous regulatory mechanisms to maintain serum potassium ($[K+]_p$) in its normal physiologic range of 3.5–5.0 mEq/L. Acutely, K^+ is shifted intracellular by means of the Na^+/K^+ ATPase and Na^+/H^+ transporter which are activated by insulin and catecholamine release in response to a meal.

Hypokalemia is defined as $K+ < 3.5$ mEq/L. There are several signs and symptoms of hypokalemia, many of which are generalized and include weakness, fatigue, tetany, paresthesias, and/or increased tendon reflexes. Patients may have nausea, vomiting, or an ileus. Myocardial conduction may be affected and manifest with classic electrocardiogram (ECG) changes including flattened T or "U" waves and ST depressions. Additionally, atrial arrhythmias (sinus bradycardia and atrial fibrillation), atrioventricular block, and premature atrial and ventricular beats can occur.

There are several causes of hypokalemia, which are usually related to excessive losses, inadequate intake, or transcellular shifts. Excessive losses of K^+ usually come from the gastrointestinal tract (diarrhea, intestinal fistula) and renal insufficiency (diabetic ketoacidosis, renal tubular acidosis, and metabolic alkalosis from Bartter and Gitelman syndromes). Medications, such as excess insulin administration, iatrogenic steroid administration, B-agonists (bronchodilators), and lithium toxicity can drive K^+ into the cell. Mineralocorticoid excess from adrenergic stimulation or hyperplasia or Cushing's disease can cause excessive renal loss.

The treatment of hypokalemia is targeted at correcting the underlying problem, whether by minimizing gastrointestinal losses, improving oral intake, or resuscitating with IVF. It is equally important to identify the offending nephrotoxic agents or mineralocorticoid excess states (refer to section on hypervolemic hypernatremia). Assessing the renal excretion of K^+ can help with determining whether the problem is primarily intrinsic or extrinsic to the kidneys. Laboratory investigations include a comprehensive serum chemistry panel, urine potassium ($[K+]_u$), and urine creatinine ($[Cr]_u$). The ratio between urine potassium and urine creatinine or $[K+]_u/[Cr]_u$ assesses the rate of potassium excretion and should generally be less than 15 mmol of K+ ions/g of creatinine in hypokalemia associated with acute intracellular shifts of potassium. Hypokalemia with $[K+]_u/[Cr]_u > 15$ mmol K+/g creatinine is suggestive of intrinsic renal disease (i.e., renal artery stenosis, Bartter, Gitelman or Liddle's syndromes, recent diuretic use).

In addition to identification and correction of the problem, potassium should be replaced orally (if tolerated) as this form has excellent bioavailability with rapid onset or IV potassium chloride (KCl). The latter is reserved for patients who cannot tolerate or absorb oral intake or who have severe hypokalemia. In the presence of ECG changes, severe muscle pains, or paralysis rapid administration of KCL should precede the detailed diagnostic endeavors. Parenteral administration of KCl should not exceed 20–60 mEq/h peripherally and 100–200 mEq/h centrally. Continuous cardiac monitoring and frequent assessment of $[K^+]_p$ response are essential. Doses range from 10 to 40 mEq and can be expected to raise $[K^+]_p$ by 1 to 1.5 mEq/L after 40 to 60 mEq.

> **Pitfalls: Replete magnesium first if it is low to potentiate potassium replacement.

Hyperkalemia is defined as K+ > 5 mEq/L and can be life-threatening with the onset of cardiac arrhythmias. Signs and symptoms of hyperkalemia are also generalized and include decreased deep tendon reflexes, paresthesias, and weakness. This can precipitate to paralysis and respiratory failure. Ventricular arrhythmia can ensue and typically occur at K+ > 7 mEq/L. ECG changes include peaked T waves, widened QRS, and shortened QT intervals. This can quickly progress to ventricular fibrillation, bradycardia, and death if left uncorrected.

There are several causes of hyperkalemia and a few causes that are more unique to surgical and trauma patients. In general, causes include acidosis, ischemia after reperfusion (particularly the extremities but also after liver transplantation and superior mesenteric artery or other main visceral artery reconstruction), rhabdomyolysis, renal failure, and succinylcholine administration (increased risk in patients with burns, crush injury, renal failure, prolonged bed rest), in addition to massive blood transfusion and hemolysis.

The treatment of hyperkalemia is expansive given its many etiologies, particularly in the trauma and surgical patient. However, initial resuscitation measures should be employed, including IV fluid resuscitation, continuous telemetry, and 12-lead ECG monitoring. Importantly, calcium IV should be given to stabilize the cardiac myocyte membrane for any patient with changes on ECG. Calcium IV (CaCl or Ca gluconate) can help prevent the depolarization effect of potassium on cardiac myocytes but remains a temporizing measure. Measures should then be taken to shift K+ intracellular or excrete excess. See Fig. 48.3 for an algorithm to manage hyperkalemia.

Shifting the K+ intracellular can be rapidly achieved by administering ten units of insulin IV with an ampule of dextrose (D50) or one ampule of sodium bicarbonate. The mechanism of action of albuterol is similar to insulin in that it stimulates release of glucose, thereby increasing insulin levels and driving potassium into the cell. Albuterol is delivered as a nebulized solution, 10–20 mg in 4 ml of sodium chloride solution.

Potassium can also be excreted via urine or stool. Renal excretion can be achieved with loop diuretics (non-potassium-sparing, i.e., furosemide) and should be given in boluses of 40–80 mg IV for furosemide. Bumetanide can also be used in patients who are not furosemide or bumetanide-naïve, with starting dose of 2–4 mg IV boluses. Dialysis (usually hemodialysis) is reserved as a last resort but may already be an option for patients who have end-stage renal disease. Stool excretion can be achieved with both sodium polystyrene sulfonate (Kayexalate) and sorbitol PO. The former acts as a potassium-binding resin that exchanges for sodium in the colon and therefore results in osmotic diarrhea. It should not be administered to patients with potential ileus or bowel obstruction as it can cause rare but devastating intestinal ischemia and necrosis.

Special Cases: Rhabdomyolysis

In patients with rhabdomyolysis, which can account for upward of 25% of acute kidney injury in adult patients, electrolyte abnormalities including hyperkalemia and kidney injury should be treated aggressively. Complete blood count, chemistry, and creatine kinase laboratory analysis should be performed, and urinalysis should be checked to look for blood in the absence of red blood cells, which is suggestive of myoglobinuria. The goal is to maintain a glomerular filtration rate (GFR) with urine output of 100–150 cc/hr. in adults.

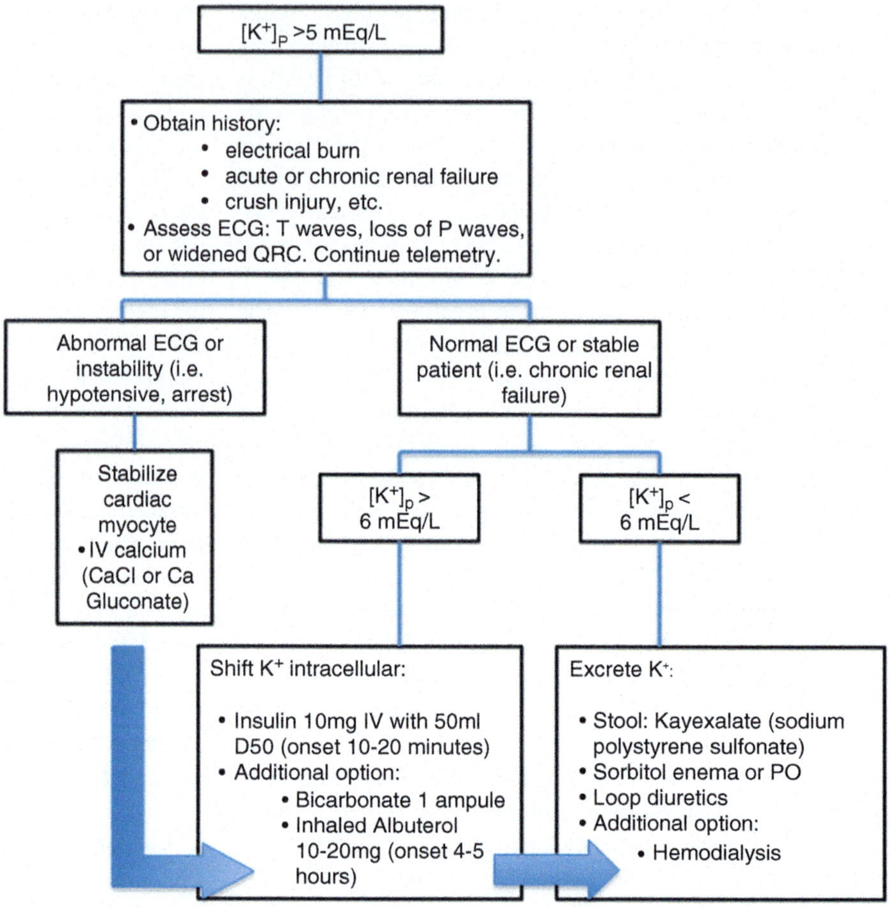

Fig. 48.3 Algorithm for approaching the patient with hyperkalemia. $[K^+]_p$ plasma potassium, CaCl calcium chloride

Most often, this can be achieved with placement of two large-bore IVs and aggressive isotonic fluid administration (i.e., 0.9% sodium chloride). The administration of bicarbonate-infused fluids is controversial and generally should be reserved for patients with creatine kinase levels >15,000–20,000 U/L, at which there is a higher risk of acute renal failure.

Take-Home Points

1. Understanding the body fluid compartments and interplay of sodium and potassium as major contributing electrolytes is essential to managing the postoperative and trauma patient in the ICU.
2. Sodium abnormalities in the surgical ICU are most frequently related to impaired volume regulation. Correction of the underlying cause (i.e., SIADH, DI, GI losses, and renal failure) and attention to the volume status will usually correct the sodium derangement.
3. Potassium derangements are common in the postoperative and trauma patient in the surgical ICU and can quickly lead to cardiac arrhythmias. As such, frequent monitoring and aggressive correction is imperative.

Suggested Readings

1. Alder SM, Verbalis JG. Disorders of body water homeostasis in critical illness. Endocrinol Metab Clin N Am. 2006;35:873–94.
2. Ayach T, Nappo RW, Paugh-Miller JL, Ross EA. Postoperative hyperkalemia. Eur J Intern Med. 2015;26:106–11.
3. Cuesta M, Thompson C. The relevance of hyponatraemia to perioperative care of surgical patients. Surgeon. 2015;13:163–9.
4. Ellison DH, Berl T. Clinical practice. The syndrome of inappropriate antidiuresis. N Engl J Med. 2007;356:2064–72.
5. Gennari FJ. Hypokalemia. N Engl J Med. 1998;339:451–8.
6. Huerta-Alardín AL, Varon J, Marik PE. Bench-to-bedside review: Rhabdomyolysis – an overview for clinicians. Crit Care. 2005;9:158–69.
7. Kamel KS, Halperin ML. Fluid, electrolyte and acid-base physiology. 5th ed. Philadelphia: Elsevier; 2017.

8. Palevsky PM, Bhagrath R, Greenberg A. Hypernatremia in hospitalized patients. Ann Intern Med. 1996;124:197–203.
9. Rhoades R, Bell DR. Regulation of fluid and electrolyte balance. In: Rhoades R, Bell DR, editors. Medical physiology: principles for clinical medicine. Baltimore: Lippincott Williams and Wilkins; 2013.
10. Rose BD, Post TW. Regulation of the effective circulating volume. In: Rose Burton D, Post TW, editors. Clinical physiology of acid-base and electrolyte disorders. New York: McGraw-Hill; 2001.
11. Rose BD, Post TW. Regulation of plasma osmolality. In: Rose BD, Post TW, editors. Clinical physiology of acid-base and electrolyte disorders. New York: McGraw-Hill; 2001.
12. Rose BD, Post TW (2001). Hypoosmolal states: hyponatremia. In Rose BD & Post TW (Eds.), Clinical physiology of acid-base and electrolyte disorders. New York: McGraw-Hill.
13. Spasovski G, et al. Clinical practice guideline on diagnosis and treatment of hyponatremia. Eur J Endocrinol. 2014;170(3):G1–47.
14. Sterns RH. Disorders of plasma sodium – causes, consequences, and correction. N Engl J Med. 2015;372:55–65.
15. Zacchia M, Abategiovanni ML, Stratigis S, Capasso G. Potassium: from physiology to clinical implications. Kidney Dis (Basel). 2016;2(2):72–9.

Other Electrolyte Abnormalities

49

Galinos Barmparas and George Paul Liao

Magnesium

Magnesium balance disorders are common in the ICU and can be observed in up to 65% of medical [1] and up to almost 50% of surgical ICU patients [2], mostly in the form of hypomagnesemia. Over 95% of critically ill surgical patients have their magnesium levels measured in the ICU [2]. The effect of magnesium imbalances on outcomes remains debatable as the available literature does not consistently and directly associate magnesium depletion or excess with a higher mortality risk or other outcomes [3]. To further complicate the matter, the "normal" values obtained for serum magnesium can be misleading and masking a chronic deficiency [4].

The total body magnesium content, approximately 24 g, is almost equally divided between bones and intracellular compartments, with less than 1% present in the serum [5]. Approximately 30% of magnesium in the plasma is bound to protein, mainly albumin, while the remaining 70% is present in ionized form that can be excreted by the kidneys. Under normal conditions, the fractional excretion of magnesium by the kidneys is approximately 4%, with the majority of ionized magnesium being reabsorbed at the thick ascending loop of Henle. The renal excretion can decrease to almost undetectable levels when plasma levels are low in order to minimize losses. The small intestine is the site of absorption of magnesium from dietary intake but also the site of loss of approximately 20 mg/day, which can increase significantly with gastrointestinal losses such as chronic diarrhea. There is no hormonal regulatory mechanism known to be responsible for magnesium balance in the body.

Magnesium is one of the most important electrolytes involved in over 300 enzymatic reactions [6]. The sodium-potassium-adenosine triphosphate (Na-K-ATPase) [7] and adenylate cyclase [8] function depends on availability of magnesium. Magnesium also regulates the intracellular calcium levels and plays a pivotal role in controlling smooth muscle tone and its deficiency might be associated with coronary vasospasm and seizures [9]. Several immunological functions are modulated by magnesium, suggesting its potential role in the inflammatory response and in sepsis [10, 11], although this role has not been determined in the clinical setting.

Magnesium is most commonly measured in the plasma. As less than 1% of the total body magnesium is present in the plasma, these measurements can be problematic and not reflective of the actual total body magnesium levels. Measuring the ionized fraction has not been proven to be superior to the total serum magnesium, as these measurements can be affected by various factors, including free calcium levels, thiocyanate, and heparin [12]. The magnesium loading test, during which magnesium is administered and the excreted amount is measured in a 24-h urine sample [13], is impractical in the ICU setting, and the results may be inaccurate as magnesium excretion can be affected by various factors including diuretics and other drugs very commonly used in the ICU.

Hypomagnesemia

Magnesium depletion is probably underestimated in the ICU as the diagnosis is currently based on magnesium levels in the plasma with all the associated confounders mentioned above [14]. Certain conditions may predispose critically ill patients to hypomagnesemia, and these include chronic alcoholism, cancer, malnutrition, and congestive heart failure requiring chronic use of loop diuretics.

Hypomagnesemia in critically ill surgical patients is usually multifactorial as it can be related to chronic deficiency, drugs, redistribution, and hypoalbuminemia. However, two systems are responsible for magnesium losses: the gastrointestinal tract and the kidneys. Emesis and nasogastric suctioning are two common causes of magnesium depletion in

G. Barmparas (✉) · G. P. Liao
Department of Surgery, Division of Acute Care Surgery and Surgical Critical Care, Cedars-Sinai Medical Center, Los Angeles, CA, USA
e-mail: galinos.barmparas@cshs.org

A. Salim et al. (eds.), *Surgical Critical Care Therapy*, https://doi.org/10.1007/978-3-319-71712-8_49

surgical patients, although diarrhea from any cause, including short-gut syndrome or due to malabsorption, and enterocutaneous fistulae and/or biliary drainage can lead to significantly higher losses [15–17]. Renal losses can also be profound in critically ill patients. Loop diuretics are the most commonly cited drugs causing hypomagnesemia, although other diuretics including anhydrase inhibitors, osmotic agents, and even thiazides have been shown to decrease magnesium resorption [18]. Other drugs implicated in hypomagnesemia include aminoglycosides, cyclosporine, cisplatin, pentamidine, amphotericin B, and colony-stimulating factor therapy [9]. Metabolic acidosis related to any underlying condition, including ketoacidosis, starvation, and alcoholism, can be another cause of hypomagnesemia. Correction of hyperglycemia in ketoacidotic patients will lead to shift of magnesium into the cells, and careful monitoring and repletion are required [9]. Lastly, it is worth mentioning that hypomagnesemia is a recognized cause of hypocalcemia. Hypocalcemic patients not responding to calcium repletion after thyroid or parathyroid surgery should be given magnesium. In these patients, magnesium stimulates parathyroid hormone (PTH) secretion, decreases bone resistance to the PTH, and, subsequently, decreases calcium losses [19, 20].

Symptoms

Low magnesium levels manifest in the form of neuromuscular, cardiovascular, and calcium/potassium derangements. Neuromuscular hyperexcitability may manifest in the form of muscular cramps, tetany, and even generalized seizures. Positive Chvostek and Trousseau signs can be elicited, even in the absence of hypocalcemia [21, 22]. Magnesium deficiency results in impaired function of the Na-K-ATPase enzyme affecting the normal cardiac repolarization. Electrocardiographic changes include prolongation of the PR interval and widening of the QRS complex, with flattening of the T wave. Ventricular tachycardia and ventricular fibrillation may also occur [23]. Torsades de pointes is a form of polymorphic ventricular tachycardia related to prolongation of the QT interval, and magnesium is implicated in its development. Digitalis cardiotoxicity may be enhanced by the presence of hypomagnesemia [24]. Severe hypomagnesemia (<1.2 mg/dl) is almost always associated with hypocalcemia, mostly due to PTH resistance [25]. Hypokalemia is very common among hypomagnesemic patients due to assumed potassium wasting in the kidneys [26, 27].

Treatment

In treating patients with hypomagnesemia, several factors should be taken into consideration, including the magnesium plasma levels, the presence of other associated electrolyte abnormalities including hypokalemia and/or hypocalcemia, the presence and severity of symptoms, and the presence of renal insufficiency and whether the gastrointestinal tract can be used for supplementation. When magnesium is repleted intravenously, the increase in the plasma levels causes inhibition of reabsorption of magnesium by the kidneys which lose their stimulus (low magnesium levels in plasma) for reabsorption. This results in a significant partial loss of the intravenously administered magnesium by the kidneys that can reach 50%. In addition, due to the absence of hormonal or enzymatic regulatory process, the magnesium uptake by the cells is slow, and repletion usually requires sustained correction of magnesium levels.

In hemodynamically unstable patients, including those with torsades de pointes and those with associated hypokalemia, magnesium sulfate is given intravenously at a dose of 1–2 g diluted in 10 ml of DW5 over 2 min [28]. Magnesium sulfate administration is unlikely to be beneficial in patients with ventricular tachycardia or inhospital cardiac arrest not related to prolonged QT interval and torsades de pointes as it hasn't been shown to affect return of spontaneous circulation [29]. Magnesium should be administered in a similar fashion in hemodynamically unstable patients with hypokalemia given the interrelationship of magnesium and potassium homeostasis [30].

Symptomatic hypomagnesemia should be treated with IV administration of magnesium sulfate at a dose of 1–2 g diluted in 10 ml of DW5 over 5–60 min. It is essential that infusion of magnesium follows this regimen as the serum magnesium levels will drop substantially in only a few hours. This infusion regimen includes administration of 4–8 g of magnesium sulfate over 12–24 h [9, 31]. For hypocalcemic patients in particular, this regimen might need to be repeated daily for at least 3 days [13, 32]. This maintenance regimen needs to be decreased by at least 50% in patients with renal insufficiency.

Treatment of preeclampsia is based on the MAGPIE trial, in which patients are given 4 g of magnesium sulfate initially, followed by 1 g/h infusion [33].

Hypermagnesemia

Hypermagnesemia is significantly less common than hypomagnesemia and is usually seen only in patients with compromised renal function and those receiving large doses of exogenous magnesium, such as patients with preeclampsia and eclampsia [34].

Symptoms

Symptoms related to hypermagnesemia vary depending on magnesium levels and can range from nausea, headache, or lethargy for magnesium levels 4–6 mEq/l to hypotension and bradycardia for levels between 6 and 10 mEq/l and paralysis with apnea and even cardiac arrest for levels exceeding 10 mEq/l.

Treatment

Mild to moderate hypermagnesemia that is associated with mild symptoms does not require any treatment, especially in patients with normal renal function. In patients with impaired renal function, saline hydration and loop diuretics might be successful in eliminating excess magnesium. Hemodialysis is probably the only mean of treatment for patients with end-stage renal disease.

Calcium

Calcium participates in the full spectrum of physiological and pathological processes that are encountered daily in the ICU, being involved in cardiovascular physiology, coagulation, and neurotransmission as well as in inflammation and cellular survival (calmodulin, apoptosis). In brief, calcium homeostasis is maintained by PTH, calcitriol, and calcitonin. PTH exerts direct renal and bone activity to increase serum calcium and has indirect action on the gastrointestinal absorption of calcium via calcitriol (1,25-dihydroxyvitamin D3), the active form of vitamin D. Calcitonin lowers calcium at each of the aforementioned sites of direct and indirect PTH action. Other electrolyte concentrations also affect calcium levels as elevated magnesium inhibits PTH release, while elevated phosphate increases PTH release.

The normal range of serum calcium is 8.5–10.5 mg/dl. In serum, 50% of calcium is ionized and biologically active. Up to 10% is complexed to organic and inorganic acids. The remaining 40% is bound to protein (80% to albumin) and is not biologically active [35–37]. Ionized calcium concentrations can vary via chelation with the flux of extracellular anions (including phosphate and bicarbonate) and also with pH, as alkaline conditions increase the affinity of albumin to ionized calcium. Free fatty acids have also been shown to increase calcium binding to albumin [38]. Hypocalcemia is defined as ionized calcium of less than 1.12 mmol/l.

Calcium levels are routinely checked in the critical care setting, often with ionized calcium levels because serum albumin levels as well as the acid base status do not affect this active form. Half of these patients will have abnormal levels. Calcium levels are often low in the critical state. The underlying etiology of hypocalcemia must be considered before correcting the calcium abnormality [39]. Studies, including a Cochrane review, show that correcting ionized calcium has not been supported in regard to outcomes and may in fact be deleterious in the setting of sepsis via calcium/calmodulin-dependent protein kinase signaling [40–43].

Hypocalcemia

Since the 1980s, investigators have recognized that critically ill patients often had transiently low ionized calcium levels, mostly due to sepsis or other unknown mechanisms rather than an underlying disease of calcium homeostasis. This was based on the observation that ionized calcium levels often normalized as patients began to improve clinically. In fact, inflammatory cytokines from sepsis and burns do impair PTH secretion [44].

Underlying diseases of calcium homeostasis include hormone-controlled conditions such as hypoparathyroidism, vitamin D deficiency, and osteoporosis. Acute diseases that cause hypocalcemia include severe acute pancreatitis where the release of free fatty acids in the acute phase sequesters calcium, and in later stages sepsis further decreases ionized calcium. Rhabdomyolysis and tumor lysis release large amounts of intracellular phosphate, which binds free serum calcium. Renal failure causes hypocalcemia via phosphate retention and impaired renal vitamin D activation. Iatrogenic causes of hypothyroidism include parathyroid surgery (hungry bone syndrome) and drugs such as cisplatin, aminoglycosides, phenobarbital, dilantin, and proton pump inhibitors. Radiologic contrast containing ethylenediaminetetraacetic acid (EDTA) and gadolinium can cause hypocalcemia. Chelation occurs with citrate, which is used as the anticoagulant in packed red blood cells and accumulates during rapid/massive transfusions, and with hemodialysis and extracorporeal membrane oxygenation (ECMO) [45].

Symptoms

Signs and symptoms are often confounding in the ICU, with patients being sedated or having neuropathy of critical illness. Classical findings related to neuromuscular dysfunction include dyspnea, stridor, carpopedal spasm (Trousseau's sign) and facial muscle hyperreflexia (Chvostek sign), QT prolongation, bradycardia, and decreased vascular tone. Neurologic signs and symptoms include confusion, hallucinations, and seizures.

Treatment

The current guidelines for correcting serum calcium in the critical care setting emphasize a targeted, selective strategy rather than normalizing a laboratory value. Studies demonstrate that attempts of intensivists to correct ionized calcium were not associated with improved outcome nor with rapid normalization of ionized calcium levels [46]. Critical care scenarios where ionized calcium should be closely monitored and corrected are cases of cardiac conductance abnormalities such as QT prolongation, iatrogenic hypocalcemia following parathyroidectomy, and severe coagulopathy.

Intravenous forms of calcium are 10% calcium chloride and 10% calcium gluconate, with the former containing three times the elemental amount of calcium (27 mg/ml). Calcium chloride should be given centrally, while calcium gluconate can be administered peripherally due to lower osmolality. Boluses of calcium gluconate 1–2 mg elemental calcium per kilogram weight transiently increases serum calcium by 0.5–1 mg/ml, but this effect declines after 30 min; therefore, an infusion of 1–2 mg/kg/h should be initiated. Calcitriol can be used at 15–50 ng/kg/day (divided into twice or three times daily) to transition to an oral regimen. Magnesium levels should be monitored and repleted in order to aid calcium normalization.

Following parathyroidectomy, symptomatic hypocalcemia can occur with hungry bone syndrome and can be controlled with oral elemental calcium of 1–2 g/day. Calcium carbonate is a readily available source of elemental calcium, containing 400 mg of elemental calcium per 1 g. Calcitriol can be added at 0.25 μg/day. Regarding coagulopathy, in vivo clot strength was studied using maximum amplitude on thromboelastography of patients at risk for or who had active bleeding, adjusting for fibrinogen, platelet counts, INR, and PTT and a target ionized calcium value of >1 mmol/l may be recommended during periods where bleeding is of concern [47].

Hypercalcemia

Hypercalcemia is much less common than hypocalcemia in the critical care setting and in hospitalized patients in general can be mostly attributed to hyperparathyroidism and malignancy with less likely causes being drugs and thyrotoxicosis.

Symptoms

Clinically, patients will present with gastrointestinal (nausea, emesis, constipation, ileus, pancreatitis), cardiac (hypovolemia, hypotension, shortened QT interval), renal (polyuria, nephrocalcinosis), and neurologic (confusion, depressed consciousness) findings. Laboratory values of total serum calcium of >12–14 mg/dl or ionized calcium of >3–3.5 mmol/l will generally reflect these clinical findings [48].

Treatment

The treatment of hypercalcemia is to address the underlying etiology and to relieve symptoms. In primary hyperparathyroidism, symptomatic patients and asymptomatic patients with age under 50 years, serum calcium levels over 1 mg/dl above the upper limit of normal, creatinine clearance <60 ml/min, clinical development of a kidney stone or by imaging and/or bone mineral density T score < −2.5 or vertebral fracture by imaging should undergo parathyroidectomy [49]. Surgery also is indicated for secondary and tertiary hyperparathyroidism. The osmotic diuresis caused by hypercalcemia should be treated with isotonic saline infusion. Diuretics, such as furosemide, administered intravenously at 40–80 mg every 2 h titrated to 100–200 ml of urine/h aid in urinary calcium excretion but must be accompanied by and replaced with isotonic saline. Calcitonin is used to treat hypercalcemia of malignancy and dosed at 4 units/kg intramuscular or subcutaneous every 12 h [50]. Corticosteroids counter neoplastic growth and enhance the activity of vitamin D. Hydrocortisone is administered at 200 mg intravenously divided into 2–3 doses per day [51]. Bisphosphonates such as zoledronate (4 mg intravenous over 15 min) and pamidronate (90 mg intravenous over 2 h) are used to inhibit bone resorption seen in malignancy-associated hypercalcemia (but can be used for other etiologies) with effects seen in 2–4 days and can be repeated every 4–10 days as needed. Lastly, hemodialysis can be used for severe levels of hypercalcemia and when fluids and bisphosphonates are ineffective.

Phosphorus

Phosphorus is an essential cellular element responsible for a variety of functions from bone structure, to energy storage and even modulation of oxygen release by hemoglobin [52]. Over 85% of the body phosphorus remains in the skeleton, with approximately 15% located in the soft tissues and less than 1% in the blood [53]. PTH, vitamin D, and fibroblast growth factor 23 (FGF23) have been recognized as the three hormones responsible for the homeostasis of phosphorus [54]. Renal reabsorption at the proximal tubule is the main determinant of a steady-state phosphate concentration [55]. The normal values for the total serum phosphate levels are 2.5–4.5 mg/dl.

Hypophosphatemia

Hypophosphatemia is common in the ICU, seen in almost 30% of surgical ICU patients. This incidence can reach 75% in trauma patients and 100% in burn and liver surgery patients [56–60]. Septic patients and patients with acute kidney injury requiring continuous renal replacement therapy have a significantly higher mortality risk when their phosphate levels are low [61, 62].

Hypophosphatemia is usually attributed to three different mechanisms: redistribution, increased renal excretion, and decreased intestinal absorption. In the ICU, the most common cause for hypophosphatemia is redistribution, which can be related to various conditions. These include respiratory alkalosis that causes increase in the intracellular pH which results in phosphate entering the cell by stimulating glycolysis [63]; administration of glucose and insulin which results in transportation of phosphate into the cells along with glucose; administration of vasopressors, including epinephrine and norepinephrine [64]; metabolic acidosis which results in increased renal excretion of phosphate; and various drugs including diuretics and glucocorticosteroids [65]. The high incidence of hypophosphatemia in sepsis might be related to the increased utilization of phosphate by the immune cells, as high levels of the cytokine IL-6 and tumor necrosis factor-a (TNF-a) are associated with decreased phosphate levels [66].

Several categories of surgical patients might be more susceptible to hypophosphatemia. These include cardiac surgery patients who are at a higher risk for respiratory alkalosis and are more likely to receive diuretic therapy [67]. It remains unclear if cardiopulmonary bypass is associated with hypophosphatemia. Another category of surgical patients includes those undergoing major hepatic resection. These patients may require large doses to replete their phosphorus for several days. The cause of this hypophosphatemia is attributed to shift of phosphate into hepatocytes and renal phosphate wasting [60, 68]. In burn patients, hypophosphatemia is related to the loss of phosphate through the skin [58]. For trauma patients, hypophosphatemia is usually attributed to the increased urinary excretion of phosphate [56]. In patients with traumatic brain injury in particular, diabetes insipidus and polyuria may lead to a higher occurrence of hypophosphatemia, especially when cooling measures are implemented [57, 69]. In patients with severe malnutrition, initiation of enteral or parenteral feeding may result in the so-called refeeding syndrome with all the associated metabolic disturbances that include severe hypophosphatemia [70]. Diabetic ketoacidosis is also associated with hypophosphatemia, especially after the initiation of treatment with insulin that causes intracellular shifting along with potassium and glucose [71]. Lastly, continuous renal replacement therapy may be associated with hypophosphatemia when low phosphate replacement solutions are utilized [72].

Symptoms

Hypophosphatemia is usually asymptomatic and can rarely be life threatening. Symptoms that may develop are related to impaired energy metabolism. Hypophosphatemia has been associated with decreased diaphragmatic muscle contractility [73], respiratory failure, and inability to wean off the ventilator [74, 75]. Impaired energy metabolism in the myocardium due to hypophosphatemia may result in decreased contractility, higher requirements for inotropic support, and arrhythmias in cardiac surgery and septic patients [59, 76–78]. Other manifestations of hypophosphatemia that have been described include insulin resistance, hemolysis, and neuromuscular effects which can range from skeletal muscle weakness to rhabdomyolysis, seizures, and central pontine myelinolysis; however, direct association cannot be established. Multiple studies have associated hypophosphatemia with a higher risk for mortality; however, whether hypophosphatemia itself predisposes to this higher risk or whether it is a marker for the severity of the patient's illness remains unknown. In addition, whether correction of hypophosphatemia in critically ill patients can decrease this mortality risk has not been established [52].

Treatment

When treating hypophosphatemia, the main factors that should be taken into consideration include the presence of symptoms, the presence of other associated electrolyte abnormalities, and the degree of phosphate depletion. In general, correction of hypophosphatemia in asymptomatic and non-ventilated patients is not supported by the available literature, and the impact of such practice on outcomes is largely unknown. Phosphate repletion is recommended, however, for symptomatic patients [79]. Given also the impact of hypophosphatemia on diaphragmatic contractility [73], achieving normal phosphate values in ventilated patients might be justified, although this is probably more relevant in chronically ventilated patients and patients with underlying respiratory pathology including chronic obstructive pulmonary disease [79, 80]. Cardiac surgery patients might benefit from phosphate repletion, independent of the presence of symptoms, as hypophosphatemia in this setting has been associated with a higher incidence of arrhythmias [76, 78, 81]. Prevention of hypophosphatemia in patients on continuous renal replacement therapy with the addition of phosphate to the hemofiltration solutions may improve outcomes [82, 83]. Lastly, phosphate repletion in septic patients might be beneficial, although direct impact of normophosphatemia on outcomes has not been established [84].

Phosphorus can be provided in enteral or parenteral form. In most patients, especially in the absence of symptoms and with a moderate degree hypophosphatemia, the enteral route will suffice, preventing volume overload and the other potential complications associated with intravenous administration. The parenteral form can be given as sodium or potassium phosphate. The sodium phosphate solution is preferable in patients at risk for hyperkalemia. High doses of intravenous phosphate administration are considered safe up to 45 mmol with up to 20 mmol/h [84]. Phosphate may complex with calcium, causing clinically significant hypocalcemia. Therefore, measuring calcium levels during phosphate administration is encouraged, especially when large doses are required.

Hyperphosphatemia

Hyperphosphatemia (phosphate > 5 mg/dl) is less common and is usually related to renal dysfunction. Elevated phosphate levels may be predictors of decreasing glomerular filtration rate (GFR) and even mortality [85, 86]. In the ICU, hyperphosphatemia is usually multifactorial and might be related to redistribution of phosphorus, increased administration, and, most importantly, decreased renal excretion.

Tumor lysis syndrome in cancer patients can cause elevated levels of phosphorus, as can rhabdomyolysis, especially when associated with acute kidney injury [87, 88]. Other quoted causes for hyperphosphatemia include pancreatitis, respiratory acidosis, and lactic acidosis, but these are rare. Pseudohyperphosphatemia can be caused by contamination of the blood sample with phosphate-buffered saline as a diluent for heparin or can be related to hyperparaproteinemia, hyperbilirubinemia, or even administration of amphotericin B [89, 90].

Symptoms

Most patients with hyperphosphatemia remain asymptomatic. Due to the creation of phosphate complexes with circulating calcium, the clinical manifestations of hyperphosphatemia are mostly related to the resulting hypocalcemia and the deposition of calcium phosphate salts in the tissues, including the myocardium. Therefore, symptoms including tetany and arrhythmias may develop.

Treatment

Hyperphosphatemia usually resolves spontaneously within a few hours in patients with normal renal function. Calcium acetate tablets may be given to patients who are hypocalcemic; however, this practice in the ICU is uncommon. Saline hydration may promote phosphaturia, especially when combined with acetazolamide. However, this is not an option in patients with impaired renal function who might require renal replacement therapy for correction of their phosphate levels.

References

1. Ryzen E, Wagers PW, Singer FR, Rude RK. Magnesium deficiency in a medical ICU population. Crit Care Med. 1985;13(1):19–21.
2. Denny JT, et al. Lower incidence of hypo-magnesemia in surgical intensive care unit patients in 2011 versus 2001. J Clin Med Res. 2015;7(4):253–6.
3. Fairley J, Glassford NJ, Zhang L, Bellomo R. Magnesium status and magnesium therapy in critically ill patients: a systematic review. J Crit Care. 2015;30(6):1349–58.
4. Elin RJ. Assessment of magnesium status for diagnosis and therapy. Magnes Res. 2010;23(4):S194–8.
5. Elin RJ. Assessment of magnesium status. Clin Chem. 1987;33(11):1965–70.
6. Noronha JL, Matuschak GM. Magnesium in critical illness: metabolism, assessment, and treatment. Intensive Care Med. 2002;28(6):667–79.
7. Hexum T, Samson FE, Himes RH. Kinetic studies of membrane (Na+-K+-Mg2+)-ATPase. Biochim Biophys Acta. 1970;212(2):322–31.
8. Grubbs RD, Maguire ME. Magnesium as a regulatory cation: criteria and evaluation. Magnesium. 1987;6(3):113–27.
9. Tong GM, Rude RK. Magnesium deficiency in critical illness. J Intensive Care Med. 2005;20(1):3–17.
10. Weglicki WB, Phillips TM. Pathobiology of magnesium deficiency: a cytokine/neurogenic inflammation hypothesis. Am J Phys. 1992;263(3 Pt 2):R734–7.
11. Nakagawa M, Oono H, Nishio A. Enhanced production of IL-1beta and IL-6 following endotoxin challenge in rats with dietary magnesium deficiency. J Vet Med Sci. 2001;63(4):467–9.
12. Cao Z, Tongate C, Elin RJ. Evaluation of AVL988/4 analyzer for measurement of ionized magnesium and ionized calcium. Scand J Clin Lab Invest. 2001;61(5):389–94.
13. Hébert P, Mehta N, Wang J, Hindmarsh T, Jones G, Cardinal P. Functional magnesium deficiency in critically ill patients identified using a magnesium-loading test. Crit Care Med. 1997;25(5):749–55.
14. Whang R. Magnesium deficiency: pathogenesis, prevalence, and clinical implications. Am J Med. 1987;82(3A):24–9.
15. Smith GA, Tompkins RK. Biliary magnesium loss in the postoperative patient. Arch Surg. 1974;109(1):77–9.
16. Nyhlin H, Dyckner T, Ek B, Wester PO. Plasma and skeletal muscle electrolytes in patients with Crohn's disease. J Am Coll Nutr. 1985;4(5):531–8.
17. Cole DE, Quamme GA. Inherited disorders of renal magnesium handling. J Am Soc Nephrol. 2000;11(10):1937–47.
18. Ryan MP. Diuretics and potassium/magnesium depletion. Directions for treatment. Am J Med. 1987;82(3A):38–47.
19. Rude RK, Oldham SB, Singer FR. Functional hypoparathyroidism and parathyroid hormone end-organ resistance in human magnesium deficiency. Clin Endocrinol. 1976;5(3):209–24.
20. Rude RK. Magnesium metabolism and deficiency. Endocrinol Metab Clin N Am. 1993;22(2):377–95.
21. Vallee BL, Wacker WE, Ulmer DD. The magnesium-deficiency tetany syndrome in man. N Engl J Med. 1960;262(4):155–61.
22. Wacker WEC, et al. Normocalcemic magnesium deficiency tetany. JAMA. 1962;180(2):161.
23. Tsuji H, Venditti FJ, Evans JC, Larson MG, Levy D. The associations of levels of serum potassium and magnesium with ventricular premature complexes (the Framingham Heart Study). Am J Cardiol. 1994;74(3):232–5.
24. Kelly RA, Smith TW. Recognition and management of digitalis toxicity. Am J Cardiol. 1992;69(18):108G–18G; disc. 118G–19G.
25. Fatemi S, Ryzen E, Flores J, Endres DB, Rude RK. Effect of experimental human magnesium depletion on parathyroid hormone secretion and 1,25-dihydroxyvitamin D metabolism. J Clin Endocrinol Metab. 1991;73(5):1067–72.
26. Whang R, Ryder KW. Frequency of hypomagnesemia and hypermagnesemia. Requested vs routine. JAMA. 1990;263(22):3063–4.
27. Whang R, Whang DD, Ryan MP. Refractory potassium repletion. A consequence of magnesium deficiency. Arch Intern Med. 1992;152(1):40–5.
28. Tzivoni D, et al. Treatment of torsade de pointes with magnesium sulfate. Circulation. 1988;77(2):392–7.
29. Thel MC, Armstrong AL, McNulty SE, Califf RM, O'Connor CM. Randomised trial of magnesium in in-hospital cardiac arrest. Duke Internal Medicine Housestaff. Lancet (London, UK). 1997;350(9087):1272–6.
30. Ryan MP. Interrelationships of magnesium and potassium homeostasis. Miner Electrolyte Metab. 1993;19(4–5):290–5.

31. Kraft MD, Btaiche IF, Sacks GS, Kudsk KA. Treatment of electrolyte disorders in adult patients in the intensive care unit. Am J Health Syst Pharm. 2005;62(16):1663–82.
32. Ryzen E, Nelson TA, Rude RK. Low blood mononuclear cell magnesium content and hypocalcemia in normomagnesemic patients. West J Med. 1987;147(5):549–53.
33. Altman D, et al. Do women with pre-eclampsia, and their babies, benefit from magnesium sulphate? The Magpie Trial: a randomised placebo-controlled trial. Lancet (London, UK). 2002;359(9321):1877–90.
34. Cao Z, Bideau R, Valdes R, Elin RJ. Acute hypermagnesemia and respiratory arrest following infusion of MgSO4 for tocolysis. Clin Chim Acta. 1999;285(1–2):191–3.
35. Baker SB, Worthley LIG. The essentials of calcium, magnesium and phosphate metabolism: part I. Physiology. Crit Care Resusc. 2002;4(4):301–6.
36. Forman DT, Lorenzo L. Ionized calcium: its significance and clinical usefulness. Ann Clin Lab Sci. 1991;21(5):297–304.
37. Kelly A, Levine MA. Hypocalcemia in the critically ill patient. J Intensive Care Med. 2013;28(3):166–77.
38. Zaloga GP, Willey S, Tomasic P, Chernow B. Free fatty acids alter calcium binding: a cause for misinterpretation of serum calcium values and hypocalcemia in critical illness. J Clin Endocrinol Metab. 1987;64(5):1010–4.
39. Aberegg SK. Ionized calcium in the ICU: should it be measured and corrected? Chest. 2016;149(3):846–55.
40. Bushinsky DA, Monk RD. Electrolyte quintet: Calcium. Lancet. 1998;352(9124):306–11.
41. Desai TK, Carlson RW, Geheb MA. Prevalence and clinical implications of hypocalcemia in acutely ill patients in a medical intensive care setting. Am J Med. 1988;84(2):209–14.
42. Forsythe RM, Wessel CB, Billiar TR, Angus DC, Rosengart MR. Parenteral calcium for intensive care unit patients. Cochrane Database Syst Rev. 2008;(4):CD006163.
43. Collage RD, et al. Calcium supplementation during sepsis exacerbates organ failure and mortality via calcium/calmodulin-dependent protein kinase kinase signaling. Crit Care Med. 2013;41(11):e352–60.
44. Lind L, et al. Hypocalcemia and parathyroid hormone secretion in critically ill patients. Crit Care Med. 2000;28(1):93–9.
45. Bai M, et al. Citrate versus heparin anticoagulation for continuous renal replacement therapy: an updated meta-analysis of RCTs. Intensive Care Med. 2015;41(12):2098–110.
46. Steele T, Kolamunnage-Dona R, Downey C, Toh C-H, Welters I. Assessment and clinical course of hypocalcemia in critical illness. Crit Care. 2013;17(3):R106.
47. Ho KM, Yip CB. Concentration-dependent effect of hypocalcaemia on in vitro clot strength in patients at risk of bleeding: a retrospective cohort study. Transfus Med. 2016;26(1):57–62.
48. Maier JD, Levine SN. Hypercalcemia in the intensive care unit: a review of pathophysiology, diagnosis, and modern therapy. J Intensive Care Med. 2015;30(5):235–52.
49. Bilezikian JP, et al. Guidelines for the management of asymptomatic primary hyperparathyroidism: summary statement from the fourth international workshop. J Clin Endocrinol Metab. 2014;99(10):3561–9.
50. Marino PL. The ICU book. 3rd ed. Philadelphia: Lippincott Williams & Wilkins; 2007.
51. Stewart AF. Clinical practice. Hypercalcemia associated with cancer. N Engl J Med. 2005;352(4):373–9.
52. Geerse DA, Bindels AJ, Kuiper MA, Roos AN, Spronk PE, Schultz MJ. Treatment of hypophosphatemia in the intensive care unit: a review. Crit Care. 2010;14(4):R147.
53. Slatapolsky E, Hruska K. Disorders of phosphorus, calcium, and magnesium metabolism. In: Schrier R, editor. Diseases of the kidneys and urinary tract. 7th ed. Philadelphia: Lippincott Williams & Wilkins; 2001.
54. Lederer E. Regulation of serum phosphate. J Physiol. 2014;592(18):3985–95.
55. Blaine J, Chonchol M, Levi M. Renal control of calcium, phosphate, and magnesium homeostasis. Clin J Am Soc Nephrol. 2015;10(7):1257–72.
56. Daily WH, Tonnesen AS, Allen SJ. Hypophosphatemia – incidence, etiology, and prevention in the trauma patient. Crit Care Med. 1990;18(11):1210–4.
57. Polderman KH, Bloemers FW, Peerdeman SM, Girbes AR. Hypomagnesemia and hypophosphatemia at admission in patients with severe head injury. Crit Care Med. 2000;28(6):2022–5.
58. Berger MM, Rothen C, Cavadini C, Chiolero RL. Exudative mineral losses after serious burns: a clue to the alterations of magnesium and phosphate metabolism. Am J Clin Nutr. 1997;65(5):1473–81.
59. Zazzo JF, Troché G, Ruel P, Maintenant J. High incidence of hypophosphatemia in surgical intensive care patients: efficacy of phosphorus therapy on myocardial function. Intensive Care Med. 1995;21(10):826–31.
60. Salem RR, Tray K. Hepatic resection-related hypophosphatemia is of renal origin as manifested by isolated hyperphosphaturia. Ann Surg. 2005;241(2):343–8.
61. Shor R, et al. Severe hypophosphatemia in sepsis as a mortality predictor. Ann Clin Lab Sci. 2006;36(1):67–72.
62. Yang Y, et al. Hypophosphatemia during continuous veno-venous hemofiltration is associated with mortality in critically ill patients with acute kidney injury. Crit Care. 2013;17(5):R205.
63. Paleologos M, Stone E, Braude S. Persistent, progressive hypophosphataemia after voluntary hyperventilation. Clin Sci (Lond). 2000;98(5):619–25.
64. Kjeldsen SE, Moan A, Petrin J, Weder AB, Julius S. Effects of increased arterial epinephrine on insulin, glucose and phosphate. Blood Press. 1996;5(1):27–31.
65. Murer H, Hernando N, Forster I, Biber J. Proximal tubular phosphate reabsorption: molecular mechanisms. Physiol Rev. 2000;80(4):1373–409.
66. Barak V, Schwartz A, Kalickman I, Nisman B, Gurman G, Shoenfeld Y. Prevalence of hypophosphatemia in sepsis and infection: the role of cytokines. Am J Med. 1998;104(1):40–7.
67. Cohen J, Kogan A, Sahar G, Lev S, Vidne B, Singer P. Hypophosphatemia following open heart surgery: incidence and consequences. Eur J Cardiothorac Surg. 2004;26(2):306–10.
68. George R, Shiu MH. Hypophosphatemia after major hepatic resection. Surgery. 1992;111(3):281–6.
69. Polderman KH, Peerdeman SM, Girbes AR. Hypophosphatemia and hypomagnesemia induced by cooling in patients with severe head injury. J Neurosurg. 2001;94(5):697–705.
70. Marinella MA. Refeeding syndrome and hypophosphatemia. J Intensive Care Med. 2005;20(3):155–9.
71. English P, Williams G. Hyperglycaemic crises and lactic acidosis in diabetes mellitus. Postgrad Med J. 2004;80(943):253–61.
72. Troyanov S, Geadah D, Ghannoum M, Cardinal J, Leblanc M. Phosphate addition to hemodiafiltration solutions during continuous renal replacement therapy. Intensive Care Med. 2004;30(8):1662–5.
73. Aubier M, et al. Effect of hypophosphatemia on diaphragmatic contractility in patients with acute respiratory failure. N Engl J Med. 1985;313(7):420–4.
74. Alsumrain MH, Jawad SA, Imran NB, Riar S, DeBari VA, Adelman M. Association of hypophosphatemia with failure-to-wean from mechanical ventilation. Ann Clin Lab Sci. 2010;40(2):144–8.

75. Agusti AG, Torres A, Estopa R, Agustividal A. Hypophosphatemia as a cause of failed weaning: the importance of metabolic factors. Crit Care Med. 1984;12(2):142–3.
76. O'Connor LR, Wheeler WS, Bethune JE. Effect of hypophosphatemia on myocardial performance in man. N Engl J Med. 1977;297(17):901–3.
77. Ognibene A, et al. Ventricular tachycardia in acute myocardial infarction: the role of hypophosphatemia. South Med J. 1994;87(1):65–9.
78. Schwartz A, et al. Association between hypophosphatemia and cardiac arrhythmias in the early stage of sepsis: could phosphorus replacement treatment reduce the incidence of arrhythmias? Electrolyte Blood Press. 2014;12(1):19.
79. Lentz RD, Brown DM, Kjellstrand CM. Treatment of severe hypophosphatemia. Ann Intern Med. 1978;89(6):941–4.
80. Fisher J, et al. Respiratory illness and hypophosphatemia. Chest. 1983;83(3):504–8.
81. Svagzdiene M, Sirvinskas E. Changes in serum electrolyte levels and their influence on the incidence of atrial fibrillation after coronary artery bypass grafting surgery. Medicina (Kaunas). 2006;42(3):208–14.
82. Demirjian S, et al. Hypophosphatemia during continuous hemodialysis is associated with prolonged respiratory failure in patients with acute kidney injury. Nephrol Dial Transplant. 2011;26(11):3508–14.
83. Bellomo R, et al. The relationship between hypophosphataemia and outcomes during low-intensity and high-intensity continuous renal replacement therapy. Crit Care Resusc. 2014;16(1):34–41.
84. Bollaert PE, Levy B, Nace L, Laterre PF, Larcan A. Hemodynamic and metabolic effects of rapid correction of hypophosphatemia in patients with septic shock. Chest. 1995;107(6):1698–701.
85. Haider DG, et al. Hyperphosphatemia is an independent risk factor for mortality in critically ill patients: results from a cross-sectional study. PLoS One. 2015;10(8):e0133426.
86. Voormolen N, et al. High plasma phosphate as a risk factor for decline in renal function and mortality in pre-dialysis patients. Nephrol Dial Transplant. 2007;22(10):2909–16.
87. Mirrakhimov AE, Ali AM, Khan M, Barbaryan A. Tumor lysis syndrome in solid tumors: an up to date review of the literature. Rare Tumors. 2014;6(2):5389.
88. Higaki M, Tanemoto M, Shiraishi T, Taniguchi K, Fujigaki Y, Uchida S. Acute kidney injury facilitates hypocalcemia by exacerbating the hyperphosphatemic effect of muscle damage in rhabdomyolysis. Nephron. 2015;131(1):11–6.
89. Larner AJ. Pseudohyperphosphatemia. Clin Biochem. 1995;28(4):391–3.
90. Bohm NM, Hoover KC, Wahlquist AE, Zhu Y, Velez JCQ. Case-control study and case series of pseudohyperphosphatemia during exposure to liposomal amphotericin B. Antimicrob Agents Chemother. 2015;59(11):6816–23.

Acid-Base Disorders

50

Jack Sava and Robel Beyene

Introduction

Under normal conditions, serum pH is the tightly controlled result of homeostatic buffering mechanisms. Mild, transient aberrations in pH may be physiologic, but if persistent, even subtle pH change may point to underlying pathology. As pH strays outside the normal range, acidemia or alkalemia may become harmful. Often this harm results from taxing attempts at compensation, such as tachypnea in response to metabolic acidosis, or through direct effects, such as systemic or pulmonary vasoregulatory changes, cerebral edema, and arrhythmias [1]. While the intensivist may rush to correct pH, acidosis or alkalosis is ultimately a marker of an underlying disease process, and correcting the pH, while important, is insufficient if the driving pathology is not also identified and corrected. In the surgical intensive care unit (SICU), both mild and significant acid-base disorders are relatively common, and an understanding of their management is key to caring for critically ill and injured patients. This chapter will review a practical approach to acid-base disorders typically encountered in the SICU.

Metabolic Acidosis

Metabolic acidosis is encountered daily in the SICU, occurring whenever acid accumulates in the extracellular space and leads to a fall in the pH below 7.35. Metabolic acidosis ranges in severity from trivial to profound – even lethal. In general, it results from excess endogenous acid production or loss of bicarbonate [2, 3]. Regardless of how the biochemistry is modeled, metabolic acidosis is most easily conceptualized as a non-respiratory accumulation of serum acids which overwhelms normal physiologic buffering capacity. The challenge of the surgical intensivist is to find and fix the underlying cause for the acidosis while also managing the physiologic consequences of abnormal pH. To the surgeon-intensivist, an additional challenge may be present, as metabolic acidosis is often the initial trigger that reveals a need for surgery. Whether it is bowel resection for mesenteric ischemia, laparotomy for trauma, or source control for sepsis, the frequent association between metabolic acidosis and operative treatment is well established [2].

Diagnosis

Metabolic acidosis may be suspected by clinical exam, which often reveals compensatory tachypnea. More often, though, the disorder will be discovered on routine or targeted laboratory testing. Bicarbonate is nearly always measured on routine metabolic panels, and a low bicarbonate is frequently the first sign of acidosis. Although frequently an arterial blood gas is ordered in order to measure the base deficit, it is important to remember that the serum bicarbonate directly correlates with base deficit, and the two can be used interchangeably [4, 5]. In the normal course of acid-base homeostasis, acidosis is buffered in the kidneys by excretion of H^+ and reabsorption and regeneration of bicarbonate [6, 7]. Respiratory compensation also buffers acidosis, but when these processes are overwhelmed, even a mild acidosis may be identified on the basis of a falling bicarbonate [6]. This change in plasma bicarbonate can be identified on both an arterial blood gas (ABG) analysis and a basic metabolic panel (BMP), and a fall below the normal range of 22–26 mEq/L deserves investigation [1]. While low serum bicarbonate on a BMP is suggestive of acidosis, it is not diagnostic of the cause.

J. Sava
Department of Trauma, MedStar Washington Hospital Center, Washington, DC, USA

R. Beyene (✉)
Division of Trauma and Surgical Critical Care, Vanderbilt University Medical Center, Nashville, TN, USA

A. Salim et al. (eds.), *Surgical Critical Care Therapy*, https://doi.org/10.1007/978-3-319-71712-8_50

Table 50.1 Acid-base disorders

Disorder	pH	PCO_2 (mm Hg)	$HCO3^-$ (mEq/L)	BDE (mEq/L)
Metabolic acidosis	<7.35	<35	<26	≤−3
Metabolic alkalosis	>7.45	>40–45	>26	≥3
Respiratory acidosis	<7.35	>45	>22	–
Respiratory alkalosis	>7.45	<35	<22	–

ABG analysis is very useful in the correct interpretation of all acid-base disorders. The telltale signs of metabolic acidosis on ABG are a pH below 7.35, a plasma bicarbonate below 22 mEq/L, worsening base deficit (less than −3 mEq/L), and a compensatory arterial partial pressure of CO_2 (PCO_2) below 35 (Table 50.1). In a simple metabolic acidosis – an acidosis without a second supervening acid-base disorder – most of these findings will be reliably present on ABG [8]. Notably, the plasma bicarbonate in an ABG is a calculated measure and is less accurate than the measured plasma bicarbonate on a metabolic panel [9]. Even in the setting of compensation, pH may not completely normalize, and metabolic acidosis will present, at least, as a pH below 7.35 and a PCO_2 less than 35 mmHg [10]. However, it is important to understand that a normal pH can be present in the setting of a metabolic acidosis (due to compensation), and the bicarbonate or base deficit is the critical laboratory measure to pay attention to.

Base deficit-excess (BDE) is a calculated value in an ABG defined as the amount of strong acid or base required to bring 1 l of blood in vitro to a pH of 7.4, assuming a PCO_2 of 40 mmHg and a temperature of 38 °C [11]. Only serum values are used in calculating BDE, so respiratory acid-base disorders do not alter the BDE. Metabolic deviations, however, do alter the BDE [11]. The severity of acidosis can be approximated by the extent of the base deficit, with mild acidosis generating a deficit of −4 to −9 mEq/L, moderate between −10 and −14 mEq/L, and severe indicated by a deficit worse than −14 mEq/L [10]. Even a mild metabolic acidosis, though, may signal potentially lethal underlying pathology.

Etiologies

Historically, metabolic acidosis is divided into two broad categories based on the existence of anion gap (AG). An anion gap is the difference in concentration between routinely measured cations (Na+ and K+) and anions (Cl^- and HCO_3^-). This difference is the anion gap – normally between 8 and 12 mEq/L. Despite what may appear to be a surplus of positively charged cations, the serum is actually electrically neutral due to numerous unmeasured anions, including sulfate and lactate [1]. An increase in these unmeasured anions produces the so-called anion gap acidosis. A normal anion gap indicates a different set of potential etiologies.

Table 50.2 Anion gap acidoses

MUDPILES	Etiology
M	Methanol
U	Uremia
D	Diabetic ketoacidosis
P	Paraldehyde
I	Infection
L	Lactic acidosis
E	Ethanol
S	Salicylates

Anion Gap Acidosis

In the SICU, the most common types of anion gap acidoses are lactic acidosis, ketoacidosis, uremia, iatrogenic acidosis, or toxins. Still, a methodical approach is important, and each event must be investigated thoroughly to confirm the etiology. "MUD PILES" has persisted as a long-standing mnemonic device for the etiologies of anion gap acidosis; this acronym includes methanol, uremia, diabetic ketoacidosis, paraldehyde, infection, lactic acidosis, ethylene glycol, and salicylates (Table 50.2). While this is helpful, it suggests each one of these etiologies is equal in standing when, in fact, some are common and others exotically rare. The two most common causes of metabolic acidosis in any surgical ICU will always be lactic acidosis (anion gap) and renal (non-gap).

Lactic Acidosis

In the SICU, lactic acidosis is the undisputed king of metabolic derangements. Lactic acidosis is not only the most common acidosis by far, but it is also used as a general screen for shock and resuscitation, and it frequently serves as a call to action [1, 8, 12, 13]. Whereas other acid-base issues may be resolved by medication or ventilator adjustments, lactic acidosis tells us – until proven otherwise – that some or all of the organism has entered a state of emergency.

Lactate is a product of anaerobic glycolysis, produced through the reduction of pyruvate by lactate dehydrogenase. Under normal physiologic conditions, only a small amount of lactate is formed in the muscle, skin, brain, intestine, and red blood cells. It is efficiently cleared by the liver, with some contribution from kidneys and other organs, and this clearance normally keeps serum lactate below 2 mmol/L [1]. When critical illness, ischemia, or trauma results in increased anaerobic metabolism, increased lactate production may overwhelm the physiologic mechanisms in place to clear or buffer it, resulting in lactic acidosis. As lactate is a strong anion, its relative increase causes an increase in the anion gap, which is why it is classified as an anion gap acidosis [14]. There is some debate regarding the actual etiology of an elevated lactate in shock states, with some arguing that it is primarily due to decreased hepatic clearance and not increased production due to anaerobic metabolism. But regardless of the etiology, it should be taken as an indicator of hypoperfusion and shock or sepsis and should prompt immediate evaluation and interventions.

Lactate exists in two isomeric molecular forms. Routine lactate labs only measure L-lactate, but its chiral opposite, D-lactate, can also be measured in serum in some laboratories [14]. Much like L-lactate, D-lactate is a product of anaerobic respiration but is thought to be produced in the GI tract through metabolism unique to gut bacteria breakdown of ingested carbohydrate. While the native acid-base state of the host may play a part, D-lactate production by gut bacteria is less easily interpreted than L-lactate (often just called "lactate") in assessing host acid-base status. D-lactic acidosis should, however, be considered in patients with anion gap acidosis in the setting of intestinal disease and confusion, especially if these symptoms worsen after a carbohydrate load [2]. Overgrowth of gut flora can be the driving force behind this uncommon occurrence. Similar gut bacterial overgrowth can be seen in patients with hyperalimentation or tube feeds, jejunoileal bypass, or short gut. Diagnosis requires an index of suspicion high enough to order a D-lactate screen, and treatment consists of treating bacterial overgrowth and avoiding carbohydrates [2].

When lactate and BDE are discordant, lactate elevation is more predictive of mortality than a base deficit [13]. In trauma and emergency general surgery patients, an elevated lactate with a normal base deficit is correlated with longer lengths of stay and higher mortality, while base deficit showed no significant correlation to mortality in the setting of normal lactate. The superiority of lactate, compared to base deficit, was confirmed in blunt trauma patients presenting in hemorrhagic shock [15]. This highlights the importance of lactate in the workup and management of metabolic acidosis.

Any unexpected rise in serum lactate should trigger clinical reevaluation and the development of a comprehensive differential diagnosis. Once a reasonable source has been identified, the intensivist should avoid "premature closure" – a type of cognitive error where a hasty conclusion is reached without full consideration of other possibilities. The causes of lactemia are not mutually exclusive. One etiology may overlap with, or lead to, another. A patient with poor cardiac output may develop superimposed bowel ischemia. Severe sepsis may be complicated by secondary cardiomyopathy.

In general, the differential diagnosis of lactic acidosis can be split into three broad categories. In the first group are those with a focal ischemia (Table 50.3) [14]. These patients may have adequate cardiac output but have a local area of impaired perfusion due to injury, infection, or vascular compromise. The most likely source depends on the clinical context, but bowel ischemia, cholecystitis, compartment syndrome, and limb ischemia are common. Focal lactate spillage often mandates surgery or other interventions to restore flow and remove necrotic tissue.

Table 50.3 Lactic acidoses treatable by intervention

Acidosis	Intervention
Occlusive acute mesenteric ischemia	Revascularization (thrombectomy, embolectomy, stent, or bypass); bowel resection
Hemorrhage	Control of bleeding; resuscitation
Soft tissue infection	Surgical debridement of infectious or necrotic tissue
Abscess	Drainage of abscess
Abdominal compartment syndrome	Decompressive laparotomy
Extremity compartment syndrome and eschar	Fasciotomy or escharotomy
Cardiogenic shock	Pathology appropriate cardiac procedure (valve repair/replacement, decompression of tamponade, reperfusion, etc.)

The next category consists of patients who are spilling lactate globally. Typically, this is due to low cardiac output, anemia, or cellular hypoxia in sepsis. As in focal ischemia, specific causes depend on patient type and will be different in the trauma ICU compared to the cardiac ICU. The intensivist must use whatever tools are available and familiar to rule in or out low flow. This may include clinical examination, looking for cool, mottled skin, altered mentation, and oliguria. A wide variety of tools and devices are available as adjuncts to this exam. When cardiac index (CI) is measured, a CI >3 is unlikely to result in lactate elevations, whereas CI < 2 commonly will do so. Intermediate lactate levels between 2 and 3 are less conclusive.

Lactic Acidosis Caused by Focal Ischemia

Acute mesenteric ischemia classically occurs secondary to four well-described mechanisms: thrombosis, embolus, venous insufficiency, and global low flow or shock causing nonocclusive mesenteric ischemia (NOMI) [16]. In the setting of a consult for mesenteric ischemia, which is often driven by an elevated lactate, the surgeon must differentiate these etiologies to conclude the best course of treatment. This can be challenging because the patients will often be otherwise complex, critically ill patients who may not be able to either give a history or cooperate with a physical exam to help narrow the surgeon's differential diagnosis. In patients who develop acute mesenteric ischemia from occlusion of arterial inflow, the cause of lactic acidosis is likely due to a localized hypoxia that is driving the bowel into anaerobic metabolism. The classic presentation is sudden onset abdominal pain out of proportion to tenderness and other findings elicited on physical exam. However, this finding is most reliably found in acute embolic mesenteric isch-

Fig. 50.1 Acidosis

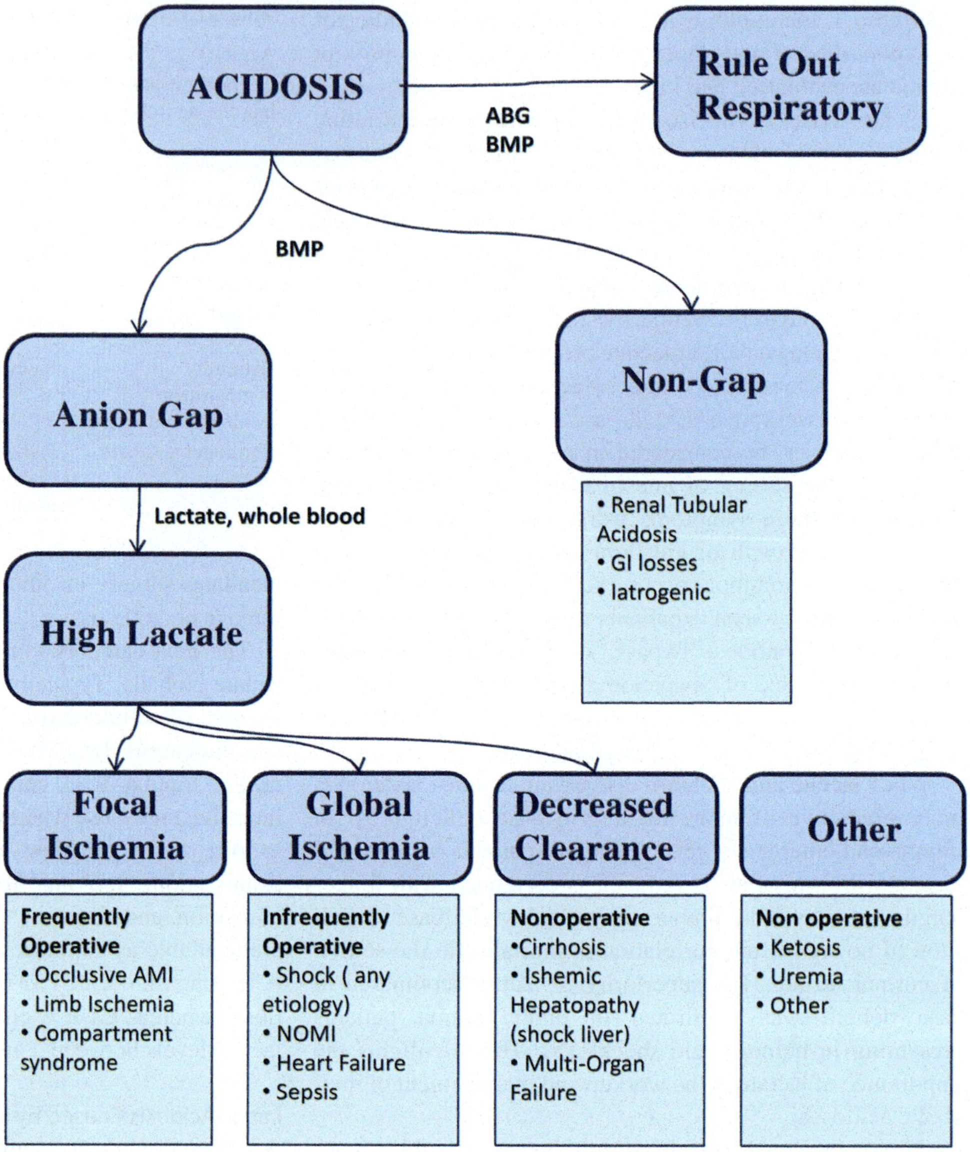

emia. Unlike the relatively distal arterial occlusion seen in embolic disease, occlusion in thrombotic disease tends to be slower and develops closer to the takeoff of the superior mesenteric artery (SMA) or celiac plexus. This leads to a prolonged course and atypical presentation [14].

In both thrombotic and embolic mesenteric ischemia, if identified early enough, there may be a role for vascular intervention to salvage bowel or other organs undergoing reversible ischemia before it progresses to irreversible necrosis (Fig. 50.1). Thrombectomy and embolectomy, however, do not obviate the need for adequate resuscitation, antibiotic coverage, and management of other critical care needs. In nonocclusive or nonmechanical causes, medical optimization, including possibly systemic heparinization, blood pressure support, and treatment of possible vasospasms, may alleviate the underlying local hypoperfusion. These etiologies require supportive care, but operative options intended to reverse or limit hypoxia are limited.

In advanced disease or delayed presentation, any of the causes of mesenteric ischemia, occlusive or otherwise, may need an exploratory laparotomy to gauge the viability of the bowel and need for bowel resection. If nonviable or frankly necrotic bowel is identified, surgical resection of the involved bowel may be warranted [16]. Patients that require resection of necrotic bowel often require multiple operations for reevaluation, with an eye toward normalization of the lactemia and acidosis to guide reoperation and eventual closure. It is also important to remember that there are other causes of bowel ischemia and necrosis, including obstruction, hernia, and iatrogenic injury to bowel or vasculature, which may cause metabolic acidosis and require operative intervention. Again, when feasible, revascularization is ideal, but resection may be necessary.

Colon ischemia less frequently requires emergent operation, primarily because it is often reversible or self-limited. In extreme cases, a nonviable or necrotic colon would also need resection to reverse the resultant acidosis [16]. Limb ischemia, much like mesenteric ischemia, causes lactic acidosis through hypoxia and anaerobic metabolism. Compartment syndrome, either abdominal or extremity, can also cause a regional hypoxia to tissue, with subsequent lactic acidosis. Abdominal compartment syndrome exists on a spectrum of intra-abdominal hypertension and can, if left undiagnosed or untreated, progress to not only visceral injury and but multi-organ system insufficiency and possibly failure. In extremity compartment syndrome, a relative rise in pressure within a restrictive compartment eventually causes compromise to the anatomy within that compartment through hypoxia. Decompression of the offending compartment, and potentially debriding nonviable tissue, is the treatment of choice in each case.

Lactic Acidosis Caused by Non-focal Ischemia

The link between sepsis, septic shock, and lactic acidosis is somewhat controversial. While tissue hypoxia may generate a certain quantity of lactate in sepsis, the full etiology is thought to be multifactorial. Contributing factors may include stimulation of increased pyruvate production, limitation of pyruvate dehydrogenase, reduced lactate clearance, hypermetabolic production of lactate from inflamed tissue, and production of lactate from indirectly related organs [14]. This is supported by the finding that, even in septic shock, resting muscle tends to utilize lactate at a higher rate than it produces it [1]. In SICU patients with sepsis, lactemia without acidosis can sometimes be seen, but this is thought to be due to hypermetabolism and has no prognostic implications [14].

In some cases, resolution of sepsis may require operative source control. While this is significantly limited in certain septic sources such as UTI or pneumonia, in cases of peripheral infection such as an abscess, wound, or necrotizing soft tissue infection, surgery or other intervention is likely to be necessary. In these cases, surgical therapy must be part of a broader strategy of supportive care for sepsis, including resuscitation and antibiotic care.

Elevation in serum lactate is common in most types of shock. A decrease in the oxygen delivery to tissues leads to increasing anaerobic glycolysis and an inability for pyruvate to enter mitochondria and undergo oxidation, a critical step in aerobic metabolism. Instead, under hypoxic conditions, pyruvate is converted to lactate, leading to a buildup of lactate [14]. This mismatch between oxygen delivery and need is thought to be present in all forms of shock as well as in severe anemia or hypoxemia [12]. Differentiating focal ischemia from global ischemia remains a substantial challenge. In cases of significant lactate elevation and unreliable clinical exam (e.g., obtundation), imaging or exploratory surgery may be necessary to exclude intra-abdominal ischemia.

Another common and confounding contributor to lactemia is diminished hepatic clearance. In cases of liver failure or cirrhosis, even normal levels of lactate production may cause lactic acidosis. This can happen through viral hepatitis but is also possible following nonviral causes such as liver toxicity, infection, or even potentially malnutrition causing intrinsic dysfunction. Ischemic hepatopathy ("shock liver") and congestive hepatopathy, if they progress to intrinsic liver dysfunction, are also possible causes or limited hepatic clearance of lactate [14]. The intensivist may be faced with a confusing circle of shock, liver dysfunction, and lactic acidosis, each of which may drive the others.

Numerous other conditions, while less common, may also cause lactic acidosis. Lung injury, in the spectrum of ARDS, has been shown to be a significant generator of lactate and subsequent acidosis. This may be due to anaerobic metabolism, glucose metabolism changes, and cytokines. Asthma has been shown to have multiple reasons to cause lactic acidosis, including elevated oxygen demand and even liver ischemia [1, 14]. Other increases in oxygen consumption, such as seizure activity, pheochromocytoma, significant burns, and neuroleptic malignant syndrome, similarly create a relative hypoxic stage through oxygen demand that outstrips delivery [2]. In cardiac surgery patients, cardiopulmonary bypass is a known cause of lactemia though inadequate perfusion similar to shock. Furthermore, the use of epinephrine can further potentiate tissue malperfusion and lactic acidosis, both in cardiac and noncardiac patients. Cancer patients have been shown to have more anaerobic metabolism and impaired hepatic lactate clearance in the setting of hepatic metastasis, making them more susceptible to lactic acidosis [14].

Even with adequate clearance and normal perfusion, there are metabolic causes of lactic acidosis to consider, including metformin and malnutrition. While it is clear that biguanides, such as metformin, can cause significant lactic acidosis, the pathophysiology is unclear, and the occurrence is rare [14]. Some HIV medications similarly have been shown to cause lactic acidosis. Malnutrition can cause thiamine and biotin deficiency, both of which are cofactors in pyruvate metabolism. In their absence, pyruvate can build up and eventually become lactate [14]. Other categorizations have been described, including differentiation of type A lactic acidosis (secondary to hypoperfusion or hypoxemia) from type B lactic acidosis (in the absence of hypoperfusion or hypoxemia). Some surgeons have found these distinctions to be of dubious value [2].

Management

As with all acid-base disorders, management of lactic acidosis must be focused on identifying and reversing the underlying etiology. Under-resuscitation is a common cause for lactate elevation, and while current surgical critical care trends point to judicious use of crystalloid, saline boluses will often resolve or improve lactic acidosis. Rapid resolution of lactemia may be reassuring, but it does not rule out focal ischemia. Sources of ongoing regional or global hypoperfusion must be addressed. For infectious etiologies, appropriate antibiotics and source control must accompany fluid resuscitation. In those cases where surgery is needed for source control, it should take place after careful but expedient optimization, generally within 2–4 h.

Uremic Acidosis

Renal failure, especially chronic renal failure with a low glomerular filtration rate (GFR), is known to cause an anion gap acidosis. The proposed pathophysiology for this is limited anion excretion in the urine, rather than increased endogenous acid production. At a GFR below 25 mL/min, there is impaired renal acidification, reduced bicarbonate reabsorption, and impaired renal homeostasis, especially concerning ammonia, phosphate, and sulfate [17, 18]. A decrease in renal ammonium excretion has been linked to a positive acid balance and reduction in bicarbonate, causing metabolic acidosis. The unexcreted anions explain the anion gap, which makes this an anion gap acidosis [18]. Unlike other metabolic acidoses, uremic acidosis can be very long standing and may take a very long time to correct.

Diagnosis of uremic acidosis should be suspected when an anion gap acidosis is identified in patients with renal failure, especially chronic renal failure. A GFR should be evaluated through a metabolic panel, as significant acidosis would not occur until GFR is critically low. Plasma bicarbonate will also generally be in the rage of 12–20 mmol/L. Other etiologies, including lactic acidosis, must also be investigated in these patients as well, as uremia does not preclude them from hypoxic or hypoperfused states [18]. Early alkali replacement to maintain adequate serum bicarbonate may be appropriate [2].

Ketoacidosis

Ketoacidosis is often understood to be pathognomonic for severe diabetes, but can also arise secondary to alcoholic and starvation ketosis [2]. Diabetic ketoacidosis occurs when fatty acid metabolism increases in the face of insulin deficiency, giving rise to acetoacetate and β-hydroxybuterate (ketoacids). This is seen after insulin is stopped in an insulin-dependent diabetic or in the face of other severe illness or infection triggers a relative increase in the insulin demand in the patient; this etiology is seen with a significant hyperglycemia. Patients will present with symptoms associated with both acidosis and hyperglycemia, including potential mental status changes, electrolyte abnormalities, and dehydration. Alcoholic ketoacidosis is seen when alcohol use is disrupted following chronic alcohol use and malnutrition. The catecholamine increase caused by alcohol withdrawal leads to increased lipolysis and a metabolic shift towards ketosis. Patients often present with nausea, vomiting, and abdominal pain. Finally, starvation ketoacidosis occurs when inadequate glucose is available for normal metabolism and the body breaks down fat and produces ketones. This may be pathologic or may be sought as a goal in certain popular weight-loss regimens. Taken to its extreme, starvation ketoacidosis can also be dangerous. In all of these cases, accumulation of ketoacids is responsible for the widening gap and acidosis seen in the patient's lab results. Serum blood tests for β-hydroxybuterate can indicate this as a potential cause of metabolic acidosis in the SICU [2].

In all ketoses management, it is important to halt the drive to ketosis. Treatment of diabetic ketoacidosis consists of low-dose insulin infusion to correct not only the hyperglycemia but also the electrolyte abnormalities, such as the total body potassium depletion that accompanies DKA. The goal of therapy is to continue insulin infusion until the anion gap has normalized, not until the hyperglycemia improves, as the insulin is treating both the hyperglycemia and the ketoacidosis. Mangement also requires fluid resuscitation to replace volume lost due to osmotic diuresis in the setting of significant hyperglycemia. Over time, chloride from the isotonic solution and renal reabsorption will replace the ketones, and the anion gap will close. Care must be taken as this correction can cause a hyperchloremic acidosis. Insulin therapy must be coupled with fluid replacement for osmotic dieresis secondary to hyperglycemia and, as always in acid-base disorders, reversal of the inciting event [2]. Alcoholic and starvation ketoses also require correction of concomitant electrolyte derangements, but rather than treating the patients with insulin (as they will not be hyperglycemic), an administration of glucose in isotonic solution is called for. It is paramount to avoid a refeeding syndrome, which can cause potentially deadly consumptive deficit in many electrolytes (most notably phosphate) when dealing with a patient in this state.

Other Anion Gap Acidoses

The other anion gap acidoses, while less common in surgical units, may occasionally be seen. Salicylate toxicity, or aspirin overdose, causes an anion gap acidosis and respiratory alkalosis by CNS-driven hyperventilation. When it is strongly suspected, gastric lavage and charcoal can be given to reverse its effects. Urine alkalinization may be offered through acetazolamide, but this must be done carefully when the patient presents with a mixed disorder, as it can exacerbate alkalosis [2].

Alcohols can cause not only an anion gap but also an osmolar gap, as they increase the osmolarity of serum. This should be suspected in patients with the appropriate history and lab findings. Methanol can also cause nervous system damage through toxic metabolites. Ethylene glycol toxicity can cause widespread organ damage and also causes an osmolar gap. In all of these cases, treatment is supportive, with possible use of alcohol dehydrogenase inhibitors or competitors to reduce toxicity. Hemodialysis must also be considered. Paraldehyde toxicity is exceedingly rare [2].

Utility of Anion Gap

Though the anion gap is one of the tenets of acid-base disorder diagnosis, there are limits to its accuracy and usefulness. As a calculated value, it rests on the reliability of its constituent parts, which may not be appropriate among critically ill patients. Electrolyte disturbances unrelated to the etiology of the acid-base disorder may alter the calculations underlying the AG. Dehydration increases the concentration of all ions, widening the apparent gap, while hypoalbuminemia narrows the gap. In the case of hypoalbuminemia, one may employ a correction of 2.5–3 mEq/L in the anion gap for every 1 g/dL decrease in the serum albumin below the normal range of 3.5–5.5 g/dL [1]. In the setting of a mixed disorder, metabolic effects may unpredictably change the AG. Exogenous acids and bases, such as certain medications and their metabolites and citrate from blood transfusion, may also increase the AG.

Non-Anion Gap Acidosis

Non-gap acidosis is defined by a normal to low anion gap. In general, it is due to a rise in measured anions (specifically Cl^-) with normal or low measured cations (specifically Na^+) or a fall in cations with stable or low anions. Known etiologies include various renal tubular acidoses, loss of cations from the GI tract, iatrogenic causes, and a few uncommon and poorly categorized etiologies [1] (Table 50.4).

While there are three types of renal tubular acidosis (RTA) with many different etiologies, from inherited and acquired disorders to medication toxicities, they all represent a disturbance of Cl^- management in the kidney. RTA types 1 and 4 result from reduced ammonia production. In RTA type 2, which presents as part of Fanconi syndrome, the issue is chloride resorption [10]. As with anion gap acidoses, treatment in all cases of RTA includes treating the underlying cause and preventing hypercalciuria. In RTA types 1 and 2, $NaHCO_3$ or citrate administration is also needed, along with management of hyperkalemia. RTA type 2 may also require thiazide diuresis. RTA type 4 may require use of furosemide and treatment of adrenal insufficiency, but alkalinization is less commonly needed.

Table 50.4 Non-gap acidoses

Non-gap acidosis	Treatment
Renal tubular acidosis	Treat underlying RTA
RTA 1 and 2	$NaHCO_3$, citrate, manage hyperkalemia; consider thiazide diuretics (alkalinize urine)
RTA 4	Furosemide and treat adrenal insufficiency
GI losses	Stop GI losses, replace volume with LR
Iatrogenic	Reverse iatrogenic causes
TPN (acetate and Cl^-)	Chang TPN formulation
Excessive normal saline	Judicious fluids, ringers lactate
Medication	Discontinue if possible

Fluid in the gut lumen contains high levels of sodium and HCO_3^- [2]. When large fluid losses occur, there is a relative loss of sodium compared to chloride. This electrolyte discrepancy is exacerbated by normal saline resuscitation that repletes these at an equal rate [10]. This presents as a non-gap acidosis. Real-world examples of this include diarrhea and proximal fistula. Treatment consists of controlling the losses and replacing volume with lactated Ringer's rather than normal saline, to avoid increasing the relative hyperchloremia.

There are many iatrogenic cause of non-gap acidosis, but the two most common are total parenteral nutrition (TPN) and 0.9% normal saline (NS) infusion [11]. TPN contains Cl^- and if an inappropriate formulation is chosen, such as insufficient bicarbonate precursors, like citrate, this may lead to a hyperchloremic acidosis. In normal saline infusion, there can be a dilutional acidosis for essentially the same reason, a relative rise in Cl^-, a measured anion. The reason this is so rarely seen, despite the ubiquitous use of normal saline, is that large amounts of NS are needed to cause clinically significant acidosis in healthy patients. In the SICU, however, it is more common for large volumes of NS to be used in resuscitation and for patients to have multiple underlying predisposing factors, including compensation-limiting respiratory failure or metabolic derangements limiting buffering capacity [10]. TPN modification and careful and appropriate fluid resuscitation, respectively, are the treatments for these etiologies.

Less common causes of non-gap acidosis include ketosis rebound, chloride ingestion (e.g., through Maalox or Mylanta), cholestyramine, carbonic anhydrase inhibitor use, hypoaldosteronism, and hyperparathyroidism. Management requires reversing the etiology and withdrawing any offending agents.

Compensation

Acid-base homeostasis requires many natural mechanisms, including compensation. In metabolic acidosis, the primary compensatory mechanism is respiratory alkalosis. The respiratory compensation, which occurs immediately, presents as an increase in minute ventilation through rising tidal volume, even to the point of dangerous, unsustainable tachypnea [3]. Central and peripheral chemoreceptors sense the falling pH of the cerebrospinal fluid and serum, respectively, and respond by triggering a rise in minute ventilation [10]. The increase in minute ventilation lowers the PCO_2, ultimately increasing the pH, but cannot completely normalize it. Maximum compensation happens at 12–24 h [10].

In managing metabolic acidosis, it is important to calculate the expected compensation and compare it to the actual compensation to determine presence of a mixed acid-base disorder. The expected acute compensation in metabolic acidosis is derived by Winter's formula - a PCO_2 equal to $(1.5 \times HCO_3^-) + 8$ [1]. A measured PCO_2 higher than calculated indicates a superimposed respiratory acidosis. If it is lower, this suggests a superimposed respiratory alkalosis [3]. These would suggest a mixed disorder rather than merely a simple, primary metabolic acidosis. The theoretical limits of compensation top out at a PCO_2 of 15 mmHg [2].

Treatment

Appropriate treatment of metabolic acidemia requires management of underlying pathology and correction of significant pH abnormality. Left untreated, acidemia and compensation may progress to the point where they both cause direct negative physiologic effects [10]. If acidemia is expected to be of short duration, supporting respiratory compensation may be the best option. This may require intubation, but after eventual resolution of acidemia, compensatory mechanisms will also normalize [1]. If a prolonged course is expected and acidemia is severe (e.g., pH <7.15), physiologic damage from acidemia alone may require treatment [2].

The physiologic effects of severe acidemia can be seen throughout the body. In the cardiovascular system, acidemia can cause venodilation, arterioconstriction, conduction abnormalities, decreased inotropy, and splanchnic vasoconstriction [10]. In the respiratory system, while compensatory mechanisms cause increase in minute ventilation, the direct effect of acidemia is respiratory depression. Documented electrolyte changes include hyperkalemia, hypercalcemia, and hyperuricemia. Metabolic changes include stimulation of many enzymes, protein wasting, bone demineralization, release of inflammatory cytokines, and insulin resistance, as well as resistance to vasoactives. Acidemia is a well-known cause of acute mental status changes [1]. In injured patients, acidemia is a part of the "lethal triad," along with hypothermia and coagulopathy, and contributes to traumatic coagulopathy [19].

Alkalinizing agents may be given in an attempt to normalize pH in severe metabolic acidosis. One such agent is $NaHCO_3$, which is indicated in sever hyperkalemia as well as metabolic acidemia secondary to toxicity from methanol, ethylene glycol, and salicylates [10]. $NaHCO_3$ (sodium is the active portion of the molecule) dosed at 1 mmol/kg may delay the effects of the acidemia. Paradoxically, this treatment may cause respiratory acidosis as compensation to its infusion, though this is unlikely if the infusion is done slowly [3, 8]. Large doses may also cause hypotension or fluid overload [1, 2]. Other formulations, such as Carbicarb® and sodium lactate, have a diminished effect, both on the pH and in inappropriate compensation. Weak acids, such as tromethamine or THAM, can help maintain electrical neutrality and shift the pH. All of these agents can potentially cause a shift in the oxygen dissociation curve and rebound alkalosis [10]. These therapies are not consistently found to improve outcome and are commonly withheld unless pH is felt to be dangerously low (e.g., <7.2) [3].

Rarely, patients with severe or refractory acidemia may require hemodialysis. Dialysis removes many ions from the plasma and can normalize pH relatively efficiently [1]. This may also be accomplished, albeit more slowly, through continuous renal replacement therapy (CRRT) [8, 11]. While these adjuncts are reasonable temporizing measures and are capable of mitigating the direct effects of acidosis, in the end, each will only buy time while the clinician investigates, identifies, and treats the true etiology of metabolic acidosis. In severe acidosis due to acute renal insufficiency, dialysis is often indicated due to a combination of acidosis and hyperkalemia that is not responsive to standard treatment.

Metabolic Alkalosis

Metabolic alkalosis is perhaps the most common acid-base disturbance in hospitalized patients [10]. A serum gain of bicarbonate or loss of acid will cause a relative accumulation of extracellular bicarbonate and a rise in pH [8]. Metabolic alkalosis is most commonly diagnosed on a basic metabolic panel and/or ABG. A primary metabolic alkalosis will appear as a measured bicarbonate level above 26 mEq/L. On blood gas analysis, the pH will exceed 7.45, HCO_3^- will be above 26 mEq/L, base excess will be greater than 3, and compensatory PCO_2 will be over 45 mmHg [10]. However, in the case of a mixed acid-base disorder, the pH may be normal or near-normal, and the diagnostic value will be the elevated bicarbonate. In patients with normal renal function, the kidneys very efficiently clear excess bicarbonate, so metabolic alkalosis requires both an etiology and a means of propagation. Common etiologies include GI fluid loss, loss of acid from the kidney, or gain of bicarbonate, though rare causes, exist.

Renal hypoperfusion and potassium depletion perpetuate the alkalosis.

Etiology

Upper and lower GI losses may both cause metabolic alkalosis. Emesis and gastric drainage contain low pH gastric fluids. Acid and electrolytes are lost, while the bicarbonate created during production of gastric acid returns to circulation. This results in hypokalemic, hypochloremic metabolic alkalosis, a cluster of abnormalities common in abdominal surgical patients. Villous adenoma generally causes metabolic acidosis through loss of bicarbonate and potassium-rich colonic fluid, but some adenomas secrete chloride instead of bicarbonate, resulting in metabolic alkalosis [20]. Laxative abuse may also cause metabolic alkalosis by this mechanism. These GI losses cause chloride-responsive metabolic alkalosis which can be treated with normal saline but may also be treated with potassium chloride (KCl) or, in severe alkalosis, hydrochloric acid [1]. As these mechanisms tend to deplete potassium as well, potassium repletion should accompany the resuscitation.

Many etiologies originate from renal pathology or insufficiency. In general, these begin as high concentration sodium delivery to the distal nephron, which increases potassium and hydrogen losses, as well as bicarbonate reabsorption. Volume contraction from renal losses also stimulates aldosterone secretion, causing a net increase of sodium and bicarbonate retention [20]. Chloride loss, in the absence of volume or potassium loss, also causes metabolic alkalosis, but it is not clear that these mechanisms are isolated in the clinical setting. Diuretics, such as chlorothiazide and furosemide, and mineralocorticoids cause metabolic alkalosis by the same mechanisms. Mineralocorticoid effects can be treated with aldosterone antagonists, such as spironolactone.

Abrupt reversal of respiratory acidosis through mechanical ventilation can also cause metabolic alkalosis [11]. Renal compensation is slower than respiratory compensation, so even after the primary disorder is stopped, persistent renal compensation continues to cause alkalosis. Bartter syndrome, Liddle syndrome, and Gitelman syndrome are congenital disorders which generate metabolic alkaloses through renal mechanisms [2].

Metabolic alkalosis can also result from an influx of bicarbonate. $NaHCO_3$ infusion is the most common cause, but other causes include citrate excess from blood transfusions or bone lytic conditions. Bicarbonate infusion is common in the SICU and can cause or potentiate alkalosis. In some patients, overcorrection of an acidosis with bicarbonate may be the inciting event leading to metabolic alkalosis. Citrate, which is found in packed red blood cells, is metabolized in the body to bicarbonate, so high volume blood resuscitation infuses a substrate of natural bicarbonate production, which leads to a metabolic alkalosis [20].

Under normal conditions, renal excretion of bicarbonate would prevent or rapidly correct metabolic alkalosis, but this protective mechanism can be impaired in a number of clinical settings. A prerenal state (insufficient renal perfusion) reduces GFR, which increases renal bicarbonate reabsorption and release of aldosterone [8]. Increased aldosterone increases reabsorption of renal sodium and water. Aldosterone also stimulates potassium and hydrogen secretion with concomitant bicarbonate reabsorption [8]. Cl^- and K^+ deficiency can lead to reduced GFR and increased HCO_3^- resorption, stimulating aldosterone secretion as well. These deficiencies support maintenance of metabolic alkalosis once it has been established [2].

Compensation

In spontaneously breathing subjects, respiratory compensation to metabolic alkalosis is almost immediate. Ventilation is suppressed, causing CO_2 retention and a fall in pH [1]. Respiratory compensation is typically not complete (pH will not completely normalize), but the impact of compensatory ventilation changes can be predicted. Respiratory compensation for metabolic alkalosis typically generates a PCO_2 equal to $0.9 \times (HCO_3^-) + 9$. If the measured PCO_2 is higher than that, there may be a respiratory acidosis as well. If the measured PCO_2 is lower than predicted PCO_2, there may be a superimposed respiratory alkalosis [10].

Treatment

Treatment is focused on reversal of the etiology of metabolic alkalosis, but severe alkalemia must also be treated to avoid its deleterious effects, many of which are the inverse of the effects of severe acidosis. These include increased hemoglobin-oxygen affinity and vasoconstriction (especially cerebral), which decrease oxygen delivery to tissues. Alkalosis causes calcium wasting, which can produce hypocalcemia symptoms including paresthesias, weakness, and tetany [8]. Other resulting electrolyte changes, such as hypokalemia and hypomagnesemia, can cause decreased cardiac contractility and arrhythmias [2, 8, 10].

The tenets of treating metabolic alkalosis include volume expansion and correction of hypochloremia and hypokalemia, which often accompany alkalosis. Volume is especially important because, even if volume loss is not the cause of alkalosis, it is often part of the secondary mechanism propagating the alkalosis. If the patient cannot tolerate the volume expansion, chloride loading with KCL may be considered as it has similar effects at lower volumes. Acetazolamide, a carbonic anhydrase inhibitor, causes bicarbonate diuresis, but it also leads to potassium losses and hypercapnia and must be managed carefully [8]. In upper GI losses, if these losses cannot be stopped, the acid production must be mitigated with an H2 blocker or proton pump inhibitor.

When the serum pH rises above 7.55, or if encephalopathy or arrhythmia occurs, hydrochloric acid infusion can be considered, though this must be administered carefully through a central venous line as it is highly caustic and blood chemistry must be regularly monitored [8].

Respiratory Acidosis

In healthy subjects, PCO_2 remains close to 40 mmHg via tight control of pulmonary ventilation [1]. Production of CO_2 is matched to minute ventilation so that the normal PCO_2 is maintained. In respiratory acidosis, CO_2 elimination is insufficient to keep up with production and therefore accumulates and is metabolized into H^+.

Diagnosis

In the absence of a mixed disorder with concomitant metabolic acidosis, pure respiratory acidosis is unlikely to be severe enough to present initially with symptoms of acidosis, so identification requires recognition of its presentation on routine laboratory results. The hallmark diagnostic feature of respiratory acidosis is the pCO2, as the other values of the blood gas can be normal or near-normal due to compensatory mechanisms or the presence of a mixed acid-base disorder. Chronic respiratory acidosis may be identified by a compesatory rise in serum bicabonate above 26 mEq/L. Blood gas analysis will reveal pH below 7.35, pCO_2 greater than 45, and a compensatory HCO_3^- above 24 [1]. In acute respiratory acidosis, clinically apparent hypoventilation and mental status changes may be present without labarotory evidence of compensation. Unlike the metabolic disorders, primary respiratory acidosis will not generate a base deficit [11].

Etiology

Hypoventilation is the common pathway for the myriad causes of respiratory acidosis [1]. Etiologies can be categorized as central nervous system suppression, neuromuscular impairment, or primary pulmonary/tracheobronchial disorders. Central nervous system depression can be pathologic or iatrogenic. Pathologic causes include cerebrovascular accidents, tumors, brain or brainstem vasculitis or infarction, encephalopathy, CNS infection, seizure activity, dementia, metabolic derangements, uremia, and other less common etiologies. When these are suspected, appropriate imaging, diagnostics, and specialty consultation must be initiated.

Traumatic injuries cause CNS depression through direct injury, decreased seizure threshold, increased intracranial pressure, or intracranial bleed. Toxicity, such as envenomation, is another consideration [10]. Iatrogenic CNS depression occurs through medications and surgical mishaps. The most common iatrogenic cause of hypoventilation in the SICU is medication overdose, including narcotics, benzodiazepines, and other anxiolytics and sleep aides. When mismanaged medication is identified, reversible causes must be reversed (naloxone for narcotics, flumazenil for benzodiazepines, etc.). Otherwise, supportive care must be offered until the patient recovers [1].

Neuromuscular impairment may result from neuromuscular diseases, such as myasthenia gravis, or electrolyte disturbances [1]. Paralytics, commonly given as a part of general anesthesia, are now frequently given in the SICU. These predictably cause a neuromuscular impairment that can lead to hypoventilation and respiratory acidosis, unless appropriate respiratory support is provided. In the postoperative patient in the SICU, it is important to consider direct nerve injury, including phrenic nerve injury, in patients presenting with respiratory acidosis [3]. Respiratory muscle fatigue may also lead to respiratory acidosis when the patient is no longer able to maintain adequate minute ventilation [1, 10].

Primary respiratory disorders can result in respiratory acidosis as well as hypoxia. This is seen in obesity hypoventilation syndrome, vocal cord paresis, tracheal stenosis, flail chest, acute lung injury/ARDS, pneumonia, pulmonary edema, and hemorrhage. This may also occur with compliance limiting pathology, such as flail segment, postoperative hypoventilation, pulmonary fibrosis, burns, pneumothorax, and compartment syndrome [1, 10]. Respiratory acidosis is seen as an acceptable consequence of permissive hypercapnia. In certain clinical settings, such as lung protective strategies employed in treating ARDS, low tidal volume is indicated, and a resultant respiratory acidosis is expected. While this is appropriate management for ARDS, it is not without risk. In these cases, the acidosis must be monitored closely, and a safe, minimum pH should not be exceeded. Typically, pH is maintained above 7.25, and a bicarbonate infusion should be initiated to keep the pH > 7.2 per the ARDSNet protocol [1].

Compensation

Metabolic compensation, unlike respiratory compensation, is not immediate but is usually effective if the patient has relatively normal renal function [10, 11]. The kidney can normalize pH for a very broad range of PCO_2, from 25 to 80 mmHg, though this happens over many days. In respiratory acidosis, the compensation will present as a metabolic alkalosis, with a base excess (over 3 mEq/L). The primary mechanism is bicarbonate reabsorption in the kidney, with a 1–3 mEq/L increase in serum bicarbonate for every 10 mmHg rise in PCO_2 [11]. Occasionally, complex mixed acid-base derangements may be found, combining multiple abnormalities as well as compensatory changes.

Treatment

When the underlying etiology is not easily or quickly reversed or when hypoxia becomes dangerous, ventilation must be directly supported. Noninvasive measures are possible when a patient does not have altered mental status. Intubation and mechanical ventilation must always be considered if the patient's condition cannot be quickly reversed and noninvasive ventilation is undesirable. In patients with chronic hypercapnia, the goal PCO_2 is the patient's baseline, rather than normal PCO_2, to avoid dangerous compensatory alkalemia. Infusion of $NaHCO_3$ may be considered, though there is a risk of respiratory failure due to increased CO_2 [1]. One final approach is to lower CO_2 production by decreasing metabolic demand through hypothermia or paralysis, for example, despite the primary respiratory nature of this disorder [1].

Respiratory Alkalosis

Respiratory alkalosis is not unusual in the SICU. It may stem from many causes but always results from the same mechanism, hyperventilation accompanied by hypocarbia [1]. Though common, mild respiratory alkalosis can be subtle and may go unidentified. Quantifying the patient's minute ventilation can be helpful in both establishing the diagnosis and in assessing the efficacy of treatment, with a decrease in minute ventilation indicating effective therapy.

Diagnosis

Obvious hyperventilation is often the first clinical finding suggestive of the diagnosis. Definitive diagnosis, however, still requires correlation with laboratory findings. Outside of an acute setting, a routine metabolic panel will typically show a measured bicarbonate below 22 mEq/L (compensatory metabolic acidosis). On blood gas analysis, pH will be above 7.45, with a PCO_2 below 35 and a HCO_3^- below 22. Base excess is not seen in respiratory alkalosis [11]. The most important diagnostic lab value for respiratory alkalosis is a low PCO_2, as the other laboratory values can be altered due to metabolic compensation or the presence of a mixed acid-base disorder.

Etiology

In surgical patients, hyperventilation is most commonly a consequence of suffering, whether due to pain, anxiety, agitation, or opiate withdrawal [10]. If the patient has effectively hyperventilated PCO_2 to subnormal levels, this is a strong indicator of either distress or of a primary CNS etiology. In some cases, hyperventilation may be due to primary respiratory compromise, hypermetabolism, or compensation for metabolic acidosis, so labs may not indicate a respiratory alkalosis. Still, the intensivist should be concerned that any hyperventilating patient may eventually fatigue and become hypercarbic [1, 10].

Central hyperventilation may be driven by sepsis, pregnancy, hepatic failure, or salicylate poisoning [1]. Salicylate toxicity primarily causes metabolic acidosis but also triggers hyperventilation, so treatment must address both mechanisms [11]. Inappropriate mechanical ventilation is an underappreciated cause of PCO_2 abnormality [3].

Compensation

Metabolic compensation for respiratory alkalosis is slower than respiratory compensation for metabolic acid-base disorders but faster than compensation for respiratory acidosis. Renal excretion of bicarbonate is very efficient, with an expected HCO_3^- fall of 1–4 mEq/L for each 10 mm Hg rise in a PCO_2 [2, 11]. This compensation takes up to 24 h to reach its full effect [3].

References

1. Kellum JA. Acid-base disorders. In: Vincent J-L, Abraham E, Kochanek P, Moore FA, Fink MP, editors. Textbook of critical care. 6th ed. Philadelphia: Elsevier Health Sciences; 2011. p. 43–52.
2. Dubose TD, Daeihagh P. Metabolic acidosis and alkalosis. In: Vincent J-L, Abraham E, Kochanek P, Moore FA, Fink MP, editors. Textbook of critical care. 6th ed. Philadelphia: Elsevier Health Sciences; 2011. p. 823–40.
3. Goldfarb S, Reilly JB. Metabolic acidoses and alkaloses. 2nd ed. Philadelphia: Elsevier Health Sciences; 2013.
4. FitzSullivan E, Salim A, Demetriades D, Asensio J, Martin MJ. Serum bicarbonate may replace the arterial base deficit in the trauma intensive care unit. Am J Surg. 2005;190(6):941–6.
5. Martin MJ, FitzSullivan E, Salim A, Berne TV, Towfigh S. Use of serum bicarbonate measurement in place of arterial base deficit in the surgical intensive care unit. Arch Surg. 2005;140(8):745–51.
6. Seifter JL. Acid-base disorders. In: Goldman L, Schafer AI, editors. Cecil textbook of medicine. 22nd ed. Philadelphia: Saunders; 2004. p. 688–99.
7. Juran P, Cheng S. Metabolic acid-base disorders. In: Kollef MH, Bedient TJ, Isakow W, editors. The Washington manual of critical care. Philadelphia: Lippincott Williams & Wilkins; 2008. p. 209–21.
8. Kline JA, Weisberg LS. Acid-base, electrolyte, and metabolic abnormalities. In: Parrillo JE, Dellinger RP, editors. Critical care medicine: principles of diagnosis and management in the adult. 4th ed. Philadelphia: Elsevier Health Sciences; 2013. p. 993–1028.
9. Ungerer J, Ungerer M, Vermaak W. Discordance between measured and calculated total carbon dioxide. Clin Chem. 1990;36(12):2093–6.
10. Morgan T. Acid-base balance and disorders. In: Bersten AD, Soni N, editors. Oh's intensive care manual. 7th ed. Philadelphia: Elsevier Health Sciences; 2013. p. 937–48.
11. Neligan PJ. How should acid-base disorders be diagnosed and managed? In: Deutschman CS, Neligan PJ, editors. Evidence-based

practice of critical care. 2nd ed. Philadelphia: Elsevier Health Sciences; 2015. p. 409–18.
12. Schmidt GA. Acid-base disorders. In: Ivy ME, Lipsett PA, editors. Adult multiprofessional critical care review. Des Plaines, Society of Critical Care Medicine; 2005. p. 279–86.
13. Martin MJ, FitzSullivan E, Salim A, Brown CVR, Demetriades D, Long W. Discordance between lactate and base deficit in the surgical intensive care unit: which one do you trust? Am J Surg. 2006;191(5):625–30.
14. Cooper JD, Higgins AM, Nichol AD. Lactic acidosis. In: Bersten AD, Soni N, editors. Oh's intensive care manual. Philadelphia: Elsevier Health Sciences; 2013. p. 158–64.
15. Gale SC, Kocik JF, Creath R, Crystal JS, Dombrovskiy VY. A comparison of initial lactate and initial base deficit as predictors of mortality after severe blunt trauma. J Surg Res. 2016;205(2):446–55.
16. O'Keefe KP, Sanson TG. Mesenteric ischemia. In: Adams JG, editor. Emergency medicine: clinical essentials. 2nd ed. Philadelphia: Elsevier Health Sciences; 2012. p. 292–8.
17. Warnock DG. Uremic acidosis. Kidney Int. 1988;34(2):278–87.
18. Kraut JA, Madias NE. Metabolic acidosis of CKD: an update. Am J Kidney Dis. 2016;67(2):307–17.
19. Cosgriff N, Moore EE, Sauaia A, Kenny-Moynihan M, Burch JM, Galloway B. Predicting life-threatening coagulopathy in the massively transfused trauma patient: hypothermia and acidoses revisited. J Trauma Acute Care Surg. 1997;42(5):857–62.
20. Galla JH. Metabolic alkalosis. J Am Soc Nephrol JASN. 2000;11(2):369–75.

Cirrhosis and End-Stage Liver Disease

51

James M. Tatum and Eric J. Ley

How Bad Is this Patient's Liver Disease and What Is the Probability of Survival?

Child-Turcotte-Pugh Score

The severity of a patient's liver disease can be quantified with one of two common grading systems. The Child-Turcotte-Pugh (CTP) score is computed by rating the severity of five contributing factors (total bilirubin, serum albumin, prothrombin time, ascites, and encephalopathy) on a scale of 1–3 with the resulting composite score ranging from 5 to 15. Scores are then grouped into one of three grades from A to C. These scores roughly correlate with the chances of mortality after major abdominal surgery with A (5–6) imparting no additional risk, B (7–9) an 81%, and C (10–15) 45% chances of survival, respectively [1]. The CTP score provides an easy way to communicate and recognize the severity of liver disease; it does however have limitations. Two of the criteria contributing to the composite score are subjective (severity of ascites and encephalopathy), and encephalopathy requires that a patient is awake for assessment. The CTP score also fails to consider renal failure or thrombocytopenia caused by hypersplenism (Table 51.1).

Model for End-Stage Liver Disease (MELD) Score

The model for end-stage liver disease (MELD) score was primarily developed to rate severity of end-stage liver disease (ESLD) among candidates for liver transplantation by predicting 90-day mortality but is now widely utilized in many ICU settings. The score is derived from a model incorporating international normalized ratio (INR), serum creatinine (Cr), total bilirubin, and now also serum sodium (Na). Of note, the two most heavily weighted variables in the MELD scoring system are the INR and the creatinine, which reflects the major morbidity associated with worsening coagulopathy or declining renal function in patients with liver disease. The model is validated in patients older than 12 years of age with liver disease longer than 6 months. There are multiple exceptions used to modify the score as it is used in attempts to equitably and pragmatically allocate livers for transplantation. Scores range from 6 to 40 which provides an indication of relative illness severity while avoiding the subjective variables in the CTP. A score of 14 carries as much risk of death after surgery as does CTP class C. The MELD score has prognostic value after specific interventions including transjugular intrahepatic portosystemic shunt (TIPS), after non-transplant major abdominal surgery, in the setting of an acute variceal bleed, and even after trauma [2–5]. A study performed in our own high-volume liver transplant center showed that including variables for organ support modalities including continue renal replacement therapy (CRRT) vasopressors or mechanical ventilation significantly increases the reliability and predictive ability of the MELD model while caring for critically ill patients with cirrhosis [6] (Table 51.2).

J. M. Tatum (✉) · E. J. Ley
Department of Surgery, Cedars-Sinai Medical Center, Los Angeles, CA, USA
e-mail: james.tatum@med.usc.edu

Neurological Challenges: Intoxication, Delirium, Cerebral Edema, and Sedation

Acute Cerebral Edema and Hepatic Encephalopathy

Acute fulminant hepatic failure can cause cerebral edema requiring medical interventions to lower intracranial pressure and even operative pressure monitor placement or decompression by a neurosurgeon. Hepatic encephalopathy is the neurological disorder more frequently encountered by the general surgeon. Hepatic encephalopathy (HE) is an incompletely understood clinical diagnosis related to impaired metabolism of amino acids and their impact on

A. Salim et al. (eds.), *Surgical Critical Care Therapy*, https://doi.org/10.1007/978-3-319-71712-8_51

Table 51.1 Child-Turcotte-Pugh scoring system

Criteria	Points assigned		
	1	2	3
Encephalopathy	Not present	Grade 1 or 2	Grade 3 or 4
Ascites	Not present	Mild/ moderate	Severe
Bilirubin (mg/dL)	<2	2–3	>3
Albumin (g/dL)	>3.5	2.8–3.5	<2.8
Prothrombin time *Seconds* *International normalized ratio*	<4 <1.7	4–6 1.7–2.3	>6 >2.3
Child-Turcotte-Pugh class			
A (5–6 points)			
B (7–9 points)			
C (10–15 points)			

Source: Pugh et al. [66]

Table 51.2 Mortality rates over 3 months following MELD/ MELD-NA

MELD[a]	*≤9*	*10–19*	*20–29*	*30–39*	*≥40*
	4%	27%	76%	83%	100%
MELD-NA	1.9%	6%	19.6%	52.6%	71.3%

Source: Kamath et al. [67]
Biggins et al. [68]
United Network for Organ Sharing (UNOS) [69]
[a]Hospitalized patients

gamma-aminobutyric acid (GABA) pathways. Encephalopathy can be graded on a scale of I–IV based on clinical findings ranging from grade I, characterized as minor sleep disorder and confusion, to grade IV, which is a comatose state. The diagnosis is supported by, although not made by, an elevated serum ammonia level. We observe little value in trending ammonia levels but do check it on admission and consider a level greater than 60 mcg/dL consistent with HE.

Any condition disturbing a patient's health can exacerbate HE. The best treatment is to address the underlying cause of the patient's illness with attention to electrolyte and fluid balance as a patient with liver disease frequently has poor nutrition—particularly those with liver disease caused by active alcoholism. In-hospital management mirrors that of treating any other delirium. Sleep hygiene, frequent reorientation, human interaction, and respect for sleep cycles especially in intensive care units (ICU) are helpful. Attention to treating infection, hypoxia, hypoglycemia renal failure, gastrointestinal bleeding, and alkalosis, all of which exacerbate HE, is necessary.

Medical treatments for HE include haloperidol for agitation and the avoidance of benzodiazepines. Lactulose either by mouth or per rectum decreases ammonia absorption from the GI tract. The antibiotic rifaximin or neomycin can be used in addition to lactulose to prevent the production of ammonia by gut bacteria. Dietary protein restriction is no longer advocated, instead there is increased emphasis on the importance of nutrition, including protein nutrition, in chronic liver disease.

Sedation and Pain Control

We strive to minimize the use of sedatives in patients with severe liver disease. Neither benzodiazepines nor dexmedetomidine should be used to achieve sedation for bedside procedures nor should they be used to maintain sedation while a patient is intubated. We prefer to provide pain control with PRN opiates whenever possible. Fentanyl is preferred as its metabolism is not significantly altered in patients with liver disease as opposed to that of morphine. Tramadol is our preferred oral pain medication. We recommend propofol to maintain sedation in intubated patients as it is effective but also short acting and not dependent on hepatic metabolism or clearance. When paralysis is required, atracurium or cisatracurium is preferred to vecuronium or rocuronium [7]. If vecuronium or rocuronium has been utilized and reversal of neuromuscular blockade is desired, then the new reversal agent sugammadex can be safely utilized in this patient population as it has no metabolites and is primarily excreted in the urine.

Disorders of the Heart and Blood Pressure Regulation

Shock Liver and Biliary Diseases

Benign elevation in liver function tests (LFT) occurs in the setting of various biliary diseases, so it is important to define the underlying etiology early in the hospital course to optimize management. Severe elevation of LFT after a systemic insult such as hemorrhage or cardiac arrest is directly related to ischemic injury [8]. These injuries generally resolve with supportive care if there is successful treatment of the underlying systemic pathology and timely reperfusion. Differentiating the relationship between liver and cardiac failure in patients with more chronic conditions can be more complex but is aided by obtaining a detailed history from the patient or family member when available and by review of the medical record.

Congestive Liver Failure and Cardiohepatic Syndrome

The heart and liver have an intertwined relationship. For example, right heart disease can lead to acute ischemic hepatitis (shock liver) or chronic congestive cirrhosis. Cirrhosis from any cause can lead to a cardiohepatic syndrome (a type of stress cardiomyopathy), and any shock can induce both stress cardiomyopathy and shock liver simultaneously [9, 10]. The treatment of congestive liver failure secondary to primary cardiac disease requires addressing the underlying cardiac disease, which can entail medical or surgical therapy including valve replacement, coronary artery bypass, the institution of mechanic circulatory support, and even heart transplantation alone or in conjunction with simultaneous liver transplantation and/or kidney transplantation [11].

Blood Pressure Regulation

Assessment of hemodynamic status and identification of shock states (such as sepsis) can be difficult in the patient with pre-existing chronic liver failure. These patients will often have a baseline hemodynamic profile characterized by relative hypotension and low systemic vascular resistance, which can be difficult to distinguish from early shock states. Maintaining adequate systemic perfusion can also be a significant challenge in severe liver disease. The systemic effects of cirrhosis include indiscriminate dilation of the splanchnic vascular beds which, in conjunction with low serum albumin levels, can lead to a profound loss of fluid into third spaces and intravascular hypovolemia with systemic hypotension [12]. This dilation can be improved with high doses of oral midodrine in patients who can swallow or have a nasogastric tube. Midodrine is not enough in some severe cases where our preferred treatment includes the judicious use of albumin for resuscitation, often guided by a Swan-Ganz catheter. Norepinephrine is our first-line vasopressor, supplemented by vasopressin receptor antagonists (vaptans) despite their debated efficacy in this setting [13].

Pulmonary and Thoracic Disorders

Hepatic Hydrothorax

The most common thoracic manifestation of cirrhosis is the hepatic hydrothorax. Treatment may include thoracentesis for cases of respiratory difficulty or prior to an urgent operative procedure. A chronic hepatic hydrothorax is a difficult problem to manage. These persistent transudative effusions are the thoracic equivalent of transudative abdominal ascites, if not actually in continuity with the abdomen through pores in the diaphragm. Like abdominal ascites, a chronic hepatic hydrothorax may resolve only when portal pressure is decreased and hypoalbuminemia improves. Thoracostomy tubes are ill-advised and invariably lead to chronic leakage from the incision, problems with fluid balance, and protein loss and expose an inherently immunosuppressed patient to the risk of intrapleural infections. In a patient with chronic effusions, the placement of indwelling tunneled pleural catheters has both been described and cautioned against in the literature, as have methods of pleurodesis and diaphragm pore closure [14–16]. Measures beyond simple thoracentesis should not be considered in most critically ill cirrhotic patients.

Pulmonary Infections

Pulmonary infections need to be considered as cirrhosis is an immunocompromising condition that places patients at high risk for both community-acquired and nosocomial pneumonias and other infections [17, 18]. Abdominal distension, autonomic dysfunction of gastrointestinal motility, altered mental status, and the frequent use of proton pump inhibitors put these patients at increased risk of micro- or macroaspiration. Invasive fungal infections while still rare can be extremely resistant to treatment, even when caught early [17, 19].

Hepatopulmonary Syndrome

Hepatopulmonary syndrome is defined by shortness of breath and hypoxemia caused by vasodilation in the lungs of patients with liver disease [20]. Severe liver dysfunction leads to inefficient distribution of blood through the lung and subsequent pulmonary vascular dilation causing shunting which leads to treatment resistant hypoxemia. When unexplained hypoxia is noted, an echocardiogram with bubble study should be ordered for possible shunting. A transjugular intrahepatic portosystemic shunt (TIPS) may be considered but may either improve or worsen the condition. The syndrome typically resolves within 1 year of successful liver transplantation, and this is currently the only effective therapy for the syndrome [21].

Airway and Ventilator Management

The threshold for intubating patients with ESLD should be very low. We advocate aggressive goal setting for these patients. One year survival in patients with ESLD who require mechanical ventilation in an intensive care unit and did not receive a liver transplant is as low as 9% [22–24]. Respiratory support when indicated must be by intubation as opposed to noninvasive ventilation. Hepatic encephalopathy combined with impaired gastrointestinal motility and increased intra-abdominal makes aspiration a constant danger. Noninvasive continuous positive airway pressure ventilation and bilevel positive airway pressure ventilation are contraindicated in this patient population and if attempted frequently result in aspiration and death. We, and others, have had early success with high-flow nasal cannula after extubation but maintain that it is contraindicated if used in attempt to delay a probable intubation [25].

Acute Respiratory Distress Syndrome

Among the most challenging of surgical ICU cases is the cirrhotic patient with acute respiratory distress syndrome (ARDS). The marginal function of multiple organ systems at baseline in these patients makes them particularly susceptible to fulminant respiratory failure [26]. It is important to set realistic goals. If there is little possibility of meaningful recovery from an acute hepatic injury, or in the case of chronic liver disease if the possibility of liver transplantation is minimal, then providing guidance on de-escalation of care is appropriate. When there is a chance of a positive outcome, we recommend maximally aggressive care as early as possible. This includes renal replacement therapy (RRT) with continuous renal replacement therapy (CRRT), pharmacological paralysis, broad-spectrum antibiotics, inhaled nitric oxide, and/or support with vasopressors. Therapies can be weaned as tolerated after the ARDS improves. We also use oscillatory ventilation, although there is no evidence for or against its use in this situation. Extracorporeal membrane oxygenation is not possible in these patients due to their thrombocytopenia and unacceptably high risk of intracranial hemorrhage.

Nutrition, Feeding, Ascites, and Intra-Abdominal Surgery

Nutrition

Attentive management of nutrition due to related challenges from ascites, gastric motility, biliary disease, and gastrointestinal bleeding is required in the care of patients with cirrhosis and ESLD. Protein and total caloric malnutrition is present in nearly all cirrhotic patients, which impacts wound healing, increases risk of infection, and contributes to the formation of ascites and extracellular fluid sequestration. In the past, protein restriction was advocated as it theoretically improved HE, although the recent studies suggest otherwise [13]. We recommend consultation with a dietician early in the ICU course and providing 1–1.5 g of protein per kg of dry body weight [27]. Vitamin K injections should be given early to any patient with poor nutrition or an obstructive biliary process especially if the initial INR is elevated. We also provide thiamine and folate to patients with active alcoholism.

Feeding and Access

We do not encourage oral nutrition in critically ill cirrhotic or ESLD patients due to the high risk of aspiration from altered mental status and increased intra-abdominal pressures which impair gastric accommodation to meals and lead to gastroparesis secondary to the autonomic dysfunction of cirrhosis [28, 29]. We avoid nasogastric tube feeds unless the patient is intubated and sparingly use post-pyloric feeding tubes in the non-intubated patient. Percutaneous gastrostomy tubes should not be placed in a patient with ascites or liver failure and should not be used unless placed well prior to the onset of cirrhosis. We advocate for early total parenteral nutrition (TPN) in hopes of preventing infection and wound breakdown and decreasing ascites despite little evidence to support or oppose its use in this setting [30]. Although many experts had previously recommended specialized nutritional formulas utilizing branched-chain amino acids for patients with chronic hepatic insufficiency, and particularly in the setting of encephalopathy, there is no evidence that this provides any benefit over the use of standard enteral formulas and medical management of the encephalopathy.

Ascites

Cirrhosis causes abdominal ascites due to increased hydrostatic pressure in the portal system combined with decreased intravascular oncotic pressure from hypoalbuminemia and hyponatremia. Ascitic fluid is protein rich and easily supports bacterial growth resulting in spontaneous or secondary peritonitis. Liver transplantation, TIPS placement, or rarely operative portal-systemic shunt creation reduce portal pressure. Improved nutrition and diuresis increase intravascular oncotic pressure and slow the leakage of fluid in the peritoneal space. Infections need to be prevented by avoiding bacterial translocation with appropriate nutrition [31, 32]. Contamination of ascites from any procedure that violates the lumen of bowel should be avoided. Contamination or infection when suspected needs to be treated with antibiotics and source control. Paracentesis as a diagnostic measure should be performed as early as possible, as delays lead to increased mortality [33].

If ascites cannot be treated medically, it can be removed by paracentesis. If more than 6 l of fluid is removed at one time, hemodynamic instability can result, and the patient should be supported with intravenous albumin at a dose of 6–8 mg per liter of ascites removed [34]. Complete drainage of large-volume (>5 l) ascites in critically ill patients without treatment of the underlying cause results in rapid reaccumulation with potential exacerbation of hepatorenal syndrome and hemodynamics [35]. Large-volume drainage should be avoided unless attempting to completely drain ascites of new onset or as a mechanism of source control after contamination.

Bleeding into the peritoneal cavity is rare as a complication of paracentesis and can be avoided by performing ultrasound-directed needle placement during thoracentesis, even in patients with profound thrombocytopenia and INR >8 [13]. It is our opinion that indwelling drain placement in a cirrhotic patient is ill-advised in general and particularly so in critically ill patients. Studies that have attempted to leave an indwelling peritoneal catheter have resulted in higher rates of bacterial peritonitis and mortality [36].

The Abdominal Wall

Abdominal wall hernias are present in 20–40% of patients with cirrhotic liver disease, most of which are umbilical [37, 38]. These can be electively repaired only in patients who have medically controlled ascites, as attempts at repair with uncontrolled ascites leak, do not heal, and rapidly recur. Patients with emergent indications (strangulation or bowel obstruction) sometimes force the surgeon's hand. Preoperative optimization with TIPS is ideal, but frequently not possible [39]. Postoperative management often occurs in the ICU given the tendency to decompensate. We recommend periodic paracentesis to minimize abdominal distension and prevent leakage around the time of repair. TIPS is advisable when the patient is stable and a candidate. We do not recommend indwelling drains in these or any other cirrhotic patients.

Elective Surgery

Elective operations on patients with cirrhosis are risky especially in patients with MELD >14 or a Child C classification. Goals of care need to be discussed with the patient and family before attempting an operation, even an emergency operation in these patients. Patients who develop cholecystitis while awaiting immediate liver transplantation of any Child's classification are best treated with a percutaneous cholecystostomy aspiration or tube placement [40]. Child A and B patients may undergo laparoscopic cholecystectomy with careful attention to hemostasis in the operating room and correcting coagulopathies during and after surgery [41]. Placement of cholecystostomy tube in the OR is preferable to opening the abdomen when a difficult gallbladder is encountered.

There are anecdotal reports of abdominal aortic aneurysm repair [42] and case series on oncologic colon resections in Child A–B patients [43]. There are also multiple studies in the cardiac literature of patients with cirrhosis undergoing complex CABG, single, or even multivalve replacement at the time of liver or simultaneous liver-kidney transplantation [11]. Major operations that are not emergent should be delayed until during or after liver transplantation.

Gastrointestinal Bleeding

Initial Stabilization and Assessment

Gastrointestinal bleeding (GIB) occurs in 20–50% of patients with cirrhosis and is a common indication for admission to an ICU. Variceal bleeds are responsible for 70% of acute bleeds in these patients [44]. When first encountered the acute GIB is treated in much the same manner as a trauma patient. The airway must be assessed and secured with intubation if necessary, circulation and hemodynamics must be stabilized, type and cross or screen and coagulation labs must be promptly obtained. Multiple large-bore intravenous lines need to be placed. A focused clinical exam to assess for jaundice or paleness, facial wasting, abdominal distention, dilated subcutaneous veins, surgical scars, and a rectal exam for black stool performed. We do not place nasogastric tubes in patients with active or suspected variceal bleeding except with endoscopic guidance. During or after stabilization, the most important action is timely consultation with supportive specialists including interventional gastroenterologists or radiologists. Patients should be transfused to a goal hemoglobin of 8 g/dL. Higher hemoglobin targets result in increased portal pressure and mortality [45, 46].

Medical Prevention and Management of Gastrointestinal Bleeding

Proton pump inhibitors should be used only when indicated for gastric ulcers or reflux disease as they do not prevent variceal bleeding and indiscriminate use is associated with higher rates of spontaneous bacterial peritonitis in patients with cirrhosis [47]. We do start patients with new GI bleeds on high-dose PPI drip until bleeding gastric or duodenal ulcer is ruled out with endoscopy. Nonselective beta-blockers (propranolol or nadolol) are indicated for primary and secondary prophylaxis against variceal bleeding although these should not be started at the time of an acute GI bleed due to concerns for hypotension. Somatostatin or an equivalent analog (octreotide, vapreotide, or terlipressin) should be started as soon as an acute variceal bleed is suspected and continued for at least 3–5 days [45]. Prophylactic antibiotics should be started when any type of GI bleed is diagnosed in these patients. Therapy should be with oral norfloxacin, intravenous ciprofloxacin, or intravenous ceftriaxone in patients with more severe liver disease. These antibiotics should be stopped if there is no other indication for use before 7 days [45].

Interventions for Acute Gastrointestinal Bleeding

Physical examination, history, and clinical judgment are necessary when faced with a cirrhotic patient with a GI bleed. If available nasogastric tube effluent or lavage should be used to determine if the most likely location of an acute GI bleed is upper or lower, endoscopy should follow. If bleeding is not found at the initial site of endoscopy, then endoscopy of the alternative site should be performed. Standard of care is for endoscopy to be performed within 12 h of diagnosis with coagulation, sclerotherapy, banding, or clipping as indicated [45]. Patients with massive bleed should have endoscopy performed as soon as possible; within an hour of consultation is a reasonable time frame in a tertiary or academic care center. Severe bleeds, ulcers with concerning features, or clinical suspicion frequently require repeat endoscopy within 24–72 h. We intubate nearly all patients who require endoscopy for acute GI bleeding.

If bleeding cannot be controlled by endoscopy, we consult additional services including interventional radiology and general or colorectal surgery as indicated for refractory gastric or hemorrhoid/colonic bleeds, respectively. TIPS is indicated for bleeds that are recurrent or refractory to endoscopic and pharmacological therapy [45]. Colonic or gastric resection is ill-advised before a TIPS procedure. We consider descriptions of esophageal transection for acute variceal bleeding to be anecdotal. Operative portal-systemic shunts are not indicated in patients with acute variceal bleeding.

Intraluminal tamponade with a self-expanding metal (SEM) stent can be attempted in cases refractory to standard endoscopic interventions [48]. Balloon tamponade can be placed in anticipation of definitive TIPS or therapeutic endoscopy within the next 24 h. Balloons carry a significant risk of esophageal necrosis and perforation so should be used with caution. We left one in place for 5 days in a bleeding patient who subsequently underwent a successful liver transplantation. Postoperatively the patient was diagnosed with a persistent effusion and esophageal perforation which was successfully managed with a covered esophageal stent.

Liver transplantation is the definitive therapy for portal hypertension, varices, and variceal bleeding. Controlled variceal bleeding is not a contraindication to liver transplantation. These patients need to be evaluated by a pretransplant team and transferred to a transplant center as soon as possible.

Renal Failure and Hyponatremia

Renal failure that results from liver failure is related to disturbances in circulation. Hypovolemia-induced renal failure is common after massive GIB if associated with hypotension or shock and is similar in presentation and treatment to any shock-related acute kidney injury. Unique to severe liver disease is the spectrum of disorders known as hepatorenal syndrome (HRS). HRS is defined by acute doubling of serum creatinine without other causes such as renal parenchymal disease, diuretic use, shock, or drug toxicity. There are two types of HRS, type I of sudden onset with a doubling of serum Cr to more than 2.5 ml/dL in less than 2 weeks from onset and type II which is more chronic [49]. In hepatorenal syndrome the kidneys are not adequately perfused secondary to decreased systemic vascular resistance and splanchnic arterial dilation. This hypoperfusion leads to a predictable response: prerenal failure leads to retaining free water to increase perfusion, which results in hyponatremia and total body fluid overload. In addition to elevation of the serum creatinine, a hallmark laboratory value seen in hepatorenal syndrome is a severely low urine sodium. Treatment includes diuretics and fluid restriction, vasopressin analogs, midodrine, norepinephrine, and even TIPS [49]. All of these therapies meet with limited success.

We routinely use a combination of Lasix, midodrine, albumin infusions, and occasionally norepinephrine to treat HRS pharmacologically. The use of terlipressin should be considered especially in patients who are awaiting liver transplantation as it may improve survival after transplant [50]. We do not routinely start patients on norepinephrine for the sole purpose of treating HRS, nor do we consider TIPS an appropriate therapy for this indication alone. Progressive and more severe HRS is best treated with RRT. CRRT is generally our modality of choice in critically ill patients given their hemodynamic instability with conventional intermittent hemodialysis. CRRT can either be slow continuous ultrafiltration (SCUF) in patients who have total body fluid overload but maintain other kidney functionality or continuous veno-venous hemofiltration dialysis (CVVHD) in patients with fluid overload and electrolyte, acid-base disturbances, or other indications for RRT.

We find the use of CRRT to be extremely helpful in optimizing volume status as patients await liver transplantation, and have not founds it use to contribute to mortality in this population, as seen in Fig. 51.1. Regardless of therapy, there is no cure for HRS other than liver or simultaneous liver-kidney transplantation, and in the absence of transplantation, prognosis is dismal with 50% survival at 1 month and 20% at 6 months [49, 51, 52].

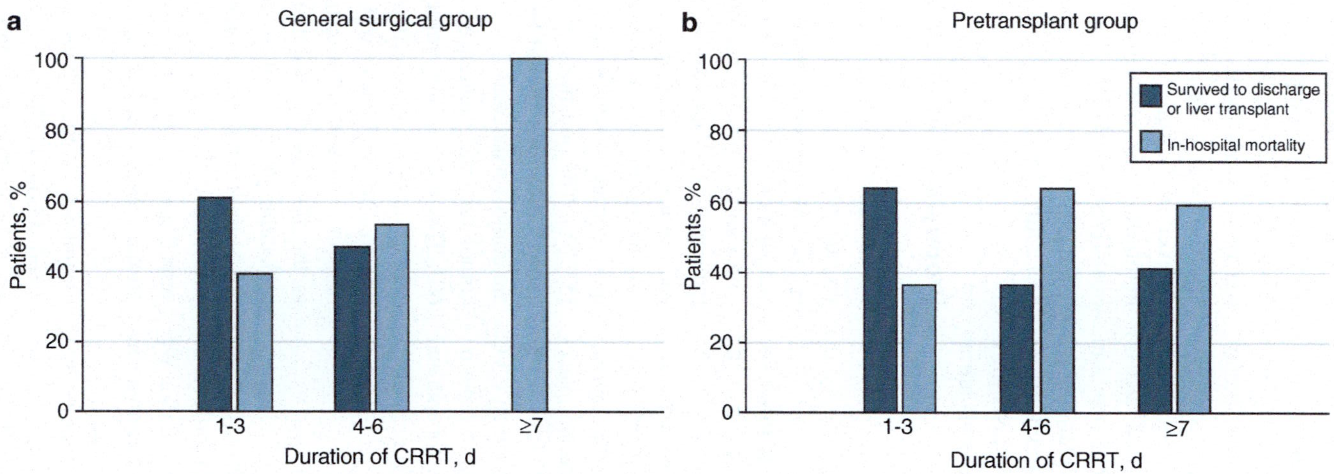

Patients included 53 in the general surgical group and 55 admitted to the surgical intensive care unit in anticipation of or for evaluation for liver transplant (pretransplant group).

Fig. 51.1 Analysis of in-hospital mortality by duration of continuous renal replacement therapy (CRRT). Patients included 53 in the general surgical group and 55 admitted to the surgical intensive care unit in anticipation of or for evaluation for liver transplant (pretransplant group) (Reproduced with permission from: Tatum et al. [65])

Coagulopathies, Transfusion, and Central Venous Access

The State of Coagulation in Acutely Ill Patients with Liver Disease

The traditional opinion is that patients with end-stage liver disease are hypocoagulable owing to the decreased production of clotting factors in the liver and a tendency to sequester platelets secondary to increased portal pressures and splenomegaly. Recent studies using thromboelastographic analysis provide a more complex picture, that of delayed clot formation and weaker thrombus strength despite decreased rates of clot lysis, owing to decreased production of both pro- and anticoagulants by the liver as well as decreased anti-Xa levels. These relationships between clot formation and degradation are not reflected in conventional coagulation tests [53]. Some studies in fact report that patients with cirrhosis are at increased risk of venous thromboembolism [54].

Line Placement and Coagulation Tests

Despite the questionable validity of conventional clotting tests, we continue to use them in most clinical scenarios, primarily the INR and fibrinogen levels. In the non-bleeding patient, we make no attempt to correct coagulation parameters. We have not observed increased rates of bleeding from the placement of central venous catheters (CVC) using this approach, although we encourage a small initial skin incision and require line placement by a senior-level resident or fellow when the INR is greater than 4. The most frequent bedside procedure other than CVC placement is paracentesis, which has been shown to have no increased risk of bleeding despite severe thrombocytopenia and elevations of INR beyond 8 at the time of the procedure [13].

Treating Coagulopathy

In the acutely bleeding patient, we initially measure conventional clotting tests and attempt to correct INR to a level of less than 3 and fibrinogen to a level of >100 mg/dL. We transfuse platelets to a level of 50×10^9/L. The treatment in these patients is to treat the source of bleeding—usually variceal bleeding. The treatment of refractory variceal bleeding or any diffuse bleeding in these patients is usually futile; however, we may order TEG to guide the therapy. All patients with cirrhosis or severe liver disease are administered therapeutic doses of vitamin K upon admission to the ICU.

Blood Transfusions

Our transfusion guidelines for fresh frozen plasma, fibrinogen, and vitamin K do not differ in the care of patients depending on whether they are awaiting liver transplantation. Our practices of red blood cell transfusion do differ between pre-transplant and non-pre-transplant patients owing to the fear of inducing antibodies in a patient who routinely requires >20 L of donor packed red blood cells during orthotropic liver transplantation. We routinely let these patients' hemoglobin level drop to a level of 6 g/dL if hemodynamically stable and the hemoglobin is not acutely dropping. Patients who are post-liver transplant recipients or who are not candidates for transplantation are managed with a hemoglobin goal of 7 g/dL [45, 46].

Prophylactic Anticoagulation

Portal vein thrombosis, peripheral venous thrombosis, and venous pulmonary emboli all occur in patients with cirrhosis, despite the appearance of coagulopathy on conventional coagulation tests [54–56]. The traditional notion of the "auto-anticoagulated" patients is simply inaccurate; these patients have complex and dynamic coagulation disorders and in some studies actually have a higher incidence of distal venous thrombosis than patients without cirrhosis, and they most certainly have higher rates of portal vein thrombosis [57, 58]. The questions of whether or not a patient without contraindications should be prophylactically anticoagulated are controversial, and there are studies showing varying outcomes regarding increased risk of significant bleeding [59, 60]. This topic is very rarely an issues in the ICU phase of care as these patients almost uniformly have a contraindication to anticoagulation while under our care. Patients who recover from acute illness and who are preparing for transfer to the floor are occasionally started on prophylactic low molecular weight heparin or unfractionated heparin, depending on their renal function, if they had a prior indication (i.e., atrial fibrillation or history of pulmonary embolus or portal vein thrombosis) after consulting with hepatology, and the primary surgeon. The management of patients with acute portal vein thrombosis, pulmonary emboli, or deep venous thrombosis is difficult and patient specific. We have recommended both TIPS for portal vein thromboses in patients not awaiting liver transplantation and also percutaneous directed thrombolysis and thrombectomy for both portal vein thrombosis and pulmonary emboli.

Infections, Disease, and Antibiotics

Patients with severe cirrhosis or ESLD all have some degree of immunosuppression owing to the loss of protein into ascites, poor nutrition, translocation of bacteria, and often multiple immunosuppressive medications. Clinicians must be vigilant for common infections such as spontaneous bacterial peritonitis and community or hospitalized pneumonias but also less common fungal infections. We frequently administer prophylactic antibiotics for acute patients with an acute GIB or a recent history of spontaneous bacterial peritonitis. Other patients are administered antibiotics on an as-needed basis. Broad-spectrum antibiotics, typically piperacillin and renal-dosed vancomycin, and antifungal medications are commonly received by patients with secondary peritonitis from a hollow viscus injury, with sepsis of unclear origin or an acute GIB. Antibiotics are narrowed as appropriate. The management of acute, chronic, or posttransplant antiviral medications is beyond the scope of this chapter.

Trauma in Patients with Liver Disease

Patients susceptible to hepatitis C or alcoholic cirrhosis are frequently victims of penetrating or blunt trauma which is poorly tolerated. In the largest study of this population, the odd ratio for death after trauma is increased to 5.56 (95% CI, 3.72–8.41) compared to patients without cirrhosis [61]. Not surprisingly, patients with higher MELD scores do worse after trauma [3]. We recommend early and aggressive correction of coagulopathy guided by TEG. The acute management of patients with penetration trauma can seldom be altered for any comorbidity, but we do advocate calling for help and additional blood products early. Severe blunt trauma in patients with Child C cirrhosis or an initial MELD score of >14 may best be treated with comfort measures and a frank discussion with family and the patient, when possible, about the dire prognosis.

The Care of Patients Awaiting Liver Transplantation

The care of patients awaiting liver transplantation is a critically important component of the topics addressed in this chapter. The idiosyncrasies of this subgroup have been carefully noted in each section above. Worth mentioning again is the importance in minimizing alloimmunization of potential organ recipients with excess blood transfusion. Equally important to the management of these patients are careful coordination and communication between the ICU, hepatology, and liver transplantation teams.

Social Work, End of Life, and Palliative Care

The long-term outcome for patients with ESLD is poor unless they receive a liver transplant. Those that are successfully discharged home frequently return to the hospital with a recurrent GIB, infections, or fluid overload, ranging between 13 and 37% within 1 month of discharge [13, 62]. Careful attention to discharge instructions, especially diuretics, is critical to maximizing the time between readmissions and may in fact prevent up to ¼ of these admissions [63, 64].

The most important recommendation that we can provide for many of these patients is guidance targeted at comfort and honesty. Caring for these patients, especially those who must be told that they are not candidates for liver transplantation, can be very difficult. We recommend the involvement of end of life service and palliative care team, where available. We also recommend frequent formal meetings between the family and the primary surgical team with frank discussion about condition, prognosis, and likely outcome.

References

1. Child CG, Turcott JGT. Surgery and portal hypertension. In: Child CG, editor. Liver and portal hypertension. Philadelphia: Saunders; 1964.
2. Befeler AS, Palmer DE, Hoffman M, Longo W, Solomon H, Di Biscegli AM. The safety of intra-abdominal surgery in patients with cirrhosis: model for end-stage liver disease score is superior to Child-Turcotte-Pugh classification in predicting outcome. Arch Surg. 2005;140:650–4.
3. Inaba K, Barmparas G, Resnick S, Browder T, Chan LS, Lam L, et al. The model for end-stage liver disease score. Arch Surg. 2011;146:1074.
4. Reverter E, Tandon P, Augustin S, Turon F, Casu S, Bastiampillai R, et al. A MELD-based model to determine risk of mortality among patients with acute variceal bleeding. Gastroenterology. 2014;146:412.
5. Northup PG, Wanamaker RC, Lee VD, Adams RB, Berg CL. Model for end-stage liver disease (MELD) predicts nontransplant surgical mortality in patients with cirrhosis. Ann Surg. 2005;242:244.
6. Annamalai A, Harada MY, Chen M, Tran T, Ko A, Ley E, et al. Predictors of mortality in the critically ill cirrhotic patient: is the model for end-stage liver disease enough? J Am Coll Surg. 2016;16:1636–42.
7. Dalal A, Lang JD. Anesthesthetic considerations for patients with liver disease. In: Abdeldayem H, editor. Hepatic surgery. Ruheja: InTech; 2013.
8. Guo G, XZ W, LJ S, Yang CQ. Clinical features of ischemic hepatitis caused by shock with four different types: a retrospective study of 328 cases. Int J Clin Exp Med. 2016;8:16670–5.
9. Fouad YM, Yehia R. Hepato-cardiac disorders. World J Hepatol. 2014;27:41–54.
10. Poelzl G, Auer J. Cardiohepatic syndrome. Curr Heart Fail Rep. 2014;12:68.
11. Tatum JM, Quinn AM, Genyk YS, Sher LS, Matsuoka LK, Hackman A, et al. Cardiac surgery at the time of simultaneous liver-kidney transplantation. J Curr Surg. 2016;6:37–40. https://doi.org/10.14740/jcs300w

12. Bolognesi M. Splanchnic vasodilation and hyperdynamic circulatory syndrome in cirrhosis. World J Gastroenterol. 2014;20:2555.
13. Ge PS, Runyon BA. Treatment of patients with cirrhosis. N Engl J Med. 2016;375:767.
14. Chen A, Massoni J, Jung D, Crippin J. Indwelling tunneled catheter for the management of hepatic hydrothorax. A pilot study. Ann Thorac Surg. 2016;13:435–8.
15. Mirrakhimov AE, Ayach T, Gray A. Indwelling tunneled pleural catheter for the management of hepatic hydrothorax: a word of caution. Ann Thorac Surg. 2016;13:1432.
16. Jung Y. Surgical treatment of hepatic hydrothorax: a "four-step approach". Ann Thorac Surg. 2016;101:1195–7.
17. Bartoletti M, Giannella M, Caraceni P, Domenicali M, Ambretti S, Tedeschi S, et al. Epidemiology and outcomes of bloodstream infection in patients with cirrhosis. J Hepatol. 2014;61:51.
18. O'Brien AJ, Fullerton JN, Massey KA, Auld G, Sewell G, James S, et al. Immunosuppression in acutely decompensated cirrhosis is mediated by prostaglandin E2. Nat Med. 2014;20:518.
19. Hassan EA, El-Rehim ASA, Hassany SM, Ahmed AO, Elsherbiny NM, Mohammed MH. Fungal infection in patients with end-stage liver disease: low frequency or low index of suspicion. Int J Infect Dis. 2014;23:69.
20. Møller S. Extrahepatic complications to cirrhosis and portal hypertension: haemodynamic and homeostatic aspects. World J Gastroenterol. 2014;20:15499.
21. Cosarderelioglu C, Cosar AM, Gurakar M, Dagher NN, Gurakar A. Hepatopulmonary syndrome and liver transplantation: a recent review of the literature. J Clin Transl Hepatol. 2016;4:47–53.
22. Levesque E, Saliba F, Ichaï P, Samuel D. Outcome of patients with cirrhosis requiring mechanical ventilation in ICU. J Hepatol. 2014;60:570.
23. Lee KC, Chiang AA. THe outcome of terminal liver cirrhosis patients requiring mechanical ventilation. Med J Free China Ed. 1997;1997:88–94.
24. Goldfarb G, Nouel O, Poynard T, Reuff B. Efficiency of respiritory assistance in cirrhotic patients with liver failure. Intensive Care Med. 1983;9:271–3.
25. Chihara Y. Use of noninvasive ventilation for pediatric patients after liver transplantation: a decrease in the need for reintubation. Liver Transpl. 18:1217–5.
26. Karcz M, Schwaiberger D, Lachmann B, Papadakos PJ. Acute respiratory failure complicating advanced liver disease. Semin Respir Crit Care Med. 2012;33:96–110.
27. Plauth M, Cabré E, Riggio O, Assis-Camilo M, Pirlich M, Kondrup J, et al. ESPEN guidelines on enteral nutrition: liver disease. Clin Nutr. 2006;25:285.
28. Galloway AC, Schwartz CF, Ribakove GH, Crooke GA, Gogoladze G, Ursomanno P, et al. A decade of minimally invasive mitral repair: long-term outcomes. Ann Thorac Surg. 2009;88:1180.
29. Kalaitzakis E. Gastrointestinal dysfunction in liver cirrhosis. World J Gastroenterol. 2014;20:14686.
30. Koretz RL, Avenell A, Lipman TO. Nutritional support for liver disease. Cochrane Database Syst Rev. 2012;(5):CD008344.
31. Benjamin J, Singla V, Arora I, Sood S, Joshi YK. Intestinal permeability and complications in liver cirrhosis: a prospective cohort study. Hepatol Res. 2012;43:200.
32. Jakubczyk M, Różowicz A, Spychalska K, Nakonowska B, Kupczyk K, Kusza K. Analysis of occurrence of bacteraemia with pathogens from gastrointestinal tract in patients fed parenterally and enterally in the intensive care unit. Gastroenterol Rev. 2016;2:127.
33. Kim JJ, Tsukamoto MM, Mathur AK, Ghomri YM, Hou LA, Sheibani S, et al. Delayed paracentesis is associated with increased in-hospital mortality in patients with spontaneous bacterial peritonitis. Am J Gastroenterol. 2014;109:1436.
34. Runyon BA. Introduction to the revised American Association for the Study of Liver Diseases Practice Guideline management of adult patients with ascites due to cirrhosis 2012. Hepatology. 2013;57:1651.
35. Nasr G, Hassan A, Ahmed S, Serwah A. Predictors of large volume paracentesis induced circulatory dysfunction in patients with massive hepatic ascites. J Cardiovasc Dis Res. 2010;1:136.
36. Kathpalia P, Bhatia A, Robertazzi S, Ahn J, Cohen SM, Sontag S, et al. Indwelling peritoneal catheters in patients with cirrhosis and refractory ascites. Intern Med J. 2015;45:1026.
37. Belghiti J, Durand F. Abdominal wall hernia in the setting of cirrhosis. Semin Liver Dis. 1997;17:219–26.
38. Carbonell AM, Wolfe LG, DeMaria EJ. Poor outcomes in cirrhosis-associated hernia repair: a nationwide cohort study of 32,033 patients. Hernia. 2005;9:353.
39. Coelho JC, Claus CM, Campos AC, Costa MA, Blum C. Umbilical hernia in patients with liver cirrhosis: a surgical challenge. World J Gastrointest Surg. 2016;8:476.
40. Curro G. Percutaneous gall bladder aspiration as an alternative to laparoscopic cholecystectomy in Child-Pugh C cirrhotic patients with acute cholecystitis. Gut. 2006;55:898.
41. Delis S, Bakoyiannis A, Madariaga J, Bramis J, Tassopoulos N, Dervenis C. Laparoscopic cholecystectomy in cirrhotic patients: the value of MELD score and Child–Pugh classification in predicting outcome. Surg Endosc. 2009;24:407.
42. Hall J, Singh G, Hood D, Mateo R, Weaver F, Selby R, et al. Management of an abdominal aortic aneurysm in a patient with end-stage liver disease. Am J Transplant. 2004;4:666.
43. Sabbagh C, Chatelain D, Nguyen-Khac E, Rebibo L, Joly J-P, Regimbeau J-M. Management of colorectal cancer in patients with cirrhosis: a retrospective, case-matched study of short- and long-term outcomes. Dig Liver Dis. 2016;48:429.
44. D'Amico G. Upper digestive bleeding in cirrhosis. Post-therapeutic outcome and prognostic indicators. Hepatology. 2003;38:599.
45. Garcia-Tsao G, Sanyal AJ, Grace ND, Carey WD. Prevention and management of gastroesophageal varices and variceal hemorrhage in Cirrhosis. Am J Gastroenterol. 2007;102:2086.
46. de Franchis R. Revising consensus in portal hypertension: report of the Baveno V consensus workshop on methodology of diagnosis and therapy in portal hypertension. J Hepatol. 2010;53:762.
47. O'Leary JG, Reddy KR, Wong F, Kamath PS, Patton HM, Biggins SW, et al. Long-term use of antibiotics and proton pump inhibitors predict development of infections in patients with cirrhosis. Clin Gastroenterol Hepatol. 2015;13:753.
48. McCarty TR, Njei B. Self-expanding metal stents for acute refractory esophageal variceal bleeding: a systematic review and meta-analysis. Dig Endosc. 2016;28:539.
49. Ginès P, Schrier RW. Renal failure in cirrhosis. N Engl J Med. 2009;361:1279.
50. Restuccia T, Ortega R, Guevara M, Ginès P, Alessandria C, Ozdogan O, et al. Effects of treatment of hepatorenal syndrome before transplantation on posttransplantation outcome. A case-control study. J Hepatol. 2004;40:140.
51. Schepke M, Appenrodt B, Heller J, Zielinski J, Sauerbruch T. Prognostic factors for patients with cirrhosis and kidney dysfunction in the era of MELD: results of a prospective study. Liver Int. 2006;26:834.
52. Alessandria C, Ozdogan O, Guevara M, Restuccia T, Jiménez W, Arroyo V, et al. MELD score and clinical type predict prognosis in hepatorenal syndrome: relevance to liver transplantation. Hepatology. 2005;41:1282.
53. Lloyd-Donald P, Vasudevan A, Angus P, Gow P, Mårtensson J, Glassford N, et al. Coagulation in acutely ill patients with severe chronic liver disease: insights from thromboelastography. J Crit Care. 2017;38:215.
54. Tripodi A, Anstee QM, Sogaard KK, Primignani M, Valla DC. Hypercoagulability in cirrhosis: causes and consequences. J Thromb Haemost. 2011;9:1713.

55. Rodríguez-Castro KI. Spontaneous bleeding or thrombosis in cirrhosis: what should be feared the most? World J Hepatol. 2015;7:1818.
56. Raja K, Jacob M, Asthana S. Portal vein thrombosis in cirrhosis. J Clin Exp Hepatol. 2014;4:320.
57. Aggarwal A. Deep vein thrombosis and pulmonary embolism in cirrhotic patients: systematic review. World J Gastroenterol. 2014;20:5737.
58. Harding DJ, Perera MT, Frederick C, Olliff S, Tripathi D. Portal vein thrombosis in cirrhosis: controversies and latest developments. World J Gastroenterol. 2015;21:6769–84.
59. Shatzel J, Dulai PS, Harbin D, Cheung H, Reid TN, Kim J, et al. Safety and efficacy of pharmacological thromboprophylaxis for hospitalized patients with cirrhosis: a single-center retrospective cohort study. J Thromb Haemost. 2015;13:1245.
60. Intagliata NM, Henry ZH, Shah N, Lisman T, Caldwell SH, Northup PG. Prophylactic anticoagulation for venous thromboembolism in hospitalized cirrhosis patients is not associated with high rates of gastrointestinal bleeding. Liver Int. 2013;34:26.
61. Georgiou C, Inaba K, Teixeira PGR, Hadjizacharia P, Chan LS, Brown C, et al. Cirrhosis and trauma are a lethal combination. World J Surg. 2009;33:1087.
62. Tapper EB, Halbert B, Mellinger J. Rates of and reasons for hospital readmissions in patients with cirrhosis: a multistate population-based cohort study. Clin Gastroenterol Hepatol. 2016;14:1181.
63. Volk ML, Tocco RS, Bazick J, Rakoski MO, Lok AS. Hospital readmissions among patients with decompensated cirrhosis. Am J Gastroenterol. 2011;107:247.
64. Tapper EB, Finkelstein D, Mittleman MA, Piatkowski G, Chang M, Lai M. A quality improvement initiative reduces 30-day rate of readmission for patients with cirrhosis. Clin Gastroenterol Hepatol. 2016;14:753.
65. Tatum JM, Barmparas G, Ko A, Dhillon N, Smith E, Margulies DR, Ley EJ. Analysis of survival after initiation of continuous renal replacement therapy in a surgical intensive care unit. JAMA Surg. 2017. https://doi.org/10.1001/jamasurg.2017.1673. [Epub ahead of print] PubMed PMID: 28636702
66. Pugh RN, Murray-Lyon IM, Dawson JL, Pietroni MC, Williams R. Transection of the oesophagus for bleeding oesophageal varices. Br J Surg. 1973;60:646–9.
67. Kamath PS, Wiesner RH, Malinchoc M, Kremers W, Therneau TM, Kosberg CL, et al. A model to predict survival in patients with end-stage liver disease. Hepatology. 2001;33(2):464–70.
68. Biggins SW, Kim WR, Terrault NA, Saab S, Balan V, Schiano T, et al. Evidence-based incorporation of serum sodium concentration into MELD. Gastroenterology. 2006;130(6):1652–60.
69. United Network for Organ Sharing (UNOS). Calculators. Accessed 11 July 2017. https://www.transplantpro.org/news/technology/policy-and-system-changes-effective-january-11-2016-adding-serum-sodium-to-meld-calculation/

52 Obesity in Critical Care

Julietta Chang and Stacy Brethauer

Introduction

Obesity, defined as a body mass index (BMI) greater than or equal to 30 m/kg^2, is increasing in incidence, with more than one-third of American adults in the United States classified as obese and numbers projected to increase [1]. Worse outcomes have been noted in both underweight (BMI <18 m/kg^2) and obese critically ill patients [2]. Other studies have associated obesity as an independent risk factor for mortality in the ICU [3]. In addition, morbid obesity is an independent risk factor for the development of organ failure after trauma in the critically ill patient [4]. Given the current obesity epidemic, the number of critically ill obese patients will continue to increase, and a greater understanding of the physiologic challenges associated with obesity in this setting will be needed.

Pulmonary

The deleterious effects of obesity on respiratory function are multifactorial. Increased work of breathing is partly mechanical, due to the upward displacement of the diaphragm resulting in suboptimal muscle contraction; increased chest wall resistance and decreased chest wall elasticity; and increased upper airway resistance due to excess parapharyngeal tissue [5], all which lead to a ventilation-perfusion mismatch and a susceptibility to hypoxemia which is exacerbated in the supine position. In addition, due to increased adipose tissue, there is a higher daily production of carbon dioxide. Chronic hypoventilation may develop in the super morbid obese patient as well. As a result, obese patients may require unplanned intubation more frequently than nonobese patients [6].

J. Chang
Massachusetts General Hospital, Department of General Surgery, Boston, MA, USA

S. Brethauer (✉)
Digestive Disease and Surgery Institute, Cleveland Clinic, Cleveland, OH, USA
e-mail: brethas@ccf.org

Airway management of the morbidly obese patient in the ICU setting can be challenging. Excess fascial fat may increase difficulty with bag-mask ventilation, while parapharyngeal fat increases upper airway resistance. These, combined with a large tongue and thick neck tissue, may account for the significant increase in difficulty in tracheal intubation [7], as well as serious complications associated with intubation such as severe hypoxia or cardiovascular collapse [8]. Adjuncts to intubation such as fiber-optic bronchoscopy are more commonly required in the obese patient. In addition, patients with BMI > 35 demonstrate a lower nadir SpO_2 during intubation, likely due to increased susceptibility to hypoxemia. Utilizing 30-degree reverse Trendelenburg position has been shown to increase preoxygenation, likely by improving the mechanics of ventilation [5].

Once intubated, tidal volumes will need to be adjusted by ideal body weight rather than actual body weight to avoid barotrauma, as lung volumes do not increase with greater BMI. One study demonstrated that while obese patients had low tidal volumes according to actual body weight (5–6 mL/kg), they were receiving high tidal volumes based on ideal body weight (10–11 mL/kg), placing them at increased risk of lung injury. As a result, the obese cohort had a significantly increased risk of developing barotrauma and acute respiratory distress syndrome [9]. In addition, in the patient with chronic hypoventilation, ventilation settings should be titrated to pH rather than pCO_2, as the latter is chronically elevated.

Obesity is also associated with higher complication rates during open tracheostomy. However, centers have reported successful implementation of percutaneous tracheostomy in super morbid obese patients without complications [10]. Data regarding whether obesity is associated with prolonged mechanical ventilation once intubated is conflicting; one meta-analysis found significantly increased duration of mechanical ventilation and resultant ICU length of stay [11], while another study showed shorter time to extubation in obese patients [12]. One study reported higher rates of postextubation stridor in obese patients, in some instances requiring reintubation [7].

A. Salim et al. (eds.), *Surgical Critical Care Therapy*, https://doi.org/10.1007/978-3-319-71712-8_52

Cardiovascular

Obesity results in increased blood volume and cardiac output due to excess tissue. This results in left ventricular hypertrophy (LVH) and hypertension [5]. However, comorbid conditions associated with obesity including diabetes, essential hypertension, and hyperlipidemia also have detrimental effects on the cardiovascular system.

Left ventricular hypertrophy associated with obesity results in diastolic dysfunction; this combined with elevated plasma volume can result in left atrial enlargement, and studies have shown that obesity is a risk factor for the development of atrial fibrillation [13]. While this may suggest the judicious use of fluids in the critically ill obese patient to prevent fluid overload and the precipitation of atrial fibrillation, studies have shown that obese patients tend to be fluid under-resuscitated for body weight, leading to persistently worse base deficit and perhaps contributing to increased mortality in the burn ICU setting [14]. Therefore, clinical judgment using clinical endpoints of resuscitation including resolution of metabolic acidosis and adequate urine output rather than weight-based fluid resuscitation volumes is advised in the obese patient.

Gastrointestinal

Physical examination of the obese patient may be somewhat limited by habitus, and x-ray imaging may be degraded by a thick abdominal wall as well, both of which can make the diagnosis of intra-abdominal pathology challenging.

Peptic ulcer disease is the product of an imbalance between acid production and mucosal barrier; in the critically ill patient, there is a defect in the latter, likely due to decreased blood flow. As obesity is a risk factor for gastroesophageal reflux disease (GERD) and hiatal hernias, many of these patients are already on some form of anti-secretory medication such as a proton pump inhibitors (PPIs) or histamine (H2) blocker. A history of bariatric surgery, especially Roux-en-Y gastric bypass, may predispose a patient to ulcer disease and upper gastrointestinal bleeding (UGIB) due to ulceration at the gastrojejunostomy (marginal ulcer) [15]. Thus, it is important to maintain a patient's home PPI or H2 blocker therapy while in the ICU, and in the setting of GI dysfunction, these may have to be converted to IV formulations.

In addition, the intensivist must be cognizant that the post-gastric bypass or duodenal switch anatomy does not allow easy endoscopic access to the biliary tree. Given that obesity is also associated with the development of biliary lithiasis [16], if the patient were to develop choledocholithiasis and sequelae such as cholangitis or gallstone pancreatitis, it is significantly more difficult to decompress the biliary tree since standard ERCP is not usually feasible. In patients who have had duodenal switch, there is no endoscopic access to the duodenum, and biliary decompression must be accomplished transhepatically (percutaneous transhepatic cholangiography, PTC) or with direct surgical access to the bile duct. Options in the gastric bypass patient include PTC decompression with interventional radiology or laparoscopic-assisted transgastric ERCP. At our institution, we favor laparoscopic-assisted transgastric ERCP as a safe and effective method to perform ERCP in these patients and particularly in cases where there is little intrahepatic ductal dilation which makes PTC more difficult or impossible. If needed, a gastrostomy tube is left in the remnant stomach to maintain access to the biliopancreatic limb and facilitate future endoscopic interventions. This remnant gastrostomy tube can also be used for enteral feeding access and is superior to a feeding jejunostomy in terms of ease of access, ability to decompress, and absorption of delivered nutrients.

Obesity is also associated with fatty infiltration of the liver, and nonalcoholic fatty liver disease (NAFLD) is the most common cause of cirrhosis in the United States [17]. More than 90% of obese patients have fatty infiltration of the liver, and one-fourth of these patients will have steatohepatitis or nonalcoholic steatohepatitis (NASH). One-third of these patients will go on to develop cirrhosis within a decade. This is relevant with regard to decreased drug clearance (see section "Pharmacology"). In the presence of cirrhosis, the patient may develop fulminant complications such as hepatorenal syndrome, spontaneous bacterial peritonitis, hepatic encephalopathy, or variceal bleeding. Ascites may be difficult to appreciate due to body habitus, and paracentesis may be especially challenging.

Renal

Obesity is associated with an increased risk of acute renal failure [2, 9] and is an established risk factor for chronic kidney disease (CKD), likely due to the existence of comorbid conditions such as hypertension, diabetes, and atherosclerotic disease as well as due to a chronic supranormal glomerular filtration rate (GFR) due to an increased blood volume and cardiac output as noted above. In addition, obesity is associated with a chronic inflammatory state with increased oxidative stress which may contribute to impaired renal function [5, 18, 19]. Local fat accumulation may cause increased intrarenal pressure with local intrarenal hypertension as well as lipotoxicity. There is marked activation of the renin-angiotensin-aldosterone system beyond expected for degree of hypertension due to enhanced angiotensinogen synthesis in fatty tissue [20]. One large retrospective study of over 16,000 patients in cardiac surgery found that obesity was significantly associated with an increased risk of postoperative renal insufficiency and that the severity of injury was proportional to the degree of obesity [18]. It should also be noted that the commonly used Cockcroft-Gault equation for calculated GFR has been shown to be inaccurate at extremes of BMI and that the Modification of Diet in Renal Disease (MDRD) study equation is less subject to inaccuracy in high-obese patients and may have implications in pharmacology in the care of the critically ill obese patient (Table 53.1) [21].

In the treatment of renal disease and hypertension in the obese patient, angiotensin-converting enzyme (ACE) inhibitors are ideal as they mitigate the overactivated RAAS. ACE inhibitors have been shown to markedly decrease proteinuria in obesity and decrease progression to renal failure [20]. However, in the acute on chronic renal failure patient, treatment is largely supportive and may include temporary hemodialysis for severe renal insufficiency [18].

Hematology

Obesity has been demonstrated to be an independent risk factor for thromboembolic disease with a hazard ratio of 1.88 compared to the nonobese population. Meta-analysis has also demonstrated a higher incidence of deep venous thromboses (DVTs) in the critically ill obese patient [2]. This may be due to decreased mobility in this patient population, thrombophilic changes related to obesity, or inadequate dosing of weight-based chemoprophylaxis [5]. The practical difficulties in obtaining high-quality duplex ultrasonography or CT angiography in patients with obesity may actually result in underdiagnosis of DVT or subsequent pulmonary embolus (PE) [2]. One study examining DVT and PE after bariatric surgery found that nearly 40% of patients with clinically significant PEs had negative lower extremity duplex studies [22]. One cohort study examining the use of heparin versus low molecular weight heparin (LMWH) in perioperative DVT prophylaxis found that the use of LMWH was more effective at preventing DVTs and not associated with a higher risk of postoperative hemorrhage [23].

Difficult vascular access should be anticipated in the critically ill obese patient as obesity results in the loss of anatomic landmarks [24]. The use of ultrasound in the ICU has been shown to aid in the placement of peripheral intravenous lines (PIVs) and help reduce the number of central venous catheters (CVC) placed in the hemodynamically stable obese patient [25]. At our institution, a dedicated vascular access nursing team places both midline catheters (not centrally positioned) and peripherally inserted central venous catheters (PICC) in patients in whom peripheral IV cannot be obtained. These types of catheters are associated with decreased bloodstream infections as well as decreased insertion-related complications such as pneumo- or hemothorax and chronic complications such as central venous stenosis compared to CVCs [26]. Although it is well established that PICC lines are associated with upper extremity DVTs, they have been shown to increase the risk of lower extremity thromboses as well, the pathogenesis of which is not well understood [27].

Table 53.1 Equations for renal function

Cockcroft-Gault equation
Creatinine clearance (male) = ((140−age)/(S_{cr})) × (weight / 72)
Creatinine clearance (female) = 0.85 × ((140−age)/(S_{cr})) × (weight / 72)
Modification of renal diseases study
GFR (mL/min/1.73 m^2) = 175 × (S_{cr})$^{-1.154}$ × (age)$^{-0.203}$ × (0.742 if female) × (1.212 if African American)

S_{cr} Serum creatinine

Infectious Disease

One prospective observational study found that obese patients in the critical care setting were significantly more likely to develop bacteremia and catheter-related bloodstream infections. The authors postulate that this related to difficult vascular access and reluctance to discontinue intravenous access even if infection is suspected, as new access may be prohibitively difficult to obtain. This series, however, did not find that there was a significant difference in the rate of pneumonia or urinary tract infections (UTIs) in the obese versus normal weight patients [28]. Other studies however have found that obesity is a risk factor for ICU admission and mortality in the setting of H1N1 influenza [29], potentially due to a disordered immune response and altered cytokine response [30]. Other studies have demonstrated that increasing BMI is a risk factor for both UTIs and pyelonephritis, with up to five times increased risk compared to nonobese patients [31].

Although obesity may be a risk factor for developing infection, outcomes of the septic obese patient is controversial. The "obesity paradox" is the observed J-shaped curve demonstrating that underweight and severely obese patients have worse outcomes, while overweight and moderately obese patients with BMI between 25 and 40 have lower mortality [32]. As these observations are based on meta-analyses of heterogeneous patient populations, it is difficult to draw conclusions about these complex associations. However, some of the observed outcomes may be due to excess adipose tissue acting as an energy reservoir [33]. Another retrospective analysis found that obese patients had the lowest 28-day mortality, followed by overweight and then normal weight patients. They hypothesize that this may be due to a blunted inflammatory response, as levels of proinflammatory IL-6 were lowest in higher

BMI patients. In addition, obese and overweight patients received less body weight-adjusted fluids and vasopressors compared to normal weight patients. The authors conclude that fluid resuscitation and vasopressor doses should be adjusted for ideal body weight, and what appeared like underresuscitation was ironically protective in this patient population [34].

Pharmacology

Considerations in drug dosing in obesity include the drug's volume of distribution (Vd), a function of its lipophilicity. Drugs with a high Vd (i.e., more lipophilic) will require higher doses in patients with increased adipose tissue with higher loading doses, while those with low Vd may require little adjustment in drug dosing [35]. Lean body weight (LBW) as calculated by the James equation (Table 53.2) is most commonly used when calculating weight-based dosing by investigators in drug trials. As it correlates to creatinine clearance, it may be more accurate than other calculations such as ideal or adjusted body weight [15]. With regard to maintenance dosing, clearance is multifactorial and depends on whether the drug is metabolized by the liver, kidney, or a combination. Rarely, drugs such as cisatracurium undergo Hoffman degradation. As noted above, obesity is associated with renal and hepatic dysfunction. Thus, the best measure of subsequent drug dosing after initial loading is clinical response. For example, antiarrhythmic medications may require breakthrough dosing, heparin drips should be titrated on coagulation studies, and antibiotics should be dosed on trough and peak serum levels after initial weight-based loading dosing. Another consideration is altered gastrointestinal anatomy in the bariatric patient in enteral dosing. For example, one study from the Netherlands found that the area under the curve (AUC) for aspirin was significantly higher after gastric bypass, while it was significantly decreased for oral omeprazole after bypass, perhaps accounting for persistent ulcer symptoms in this patient population [36]. This issue can be avoided by administering parenteral formulations.

Table 53.2 Common weight equations

Lean body weight (LBW)
LBW (men) = (1.10 × weight in kg)−120 × (weight 2 / (100 × height in m) 2)
LBW (women) = (1.07 × weight in kg)−148 × (weight 2 / (100 × height in m) 2)
Ideal body weight (IBW) in kg
IBW (men) = 50 kg + 2.3 kg for each inch in height over 60 inches
IBW (women) = 45.5 kg + 2.3 kg for each inch in height over 60 inches
Adjusted body weight (ABWadj) in kg
ABWadj = IBW + 0.4 (actual weight−IBW)

Pearls in the Management of the Morbidly Obese Patient

Venous access as noted above, peripheral line placement is more difficult in the obese patient [24]. Preemptive use of the ultrasound in placement of peripheral intravenous catheters (PIV) is recommended. We recommend avoiding routine placement of central venous catheters due to increased complications compared to PIVs.

Intubation placement of obese patients in a "ramped" position rather than the standard "sniff" position allows for easier laryngoscopy. A high index of suspicion should be maintained for all obese patients with regard to difficult intubation, and an awake fiber-optic intubation should be considered for those with a history of difficult intubation [37].

Chest tube placement normal anatomic landmarks may be impossible to palpate in the obese patient. The intersection of the anterior axillary line and inframammary folds, even in the obese patient, will reliably lead to the placement of an intrathoracic tube. In patients with prohibitively thick chest walls, the use of a 12 or 15 mm optical trocar and a 0-degree laparoscope has been described [38]. This allows for visualization of the soft tissue, intercostal muscles, and lung parenchyma. The laparoscope is removed, and a 28 French chest tube is inserted through the trocar into the chest cavity, and the trocar is removed over the chest tube. The use of a smaller-diameter optical trocar could be used for thoracentesis as well, if ultrasound image guidance is unsuccessful.

Bedside ultrasonography due to poor tissue penetration, the use of bedside ultrasound may be limited in the evaluation of the obese patient. Obesity has been shown to be associated with increased rates of false-negative FAST (focused assessment with sonography for trauma) [39]. Lower-frequency ultrasound probes will allow for greater tissue penetration at the expense of image quality, while higher-frequency probes will do the opposite [40]. Multiple probes may need to be utilized in the same patient. Placing the patient on their side contralateral to the organ of interest will help displace adipose tissue in those with truncal obesity. The pannus should be elevated when scanning the suprapubic region.

Paracentesis due to the increased number of patients presenting with cirrhosis from nonalcoholic fatty liver disease, there has been interest in finding the ideal site for paracentesis. The infraumbilical midline is associated with increased abdominal wall thickness compared with the left lower quadrant. The right lower quadrant is avoided due to proximity to a thin-walled, gas-filled cecum. Placing the patient in a left lateral oblique position will increase the depth of ascites as well, increasing the chance of successful aspiration [41].

Conclusions

Obesity is an increasing epidemic and a major public health problem globally, and there are specific challenges in the management of the obese critically ill patient. Evidence currently suggests that the disparate outcomes between obese and normal weight patients in the critical care setting are not due to weight alone but are due to complex alterations in physiology and organ dysfunction, hormone regulation, and interactions between cytokines. Evidence is lacking as to whether obesity is protective in critical illness, and further studies are required to refine the best management practices in the care of these patients.

References

1. Flegal KM, Carroll MD, Kit BK, Ogden CL. Prevalence of obesity and trends in the distribution of body mass index among US adults, 1999–2010. JAMA. 2012;307:491–7. https://doi.org/10.1001/jama.2012.39.
2. Hogue CW, Stearns JD, Colantuoni E, Robinson KA, Stierer T, Mitter N, et al. The impact of obesity on outcomes after critical illness: a meta-analysis. Intensive Care Med. 2009;35:1152–70. https://doi.org/10.1007/s00134-009-1424-5.
3. Bercault N, Boulain T, Kuteifan K, Wolf M, Runge I, Fleury J-C. Obesity-related excess mortality rate in an adult intensive care unit: a risk-adjusted matched cohort study. Crit Care Med. 2004;32:998–1003.
4. Ciesla DJ, Moore EE, Johnson JL, Burch JM, Cothren CC, Sauaia A. Obesity increases risk of organ failure after severe trauma. J Am Coll Surg. 2006;203:539–45. https://doi.org/10.1016/j.jamcollsurg.2006.06.029.
5. Shashaty MGS, Stapleton RD. Physiological and management implications of obesity in critical illness. Ann Am Thorac Soc. 2014;11:1286–97. https://doi.org/10.1513/AnnalsATS.201404-159FR.
6. Tafelski S, Yi H, Ismaeel F, Krannich A, Spies C, Nachtigall I. Obesity in critically ill patients is associated with increased need of mechanical ventilation but not with mortality. J Infect Public Health. 2016;9:577. https://doi.org/10.1016/j.jiph.2015.12.003.
7. Frat J-P, Gissot V, Ragot S, Desachy A, Runge I, Lebert C, et al. Impact of obesity in mechanically ventilated patients: a prospective study. Intensive Care Med. 2008;34:1991–8. https://doi.org/10.1007/s00134-008-1245-y.
8. De Jong A, Molinari N, Pouzeratte Y, Verzilli D, Chanques G, Jung B, et al. Difficult intubation in obese patients: incidence, risk factors, and complications in the operating theatre and in intensive care units. Br J Anaesth. 2015;114:297–306. https://doi.org/10.1093/bja/aeu373.
9. Anzueto A, Frutos-Vivar F, Esteban A, Bensalami N, Marks D, Raymondos K, et al. Influence of body mass index on outcome of the mechanically ventilated patients. Thorax. 2011;66:66–73. https://doi.org/10.1136/thx.2010.145086.
10. Kaese S, Zander MC, Lebiedz P. Successful use of early percutaneous dilatational tracheotomy and the no sedation concept in respiratory failure in critically ill obese subjects. Respir Care. 2016;61:615. https://doi.org/10.4187/respcare.04333.
11. Akinnusi ME, Pineda LA, El Solh AA. Effect of obesity on intensive care morbidity and mortality: a meta-analysis. Crit Care Med. 2008;36:151–8. https://doi.org/10.1097/01.CCM.0000297885.60037.6E.
12. O'Brien JM, Philips GS, Ali NA, Aberegg SK, Marsh CB, Lemeshow S. The association between body mass index, processes of care, and outcomes from mechanical ventilation: a prospective cohort study. Crit Care Med. 2012;40:1456–63. https://doi.org/10.1097/CCM.0b013e31823e9a80.
13. Wang TJ, Parise H, Levy D, D'Agostino RB, Wolf PA, Vasan RS, et al. Obesity and the risk of new-onset atrial fibrillation. JAMA. 2004;292:2471–7. https://doi.org/10.1001/jama.292.20.2471.
14. Rae L, Pham TN, Carrougher G, Honari S, Gibran NS, Arnoldo BD, et al. Differences in resuscitation in morbidly obese burn patients may contribute to high mortality. J Burn Care Res. 34:507–14. https://doi.org/10.1097/BCR.0b013e3182a2a771.
15. El Solh AA, editor. Critical care management of the obese patient. Oxford: Wiley-Blackwell; 2012. https://doi.org/10.1002/9781119962083.
16. Chang J, Corcelles R, Boules M, Jamal MH, Schauer PR, Kroh MD. Predictive factors of biliary complications after bariatric surgery. Surg Obes Relat Dis. 2015. https://doi.org/10.1016/j.soard.2015.11.004.
17. Diehl AM. Hepatic complications of obesity. Gastroenterol Clin North Am. 2010;39:57–68. https://doi.org/10.1016/j.gtc.2009.12.001.
18. Virani SS, Nambi V, Lee V-V, Elayda MA, Pan W, Petersen LA, et al. Obesity: an independent predictor of in-hospital postoperative renal insufficiency among patients undergoing cardiac surgery? Texas Hear Inst J. 2009;36:540–5.
19. Cignarelli M, Lamacchia O. Obesity and kidney disease. Nutr Metab Cardiovasc Dis. 2007;17:757–62. https://doi.org/10.1016/j.numecd.2007.03.003.
20. Rutkowski P, Klassen A, Sebekova K, Bahner U, Heidland A. Renal disease in obesity: the need for greater attention. J Ren Nutr. 2006;16:216–23. https://doi.org/10.1053/j.jrn.2006.04.017.
21. Cirillo M, Anastasio P, De Santo NG. Relationship of gender, age, and body mass index to errors in predicted kidney function. Nephrol Dial Transplant. 2005;20:1791–8. https://doi.org/10.1093/ndt/gfh962.
22. Jamal MH, Corcelles R, Shimizu H, Kroh M, Safdie FM, Rosenthal R, et al. Thromboembolic events in bariatric surgery: a large multi-institutional referral center experience. Surg Endosc. 2015;29:376–80. https://doi.org/10.1007/s00464-014-3678-4.
23. Birkmeyer NJO, Finks JF, Carlin AM, Chengelis DL, Krause KR, Hawasli AA, et al. Comparative effectiveness of unfractionated and low-molecular-weight heparin for prevention of venous thromboembolism following bariatric surgery. Arch Surg. 2012;147:994–8. https://doi.org/10.1001/archsurg.2012.2298.
24. Juvin P, Blarel A, Bruno F, Desmonts J-M. Is peripheral line placement more difficult in obese than in lean patients? Anesth Analg. 2003;96:1218. table of contents
25. Gregg SC, Murthi SB, Sisley AC, Stein DM, Scalea TM. Ultrasound-guided peripheral intravenous access in the intensive care unit. J Crit Care. 2010;25:514–9. https://doi.org/10.1016/j.jcrc.2009.09.003.
26. Moureau N, Chopra V. Indications for peripheral, midline and central catheters: summary of the MAGIC recommendations. Br J Nurs. 2016;25:S15–24. https://doi.org/10.12968/bjon.2016.25.8.S15.
27. Greene MT, Flanders SA, Woller SC, Bernstein SJ, Chopra V. The association between PICC use and venous thromboembolism in upper and lower extremities. Am J Med. 2015;128:986–993.e1. https://doi.org/10.1016/j.amjmed.2015.03.028.
28. Dossett LA, Dageforde LA, Swenson BR, Metzger R, Bonatti H, Sawyer RG, et al. Obesity and site-specific nosocomial infection risk in the intensive care unit*. Surg Infect (Larchmt). 2009;10:137–42. https://doi.org/10.1089/sur.2008.028.
29. Fezeu L, Julia C, Henegar A, Bitu J, FB H, Grobbee DE, et al. Obesity is associated with higher risk of intensive care unit admis-

sion and death in influenza A (H1N1) patients: a systematic review and meta-analysis. Obes Rev. 2011;12:653–9. https://doi.org/10.1111/j.1467-789X.2011.00864.x.
30. Huttunen R, Syrjänen J. Obesity and the risk and outcome of infection. Int J Obes (Lond). 2013;37:333–40. https://doi.org/10.1038/ijo.2012.62.
31. Semins MJ, Shore AD, Makary MA, Weiner J, Matlaga BR. The impact of obesity on urinary tract infection risk. Urology. 2012;79:266–9. https://doi.org/10.1016/j.urology.2011.09.040.
32. Marik PE, Desai H. Characteristics of patients with the "malignant obesity hypoventilation syndrome" admitted to an ICU. J Intensive Care Med. 28:124–30. https://doi.org/10.1177/0885066612444261.
33. Gharib M, Kaul S, LoCurto J, Perez M, Hajri T. The obesity factor in critical illness: between consensus and controversy. J Trauma Acute Care Surg. 2015;78:866–73. https://doi.org/10.1097/TA.0000000000000597.
34. Wacharasint P, Boyd JH, Russell JA, Walley KR. One size does not fit all in severe infection: obesity alters outcome, susceptibility, treatment, and inflammatory response. Crit Care. 2013;17:R122. https://doi.org/10.1186/cc12794.
35. Lemmens HJM, Ingrande J. Pharmacology and obesity. Int Anesthesiol Clin. 2013;51:52–66. https://doi.org/10.1097/AIA.0b013e31829a4d56.
36. Mitrov-Winkelmolen L, van Buul-Gast M-CW, Swank DJ, Overdiek HWPM, van Schaik RHN, Touw DJ. The effect of roux-en-Y gastric bypass surgery in morbidly obese patients on pharmacokinetics of (acetyl)salicylic acid and omeprazole: the ERY-PAO study. Obes Surg. 2016;26:2051–8. https://doi.org/10.1007/s11695-016-2065-8.
37. Donohoe CL, Feeney C, Carey MF, Reynolds JV. Perioperative evaluation of the obese patient. J Clin Anesth. 2011;23:575–86. https://doi.org/10.1016/j.jclinane.2011.06.005.
38. Schaefer GP, Pender J, Toschlog EA, Waibel BH, Cohen KC. Endoscopically-assisted tube thoracostomy placement in a super-morbidly obese patient with penetrating thoracoabdominal trauma. Am Surg. 2011;77:119–20.
39. Gaarder C, Kroepelien CF, Loekke R, Hestnes M, Dormage JB, Naess PA. Ultrasound performed by radiologists-confirming the truth about FAST in trauma. J Trauma. 2009;67:323–7. ; discussion 328-9. https://doi.org/10.1097/TA.0b013e3181a4ed27.
40. Tsai P-JS, Loichinger M, Zalud I. Obesity and the challenges of ultrasound fetal abnormality diagnosis. Best Pract Res Clin Obstet Gynaecol. 2015;29:320–7. https://doi.org/10.1016/j.bpobgyn.2014.08.011.
41. Sakai H, Sheer TA, Mendler MH, Runyon BA. Choosing the location for non-image guided abdominal paracentesis. Liver Int. 2005;25:984–6. https://doi.org/10.1111/j.1478-3231.2005.01149.x.

53 Care of the Elderly Critical Care Patient

Christos Colovos, Nicolas Melo, and Daniel Margulies

Introduction

Critical care poses significant challenges for all patients. However, the elderly population requires extra vigilance owing to age-related changes in physiology, multiple medical comorbidities, polypharmacy, and deconditioning. The elderly, defined here as persons 65 years or older, account for 14.5% of the population and account for 42–52% of ICU admissions. The impact of the elderly will dramatically increase as their population will double to 70 million in 2030. Given increasing life expectancy (78.8 years in the United States), and the fact that this segment of the population accounts for 42–52% of ICU admissions [1, 2], the impact on health care and critical care is immense. Mortality is increased in the elderly, and studies demonstrate an 18.7% mortality for surgical patients, up to 26.5% ICU mortality for medical cause, and up to 50% mortality 1 year after discharge [1–3]. Aging affects every system in the body, and combined with comorbidities, multiple medications, and frequent end-of-life ethical issues, caring for these patients poses significant challenges in today's health-care environment [4–13]. Knowing how to care for this special population with age-related physiologic changes and a lack of physiologic reserve compared to the general population is of paramount importance.

C. Colovos
Department of Surgery, Cedars-Sinai Medical Center, Los Angeles, CA, USA

N. Melo
Department of Surgery, Division of Acute Care Surgery, Cedars-Sinai Medical Center, Los Angeles, CA, USA

D. Margulies (✉)
Section of Trauma, Emergency Surgery & Surgical Intensive Care and Professor of Surgery, Cedars-Sinai Medical Center, Los Angeles, CA, USA

University of California at Los Angeles David Geffen School of Medicine, Los Angeles, CA, USA
e-mail: daniel.margulies@cshs.org

Cardiovascular

Cardiovascular comorbidities are prevalent in the elderly. In the United States, 50% of all heart failure patients occur in patients aged over 70, with 90% of deaths due to heart failure in patients older than 65 years old [14]. Coronary artery disease occurs in 21.1% of men and 10.6% of women aged 60–79 – increasing for those older than 80 to 34.6% of men and 18.6% of women [15, 16]. Ventricular changes from impaired contractility and relaxation result in reduced systolic and diastolic function with an increased atrial dependence for stroke volume augmentation. There is a blunted baroreceptor reflex and decreased adrenergic responsiveness with a decreased reliance on heart rate in times of physiologic stress. Furthermore, medication used to treat chronic medical conditions in the elderly can further blunt compensatory mechanisms. Conduction abnormalities arise from changes in surrounding autonomic tissue and lead to an increased incidence of sick sinus syndromes, atrial arrhythmias, and bundle branch blocks [6]. Understanding these physiologic changes due to aging combined with systemic stress responses from critical illness is vital in improving outcomes and quality of care.

Changes in Cardiac Function

Structural and functional cardiovascular changes occur in aging and have implications for critical care management. With aging, there is a depressed myocardial contractility and decreased ventricular compliance from progressive muscular degeneration and increased collagen deposition [17]. Myocardial thickness increases due to cardiomyocyte hypertrophy from increased collagen deposition with an overall depletion of myocytes [18]. This is predominantly focused in the intraventricular septum and results in the heart changing shape from elliptical to spheroid – affecting ventricular compliance and intraventricular dependence [18]. Cardiac reserve is substantially diminished and contributes to

A. Salim et al. (eds.), *Surgical Critical Care Therapy*, https://doi.org/10.1007/978-3-319-71712-8_53

increased cardiac dysfunction in types of physiologic stress (e.g., sepsis, acute blood loss, hypoxia, or hypovolemia).

Cardiac output (CO) and ejection fraction (EF) are maintained in times of rest. In the elderly, hypertension, ventricular myocyte hypertrophy, and increased resistance to ventricular emptying owing to stiffening of the ventricular outflow tract and arteries exacerbate heart failure in times of stress [6, 19]. Acute stress response from illness, trauma, or even with exercise result can result in decreased cardiac output [6, 20]. Oxygen delivery (VO_2max) progressively decreases with age starting between 20 and 30 years old and continues to decrease by 10% per decade [21]. Although it is observed that stroke volume (SV) is generally preserved with aging, decreased CO is predominantly due to impaired heart-rate acceleration (or maximal heart rate). Multiple factors including increased vascular afterload, reduced myocardial contractility, impaired autonomic regulation, and physical deconditioning contribute to the reduction of cardiac reserve as evidenced by decreased VO_2max.

Although systolic function at rest is preserved with aging, diastolic dysfunction worsens with age and is responsible of nearly 50% of heart failure cases in the aged [22, 23]. Since ventricular relaxation is more energy dependent than ventricular contraction, myocardial hypoxia increases end-diastolic pressure (EDP), exacerbates pulmonary congestion, and results in increasing hypoxia. Cardiac filling decreases with age, primarily from impaired diastolic filling and increased isovolumic relaxation time [24]. This contributes to significant atrial enlargement contributing a greater proportion of total end-diastolic volume as ventricular filling shifts to later in diastole.

Compensatory sympathetic stimulation from β-adrenergic stimulation decreases with age as the myocardium has a blunted response to catecholamines [19, 25]. Changes in cardiac conduction system develop with the age-related increase in collagen and from cardiac myocyte fibrosis. This can result in AV nodal conduction abnormalities and AV block. Lipomatous deposition around the SA node with age can lead to bradyarrhythmias. Additionally, there is a decrease in pacemaker cells that can limit compensatory sympathetic stimulation and a reduction in calcium channel proteins which suppress action potentials and propagation [19, 26]. In addition to a blunted response to catecholamines, with aging, the baroreceptor reflux is blunted and may contribute to syncope from orthostatic hypotension with the loss of compensatory cardiac chronotropy [27–29].

With aging, CO becomes dependent upon preload which is augmented by increasing ventricular filling and stroke volume [4]. Preload dependence makes CO sensitive to volume status. In critical illnesses, fluid resuscitation for hypovolemia to preserve CO is essential. However, avoidance of hypervolemia is equally essential since the elderly are particularly at risk of developing pulmonary congestion and subsequent heart failure. Complicating the care of the elderly is that a significant number take medications (e.g., β-blockers, calcium channel blockers, digoxin) that can further blunt or inhibit compensatory tachycardia from hypovolemia. Autoregulation of coronary blood flow is affected by a coronary artery disease. With increased myocardial activity from critical illness, increased myocardial oxygen demand with decreased VO_2max can result in cardiac ischemia and heart failure.

Arrhythmias

The prevalence of clinically significant arrhythmias increases with age [15]. The most common arrhythmia is atrial fibrillation (AF), occurring in up to 12% of individuals above 85 years of age [15]. Numerous factors likely contribute to the increase in AF prevalence with age, including an increased prevalence of comorbid conditions, such as hypertension, diabetes, thyrotoxicosis, and mitral valve disorders. Age-related increase in left ventricular stiffness, with resulting diastolic dysfunction and elevated left atrial pressure contributes to age-related changes in the cardiac conduction system.

As a result of the previously described changes in the cardiac conduction system, a number of changes occur in cardiac electrical properties as demonstrated by EKG. Although the R-R interval does not change with age, there is a decrease in its variation with respiration and an increase in sinus bradycardia due to decreased parasympathetic activity and pathologic sick sinus syndrome [30]. The P-R interval increases with age, while the QRS axis shifts left secondary to increased LV wall thickness, and although not clinically significant, there is an increase in nonspecific ST-T [15, 31, 32].

With increased age, atrial arrhythmias, atrial fibrillation (AF), paroxysmal supraventricular tachycardia (pSVT), and ventricular arrhythmias (VA) are more frequently observed [15, 31]. AF afflicts approximately 4% of patients over 60 and 15% over 85, representing a tenfold increased rate over the general population. The increased rate of AF in the elderly arises from atrial distention from large-volume resuscitation, acute changes in inflammatory cytokines (IL-6, IL-8), changes in endogenous catecholamine release, fluid and electrolyte shifts, hypoxia, and hypercarbia [33–35]. As a consequence of increased rates of atrial fibrillation in the elderly, these patients are often on chronic anticoagulation and can pose challenges in the acutely bleeding patient or in traumas.

Arterial Changes in Aging

Arteries are dynamic structures that can adapt to stimuli, remodel, repair, and age. With aging, large arteries dilate and thicken. For example, the aortic root dilates by ~6% between 40 and 80 years old and stimulates LV hypertrophy given increased afterload [19]. It is recognized that the aorta thickens with time in healthy individuals by up to three times from adolescence to age 90. At the microscopic level, structural and functional changes occur with aging. Increases in arterial medial collagen content, nonenzymatic collagen cross-linking, and fraying of elastin fibrils result in hypertrophy and extracellular matrix accumulation and ultimately decreased distenisbility [36]. Additionally, calcium deposition and changes in the vascular endothelium also contribute to increased vascular stiffness [37, 38].

Further contributing to arterial age-relate are inflammatory stress responses from acute and chronic illnesses. Hypertension, hypercholesterolemia, and coronary/peripheral atherosclerosis result from endothelial dysfunction. Decreased concentrations of NO and expression of endothelial nitric oxide synthase (eNOS) reduce the ability of the arterial system to vasodilate further contributing to increases in hypertension and afterload [36, 37, 39]. With age, changes in the renin-angiotensin system (RAS) include increases of angiotensinogen, renin, angiotensin I and II, angiotensin-converting enzyme (ACE), angiotensin, and angiotensin II receptor (AT1) [40, 41]. For example, it is thought that increased angiotensin II level in aging arterial walls contributes to decreased plasma concentrations and increased expression of proteins important in extracellular remodeling including matrix metalloproteinase 2 and 9 (MMP-2 and MMP-9), monocyte chemotactic protein-1 (MCP-1), and transforming growth factor-beta 1 (TGF-β1) [40, 42].

Functionally, increased arterial stiffness and loss of wall compliance results increased systolic blood pressure (SPB), decreased diastolic blood pressure (DPB), and ultimately results in an increased pulse pressure. According to some studies, this increase in pulse pressure may be a more powerful predictor of cardiovascular events in older adults than changes in SBP or DBP [43]. Another consequence of arterial stiffness and loss of compliance is increasing arterial pulse wave velocity (PWV) [44]. It is recognized that reflected waves assist with coronary artery diastolic filling. However, with increased arterial stiffness, the reflected waves arrive at the coronary ostia during late systole, increasing ventricular afterload, failing to augment DBP, and compromising coronary blood flow. Studies reveal that PWV may be a predictor of future CV events, independent of blood pressure [45].

Critical Care Considerations

As described above, the aged patient lacks physiologic reserve. Maintenance of adequate preload, cardiac contractility, and afterload is paramount. Assessment of the patient begins with physical exam to determine signs and symptoms consistent with a shock state. This is complicated by the presence of age-related conditions that affect mental status including delirium and dementia. Chronic renal insufficiency and loss of glomerular function (described in the following sections) limit the use of urine output as an endpoint of resuscitation. Peripheral vascular and arterial disease can compound physical findings of cool extremities and weak pulses. Laboratory evaluation includes CBC with differential, ABG, and lactic acid to assist with diagnosing shock.

A strong consideration for invasive arterial blood pressure monitoring with an arterial line should be given to elderly patients with a diagnosis of shock or questionable hemodynamic status [46]. In a study by Scalea and co-workers, up to 50% of patients with "normal" blood pressure showed evidence for occult cardiogenic shock with invasive pulmonary artery monitoring [47]. Although numerous studies have questioned the benefit of pulmonary artery catheterization in light of increased complication rates, the interpretation of pulmonary artery pressures and cardiac function are vital to its successful use in determining a therapeutic plan. Pulmonary artery catheters are useful in patients with a concern for cardiogenic shock, the inability to confidently determine the patient's intravascular volume status, and actively make management decisions based upon pulmonary artery catheter parameters. Alternatively, bedside echocardiography is a quick, noninvasive test that can illuminate the intensivist toward cardiac function and volume status. Noninvasive monitoring devices that calculate stroke volume variance can also offer guidance to volume resuscitation. Some clinical studies comparing the accuracy of pulmonary artery catheters and noninvasive techniques measuring change in stroke volume variation (ΔSVV), SvO2, and change in pulse pressure variation (ΔPPV) show equivalence and possibly improved outcomes in the elderly and surgical patients [48–52].

Pulmonary

In the elderly, several morphological changes reduce the respiratory efficiency of the chest wall and diaphragm. Most of the aging-associated changes in the respiratory system evolve from a decrease in chest wall compliance, reduced static elastic lung recoil, and weakened respiratory muscles. The cross-sectional areas of the intercostal muscles start to decrease after the age 50. There appears to be no change in the thickness of the diaphragm with age. However, structural changes in the chest wall reduce the curvature of the diaphragm and maximal transdiaphragmatic pressure which results in a reduction in respiratory muscle strength. Decreased intercostal muscle mass and strength, calcification of rib cage cartilage and vertebral articulations, narrowing of intervertebral disk spaces, and osteoporosis contribute to reduced chest wall compliance. Increasing thoracic kyphosis results in decreased mechanical advantage for the diaphragm further impeding inspiration [53–56]. At rest, this can predispose the elderly to muscle fatigue resulting in nearly at 50% decrease in maximal inspiratory and expiratory force. In spite of accessory muscle use, these changes can significantly affect pulmonary function in acute illnesses [57–59].

Decreased static elastic recoil of the lung with age contributes to decreased tidal volume (Vt) and an increase in respiratory rate (RR) that increases breathing-related energy expenditure by 20% [53]. Sarcopenia with aging results in loss of fast-twitch muscle mass, decreased muscle energy production, and decreased muscle protein synthesis [60–64]. As a result, during stress there is an impaired ability to maintain minute ventilation that is exacerbated by decreased maximum inspiratory and expiratory pressures generated [53]. In trauma patients, 71% of 149 severely injured elderly patients (median age 79 years) were sarcopenic [65]. Multivariate linear regression demonstrated that sarcopenia was associated with decreased ventilator-free ($P = 0.004$) and ICU-free days ($P = 0.002$) [65].

Tracheobronchial and pulmonary parenchyma change with aging in addition to the previously described chest wall changes. The diameter of bronchioles decreases, while alveolar diameter increases resulting in an increased resistance to airflow and reduction of alveolar surface area, respectively [53, 61]. A form of obstructive airway disease known as "senile emphysema" arises from dynamic collapse of bronchioles <2 mm in diameter owing to a decrease in supporting tissue. In association with structural remodeling, pulmonary arterial pressure and pulmonary wedge pressure become significantly elevated after 50 years. Gas exchange is also compromised with reduced pulmonary capillary volume and number. These changes result in predictable changes in P_aO_2, decreased DLCO, and increased work of breathing.

Compensation for increased pulmonary demands is decreased in the elderly. Responses to hypoxia and hypercapnia are blunted due to changes in chemoreceptor function. The response to hypoxemia and hypercapnia is significantly reduced as compared to younger patients. This may permit elderly patients who are hypoxic or hypercapnic not to manifest clinical signs such as tachypnea through age-related CNS changes [58]. As a result of decreased pulmonary function and a lack of adequate compensatory mechanisms, the elderly require careful monitoring and vigilance for respiratory collapse.

Centrally, cough reflexes are less forceful and productive in the elderly. Cough sensation is suppressed, and due to decreased muscle strength, the motor component of the cough reflex that aids in airway clearance is also less effective. Weakening of the cough reflex could be a factor in the higher incidence of aspiration pneumonia in older patients [66, 67]. Additionally, loss of fast-twitch muscle fibers and decreased maximum expiratory pressure combined with decreased ciliary motility and mucus production from the tracheobronchial tree further diminish clearance of mucus [53, 67]. Impaired clearance of mucus and secretions along with blunting of an immune response to pathogens predisposes geriatric patients to increased frequency of pulmonary infections [54]. Pneumonia in the elderly is associated with a sixfold increased mortality and 16% lower quality of life in the post-discharge year among patients surviving hospitalization for community-acquired pneumonia [68]. In ventilator-associated pneumonia (VAP), mortality among patients was higher among elderly patients accounting for a 20% increase in the elderly (35% vs. 51%). Thus strategies to prevent, identify, and treat VAP is paramount [69]. Acute respiratory distress syndrome (ARDS) has also become increasingly prevalent in the geriatric population, and historically the mortality rate was up to 80%, but with protocol-driven treatment and early recognition, recent studies demonstrate mortality as low as 50% [70].

Critical Care Considerations

Foremost in managing elderly patients with pulmonary pathology is optimizing gas exchange. Every decade there is an age-related decrease of PaO2 due to decreased efficiency of gas exchange. Simple maneuvers to prevent atelectasis can improve ventilation-perfusion matching (V/Q matching) and include (a) raising the head end of the bed 30° [71, 72], (b) incentive spirometry to promote alveolar re-expansion [73–75] and pulmonary toilet to clear secretions [76, 77], and (c) minimizing sedation adequately – emphasizing non-narcotics, local nerve blocks, and epidural anesthesia. These maneuvers also can decrease the incidence of aspiration that is a common cause of respiratory failure. Additionally, evidence suggests early gastrostomy, avoidance of long-term nasogastric tubes [78], and early detection of high gastric residuals [79–82] from tube feedings can decrease aspiration risks. Avoiding prolonged intubation may decrease the risk for microaspiration [83] as does oral decontamination with chlorhexidine gluconate [84]. The IHI VAP bundle which includes elevation of the head of the bead, daily sedation holidays, appropriate PUD and DVT prophylaxis, and oral hygiene studies demonstrate statistically significantly decreased VAP rates [85].

The decision to provide supplemental noninvasive or invasive positive-pressure ventilation is based on early detection of respiratory compromise. Factors independent of surgical considerations should be evaluated when deciding to provide invasive positive-pressure ventilation versus noninvasive ventilation such as BiPAP or CPAP. Should mechanical ventilation be required, this decision must be tempered by life expectancy, patient/family wishes, advanced directives, and prognosis [86]. Intubated elderly patients have a significant mortality – up to 30–67% for patients aged 85–89 and up to 75% for those over 90 [87]. In a study of ARDS patients, age > 70 was associated with increased overall mortality, increased in-hospital mortality, increased ICU stay, and decreased ventilator-free days [88]. Failure to liberate from mechanical ventilation can be improved with tracheostomy but is associated with a mortality rate upward of 75% in 3 months and 93% in a year [89, 90]. Decision to perform a tracheostomy must be in line with the patient's wishes, goals of care, and minimal acceptable outcomes. Noninvasive mechanical ventilation in select patient populations may act as a palliative bridge avoiding endotracheal intubation and is associated with decreased mortality in COPD patients [91–93].

Signs such as changes in mental status and vital signs may be subtle and are exacerbated by pulmonary infections. Often only subtle mental status changes and increasing agitation are noted. When there is a clinical suspicion for infection, early identification of sources including pneumonia, tracheobronchitis, pharyngitis, or sinusitis should be undertaken. If clinical suspicion is high for a respiratory infection, deep tracheal aspirates for cultures should be obtained and empiric antibiotics started based upon hospital antibiograms. Consideration to cover methicillin-resistant *Staphylococcus aureus* (MRSA) and hospital-acquired multidrug-resistant gram-negative organisms (MDRO) should be strongly considered in patients with recent hospitalizations, skilled nursing facility boarding, and recent antibiotic use.

Renal

In the absence of an intrinsic disease, the kidney undergoes age-dependent structural and functional alterations leading to a significant decrease in renal mass, functioning nephrons, and baseline kidney function. The incidence of sclerotic glomeruli rises with advancing age, increasing from less than 5% of the total glomeruli at the age of 40 years to 10–30% by the eighth decade of life. Overall the incidence of acute kidney injury (AKI) has increased with increasing life expectancy and the use of nephrotoxic therapies [94–97]. Renal dysfunction is common (~66%) in the ICU, and upwards of 5% of patients will require some sort of renal replacement therapy (RRT) [98]. Multiples studies confirm increased mortality, hospital length of stay, ventilator days, and costs in patients with AKI [99–102]. One in five patients that require RRT in the ICU becomes dialysis dependent with a 50–60% mortality rate [98, 103–105].

In critical illnesses or trauma, hypovolemia, malnourishment, shock and baseline cardiovascular disease, congestive heart failure, and pre-existing kidney disease can further increase AKI risk [106, 107]. With aging, there is a variable decrease in glomerular filtration rate (GFR) [16, 108, 109]. The number of functioning glomeruli declines roughly in proportion with the changes in renal weight, whereas the size of the remaining glomeruli increases. As renal mass declines, the ability to clear creatinine is reduced. Measuring serum creatinine (SrCr) as a surrogate for renal function is difficult to interpret in the elderly as decreasing total lean body mass reduces SrCr – which is further reduced in critical illness [110–112].

The ability to regulate electrolyte homeostasis decreases as the kidney ages. Sodium reabsorption decreases with age – affecting up to 85% of the aged – and results in inability to maximally concentrate urine and promoting dehydration. Decreased responsiveness to antidiuretic hormone (ADH) can result in chronic hyponatremia and is more susceptible to becoming hyperkalemic [106, 107, 109]. This hypovolemic state can be exacerbated by underlying congestive heart disease and increases the risk of ischemic and nephrotoxic-induced nephropathy [106, 109, 113]. In resuscitation for hypovolemia, the goal is euvolemia to minimize tissue edema which can further exacerbate end-organ dysfunction [114–116]. Furthermore, infection or sepsis is associated with nearly 50% of ICU patients developing AKI [117–121]. As a consequence, understanding age-related changes in kidney function can augment strategies aimed at minimizing renal insults resulting in AKI and maximizing outcomes.

Critical Care Considerations

Treatment is supportive, as summarized by the Kidney Disease: Improving Global Outcomes (KDIGO) clinical practice guidelines that recommend avoiding nephrotoxins, maintaining euvolemia, avoiding the use of diuretics, avoiding hyperglycemia, and providing adequate nutrition [122]. Although it may be beneficial to use diuretics in managing pulmonary edema, studies reveal that there is neither decreased mortality nor RRT utilization, with the use of diuretics [123, 124]. The indications for RRT are renal support for conditions including severe electrolyte derangements, acidosis, congestive heart failure, liver failure, and multi-organ failure [125–127]. Early initiation of RRT may have superior outcomes and be associated with decreased mortality, shorter lengths of stay, and decreased RRT utilization [118, 128]. Survival rates between intermittent hemodialysis (iHD) and continuous renal replacement therapy (RRT) are similar [126, 128, 129].

Endpoints to discontinue RRT, especially CRRT, are ill-defined. Failure to recover renal function in the elderly following RRT is increased when compared to younger patients [130], is associated with 33% in-hospital mortality [131], and carries approximately 8 months median survival [132]. Long-term use of CRRT (>7d) was observed to carry a 100% mortality rate in non-liver transplant surgical ICU patients and was associated with an increased adjusted odds ratio of death [OR:1.39 (95% CI, 1.01–1.90; $P = 0.04$)] [133]. Because of the morbidity and mortality associated with AKI and RRT in the elderly, the decision to initiate and withdraw RRT is a challenging ethical consideration. Supportive or hospice care may be a consideration in elderly patients with a limited life expectancy or with an expected unacceptable quality of life, while transitioning to iHD may be acceptable for others [134–136].

Gastrointestinal and Nutrition

With aging there are profound changes in motility, nutrient absorption, and gut-associated immunity. Esophageal function displays impaired motility, increased esophageal pressurization, and decreased LES relaxation and results in dysphagia [137, 138]. Gastric acid secretion decreases, affecting the absorption of iron and other vitamins. Gastric emptying appears to be unaffected with age. Small-bowel motility transit time is unaffected by aging, but migrating motor complexes become less frequent. It is at the colon, however, that motility decreases in the elderly and results in constipation [139]. Enteral absorption of nutrients is hampered by mucosal atrophy. The gut microbiome has been postulated to change with aging, and may attenuate mucosal immunity [140–142]. Taken together these changes contribute to malnutrition and pathology in the elderly.

Elderly patients are more sensitive to changes in intestinal motility and are subjected to higher rates of postoperative and narcotic-induced ileus [143–146]. Ogilvie syndrome, also known as acute intestinal pseudo-obstruction, is attributed to enteric dysautonomia and results in a severe ileus of the large bowel and is not uncommon in the elderly and critically ill [147, 148]. Bowel perforation from Ogilvie's can result in mortality rates as high as 40% [149, 150]. Management is supportive, but care must be made to initiate bowel decompression prior to impending perforation. Neostigmine is used to treat Ogilvie's owing to a parasympathomimetic stimulation of colonic intestinal motility [151]. Side effects of neostigmine include potentiation of baseline cardiac arrhythmias including severe bradyarrhythmias. When administering neostigmine, the patient must be placed on continuous telemetry, and atropine should be readily available.

Malnutrition can be defined as weight loss ≥5% in 1 month or ≥10% in 6 months, body mass index <21 (note: BMI ≥21 does not exclude malnutrition), and serum albumin concentrations <3.5 mg/l. Severe malnutrition can be defined as weight loss of ≥10% in 1 month or ≥15% in 6 months, BMI <18, and serum albumin <3.0 mg/l. The elderly have impaired ability to maintain weight via increased food intake, even after periods of starvation, owing to changes in metabolism. Loss of skeletal muscle, or sarcopenia, is a well-known consequence of aging. Patients may lose up to 6 pounds of lean mass per decade after age 50 [152, 153].

Depending on criteria used, the prevalence of malnutrition ranges from as low as 5% to 12% among elderly patients in the general population to as high as 52–85% among institutionalized geriatric patients [154, 155]. Elderly patients at higher risk for malnutrition include those with poor social and financial situations, dementia, and neurological disorders. Depression is thought to be the most common cause of involuntary weight loss and malnutrition in older adults.

The causes are multifactorial and include limitations in activities of daily living and functional limitations in addition to physiologic changes. With age, the basal metabolic rate (BMR) decreases, total body fat increases, and protein content decreases [156]. Patients with swallowing and mastication impairment are at risk from malnutrition due to dietary modification or food avoidance. Impaired cognition can also be a result of malnutrition. Dementia can cause impairment of food intake by failure to remember to eat or prepare meals. Dementia can be complicated by swallowing difficulties. Caloric and protein intake are affected with changes in taste, smell, and regulation of the hunger response. These changes are further exacerbated with chronic medical conditions and critical illnesses. Dysphagia, early satiety, and altered bowel habits are common and are related to esophageal and colonic dysmotility, dyspepsia, reflux, atrophic gastritis, lactose intolerance, bacterial overgrowth, and the use of laxatives to treat chronic constipation.

Assessing nutritional status in the elderly is challenging. The utility of body mass index in assessing nutritional status has its limitations in the elderly due to loss of muscle mass owing to an age-related decrease in appetite and energy intake, where the average daily energy intake decreases by 30% up until 80 years of age. This decrease in energy intake coincides with the age-associated decline in energy expenditure and contributes to weight loss in this population. Body weight and BMI increase until age 60 and then decline. BMR can be estimated through a variety of equations that estimate resting energy expenditure such as the Harris-Benedict equation. These equations are confounded by a number of factors including obesity/cachexia, volume overload, metabolic stress from infection, surgery, or other critical illnesses. The most accurate method to determine BMR is indirect calorimetry [157, 158]. Screening tools described in the literature for the elderly include the Mini Nutritional Assessment (MNA) and the Nutrition Risk in the Critically Ill (NUTRIC) [159]. Standard markers for malnutrition include albumin ($t_{1/2}$ = 20–21 days) and prealbumin ($t_{1/2}$ = 2 days). Transferrin ($t_{1/2}$ = 8–10 days) is not accurate in the elderly owing to falsely normal levels in malnourished elderly patients with low iron stores. The use of C-reactive protein can distinguish between decreased levels of nutritional markers owing to an inflammatory state.

Owing to malnutrition, changes in BMR, anorexia to food, and impaired GI function, protein, calorie, and vitamin deficiencies are common. Decreased appetite, the inability to chew certain foods (e.g., fresh fruits and vegetables), and the increased incidence of lactose intolerance contribute to these deficiencies. Iron, folate, and vitamin B12 are the predominant vitamins found to be deficient. Up to 20% of geriatric patients are deficient in vitamin B12 – thought to be caused by achlorhydria that decreases secretion of intrinsic factor. Vitamin D is often deficient owing to limited exposure to sunlight, decreased consumption of dairy products, and lactose intolerance. In addition to vitamin C deficiency, elderly patients with a poor diet are at risk for vitamin K deficiency, which is important for clotting factors and the mechanism of vitamin K antagonists such as warfarin [160–162].

Critical Care Considerations

All patients admitted to the ICU should be assessed for the risk of malnutrition. A careful history detailing prehospitalization/illness nutritional intake, assessment of anthropometric data, and nutrition laboratories (albumin, prealbumin, iron panel, vitamin B12, folate, vitamin D) should be performed. Nutritional supplementation with protein-rich liquids is routinely used in the inpatient setting and has demonstrated benefits in the postoperative period in hospitalized patients. Appetite stimulants (e.g., megestrol acetate) can improve appetite and well-being with no overall increase in weight gain or survival. It must be used with caution as side effects such as deep vein thrombosis, adrenal suppression, and hypoglycemia are not uncommon. In patients unable to tolerate enteral nutrition, parental nutrition can be offered.

Enteral feeding is common in the elderly patients and has shown to improve outcome in non-demented and malnourished patients; its role in elderly patient with dementia is still controversial. There is no evidence that tube feeding would prevent aspiration pneumonia, prolong survival, or provide palliation in patients with advanced dementia [108, 163–170]. The decision to offer nutrition in the terminally ill should only be used when it would improve the quality of life.

Advanced directives and discussions with surrogate decision-makers are important prior to any permanent enteral access is established as to be in line with the wishes of the patient [171].

Hematologic

Given the physiologic changes that occur with aging, it is not surprising that anemia and thrombocytopenia are seen in the elderly population–occuring in more than 10% of adults age 65 years and older and exceeding 20% in those 85 years and older. In nursing homes, anemia is present in 48–63% of residents. Though anemias are multifactorial resulting from iron, folate, vitamin B12 deficiency, and renal insufficiency or chronic inflammation. The predominant cause of anemia in the elderly is decreased stem cell proliferation [172–174]. This decreased stem cell proliferation results in elevated erythropoietin levels in the eldery [174]. As a result of anemia, the physiologic response to acute blood loss in the aged is compromised.

Pharmacologic anticoagulation and antiplatelet therapy is commonly seen in the elderly population, as atrial fibrillation, coronary artery disease, deep vein thrombosis (DVT), and strokes are some of the more common comorbidities present. It doesn't help that this population is also more prone to accidents secondary to falls and have bones that are less dense, making the elderly patient more prone to bleeding when these agents are present [175]. Interestingly, age is a risk factor for DVT, and if combined with a traumatic injury, the risk increases [176].

Warfarin can be readily reversed by administering prothrombin concentrates (PCC), fresh frozen plasma (FFP), and vitamin K. FFP has a disadvantage in that it has to be thawed and is colloid, which delays reversal and for older frail patients accounts for a significant volume challenge for the aging heart. Aspirin and clopidogrel irreversibly bind to platelets, and thus administration of platelets is the only reversal agent available in the emergency setting. Heparin can be reversed with protamine, and the low molecular weight heparins do not have specific reversal agents [177].

The non-vitamin K antagonist oral anticoagulants (NOACs) can pose challenges in the bleeding geriatric ICU patient. NOACs are approved for the treatment of atrial fibrillation and venous thromboembolic disease and in studies revealed equivalence or increased efficacy in preventing CVAs in atrial fibrillation patients and venous thromboembolic disease [178–185]. The documented benefits, in addition to decreased bleeding events, are as follows: there is often no need for bridging therapy, they have limited drug interactions, they do not require routine laboratory monitoring, and they have predictable pharmacokinetic/pharmacodynamic profiles [186, 187].

In the geriatric trauma patient population, there is an increased utilization of NOACs and until recently presented a challenge to reverse NOAC anticoagulation. Dabigatran can now be reversed with the use of idarucizumab and its effectiveness monitored with thrombin time or ecarin clotting time. Direct factor Xa inhibitors have no specific reversal agent, but their effects can be used with inactivated 3- or 4-factor protein C concentrate (PCC) or activated PCC (aPCC; factor VIII inhibitor activity bypassing agent (FEIBA)) [188–190]. Other therapies to decrease pharmacologic-based bleeding include the use of recombinant activated factor VII (rFVIIa), tranexamic acid, or vasopressin (DDAVP) with limited efficacy.

Neurological and Psychiatric Changes

As persons are living longer, the prevalence of dementia and other neurodegenerative disorders increase in prevalence. In addition, the degree of polypharmacy and the degree of drug interactions, and impaired hepatic and renal clearance of all classes of medications, increase the risk of delirium. ICU delirium. This results in a prevalence of up to 28% in the elderly population, increases both morbidity and mortality [191, 192]. Strategies such as lessening centrally acting medications are potentially of benefit to this population [191, 193–195]. In addition, this population is at higher risk of aspiration and falls. Even a mild traumatic brain injury, regardless of gender, has a significant mortality [195–197].

Delirium can occur in up to 60% of elderly patients and up to 70% of surgical ICU patients [198, 199]. It is defined as an acute, fluctuating, transient, reversible syndrome of impairment of consciousness, attention, and perception Delirium is divided into three subtypes (hyperactive, hypoactive, and mixed). Delirium may occur following cognitive disorders, immobilization, metabolic derangements, sleep deprivation, age >65, hyper-/hypothermia, hypoxia, hypoglycemia, encephalopathy, CNS infections, seizures, or medications [200, 201]. Medications particularly linked to delirium are psychoactive drugs especially with anticholinergic mechanism of action [202]. Narcotics and sedatives can exacerbate delirium – especially when used to treat postoperative pain which also is an independent risk factor for delirium [203–205].

ICU delirium increases morbidity and mortality rates and results in significant increases in health-care costs [206, 207]. It is an independent predictor of worse global cognition and decreased functional status as measured by activities of daily living and impaired perception of motor sensory function [199, 208, 209]. A meta-analysis by Salluh et al. revealed that ICU patients who develop delirium have increased mortality (OR 2.19 (CI 1.78–2.70)), trend toward longer ICU lengths of stay (OR 1.38 (CI 0.99–1.77)), and trend toward longer ventilator dependence [210].

Diagnosis of delirium is challenging and results in underdiagnosis. All elderly patients should be screened for risk factors and the presence of delirium. Recommended tools include clinical assessment by DSM-IV criteria (disturbance of consciousness, change in cognition, development over a short period, and fluctuation) [211] or the use of the *Confusion Assessment Method* (*CAM*). Intubated or postoperative patients should be screened with CAM-ICU [212–214].

Treatment of delirium is also challenging. It is often preferable to minimize risk factors that may result in a delirious state rather than initiate pharmacologic therapy as a front-line therapy. These maneuvers include frequent reorientations to time, place, and condition, continuity of caregivers, maintenance of circadian rhythms, and avoiding medications associated with delirium. Analgesia should be tailored and minimize the use of opioids and sedatives [215]. Elderly patients should be monitored for hypoxia and infections which also can manifest as delirium. Functional impairments, visual, auditory, and mobility should be addressed and optimized. Should the patient remain delirious despite non-pharmacologic treatment, short-term medications may be indicated. Medications useful in the management of delirium include haloperidol or olanzapine. Should the delirium be caused by alcohol withdrawal, dexmedetomidine rather than benzodiazepine infusions are recommended, as benzodiazepines in the geriatric patient may exacerbate delirium [216].

Dementia is defined as multiple severe cognitive deficits representing a persistent declining functional status. It encompasses a spectrum of diseases including Alzheimer's disease, vascular disease, frontal lobe dementia, and Lewy body dementia. Alzheimer's disease (AD) affects more than 5 million people in the United States, affects one in ten people over 65 and 32% over 85, is the sixth leading cause of death in adults and the fifth leading cause of adults over 65, and results in increasing direct medical costs [217]. It is a progressive and irreversible disease resulting from neurofibrillary tangles and neuritic plaques [218]. Vascular dementia includes multi-infarct dementia and small vessel disease. Cardiovascular risk factors such as diabetes, hypertension, dyslipidemia, smoking, and inactivity increase the risk for vascular dementia. Defects are related to the location of infarction and include language problems (left-sided lesions), visuospatial deficits (right-sided lesions), mood/memory deficits, and neurocognitive deficits. Lewy body dementia accounts for 20% of dementia and is characterized by visual hallucinations, fluctuating cognition, falls or syncope, and loss of consciousness. This form of dementia is characterized by hallmark protein located in the cortex and amygdala disrupting cholinergic and dopaminergic systems.

Degeneration of the frontotemporal lobe results in a heterogeneous group of dementias known as frontal lobe dementia affecting behavior and personality.

To diagnose dementia, reversible cognitive deficits must be first ruled out resulting from hypercapnia, hypoxemia, hypoglycemia, electrolyte disturbances, sepsis, and traumatic brain injury. The Mini-Mental State Examination (MMSE) is a short questionnaire that evaluates for dementia [219]. Mini-Cog is a shorter questionnaire including a three-item recall and clock drawing, with a higher sensitivity at 99% than the MMSE [220].

Treatment depends on the type of dementia and ideally includes a multidisciplinary approach with internists and neurologists, among others. Progression of AD and Lewy body dementia cognitive symptoms can be slowed with the use of cholinesterase inhibitors and memantine. Although Lewy body dementia motor symptoms may be improved with levodopa, this can exacerbate neuropsychiatric symptoms. Frontal lobe and vascular dementias have no specific treatment, and management is aimed at reducing risk factors. Acute treatment should be non-pharmacologic and includes frequent reorientation, preservation of the sleep-wake cycle, and regular meals. When medication is needed, atypical antipsychotics are preferred but carry a risk of extrapyramidal symptoms [221, 222]. Benzodiazepines and tricyclic antidepressants should be avoided as this may exacerbate agitation, sedation, confusion, motor impairment and result in anticholinergic effects.

Depression in the aged is common occurring over 5 million or 1 of 20 elderly adults and is increased in hospitalized patients or those receiving home health care [223]. Diagnosis includes depressed mood or anhedonia that cause decreased functional capacity. Risk factors for depression include dementia, stroke, Parkinson's disease, and cancer. Screening for depression is facilitated with a variety of tools including the Geriatric Depression Scale or diagnosis based on DSM-IV-TR criteria [211]. Patients at risk for depression should be evaluated by a psychiatrist to assist with medical management, cognitive and behavioral therapy, and psychotherapy.

Ethics, End-of-Life Care, and Advanced Directives

The principles of non-maleficence, confidentiality, beneficence, autonomy, and justice are the core pillars to medical ethics. In the elderly, these factors, along with severity of illness/injury, recuperative potential, and minimal expected outcome, shape discussions with family and patients alike regarding end-of-life care. Elderly patients should be assessed for cognition. This is important in determining if the patient has capacity to provide informed consent or if a surrogate decision-maker is needed to guide care [224, 225].

Decision-making capacity is central to patient autonomy, and determining if an elderly individual possesses capacity can be challenging. Capacity can be determined if the patient demonstrates understanding of the planned therapeutic course, ability to express a clear choice and rational for a choice when multiple options are presented, and appreciation of how these choices could affect the patient [226]. Unfortunately, with aging changes in cognition including delirium and dementia can limit decision-making capacity and competency to provide informed consent. When capacity is limited, advance directives and surrogate decision-makers are paramount to providing high-quality, ethical care to the geriatric patient.

The purpose of advance directives is to honor and respect a patient's values and beliefs in relationship to medical care. Advance directives include living wills, durable power of attorney (DPOA), and Physician Orders for Life-Sustaining Treatment (POLST). Living wills are a legal document outlining goals for medical therapy, resuscitation, and end-of-life care. Often, living wills name a DPOA as a medical decision-making surrogate to assist with decisions not specifically addressed in a living will when the patient lacks capacity or to address the patient's expressed minimal acceptable outcome following a critical illness.

In-line with honoring a patient's minimal acceptable outcome, the concepts of "do not resuscitate" and "medical futility" are important to understand. Patients have the right to refuse medical treatment given that they demonstrate capacity and informed consent is given including the risks, benefits, alternatives, complications, and expected outcomes. "Do not resuscitate" (DNR) limits resuscitation efforts including chest compressions, electrical defibrillation, medical interventions and endotracheal intubations. The patient, or decision-making surrogate, can limit all or some of these interventions for a cardiopulmonary arrest. Of note, physicians are not obligated to perform CPR in patients with a chronic, fatal, medical illness, or medical futility.

Futility is defined as the lack of significant medical benefit for a patient undergoing a medical intervention. Generally, futility is applied to specific interventions (i.e., continuation of CRRT, applying CPR to a moribund patient, etc.) that will not offer benefit to the person as a whole. In determining futility, there are multiple definitions including physiologic futility (intervention cannot achieve its desired clinical effect due to underlying physiologic derangements), clinical futility (clinical benefit will not achieve a minimal acceptable outcome regarding interaction of the patient with the surrounding environment), and qualitative futility (if the intervention could be physiologically and clinically effective but with significant morbidity that would limit future functional status and quality of life) [227]. A multidisciplinary approach is needed including the patient/medical decision surrogate, family, treating physicians, supportive care/palliative care providers, medical ethics, and occasionally risk management.

References

1. Ball IM, et al. Outcomes of elderly critically ill medical and surgical patients: a multicentre cohort study. Can J Anesth Can d'anesthésie. 2017;64:260–9.
2. Federal Interagency Forum on Aging-Related Statistics. Older Americans 2016: Key Indicators of Well-Being. U.S. Gov. Print. Off; 2016..
3. Sacanella E, et al. Functional status and quality of life 12 months after discharge from a medical ICU in healthy elderly patients: a prospective observational study. Crit Care. 2011;15:R105.
4. Menaker J, Scalea TM. Geriatric care in the surgical intensive care unit. Crit Care Med. 2010;38:S452–9.
5. Happ MB. Individualized care for frail older adults: challenges for health care reform in acute and critical care. Geriatr Nurs. 2010;31:63–5.
6. Marik PE. Management of the critically ill geriatric patient. Crit Care Med. 2006;34:S176–82.
7. Nagappan R, Parkin G. Geriatric critical care. Crit Care Clin. 2003;19:253–70.
8. Woll MM, Maerz LL. Surgical Critical Care for the Trauma Patient with Cardiac Disease. Anesthesiol Clin. 2016;34:669–80.
9. Walker M, Spivak M, Sebastian M. The impact of aging physiology in critical care. Crit Care Nurs Clin North Am. 2014;26:7–14.
10. Joyce MF, Reich JA. Critical care issues of the geriatric patient. Anesthesiol Clin. 2015;33:551–61.
11. Sjoding MW, Prescott HC, Wunsch H, Iwashyna TJ, Cooke CR. Longitudinal changes in ICU admissions among elderly patients in the United States. Crit Care Med. 2016;44:1353–60.
12. Moitra VK, Guerra C, Linde-Zwirble WT, Wunsch H. Relationship Between ICU Length of Stay and Long-Term Mortality for Elderly ICU Survivors. Crit Care Med. 2016;44:655–62. https://doi.org/10.1097/CCM.0000000000001480.
13. Neuman MD, Eckenhoff RG. Functional outcomes after critical illness in the elderly. Crit Care Med. 2015;43:1340–1.
14. Sandstede J, et al. Age- and gender-specific differences in left and right ventricular cardiac function and mass determined by cine magnetic resonance imaging. Eur Radiol. 2000;10:438–42.
15. Chow GV, Marine JE, Fleg JL. Epidemiology of arrhythmias and conduction disorders in older adults. Clin Geriatr Med. 2012;28:539–53.
16. Rangel EL. Future directions of geriatric trauma care: function and quality of life beyond survival. JAMA Surg. 2017;152:e164642.
17. Morley JE, Reese SS. Clinical implications of the aging heart. Am J Med. 1989;86:77–86.
18. Olivetti G, Melissari M, Capasso JM, Anversa P. Cardiomyopathy of the aging human heart. Myocyte loss and reactive cellular hypertrophy. Circ Res. 1991;68:1560–8.
19. Strait J, Lakatta E. Aging-associated cardiovascular changes and their relationship to heart failure. Heart Fail Clin. 2012;8:143–64.
20. Stratton JR, Levy WC, Cerqueira MD, Schwartz RS, Abrass IB. Cardiovascular responses to exercise. Effects of aging and exercise training in healthy men. Circulation. 1994;89:1648–55.
21. Schulman SP, et al. Age-related decline in left ventricular filling at rest and exercise. Am J Phys. 1992;263:H1932–8.
22. McGough MF. Heart failure with normal systolic function: a common disorder in older people. J Am Geriatr Soc. 1995;43:1035–42.
23. Kitzman DW, et al. Importance of heart failure with preserved systolic function in patients ≥65 years of age. Am J Cardiol. 2001;87:413–9.
24. Bryg RJ, Williams GA, Labovitz AJ. Effect of aging on left ventricular diastolic filling in normal subjects. Am J Cardiol. 1987;59:971–4.
25. Lakatta EG. Age-related alterations in the cardiovascular response to adrenergic mediated stress. Fed Proc. 1980;39:3173–7.
26. Kistler PM, et al. Electrophysiologic and electroanatomic changes in the human atrium associated with age. J Am Coll Cardiol. 2004;44:109–16.
27. Gribbin B, Pickering TG, Sleight P, Peto R. Effect of age and high blood pressure on Baroreflex sensitivity in man. Circ Res. 1971;29:424–31.
28. Shannon R, Wei J, Rosa R, Epstein FH. The effect of age and sodium depletion on cardiovascular response to Orthostasis. Hypertension. 1986;8:438–43.
29. Shimada K, Kitazumi T, Sadakane N, Ogura H, Ozawa T. Age-related changes of baroreflex function, plasma norepinephrine, and blood pressure. Hypertension. 1985;7:113–7.
30. Hiss RG, Lamb LE. Electrocardiographic findings in 122,043 individuals. Circulation. 1962;25:947–61.
31. Fleg JL, Das DN, Wright J, Lakatta EG. Age-associated changes in the components of atrioventricular conduction in apparently healthy volunteers. J Gerontol. 1990;45:M95–100.
32. Mihalick MJ, Fisch C. Electrocardiographic findings in the aged. Am Heart J. 1974;87:117–28.
33. Hadi HAR, Alsheikh-Ali AA, Mahmeed WAL, Al Suwaidi JM. Inflammatory cytokines and atrial fibrillation: current and prospective views. J Inflamm Res. 2010;3:75–97.
34. Solti F, Vecsey T, Kékesi V, Juhász-Nagy A. The effect of atrial dilatation on the genesis of atrial arrhythmias. Cardiovasc Res. 1989;23:882–6.
35. Amar D, Zhang H, Leung DHY, Roistacher N, Kadish AH. Older age is the strongest predictor of postoperative atrial fibrillation. Anesthesiology. 2002;96:352–6.
36. Lakatta EG, Levy D. Arterial and cardiac aging: major shareholders in cardiovascular disease enterprises: part I: aging arteries: a 'set up' for vascular disease. Circulation. 2003;107:139–46.
37. Ungvari Z, Kaley G, De Cabo R, Sonntag WE, Csiszar A. Mechanisms of vascular aging: new perspectives. J Gerontol A Biol Sci Med Sci. 2010;65A:1028–41.
38. Zieman SJ, Melenovsky V, Kass DA. Mechanisms, pathophysiology, and therapy of arterial stiffness. Arterioscler Thromb Vasc Biol. 2005;25:932–43.
39. Tschudi MR, et al. Effect of age on kinetics of nitric oxide release in rat aorta and pulmonary artery. J Clin Invest. 1996;98:899–905.
40. Wang M, et al. Aging increases aortic MMP-2 activity and angiotensin II in nonhuman primates. Hypertension. 2003;41:1308–16.
41. Wang M, Monticone RE, Lakatta EG. Arterial aging: a journey into subclinical arterial disease. Curr Opin Nephrol Hypertens. 2010;19:201–7.
42. Wang M, et al. Matrix metalloproteinase 2 activation of transforming growth factor-beta1 (TGF-beta1) and TGF-beta1-type II receptor signaling within the aged arterial wall. Arterioscler Thromb Vasc Biol. 2006;26:1503–9.
43. Roman MJ, et al. High central pulse pressure is independently associated with adverse cardiovascular outcome. The strong heart study. J Am Coll Cardiol. 2009;54:1730–4.
44. Vaitkevicius PV, et al. Effects of age and aerobic capacity on arterial stiffness in healthy adults. Circulation. 1993;88:1456–62.
45. Williams B, Lacy PS. Central haemodynamics and clinical outcomes: going beyond brachial blood pressure? Eur Heart J. 2010;31:1819–22.
46. Oleske DM, Wilson RS, Bernard BA, Evans DA, Terman EW. Epidemiology of injury in people with Alzheimer's disease. J Am Geriatr Soc. 1995;43:741–6.
47. Scalea TM, et al. Geriatric blunt multiple trauma: improved survival with early invasive monitoring. J Trauma-Injury Infect Crit Care. 1990;30:129–36.

48. Goedje O, et al. Continuous cardiac output by femoral arterial thermodilution calibrated pulse contour analysis: comparison with pulmonary arterial thermodilution. Crit Care Med. 1999;27:2407–12.
49. Halvorsen PS, et al. Agreement between PiCCO pulse-contour analysis, pulmonal artery thermodilution and transthoracic thermodilution during off-pump coronary artery by-pass surgery. Acta Anaesthesiol Scand. 2006;50:1050–7.
50. Brown CVR, Shoemaker WC, Wo CCJ, Chan L, Demetriades D. Is noninvasive hemodynamic monitoring appropriate for the elderly critically injured patient? J Trauma. 2005;58:102–7.
51. Shoemaker WC, et al. Noninvasive physiologic monitoring of high-risk surgical patients. Arch Surg (Chicago, Ill 1960). 1996;131:732–7.
52. Lopes MR, et al. Goal-directed fluid management based on pulse pressure variation monitoring during high-risk surgery: a pilot randomized controlled trial. Crit Care. 2007;11:R100.
53. Janssens J-P, Pache J-C, Nicod LP. Physiological changes in respiratory function associated with ageing. Eur Respir J. 1999;13:197–205.
54. Lowery EM, Brubaker AL, Kuhlmann E, Kovacs EJ. The aging lung. Clin Interv Aging. 2013;8:1489–96.
55. DeLorey DS, Babb TG. Progressive mechanical ventilatory constraints with aging. Am J Respir Crit Care Med. 1999;160:169–77.
56. Zeleznik J. Normative aging of the respiratory system. Clin Geriatr Med. 2003;19:1–18.
57. El Solh AA, Ramadan FH. Overview of respiratory failure in older adults. J Intensive Care Med. 2006;21:345–51.
58. Rosenthal RA, Kavic SM. Assessment and management of the geriatric patient. Crit Care Med. 2004;32:S92–S105.
59. Cheng S, et al. Age-related left ventricular remodeling and associated risk for cardiovascular outcomes: the multi-ethnic study of atherosclerosis. Circ Cardiovasc Imaging. 2009;2:191–8.
60. Hanna JS. Sarcopenia and critical illness: a deadly combination in the elderly. J Parenter Enter Nutr. 2015;39:273–81.
61. Janssens JP. Aging of the respiratory system: impact on pulmonary function tests and adaptation to exertion. Clin Chest Med. 2005;26:469–84.
62. Kaya RD, Nakazawa M, Hoffman RL, Clark BC. Interrelationship between muscle strength, motor units, and aging. Exp Gerontol. 2013;48:920–5.
63. Luff AR. Age-associated changes in the innervation of muscle fibers and changes in the mechanical properties of motor units. Ann N Y Acad Sci. 1998;854:92–101.
64. Galea V. Changes in motor unit estimates with aging. J Clin Neurophysiol. 1996;13:253–60.
65. Moisey LL, et al. Skeletal muscle predicts ventilator-free days, ICU-free days, and mortality in elderly ICU patients. Crit Care. 2013;17:R206.
66. Watsford ML, Murphy AJ, Pine MJ. The effects of ageing on respiratory muscle function and performance in older adults. J Sci Med Sport. 2007;10:36–44.
67. Lalley PM. The aging respiratory system-pulmonary structure, function and neural control. Respir Physiol Neurobiol. 2013;187:199–210.
68. Mangen M-JJ, Huijts SM, Bonten MJM, de Wit GA. The impact of community-acquired pneumonia on the health-related quality-of-life in elderly. BMC Infect Dis. 2017;17:208.
69. Blot S, et al. Prevalence, risk factors, and mortality for ventilator-associated pneumonia in middle-aged, old, and very old critically ill patients*. Crit Care Med. 2014;42:601–9.
70. Eachempati SR, Hydo LJ, Shou J, Barie PS. Outcomes of acute respiratory distress syndrome (ARDS) in elderly patients. J Trauma. 2007;63:344–50.
71. Kollef MH. Prevention of ventilator-associated pneumonia or ventilator-associated complications: a worthy, yet challenging, goal. Crit Care Med. 2012;40:271–7.
72. Niël-Weise BS, et al. An evidence-based recommendation on bed head elevation for mechanically ventilated patients. Crit Care. 2011;15:R111.
73. Lawrence VA, Cornell JE, Smetana GW, American College of Physicians. Strategies to reduce postoperative pulmonary complications after noncardiothoracic surgery: systematic review for the American College of Physicians. Ann Intern Med. 2006;144:596–608.
74. Pelus S. What the new guidelines offer for preoperative risk reduction. Patient Care. 2006;40:18–25.
75. Westwood K, et al. Incentive spirometry decreases respiratory complications following major abdominal surgery. Surgeon. 2007;5:339–42.
76. Allen GS, Coaxes NE. Pulmonary contusion: a collective review. Am Surg. 1996;62:895–900.
77. Michaels AJ. Management of post traumatic respiratory failure. Crit Care Clin. 2004;20:83–99.
78. Kostadima E, Kaditis AG, Alexopoulos EI, Zakynthinos E, Sfyras D. Early gastrostomy reduces the rate of ventilator-associated pneumonia in stroke or head injury patients. Eur Respir J. 2005;26:106–11.
79. Metheny NA, Schallom L, Oliver DA, Clouse RE. Gastric residual volume and aspiration in critically ill patients receiving gastric feedings. Am J Crit Care. 2008;17:512–9.
80. Pinilla J, Samphire J, Arnold C, Liu L, Thiessen B. Comparison of gastrointestinal tolerance to two enteral feeding protocols in critically ill patients: a prospective, randomized controlled trial. J Parenter Enter Nutr. 2001;25:81–6.
81. Bankhead R, et al. Enteral nutrition practice recommendations. J Parenter Enter Nutr. 2009;33:122–67.
82. Mcclave SA, et al. Guidelines for the provision and assessment of nutrition support therapy in the adult critically ill patient : Society of Critical Care Medicine (SCCM) and American. J Parenter Enter Nutr. 2016;33:277–316.
83. Hamilton VA, Grap MJ. The role of the endotracheal tube cuff in microaspiration. Heart Lung J Acute Crit Care. 2012;41:167–72.
84. Scannapieco F a, et al. A randomized trial of chlorhexidine gluconate on oral bacterial pathogens in mechanically ventilated patients. Crit Care. 2009;13:R117.
85. IHI. How-to guide: prevent ventilator–associated pneumonia. IHI, Ed. EUA;2006.
86. Nguyen Y-L, Angus DC, Boumendil A, Guidet B. The challenge of admitting the very elderly to intensive care. Ann Intensive Care. 2011;1:29.
87. Cohen IL, Lambrinos J. Investigating the impact of age on outcome of mechanical ventilation using a population of 41,848 patients from a statewide database. Chest. 1995;107:1673–80.
88. Ely EW, et al. Recovery rate and prognosis in older persons who develop acute lung injury and the acute respiratory distress syndrome. Ann Intern Med. 2002;136:25–36.
89. Drendel M, et al. Outcome of tracheostomy in patients over 85 years old (oldest-old patients). Otolaryngol Head Neck Surg. 2009;140:395–7.
90. Baskin JZ, Panagopoulos G, Parks C, Rothstein S, Komisar A. Clinical outcomes for the elderly patient receiving a tracheotomy. Head Neck. 2004;26:71–5.
91. Chandra D, et al. Outcomes of noninvasive ventilation for acute exacerbations of chronic obstructive pulmonary disease in the United States, 1998–2008. Am J Respir Crit Care Med. 2012;185:152–9.
92. Piroddi IMG, et al. Non-invasive mechanical ventilation in elderly patients: a narrative review. Geriatr Gerontol Int. 2017;17:689.

93. Bülow HH, Thorsager B. Non-invasive ventilation in do-not-intubate patients: five-year follow-up on a two-year prospective, consecutive cohort study. Acta Anaesthesiol Scand. 2009;53:1153–7.
94. Coca SG, Cho KC, Hsu C-Y. Acute kidney injury in the elderly: predisposition to chronic kidney disease and vice versa. Nephron Clin Pract. 2011;119(Suppl):c19–24.
95. Jacobson PA, et al. Genetic and clinical determinants of early, acute calcineurin inhibitor-related nephrotoxicity: results from a kidney transplant consortium. Transplantation. 2012;93:624–31.
96. Kuypers DRJ. Immunotherapy in elderly transplant recipients: a guide to clinically significant drug interactions. Drugs Aging. 2009;26:715–37.
97. Haase M, Story DA, Haase-Fielitz A. Renal injury in the elderly: diagnosis, biomarkers and prevention. Best Pract Res Clin Anaesthesiol. 2011;25:401–12.
98. Hoste E a J, Schurgers M. Epidemiology of acute kidney injury: how big is the problem? Crit Care Med. 2008;36:S146–51.
99. Chertow GM, Burdick E, Honour M, Bonventre JV, Bates DW. Acute kidney injury, mortality, length of stay, and costs in hospitalized patients. J Am Soc Nephrol. 2005;16:3365–70.
100. Brandt M-M, et al. Renal dysfunction in trauma: even a little costs a lot. J Trauma. 2007;62:1362–4.
101. Himmelfarb J. Acute kidney injury in the elderly: problems and prospects. Semin Nephrol. 2009;29:658–64.
102. Hobson C, et al. Cost and mortality associated with postoperative acute kidney injury. Ann Surg. 2015;261:1207–14.
103. Bagshaw SM, et al. Review article: renal support in critical illness. Can J Anesth. 2010;57:999–1013.
104. Palevsky PM, et al. Intensity of renal support in critically ill patients with acute kidney injury. N Engl J Med. 2008;359:7–20.
105. Linder A, et al. Small acute increases in serum creatinine are associated with decreased long-term survival in the critically ill. Am J Respir Crit Care Med. 2014;189:1075–81.
106. Rosner MH. Acute kidney injury in the elderly. Clin Geriatr Med. 2013;29:565–78.
107. Baldea AJ. Effect of aging on renal function plus monitoring and support. Surg Clin N Am. 2015;95:71–83.
108. Park JY, et al. Early initiation of continuous renal replacement therapy improves survival of elderly patients with acute kidney injury: a multicenter prospective cohort study. Crit Care. 2016;20:260.
109. Chronopoulos A, Rosner MH, Cruz DN, Ronco C. Acute kidney injury in elderly intensive care patients: a review. Intensive Care Med. 2010;36:1454–64.
110. Swaminathan R, Major P, Snieder H, Spector T. Serum creatinine and fat-free mass (lean body mass). Clin Chem. 2000;46:1695–6.
111. Baxmann AC, et al. Influence of muscle mass and physical activity on serum and urinary creatinine and serum cystatin C. Clin J Am Soc Nephrol. 2008;3:348–54.
112. Pannarale G, et al. The aging kidney: structural changes. J Nephrol. 2010;23:S37.
113. Rosner MH. The pathogenesis of susceptibility to acute kidney injury in the elderly. Curr Aging Sci. 2009;2:158–64.
114. Nadeau-Fredette A-C, Bouchard J. Fluid management and use of diuretics in acute kidney injury. Adv Chronic Kidney Dis. 2013;20:45–55.
115. Godin M, Bouchard J, Mehta RL. Fluid balance in patients with acute kidney injury: emerging concepts. Nephron Clin Pract. 2013;123:238–45.
116. Yerram P, Karuparthi PR, Misra M. Fluid overload and acute kidney injury. Hemodial Int. 2010;14:348–54.
117. Strausbaugh LJ. Emerging health care-associated infections in the geriatric population. Emerg Infect Dis. 2001;7:268–71.
118. Uchino S, et al. Acute renal failure in critically ill patients: a multinational, multicenter study. JAMA. 2005;294:813–8.
119. Bagshaw SM, et al. Septic acute kidney injury in critically ill patients: clinical characteristics and outcomes. Clin J Am Soc Nephrol. 2007;2:431–9.
120. White LE, et al. Acute kidney injury is surprisingly common and a powerful predictor of mortality in surgical sepsis. J Trauma Acute Care Surg. 2013;75:432–8.
121. Bellomo R, Wan L, Langenberg C, May C. Septic acute kidney injury: new concepts. Nephron Exp Nephrol. 2008;109:e95.
122. Kidney Disease: Improving Global Outcomes (KDIGO) Acute Kidney Injury Work Group. KDIGO Clinical Practice Guideline for Acute Kidney Injury. Kidney Int Suppl. 2012;2:1–138.
123. Karajala V, Mansour W, Kellum JA. Diuretics in acute kidney injury. Minerva Anestesiol. 2009;75:251–7.
124. Dennen P, Douglas IS, Anderson R, M. & Objective. Acute kidney injury in the intensive care unit: an update and primer for the intensivist. Crit Care Med. 2010;38:261–75.
125. Mehta RL. Indications for dialysis in the ICU: renal replacement vs. renal support. Blood Purif. 2001;19:227–32.
126. Ronco C, Bellomo R, Ricci Z. Continuous renal replacement therapy in critically ill patients. Nephrol Dial Transplant. 2001;16(Suppl 5):67–72.
127. Ricci Z, et al. Practice patterns in the management of acute renal failure in the critically ill patient: an international survey. Nephrol Dial Transplant. 2006;21:690–6.
128. Pakula AM, Skinner RA. Acute kidney injury in the critically ill patient: a current review of the literature. J Intensive Care Med. 2015:4–9. https://doi.org/10.1177/0885066615575699.
129. Akcay A, Turkmen K, Lee D, Edelstein CL. Update on the diagnosis and management of acute kidney injury. Int J Nephrol Renov Dis. 2010;3:129–40.
130. Schmitt R, et al. Recovery of kidney function after acute kidney injury in the elderly: a systematic review and meta-analysis. Am J Kidney Dis. 2008;52:262–71.
131. Xue JL, et al. Incidence and mortality of acute renal failure in Medicare beneficiaries, 1992 to 2001. J Am Soc Nephrol. 2006;17:1135–42.
132. Wong SPY, Kreuter W, O'Hare AM. Healthcare intensity at initiation of chronic dialysis among older adults. J Am Soc Nephrol. 2014;25:143–9.
133. Tatum JM, et al. Analysis of survival after initiation of continuous renal replacement therapy in a surgical intensive care unit. JAMA Surg. 2017. https://doi.org/10.1001/jamasurg.2017.1673.
134. Williams AW, et al. Critical and honest conversations: the evidence behind the "Choosing Wisely" campaign recommendations by the American Society of Nephrology. Clin J Am Soc Nephrol. 2012;7:1664–72.
135. Koncicki HM, Swidler MA. Decision making in elderly patients with advanced kidney disease. Clin Geriatr Med. 2013;29:641–55.
136. Cohen LM, Moss AH, Weisbord SD, Germain MJ. Renal palliative care. J Palliat Med. 2006;9:977–92.
137. Bitar K, Greenwood-Van Meerveld B, Saad R, Wiley JW. Aging and gastrointestinal neuromuscular function: insights from within and outside the gut. Neurogastroenterol Motil. 2011;23:490–501.
138. Besanko LK, et al. Lower esophageal sphincter relaxation is impaired in older patients with dysphagia. World J Gastroenterol. 2011;17:1326–31.
139. Britton E, McLaughlin JT. Ageing and the gut. Proc Nutr Soc. 2013;72:173–7.
140. Shaw AC, et al. Dysregulation of human toll-like receptor function in aging. Ageing Res Rev. 2011;10:346–53.
141. Desai A, Grolleau-Julius A, Yung R. Leukocyte function in the aging immune system. J Leukoc Biol. 2010;87:1001–9.
142. Salminen A, et al. Activation of innate immunity system during aging: NF-kB signaling is the molecular culprit of inflamm-aging. Ageing Res Rev. 2008;7:83–105.

143. Story SK, Chamberlain RS. A comprehensive review of evidence-based strategies to prevent and treat postoperative ileus. Dig Surg. 2009;26:265–75.
144. Thomson ABR. Small intestinal disorders in the elderly. Best Pract Res Clin Gastroenterol. 2009;23:861–74.
145. Holt PR. Gastrointestinal diseases in the elderly. Curr Opin Clin Nutr Metab Care. 2003;6:41–8.
146. Tu CP, et al. Postoperative ileus in the elderly. Int J Gerontol. 2014;8:1–5.
147. Kaiser AM. Ogilvie transition to colonic perforation. Am J Surg. 2010;200:e15.
148. Hsu HL, Wu YM, Liu KL. Ogilvie syndrome: acute pseudo-obstruction of the colon. CMAJ. 2011;183:E162.
149. Tack J. Acute colonic pseudo-obstruction (Ogilvie's syndrome). Curr Treat Options Gastroenterol. 2006;9:361–8.
150. Saunders MD, Kimmey MB. Systematic review: acute colonic pseudo-obstruction. Aliment Pharmacol Ther. 2005;22:917–25.
151. Ponec RJ, Saunders MD, Kimmey MB. Neostigmine for the treatment of acute colonic pseudo-obstruction. N Engl J Med. 1999;341:137–41.
152. Wilson D, Jackson T, Sapey E, Lord JM. Frailty and sarcopenia: the potential role of an aged immune system. Ageing Res Rev. 2017;36:1–10.
153. Wallace JD, et al. Sarcopenia as a predictor of mortality in elderly blunt trauma patients: comparing the masseter to the psoas using computed tomography. J Trauma Acute Care Surg. 2017;82:65–72.
154. Interagency Forum on Aging-Related Statistics, F. Older Americans 2016: Key Indicators of Well-Being; 2016.
155. Dorner B, Posthauer ME, Friedrich EK, Robinson GE. Enteral nutrition for older adults in nursing facilities. Nutr Clin Pract. 2011;26:261–72.
156. Cutugno CL. The 'graying' of trauma care: addressing traumatic injury in older adults. Am J Nurs. 2011;111:40–850.
157. Cooney RN, Frankenfield DC. Determining energy needs in critically ill patients: equations or indirect calorimeters. Curr Opin Crit Care. 2012;18:174–7.
158. Walker RN, Heuberger RA. Predictive equations for energy needs for the critically ill. Respir Care. 2009;54:509–21.
159. Heyland DK, Dhaliwal R, Jiang X, Day AG. Identifying critically ill patients who benefit the most from nutrition therapy: the development and initial validation of a novel risk assessment tool. Crit Care. 2011;15:R268.
160. Zulfiqar AA, Sui Seng X, Gillibert A, Kadri N, Doucet J. Anemia and frailty in the elderly hospitalized in an acute unit: preliminary results. Eur J Intern Med. 2017;38:e8–9.
161. Patel KV. Epidemiology of anemia in older adults. Semin Hematol. 2008;45:210–7.
162. Bron D, Ades L, Fulop T, Goede V, Stauder R. Aging and blood disorders: new perspectives, new challenges. Haematologica. 2015;100:415–7.
163. Barkoukis H. Nutrition recommendations in elderly and aging. Med Clin N Am. 2016;100:1237–50.
164. Wade CE, et al. Evaluation of nutrition deficits in adult and elderly trauma patients. J Parenter Enter Nutr. 2015;39:449–55.
165. Tripathy S, Mishra J. Assessing nutrition in the critically ill elderly patient: a comparison of two screening tools. Indian J Crit Care Med. 2015;19:518.
166. Shiozu H, Higashijima M, Koga T. Association of sarcopenia with swallowing problems, related to nutrition and activities of daily living of elderly individuals. J Phys Ther Sci. 2015;27:393–6.
167. van Stijn MFM, et al. Preoperative nutrition status and postoperative outcome in elderly general surgery patients: a systematic review. JPEN J Parenter Enteral Nutr. 2013;37:37–43.
168. Kuroda Y, Kuroda R. Factors affecting the decision to provide artificial nutrition for elderly adults with oral intake difficulty. J Am Geriatr Soc. 2013;61:1835–6.
169. Monod S, Chiolero R, Büla C, Benaroyo L. Ethical issues in nutrition support of severely disabled elderly persons: a guide for health professionals. JPEN J Parenter Enteral Nutr. 2011;35:295–302.
170. Sheean PM, et al. Utilizing multiple methods to classify malnutrition among elderly patients admitted to the medical and surgical intensive care units (ICU). Clin Nutr. 2013;32:752–7.
171. Mohanty S, et al. Optimal perioperative Management of the Geriatric Patient: a best practices guideline from the American College of Surgeons NSQIP and the American Geriatrics Society. J Am Coll Surg. 2016;222:930–47.
172. Gershoff SN, Brusis OA, Nino HV, Huber AM. Studies of the elderly in Boston. I. The effects of iron fortification on moderately anemic people. Am J Clin Nutr. 1977;30:226–34.
173. Lipschitz DA, Udupa KB, Milton KY, Thompson CO. Effect of age on hematopoiesis in man. Blood. 1984;63:502–9.
174. Ershler WB, et al. Serum erythropoietin and aging: a longitudinal analysis. J Am Geriatr Soc. 2005;53:1360–5.
175. Kämpfen P, et al. Risk of falls and bleeding in elderly patients with acute venous thromboembolism. J Intern Med. 2014;276:378–86.
176. Kim DY, et al. Venous thromboembolism in the elderly: the result of comorbid conditions or a consequence of injury? J Trauma Acute Care Surg. 2012;72:1286–91.
177. Bauersachs RM. Managing venous thromboembolism with novel oral anticoagulants in the elderly and other high-risk patient groups. Eur J Intern Med. 2014;25:600–6.
178. Connolly SJ, et al. Dabigatran versus warfarin in patients with atrial fibrillation. N Engl J Med. 2009;361:1139–51.
179. Connolly SJ, et al. Apixaban in patients with atrial fibrillation. N Engl J Med. 2011;364:806–17.
180. Schulman S, et al. Dabigatran versus warfarin in the treatment of acute venous thromboembolism. N Engl J Med. 2009;361:2342–52.
181. Schulman S, et al. Treatment of acute venous thromboembolism with dabigatran or warfarin and pooled analysis. Circulation. 2014;129:764–72.
182. Patel MR, et al. Rivaroxaban versus warfarin in nonvalvular atrial fibrillation. N Engl J Med. 2011;365:883–91.
183. Prins MH, et al. Oral rivaroxaban versus standard therapy for the treatment of symptomatic venous thromboembolism: a pooled analysis of the EINSTEIN-DVT and PE randomized studies. Thromb J. 2013;11:21.
184. Investigators*, T. E. Oral rivaroxaban for symptomatic venous thromboembolism. N Engl J Med. 2010:2499–510. https://doi.org/10.1056/NEJMoa1007903.
185. Granger CB, et al. Apixaban versus warfarin in patients with atrial fibrillation. N Engl J Med. 2011;365:339–54.
186. Gallego P, Roldan V, Lip GYH. Novel oral anticoagulants in cardiovascular disease. J Cardiovasc Pharmacol Ther. 2014;19:34–44.
187. Lauffenburger JC, et al. Factors driving anticoagulant selection in patients with atrial fibrillation in the United States. Am J Cardiol. 2015;115:1095–101.
188. Sharma M, Cornelius VR, Patel JP, Davies JG, Molokhia M. Efficacy and harms of direct oral anticoagulants in the elderly for stroke prevention in atrial fibrillation and secondary prevention of venous thromboembolism: systematic review and meta-analysis. Circulation. 2015;132:194–204.
189. Insam C, et al. Anticoagulation management practices and outcomes in elderly patients with acute venous thromboembolism: a clinical research study. PLoS One. 2016;11:e0148348.
190. Geldhof V, Vandenbriele C, Verhamme P, Vanassche T. Venous thromboembolism in the elderly: efficacy and safety of non-VKA oral anticoagulants. Thromb J. 2014;12:21.
191. Warshaw G, Mechlin M. Prevention and management of postoperative delirium. Int Anesthesiol Clin. 2009;47:137–49.

192. Pisani MA, et al. Days of delirium are associated with 1-year mortality in an older intensive care unit population. Am J Respir Crit Care Med. 2009;180:1092–7.
193. Balas MC, et al. Delirium in older patients in surgical intensive care units. J Nurs Scholarsh an Off Publ Sigma Theta Tau Int Honor Soc Nurs. 2007;39:147–54.
194. Gaspardo P, et al. Delirium among critically ill adults: evaluation of the psychometric properties of the Italian 'confusion assessment method for the intensive care unit'. Intensive Crit Care Nurs. 2014;30:283–91.
195. Albrecht JS, McCunn M, Stein DM, Simoni-Wastila L, Smith GS. Sex differences in mortality following isolated traumatic brain injury among older adults. J Trauma Acute Care Surg. 2016;81:486–92.
196. Almeida OP, Hankey GJ, Yeap BB, Golledge J, Flicker L. Prevalence, associated factors, mood and cognitive outcomes of traumatic brain injury in later life: the health in men study (HIMS). Int J Geriatr Psychiatry. 2015;30:1215–23.
197. Bo M, et al. Predictive factors of in-hospital mortality in older patients admitted to a medical intensive care unit. J Am Geriatr Soc. 2003;51:529–33.
198. Francis J, Martin D, Kapoor WN. A prospective study of delirium in hospitalized elderly. JAMA. 1990;263:1097–101.
199. Pandharipande P, et al. Prevalence and risk factors for development of delirium in surgical and trauma intensive care unit patients. J Trauma. 2008;65:34–41.
200. Reade MC, Finfer S. Sedation and delirium in the intensive care unit. N Engl J Med. 2014;370:444–54.
201. Garpestad E, Devlin JW. Polypharmacy and delirium in critically ill older adults: recognition and prevention. Clin Geriatr Med. 2017;33:189–203.
202. Tune L, Carr S, Cooper T, Klug B, Golinger RC. Association of anticholinergic activity of prescribed medications with postoperative delirium. J Neuropsychiatry Clin Neurosci. 1993;5:208–10.
203. Vaurio LE, Sands LP, Wang Y, Mullen EA, Leung JM. Postoperative delirium: the importance of pain and pain management. Anesth Analg. 2006;102:1267–73.
204. Gaudreau JD, Gagnon P, Roy MA, Harel F, Tremblay A. Opioid medications and longitudinal risk of delirium in hospitalized cancer patients. Cancer. 2007;109:2365–73.
205. Fong HK, Sands LP, Leung JM. The role of postoperative analgesia in delirium and cognitive decline in elderly patients: a systematic review. Anesth Analg. 2006;102:1255–66.
206. Leslie DL, Marcantonio ER, Zhang Y, Leo-Summers L, Inouye SK. One-year health care costs associated with delirium in the elderly population. Arch Intern Med. 2008;168:27.
207. Ely EW, et al. Delirium as a predictor of mortality in mechanically ventilated patients in the intensive care unit. JAMA. 2004;291:1753–62.
208. Girard TD, et al. Delirium as a predictor of long-term cognitive impairment in survivors of critical illness. Crit Care Med. 2010;38:1513–20.
209. Pandharipande PP, et al. Long-term cognitive impairment after critical illness. N Engl J Med. 2013;369:1306–16.
210. Salluh JIF, et al. Outcome of delirium in critically ill patients: systematic review and meta-analysis. BMJ. 2015;350:h2538.
211. American Psychiatric Association. Diagnostic and Statistical Manual of Mental Disorders 4th ed, text revision (DSM-IV-TR). Diagnostic and Statistical Manual of Mental Disorders 4th ed TR; 2000.
212. Ely EW, et al. Evaluation of delirium in critically ill patients: validation of the confusion assessment method for the intensive care unit (CAM-ICU). Crit Care Med. 2001;29:1370–9.
213. Reade MC, Eastwood GM, Peck L, Bellomo R, Baldwin I. Routine use of the confusion assessment method for the intensive care unit (CAM-ICU) by bedside nurses may underdiagnose delirium. Crit Care Resusc. 2011;13:217–25.
214. Inouye SK, et al. Clarifying confusion: the confusion assessment method: a new method for detection of delirium. Ann Intern Med. 1990;113:941–8.
215. Wang J, et al. Risk factors contributing to postoperative delirium in geriatric patients postorthopedic surgery. Asia Pac Psychiatry. 2015;7:375–82.
216. Barr J, et al. Clinical practice guidelines for the Management of Pain, agitation, and delirium in adult patients in the intensive care unit. Crit Care Med. 2013;41:263–306.
217. Association, A. 2017 Alzheimer's disease facts and figures. Alzheimers Dement. 2017;13:325–73.
218. Selkoe DJ. Aging, amyloid, and Alzheimer's disease: a perspective in honor of Carl Cotman. Neurochem Res. 2003;28:1705–13.
219. Folstein MF, Folstein SE, McHugh PR. 'Mini-mental state'. A practical method for grading the cognitive state of patients for the clinician. J Psychiatr Res. 1975;12:189–98.
220. Borson S, Scanlan J, Brush M, Vitaliano P, Dokmak A. The mini-cog: a cognitive 'vital signs' measure for dementia screening in multi-lingual elderly. Int J Geriatr Psychiatry. 2000;15:1021–7.
221. Carson S, McDonagh MS, Peterson K. A systematic review of the efficacy and safety of atypical antipsychotics in patients with psychological and behavioral symptoms of dementia. J Am Geriatr Soc. 2006;54:354–61.
222. McManus DQ, Arvanitis LA, Kowalcyk BB. Quetiapine, a novel antipsychotic: experience in elderly patients with psychotic disorders. Seroquel trial 48 study group. J Clin Psychiatry. 1999;60:292–8.
223. Hybels CF, Blazer DG. Epidemiology of late-life mental disorders. Clin Geriatr Med. 2003;19:663–96.
224. Giampieri M. Communication and informed consent in elderly people. Minerva Anestesiol. 2012;78:236–42.
225. Appelbaum PSC p. Assessment of patients' competence to consent to treatment. N Engl J Med. 2007;357:1834–40.
226. Moye J, Marson DC. Assessment of decision-making capacity in older adults: an emerging area of practice and research. J Gerontol B Psychol Sci Soc Sci. 2007;62:P3–P11.
227. McCullough LB, Jones JW. Postoperative futility: a clinical algorithm for setting limits. Br J Surg. 2001;88:1153–4.

Burns

54

Gary Vercruysse

Introduction

This chapter was written to guide the general surgeon through the thought processes used by burn surgeons that guide patient care, specifically in the ICU. It is divided into sections covering the initial care of the burn patient, and ICU management, which goes hand in hand with the initial care. It is not designed as a stand-alone guide for all of burn care but more of a guide to the special problems faced by burn surgeons in the management of complex burn patients in the ICU.

How to Decide if a Patient Needs to Be Admitted

As burn surgeons, we look at patients in terms of what they can and cannot accomplish if left to their own devices. We admit anyone who cannot adequately care for their burn by themselves, or with a relative, or friend's help at home. It is much easier to admit a patient, teach them wound care, and send them home than to readmit the same patient a few days later with an infected burn wound, bacteremia, and SIRS and then to be forced to care for the now sicker and more complicated burn patient.

As a general rule, we will admit:

1. Full-thickness (third-degree) burns >3% TBSA
2. Burns with possible inhalation injury
3. Infected burns (those who did not seek care until their burn became infected)
4. Electrical burns
5. Hydrofluoric acid burns
6. Suspicion of child or elder or spousal/significant other abuse
7. Perianal and/or buttock burns
8. Lower extremity burns in diabetic patients or patients with peripheral vascular disease
9. Any significant chemical burns
10. New circumferential extremity burns
11. Any burn in a child greater than 10% TBSA
12. Any burn in an adult greater than 20% TBSA
13. Any burn in an "elderly" (more than 50 years old) person greater than 10% TBSA

Who Should Be Admitted to the ICU

As a general rule, burn patients are sicker than they may appear. A patient with a 90% burn who is 60 years old can have a normal conversation with you and be in only moderate distress for about 4 h post-burn. It is important that you remember that this is a temporary phenomenon. The cytokine release that is occurs during this period will cause shock to begin about 6 h post-burn, and the patient will soon become much sicker.

In a similar fashion, a patient with a much smaller burn (~20% TBSA) can look relatively well for a couple of days before developing an infection that will become life-threatening in a matter of hours. These patients are severely immunosuppressed and are prone to acute deterioration [1, 2]. Our current theories of multisystem organ failure suggest that ARDS (acute respiratory distress syndrome) results from under resuscitation of shock [3, 4]. For these reasons, we routinely admit the following patients to the ICU:

A. Burns 20% TBSA or greater, any age patient
B. Burns 10–20% TBSA if the patient is >50 or <5 years old, or if most of the burn is full thickness (third degree)
C. Burns <10% TBSA if there is a significant history of smoke inhalation
D. Any burn patient with severe medical problems
E. Any patient with toxic epidermal necrolysis or Stevens-Johnson syndrome

G. Vercruysse (✉)
Director of Emergency General Surgery,
University of Michigan, Ann Arbor, MI, USA
e-mail: vercruys@med.umich.edu

A. Salim et al. (eds.), *Surgical Critical Care Therapy*, https://doi.org/10.1007/978-3-319-71712-8_54

F. Any patient that has to be sedated to the point of unconsciousness to do wound care
G. Any patient that requires more than 4 l nasal cannula oxygen

Keep in mind that ARDS can start in a burn patient at almost any time. It can be triggered by something as simple as an infected IV site. Whenever a patient does not "look right" on the floor, check a pulse ox. It is difficult to tell when a patient has ARDS. A patient can be at rest and have an oxygen saturation of 80–85% without clinical symptoms [5].

Anyone who needs ICU care for a burn should be admitted to the ICU at a burn center. That being said, due to EMS triage, inclement weather, or other complications, critically ill burn patients may reside in hospitals without burn centers for a period of time. If a burn patient is initially triaged to a trauma center, they should be assessed in the trauma bay and other life-threatening injuries ruled out. Once this is accomplished, formal burn resuscitation should begin, and the patient should receive ICU-level care, while arrangements are being made for transfer to a burn center. If ICU-level care cannot be rendered in the emergency center due do patient volume and nursing limitations, the patient should be transferred to the ICU and resuscitated until a time at which they can be transferred to a burn center.

Initial Care in the ED

When a major burn victim first arrives in the ED:

1. Check airway and breathing.
2. Check blood pressure and establish IV access.
3. Draw electrolytes, CBC, ABG with carboxyhemoglobin, coags, and type and cross.
4. Obtain relevant history quickly:
   (a) Cause and type of fire.
   (b) Location, smoke exposure, loss of consciousness?
   (c) Time burn occurred.
   (d) Other trauma: does patient need a trauma workup?
   (e) Allergies.
   (f) PMH and PSH.
5. Obtain CXR (chest X-ray) and other needed films.
6. Estimate wound size (%TBSA).
7. Call burn center to begin transfer arrangements.
8. Wash the patient with warm saline solution and towel dry, and then place in dry sheets and blankets to avoid hypothermia.
9. Photograph all burns pre- and post-debridement for the medical record and subsequent communication with the burn center.
10. Include all films and labs obtained to transfer with the patient.
11. Prepare for transport to burn center.

Initial Debridement

As burn surgeons, we need to assess the burn to determine depth (deep or superficial burn) in order to determine if the burn is likely to heal or if it will require surgery to close. To this effect, we debride all blisters and cleanse the wound to remove all possible dirt and debris to try to prevent eventual burn wound cellulitis or burn wound sepsis.

Burn wounds are debrided with warm or room temperature saline, mild soap, and a washcloth. Titrate IV ketamine and morphine or fentanyl for analgesia and IV versed for amnesia after being sure that the patient has a working pulse oximeter, working NC oxygen, oral airway, and bag valve mask in proximity. It is a good idea to have Narcan available. Always check blood pressure before giving more narcotic. Remove all loose epidermis, open and debride all blisters, and reestimate the size and depth of the burn after debridement. If the patient is to be transferred to a burn center in the near future, it would be reasonable to simply place the patient in clean dry sheets as they will be reassessed upon arrival to the burn center. If transfer will take a relatively long time due to distance or availability of transportation, wrap the burns in Silvadene and Kerlix gauze. These patients will get hypothermic very quickly, so try to keep the patient warm by increasing the room temperature, warming IV fluids, French fry lights, blankets, and Bair Hugger as needed.

IV Access

It is imperative that patients with major burns have reliable IV access, especially during the resuscitation period. These guidelines are designed to help provide for this access while minimizing the risk of infection and complications.

Resuscitation Phase (First 72 h)

This is the time that reliable IV access is the most important and sometimes the most difficult to achieve. Peripheral IV lines placed through burned areas often will infiltrate 5–8 h after being placed, and they are difficult to secure. They should be replaced with IVs through unburned areas as soon as possible. IVs placed through the burn or near the wounds have a very high infection rate and should always be changed to a site away from the burn or to a central line. It is reasonable to change lines that are placed in the ER or in the field within 24 h (This includes IVs placed at other institutions).

In burn patients with TBSA burns larger than 30% or so, it is a good idea to place a central line to provide for reliable access for the large volume of fluid that is required. Do not place Cordis catheters as large bore lines. These catheters are relatively short and will often be pulled out of the vein by the swelling of the patient and the frequent turning that is required. The best choice is a 7 French triple-lumen catheter; it provides separate ports for sedation/analgesia, antibiotics (when necessary), and fluids. Initially, the best approach is probably the femoral route. It has the advantages of being easy to place and not requiring an X-ray to rule out pneumothorax and confirm placement. In addition, the groins are often spared from the burning process. Although a femoral line can be threaded into the thorax to measure the CVP, this is seldom done because the volume and rate of fluids are titrated to markers of perfusion and not to a specific CVP.

In pediatric burn patients, use a 5.5 French triple-lumen catheters for children <25 kg. The largest port these catheters have is 20 gauge. Do not use other pediatric multi-lumen catheters that have ports smaller than 20 gauge because the IV pumps may not be able to pump the fluids through them at the required rate and unless fluid is running through them constantly, or they are filled with heparinized saline, the lumens tend to become thrombosed.

Intraosseous lines are often placed in the ECC for large burns in small children. Unfortunately, these lines are unreliable and may not able to accept the relatively high rates of fluids that are required to resuscitate large burns. These lines should be replaced immediately with percutaneous femoral lines. If a percutaneous femoral line cannot be placed, then a cutdown may have to be performed. The most reliable cutdown is the groin at the saphenous-femoral junction. Saphenous vein cutdowns at the ankle are very difficult to do because the vein is so small, the area is difficult to immobilize, and the subsequent line that is placed is small. Cutdowns are seldom if ever needed in adults but, on occasion, can be lifesaving. Occasionally the burn eschar may need to be incised in an adult to feel the appropriate landmarks in a badly burned individual.

Basic Initial Fluid Resuscitation

There have been many formulae developed for the resuscitation of the burn patient. Fluid resuscitation is necessary in those who have a burn large enough for them to be unable to meet their fluid needs orally. That is, not all burn patients will require fluid resuscitation. It is quite common for referring centers to give large amounts of fluids (often normal saline) to burn patients before and during transport to the burn center without taking the patient's needs into consideration.

Burn patients who require fluid resuscitation include the following:

1. Children (<5 years old) with burns larger than 10% TBSA
2. Adults with burns larger than 20% TBSA
3. Elderly (> 50 years old) with burns larger than 10% TBSA

Generally fluid is given as a rate, not a bolus. If given in bolus form, this fluid is likely to extravasate into the interstitial space very quickly and increase the amount of generalized and pulmonary edema the patient will experience.

The goals of fluid resuscitation are to prevent dehydration and hypotension. This is important because if the patient experiences either of these things for a prolonged period of time, areas of burn that are initially partial thickness may become full thickness due to a lack of blood supply (blood is shunted centrally away from skin and soft tissue to perfuse the brain, heart, etc.). This is known as extension of the burn.

Conversely, if large amounts of fluid are given without regard to patient requirements, resuscitation morbidity may occur. This is a phenomenon by which too much fluid causes excessive pulmonary edema, abdominal, and secondary extremity compartment syndromes necessitating opening of the abdomen and extremity fasciotomies [6–8]. If a patient with a large burn suffers resuscitation morbidity, mortality is in the range of 95% or greater.

Several long-standing formulae exist for the resuscitation of burn patients. Below are some examples.

For burns in Adults >20% TBSA or the Elderly >10% TBSA

The Parkland Formula:

4 cc × (% TBSA of second- and third-degree burn) × kg wt = cc/24 h.

Give one-half of this fluid in the first 8 h and the other half over the next 16 h; use Ringer's lactate.

Or

The Rule of Tens for Burn Resuscitation:

This formula was developed by military surgeons for use on burn patients. It has the advantage of being easy to calculate and gives you an initial fluid rate that can be titrated up or down to urine output [9].

Using Lactated Ringer's

1. Estimate burn size to the nearest 10%.
2. Multiply %TBSA × 10 = Initial fluid rate in ml/h (for adult patients weighing 40–80 kg).
3. For every 10 kg above 80 kg, increase the rate by 100 ml/h.

If the patient is an adult and weighs less than 40 kg, use the Parkland formula.

For children: burns >10% TBSA

The Galveston Formula (Pediatric Burns <40 kg):

1. 3–4 ml/kg/%TBSA burn
2. 1/2 volume over the first 8 h, second half over the next 16 h

3. Also infuse maintenance fluid at:
   - 4 ml/kg for the first 10 kg body weight
   - 2 ml/kg for the second 10 kg body weight
   - 1 ml/kg for the remaining kilogram body weight

Use D5LR for the maintenance component to avoid hypoglycemia in small children.

We always use Ringer's lactate for initial resuscitation. If NS is used, within a few hours, the patient will predictably develop a severe hyperchloremic metabolic acidosis in addition to the already serious lactic acidosis driven by the dehydration experienced by those with large burns. We do not resuscitate children with large volumes of hypotonic fluids. It is important to understand that these formulas are for initial IV fluid rates only. If a patient is making adequate urine, and not physiologically deranged, (not hyperglycemic or acidotic) you should tailor the fluid rate to urine output. During pediatric burn resuscitation, remember that children may have limited glycogen stores, so give part of the Galveston formula (the maintenance fluid component) as D5 LR to avoid hypoglycemia. As stated before, always adjust the IVF rates such that adults have a urine output of at least 40 cc/h; and children have an output of 1 cc/kg/h but not 3 cc/kg/h. Also make certain that if present, the patients' metabolic acidosis is resolving. Remember, some patients require more fluid; some require less. On post-burn day #2 for larger burns (>30% TBSA), a 5% albumin drip can be started at 1 cc/kg % TBSA burn for 24 h. This will help to mitigate unnecessary interstitial edema [10, 11].

Exceptions to the 30 cc/h or (1 cc/kg/h) urine output rule:

A. *Chronic Renal Failure* – these patients require a CVP, Swan-Ganz catheter, or other objective measure of endpoints of resuscitation.
B. *Myoglobinuria* – not uncommon in large burns or electrical burns; in this case you should try to achieve 100 cc/h of urine output in adults and 2 cc/kg/h of urine output in children.
C. *Hyperglycemia* – more common in young patients. Glycosuria causes a high urine output in face of hypovolemia. If this is persistent, it would be reasonable to reduce (not eliminate D5LR given as maintenance in pediatric resuscitation.)

The Difficult Resuscitation

The difficult resuscitation is defined by oliguria despite optimal fluid delivery. This may be the result of underestimate of burn size or a missed injury leading to early sepsis (hollow viscus injury) or hypotension due to hemorrhagic shock. Once these alternatives have been excluded, an escalation in basic resuscitation strategy should follow.

Difficult Resuscitation Guidelines

- Switch intravenous fluid to 5% albumin to attempt to maintain more volume within the intravascular space.
- Check bladder pressures every 4 h to rule out abdominal compartment syndrome.
- If urine output (UOP) <30 ml/h in a >30 kg patient or <1 ml/kg/h in a ≤30 kg patient, strongly consider monitoring central venous pressures (CVP) from a subclavian or IJ line along with central venous (ScvO2) saturations (goal CVP 8–10 mmHg, ScvO2 60–65%):
  (a) If CVP is not at goal, then increase fluid rate by 33%.
  (b) If CVP is at goal, then consider dobutamine 5 μg/kg/min (titrate until ScvO2 (if available) at goal). Max dose of dobutamine is 20 μg/kg/min.
  (c) If both CVP and ScvO2 (if available) are at goal, then stop increasing fluids (even if UOP < target). In these instances, the patient should be considered hemodynamically optimized, and the oliguria is likely a result of established renal insult. Some degree of renal failure should be tolerated and expected. Continued increases in fluid administration despite optimal hemodynamic parameters will only result in "resuscitation morbidity" that is oftentimes more detrimental than renal failure.

Every attempt should be made to minimize fluid administration while maintaining organ perfusion. If UOP >70 ml/h and patient >30 kg, then decrease the fluid rate by 33%. If UOP >2 ml/kg/h and patient is ≤30 kg, then decrease the fluid rate by 33%. Do not decrease below the maintenance IVF rate based on the patients' weight. After 24 h, infusion of lactated Ringer's should be titrated down to maintenance levels, and 5% albumin continued until the 48-h mark.

Resuscitation Morbidity

If guidelines for resuscitation are not followed and patients are simply repeatedly bolused large amounts of crystalloid, they will continue extravasate fluid into the interstitial space [7]. If this mode of resuscitation continues unchecked, it may eventually lead to resuscitation morbidity, a consequence of over resuscitation. It is characterized by pulmonary edema, difficult oxygenation despite elevated ventilatory pressures, distended abdomen, and edematous extremities [12]. If not recognized and fluid management optimized, it may lead to abdominal compartment syndrome necessitating laparotomy and an open abdomen and secondary extremity compartment syndrome requiring fasciotomy for limb salvage [13]. It is important to carefully avoid this complication as patients with a large burn and resuscitation morbidity requiring laparotomy and fasciotomy have a very high mortality rate [8].

Airway/Intubation

Managing the airway of an acute burn patient is one of the most difficult aspects of the first 24 h of care. Major decisions involve which patients will need intubation, and when and where is the best location to intubate [14].

A. Which patients to intubate:

Very strong indications:

1. COHb >10% with depressed mental status (note COHb >10% with fairly normal (talking) mental status is in itself not an indicated to intubate.)
2. Burns >50% – especially in children.
3. Burns > with full-thickness facial component.
4. The entire head is burned (both face and scalp) even if it is all just second degree.

Relative indications:

(a) Burn occurred indoors with significant smoke inhalation.
(b) Hoarseness.
(c) Carbonaceous sputum.
(d) Partial thickness burns to the face.
(e) Very young <1 or very old >75.

Patients with the above findings who have relatively large burns, 40–50%, often need to be intubated. Patients with the same findings, and smaller burns, can often be successfully observed without intubation.

Findings that are generally not helpful:

(a) Singed Nasal Hairs. This occurs frequently with home oxygen burns, where a patient smokes a cigarette while on oxygen for COPD. This type of burn, by definition, does not have an inhalational component. The patient may have a low pulse oximetry reading, but it is due to the fact that the person is on chronic O_2 for lung disease, not because of an inhalation injury.
(b) CXR.
(c) Bronchoscopy findings are relatively unhelpful (Fig. 54.1a–c).

B. Thought process: when and where to intubate

In most patients, there is a 4–6-h period of time post-burn before edema will occlude the airway. We will generally establish good IV access, check vital signs, and then get anesthesia or the ED to help intubate the patients in a relatively elective fashion:

(a) We always do a pre-intubation physical exam, especially a neurological exam focusing on other possible injuries beside the burn.
(b) Oral tracheal intubation is preferred. Try to put in as large an ET tube as possible. It is not possible to perform bronchoscopy on an adult with an endotracheal tube smaller than a size 7 in an adult or a 4.5 in a child.

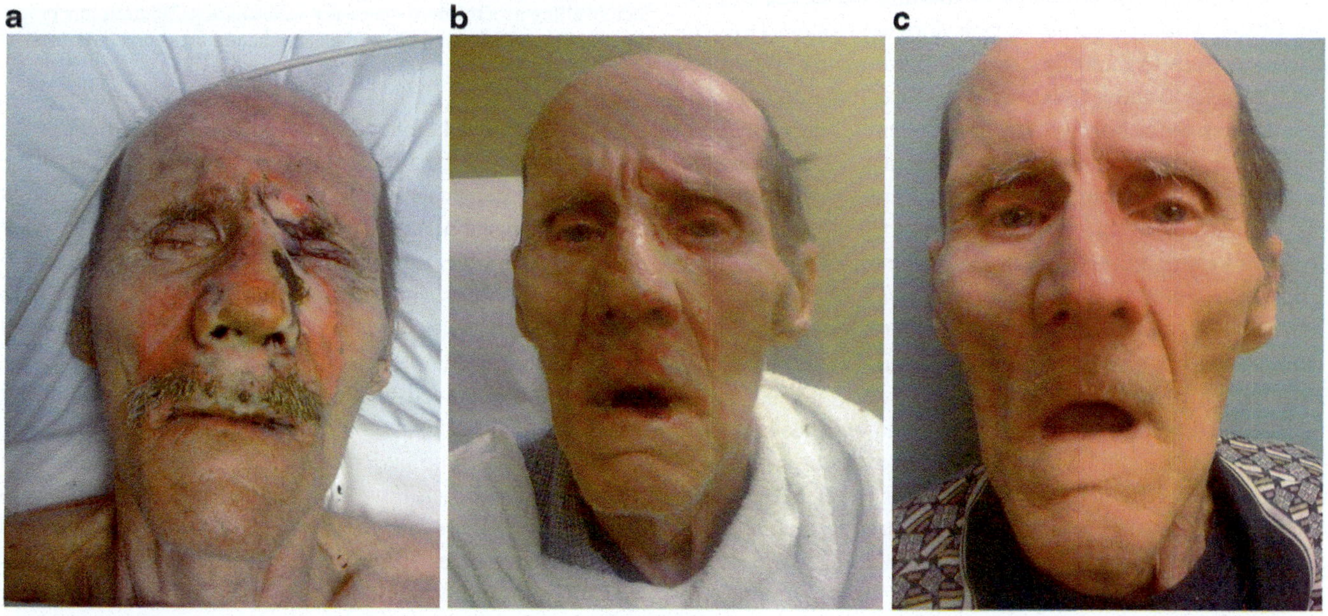

Fig. 54.1 (a–c) Singed nasal and facial hair in a patient after suffering a home oxygen burn. He had a pulse oximetry reading in the high 80s (due to COPD) which improved with oxygen. He was managed conservatively and did quite well. Six weeks later, his burn was completely healed

Tips on intubation:

A. Size of pediatric ET tube: Age + 16 = Size of ET tube/4. Remember: pediatric ET tubes traditionally were uncuffed. Recently high-volume, low-pressure, cuffed endotracheal tubes have become available. Use a cuffed tube if possible. If an adequate seal does not form between the trachea and ET tube, ventilation will be difficult. Additionally, smaller ET tubes interfere with the removal of secretions and occlude easier. Try to use a 4.5 ET tube or larger when possible. Cuffed pediatric ET tubes offer better seals when dealing with advanced modes of ventilation.
B. Always listen carefully for breath sounds to avoid a right mainstream intubation. Record the position of the ET tube at the teeth.
C. Carefully secure the ET tube with adhesive tape or umbilical tape. Heavy sedation and/or paralytic drugs and restraints are essential to make certain that the airway is not dislodged. If the patient has a facial burn, tape will not stick to the fa; however, it can be used to secure an airway if it is laid on the skin above the upper lip and stapled in place. This offers a secure airway and allows for facial swelling. A second piece of tape is then often placed over the staples to mitigate family discomfort.

a

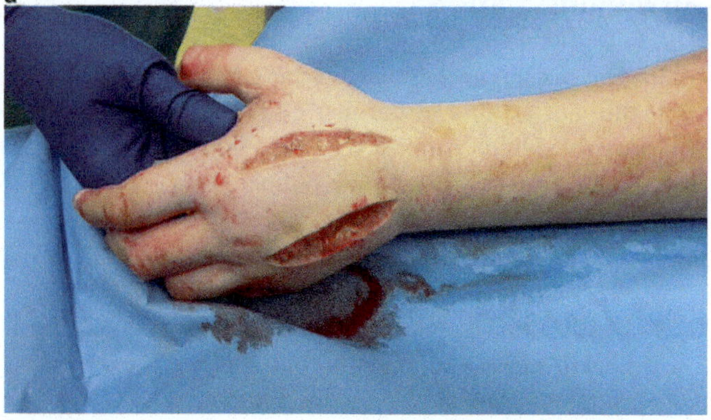

b

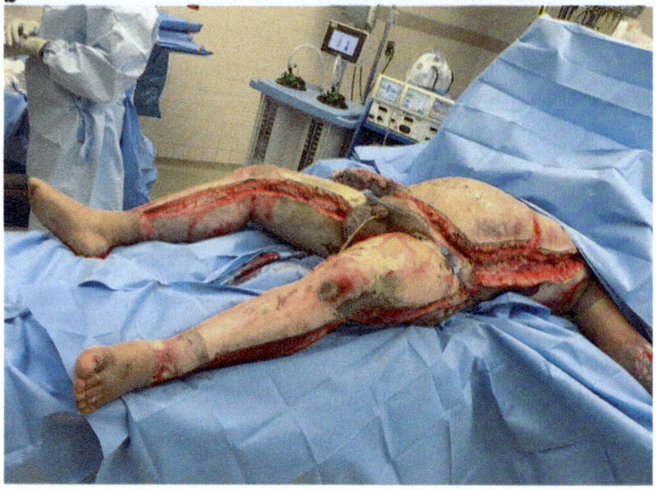

Fig. 54.2 (a, b) Demonstration of hand, chest, abdomen, and lower extremity escharotomies through clearly dead dermis to allow for further swelling as a result of necessary resuscitation. Without this procedure, these patients would have developed compartment syndromes

Escharotomies

In patients with circumferential extremity burns, the arm or leg swells, while the burned dermis does not stretch. This can allow pressure to build up under the burn eschar. When the pressure rises to above tissue perfusion, pressure ischemia will result. First, the nerves will become ischemic, and patients, if conscious, will note tingling. Next, the muscles will become ischemic, and if nothing is done, rhabdomyolysis and necrosis will result. If left under compression, the patient will develop a compartment syndrome of the effected extremity. This is prevented by cutting the eschar and letting the swollen tissue expand. Escharotomies are done for patients with deep 2 and 3° burns that are circumferential around the chest, extremities, abdomen, penis, or neck [15–17].

The most common indication for escharotomies is loss of the palmar arch Doppler signal for upper extremities and loss of the posterior tibial Doppler signal for lower extremities. Other indications are cyanosis of the extremity paresthesias and loss of capillary refill/loss of pulse-ox signal from the extremity. It is important to note that this "compartment syndrome" is due to the burned skin and dermis and not to pathology of the actual muscular compartments. Therefore it is escharotomy that will relieve the compartment syndrome, and a deeper fasciotomy is not required unless there is some coexistent pathology (such as a fracture or vascular injury) that creates a true compartment syndrome.

After giving sedation, cut the eschar with a knife or bovie cautery. This can be very painful, so make certain that the patient has received sufficient narcotics. Classically, a medial and lateral incision is made on the arms or legs. It is carried down to the subcutaneous fat to allow the extremity to expand. After ensuring hemostasis, wrap the limb with Silvadene after the procedure. Avoid cutting through normal skin during escharotomies if burned skin is available. Incisions do not need to be strictly medial and lateral but should be adjusted to avoid non-burned skin when possible.

Always check the patient after an escharotomy has been done to make certain flow has been reestablished. Rarely, a fasciotomy will be needed to reestablish adequate blood flow. Escharotomies are most commonly needed in patients who have circumferential deep 2 or 3° burns on the chest or extremity and who will receive large volumes of fluid for their resuscitation. If it is apparent that the patient will eventually need an escharotomy, do not wait until Doppler signals are lost. The most advantageous time to do this procedure is when the patient is in his room with good IV access and fully monitored (Fig. 54.2a, b).

Basic Wound Care and Dressings

Antimicrobial Dressings

After the initial debridement of the epidermis, topical antimicrobial dressings are started on all burns. The goal of the antimicrobials is to limit bacterial overgrowth on and under the eschar and thus prevent or limit burn wound cellulitis and burn wound sepsis:

A. *1% Silver Sulfadiazine Cream (Silvadene)* – A combined agent sulfonamide and silver ion. SSD has fair eschar penetration. Apply once a day, and cover with gauze. Not used on face or ears. SSD has good gram-positive, gram-negative, and antifungal properties. It is painless but can cause leukopenia that usually spontaneously resolves. It is contraindicated in true sulfa allergies. The sulfonamide component of silver sulfadiazine can be absorbed through the skin. This is especially true in small children who have a greater area-to-mass ratio. Sulfonamides can cause kernicterus in newborns. For these reasons silver sulfadiazine is contraindicated in children under 2 months of age. For these patients, gentamicin or bacitracin ointment should probably be used. As an ointment, it does not contain propylene glycol and the absorption can easily be monitored by checking gentamicin levels. Silver sulfadiazine cream is the most common dressing used for initial wound care. It can also be used on donor sites [18–20].

B. *Mafenide Acetate (Sulfamylon)* – A 2% solution of sulfonamide that penetrates eschar well and is rapidly absorbed. Sulfamylon has broad spectrum antimicrobial qualities and is bactericidal at wound concentration. It has good gram-positive and gram-negative activity, including *Clostridia*, but has little antifungal activity. It can be used BID because wound levels fall as it is absorbed. It causes pain when applied, and it is a strong carbonic anhydrase inhibitor, causing loss of bicarbonate in the urine and if used in great amounts can cause polyuria [21]. It is mainly used to control invasive wound infections (until surgery can be done). It is often used alternately with Silvadene. Patients who are getting Sulfamylon dressings need close monitoring of their pH and often need supplemental bicarbonate. This is often used on ear burns because it penetrates into the cartilage and helps prevent chondritis [22].

C. *0.5% Silver Nitrate Solution* – Prepared in distilled water (because of the solubility of silver salts). Broad spectrum antimicrobial action resistance is uncommon. Minimal absorption occurs, and it does not penetrate eschar. It is used by placing the patient in large bulky dressings of gauze and pouring the silver nitrate Solution on them Q2-3H to keep the dressings moist. The bulky dressings are changed Q8-12H. This dressing is more of a historic footnote, but it can be used if other preparations are not available. These dressings can cause hyponatremia and hypokalemia due to the distilled water washing out electrolytes. BMP should be checked at least Q8H initially. In addition, the nitrate ion can cause methemoglobinemia (the iron atom is oxidized), which will impair oxygen delivery. Methemoglobinemia levels should be checked Q4-6H. If above 10%, 1 amp of methylene blue (up to 1 mg/kg) (a reducing agent) should be given. Vitamin C (another reducing agent) should be given 500 mg BID for patients on silver nitrate dressings over a large part of their body. This type of dressing is used only for documented sulfonamide allergy, patients with toxic epidermal necrolysis (Stephens-Johnson syndrome), or sometimes on fresh skin grafts for a couple of days [23–25].

D. *Bacitracin Ointment* – Used on the face burns or on small burns <5% because it is clear. It probably does not inhibit epithelialization as much as Silvadene. It is useful for superficial partial thickness burns or clean donor sites where the opsite or xeroform dressing has come off. It is best if used with nonstick gauze.

E. *Nystatin-Silvadene* – 50–50 mixture. Nystatin is a polyene antibiotic structurally similar to amphotericin B. They bind ergosterol in the fungus cell membrane. It has broad spectrum antifungal effect but little antibacterial effect. It is used with Silvadene in cases of heavy fungal colonization of the burn wound or in invasive fungal burn wound infections. It is not systemically absorbed, and resistance is rare.

Once the wound is washed and debrided and antimicrobials have been applied, we dress the wound with Kerlix gauze and either loosely applied elastic netting or ace wraps. Dressings are then changed daily until a decision to operate, or manage nonoperatively has been determined. All along, patients and their families are encouraged to participate in dressing changes as much as possible, so as to learn to care for the wound once the patient is discharged.

Antibiotics and Infections

Burn injury causes suppression of all components of the immune system. Furthermore, when burned, patients have lost the barrier function that the skin provides. This makes burn patients very prone to infection [26, 27]. Early diagnosis and intervention are essential to care for the burn patient. Antibiotics should be directed as specifically as possible at the known or most likely pathogens. The most common types of infections are:

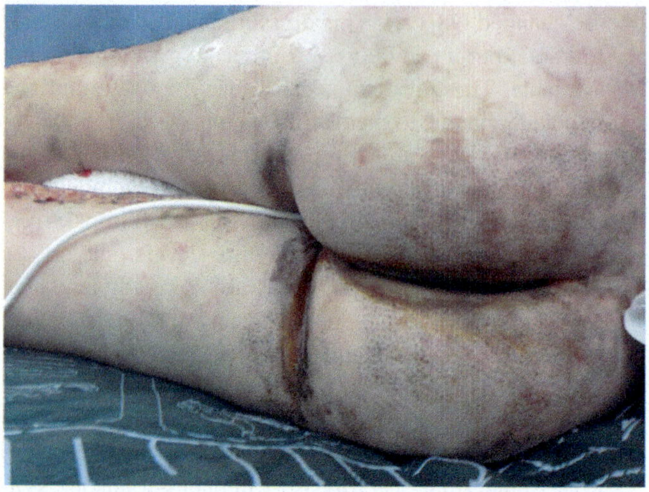

Fig. 54.3 Severe burn wound infection in a 5-year old with a 73% TBSA burn. Note the obvious bacterial invasion of the dead dermis as black stippling within the hair follicles. This type of wound requires broad spectrum IV antibiotics and immediate debridement to viable tissue

A. *Burn Wound Cellulitis* – This usually occurs in the first 3–5 days after the burn injury (but it can occur within 24 h of injury). The burn acts as a portal of entry for Gram (+) organisms (usually streptococcus and, less commonly, staph). The patient develops an erythema extending several centimeters from the wound edge. There is swelling, especially if an extremity is involved. The patient will almost always have a fever to 38–39.5°C. Treatment is with a beta-lactamase-resistant penicillin or a first generation cephalosporin (Ancef). The patients usually respond to therapy within 48–72 h, and then they can be switched to PO antibiotics. If penicillin allergic, clindamycin is a good alternative. Rarely, the cellulitis will not respond to these measures, and gentamicin can be added, or the burn may need to be excised [28].

B. *Burn Wound Sepsis* – This is a systemic infection caused by proliferation of bacteria in the burn wound. It has a high mortality. The diagnosis is usually made clinically by the appearance of the wound. The diagnosis can be confirmed by wound biopsy and frozen section. The treatment is broad spectrum antibiotics and excision of the necrotic part of the wound. Burn wound sepsis can attack normal tissue and thus cause portions of the burn wound that were initially superficial to "extend" and become full-thickness burn. It can also infect donor sites and convert them to full-thickness wounds. On a large wound, these infections can have a very rapid course [29–31] (Fig. 54.3).

C. *Pneumonia* – This is the most common infection occurring in the ICU, usually in intubated patients. It is difficult to diagnose. The patients need to have three of the following: (1) a new infiltrate on CXR, (2) numerous white blood cells on gram's stain of sputum, (3) a predominant pathogen on sputum culture, and (4) some of the signs of sepsis (see signs of sepsis in the burn patient). This infection most often occurs after the patients have been intubated for 5–7 days. The pathogen is almost always a gram-negative rod (*Acinetobacter* or *Pseudomonas* are common). There is no one antibiotic or combination of antibiotics that kills all of the gram-negative pathogens, so it is essential that you check the cultures and sensitivities daily. In the past, antibiotics such as ticarcillin/clavulanic acid, or imipenem/cilastatin with an aminoglycoside such as tobramycin or amikacin, have been effective [32]. It is important to recognize and treat pneumonia early as it may lead to septic shock, which may result in further extension of the burn, or conversion of donor site (which are by definition partial thickness wounds) to full-thickness wounds due to hypotension resulting in shunting of blood to the central circulation and exclusion of oxygen-rich blood to the subcutaneous tissue and skin.

D. *Peripheral and Central Line Infection* – Intravenous catheters are both essential to the burn patient and one of the most frequent portals of infection [33].

Line Changes

Central lines are changed to prevent infection. The longer the lines stay in, the greater incidence of infection. Line sepsis is a clinical diagnosis. To prevent sepsis, the site of the line should be changed if the patient has a fever, elevated white cell count, and without an obvious source. If the line site is purulent or erythematous, change the line. In general, do not do changes over a guide wire unless you have tried three times to change a line and have not met with success. There is little to be gained by culturing the tip or the intracutaneous portion of the catheter. Never draw a blood culture from a central line unless you do it as you are inserting it [34, 35].

Peripheral lines should be changed when the patient arrives in the unit (field lines) and if they become erythematous, or a palpable cord is present.

E. *Suppurative Thrombophebitis*

When a peripheral line becomes infected, pus can accumulate inside the cannulated vein, forming what amounts to an intravascular abscess. The infection subsequently progresses up the vein. The patients develop a fever, leukocytosis, and a painful swollen IV site. Sometimes pus can be expressed from the insertion site. This is a common hospital acquired infection in burn patients. The organism responsible is usually a gram-positive, though gram-negatives and yeast can also cause it. Remember that suppurative thrombophlebitis can occur in veins where the IV had been removed. The treatment is to administer antibiotics and to excise the infected vein up to the point where it becomes normal again.

Rarely, suppurative thrombophlebitis can occur in a deep vein. Keep in mind that suppurative thrombophlebitis or an infection in a site of an infiltrated IV can be a life-threatening infection in a burn patient.

Special Problems/Nontypical Burns that May Require ICU Care

Ear Burns

The ear is unique in that it contains cartilage that is just under thin skin. This cartilage can easily be exposed or injured by a deep second- or third-degree burn. Because the cartilage has a poor blood supply, it is very susceptible to infection, and these infections are very difficult to cure. Sulfamylon penetrates into the cartilage better than any other topical antibiotic, so it is always used on ear burns. It is important that ear cartilage infections, auricular chondritis, be recognized promptly and be properly treated. The diagnosis is made by history and physical exam. The patient will report new pain or an increase of pain in the ear; the ear will be erythematous and tender to palpation; and there will be an increase in the auriculocephalic angle (the ear will protrude laterally from the head). Chondritis usually occurs 2–6 weeks after the burn, often after the patient has gone home. It can occur after a superficial second-degree burn, as well as a third-degree burn. The ear must be carefully examined for small abscesses. If any are present, they must be incised and drained in the OR, and any necrotic cartilage must be debrided. Sometimes, an irrigation catheter is left in the ear, and antibiotic irrigation is used post-op. The patients should be started on IV antibiotics. There is a technique for making antibiotics go into the cartilage with a low-voltage electric current (ionophoresis). This technique can be used for refractory cases. The most common organism is *Pseudomonas aeruginosa*, but gram-positive infections are possible, and cultures should always be sent. The infection in the cartilage can be very difficult to eliminate. Often it recurs after appearing initially to be eradicated. The patients occasionally develop chronic severe pain that can only be cured by amputating the ear [36].

Tar Burns

Tar or pitch blend is used in sealing roofs. It is heated to about 450°F to melt. Burns are usually on the hands and forearms. Patients present with a thick layer of adherent tar. Do not try to peel it off. Apply petroleum ointment or a fleet's oil retention enema. This will slowly dissolve the tar so that it can be removed. The burns are then treated with Silvadene [37, 38].

Electrical Burns

There are two kinds of electrical burns:

1. Arc burns – flash burns produced by heat generated by an electrical arc
2. Current burns – tissue destruction caused by electricity passing through the human body

It is very important that you be able to distinguish between these two types of burns.

Arc burns are essentially thermal burns caused by electrically generated heat. They are much more common than current burns. There usually is no history of tetany in involved muscle groups. The neurological exam of the affected extremity is usually normal. There is no entrance and exit wound. There is no deep tissue damage and no rise in compartment pressures, and urine myoglobin does not need to be checked. Arc burns are treated just like thermal burns [39].

Current burns represent direct tissue destruction by electricity. There is a characteristic deep well-circumscribed entrance and exit wound. The entrance and exit wounds are usually on widely different areas of the body (i.e., entrance hand; exit feet). There is usually a history of tetanus muscle contracture. The neurological exam of the involved extremity is usually not normal [40].

Management:

1. Document and careful neurological exam.
2. Watch closely for compartment syndrome. If there is any doubt, measure compartment pressures directly with Stryker soft tissue pressure monitor.
3. If myoglobin is present in the urine, maintain urine output of 100 cc/h.
4. Most of the patients will need operative debridement within 48 h of admission. Often, multiple procedures are done with eventual soft tissue coverage of the defect.

Chemical Burns that Usually Require ICU Care

Burns from caustic chemicals are uncommon. It is important to ascertain exactly what the offending chemical was, how the exposure occurred, whether or not any of the chemical was swallowed or inhaled, and how long the chemical was in contact with the skin before being irrigated.

The first aid for all chemical burns is copious irrigation in shower for adults and with normal saline for small children. Remove and dispose of contaminated clothing. Be careful not to get any chemical on yourself.

Chemical exposures to the eyes should be irrigated with 1 liter normal saline, and then a visual acuity test and a fluorescein dye test should be performed. Ophthalmology should be consulted on any patient with a significant eye chemical exposure.

After irrigation, the burn should be debrided and dressed like any other burn. Some chemical exposures cause unique problems and require specific therapy. These are hydrofluoric acid (HF), phenol, and white phosphorus burns.

HF Concentration Symptoms and Systemic Toxicity

Hydrofluoric acid (HF) is used in chrome or rust cleaners and in industry for etching other metals or glass. It is corrosive and the fluoride ion penetrates deeply into tissues to cause progressive tissue destruction. Burns are usually seen when HF concentrations are >20%. The fluoride ion is inactivated by calcium ions.

Hydrofluoric acid is toxic. Even small amounts swallowed, inhaled, or absorbed through the skin can cause systemic symptoms. Toxicity from isolated dermal exposure is uncommon when the HF concentration is less than 50%. For HF concentrations above 50%, even small burns can be fatal.

The toxicity of HF is related to its ability to bind Ca^{++} and Mg^{++} ions and remove them from the blood. The classic physical signs of hypocalcemia do not usually occur. The patients develop ventricular arrhythmias (V-tach, V-fib) that are remarkably resistant to antiarrhythmic drugs and tend to recur after cardioversion. The arrhythmias occur even after the ionized calcium, and magnesium have been corrected. It is thought that the fluoride ion is directly cardiotoxic [41].

Patients who present with acute HF burns that are obviously full thickness and are >1% TBSA should be taken immediately to surgery to excise the wound and thus remove the toxin. Intravenous doses of calcium chloride and magnesium sulfate should be given to prevent cardiac arrhythmias. Magnesium and ionized calcium levels should be followed.

Inhaled HF causes severe pulmonary edema and lung parenchymal destruction. The patients develop an ARDS-like syndrome that is rapidly progressive. Aerosolized calcium gluconate has been used to treat the condition with mixed results. Dilute the calcium gluconate with saline to 2.5–3.0% and aerosolize it with a nebulizer.

HF Hand Burns

HF hand burns are typically seen in those who use industrial strength chrome cleaner at home without gloves to wash the chrome on their car (wheels). The hallmark of ongoing tissue destruction is pain. If the patient has persistent pain after rinsing the involved part, begin calcium therapy. If there is no bleb formation or tissue blanching, calcium gluconate gel (2.5%) (available from the pharmacy) can be rubbed over the affected area and put into rubber gloves and worn by the patient. The glove is left in place until the pain and tenderness resolves or progresses to a more severe burn.

For more severe burns (tissue blanching or bleb formation) not on the digits, calcium gluconate 10% solution is injected into the subcutaneous tissues with a 25 gauge needle, 0.5 cc/cm^2 of burned tissue.

For HF digital burns that progress to bleb formation or blanching, an intra-arterial calcium infusion may be used. 10 cc of 10% calcium gluconate is mixed with 40 ml of D5W. Place either a radial or brachial art line. Infuse at 12 cc/h (4 h for the entire mixture) and then reevaluate. If the symptoms have not resolved, infuse for another 4 h. These burns will rarely be severe enough to need palmer or digital fasciotomies [42].

Phenol Burns

Phenol is a solvent used by industry. It acts as a local anesthetic, so the patient may not realize that he is burned. If removed promptly, it causes a partial thickness burn. Phenol is rapidly absorbed through the skin and has systemic toxicity. The burn should be cleaned with polyethylene glycol (PE6 300 or 400), propylene glycol, or vegetable oil to remove the phenol. Eucerin lotion contains these substances. Rinse off the lotion and apply Silvadene. Delayed toxicity from the absorbed phenol can cause renal failure, intravascular hemolysis, and altered hepatic function [43, 44].

White Phosphorus Burns

White phosphorus is an incendiary agent used in fireworks and military ammunitions. White phosphorus is used primarily by the military in bullets, mortars, rockets, improvised explosive devices, or bombs. Its' use was outlawed by the Geneva Conventions years ago, but old stockpiles exist, and it is used by terrorist groups and rogue states and non-state actors. The burn is progressive as long as oxygen is available. This thermogenic reaction generates a number of phosphates and oxidates, which bind calcium ions producing hypocalcaemia. It causes potentially lethal deep burns. It is highly lipolytic, which penetrate the tissue producing systemic effects. If still burning, soft tissue may need rapid debridement until all visible white phosphorus has been removed. It is important to remember that water application will not "extinguish" the white phosphorus and in fact may only exacerbate the chemical burn. Physical removal (via debridement) of the white phosphorus is what will be effective. Then soak the wounds with saline or water to avoid exposure to oxygen and then 2% copper sulfate solution if available. Monitor calcium and phosphorus levels closely. Debride the wounds until no more white phosphorus can be found in the wound. Sudden death from electrolyte abnormalities has been seen for burns more than 10% TBSA. Delayed hepatotoxicity is possible [45, 46].

References

1. Ryan CM, et al. Objective estimates of the probability of death from burn injuries. N Engl J Med. 1998;338:362–6.
2. Wolf SE, et al. Mortality determinants in massive pediatric burns - an analysis of 103 children with >=80% TBSA burns (>=70% full-thickness). Ann Surg. 1997;29:2075–80.
3. Till GO, et al. Oxygen radical dependent lung damage following thermal-injury of rat skin. J Trauma. 1983;23:269–77.
4. Allison F, et al. Studies on the pathogenesis of acute inflammation. 1. The inflammatory reaction to thermal injury as observed in the rabbit ear chamber. J Exp Med. 1955;102:655–68.
5. Wilmore DW, et al. Influence of the burn wound on local and systemic responses to injury. Ann Surg. 1977;186:444–58.
6. Pruitt BA Jr. Protection from excessive resuscitation: "pushing the pendulum back". J Trauma. 2000;49(3):567–8.
7. Saffle JR. The phenomenon of "fluid creep" in acute burn resuscitation. J Burn Care Res. 2007;28(3):382–95.
8. Chung KK, Wolf SE, Cancio LC, et al. Resuscitation of severely burned military casualties: fluid begets more fluid. J Trauma Crit Care. 2009;67:231–7.
9. Chung KK, Salinas J, Renz EM, et al. Simple derivation of the initial fluid rate for the resuscitation of severely burned adult combat casualties: in silico validation of the rule of 10. J Trauma. 2010;69(suppl 1):S49–54.
10. Goodwin CW, et al. Randomized trial of efficacy of crystalloid and colloid resuscitation on hemodynamic-response and lung water following thermal-injury. Ann Surg. 1983;197:520–31.
11. Navar PD, et al. Effect of inhalation injury on fluid resuscitation requirements after thermal-injury. Am J Surg. 2004;363:1895–902.
12. Ivy ME, Atweh NA, Palmer J, et al. Intra-abdominal hypertension and abdominal compartment syndrome in burn patients. J Trauma. 2000;49:387–91.
13. Brownson EG, Pham TN, Chung KK. How to recognize a failed burn resuscitation. Crit Care Clin. 2016;32:567–75.
14. Smith DL, et al. Effect of inhalation injury, burn size, and age on mortality—a study of 1447 consecutive burn patients. J Trauma. 1994;37:655–9.
15. Bennett JE, Lewis E. Operative decompression of constricting burns. Surgery. 1958;43:949–55.
16. Kaplan I, White W. Incisional decompression of circumferential burns. Plast Reconstr Surg. 1961;28:609–18.
17. Pruitt BA, Dowling JA, Moncrief JA. Escharotomy in early burn care. Arch Surg. 1968;96:502–7.
18. Fox CL Jr. Silver sulfadiazine—a new topical therapy for *Pseudomonas* in burns. Arch Surg. 1968;96:184–8.
19. Stanford W, Rappole BW, Fox CL Jr. Clinical experience with silver sulfadiazine, a new topical agent for control of *Pseudomonas* infections in burns. J Trauma. 1969;9:377–88.
20. Fox CL Jr, Modak SM. Mechanism of silver sulfadiazine action on burn wound infections. Antimicrob Agents Chemother. 1974;5:582–8.
21. White MG, Asch MJ. Acid-base effects of topical mafenide acetate in the burned patient. N Engl J Med. 1971;284:1281–6.
22. Harrison HN, Bales H, Jacoby F. The behavior of mafenide acetate as a basis for its clinical use. Arch Surg. 1971;103:449–53.
23. Klasen HJ. A historical review of the use of silver in the treatment of burns. II. Renewed interest for silver. Burns. 2000;26:131–8.
24. Lindberg RB, Moncrief JA, Switzer WE, Order SE, Mills W Jr. The successful control of burn wound sepsis. J Trauma. 1965;5:601–16.
25. Moyer CA, Brentano L, Gravens DL, Margraf HW, Monafo WW Jr. Treatment of large burns with 0.5% silver nitrate solution. Arch Surg. 1965;90:812–67.
26. Pruitt BA Jr. The diagnosis and treatment of infection in the burn patient. Burns. 1984;11:79–83.
27. Brown TP, Cancio LC, McManus AT, Mason AD Jr. Survival benefit conferred by topical antimicrobial preparations in burn patients: a historical perspective. J Trauma. 2004;56:863–6.
28. Mayhall GC. The epidemiology of burn wound infections: then and now. Clin Infect Dis. 2003;37:543–50.
29. Richard P, et al. *Pseudomonas aeruginosa* outbreak in a burn unit—role of antimicrobials in the emergence of multiply resistant strains. J Infect Dis. 1994;170:377–83.
30. Pruitt BA, et al. Burn wound infections: current status. World J Surg. 1998;22:135–45.
31. Pruitt BA Jr, O'Neill JA Jr, Moncrief JA, Lindberg RB. Successful control of burn-wound sepsis. JAMA. 1968;203:1054–6.
32. Shirani KZ, et al. The influence of inhalation injury and pneumonia on burn mortality. Ann Surg. 1987;205:82–7.
33. van Duin D, Jones SW, Dibiase L, et al. Reduction in central line-associated bloodstream infections in patients with burns. Infect Control Hosp Epidemiol. 2014;35(8):1066–8. Epub 2014 Jun 20
34. O'Mara MS, Reed NL, Palmieri TL, Greenhalgh DG. Central venous catheter infections in burn patients with scheduled catheter exchange and replacement. J Surg Res. 2007;142(2):341–50.
35. King B, Schulman CI, Pepe A, Pappas P, Varas R, Namias N. Timing of central venous catheter exchange and frequency of bacteremia in burn patients. J Burn Care Res. 2007;28(6):859–60.
36. Purdue GF, Hunt JL. Chondritis of the burned ear: a preventable complication. Am J Surg. 1986;152:257–9.
37. Baruchin AM, Schraf S, Rosenberg L, Sagi AA. Hot bitumen burns: 92 hospitalized patients. Burns. 1997;23:438–41.
38. Carta T, Gawaziuk J, Liu S, Logsetty S. Use of mineral oil Fleet enema for the removal of a large tar burn: a case report. Burns. 2015;41(2):e11–4. https://doi.org/10.1016/j.burns.2014.07.007. Epub 2014 Oct 11
39. Buja Z, Arifi H, Hoxha E. Electrical burn injuries. An eight-year review. Ann Burns Fire Disasters. 2010;23(1):4–7.
40. Simmons R. Emergency management of electrical burns. J Emerg Nurs. 1977;3(2):13–5.
41. Burd A. Hydrofluoric acid burns: rational treatment. J Burn Care Res. 2009;30:908.
42. Dalamaga M, Karmaniolas K, Nikolaidou A, et al. Hypocalcemia, hypomagnesemia, and hypokalemia following hydrofluoric acid chemical injury. J Burn Care Res. 2008;29:541–3.
43. Lin TM, Lee SS, Lai CS, et al. Phenol burn. Burns. 2006;32:517–21.
44. Parikh TJ. Acute concentrated phenol dermal burns: complications and management. Indian J Crit Care Med. 2015;19(5):280–2.
45. Davis KG. Acute management of white phosphorus burn. Mil Med. 2002;167:83–4.
46. Barillo DJ, Cancio LC, Goodwin CW. Treatment of white phosphorus and other chemical burn injuries at one burn center over a 51-year period. Burns. 2004;30:448–52.

Care of the Patient with Liver Failure Requiring Transplantation

55

Caroline Park and Damon Clark

Introduction and Preoperative Care

Patients undergo liver transplantation to address chronic liver failure, acute fulminant liver failure, or primary liver cancer. Depending on acuity, patients with decompensated chronic or acute fulminant liver failure generally require preoperative intensive care unit (ICU) admission to manage organ dysfunction.

Those with chronic liver failure are allocated an organ based on waiting list position determined by their local organ procurement organization (OPO). This position is dependent upon blood type and Model for End-Stage Liver Disease (MELD) score. MELD is determined by a weighting of serum bilirubin, creatinine, and international normalization ratio (INR). Those with a high MELD score have a greater risk of mortality and thus are given priority to transplantation. Patients with a MELD score of 40 have a 75% chance of death within 3 months. This is particularly important given the transplantation is typically performed on those with high MELD scores in large urban areas such as ours in the greater Los Angeles area. These patients thus are critically ill and require preoperative ICU monitoring and care.

Patients with hepatocellular carcinoma (HCC) who require liver transplantation are given a MELD exception and rarely require preoperative ICU care. The patient's ability to undergo liver transplant in the setting of HCC is determined by the Milan criteria or the University of California, San Francisco (UCSF) criteria. HCC patients with a single tumor <5 cm, up to three tumors <3 cm, absence of macroscopic vascular invasion, and absence of extrahepatic spread may undergo liver transplantation based on the Milan criteria.

C. Park · D. Clark (✉)
University of Southern California Keck School of Medicine, Keck Hospital, Norris Cancer Hospital and LAC-USC, Department of Surgery, Acute Care Surgery and Surgical Critical Care, Los Angeles, CA, USA
e-mail: Caroline.Park2@med.usc.edu; Damon.Clark@med.usc.edu

Preoperative Care of Patients with Decompensated Chronic Liver Failure

Neurologic

Altered level of consciousness is common in patients with decompensated cirrhosis. This is a result of portosystemic shunting and hepatocellular dysfunction/toxin production that results in hepatic encephalopathy. Most severe or accelerated changes in the level of consciousness are the result of a precipitating event such as a significant upper gastrointestinal bleed and resultant uremia or a new infection. Encephalopathy can be exacerbated by the administration of medications such as benzodiazepines that are generally avoided in the routine treatment of this patient population. Those with low-grade encephalopathy, manifested by mild confusion and tremors, are administered agents such as lactulose to decrease ammonia absorption by acidifying bowel content and increase transit of the bowel contents. Rifaximin is also commonly used to diminish the presence of urease and protease-splitting bacteria. It is important to remember to discontinue lactulose therapy in advance of anticipated liver transplantation to avoid intraoperative diarrhea and possible bowel distention.

Cardiac

Systemic and splanchnic arteriolar vasodilation is a well-known physiologic derangement in patients with end-stage liver disease. As a result, these patients have hyperdynamic and low systemic vascular resistance cardiac profiles and often require vasopressor therapy—whether oral (e.g., midodrine) or intravenous (e.g., norepinephrine)—to maintain adequate mean arterial pressures (MAP) of >65 mmHg. It is important to consider that hypotension may be multifactorial, resulting from active hemorrhage, infection, and/or systemic inflammatory response (SIRS). Further, cardiac contractile function may be impaired in patients with long-standing cirrhosis or in those with associated ischemic cardiac disease. Routine use of beta blockade as prophylaxis in those with varices may also cause hypotension. If hemor-

A. Salim et al. (eds.), *Surgical Critical Care Therapy*, https://doi.org/10.1007/978-3-319-71712-8_55

rhage and SIRS response have been addressed and ruled out, refractory hypotension could be a result of adrenal insufficiency; this is a common pathophysiology in end-stage liver disease patients. There is little additional role for invasive cardiac monitoring in cirrhotic patients for the diagnosis and treatment of shock over echocardiography and other noninvasive means. In general, the treatment of shock does not depart much from that in other patients. Patients should be approached similarly with crystalloid resuscitation and early goal-directed therapy; there is little evidence that albumin should be the resuscitative fluid of choice. Monitoring base deficit and lactate is as prognostic and useful to guide resuscitative efforts in patients with decompensated liver disease as it is for the general ICU population.

Pulmonary

Patients with advanced liver disease may have other associated pulmonary disorders, including hepatic hydrothorax, emphysema from alpha-1-antitrypsin deficiency, hepatopulmonary syndrome (HPS), and portopulmonary hypertension (PPH).

Hydrothorax is typically the result of tense abdominal ascites and should be addressed by paracentesis, thoracentesis, and total body volume management. Draining of pulmonary effusions should be limited to those with impending respiratory failure due to the risk of infection and hemorrhage associated with invasive procedures and re-accumulation. Definitive treatment of pulmonary effusions is with liver transplantation.

HPS is caused by intrapulmonary shunting and does not result in right heart failure. Patients with HPS will classically experience positional hypoxia. PPH on the other hand results from pulmonary vascular vasoconstriction and can ultimately lead to thrombosis and fibrosis. In contrast to HPS, right heart failure is typical in PPH.

It is important to distinguish between HPS and PPH. In general, liver transplantation is curative of the former and, until recently, was contraindicated in the latter. However, the introduction of many new agents and classes of agents to treat pulmonary hypertension may render liver transplantation possible in centers of excellence with careful pre- and intraoperative monitoring. Although noninvasive monitoring is helpful and new modalities are being developed, the most expeditious and accurate modality to differentiate between HPS and PPH is right heart catheterization. HPS, PPH, and CHF can all cause elevated pulmonary artery pressures. However, pulmonary artery wedge pressure (PAWP) is low in HPS and PPH (and elevated in CHF). Pulmonary vascular resistance (PVR) is normal to decreased in HPS but elevated in PPH. Thus, cardiac output is elevated in HPS and normal to decreased in PPH.

Renal

One of the major causes of AKI in patients with advanced cirrhosis and ascites is the phenomenon of hepatorenal syndrome (HRS) or acute renal failure without other etiology. There are two subtypes of HRS, types I and II. The first type generally progresses with a rapid decrease in renal function and is characterized with doubling in serum creatinine within that period of time. It may be precipitated by spontaneous bacterial peritonitis, gastroenteritis with high-volume diarrhea, volume loss from gastrointestinal bleed, or large-volume paracentesis without appropriate volume repletion. Type I HRS can be fatal and often leads to multi-system organ failure. Type II HRS demonstrates a more indolent course of renal failure, often precipitated by ascites refractory to diuretic treatment [1]. HRS develops due to splanchnic circulation vasodilation, intravascular hypovolemia, and renal vasoconstriction and is most often a diagnosis of exclusion after investigating for other causes of renal failure. The treatment approach includes strict intake and output monitoring, serum creatinine monitoring, and following changes from baseline or within the past 48 h. If the patient develops oliguria with elevated serum creatinine greater than 50% from a reference value or baseline serum creatinine level, suspect AKI. Multiple diagnostic variable are used to diagnose HRS in patients with cirrhosis (Fig. 55.1). These patients may require combined liver and renal transplant and/or intraoperative renal replacement therapy to assist with volume status, correcting acidosis, and electrolyte abnormalities. The mainstay of treatment for HRS is liver transplantation, after which a majority of patients demonstrate a return to adequate renal function. Consideration should be given to a combined liver/kidney transplantation in those who have required dialysis for greater than 2 months, although this time period is controversial. A variety of approaches can be used to increase intravascular volume and MAP including albumin and vasopressors (norepinephrine, terlipressin). Intermittent paracentesis may be necessary to manage third spacing of fluids in hepatorenal syndrome prior to liver transplant [2, 3]. Type 1 HRS requires multiple therapeutic strategies and therapies; please refer to Fig. 55.2 for a detailed algorithm.

Infectious Disease

The presence of infection in a cirrhotic patient quadruples mortality and worsens liver function. Those with chronic liver failure are functionally immunosuppressed and are often colonized with multiresistant organisms. The most common infection in these patients is spontaneous bacterial peritonitis. Strict attention should be paid to removing unnecessary catheters and avoiding intubation/mechanical ventilation, when possible. Patients require prophylactic antibiotics for spontaneous bacterial peritonitis after a variceal bleed; however, there is little need for general broad-spectrum antimicrobial therapy.

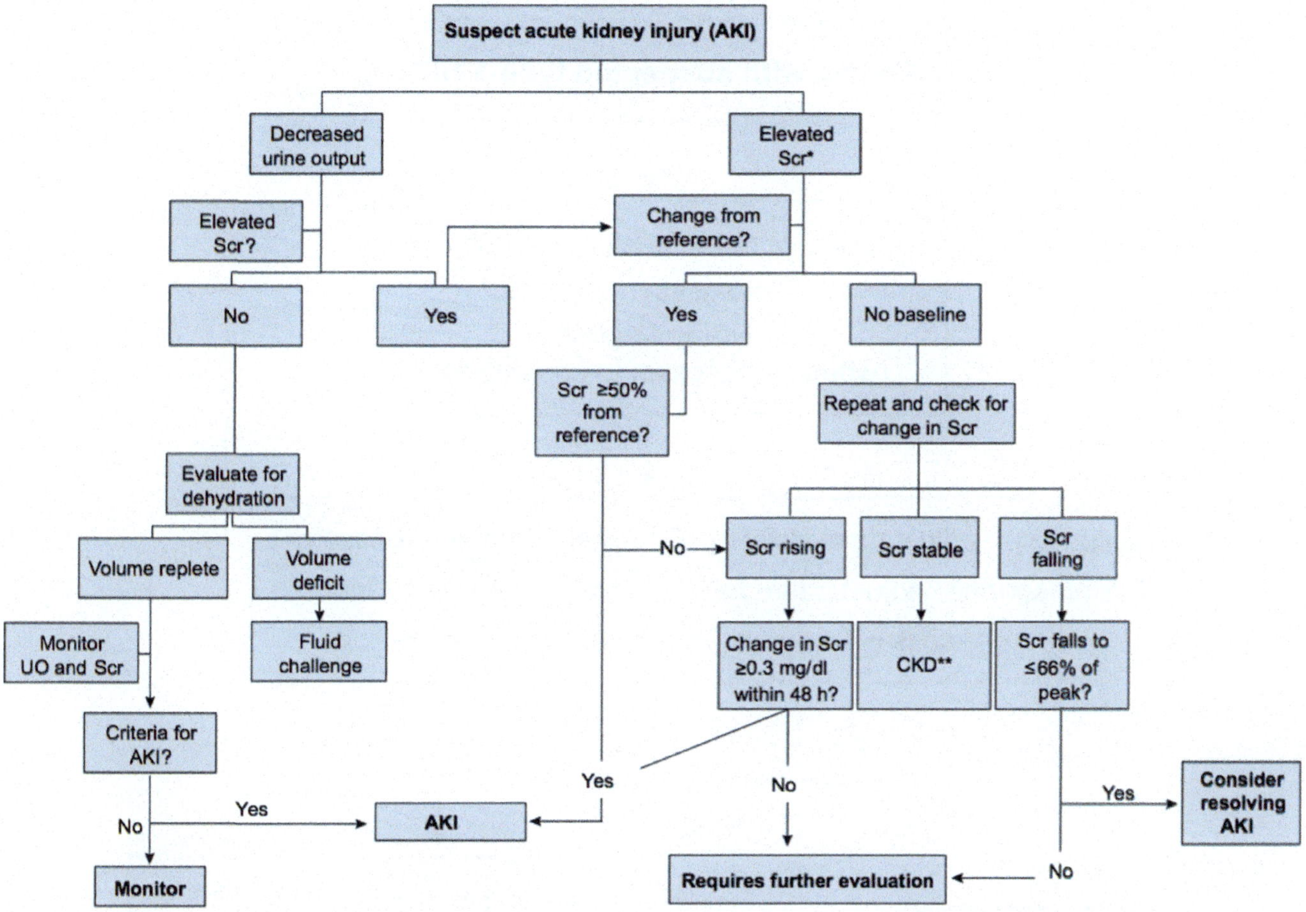

Fig. 55.1 Diagnostic algorithm to evaluate acute kidney injury in the hospitalized patient with cirrhosis. AKI acute kidney injury, Scr serum creatinine, UO urine output, CKD chronic kidney disease, RRT renal replacement therapy, Na sodium (Reproduced with permission from Nadim et al. "Management of the critically ill patient with cirrhosis: A multidisciplinary perspective")

Preoperative Care of the Patient with Acute Fulminant Liver Failure

Patients with fulminant liver failure receive a MELD exemption in listing—the appropriateness of transplantation may be determined by King's criteria (Table 55.1). In general, patients experience toxic necrosis of the liver on a baseline of normal function, most commonly due to intentional or inadvertent ingestion of large doses of acetaminophen. Thus, the abnormalities noted are lactic acidosis, marked elevation of INR, and high-grade encephalopathy. Ascites and hepatorenal syndrome are often not present given the acuity of presentation. Creatinine, however, is often elevated due to ATN. If time of ingestion is known, and within 8 h, N-acetylcysteine should be administered to prevent further toxicity in acute liver failure patients. If the patient fails medical management with progression of liver failure, liver transplantation will be required. The most significant risk of mortality to a patient with fulminant liver failure is that of cerebral edema and subsequent death from cerebral herniation. Intracranial monitoring remains controversial given severe coagulopathy, thrombocytopenia, and risk of infection. Serum sodium of 145–150 meq/L should be maintained with hypertonic saline to decrease the amount of cerebral edema. If renal dialysis is required, a continuous mode is preferred to avoid rapid fluid shifts that may exacerbate cerebral edema.

Postoperative Care

Patients having undergone liver transplantation will require postoperative intensive care unit (ICU) admission. Close communication and coordination of care between the surgeons, anesthesiologists, intensivists, and nursing staff are essential to the management of the patient in this setting. Liver transplantation typically entails a lengthy surgical procedure requiring significant amounts of blood product transfusion and risk of postoperative respiratory insufficiency. Preoperatively, many of these patients have neurologic, cardiopulmonary, and renal dysfunction requiring

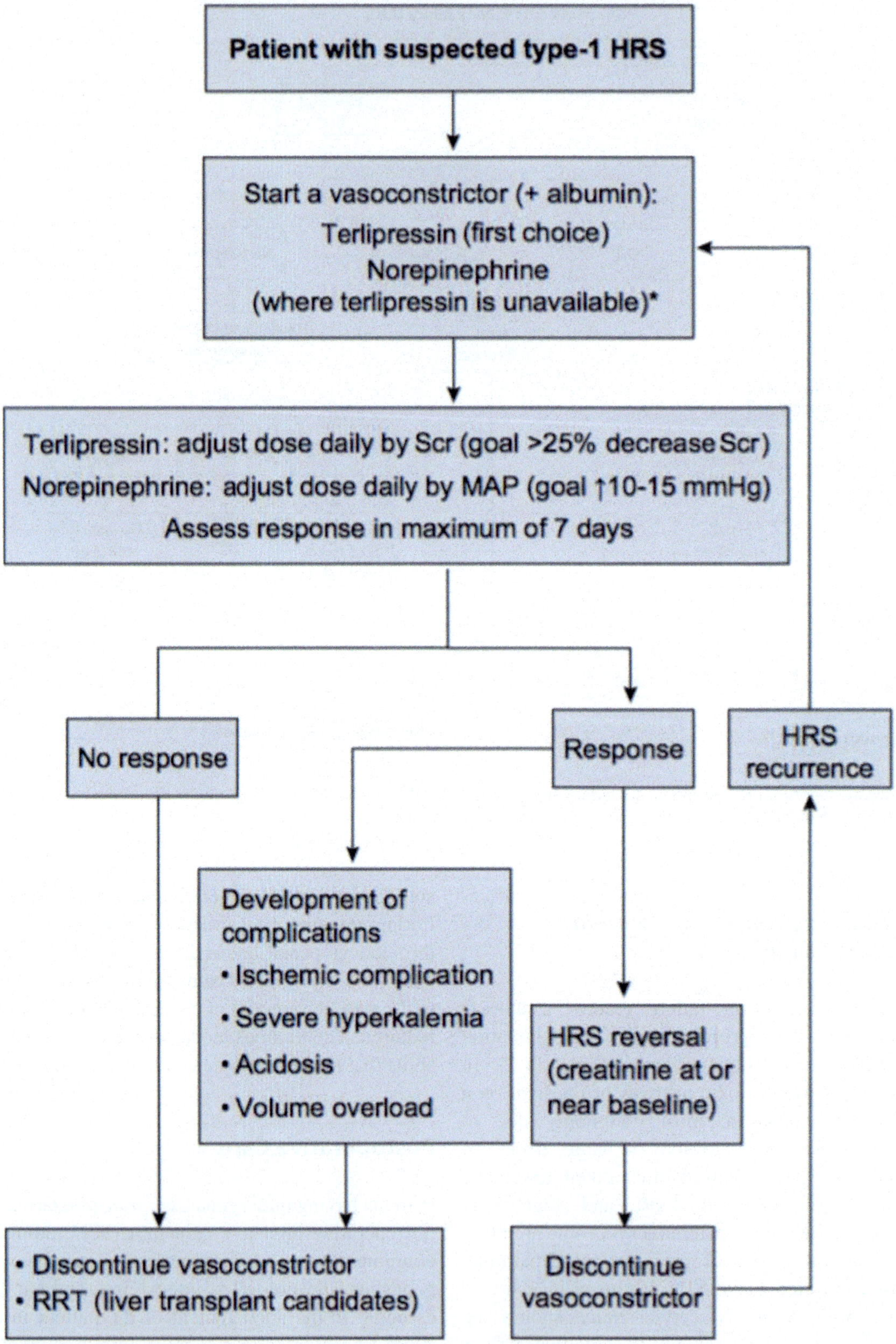

Fig. 55.2 Algorithm for patients with suspected type 1 HRS. HRS hepatorenal syndrome, RRT renal replacement therapy. *The authors recommend a trial of octreotide IV and midodrine for a maximum of 3 days prior to the initiation of norepinephrine (Reproduced with permission from Nadim et al. "Management of the critically ill patient with cirrhosis: A multidisciplinary perspective")

Table 55.1 King's College criteria for patients with acute liver failure

Acetaminophen	Non-acetaminophen
Lactate >3.5	INR > 6.5 regardless of encephalopathy
pH < 7.3	3 out of 5 of the following
Grade 3 or 4 encephalopathy	Bilirubin >3.0
INR > 6.5	INR > 3.5
Creatinine >3.0	Age < 10 or >40
	Cause indeterminate or drug induced
	Jaundice to encephalopathy >7 days

ICU admission prior to the transplant. Pre-liver transplant patients that are in renal failure requiring dialysis, in respiratory failure requiring mechanical ventilation, and/or admitted to the ICU prior to transplant have a higher risk of postoperative complications and prolonged ICU length of stay (LOS) [4].

Neurologic

Fentanyl, a narcotic, is the first-line agent for the treatment of pain and agitation given its rapid onset and short duration of action in postoperative transplant patient. Those who require additional sedation for agitation not controlled with narcotic analgesia benefit from the use of dexmedetomidine over benzodiazepines given a decreased risk of iatrogenic delirium and decreased length of mechanical ventilation [5]. Dexmedetomidine is an alpha-2 adrenoreceptor agonist and should be used in caution with patients with hypotension and baseline bradycardia as it can exacerbate both conditions. With the use of spontaneous awakening trials (SATs), Richmond Agitation and Sedation Score (RASS), and Confusion Assessment Method for the ICU (CAM-ICU), patients have decreased episodes of delirium, duration of mechanical ventilation, and ICU and hospital length of stay [6]. In this particular population, however, sustained delirium and encephalopathy may be the result of poor functioning of liver transplant graft, infection, intracranial hemorrhage or cerebral ischemia, seizures, and/or immunosuppressant toxicity. There should be a low threshold to pursue diagnostic CT scan of head, cultures including cerebral spinal fluid, and electroencephalography (EEG) in the posttransplant patient with change in mental status.

Encephalopathy due to cerebral edema associated with fulminant liver failure and elevated ammonia levels in patients with end-stage liver disease should be corrected with an adequately functioning liver transplant graft. If an intracranial monitor was placed preoperatively, it should be maintained until the INR is corrected and the liver is functioning well.

Respiratory Failure and Insufficiency

In the past decade, early recovery after surgery or "fast-track" programs have been implemented in a variety of disciplines, including hepatobiliary and colorectal patients after elective surgery with no worsening of postoperative outcomes and improvement in patient satisfaction. Liver transplant patients may be eligible for fast-track extubation immediately postoperative in the operating room and upon arrival to the ICU. Patients that successfully undergo fast-track extubation have been shown to benefit from decreased rates of re-intubation and tracheostomy along with improved survival [7]. Patients that are likely not candidates for fast-track extubation include those with preoperative acute liver failure, re-transplantation, Child's C cirrhosis, and intraoperative red blood cell transfusion >6 units [7]. Patients that require continued mechanical ventilation upon arrival to the ICU should be placed on ventilator settings of tidal volume 6 mL/kg and FiO2 < 0.4 [8]. Patients who may exhibit transfusion-related lung injury after receiving a significant amount of blood products require ventilation strategies similar to patients with acute respiratory distress syndrome (ARDS); in this case, target tidal volumes of 6 mL/kg with supplemental oxygen and positive end-expiratory pressure (PEEP) [9]. Infections of the lower respiratory tract require broad-spectrum antibiotics and antifungals until species and sensitivities are established. The liver transplant patients who remain hemodynamically stable and require minimal mechanical ventilation settings with resolved encephalopathy should undergo daily spontaneous breathing trials (SBT) and subsequent evaluation for possible extubation to reduce the duration of mechanical ventilation and ICU length of stay [10]. Early mobilization and aggressive chest physiotherapy are performed to prevent complications of atelectasis and inadequate ventilation.

Cardiovascular

Centers may opt to monitor patients intraoperatively with pulmonary artery catheters and/or transesophageal echocardiography. Once stable and resuscitated, patients should be liberated from these devices. Steroids are routinely administered as a part of early immunosuppression regimen after liver transplant and may require a prolonged course in treating hypotension secondary to adrenal insufficiency.

Hematology

Liver transplantation patients remain at risk for postoperative hemorrhage due to thrombocytopenia, fibrinolysis, and deficiency of coagulation factors. Abnormal coagulation tests and platelet count are not good predictors of bleeding; thus aggressive correction of these coagulopathies should be avoided. Therapy should also include practical measures as avoiding hypothermia and persistent acidosis. Aggressive correction of coagulopathy and thrombocytopenia may also put patients at higher risk of hepatic artery, portal vein, and deep vein thrombosis. Typical target ranges include hemoglobin of 8 g/dl and platelet count >20 × 10^9/l [11]. Thromboelastography (TEG) may be useful in dictating guided blood product resuscitation in the post-liver transplant patients to decrease blood loss and transfusion requirements [12]. Liver transplant patients with hemorrhage that are undergoing appropriate blood product resuscitation and become hemodynamically unstable or develop abdominal compartment syndrome should return immediately to the operating room.

Nutrition

Patients with advanced cirrhosis are often malnourished and as such are at higher risk for infections, worsening encephalopathy, and decompensation. Though these patients may appear grossly overweight, their usual or dry weight is often masked by massive ascites and edema secondary to hypoalbuminemia. The American and European Society for Clinical Nutrition and Metabolism and the European Society for Clinical Nutrition and Metabolism (ASPEN [13] and ESPEN [14], respectively) have compiled an extensive set of guidelines, both of which provide a subset of consensus statements for patients with hepatic failure.

The primary goals of nutrition for patients with hepatic failure include (1) identifying and assessing patients at risk for undernutrition, (2) calculating nutritional needs and incorporating adequate protein and high-calorie formulas, and (3) considering dobhoff placement if encephalopathy precludes voluntary enteral nutrition or short-term parenteral nutrition if unable to provide enteral feeds secondary to ileus or malabsorption.

Dry or usual weight may be difficult to ascertain given the chronicity of liver disease, thus complicating calculations for caloric needs. Poor oral intake may be a result of underlying encephalopathy, gastroparesis, and overall decreased gastrointestinal motility. In prior years, protein restriction was emphasized to mitigate the effects on worsening hepatic encephalopathy. However, given the already reduced lean muscle mass of this vulnerable patient population, protein-restricted diets can worsen hepatic failure. Recommended protein intake is 1.2–1.5 g/kg/day, with a total energy intake of 35–40 kcal/kg/day. Dobhoff placement is recommended if the patient is unable to meet his/her caloric needs per os; percutaneous endoscopic gastrostomy or open gastrostomy tube is otherwise not recommended given an increased risk of complications [14].

Renal

Post-liver transplant acute kidney injury (AKI) is a frequent event with reports of up to 52% of patients developing AKI [15]. Factors such as increased Child-Pugh score, pre-existing diabetes, and large number of intraoperative transfusions increase the risk of AKI in the post-liver transplant. The development of post-liver transplant AKI leads to prolonged ICU and hospital length of stay, increased mortality, and decreased duration of liver graft function [15]. In patients that develop AKI post-liver transplantation, treatment includes the prevention of hypotension and decreased use of unnecessary blood products. The use of renal replacement therapy is reserved for patients that develop significant volume overload, uremia, and electrolyte abnormalities. The most effective treatment of postoperative liver transplant AKI is prevention. Preventive strategies include delayed initiation of calcineurin inhibitors, avoiding nephrotoxic agents such as IV contrast, and ensuring adequate control of hyperglycemia [15].

Infection

The most common cause of morbidity and mortality after liver transplantation is infection, accounting for 60% of the deaths after liver transplantation [16]. Prolonged and complicated operations, multiple catheter insertions, immunosuppression, and large quantities of fresh frozen plasma can all increase the risk of infectious complications [17]. Diagnosis of infections in this patient population may be difficult due to the lack of signs and symptoms such as fever, chills, cellulitis, and leukocytosis due to an immunosuppressed status. Early postoperative infections in liver transplant patients are typically bacterial and related to the donor's status (previous infections from advanced cirrhosis), the surgical procedure itself, prolonged use of invasive catheters, and duration of mechanical ventilation. Perioperative antibiotics are typically broad spectrum and may include third-generation cephalosporins. Early removal of invasive catheters, early mobility, pulmonary toilet, vigilant monitoring of patient's surgical wounds and drains, and early discharge from the ICU may decrease these infectious complications. Liver transplant patients are at risk of developing opportunistic infections given the initial burst of immunosuppression with high-dose steroid therapy and, as such, should be initiated on prophylactic trimethoprim-sulfamethoxazole (TMP-SMX) to prevent *Pneumocystis carinii* pneumonia and ganciclovir to prevent cytomegalovirus infection.

Complications

Technical Errors

Besides surgical and coagulopathic bleeding, other postoperative complications can occur; these include postoperative hepatic artery thrombosis (3%) or portal vein thrombosis (< 1%) [11]. The resulting lack of blood flow and developing ischemia and necrosis from hepatic artery thrombosis present with signs and symptoms similar to fulminant liver failure patients with elevated liver serum tests, coagulopathy, and severe metabolic acidosis. Doppler ultrasound of the hepatic artery and portal vein is routinely employed within the first 24–48 h after liver transplant to diagnose possible vascular complications prior to the development of ischemia and necrosis of the liver transplant graft. These patients are at high risk for continued ischemia and necrosis of the graft with the need for urgent relisting and re-transplantation. Compared to patients with hepatic artery thrombosis, those with portal vein thrombosis do not present with such critical signs and symptoms as a rapid rise in liver function tests and disruption in synthetic function. Although portal vein thrombosis leads to elevation in liver serum tests, signs and symptoms are less dramatic and may consist of mesenteric venous congestion, gastrointestinal hemorrhage, and the development of ascites. Although these patients may require re-transplantation, they can typically be managed with thrombectomy, shunt, or revision of the portal vein anastomosis. Biliary duct complications, which include anastomosis stricture or leak, affect 5–25% of liver transplant patients and are often delayed diagnoses [18]. Thrombosis of the liver transplant hepatic artery can also lead to non-anastomotic stricture [18]. Biliary duct complications can be evaluated with ultrasound of the liver transplant graft looking for biloma and biliary duct dilation. Similarly, internal to external drains placed during the liver transplantation may show biliary drainage during the first several postoperative days. Elevated serum liver tests specifically bilirubin will elevate or fail to appropriately decrease after liver transplant, and the patients may develop signs and symptoms of infection. Magnetic resonance cholangiopancreatography (MRCP) may be used as a noninvasive diagnostic modality to look for biliary anastomosis complications. Endoscopic retrograde cholangiopancreatogram (ERCP) can be used for the diagnosis of biliary anastomosis leak and stricture, in addition to possible treatment with sphincterotomy and/or biliary stent [19]. Endoscopic treatment is often preferred over percutaneous management of biliary leaks and stricture. Treatment options include endoscopic dilation and stenting and have excellent success rates approaching 75% [20]. Surgical revision of the biliary anastomosis due to stricture or leak may be required in 10–20% of patients [18, 21]. The use of broad-spectrum antibiotics for treatment or prophylaxis is recommended due to the high risk of cholangitis and intra-abdominal sepsis [22]. 30–50% of patients with biliary stricture will have to undergo re-transplantation due to chronic biliary cirrhosis due to obstruction even with adequate treatment [19, 22].

Nontechnical

Primary graft nonfunction and hyperacute rejection can occur in the immediate or acute postoperative setting. Primary graft nonfunction occurs in 2–14% of orthotopic liver transplants and typically presents similar to fulminant liver failure with significant metabolic acidosis, elevated liver enzymes, coagulopathy, and lack of bile production [11, 23]. Intraoperative hemodynamic instability, reperfusion injury of the liver transplant graft, marginal livers, and advanced age of donors and recipient are factors that may lead to primary graft nonfunction. Once diagnosed, the only treatment indicated is for relisting and liver re-transplantation. Development of hyperacute rejection (HAR) after liver transplant is a rare complication that may develop intraoperatively or in the immediate postoperative period, which is antibody-mediated and due to ABO crossmatch incompatibility. Patients with HAR typically present with progressive encephalopathy and weakness, elevated bilirubin, severe coagulopathy, thrombocytopenia, metabolic acidosis, and shock. Diagnosis is confirmed with Doppler ultrasound that displays portal vein thrombosis and absence of biliary duct stricture. Along with critical care supportive therapy, patients can be managed with plasma exchange for antibody removal and intravenous immunoglobulin [11]. Overall, patients that develop HAR will need immediate relisting and re-transplantation. Acute cellular rejection after liver transplant may occur within the first 6–8 weeks, and the patients are often out of the ICU and no longer critically ill. Patients with acute cellular rejection typically are not critically ill and may present with fever, weakness, and elevated liver function tests. Prior to treating the patients for acute cellular rejection, one must rule out all possible acute infections that could account for the signs and symptoms given that the treatment of acute cellular rejection requires immunosuppression with pulse-dose glucocorticoids and adjustment of other immunosuppression medications.

Immunosuppression

Glucocorticoids are the first-line therapy for the prevention and treatment of acute cellular rejection. Common glucocorticoids used for liver transplant include prednisone, hydrocortisone, and methylprednisolone with the first dose given while in surgery. Intravenous hydrocortisone is typically administered in the immediate postoperative period until the patient is taking enteral nutrition and can transition to oral prednisone. Most patients will undergo a glucocorticoid taper and either transitioned off of glucocorticoids or to a low maintenance dose, typically over a 6-month to 2-year period [24]. Glucocorticoids have a significant number of side effects including poor wound healing, increased infection risks, hyperglycemia, and hypertension; these patients may need judicious adjustment of insulin sliding scale for hyperglycemia. Glucocorticoid-free immunosuppression is possible and may be of benefit in patients with cirrhosis due to hepatitis C virus. [25, 26]

Calcineurin inhibitors (CNI), including cyclosporine and tacrolimus, are used to prevent and treat acute rejection and liver transplant graft loss. Both provide immunosuppression by inhibiting interleukin-2 and interferon-gamma production and require monitoring of blood levels to reach appropriate therapeutic levels. Potential side effects including altered mental status, seizures, neuropathy, renal failure, electrolyte abnormalities, and others should be monitored for and treated appropriately. Tacrolimus is currently the CNI of choice and has demonstrated superiority in preventing acute rejection and graft loss with decreased mortality [27, 28]. Posterior reversible encephalopathy syndrome (PRES) is a rare syndrome and side effect of CNI that is diagnosed with clinical exam and CT or MRI. Patients with PRES most commonly present with seizures but may also have symptoms such as headache, delirium, and visual changes. Head CT or MRI typically demonstrates vasogenic edema of the parietal or occipital lobes; however MRI may be more sensitive in diagnosing PRES. Treatment of PRES most often involves discontinuing the offending CNI and supportive care.

Mycophenolate mofetil (MMF, CellCept) is an antimetabolite that inhibits purine and pyrimidine synthesis with the active by-product of mycophenolic acid (MPA). MPA ultimately inhibits the proliferation of T lymphocytes for immunosuppression. MMF is typically used long term to reduce the dose or replace glucocorticoids. As such, the use of MMF will avoid common CNI side effects, such as nephrotoxicity and neurotoxicity, though it can cause other side effects, including abdominal pain, nausea, vomiting, anorexia, diarrhea, and bone marrow suppression. MMF as a monotherapy after the acute phase of liver transplant has shown similar results to glucocorticoids and CNI for prevention of chronic rejection and mortality [29, 30].

Mammalian target of rapamycin (mTOR) inhibitors (everolimus and sirolimus) inhibit the proliferation of lymphocytes. The use of mTOR inhibitors allows for immunosuppression while avoiding renal dysfunction and has shown potential benefit in patients undergoing liver transplant for HCV. Common complications of dyslipidemia and oral ulcers are typically easy to manage.

References

1. Yeboah MM. Hepatorenal syndrome. In: Liver disorders. Switzerland: Springer; 2017.
2. Durand F, Graupera I, Gines P, et al. Pathogenesis of Hepatorenal Syndrome: Implications for Therapy. Am J Kidney Dis. 2016;67(2):318–28.
3. Gluud LL, Christensen K, Christensen E, et al. Systematic review of randomized trials on vasoconstrictor drugs for hepatorenal syndrome. Hepatology. 2010;51(2):576–84.
4. Nadim MK, Durand F, Kellum JA, et al. Management of the critically ill patient with cirrhosis: a multidisciplinary perspective. J Hepatol. 2016;64:717–35.
5. Dale CR, Kannas DA, Fan VS, et al. Improved analgesia, sedation and delirium protocol associated with decreased duration of delirium and mechanical ventilation. Ann Am Thorac Soc. 2014;11(3):367–74.
6. Jakob SM, Ruokonene E, Grounds RM, et al. Dexmedetomidine vs. midazolam or propofol for sedation during prolonged ventilation. JAMA. 2012;307(11):1151–60.
7. Glanemann M, Hoffmeister R, Neumann U, et al. Fast tracking in liver transplanatation: which patient benefits from this approach? Transplant Proc. 2007;39(2):535–6.
8. Futier E, Constantin JM, Paugam-Burtz C, et al. A trial of intraoperative low-tidal-volume ventilation in abdominal surgery. N Engl J Med. 2013;369(5):428–37.
9. The Acute Respiratory Distress Syndrome Network. Ventilation with lower tidal volumes as compared with traditional tidal volumes for acute lung injury and the acute respiratory distress syndrome. N Engl J Med. 2000;342(18):1301–8.
10. Blackwood B, Burns KE, Cardwell CR, et al. Protocolized versus non-protocolized weaning for reducing the duration of mechanical ventilation in critically ill adult patients. Cochrane Database Syst Rev. 2014;6(11):CD006904.
11. Bates E, Martin D. Immediate postoperative management and complications on the intensive care unit. Br J Hosp Med. 2017;78(5):273–7.
12. Gurusamy KS, Pissanou T, Pikhart H, et al. Methods to decrease blood loss and transfusion requirements for liver transplantation. Cochrane Database Syst Rev. 2011;12:CD009052.
13. McClave SA, Taylor BE, Martindale RG, et al. Guidelines for the provision and assessment of nutrition support therapy in the adult critically ill patient: Society of Critical Care Medicine (SCCM) and American Society for Parenteral and Enteral Nutrition (A.S.P.E.N). J Parenter Enter Nutr. 2016;40(2):159–211.
14. Plauth M, Cabre E, Riggio O, et al. ESPEN guidelines on enteral nutrition liver disease. Clin Nutr. 2006;25(2):285. Epub 2006 May 16
15. Hilmi D, Damian A, Al-Khafaji R, et al. Acute kidney injury following orthotopic liver transplantation: incidence, risk factors and effects on patient and graft outcomes. Br J Anaesth. 2015;114(6):919–26.
16. Torbenson M, Wang J, Nichols L, et al. Causes of death in autopsied liver transplantation patients. Mod Pathol. 1998;11(1):37.
17. Paya CV, Wiesner RH, Hermans PE, et al. Risk factors for cytomegalovirus and severe bacterial infections following liver transplantation: a prospective multivariate time-dependent analysis. J Hepatol. 1993;18(2):185.
18. Memeo R, Piardi T, Sangiuolo F, et al. Management of biliary complications after liver transplantation. World J Hepatol. 2015;7(29):2890–5.

19. Thuluvath PJ, Pfau PR, Kimmey KB, et al. Biliary complications after liver transplantation: the role of endoscopy. Endoscopy. 2005;37:857–63.
20. Park JS, Kim MH, Lee SK, et al. Efficacy of endoscopic and percutaneous treatments for biliary complications after cadaveric and living donor liver transplantation. Gastrointest Endosc. 2003;57:78–85.
21. Verdonk RC, Buis CI, Porte RJ, et al. Anastomotic biliary strictures after liver transplantation: causes and consequences. Liver Transpl. 2006;12:726–35.
22. Verdonk RC, Buis CI, van der Jagt EJ, et al. Nonanastomotic biliary strictures after liver transplantation, part 2: management, outcome and risk factors for disease progression. Liver Transpl. 2007;13:725–32.
23. Al-Freah MAB, McPhail MJW, Dionigi E, et al. Improving the diagnostic criteria for primary liver graft nonfunction in adults utilizing standard and transportable laboratory parameters: an outcome-based analysis. Am J Transplant. 2017;17:1255–66.
24. Vivarelli M, Burra P, La Barba G, et al. Influence of steroids on HCV recurrence after liver transplantation: a prospective study. J Hepatol. 2007;47:793.
25. Klintmalm GB, Davis GL, Teperman L, et al. A randomized, multicenter study comparing steroid free immunosuppression and standard immunosuppression for liver transplant recipients with chronic hepatitis C. Liver Transpl. 2011;17:1394.
26. Takada Y, Kaido T, Asonuma K, et al. Randomized, multicenter trial comparing tacrolimus plus mycophenolate mofetil to tacrolimus plus steroids in hepatitis C virus-positive recipients of living donor liver transplantation. Liver Transpl. 2013;19:896.
27. O'Grady JG, Hardy P, Burroughs AK, et al. Randomized controlled trial of tacrolimus versus microemulsified cyclosporine (TMC) in liver transplantation: poststudy surveillance to 3 years. Am J Transplant. 2007;7:137.
28. Haddad EM, McAlister VC, Renouf E, et al. Cyclosporin versus tacrolimus for liver transplanted patients. Cochrane Database Syst Rev. 2006;4:CD005161.
29. O'Grady JG. Corticosteroid-free strategies in liver transplantation. Drugs. 2006;66:1853.
30. Hebert MF, Ascher NL, Lake JR, et al. Four-year follow-up of mycophenolate mofetil for graft rescue in liver allograft recipients. Transplantation. 1999;67:707.

Care of the Critically Ill Pregnant Patient

56

Alexandra Edwards and Wendy F. Hansen

Introduction

While pregnancy and childbirth are common, trauma and critical illness during pregnancy are relatively rare. This chapter will review the evaluation and management of a critically injured or critically ill pregnant woman when a fetus is considered viable: the gestational age in which a premature infant is able to survive outside the womb with modern neonatal care. It will start with a review of pregnancy epidemiology with a focus on trauma and the critically ill. It will review the profound maternal physiologic changes that accompany pregnancy as nearly every organ system is altered. It will explore the concept of the fetus as a patient and discuss mechanisms of injury to the maternal-fetal unit that are unique to pregnancy. Lastly it will provide a template for evaluation of the fetus and the mother whether in the setting of trauma or an ICU setting.

Epidemiology of Injury Pregnancy

Each year more than four million American women give birth. In 2014, in most recent reported data by the CDC, there were 2,699,951 vaginal deliveries and 1,284,551 cesarean deliveries for a national cesarean rate of 32.2% [1]. The CDC defines pregnancy-related maternal deaths as the death of a woman while pregnant or within 1 year of pregnancy termination – regardless of the duration or site of the pregnancy – from any cause related to or aggravated by the pregnancy or its management, but not from accidental or incidental causes. These maternal deaths are reported per 100,000 live births and are called pregnancy mortality ratios.

A. Edwards (✉)
Department of Surgery, University of Kentucky, Lexington, KY, USA
e-mail: Alexandra.edwards@uky.edu

W. F. Hansen
Department of Obstetrics and Gynecology, University of Kentucky College of Medicine, Lexington, KY, USA

Like infant deaths, pregnancy mortality is often used as a general indicator of a nation's health. Pregnancy-related mortality ratios increased from 7.2 deaths per 100,000 live births in 1987 to 17.8, 15.9, and 17.3 deaths per 100,000 live births in 2011 through 2013, respectively [2].

Although maternal mortality has significantly improved over the last 50 years, there is significant concern that maternal mortality is increasing over the past decade. The causes are likely multifactorial with authors pointing to a new broader definition, improved reporting capabilities on death certificates, continued problems with access to prenatal care, rising cesarean rates, older age at first birth, the rising obesity epidemic, and the increase in comorbid chronic diseases such as hypertension and diabetes.

Considerable racial disparities in pregnancy-related mortality continue to exist. Black women continue to have the highest rates of pregnancy-related mortality; over three times that of white women. During 2011–2013, the pregnancy-related mortality ratios were:

12.1 deaths per 100,000 live births for white women
40.4 deaths per 100,000 live births for black women
16.4 deaths per 100,000 live births for women of other races [2]

In 2014, the all-cause maternal mortality ratio in the United States was 24/100,000. Trauma is the leading cause of non-obstetric maternal death with motor vehicle collisions leading the list. In a recent systematic review of trauma in pregnancy, the overall incidence rate of MVC during pregnancy was estimated at 207 cases per 100,000 pregnancies [3]. It is one of the leading causes of maternal and fetal mortality with estimated maternal mortality rates of 1.4/100,000 and fetal mortality 3.7/100,000 pregnancies. The fetus is disproportionately harmed in comparison with the mother in all reports of trauma in pregnancy; ranging from 3:1 to 9:1 fetal mortality/maternal mortality [4]. One of the traditional teachings in obstetric trauma care is that when a mother is severely injured, the fetus is almost always severely injured;

A. Salim et al. (eds.), *Surgical Critical Care Therapy*, https://doi.org/10.1007/978-3-319-71712-8_56

however when the mother is only mildly injured, the fetus is often severely injured, deliberately communicating a sense of urgency and due diligence for the fetus in all trauma cases.

Prevention strategies and reduction in injury to both mother and fetus come with proper seat belt use during pregnancy. Several studies have shown that proper seat belt use reduces the risk of adverse maternal and fetal outcomes. Their use throughout pregnancy is recommended by the American College of Obstetricians and Gynecologists (ACOG). The recommendation is very specific to wearing the shoulder belt between the breasts and wearing the lap belt below the uterus and across the lap. This three-point restraint system distributes the force of the impact and reduces the risk of injury to both the mother and fetus [5]. The safety of airbags in pregnancy has also been studied. Two reports have confirmed the safety of front airbags in pregnancy [6, 7]. There are no reports of side airbags on pregnancy outcomes.

Domestic violence or intimate partner violence (IPV) is the most common cause of trauma. Injury in pregnant women is not uncommon with a prevalence of 8307/100,000 pregnancies, a considerable increase from 5239/100,000 in nonpregnant women [3]. Reported incidences have a broad range depending on the population studied and the definition applied. Several studies have identified pregnancy as a high-risk time for the acceleration of IPV. A high index of suspicion for IPV must be maintained when caring for pregnant patients with traumatic injuries. Slips and falls are another common cause of trauma. Up to one in four pregnant women will fall during pregnancy [3]. Gravid women have increased joint laxity, weight gain, and disturbed balance leading to the increased incidence. Most falls are not major issues but are a frequent cause of maternal and fetal evaluation.

Epidemiology of Critical Care

About 200–700 per 100,000 pregnant women require admission to an ICU during pregnancy or the postpartum period. Most admissions occur in the immediate postpartum period (60–70%). The majority of ICU admissions are related to obstetric complications including hemorrhage, hypertensive diseases of pregnancy (preeclampsia and eclampsia), sepsis, thromboembolism, and cardiac disease [8]. Non-obstetric causes are the same as for the nonpregnant state. It is important to remember that any disease or injury that can happen in a nonpregnant woman can happen in a pregnant woman.

Prediction of mortality risk for pregnant patients is difficult. APACHE scores do not adequately predict mortality in pregnant women. No scoring system adequately adjusts for the physiologic changes and other unique pregnancy characteristics. Of obstetric patients admitted to the ICU, the rate of mortality ranges from 0% to 20% with most series report a mortality rate near 5%.

The Physiologic and Maternal Adaptation to Pregnancy

Pregnancy brings profound hemodynamic, cardiopulmonary, and hematologic changes to maternal physiology (Table 56.1). These changes are perhaps easiest understood using a developmental biology model and asking the question: "What adaptation in maternal physiology is needed in order to make a baby and survive childbirth in order to ensure continuation of the species?"

Once fertilization occurs, the fetus must be nourished for the next 40 weeks. Although the maternal and fetal blood systems are separate and parallel, complex mechanisms have evolved that transport oxygen and nutrients from mother to fetus and in return transport carbon dioxide and metabolic waste from fetus to mother. These complex mechanisms transport across fragile boundaries at the uterine-placental interface. By 30 weeks gestation the maternal body has profoundly changed. Blood flow to the uterus has increased from 80 ccs/min in the nonpregnant state to 500–800 ccs/min in the gravid uterus. This increase is essential in order to perfuse the uterine-placental interface and support the growth and well-being of the fetus. In order to bring this much blood to the uterine-placental interface, the maternal body must make more blood, pump more blood, and accommodate more blood. Blood volume increases by 30–50%, cardiac output increases by 50%, and vascular resistance decreases throughout the body in order to accommodate this increased volume. Normal adaptation results in a small but measurable decrease in maternal blood pressure of 3–5 mmHg systolic and 5–10 mmHg diastolic and an increase in normal resting pulse rate by 10–15 bpm.

The uterine-placental circulation is maximally dilated during pregnancy and does not have the capacity to vasoconstrict. This circulation is dependent on having adequate blood pressure, adequate blood volume, and adequate cardiac output. If any of these three are reduced, the maternal compensatory response (no matter the cause) is to selectively direct blood flow to the vital organs. The pregnant uterus is

Table 56.1 Normal adaptation to pregnancy

Cardiac	Increased cardiac output (30–50%), increased heart rate 10–15 bpm
Pulmonary	Increased minute ventilation (20–50%), increased tidal volume, decreased functional residual capacity, respiratory alkalosis
Hematologic	Increased blood volume RBC > plasma, physiologic decrease in hct
Renal	Increased renal blood flow (50%), decreased creatinine, uric acid
Gastrointestinal	Decreased peristalsis, gastric emptying
Coagulation	Increased clotting factors
Breasts	Increased glandular tissue, increased blood flow
Vascular	Decreased resistance, vasodilation

NOT a vital organ. Blood will be shunted from the uterine-placental interface circulation (away from the fetus) with a resultant fetal distress. If this is not remedied quickly, delivery of a viable fetus will be urgent.

The coagulation cascade is skewed toward coagulation, placing a pregnant and a postpartum woman at increased risk for thromboembolism especially when other comorbidities such as obesity, genetic predisposition, cesarean delivery, and/or trauma are present. The highest risk time for thromboembolism is postoperative cesarean that persists for 4–6 weeks.

The mother completes basic respiratory exchange for the fetus with the placenta acting as an ECMO circuit for the baby. Any disruption in oxygen to the fetus because of an alteration of oxygen or blood flow at the uterine-placental interface as found in trauma with either a placental abruption, a fetal-maternal hemorrhage, or maternal shock from hemorrhage or in a critically ill woman with hypoxemia or shock (regardless of the cause) will also be life-threatening to the fetus.

These basic maternal physiologic changes that occur in pregnancy, summed up in Table 56.1, coupled with an understanding of the uterine-placental unit, are essential in order to optimize resuscitation and manage the critically injured or critically ill gravida in the ICU.

The Fetus as a Patient

Trauma in a pregnant woman is a paradigm shift for the trauma team. Taught to focus on the ABCDE of resuscitation on a single human, the trauma team must now consider two humans, the mother and fetus, intimately dependent on one another. The mother is readily identifiable by approximate age and weight and easily evaluated with vital signs, whereas the fetus is hidden, not readily identifiable and not as easily evaluated.

Mother always first has been the long-standing mantra and tradition and a common belief by many. However, as we understand better the close interdependency of both mother and fetus, it is hard to define them as separate. The decision to separate them by a cesarean delivery may benefit both mother and fetus. Their interdependence is reflected in that delivery may very well help with resuscitation of the mother with a cardiopulmonary arrest and in certain circumstances emergency delivery is the only alternative for fetal survival. In terms of priorities and initial resuscitation goals, the focus should be on the mother first and the fetus second. Fortunately, what is good for the mother in terms of resuscitation and reversal of shock is usually also what is best in the acute stage for the fetus.

Modern-day neonatology has brought significant improvements to the morbidity and mortality for premature infants. By 28 weeks gestation, 99% of preterm infants survive, and the vast majority are without any major impairment. At 24 weeks, all infants are standardly resuscitated. The most recent review of survival and neurodevelopmental outcomes in neonates born at 24 weeks gestation and followed out to 18–22 months reports a 55% survival rate with 32% of neonates without neurodevelopmental impairment and 23% with neurodevelopment impairment [9]. Current obstetric practice now counsels women about fetal survival at 23 weeks, although the 23–24-week period remains a gray zone. This period of peri-viability is certain to slowly change over time.

These changes in outcomes for preterm infants have shaped our thinking and our ethics regarding the fetus as a patient.

If the mother is indeed first, then the fetus is a very close second. Obstetricians think of them simultaneously in both the evaluation and management. It's a change in thinking for some but one that reflects modern-day best obstetric practice.

Mechanisms of Fetal Injury/Harm During Maternal Trauma and Critical Illness

General Considerations

The maternal-fetal unit is two separate circulatory systems, intimately interdependent, and physiologically defined by the uterine-placental unit. At term 15% of cardiac output goes to the uterus (500–800 cc/min). The uterine-placental vascular bed is maximally dilated and completely dependent on maternal cardiac output and volume. There is no known autoregulation of this vascular bed. The uterine-placental unit is not necessary for maternal survival. Any maternal disease state or injury that disrupts the basic circulatory requirements of the maternal uterine-placental unit has the potential to bring harm to a fetus.

Maternal Shock

In the setting of maternal shock, whether it is from hemorrhage (trauma), sepsis, severe allergic reaction, or primary cardiac failure (regardless of the reason,) the maternal uterine-placental unit will not be perfused adequately with significant consequent harm to the fetus. This would be detected by continuous fetal heart rate (FHR) monitoring with changes in the FHR pattern whether in the immediate resuscitation of trauma or during maternal decompensation in the ICU.

Placental Abruption

Placental abruption is the premature separation of the placenta from the uterus and has a wide spectrum of clinical significance. It can be mild or partial or at its worst severe and complete causing life-threatening consequences for the mother and fetus. Risk factors for abruption include chronic hypertension; hypertensive disorders of pregnancy such as preeclampsia and eclampsia; tobacco, alcohol, and cocaine use; trauma; maternal age multiple pregnancy; and a previous abruption.

Abruption accounts for 50–70% of fetal death following trauma and is more common among women with higher injury severity [10]. However, major placental abruptions are seen even when the mother has relatively minor injuries. The uterus is muscular and can change shape to accommodate external forces (blunt trauma or a deceleration from a MVC); however, the placenta contains no elastic tissue leading to a shearing effect of the placenta from the uterus. Abruption may result from shearing forces, tensile failure, or contrecoup injury.

Abruption is clinically characterized by painful vaginal bleeding from the maternal placental site. The placenta is abundant in tissue factor. When a significant disruption of the uterine-placental interface occurs, tissue factor is exposed to maternal circulation. Tissue factor initiates the extrinsic system of the coagulation cascade causing thrombin to form. Thrombin acts as a uterotonic or irritant by initiating a cascade of chemical changes that induce labor. Continued exposure to tissue factor propels the cascade causing life-threatening bleeding. The coagulopathy is marked by hypofibrinogenemia, thrombocytopenia, and an elevated INR. The coagulopathy will continue until the placenta is removed (delivery). Blood component therapy with attention to immediate delivery is lifesaving. An abruption that is major enough to cause a fetal death in the late second and third trimester is highly likely to cause a life-threatening maternal coagulopathy.

Abruption continues to be a clinical diagnosis and not an ultrasound diagnosis. The role of ultrasound is largely confirmatory in major abruptions in the setting of trauma. Ultrasound fails to detect up to 50% of all placenta abruptions especially those that are more partial. Therefore, a negative ultrasound does not rule out abruption. Abruption has a wide range of ultrasonographic appearances as the initial bleeding undergoes the normal changes of clot formation, inflammation, and resolution.

Management of abruption depends upon maternal and fetal status. Abruption does not preclude a vaginal delivery; however, a cesarean delivery may be indicated if the maternal or fetal status is unstable as it allows for immediacy. Once delivery occurs, the coagulopathy will begin to resolve.

When the mother is severely injured, the fetus is almost always severely injured. However, a fetus is often severely injured even when the mother has relatively minor injuries. Most case series of trauma in pregnancy report fetal injury far more common than maternal injury. Major placental abruptions are seen in women with minor injuries who have incurred a MVC or a direct hit to the abdomen.

Penetrating Trauma

The gravid uterus protects maternal viscera. The uterus, amniotic fluid, and fetus decrease missile velocity and transfer of energy. Gastrointestinal injuries are less common in pregnancy because of the force absorbed by the uterus. As the pregnancy advances and the uterus grows, the risk to the uterus increases. Laceration and/or perforation of the uterus occurs with increasing uterine size. Direct injury to the fetus has been reported in gunshot wounds, stab wounds, and shrapnel injuries.

Traumatic Uterine Rupture

Traumatic uterine rupture is rare. It is the catastrophic sequelae after penetrating or high-energy blunt abdominal trauma. When traumatic rupture of the uterus occurs, fetal mortality approaches 100%. Open pelvic fractures carry a high risk of maternal and fetal mortality rate. Fetal head injuries are more common when a pelvic fracture is sustained. Pelvic vasculature increases during pregnancy as the near-term uterine arteries carry 500–800 cc/min. Thus the risk for more significant hemorrhage in the pelvis after pelvic fracture is increased. Uterine artery injury or avulsion can lead to retroperitoneal hemorrhage. Emergency surgery is the only response.

Maternal-Fetal Hemorrhage

Fetal-maternal hemorrhage (FMH) is the loss of fetal red blood cells into the maternal circulation. Although this can happen in normal pregnancies, trauma is thought to be one of the inciting causes. In rare instances, FMH can cause a significant anemia in a fetus. There is typically no vaginal bleeding or contractions. It is detected by an abnormal fetal heart rate tracing during continuous monitoring. If a sinusoidal pattern or a Category 3 tracing is noted, cesarean delivery is indicated urgently with preparations for immediate transfusion of the infant.

Kleihauer-Betke and flow cytometry are quantitative laboratory tests that estimate the percentage of fetal hemoglobin that has been lost into the maternal circulation. These test results typically return far too late for clinical decision-making. However, they are helpful for dosing anti-D immunoglobulin in order to prevent future alloimmunization in an Rh-negative mother.

Management of the Fetus as a Patient (ABCDE)

In keeping with the spirit of trauma and critical care, these authors would like to propose an ABCDE algorithm for the fetus as a patient:

Age: How to assess gestational age.
Beating/Breathing: Is the heart beating? In a fetus breathing (oxygenation) is consistent with body movement and cardiac activity.
Continuous cardiac fetal monitoring.
Determine need for immediate delivery.
Effect a plan.

Age

It is generally accepted that a fetus is able to survive outside a mother at 24 weeks gestation. Given that the trauma team cannot see the fetus, there are only three ways to assess age:

1. History: If the mother is able to give a reliable history, use her stated due date. Be careful in trying to equate layman months with weeks. The most reliable history comes from prenatal ultrasound and due date based on an early scan.
2. Measurement of fundal height remains a cornerstone of the obstetric physical exam with the umbilicus acting as the traditional milestone marker for 20 weeks gestational age. Every centimeter above the umbilicus represents another week of gestation. This is limited in obese women, in women with fibroids, and in twins and frankly can be difficult to ascertain in some women. However, if the top of the uterus is palpated two fingerbreadths above the umbilicus, you are close to 24 weeks gestation in a singleton fetus. This is good enough in an emergent situation without history or an ultrasound
3. Ultrasound: All modern-day emergency departments have point-of-care ultrasound. Assessing the age of a fetus can be done with a single biparietal diameter, a femur length, or an abdominal circumference. The first two are preferred.

Breathing/Beating

Clearly a fetus does not breathe as we commonly think of breathing. Instead the mother via the placenta acts as the lungs of the fetus. Cardiac activity and fetal movement are indirect measures of a well-oxygenated fetus. A normal FHR is 120–160 bpm. If the expertise is present, evaluation of amniotic fluid and placentation can be very helpful.

Continuous Fetal Monitoring

Once the fetus is thought to be 24 weeks and alive, continuous FHR monitoring should be immediately started. Fetal well-being cannot be fully assessed without continuous monitoring. If this is not possible for whatever the reason, the fetus needs to have some form of ongoing assessment. This is essential in order to understand if an intervention such as delivery is needed.

Decision for Delivery

If the fetus were to have a Category 3 FHR tracing and a major clinical abruption or is having repetitive FHR decelerations, an emergent cesarean is needed, and the team should move urgently toward delivery. Sometimes it is necessary to proceed with delivery in the trauma bay, while at other times it can be done in the main operating rooms. If the mother is so severely injured that a cardiac arrest is witnessed, a perimortem cesarean delivery is indicated.

Effect a Plan

If delivery is not needed immediately, full evaluation of maternal injuries should be completed with simultaneous continuous fetal monitoring. Decisions will need to be made concerning admitting service, need for a planned delivery, length of continuous monitoring, and more. As the uterus is a nonessential organ bed, hypovolemia will affect the uterus early and moreover the fetus. If the fetus is viable and monitored, maternal hypoperfusion will manifest as changes in the fetal heart rate. A fetus with reassuring tracing is often a reassuring measure of maternal status as hypoperfusion will often lead to changes in FHR before maternal vital sign changes. The fetus is an occult barometer of maternal status. It is important to remember that fetal distress and demise may occur with relatively minor maternal trauma. Fetal monitoring following trauma is often indicated for 4–24 h depending on clinical scenario. A minimum of 4 h of fetal heart rate and contraction monitoring is recommended after blunt trauma to pregnant women regardless of maternal injury. If contractions are present or other concerns arise, a 24-h period of continuous fetal monitoring is common practice.

Special Considerations for Initial Management of the Critically Injured Pregnant Patient

Initial Management

Pregnant traumatically injured patients should be managed via Advanced Trauma Life Support (ATLS) algorithms. A multidisciplinary team approach including obstetrics, neonatology, emergency medicine, and trauma surgery can allow for best care of the patient. Advance notice if available is ideal to assemble teams and equipment. The clinician should perform necessary tests and procedures on the traumatically injured obstetric patient that are indicated including but not limited to radiographic studies, intubation, vascular access, and surgical intervention. Caring for the mother is caring for the pregnancy, and maternal care should not be compromised due to pregnancy. ATLS emphasizes the ABCDE mnemonic – airway, breathing, circulation, disability, and exposure. Following the assessment and stabilization of airway, breathing, and circulation, rapid confirmation of gestational age and viability of the fetus is imperative. If gestational age is greater than 24 weeks, continuous fetal monitoring is imperative. This ABCDE assessment of the fetus can be performed simultaneously with maternal resuscitative or stabilization techniques. This simultaneous evaluation will allow decision-making regarding the need for immediate delivery (Fig. 56.1).

Airway

Obtaining a definitive airway in an obstetric patient may prove more difficult. Airway edema is increased as well as the risk for aspiration secondary to delayed gastric emptying. Avoiding maternal hypoxia and maintaining pulse oximetry saturations greater than 92% are ideal for the fetus. However, short-duration hypoxia is tolerated if utero-placental blood flow is maintained [11]. Respiratory failure may manifest as tachypnea and should not be mistaken for normal pregnancy physiology. If rapid sequence intubation is required, bear in mind that sedatives cross the placenta readily. A delivery following general anesthesia often leads to a depressed infant for which the neonatal resuscitation team should prepare.

Breathing

Pregnant women increase minute ventilation by 40% in tidal volume and small increase in respiratory rate. The end result is a respiratory alkalosis. A pCO_2 of >35 in a pregnant woman is often an indicator of impending respiratory failure.

If a chest tube is required, care should be taken to avoid the elevated diaphragm. As pregnancy continues, the chest widens at the subcostal angle to accommodate the elevation of the gravid uterus. Consequently the diaphragm is elevated. If tube thoracostomy is required, it should be placed two costal margins higher than typically placed [12]. After airway and breathing are assessed, during assessment of circulation, is it quick and easy to displace the uterus.

Circulation

Pregnancy brings profound changes in the cardiovascular system. The natural increase in blood volume can cause a delay in tachycardia and hypotension until the patient loses nearly 30% of her blood volume [13]. The growing uterus at two fingerbreadths above the umbilicus, typically at 24–25 weeks, causes a aortocaval compression and decreased venous return to the heart when lying supine. To improve maternal venous return and cardiac output, the uterus should be displaced off the vena cava. Place a blanket or towel underneath the backboard at hip level on either side of the patient to allow for displacement off of the inferior vena cava. Emphasis is often placed on tilting away from the IVC, but this is sometimes impractical. If a pregnant patient requires emergent transfusion, Rh-negative blood should be administered.

Laboratory

Typical trauma blood work is indicated in the pregnant trauma patient along with obstetric-specific blood work such as fibrinogen and a Kleihauer-Betke or flow cytometry. A fibrinogen level that is normal in a nonpregnant patient may be abnormal for pregnancy and a potential early indicator of placental abruption with consumptive coagulopathy. A Kleihauer-Betke and flow cytometry are qualitative tests that allow for evaluation of a fetal-maternal hemorrhage.

Radiology

Indicated diagnostic imaging studies should be obtained in the obstetric trauma patient. No study to date has shown any increase in teratogenicity for a fetus exposed to less than 100 mGy or 0.1 Gy. Risks for teratogenicity of radiation to the pregnancy are well above typical diagnostic imaging doses. However, the risk of childhood cancer in the fetus may be increased. The risk of carcinogenesis as a result of in utero exposure to radiation is unclear but probably very small. A 10–20 mGy fetal exposure (the amount of radiation in a CT scan) may increase the risk of childhood leukemia

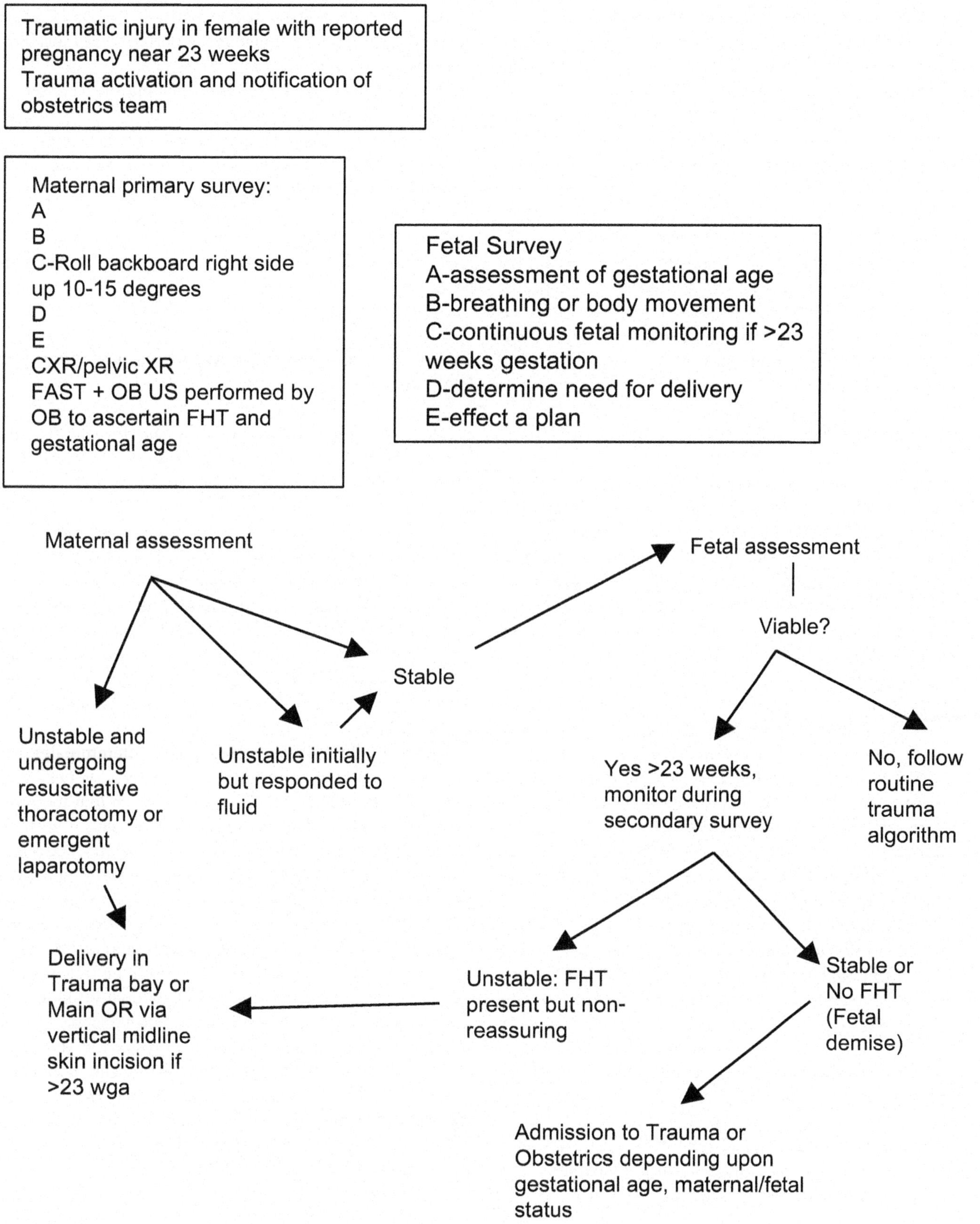

Fig. 56.1 Flow diagram of trauma protocol for pregnant women

by a factor of 1.5–2 to an existing risk of 1 in 3000. The fetus is exposed to a background of 1 mGy of radiation during the pregnancy from the environment alone. The American College of Obstetrician Gynecologists has published guidelines on use of radiographic imaging in pregnancy [14]. Pregnant women who have incurred serious traumatic injury should have the same imaging as a non-pregnant woman.

MRI is a safe alternative to CT scan to avoid ionizing radiation if accessible in a timely manner. Magnetic resonance imaging is able to penetrate soft tissues without the use of ionizing radiation. There are no precautions or specific contraindications for MRI in pregnancy. However, MRI has not been evaluated in the setting of trauma likely due to time burden, feasibility, and availability.

Non-obstetric Surgical Intervention

If non-obstetric surgery is indicated but delivery is not indicated, attention should be paid to maternal positioning, oxygenation, and intravascular volume in order to optimize uterine perfusion to maintain fetal oxygenation. Surgical decisions must be based on maternal and fetal clinical status. Whether to perform fetal heart monitoring during a surgical operation is dependent on several variables. ACOG has established the following guidelines:

- No currently used anesthetic agents have been shown to have any teratogenic effects in humans when using standard concentrations at any gestational age.
- Fetal heart rate monitoring may assist in maternal positioning and cardiorespiratory management and may influence a decision to deliver the fetus.
- If the fetus is considered previable (<24 weeks gestation), it is generally sufficient to ascertain the fetal heart rate by Doppler before and after the procedure.
- At a minimum, if the fetus is considered to be viable, simultaneous electronic fetal heart rate and contraction monitoring should be performed before and after the procedure to assess fetal well-being and the absence of contractions [15].

Intraoperative electronic fetal monitoring may be appropriate when all of the following apply:

1. The fetus is viable.
2. It is physically possible to perform intraoperative electronic fetal monitoring.
3. A healthcare provider with obstetric surgery privileges is available and willing to intervene during the surgical procedure for fetal indications.
4. When possible, the woman has given informed consent to emergency cesarean delivery.
5. The nature of the planned surgery will allow the safe interruption or alteration of the procedure to provide access to perform emergency delivery.

If there is some concern about deteriorating maternal or fetal status during the procedure, delivery via cesarean may be required.

Perimortem Cesarean Delivery/Resuscitative Hysterotomy

It is clear that a cesarean can be lifesaving for a fetus. What is not as clear is whether a cesarean can be lifesaving for a mother in the setting of a cardiac arrest, regardless of the cause.

Steeped within the obstetric literature is the concept of the "4-min rule" which refers to 4 min from the time of a witnessed cardiac arrest to delivery of the fetus by emergent cesarean whether in the trauma bay or in labor and delivery. This "4-min rule" allows for a fetus to be delivered with the least harm, although normal infants are reported as far as 30 min after an arrest. So, even if it has been longer than 4 min, an immediate cesarean should be completed [16, 17].

There are multiple case reports in the literature describing successful resuscitation of a pregnant woman only after delivery of the fetus. It is well known that the pregnant uterus, after 24–25 weeks gestation, causes aortocaval compression when the woman is supine. Cardiac output has been shown to decrease by 60% in the supine position limiting preload and in the setting of cardiac arrest limiting the effectiveness of chest compressions. Emptying the uterus by way of an emergent cesarean allows relief of the aortocaval compression and restoration of circulation with effective chest compressions and hopefully successful resuscitation. The concept of perimortem cesarean has transitioned to resuscitative hysterotomy and should be part of the algorithm and included in the ABCDE of the fetus when a cardiac arrest, whatever the cause, occurs. The steps of an emergency cesarean delivery have been outlined in Fig. 56.2 and further described in Box 56.1.

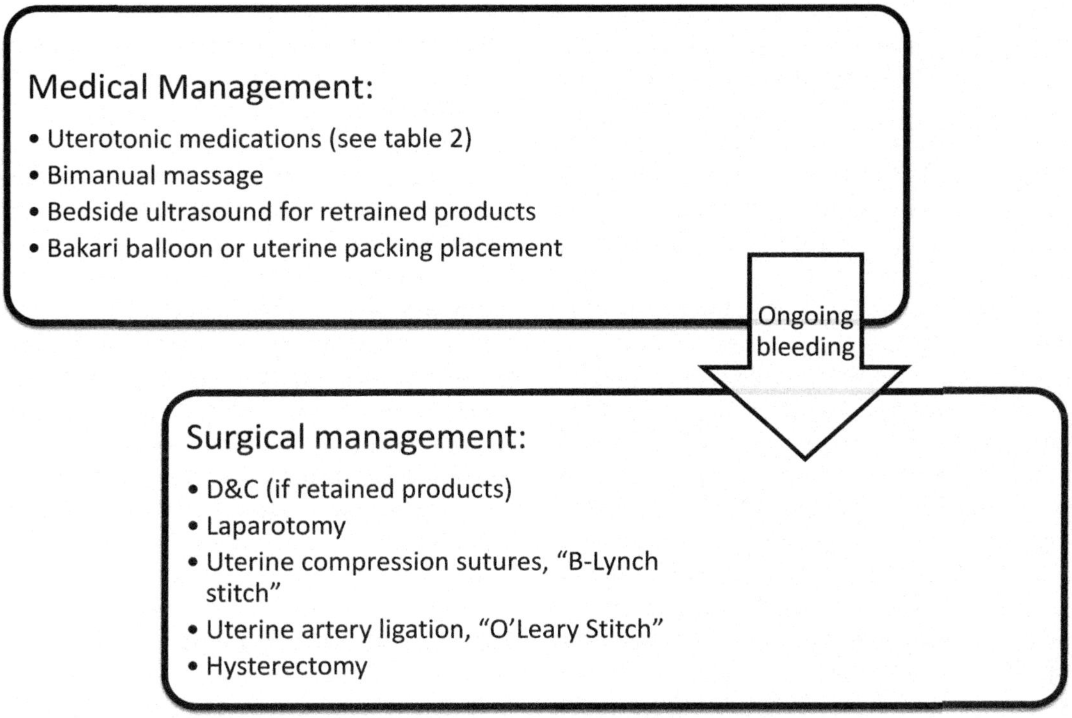

Fig. 56.2 Flow diagram of stepwise management of uterine atony

Box 56.1 Emergency C/S Steps

1. Prep abdomen as much as possible.
2. Enter abdomen; generally obstetricians are most comfortable or quickest with Pfannenstiel incisions, but the clinically scenario (i.e., traumatic vs medical code) should dictate the incision.
3. Enter uterus:
   (a) If near term, create a low transverse hysterotomy above the vesicouterine peritoneum avoiding the bladder. The incision should enter the musculature of the uterus; bleeding will be encountered. Ideally the surgeon would use their finger to enter the uterus after the initial incision to avoid fetal injury. Extend hysterotomy by placing two fingers in the uterus and applying traction superiorly and inferiorly taking care not to extend the incision directly laterally into uterine vasculature.
   (b) If fetus is preterm, create a vertical incision on the uterus. A vertical incision is preferred to avoid uterine vasculature as the lower uterine segment is underdeveloped early in gestation. It is also a preferable incision for a small fetus with an unknown lie as delivery could be more difficult. This incision will traverse the thickest part of the myometrium and will take several passes with a scalpel to create an area thin enough to enter with a finger. Once uterus has been entered, place two fingers within the incision and pull the uterus toward the operator using the other hand to extend the incision with bandage scissors.
4. Deliver fetus:
   (a) Near term the vast majority of fetuses will be in cephalic or head down presentation. Delivery requires elevation of the fetal head to the level of the hysterotomy while the assistant gives fundal pressure. Once the fetal head is delivered, attention turns to shoulders and the rest of the body follows.
   (b) If preterm, position is variable and a breech delivery may be necessary. Breech deliveries vary based on the type of breech, but the final pathway once hips are out is the same. For a footling breech (both feet presenting first): grasp feet and pull through incision ideally

(continued)

Pathogenesis

The pathogenesis is not known with certainty, but the most common theory is defective decidualization related to incomplete healing from prior insult (cesarean, surgery, etc.). Trophoblastic invasion must then occur in the lower uterine segment to include the area of defective decidualization [24]. Some have speculated that abnormal or excessive trophoblastic invasion is necessary for development of a morbidly adherent placenta beyond just defective decidualization [25].

Diagnosis

Ideally, invasive or morbidly adherent placenta is diagnosed before delivery on prenatal ultrasound. Ultrasound is a reliable modality, and the reported sensitivity and specificity based on meta-analysis for the diagnosis of invasive placenta are 97% and 90%, respectively [26]. The ultrasound findings considered to be consistent with invasive placentation include the following:

1. Obliteration of the bladder-uterine interface with loss or irregularity of the normal hyperechoic area representing the bladder wall-uterine serosa junction ("bladder line")
2. Loss of placenta homogeneity aka placental sonolucencies
3. Increases in vascularity noted between the uterus and bladder seen on color Doppler
4. Loss or irregularity of the normal hypoechoic retroplacental line or "clear space"
5. Obvious protrusion of the placenta into the bladder

The presence of any one of these findings in the setting of a previa with prior cesarean is characteristic of invasive placentation. MRI may be a useful adjunct to ultrasound for operative planning or when ultrasound is inconclusive [27]. Postnatal diagnosis is definitively made on histological examination.

Presentation

Placenta accreta can present with similar symptoms to placenta previa as most are previae as well. However, what distinguishes a morbidly adherent placenta is the loss of plane between the uterus and the placenta. This leads to an inability to manually separate the placenta with ease and profuse hemorrhage in the area of placental invasion where the uterus cannot contract. Placenta increta and percreta may present with abnormal vasculature in the lower uterine segment noted on initial entry to the abdomen. Women with placenta percreta which have invaded the bladder may present with hematuria.

Complications and Management

Management of a morbidly adherent placenta varies as there are no randomized trials to define the best practice [28]. As such, recommendations for management are based on case series, expert opinion, and good clinical judgment. In general the diagnosis of invasive placentation requires a cesarean hysterectomy; there are rare cases in which uterine conservation may be attempted, and those will not be discussed here. Moreover some of the most severe percreta may be managed conservatively with placenta in situ [29].

Once invasive placentation of any kind is suspected, patient should be counseled about the diagnosis and potential complications including hemorrhage, blood transfusion, preterm birth, bladder resection, and hysterectomy. The American College of Obstetricians and Gynecologists recommends a multidisciplinary approach to cases of suspected invasive placentae. Management by a multidisciplinary team at a tertiary care center has been shown to improve maternal morbidity [30]. Moreover, an aggressive standardized institutional multidisciplinary approach at Baylor Houston has been shown to improve patient outcomes [31].

All patients with placenta previa and/or invasive placentation should be placed on pelvic rest. Admission to the hospital should ideally occur prior to becoming symptomatic. Hospitalization may occur anytime within the third trimester or if the patient becomes symptomatic. If the patient is asymptomatic, delivery should occur electively at 34 weeks which reduces maternal morbidity [32]. Preparation may include consultation with other services such as neonatology, anesthesiology, urology, IR, blood bank, and surgical or critical care services. If bladder invasion is suspected, consultation with urology or gynecologic oncology should be obtained.

Delivery Technique

Preparation should be made for massive hemorrhage including notification of blood bank. Before induction of anesthesia, placement of large-bore intravenous catheters as well as arterial or central lines may be indicated. Patients are positioned in low lithotomy with Allen stirrups to allow access to bladder for potential urologic interventions as well as observation of vaginal bleeding. Low lithotomy also allows for a third co-surgeon to have access to the surgical field. Anesthesia for delivery must be individualized; however, it has been shown to be safe to use spinal-epidural for scheduled deliveries [33]. This minimizes fetal exposure to general anesthesia and facilitated postoperative pain management. If feasible or necessary, endotracheal intubation and general anesthesia can follow delivery of the neonate. In emergency cases, general anesthesia is preferred.

A vertical midline laparotomy allows more access to the abdomen for hysterectomy. A fundal or classical hysterotomy is recommended as it allows for avoidance of the placenta which results in better maternal outcomes [34]. Following the clamping of the cord, a quick closure of the hysterotomy is completed as preparations are made to complete the hysterectomy. Cesarean hysterectomy in the setting of a morbidly adherent placenta requires access to the retroperitoneum and identification of the ureters and iliac vessels, and this is often accomplished with initial division of the round ligaments. There have been multiple techniques described to accomplish this complicated cesarean hysterectomy when anatomy is distorted and highly vascular.

Postpartum Hemorrhage

Introduction

Postpartum hemorrhage (PPH) is a potentially life-threatening complication after delivery. The term postpartum hemorrhage is used to describe an etiologically heterogeneous event but does not define a cause and is not a diagnosis. The most common causes of postpartum hemorrhage include uterine atony, retained or abnormal placenta, and lacerations of the genital tract. The mean blood loss for a vaginal delivery is 500 ml, and for a cesarean delivery is 1000 ml. The definition of PPH is variable in literature. ACOG defines postpartum hemorrhage as >500 ml. Uterine atony complicates 1 in 20 deliveries and is the most common cause of PPH.

Definition/Pathogenesis

Postpartum hemorrhage is generally divided into early and late. Early PPH refers to excessive bleeding within the first 24 h after delivery, while late may occur up to 12 weeks following delivery. Uterine atony is the most common cause of PPH. The term atony refers to inability of the uterine myometrium or musculature to contract effectively to stop bleeding. After the placenta is delivered, contraction of the uterus is required to decrease blood flow through the dilated spiral arterioles, which have been bringing 500–800 cc each minute to this area. Without contraction, bleeding can become profuse. Many risk factors have been identified for uterine atony including induction of labor, rapid or prolonged labor, grand multiparity, uterine overdistension, use of uterine relaxants or certain anesthetics, retained products of conception, and abnormal placentation.

Presentation

PPH is recognized with excessive bleeding following delivery of the placenta. A vaginal examination is completed, and the source of the hemorrhage is typically readily apparent on examination. Uterine atony will present with an enlarged and boggy uterus with brisk bleeding from the cervical os. Retained products of conception may lead to uterine atony, and manual exploration of the uterus will reveal a roughened area of the endometrium. Genital lacerations of the vaginal mucosa are readily recognizable; however cervical lacerations are more difficult to identify.

Management

Prevention of PPH may be accomplished with active management of the third stage of labor as well as routine oxytocin infusion following placental delivery. Active management of the third stage includes controlled cord traction, uterine massage, and administration of oxytocin prior to removal of the placenta [35]. Prolonged oxytocin infusion has been shown to be effective in preventing postpartum hemorrhage, and data supports infusion of oxytocin 4–8 h following delivery [36]. Once preventative measures have failed and bleeding is continued, management of PPH typically begins with medical therapy and uterine massage.

ACOG and the California Maternal Quality Care Collaborative (CMQCC) have published guidelines on management of obstetric hemorrhage, and most institutions have specific protocols. However, PPH management has some generalizable tenants, organized in a flow diagram in Fig. 56.3. Once PPH has been identified, it is practical to call for further assistance from nurses, scrub techs, and anesthesia. The patient will require adequate intravenous access, frequent vital sign monitoring, volume resuscitation, and potentially administration of blood product. Prompt review of potential sources of hemorrhage should be completed.

Uterine atony is the most common source of hemorrhage; oxytocin should be administered either IV infusion or IM. Oxytocin should not be bolused as it can cause hypotension. Other uterotonics such as methylergonovine maleate (Methergine) and 15-methyl analogue of prostaglandin F-2alpha (Hemabate) may be given intramuscularly. Both have contraindications for hypertension and asthma, respectively. Misoprostol is another prostaglandin which can be administered orally, rectally, or vaginally (Table 56.2). If bleeding is uncontrolled after medical management, uterine tamponade may be attempted using a Bakri balloon or sterile gauze packing. In rare cases, bleeding will persist and exploratory laparotomy is required. Surgical management of

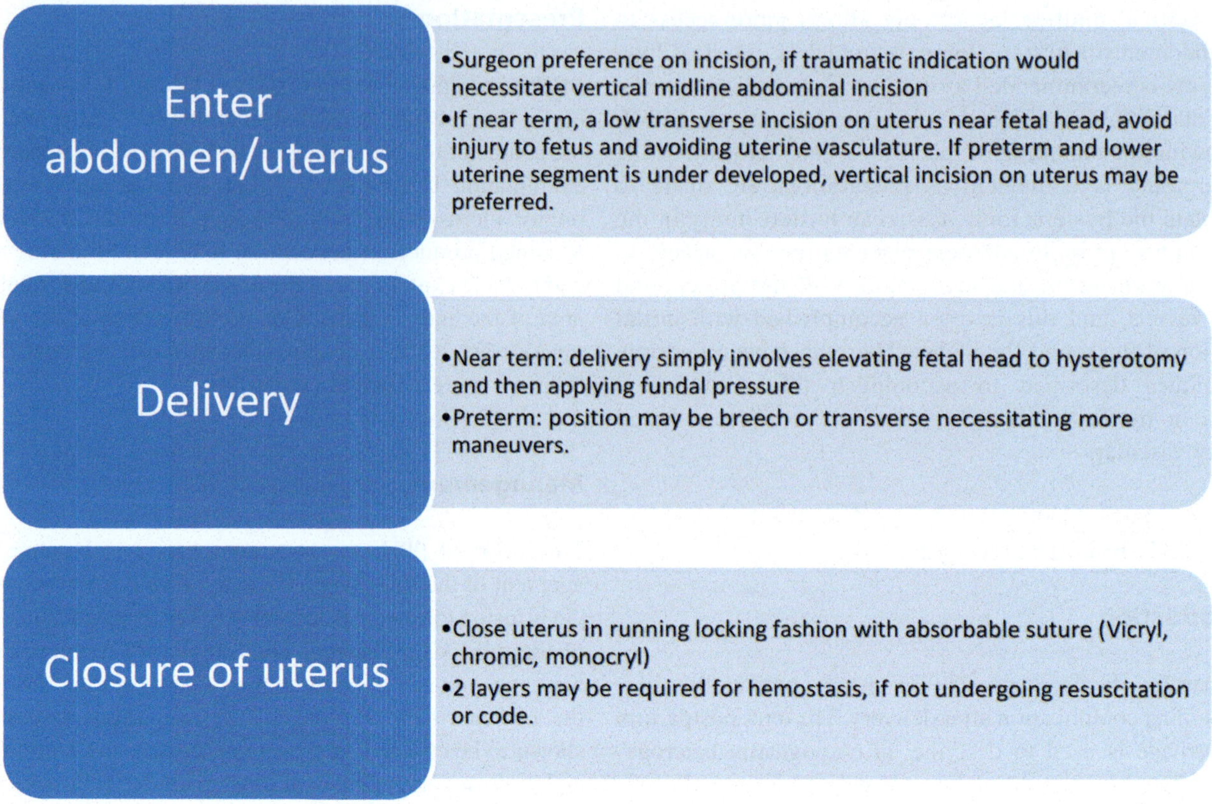

Fig. 56.3 Emergency cesarean delivery steps

Table 56.2 Medical management of postpartum hemorrhage

Drug	Dose/route	Frequency	Comment
Oxytocin (Pitocin)	IV, 10–40 units in 1 l normal saline or lactated Ringer's solution IM, 10 units	Continuous	Avoid undiluted rapid IV infusion, which causes hypotension
Methylergonovine (Methergine)	IM: 0.2 mg	Every 2–4 h	Avoid if patient is hypertensive
15-Methyl PGF2α (carbopost) (Hemabate)	IM: 0.25 mg	Every 15–90 min, eight doses maximum	Avoid in asthmatic patients; relative contraindication if hepatic, renal, and cardiac disease. Diarrhea, fever, and tachycardia can occur
Dinoprostone (Prostin E2)	Suppository: vaginal or rectal 20 mg	Every 2 h	Avoid if patient is hypotensive. Fever is common. Stored frozen, it must be thawed to room temperature
Misoprostol (Cytotec, PGE1)	800–1000 mcg rectally		

Modified from Ref. [59]
Abbreviations: *IV* intravenously, *IM* intramuscularly, *PG* prostaglandin
All agents can cause nausea and vomiting

uterine atony includes compression sutures, uterine artery ligation, and ultimately hysterectomy.

Management of severe hemorrhage in the obstetric patient will occasionally include utilization of massive transfusion protocols. A 1:1:1 ratio of pRBC to plasma to platelet concentrate has been shown to improve mortality in the first 24 h for trauma patients [37]. No evidence exists for component ratios in the obstetric population as MTP activation is uncommon in the obstetric population [38].

Amniotic Fluid Embolism

Amniotic fluid embolism (AFE) is a rare and potentially catastrophic event. AFE has been recognized as a spectrum disorder ranging from subclinical to fatal. The mechanism underlying AFE is uncertain; despite its name AFE is no longer theorized to be embolic but an anaphylactoid reaction. Registries have been set up in the United States and the United Kingdom to further characterize AFE. The incidence ranges from 1 in 8000 to 1 in 83,000 live births. Mortality ranges from 26% to 86% [39]. AFE may occur during labor and delivery or postpartum. In many cases delivery has not yet occurred [40]. The diagnosis of AFE is a clinical diagnosis of exclusion. The cardinal signs are cardiovascular collapse, acute left ventricular failure with pulmonary edema, DIC, and altered mental status. Early recognition is critical to a successful outcome. Management is primarily supportive and resuscitative. Therefore, airway management is the first step in care, typically with endotracheal intubation and administration of 100% O_2 with positive pressure ventilation. If still pregnant, delivery of the fetus should be expeditious to avoid hypoxic injury and increase chances of survival. Inotropes and vasopressors are generally needed for hemodynamic support. Echocardiography is a sensitive tool for evaluation of cardiac function and volume status and can be useful in the acute phase of resuscitation for AFE. Cardiopulmonary bypass and VA ECMO have been used with good effect for supportive treatment during AFE [41, 42]. Maternal morbidity is high with historically reported case fatality of 50% with only 15% of survivors being neurologically intact. Most recently a population-based cohort study from the UK registry showed a maternal mortality of 37% [43].

Critical Care in Obstetric Patients

Access

Central venous catheter (CVC) access is commonly used in critically ill patients for various reasons including reliable access, delivery of parenteral therapies (drugs, nutrition), or infusion of vesicants (vasopressors). Standardized insertion technique, ultrasound utilization, catheter design, and site maintenance have reduced complication rates. The rate of complication with CVCs is difficult to estimate depending upon the anatomic site, operator experience, and the amount of time the catheter which has been in place. Mechanical complications such as failure to place, arterial puncture, and line malposition occur in about 1/3 of catheter placements [44]. There are no complications specific to pregnancy. However, one retrospective series examined CVC complications in pregnancy and found that infection is the most frequent complication and mechanical complications occurred less frequently [45].

Nutrition

Critical illness and pregnancy are states of hypermetabolism. Nutritional support is now considered a key component in the care of critically ill patients. Moreover, early enteral support has been shown to improve outcomes in critical illness. The American Society of Parenteral and Enteral Nutrition (ASPEN) has put forth straightforward recommendations for nutrition in critically ill patients. It is important to keep in mind that in pregnancy there are additional caloric and vitamin requirements. The total maternal energy requirements for a full-term pregnancy are 80,000 kcal. When divided into 250 days of pregnancy, energy requirements are about 300 kcal additional daily. Protein requirements increase in pregnancy from 0.8 g/kg/day to 1.1 g/kg/day [46]. Folate supplementation is recommended to reduce the risk of neural tube defects [47, 48]. Women of childbearing age should consume 400 μg of folate daily as well as low-risk pregnant women. Women who are high risk of NTD or who have had a previous NTD should take 4000 μg or 4 mg of folate daily [49]. Lastly, iron supplementation (30–60 mg elemental iron) should be provided to pregnant women for prevention of anemia, maternal sepsis, low birth weight, and preterm birth [50].

Respiratory Failure

Acute respiratory failure is a rare complication of pregnancy. As such, the body of evidence surrounding ARF in pregnancy is limited, and there are no randomized controlled trials of ventilator strategies in pregnant women. Dyspnea is a common symptom within pregnancy, and it is important to distinguish from pathological shortness of breath. Causes of acute respiratory failure in pregnancy include pulmonary edema, infection, and pulmonary embolus [51]. It is important to be mindful of anatomic and physiologic changes during pregnancy. Appropriate management of a difficult intubation in pregnancy is essential in reducing maternal and fetal morbidity and mortality.

Airway anatomy alteration can result in difficult airway and lead to a potential failed intubation. Upper airway edema is the result of increased blood volume and capillary engorgement of the mucosa throughout the respiratory tract [52]. These changes can be made worse by pathology such as edema associated with preeclampsia or infection. Decreased tone at the lower esophageal sphincter as well as displacement of the stomach superiorly places pregnant women at increased risk of aspiration. Preoxygenation was 100%; O_2 is ideal. Equipment for difficult airway management, surgical airway, and suctioning devices should be immediately available.

Physiologic Considerations

Oxygen delivery to the fetus is accomplished via uterus blood flow, maternal blood oxygen content, and concentration of maternal hemoglobin. The placenta exchanges gas between mother and fetus driven by a gradient of oxygen and carbon dioxide. Even in the setting of mild maternal hypoxemia, the low oxygen content within fetal blood preserves the gradient between mother and fetus. In an experimental trial of hypoxia in term pregnancy, fetal parameters including heart rate, variability, and umbilical artery, Doppler indices were unchanged during maternal hypoxia. These values are considered representative of fetal oxygenation [11]. The umbilical venous blood returning to the fetus has only a PaO_2 of 25–33 mmHg. Therefore, the most highly oxygenated blood on the fetal side is still lower than the least oxygenated blood in maternal circulation. Maternal venous oxygen content is accessible by testing the mixed venous saturation of oxygen (SvO_2). It is a common recommendation to maintain maternal oxygen saturation by pulse oximetry at 92% or greater due to the fetal hemoglobin oxygen dissociation curve. However, uteroplacental blood flow rather than maternal oxygenation is the major determinant in fetal oxygen delivery. The fetus is specifically adapted to this environment with a higher hemoglobin affinity for oxygen and higher cardiac output relative to fetal size.

Traditional higher tidal volumes were previously utilized in a pregnant population with ARDS, and barotrauma rates were notably high [53]. Lower tidal volumes in patients with ARDS (6–8 ml/kg) are associated with improved mortality and morbidity [54]. This benefit is presumed in pregnancy as well. In the era of low tidal volume ventilation, permissive hypercapnia is a common strategy in treating patients with ARDS. However, the effects of maternal hypercapnia are less well understood. Hypocapnia results in decreased uterine blood flow, while mild hypercapnia, in a pig model, leads to decreased uterine vascular resistance [55]. However, an elevated maternal pCO_2 may impede transfer from fetal CO_2 to into maternal circulation as this is gradient driven. Retention of CO_2 within the fetus could lead to potential worsened acidosis, and thus monitoring would be imperative in monitoring fetal well-being. Hypercapnia has been associated with loss of fetal heart rate variability, but normalization to moderate variability occurred when normocapnia is returned [56]. Thus, if fetal heart rate tracing is consistent with fetal acidosis, attempts to improve maternal pCO_2 may lead to improvement in the tracing and fetal acid-base status. Options to reduce maternal pCO_2 would include increasing TV, increasing releases, or breaths.

Prone Position

Prone positioning may be required to improve oxygenation in a patient with ARDS. This strategy has been used in pregnant patients. Fetal concerns regarding sedation medication should not interfere with adequate care of a mother. NMB agents do not cross the placenta.

ECMO

ECMO is becoming a more common technique in patients with ARDS or cardiogenic shock who fail conventional strategies. The CESAR trial demonstrated mortality benefit in an ARDS, non-obstetric population. In pregnancy and recently postpartum patients, ECMO use in the literature has been reported with increasing frequency though it is still uncommon. In obstetric and recently postpartum women, no specific maternal or fetal morbidity or mortality has been reported. Among pregnant and postpartum women who underwent ECMO for ARDS, maternal and fetal survival on ECMO were 80% and 70%, respectively [57]. One report of catastrophic bleeding was noted in the peripartum period.

Delivery

There are a multitude of indications for delivery in pregnancy. Specifically if delivery improves, maternal respiratory status in the setting of ARF or ARDS is unknown. Several studies have asked this question all to no avail, with small numbers. Delivery itself utilizes additional oxygen and increase in cardiac output.

Fetal survival in ARDS is directly related to gestational age at delivery which would imply that the fetus gains the most benefit from staying in utero if feasible and safe after consideration of maternal and fetal status. Maternal respiratory parameters may only improve slightly with delivery [58]. However, consideration of the pathology which leads to maternal respiratory decompensation may alter decision to deliver. If respiratory decline is related to preeclampsia or amniotic fluid embolism, delivery would likely be indicated. But, the decision to delivery is typically a multifaceted one and requires a discussion among maternal-fetal medicine, intensivist, anesthesiologist, and neonatologist.

Summary

Although uncommon, pregnancy can become complicated by trauma and critical illness. Trauma remains the leading cause of mortality in pregnant women, while obstetric causes are the leading indication for ICU admission. Regardless of etiology, there are several important points to bear in mind when caring for a traumatically injured or critically ill pregnant woman.

1. If mom is hurt badly, baby is certainly hurt badly. Conversely, if the mother is uninjured, the fetus may be severely injured.

2. Blood flow to the uterus is everything for baby, as such maternal physiologic changes are directed at the goal of bringing blood supply to growing fetus. Maintaining adequate maternal hemodynamics and oxygenation is crucial for a good fetal outcome.
3. Modern-day obstetrics and neonatology have improved fetal outcomes; mom is always first, but baby is a very close second. We propose an ABCDE mnemonic for the care of the fetus as well.
   (a) A – assessment of gestational age
   (b) B – breathing or body movement
   (c) C – continuous monitoring
   (d) D – determine need for immediate delivery
   (e) E – effect a plan
4. Perimortem cesarean section, now termed resuscitative hysterotomy, is a procedure initially intended for improved fetal survival but importantly improves maternal survival as well. The 4-min rule is gone; if maternal cardiac arrest occurs, resuscitation of the mother should include a simultaneous cesarean section when the fetus is greater than 23 weeks gestational age.

References

1. Centers for Disease Control and Prevention. National center for health statistics. Births – method of delivery. 2017. https://www.cdc.gov/nchs/fastats/delivery.htm.
2. Centers for Disease Control and Prevention. Pregnancy mortality surveillance system. 2017. https://www.cdc.gov/reproductivehealth/maternalinfanthealth/pmss.html.
3. Mendez-Figueroa H, Dahlke J, Vrees R, et al. Trauma in pregnancy: an updated systematic review. Am J Obstet Gynecol. 2013;209:1–10.
4. Pearlman M, Tintinalli J, Lorenz R. Blunt trauma during pregnancy. N Engl J Med. 1990;323:1609–13.
5. U.S. Department of Justice. Extent, nature, and consequences of intimate partner violence. 2000. https://www.ncjrs.gov/pdffiles1/nij/181867.pdf. Accessed 12 June 2012.
6. Wolf M, Alexander B, Rivara F, et al. A retrospective cohort study of seatbelt use and pregnancy outcome after a motor vehicle crash. J Trauma. 1993;34:116–9.
7. Schiff M, Mack C, Kaufman R, et al. The effect of air bags on pregnancy outcomes in Washington State: 2002-2005. Obstet Gynecol. 2010;115:85–92.
8. Zwart J, Dupuis J, Richters A, et al. Obstetric intensive care unit admission: a 2-year nationwide population-based cohort study. Intensive Care Med. 2010;36:256–63.
9. Younge N, Goldstein R, Eunice Kennedy Shriver National Institute of Child Health and Human Development Neonatal Research Network, et al. Survival and neurodevelopmental outcomes among periviable infants. N Engl J Med. 2017;376:617–28.
10. Gunter J, Pearlman M. Emergencies during pregnancy: trauma and non obstetric surgical conditions. In: Ling F, Duff P, editors. Obstetrics and gynecology: principles for practice. New York: McGraw-Hill; 2001.
11. Erkkola R, Pirhonen J, Polvi H. The fetal cardiovascular function in chronic placental insufficiency is different from experimental hypoxia. Ann Chir Gynaecol Suppl. 1994;208:76–9.
12. Brown HL. Trauma in pregnancy. Obstet Gynecol. 2009;114:147–60.
13. Sanghavi M, Rutherford J. Cardiovascular physiology of pregnancy. Circulation. 2014;130:1003–8.
14. American College of Obstetricians and Gynecologists' Committee on Obstetric Practice. Committee opinion no. 656: guidelines for diagnostic imaging during pregnancy and lactation. Obstet Gynecol. 2016;127:e75–80.
15. Committee on Obstetric Practice and the American Society of Anesthesiologists. Committee opinion no. 696: nonobstetric surgery during pregnancy. Obstet Gynecol. 2017;129:777–8.
16. Katz V, Balderston K, DeFreest M. Perimortem cesarean delivery: were our assumptions correct? Am J Obstet Gynecol. 2005;192:1916–20.
17. Katz V. Perimortem cesarean delivery: its role in maternal mortality. Semin Perinatol. 2012;36:68–72.
18. Say L, Chou D, Gemmill A, et al. Global causes of maternal death: a WHO systematic analysis. Lancet Glob Health. 2014;2:e323–33.
19. Pritchard J, Brekken A. Clinical and laboratory studies on severe abruptio placentae. Am J Obstet Gynecol. 1967;97:681–700.
20. Reddy U, Abuhamad A, Levine D, Fetal Imaging Workshop Invited Participants, et al. Fetal imaging: executive summary of a joint Eunice Kennedy Shriver National Institute of Child Health and Human Development, Society for Maternal-Fetal Medicine, American Institute of Ultrasound in Medicine, American College of Obstetricians and Gynecologists, American College of Radiology, Society for Pediatric Radiology, and Society of Radiologists in Ultrasound Fetal Imaging Workshop. Am J Obstet Gynecol. 2014;210:387–97.
21. Smith R, Lauria M, Comstock C, et al. Transvaginal ultrasonography for all placentas that appear to be low-lying or over the internal cervical os. Ultrasound Obstet Gynecol. 1997;9:22–4.
22. Wu S, Kocherginsky M, Hibbard J. Abnormal placentation: twenty-year analysis. Am J Obstet Gynecol. 2005;192:1458–61.
23. Silver R, Landon M, Rouse D, National Institute of Child Health and Human Development Maternal-Fetal Medicine Units Network, et al. Maternal morbidity associated with multiple repeat cesarean deliveries. Obstet Gynecol. 2006;107:1226–32.
24. Tantbirojn P, Crum C, Parast M. Pathophysiology of placenta creta: the role of decidua and extravillous trophoblast. Placenta. 2008;29:639–45.
25. Jauniaux E, Jurkovic D. Placenta accreta: pathogenesis of a 20th century iatrogenic uterine disease. Placenta. 2012;33:244–51.
26. D'Antonio F, Iacovella C, Bhide A. Prenatal identification of invasive placentation using ultrasound: systematic review and meta-analysis. Ultrasound Obstet Gynecol. 2013;42:509–17.
27. Warshak C, Eskander R, Hull A, et al. Accuracy of ultrasonography and magnetic resonance imaging in the diagnosis of placenta accreta. Obstet Gynecol. 2006;108:573–81.
28. Jolley J, Nageotte M, Wing D, et al. Management of placenta accreta: a survey of Maternal-Fetal Medicine practitioners. J Matern Fetal Neonatal Med. 2012;25:756–60.
29. Fox K, Shamshirsaz A, Carusi D, et al. Conservative management of morbidly adherent placenta: expert review. Am J Obstet Gynecol. 2015;213:755–60.
30. American College of Obstetricians and Gynecologists. ACOG practice bulletin: clinical management guidelines for obstetrician-gynecologists number, 76: postpartum hemorrhage. Obstet Gynecol. 2006;108:1039–47.
31. Shamshirsaz A, Fox K, Salmanian B, et al. Maternal morbidity in patients with morbidly adherent placenta treated with and without a standardized multidisciplinary approach. Am J Obstet Gynecol. 2015;212:218.e1–9.
32. Belfort M. Indicated preterm birth for placenta accreta. Semin Perinatol. 2011;35:252–6.
33. Lilker S, Meyer R, Downey K, et al. Anesthetic considerations for placenta accreta. Int J Obstet Anesth. 2011;20:288–92.

34. Wong H, Hutton J, Zuccollo J, et al. The maternal outcome in placenta accreta: the significance of antenatal diagnosis and non-separation of placenta at delivery. N Z Med J. 2008;121:30–8.
35. Begley C, Gyte G, Devane D, et al. Active versus expectant management for women in the third stage of labour. Cochrane Database Syst Rev. 2015;2:CD007412.
36. Dahlke J, Mendez-Figueroa H, Rouse D, et al. Evidence-based surgery for cesarean delivery: an updated systematic review. Am J Obstet Gynecol. 2013;209:294–306.
37. Holcomb J, Tilley B, Baraniuk S, PROPPR Study Group, et al. Transfusion of plasma, platelets, and red blood cells in a 1:1:1 vs a 1:1:2 ratio and mortality in patients with severe trauma: the PROPPR randomized clinical trial. JAMA. 2015;313:471–82.
38. Gutierrez M, Goodnough L, Druzin M, et al. Postpartum hemorrhage treated with a massive transfusion protocol at a tertiary obstetric center: a retrospective study. Int J Obstet Anesth. 2012;21:230–5.
39. Gilbert W, Danielsen B. Amniotic fluid embolism: decreased mortality in a population-based study. Obstet Gynecol. 1999;93:973–7.
40. Moore J, Baldisseri M. Amniotic fluid embolism. Crit Care Med. 2005;33:S279–85.
41. Stanten R, Iverson L, Daugharty T, et al. Amniotic fluid embolism causing catastrophic pulmonary vasoconstriction: diagnosis by transesophageal echocardiogram and treatment by cardiopulmonary bypass. Obstet Gynecol. 2003;102:496–8.
42. Wiznitzer A, Gabbay-Benziv R, Alman E, et al. Amniotic fluid embolism: combined treatment with surgery and extracorporeal membrane oxygenation support – a case report. Obstet Gynecol Cases Rev. 2016;3:082.
43. Tuffnell D. United Kingdom amniotic fluid embolism register. BJOG. 2005;112:1625–9.
44. Eisen L, Narasimhan M, Berger J, et al. Mechanical complications of central venous catheters. J Intensive Care Med. 2006;21:40–6.
45. Nuthalapaty F, Beck M, Mabie W. Complications of central venous catheters during pregnancy and postpartum: a case series. Am J Obstet Gynecol. 2009;201:311.e1–5.
46. Institute of Medicine. In: Meyers LD, Hellwig JP, editors. Dietary reference intakes: the essential guide to nutrient requirements. Washington, DC: National Academies Press; 2006.
47. Mulinare J, Cordero J, Erickson J, et al. Periconceptional use of multivitamins and the occurrence of neural tube defects. JAMA. 1988;260:3141–5.
48. US Preventive Services Task Force, Bibbins-Domingo K, Grossman D, et al. Folic acid supplementation for the prevention of neural tube defects: US Preventive Services Task Force recommendation statement. JAMA. 2017;317:183–9.
49. Cheschier N, ACOG Committee on Practice Bulletins-Obstetrics. ACOG practice bulletin. Neural tube defects. Number 44, July 2003. Int J Gynaecol Obstet. 2003;83:123–33.
50. World Health Organization (WHO). Guideline: daily iron and folic acid supplementation in pregnant women. Geneva: World Health Organization; 2012.
51. Jenkins T, Troiano N, Graves C, et al. Mechanical ventilation in an obstetric population: characteristics and delivery rates. Am J Obstet Gynecol. 2003;188:549–52.
52. Norwitz E. Pregnancy induced physiologic alterations. In: Belfort M, editor. Critical care obstetrics. 5th ed. Oxford, UK: Wiley-Blackwell; 2012.
53. Catanzarite V, Willms D, Wong D, et al. Acute respiratory distress syndrome in pregnancy and the puerperium: causes, courses, and outcomes. Obstet Gynecol. 2001;97:760–4.
54. Acute Respiratory Distress Syndrome Network, Brower R, Matthay M, et al. Ventilation with lower tidal volumes as compared with traditional tidal volumes for acute lung injury and the acute respiratory distress syndrome. N Engl J Med. 2000;342:1301–8.
55. Levinson G, Shnider S, DeLorimier A, et al. Effects of maternal hyperventilation on uterine blood flow and fetal oxygenation and acid-base status. Anesthesiology. 1974;40:340–7.
56. Fraser D, Jensen D, Wolfe L, et al. Fetal heart rate response to maternal hypocapnia and hypercapnia in late gestation. J Obstet Gynaecol Can. 2008;30:312–6.
57. Sharma N, Wille K, Bellot S, et al. Modern use of extracorporeal life support in pregnancy and postpartum. ASAIO J. 2015;61:110–4.
58. Tomlinson M, Caruthers T, Whitty J, et al. Does delivery improve maternal condition in the respiratory-compromised gravida? Obstet Gynecol. 1998;91:108–11.
59. Dildy GA, Clark SL. Postpartum hemorrhage. Contemp Ob Gyn. 1993;38(8):21–9.

Unique Aspects of Surgical Critical Care for Children

57

Jamie Golden, Aaron R. Jensen, David W. Bliss, and Jeffrey S. Upperman

Introduction

The care of critically ill children can differ significantly from their adult counterparts by virtue of the differences in anatomy, physiology, behavioral development, and family factors. It is also important to understand that although the terms "children" and "pediatric" are often used as if they represent a relatively homogenous group, they are general catchall terms that have little validity for directing evaluation or ICU management. With the wide variations in anatomy, physiology, metabolism, and response to injury/illness that are present along the age spectrum from neonate to adolescence, it is more important to characterize the patient by their specific age or developmental category. While the care and considerations for a neonate will be entirely different than care for a similar illness or injury in an adult, the care of an older adolescent will essentially be identical to that for non-elderly adults. But for all true "children," the multiple significant differences will impact choices of monitoring tools, therapeutic interventions, and operations that may differ substantially from those applied in adult patients. In this chapter, we review the key differences in critical care between children and adults using a systems-based approach.

J. Golden · A. R. Jensen · D. W. Bliss · J. S. Upperman (✉)
Department of Surgery, Keck School of Medicine of the University of Southern California, Division of Pediatric Surgery, Children's Hospital Los Angeles, Los Angeles, CA, USA
e-mail: jupperman@chla.usc.edu

Anatomic, Physiologic, and Behavioral Differences in Children as Compared to Adults

Vital Signs

Normal vital signs and urine output vary by patient age and are summarized in Table 57.1 [2]. For providers that rarely care for children, age-normal references for vital signs and urine output can be rapidly obtained from either a color-coded length-based estimation tape (Broselow tape) or a digital reference card that can be downloaded to a mobile device (Fig. 57.1) [3]. The pediatric surgical intensivist must realize that hypotension is a late finding for children in shock and that bradycardia is an ominous sign in the progression toward cardiac arrest. Moreover, young children are more prone to rapid development of hypoxia due to increased metabolic rate, anatomic and physiologic shunts, and pulmonary immaturity.

Pediatric Airway

Anatomic differences present unique airway management challenges in children – especially neonates and children with craniofacial anomalies related to genetic syndromes. Younger children have a relative large occiput, redundant soft tissue, a large tongue, adenotonsillar hypertrophy, a long and narrow epiglottis, and a laryngeal inlet that appears more anterior [4, 5]. A straight miller blade and a shoulder bump to better align the airway can be used to facilitate successful intubation. Videolaryngoscopy may improve visualization of the anterior airway, but the practitioner must anticipate tremendous difficulty in maneuvering the tube through the anterior structures and bend the stylet accordingly [6]. The airway of a child is both smaller in diameter and shorter in length than that of an adult and is therefore more prone to obstruction with secretions or foreign bodies and more prone to endotracheal tube positional changes such as mainstem intubation or dislodge-

A. Salim et al. (eds.), *Surgical Critical Care Therapy*, https://doi.org/10.1007/978-3-319-71712-8_57

Table 57.1 Normal vital signs by age [1]

Age	Heart rate (beats/min)	Systolic BP (mmHg)	Diastolic BP (mmHg)	Respiratory rate (breaths/min)	Urine output (mL/kg/hr)
Newborn	90–180	50–70	27–47	30–50	1–2
1–5 months	100–180	70–90	30–60	30–40	1–2
6–11 months	100–150	60–120	50–70	25–35	1–2
1 year	100–150	65–125	40–90	20–30	0.5–1
2–3 years	65–150	75–125	40–90	15–25	0.5–1
4–5 years	65–140	80–120	50–80	15–25	0.5–1
6–9 years	65–120	80–120	50–80	12–20	0.5–1
10–12 years	65–120	90–130	55–85	12–20	0.5–1
≥ 13 years	55–110	100–140	60–90	12–28	0.5–1

ment. Particular attention must be paid by the respiratory care practitioner (RCP) to frequent suctioning and careful securement of the tube (especially in an active child). Critical airways in children often require deep levels of sedation to prevent accidental dislodgement, disconnection, or obstruction – particularly in children that may be adept at getting out of restraints. Generally, uncuffed endotracheal tubes are preferred for children less than 8 years old due to historical concerns for the development of subglottic stenosis, though more recent data suggests this risk may be overstated. Endotracheal tube size can be approximated to the size of a child's fifth finger or can be calculated using the formula (age in years +4)/4 or, again, can be referenced from a color-coded tape or smartphone app [5]. The depth of endotracheal intubation for children >1 year old is outlined in the PALS guidelines and can be estimated by (age in years / 2) + 12 cm [7, 8].

A difficult airway should be anticipated in patients with facial dysmorphia or genetic syndromes such as Pierre Robin, Goldenhar, Freeman-Sheldon, Apert, Hunter and Hurler, and Beckwith-Wiedemann syndrome, and a practitioner with expertise in advanced airway management for pediatric difficult airway should be present for intubation [4, 9]. If an airway cannot be established by other means, an emergency cricothyroidotomy may be performed in older children. A needle cricothyroidotomy is preferred in young children due to the small size of the cricothyroid membrane and the larynx and risk of injury and total loss of the airway with the surgical technique. The absolute age with which needle cricothyroidotomy is preferred over the surgical technique is controversial, but a conservative age cutoff is less than 12 years old [8]. Formal tracheostomy techniques are similar to those in adults but require short, pediatric cannulas.

Vascular Access

While often straightforward in older children, vascular access can be challenging in very young children, particularly neonates. Peripheral venous access can be attempted in traditional sites in the upper or lower extremity veins but can also be attained using the scalp veins (frontal superficial, temporal posterior, auricular, supraorbital, and posterior facial veins) in infants and toddlers. The femoral, internal jugular, external jugular, and subclavian veins can be used for central venous access, but the disproportion of vessel size must be considered [8]. Babies have large heads with small arms and legs in relation to the torso and head, which in practice makes the internal or external jugular the preferred site for access in smaller children. Femoral vessels, in particular, can be quite small and are at risk for vascular thrombosis if large catheters are placed in the groin. Children under 1 year of age are at particular risk of arterial thrombosis with femoral arterial lines, and these should be avoided if at all possible [10]. In neonates at or shortly after birth, umbilical vessel cannulation can be performed for venous access or arterial monitoring [11]. While this site is attractive in this population, lines generally are not maintained in place for longer than 1 week due to the risk of mesenteric vascular and portal venous thrombosis [12–15]. Establishing intravenous access, peripheral or central, can be particularly challenging in hypovolemic children. Early resuscitation can be effectively administered via intraosseous (IO) access in the larger long bones (humerus, femur, tibia) or the iliac wings. Although sternal IO is increasingly used in adults, it is absolutely contraindicated in children (age < 14). Laboratory studies may be obtained from intraosseous cannulas including serum chemistries, coagulation studies, venous blood gas, and blood typing and crossmatch, though traditional blood counts are generally unreliable. The main drawback of IO use is the propensity for the IO to become dislodged with resulting risks of extravascular infusion and the attendant complications. Once intravascular volume has been restored, attempts at durable vascular access with peripheral IV placement, percutaneous central access, or saphenous cutdown (at the ankle peripherally or in the groin centrally) should be attempted. Unlike adults, children do not tolerate central venous catheterization awake and should be anesthetized for central line placement because it can be technically challenging with perhaps only a few millimeter margin of error and because children will not hold still reliably. Careful selection of anesthesia and sedation should be balanced with the putative benefits of central venous cannulation.

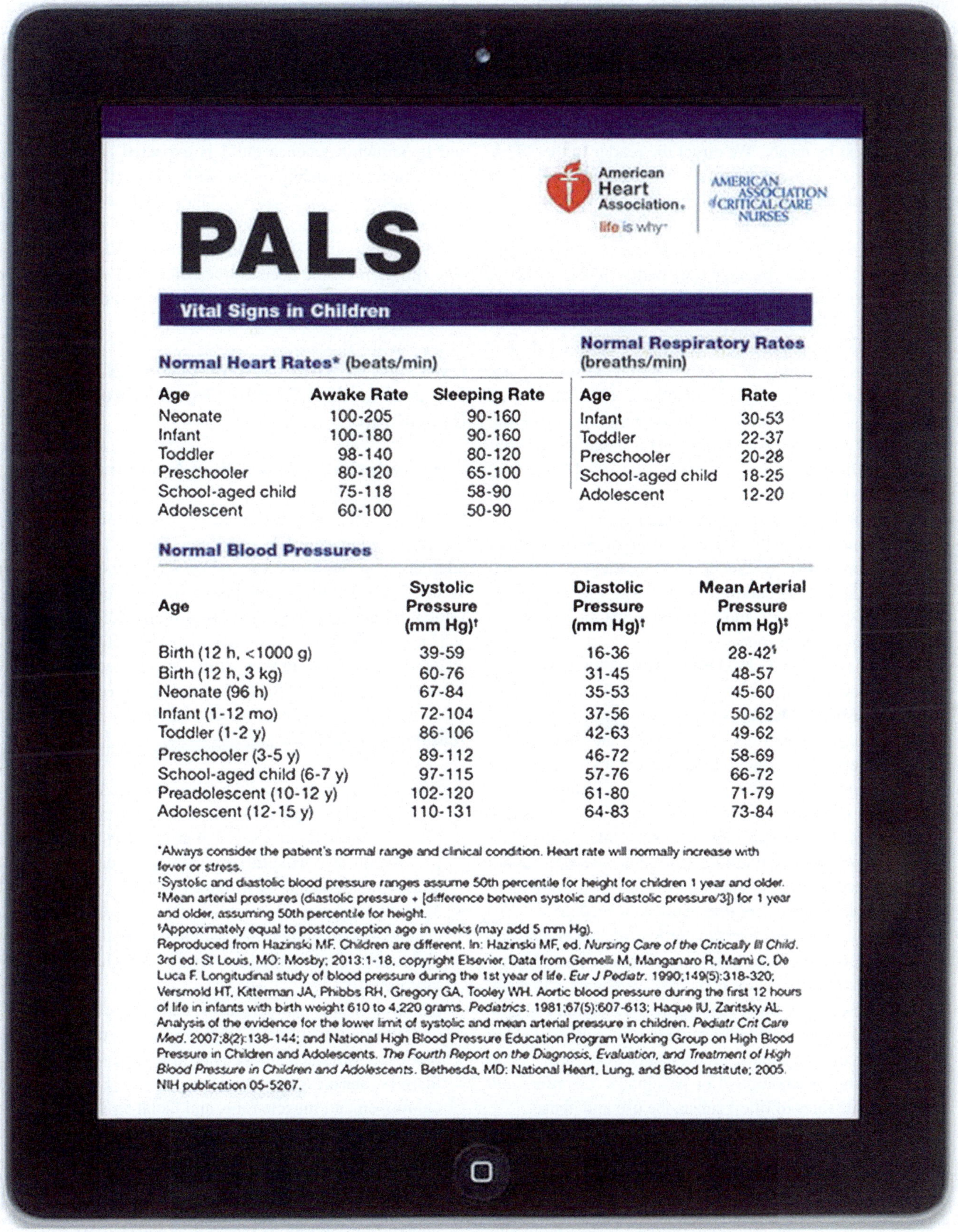

American Heart Association. life is why

AMERICAN ASSOCIATION of CRITICAL-CARE NURSES

PALS

Vital Signs in Children

Normal Heart Rates* (beats/min)

Age	Awake Rate	Sleeping Rate
Neonate	100-205	90-160
Infant	100-180	90-160
Toddler	98-140	80-120
Preschooler	80-120	65-100
School-aged child	75-118	58-90
Adolescent	60-100	50-90

Normal Respiratory Rates (breaths/min)

Age	Rate
Infant	30-53
Toddler	22-37
Preschooler	20-28
School-aged child	18-25
Adolescent	12-20

Normal Blood Pressures

Age	Systolic Pressure (mm Hg)†	Diastolic Pressure (mm Hg)†	Mean Arterial Pressure (mm Hg)‡
Birth (12 h, <1000 g)	39-59	16-36	28-42§
Birth (12 h, 3 kg)	60-76	31-45	48-57
Neonate (96 h)	67-84	35-53	45-60
Infant (1-12 mo)	72-104	37-56	50-62
Toddler (1-2 y)	86-106	42-63	49-62
Preschooler (3-5 y)	89-112	46-72	58-69
School-aged child (6-7 y)	97-115	57-76	66-72
Preadolescent (10-12 y)	102-120	61-80	71-79
Adolescent (12-15 y)	110-131	64-83	73-84

*Always consider the patient's normal range and clinical condition. Heart rate will normally increase with fever or stress.

†Systolic and diastolic blood pressure ranges assume 50th percentile for height for children 1 year and older.

‡Mean arterial pressures (diastolic pressure + [difference between systolic and diastolic pressure/3]) for 1 year and older, assuming 50th percentile for height.

§Approximately equal to postconception age in weeks (may add 5 mm Hg).

Reproduced from Hazinski MF. Children are different. In: Hazinski MF, ed. *Nursing Care of the Critically Ill Child*. 3rd ed. St Louis, MO: Mosby; 2013:1-18, copyright Elsevier. Data from Gemelli M, Manganaro R, Mami C, De Luca F. Longitudinal study of blood pressure during the 1st year of life. *Eur J Pediatr*. 1990;149(5):318-320; Versmold HT, Kitterman JA, Phibbs RH, Gregory GA, Tooley WH. Aortic blood pressure during the first 12 hours of life in infants with birth weight 610 to 4,220 grams. *Pediatrics*. 1981;67(5):607-613; Haque IU, Zaritsky AL. Analysis of the evidence for the lower limit of systolic and mean arterial pressure in children. *Pediatr Crit Care Med*. 2007;8(2):138-144; and National High Blood Pressure Education Program Working Group on High Blood Pressure in Children and Adolescents. *The Fourth Report on the Diagnosis, Evaluation, and Treatment of High Blood Pressure in Children and Adolescents*. Bethesda, MD: National Heart, Lung, and Blood Institute; 2005. NIH publication 05-5267.

Fig. 57.1 A digital reference sheet for age-specific vitals can be downloaded from the American Heart Association for quick reference on one's mobile device

Other Anatomic, Physiologic, and Behavioral Vulnerabilities Specific to Traumatically Injured Children

This chapter focuses mostly on ICU care of children, but there are a number of vulnerabilities of which the surgical intensivist must be aware. We direct the reader to the ATLS student guide for a more thorough discussion of these vulnerabilities but will summarize highpoints below [16].

- The large, relatively heavy head of young children and the associated cervical ligamentous laxity place them at increased risk of traumatic brain injury and cervical spine injury.
- The pliable cartilaginous ribs of young children do not confer the same degree of rigid protection of the chest and upper abdominal structures that those ossified ribs of adults provide. Pulmonary injuries may occur in the absence of rib fractures and may not be apparent on initial trauma radiography until after the first 24–48 h in the ICU. The surgical intensivist must monitor for this even in the absence of bony thoracic cage injuries.
- The abdomen in young children is larger, more rotund, and less protected by the horizontal oriented ribs and small pelvis in these children. Abdominal viscera (particularly the spleen, liver, and bladder) are at increased risk of blunt injury in this population.
- Children have smaller circulating blood volume (see later section – hematology) and a remarkable ability to compensate for blood loss.
- Children have higher relative metabolic rates that require higher levels of substrate administration and that predispose them to hypoperfusion, hypoxia, and acidosis.
- Due to their higher ratio of body surface area to weight than adults and relative lack of brown fat, children are prone to hypothermia if left uncovered or if cold fluids are administered. Particular attention to active warming measures in cold pediatric trauma patients is needed.
- Psychologic response to trauma or loss of a loved one can be quite variable in children and can range from regression to nonverbal behavior to aggressive behavior that can be quite disruptive. Early engagement of a child life specialist to assist the healthcare team can be quite helpful in caring for these patients. Adolescents may have occult and evolving psychological or psychiatric disorders and have notable rates of illicit substance use and abuse.

Expected Neurodevelopmental Milestones

The care of infants and children requires a basic knowledge of expected stages of neurodevelopment. Table 57.2 includes an overview of basic developmental milestones that are attained by 50–90% of children [17]. While these milestones may not seem relevant to a trauma surgeon or surgical intensivist on the surface, one must remember that a knowledge of appropriate motor activities is essential in recognizing nonaccidental trauma (e.g., a 1-month-old will not roll off a bed) and in knowing when a child is expected to follow commands or have reliable verbal skills to calculate a Glasgow coma score (GCS). Moreover, stages of development should be considered when the clinician interacts with the child, designs therapeutic interventions, and evaluates responses over time. This table need not be committed to memory, but should be kept as a reference for instances such as these.

Overview of Unique Aspects of Pediatric Surgical Critical Care by Organ System Neurologic

Pain, Sedation, and Delirium Assessment

Evaluation of pain management, sedation, withdrawal symptoms, and delirium in infants and children to assess adequate interventions for pain and distress is a critical component of their care and is particularly challenging for intubated, nonverbal, or developmentally delayed children. Various standardized tools have been developed to assess infants and children in this setting. A detailed review of all of these assessments is beyond the scope of this chapter, but we present examples of an assessment in each of the four domains [18]:

- *Withdrawal Assessment*: The WAT-1 scale for withdrawal in children is a validated instrument that maps 11 factors tracked by bedside nurses to four domains (gastrointestinal symptoms, wakefulness, return to calm state, and autonomic evidence of withdrawal) [19].
- *Pain Management Assessment*: The FLACC scale is an established instrument for pain assessment in infants and children evaluating the face, legs, activity, cry, and consolability [20].
- *Sedation Assessment*: Sedation can be assessed in infants and children using the COMFORT behavior scale which has been validated for bedside use. The scale evaluates distress, alertness, agitation, respiratory response, physical movement, muscle tone, and facial tension [21, 22].
- *Delirium Assessment*: The Cornell Assessment of Pediatric Delirium (CAPD) tool has been validated for the assessment of delirium. Eye contact, purposefulness, awareness, ability to community needs, restlessness, inconsolability, and responsiveness to interaction and activity are evaluated and can be used for bedside assessment [23].

Table 57.2 Developmental milestones (taken from Bright Futures Handbook) for 50–90% of children [17]

Age	Gross motor	Fine motor	Cognitive, linguistic, and communication	Social-emotional
2 months	Head up 45 degrees	Follow past midline	Laugh	Smile spontaneously
4 months	Roll over	Follow to 180 degrees	Turn to rattling sound	
6 months	Sit without support	Look for dropped yarn	Turn to voice	Feed self
9 months	Pull to stand	Take 2 cubes	Dada/mama, nonspecific	Wave bye-bye
1 year	Stand alone	Put block in cup	1 word	Imitate activities
15 months	Walk backward	Scribble	3 words	Drink from cup
18 months	Walk up steps Run	Dump raisin Tower of 2 cubes	Point to at least 1 body part 6 words	Remove garment
2 years	Throw ball overhand Jump up	Tower of 6 cubes	Name 1 picture Combine words	Put on clothing
2.5 years	Throw ball overhand	Imitate vertical line Tower of 8 cubes	Know 2 actions Speech half understandable	Wash and dry hands
3 years	Balance on each foot (1 second) Broad jump	Thumb wiggle Imitate vertical line Tower of 8 cubes	Speech all understandable Name 1 color Know 2 adjectives	Name friend
4 years	Hop	Draw a person with 3 parts	Define 5 words Name 4 colors	Copy a cross (+)

There are several additional assessments available, and this field is developing continually as more research efforts are becoming focused on neurodevelopmental outcomes in children with prolonged ICU courses that develop ICU delirium [24–26]. This is a rapidly evolving field, and the long-term impact of delirium in the pediatric ICU is currently being elucidated. We do suspect that the impact is greater than we currently understand and particular attention should be paid to treatment of delirium in children. Involving pediatric mental health providers in the management of PICU patients at risk for delirium is warranted.

Pediatric Traumatic Brain Injury and Blunt Cerebrovascular Injury

Pediatric traumatic brain injury (TBI) warrants special consideration for critical care physicians as it is the leading cause of morbidity and mortality in infants and children [27]. Infants and children with TBI may be more difficult to assess in the trauma bay and ICU due to differences in their neurodevelopment. In particular, orientation or ability to follow commands cannot be assessed in nonverbal trauma patients. Infant and pediatric Glasgow coma scores (GCS) have been developed to assist in the assessment of young trauma patients (Table 57.3). Evidence-based criteria for obtaining head CT in the work-up of both verbal and nonverbal children have been developed and validated to decrease the overuse of CT in children with minor head trauma (Fig. 57.2) [29, 30]. Furthermore, there is increasing evidence that argues against the use of empiric repeat head CT for children admitted with intracranial hemorrhage in the absence of progressive neurologic symptoms [31–34].

In addition to the typical subdural, epidural, or subarachnoid hemorrhages seen in adults, children are more susceptible to diffuse cerebral edema and parenchymal injuries than their adult counterparts due to anatomic differences in their cranial vault [35]. Infants in particular can bleed large volumes into their head due to their open fontanelles, and serial head circumference should be measured in these patients to assess for the development of hydrocephalus or chronic hygromas that may require drainage. Skull fractures are identified in up to 21% of children with head trauma – most of which are nondepressed and do not require treatment [35]. Children with minor head trauma and an asymptomatic linear skull fracture can be safely discharged from the emergency room following observation unless there is a suspicion of nonaccidental trauma that requires further inpatient forensic work-up [36, 37]. Depressed skull fractures requiring operative intervention and skull base fractures are uncommon in children [35]. However, a basilar skull fracture involving the carotid canal along with a cervical vertebral body fracture, soft tissue injury of the anterior neck, near hanging, and severe cervical hyperextension or hyperflexion should prompt consideration of blunt cerebrovascular injury (BVCI) screening as part of the Denver and Memphis screening criteria [38]. Although these screening criteria are well validated in the adult trauma population, this practice is highly controversial in children. There is a lack of data on BCVI in the pediatric population, and no evidence-based pediatric screening criteria exist at this time.

Another controversial area in pediatric traumatic brain injury is the use of intracranial pressure (ICP) monitoring. The second edition of the guidelines for the acute medical management of severe traumatic brain injury in infants, children, and adolescents supports the use of ICP monitoring in children with severe traumatic brain injury but reports it is

Table 57.3 Infant and pediatric Glasgow coma score [28]

Infant	Pediatric	Adult	Score
Eye opening			
Spontaneous	Spontaneous	Spontaneous	4
To verbal stimuli	To verbal stimuli	To verbal stimuli	3
To pain only	To pain only	To pain only	2
No response	No response	No response	1
Verbal			
Coos and babbles	Oriented, appropriate	Oriented	5
Irritable cries	Confused	Confused	4
Cries to pain	Inappropriate words	Inappropriate words	3
Moans to pain	Incomprehensible/nonspecific sounds	Incomprehensible/nonspecific sounds	2
No response	No response	No response	1
Motor			
Moves spontaneously and purposefully	Obeys commands	Obeys commands	6
Withdraws to touch	Localizes to painful stimulus	Localizes to painful stimulus	5
Withdraws in response to pain	Withdraws in response to pain	Withdraws in response to pain	4
Decorticate posturing to pain	Flexion in response to pain	Flexion in response to pain	3
Decerebrate posturing to pain	Extension in response to pain	Extension in response to pain	2
No response	No response	No response	1

not routinely indicated in mild or moderate injury [39]. The Brain Trauma Foundation further outlines recommendations for the monitoring of ICP following trauma [40]. Despite these recommendations, randomized international data suggests that ICP monitoring may not actually improve outcomes [41].

Post-traumatic Seizures

Early post-traumatic seizures are more common in children – usually occurring within the first 7 days following injury – and are associated with an increased risk of late post-traumatic seizures [35]. The incidence of early seizures in severe TBI patients has been reported to be as high as 30% [42]. Age less than 2 years, initial GCS less than or equal to 8, and non-accidental trauma have been identified as independent risk factors for the development of early post-traumatic seizures [43]. Current recommendations for the prophylaxis of pediatric post-traumatic seizures are based on the severity of TBI, with antiepileptics recommended for the first 7 days following severe TBI in children. However actual practice among neurosurgeons and neurointensivists is not uniform [42]. Clinical trials for antiepileptic drugs for post-traumatic seizures in children have used either phenytoin or levetiracetam and range in treatment duration from 30 days to 18 months [42, 44–46].

Febrile Seizures and Status Epilepticus

Febrile seizures are unique to children and must be differentiated from seizures of other etiologies that may have more severe ramifications. Febrile seizures occur in children between 3 months and 5 years of age and are associated with fever without evidence of a central nervous system infection [47]. The reported incidence ranges from 2 to 10% of the population and is associated with a family history of febrile seizures [48]. The fever is typically due to a self-limited viral illness with seizures usually occurring at home [49]. The diagnosis can usually be established with a thorough history and physical examination, and the seizures are usually self-limiting. Simple febrile seizures are generalized, last for less than 15 minutes, and only occur once in 24 h, while complex febrile seizures are prolonged, focal, or occur more than once in 24 h [50]. If the child is still seizing on presentation, management is similar to other nonfebrile seizures and involves stabilization and anticonvulsive and antipyretic administration. It is important to rule out metabolic abnormalities and central nervous system infection in the evaluation of children presenting with seizures [48]. A lumbar puncture should be performed in patients with signs or symptoms of meningitis or intracranial infection (e.g., nuchal rigidity or photophobia) and is considered an option in infants who are not immunized against *Haemophilus influenzae* type b or *Streptococcus pneumoniae* or who have been pretreated with antibiotics [51]. In most children presenting with a simple febrile seizure, minimal intervention is recommended and prophylactic antipyretics and antiepileptics are not needed [52].

Pediatric status epilepticus also presents a unique challenge to the critical care physician. New-onset convulsive status epilepticus is most commonly caused by febrile seizures followed by CNS infection, stroke, and trauma. Children admitted to the PICU with acute encephalopathy have been increasingly recognized to have nonconvulsive

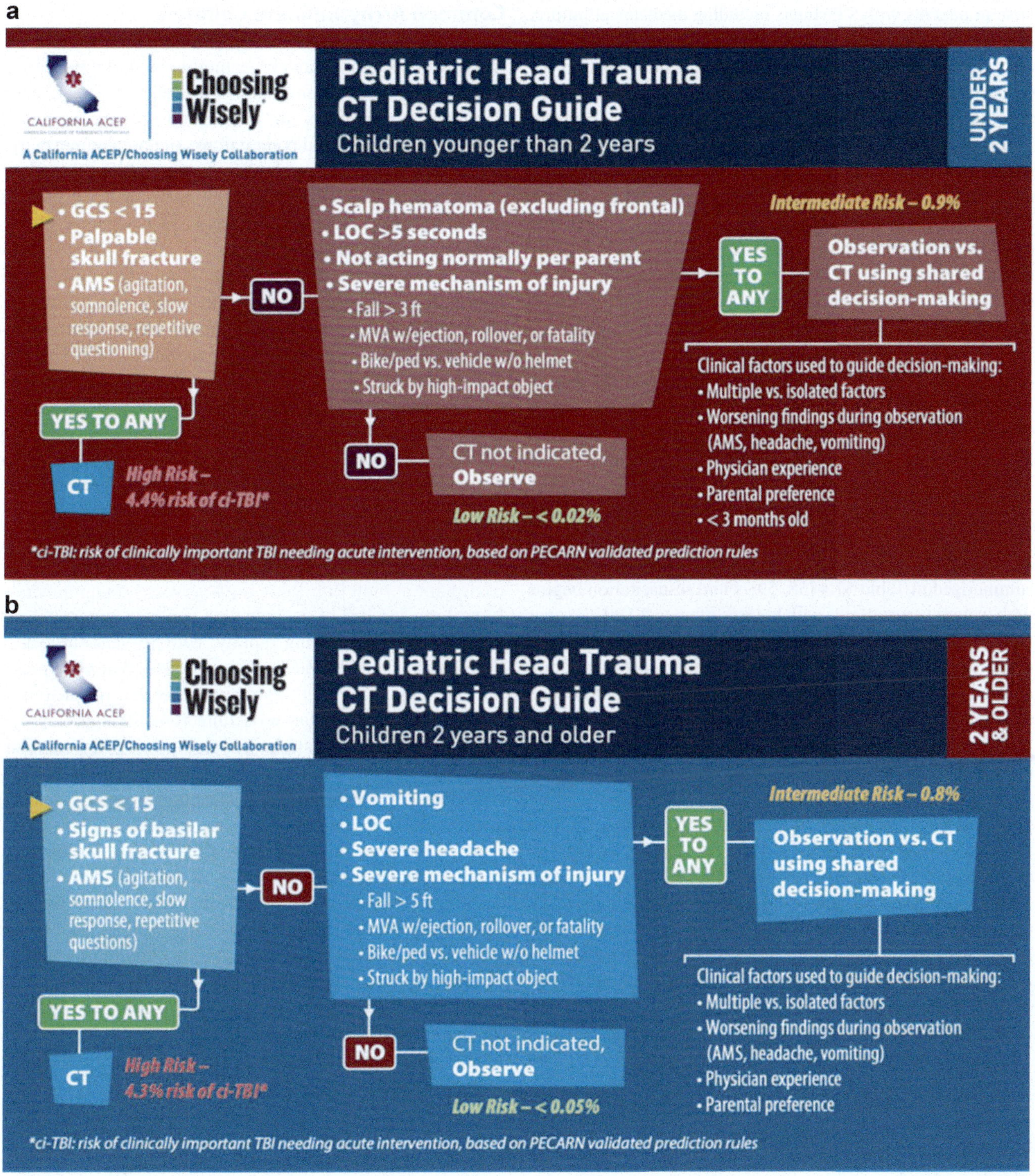

Fig. 57.2 (**a**, **b**) PECARN clinical decision algorithms for identification of children at risk for clinically important traumatic brain injury (TBI) for ages less than (nonverbal) and greater than (verbal) 2 years old

status epilepticus. The recommended work-up for convulsive and nonconvulsive status epilepticus in children was recently outlined by Freilich et al. and includes neuroimaging, electroencephalogram, blood work, lumbar puncture, and potentially genetic testing [53]. We recommend early involvement of a pediatric neurologist in these cases.

Ventriculoperitoneal Shunts

Drainage of cerebrospinal fluid using a ventriculoperitoneal (VP) shunt may be indicated in pediatric patients with hydrocephalus (either from trauma or congenital causes). The critical care physician should be aware of complications that may arise in patients with VP shunts including mechanical failure, infection, and functional failure [54]. Concern for VP shunt complications should prompt a neurosurgical evaluation for proper shunt positioning and function as well as infectious work-up. It is not uncommon for a trauma patient with severe TBI to require a VP shunt and a gastrostomy tube. Data are limited to small retrospective studies, and outcomes are controversial with shunt infection rates reported to be 2–23% [55–57]. Our practice is to place the gastrostomy at least 48 h prior to VP shunt placement with 24 h of post-gastrostomy cefazolin plus vancomycin whenever possible though a recent study of the inpatient KIDS database submitted by our research group suggests that simultaneous placement may be safe.

Cardiovascular

End Points of Resuscitation

A detailed guide for pediatric end points of resuscitation was published by the Surviving Sepsis Campaign and by the American College of Critical Care Medicine and is summarized in Table 57.4 [58, 59]. Fluid resuscitation begins with isotonic crystalloids with boluses of up to 20 mL/kg over 5–10 min and should be titrated to heart rate, blood pressure, urine output, capillary refill, and peripheral pulses. Albumin can be used in bolus aliquots of 5–10 cc/kg but should not be used in patients with TBI [60]. If a patient is showing signs of hepatomegaly, pulmonary edema, or refractory shock, inotropic support should be initiated [58]. Dopamine, dobutamine, or epinephrine can be used in children, with dopamine being preferred as a first-line agent in infants and children [59, 61]. Patients who are normotensive with low cardiac output and elevated systemic vascular resistance may require inodilators such as milrinone for additional cardiac output support [58, 61]. Though central venous pressures may be useful in guiding resuscitation, pulmonary artery (Swan-Ganz) catheters are only rarely used in infants or children with complex cardiac anomalies and are in general placed in the cardiac catheterization lab when required [11].

Table 57.4 End points of resuscitation (Dellinger Surviving Sepsis Campaign)

Surviving sepsis end points of resuscitation
Capillary refill <2 s
Normal blood pressure for age
Normal pulses with no differential between peripheral and central pulses
Warm extremities
Urine output >1 mL/kg/hr
Normal mental status
$ScvO_2$ saturation ≥ 70%
Cardiac index 3.3–6 L/min/m²

Common Arrhythmias in Children

Dysrhythmias are relatively common in children without underlying cardiac disease admitted to the PICU. The most common dysrhythmias in this group include junctional rhythm, premature atrial contractions, and premature ventricular contractions followed by low atrial rhythm, sinus pause, supraventricular tachycardia, ventricular tachycardia, and other AV block. Bradycardia, particularly in neonates, may be ominous and can be followed by asystole. Risk factors for cardiac rhythm disturbances in the ICU include hypoxemia, hypercarbia, sepsis, inflammation, inotropes, prolonged mechanical ventilation, and central venous access [62]. For the management of pediatric arrhythmias, the Pediatric Cardiac Intensive Care Society consensus statement highlighting arrhythmias in pediatric critical care patients and relevant pharmacotherapy can be referenced [63]. We generally involve a pediatric cardiologist with particular expertise in electrophysiology in the management of these patients.

Complex Congenital Heart Disease

Long-term survival of patients with complex congenital cardiac lesions is improving rapidly, with 15-year survival of 70% among patients undergoing successful Norwood procedure for hypoplastic left heart syndrome and proceeding to the final stage or Fontan procedure [64]. Recognition of a child with single-ventricle physiology is of paramount importance as these patients should be transferred to centers with expertise in complex cardiac management. Patients with single-ventricle physiology are exceedingly sensitive to changes in pulmonary vascular resistance and in filling pressures as their pulmonary blood flow is in parallel after the first-stage Norwood and is entirely passive after the final Fontan procedure. Children with congenital heart disease are generally classified as cyanotic (with impaired pulmonary circulation and central right to left shunt) or overcirculating (with left to right shunt). Management of children with these lesions requires special expertise, and early engagement of a cardiologist with specific expertise in management of single-ventricle patients is warranted.

Heart Failure Following Chemotherapy and Radiation

It is important for critical care physicians to obtain a thorough history on pediatric patients who have a history of cancer treated with chemotherapy and/or radiation. Chemotherapeutic agents such as anthracyclines (doxorubicin/Adriamycin™) as well as thoracic radiation can lead to subclinical cardiomyopathies at varying intervals following treatment with increasing prevalence up to 20 years after exposure [65–73]. Other agents may affect pulmonary function (bleomycin), renal function (cis-platinum, carboplatinum), bone marrow (antimetabolites), and other organ systems. Children with a history of relevant exposures should be expeditiously evaluated with echocardiography, chest radiography, and laboratory assessments to determine the quality of cardiac and other major organ functions on ICU admission and should undergo careful monitoring during critical illness or prior to undergoing general anesthesia [74, 75].

Extracorporeal Life Support in Infants and Children

Often referred to as extracorporeal membrane oxygenation (ECMO), extracorporeal life support (ECLS) provides for respiratory or full cardiopulmonary bypass in patients with reversible cardiac or respiratory failure who do not respond to conventional methods [76]. ECLS and the components of the circuit are discussed in detail in Chap. 67, and here we will focus on issues specific to infants and children.

Indications for ECLS in pediatrics can be broadly divided into endogenous causes (congenital diaphragmatic hernia and persistent pulmonary hypertension of the newborn) or acquired causes (sepsis, pneumonia, or meconium aspiration). The 2016 international report from the Extracorporeal Life Support Organization Registry provides an overview of most common ECLS indications outlined in Table 57.5 [77]. ECLS can be either venoarterial (VA) or venovenous (VV). VA ECLS is the most commonly used mode in neonates and children [76]. In infants, ECLS cannulation is usually performed using the jugular vein for VV and the jugular vein and carotid artery for VA access. The SICU provider should be aware that in patients with prior right-neck access for VA or VV ECMO, the vessels were likely ligated at the time of cannula removal and right IJ access for central venous catheterization is likely no longer possible. The internal jugular and femoral veins can be used in children over the age of 3; however, the femoral vein is not large enough to accept a double-lumen cannula for VV ECLS or to be the primary drainage site for VA ECLS in children less than 5 years old [78, 79]. The femoral artery or axillary artery can be used for arterial access in children over the age of 5, although an antegrade perfusion cannula may be needed in children to prevent limb ischemia [76].

Table 57.5 Common indications for infant and pediatric ECLS

Infants	Children
Respiratory Meconium aspiration syndrome Persistent pulmonary hypertension of the newborn Congenital diaphragmatic hernia Respiratory distress syndrome of the newborn Sepsis	Respiratory Infection Pneumonia Acute respiratory failure
Cardiac Congenital heart disease Cardiomyopathy Myocarditis	Cardiac Congenital cardiac defect Cardiomyopathy Myocarditis

Outcomes of ECLS in infants and children vary by age and indication with reports of 70% of patients successfully weaned off ECLS and 58% surviving to hospital discharge. The highest survival rate was found in patients who underwent ECLS for respiratory indications. The most common complications of ECLS include hemorrhage, cerebral or visceral infarction from thromboembolism, mechanical failure or malfunction, renal failure, infection, and hyperbilirubinemia [77]. Intraventricular hemorrhage (IVH) is of particular concern in premature infants on ECLS due to an immature germinal matrix. IVH can occur in up to 13% of neonates on ECLS, and routine cranial ultrasound is often performed prior to cannulation and daily throughout the ECLS run [76].

Pulmonary

Management of respiratory failure in infants and children requires the consideration of two major differences in physiology (pulmonary vascular response to sepsis) and anatomy (circuit dead space relative to tidal volume).

Pulmonary Hypertension

Pulmonary hypertension (PH) is an important cause of hypoxemia in critically ill infants and children and can lead to significant morbidity and mortality. It is generally defined as a mean pulmonary artery pressure greater than or equal to 25 mmHg at rest or greater than 30% of mean systemic arterial pressure (usually estimated in children with echocardiography using the tricuspid regurgitation velocity to estimate RV pressure gradient). PH affects approximately 64 cases per 1 million children and can be transient or persistent with the course and prognosis determined by underlying cause. The most common causes are sepsis, persistent pulmonary hypertension of the newborn, congenital heart disease, and idiopathic PH [80]. Patients with a history of congenital diaphragmatic hernia (CDH) repair or a history of chronic lung disease of prematurity (sometimes referred to as bronchopulmonary dysplasia or BPD) have increased pulmonary vascular reactivity and are at risk of pulmonary hypertensive exacerbation well into their childhood years, and a high index of suspicion for PH as a cause of hypoxemia is needed. Pediatric patients with a history of pulmonary hypertension, congenital diaphragmatic hernia repair, or chronic lung disease of prematurity should have an echocardiogram prior to scheduling of anesthesia, though this may significantly underestimate pulmonary pressures in high-risk groups such as diaphragmatic hernia. If there is evidence of elevated RV pressures, an anesthesiologist with expertise in management of these patients should be involved in the anesthetic management of these patients [81].

Pediatric Mechanical Ventilation

Conventional forms of mechanical ventilation are used commonly in infants and children, but attention must be paid to tidal volumes and pressures being delivered. Pediatric ventilators should be used in infants and children due to the narrow therapeutic window for tidal volume delivery. The ventilator circuit and tubing represents a large dead space relative to the actual tidal volume of the child's lungs. For this reason, many pediatric and neonatal intensive care units utilize pressure control ventilation as the pressure is easier to regulate than volume in these small children. If volume control ventilation is going to be utilized, a flow sensor placed on the endotracheal tube can be utilized to more precisely measure tidal volumes (Fig. 57.3). Pressure-regulated volume control (PRVC) is a hybrid of pressure and volume control and is commonly used in stable pediatric patients, particularly as they approach liberation from mechanical ventilation [82]. Pressure-regulated ventilator modes are generally preferred in order to adjust for rapid and significant changes in pulmonary and thoracic compliance that attend many pediatric disorders.

Non-conventional ventilation such as high-frequency oscillatory ventilation (HFOV), high-frequency jet ventilation (HFJV), or high-frequency percussive ventilation is used when conventional modes are not able to adequately oxygenate or ventilate pediatric patients [83]. While we present an overview of these modalities in this section, specific expertise and familiarity is needed to effectively manage children with refractory respiratory failure using these modalities, and consultation with a pediatric surgical intensivist should be obtained in these scenarios. HFOV is thought to decrease barotrauma and maximize lung recruitment in noncompliant lungs by delivering a constant mean airway pressure while ventilating with small "subtidal" volumes instead of conventional peak inspiratory pressure [84]. This strategy maintains constant alveolar recruitment and minimizes the "opening pressure" that is required to open alveoli with conventional ventilation. Mean airway pressure and FiO_2 can be titrated to maintain oxygenation, while amplitude and frequency of oscillation can be adjusted to achieve optimal CO_2 clearance. A common pitfall when using HFOV is continuing to increase the mean airway pressure in response to hypoxemia, which in a hypovolemic patient can lead to impaired pulmonary blood flow and worsening hypoxemia. Disconnecting the patient from the ventilator circuit and handbag ventilating to ascertain the optimal mean airway pressure (sometimes lower than previously set) is often required in this scenario. HFJV delivers high-frequency low-volume pulses of gas in combination with positive end-expiratory pressure to allow for active inspiration and passive expiration [85]. High-frequency percussive ventilation has been used with good outcomes in burned children with inhalational injury [86, 87].

The general practice of pediatric intensive care unit practitioners related to tracheostomy placement is divergent to their adult counterparts. This is due to two factors in children: 1) the incidence of subglottic stenosis with prolonged intubation is lower in children compared to adults [88–90], and 2) tracheostomy-related mortality is substantially higher

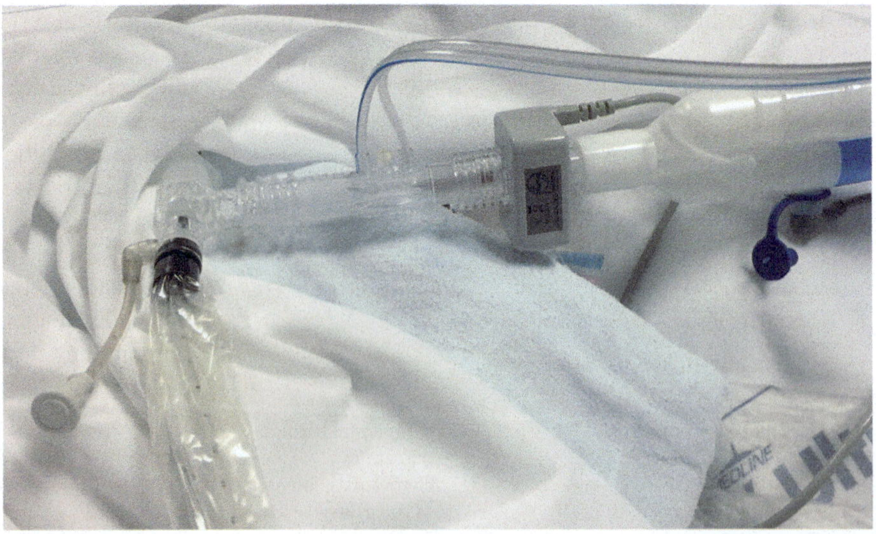

Fig. 57.3 A proximal inline flow sensor can be placed between the ventilator tubing and endotracheal tube in small children to more precisely measure tidal volumes without the large residual dead space of the ventilator circuit

in children, especially children less than 1 year of age, so the potential benefit of early tracheostomy in children may not outweigh the risks associated with it. [91–95]

Gastrointestinal

Nutrition

Children have an increased baseline metabolic rate up to fourfold that of adults in newborn infants, require substrate for ongoing growth and development, and have decreased body fat, carbohydrate, and protein stores. These three factors place an increased importance on attention to nutritional factors in critically ill pediatric patients. The prevalence of malnutrition in critically ill children is quite high (up to 47%) and is associated with longer ICU stay, prolonged mechanical ventilation, and higher mortality [96]. Infants in particular may have decreased enteral intake and have the highest metabolic demands, placing them at risk for hazards of malnutrition such as slow growth, delayed mental and psychomotor development, and bone demineralization [96, 97]. Measurement of serum albumin, transferrin, prealbumin, and retinol-binding protein (Table 57.6) or nutritional assessment scores may aid in the assessment of a patient's nutritional status, but the clinical outcomes associated with these markers are not well validated in children [94].

Enteral nutritional support is preferred for critically ill patients that will tolerate oral or enteric feeds. Infant formulas should be used in children less than 1 year of age as the caloric content (0.67 kcal/mL for breast milk or non-fortified infant formula) and osmotic load are less than found in pediatric or adult formulas. Many pediatric formulas are available for oral or tube feeding, and most formulas are similar to adult formula in caloric content (1.0–1.5 kcal/ml). Parenteral nutrition (PN) is heavily utilized in neonates and judiciously utilized in older children that cannot tolerate enteral nutrition. Evidence to guide timing of initiation PN in neonates is limited to expert opinion and nitrogen balance studies, but current practice is that PN should be initiated early due to their increased energy requirements and development of negative nitrogen balance [97]. For older children (age 1–17 years), the evidence is similar to that found in adult patients and supports withholding parenteral nutrition for 1 week due to decreased rates of infection, decreased ICU stay, and shorter duration of mechanical ventilation compared to early initiation [98]. Pediatric patients have higher fluid and caloric requirements than adults, and as such, PN can generally be started at a higher initial rate (25–30 kcal/kg/day in young children) and can be advanced to goal nutrition over 2–3 days. Caloric intake in infants should be 80–110 kcal/kg/day, while intake in adults should be 35 kcal/kg/day [97]. Daily energy requirements are variable by age and are summarized in Table 57.7 [99].

Table 57.6 Serum markers of nutrition

Serum protein	Half-life	Normal range
Albumin	18 days	3.5–5.5 g/dL
Transferrin	8 days	170–370 mg/dL
Prealbumin	3 days	<5 days old, 6–21 mg/dL 1–5 years old, 14–30 mg/dL 6–9 years old, 15–33 mg/dL 10–19 years old, 22–45 mg/dL
Retinol-binding protein	12 h	40–60ug/mL

Table 57.7 Pediatric energy requirements (From Coran Table 12–1)

	Daily energy requirements (total kcal/kg)
Preterm neonate	90–120
<6 months	85–105
6–12 months	80–100
1–7 years	75–90
7–12 years	50–75
>12–18 years	30–50

Stress Ulcer Prophylaxis

There is limited data on the use of gastrointestinal prophylaxis in critically ill infants and children. Early initiation of enteral nutrition is preferred, but when this is not possible, children in the PICU are generally treated with the same indications for ulcer prophylaxis as adults as pediatric-specific data is lacking. Ranitidine is the most commonly used drug for prophylaxis in the PICU, with mechanical ventilation, sepsis, coagulopathy, corticosteroid therapy, high-risk injuries such as TBI and burns, PRISM score > 10, inotrope use, and informal routine use as reported indications [100–105]. Infants in the NICU generally do not receive gastrointestinal prophylaxis even in the context of prolonged mechanical ventilation or prolonged NPO status, as acid suppression in this population can lead to increased rates of infection, necrotizing enterocolitis, and death [106, 107].

Bilious Emesis

Bilious vomiting in an infant or child warrants special consideration as it usually constitutes a surgical emergency, and delay in management can result in intestinal ischemia and loss. Urgent pediatric surgical consultation should be obtained in any child with bilious emesis. In the neonatal period, these patients should be evaluated for intestinal obstruction potentially caused by intestinal atresia or Hirschsprung's disease; but more notably, malrotation and midgut volvulus can occur in any age. A recent study evaluating neonates transferred to a neonatal surgical center with bilious vomiting in the first week of life found that 46% of patients had a surgical diagnosis and 14% required an urgent operation [108]. The most common diagnoses in these patients were malrotation, volvulus, and intestinal perforation. Outside of the neonatal period, one must consider intussusception (typical age 6 months–3 years), internal hernia, and congenital bands, as well as postsurgical problems such as adhesive bowel obstruction, foreign bodies, and occult injury.

Renal

Pediatric Renal Replacement Therapy

The most common indications for chronic renal replacement therapy (RRT) in infants are obstructive uropathy, autosomal recessive polycystic kidney disease, cortical necrosis, and hypoplastic or dysplastic kidneys, while indications in young children also include congenital nephrotic syndrome, hemolytic uremic syndrome, and renal infarction [109, 110]. In infants and children with kidney failure, peritoneal dialysis (PD) is the modality of choice for renal replacement therapy and is used in over 90% of children under the age of 2 requiring long-term dialysis [110, 111]. Compared with hemodialysis (HD), PD does not require accessing small blood vessels, preserves blood vessels for HD later in life, can be performed in a wide range of patient ages, can be performed at home, and leads to improved growth and residual renal function [110–113].

Renal replacement therapy is also used therapeutically in pediatric critical care for the correction of electrolyte disturbances and the removal of fluid, urea, toxins, and inflammatory mediators. Continuous renal replacement therapy (CRRT) is preferred over PD in most cases for treating pediatric acute kidney injury (AKI) [114]. CRRT can be used in the setting of acute renal failure associated with cardiac surgery, sepsis, burns, acute tubular necrosis, hematologic-oncologic complications, inborn errors of metabolism, hyperthermia, hepatic dysfunction, bone marrow transplantation, and respiratory failure [115]. A prospective pediatric CRRT registry group reported that overall survival with CRRT was 58%. Although infant survival was worse than pediatric patients with AKI, they found that CRRT was feasible even in the smallest patients [114]. The large circulating volume of the CRRT circuit can make initiation a challenge in neonates and infants as the volume of the circuit can exceed the blood volume of the baby. In the youngest children, our preference is to proceed with acute peritoneal dialysis as first-line therapy whenever possible for infants under 1 year of age.

Intravenous Fluids

Intravenous fluids for infants and children are based on patient age and weight. Daily fluid requirements for pediatric patients are outlined in Table 57.8. It is important to note that infants are born with a fluid reserve and are expected to lose 10–15% of their body weight in the first week of life [97]. Aggressively replacing these normal fluid and sodium losses can predispose to fluid overload, persistent ductus arteriosus, cardiac failure, necrotizing enterocolitis, and bronchopulmonary dysplasia. Infants also have limited ability to concentrate urine due to immature proximal tubules, poor interstitial reabsorptive capacity, and immature sodium transporters [2]. For this reason, $D_{10}W$ is used for maintenance fluids at birth in euvolemic patients not in shock and changed to $D_{10}W$ 0.2% normal saline with 20 meq KCl/L on day of life 2. This concept is often misunderstood by practitioners that rarely care for neonates. If a neonate is in shock, the baby will require isotonic volume expansion with normal saline, followed by sodium-containing fluids (usually D_5- or D_{10}–1/2 normal saline) with close monitoring of sodium levels. Urine output and serum electrolytes should guide ongoing fluid management and to avoid hyponatremia. After 3–4 weeks of life, D_5W 0.45 normal saline with 20 meq KCl/L can be used as maintenance intravenous fluids. If albumin is utilized in young babies, particular attention must be paid to sodium levels as the sodium concentration in standard albumin can be quite high (130–160 mEq/dL).

Hematology

Blood Transfusion

Clear evidenced-based guidelines for term infants and older children (age range 3 days–14 years) are similar to adults, with a 7 g/dL transfusion threshold in stable euvolemic patients associated with decreased transfusion requirements without altering adverse outcomes for critically ill children [116]. Guidelines for a transfusion threshold in premature neonates are lacking, however, leaving clinical judgment and patient hemodynamic status and key factors in the decision-making process. Premature neonates are commonly transfused in the presence of apnea or inability to wean from a

Table 57.8 Daily fluid requirements for pediatric patients (Coran Table 12–2)

Body weight	Volume per day
<1500 g	130–150 mL/kg
1500–2000 g	110–130 mL/kg
2–10 kg	100 mL/kg
>10–20 kg	1000 mL for first 10 kg + 50 mL/kg for each kg >10
>20 kg	1500 mL for first 20 kg + 20 mL/kg for each kg >20

ventilator [117]. The estimated circulating blood volume is 90 ml/kg in a newborn and in 80 ml/kg in a child, reaching adult levels of 70 ml/kg by late childhood [117]. Neonates are commonly transfused due to anemia of prematurity or blood loss from multiple lab draws [117]. As with all dosing in children, transfusion is also weight-based, rather than giving "units" of blood products. A general rule of thumb is that a 5 cc/kg transfusion of RBCs in a child is the equivalent of one "unit" in an adult (and, as such, would be expected to raise the hemoglobin 1 g/dL or hematocrit by 3%). Table 57.9 shows the recommended transfusion aliquot volumes for packed red blood cells, platelets, fresh frozen plasma, and cryoprecipitate in children [117]. If a small child is being transfused and is expected to potentially require further transfusion, the blood bank can set aside the whole adult unit of product the transfusion aliquot was taken from to use for future transfusion aliquots in that child to limit antigen exposure in each child [118].

Thromboembolic Disease

Venous thromboembolic (VTE) disease is being reported at an increasing frequency in infants and children with an estimated incidence of 0.07 per 10,000 children and 58 per 10,000 pediatric admissions [119, 120]. High-risk groups for deep venous thrombosis (DVT)/pulmonary embolism (PE) include those with central venous access, with malignancy, and with recent trauma, undergoing solid organ transplantation, or who are obese [121–124]. Recent studies have sought to properly diagnose and treat those affected, but quality evidence around prophylaxis and management of VTE in the pediatric population is still lacking. The American College of Chest Physicians published evidenced-based guidelines for the treatment and prevention of thromboembolism in neonates and children, but these guidelines are unfortunately primarily grade 2C recommendations [125]. These recommendations include the involvement of pediatric hematologists in anticoagulant management and the use of unfractionated heparin titrated to anti-Xa and activated partial thromboplastin time. Our practice for trauma patients with catheter-associated DVT is to remove the catheter and repeat the duplex ultrasound in 1 week and only anticoagulate those patients with clot propagation after the line has been removed. Post-thrombotic syndrome can occur in approximately 15% of patients and does not seem to be impacted by anticoagulation [124]. Evidence to guide practice in catheter-associated DVT (especially for very young children) is desperately needed. VTE prophylaxis in pediatric trauma patients is generally reserved for postpubescent children.

Table 57.9 Pediatric transfusion volume and indications

Product	Volume	Indication/expected response
Packed red blood cells	10 ml/kg	Blood loss, increase hematocrit 6%
Platelets	1 unit/10 kg	Raise platelets by 25,000
Fresh frozen plasma	10 ml/kg	Coagulopathy
Cryoprecipitate	1 unit/5 kg	Replace fibrinogen

Disorders of Coagulation

An overview of the coagulation cascade and all disorders of coagulation is beyond the scope of this chapter, but a surgical intensivist caring for children must have a heightened awareness of this possibility. While most disorders of coagulation have been diagnosed prior to adulthood, pediatric patient may have a yet undiagnosed coagulopathy. Even though unexplained intracranial hemorrhage may be related to abuse, a thorough work-up for coagulation disorders is warranted. Pathologic bleeding may be differentiated from non-pathologic bleeding by age at first episode, frequency and duration of bleeding, history of recurrent spontaneous or procedure-related bleeding, and family history of bleeding disorders [126].

Infectious Disease

Sepsis

Sepsis was recently redefined as life-threatening organ dysfunction caused by a dysregulated host response to infection [127]. The diagnosis depends on age-adjusted vital signs and laboratory markers, with the overall mortality of pediatric sepsis lower than in adults. The Surviving Sepsis Campaign International Guidelines have considerations specifically for children, including age-adjusted initial end points of resuscitation (vital signs and urine output), a hemoglobin target of 10 g/dL if central venous oxygen saturation is low, closely monitoring for drug toxicity, and using a continuous glucose infusion during insulin therapy (Table 57.4) [58]. The classic vasodilatory response seen in adult septic shock is often not seen in children, with vasoconstrictive "cold shock" associated with low cardiac output and elevated systemic vascular resistance more commonly seen. These children may require inodilators (milrinone) in addition to inotropic therapy [58].

Sepsis in neonates is specifically divided into early-onset sepsis (EOS) and late-onset sepsis (LOS). Early-onset sepsis occurs within 72 h of delivery and is thought to be due to infection during gestation or delivery. Risk factors for EOS include chorioamnionitis, prolonged rupture of membranes, premature rupture of membranes, prematurity, and maternal group B strep colonization [128]. Late-onset sepsis occurs between 72 h and 28 days of life, is more common than EOS, and is thought to be due to nosocomial or community pathogens. Risk factors include low birth weight, newborn jaundice, intraventricular hemorrhage, prematurity, indwelling catheters, and invasive procedures [129].

Fever Work-Up

One of the most common signs of illness in infants and children is fever, though hypothermia may be the first manifestation of sepsis. Patients in the first 4 weeks of life require special consideration due to the incomplete development of the meninges and increased susceptibility to CNS infection. It is recommended that fever in any child younger than 29 days of age or any child with a toxic appearance undergo a full sepsis work-up of blood, urine, and cerebrospinal fluid [130, 131]. Positive blood cultures in a neonate mandate a lumbar puncture. Empiric antibiotic treatment with meningitic dosing using a drug that penetrates the CNS (such as a third-generation cephalosporin) should be started in any child suspected of having a possible CNS infection. Infants 29 days to 3 months with a normal complete blood cell count with differential and a normal urinalysis can be re-evaluated in 24 h with either ceftriaxone or no antibiotics, and nontoxic infants 3–36 months old with a fever lower than 39 °C can be observed with close follow-up alone [130].

Special Considerations

Pediatric Trauma and Non-accidental Trauma

Trauma is the leading cause of morbidity and mortality in infants and children [132]. System-specific trauma considerations in children are discussed above. While a full review of the management of pediatric trauma is beyond the scope of this chapter, the Pediatric Advanced Life Support Provider Manual and the Advanced Trauma Life Support Manual are references for the full initial evaluation of pediatric trauma patients [16, 133].

We would like to highlight in this chapter the importance of considering non-accidental trauma (NAT) for children admitted to the trauma ICU – particularly young nonverbal children and children with complex medical needs. A review of the KIDS database found that 25% of infants with abdominal trauma had been abused and that morbidity and mortality were higher in the NAT population than in the accidental trauma population [134, 135]. Some presenting signs that should be concerning for NAT include bruises that are not over bony prominences, scald or thermal burns, spiral or oblique long-bone fractures, spine fractures, posterior rib fractures, retinal hemorrhages, and skull fractures. Evaluation of patients with suspected NAT should include a full history and physical examination, social work evaluation, coagulation studies, a skeletal survey, intracranial imaging, and an ophthalmologic examination in addition to any warranted injury-specific trauma work-up [136]. Engagement of a child abuse specialist or referral to a center with this expertise is warranted if there is a suspicion of NAT.

Parental Involvement in the Care of Infants and Children

A special consideration in the care of critically ill infants and children is attention to the needs of parents and caretakers. Parents play an essential role in a child's healthcare as they are generally the child's best resource for support, coping with stress, recovery, and follow-up care [137]. However, a child's injury or illness can be a significant stressor for parents who can experience symptoms of acute stress disorder or post-traumatic stress disorder during or after a child's admission to the intensive care unit [138, 139]. Empathetic communication and multidisciplinary care involving social work and child life can reduce anxiety in the ICU setting [137]. The Guidelines for Family-Centered Care in the Neonatal, Pediatric, and Adult ICU can be used for more detailed recommendations [140]. The impact of a child's ICU admission on a parent should not be underestimated nor the impact of a parent functioning as an ally to the physician on the child's treatment plan.

Conclusion

The critical care management of severely injured children or children with primary surgical disorders follows many of the same principles as adult surgical critical care. There are many pediatric-specific nuances, however, that impact treatment decisions in critically ill children. The adult surgical intensivist should maintain a working relationship with a colleague with expertise in caring for critically ill infants and children in order to provide optimal care for this cohort of patients. This chapter aimed to provide an overview of particular pediatric-specific issues and the importance of maintaining expertise in these realms if one intends to care for pediatric patients in the ICU.

References

1. Silverman AM, Wang VJ. Shock: a common pathway for life-threatening pediatric illnesses and injuries. Pediatr Emerg Med Pract. 2005;2:1–22.
2. Quareshi F, Blanco FC. Renal physiology, acute renal failure and renal replacement therapy in children. Handbook of pediatric surgical critical care. Arca MJ, editor. 1st ed. 2013. https://www.eapsa.org/apsa/media/Documents/APSAHandbookofSurgicalCriticalCare_Jun52014.pdf.
3. Association AH. Pediatric advanced life support (PALS) digital reference card. 2016. https://www.acls.net/pals-algorithms.htm.
4. Sunder RA, Haile DT, Farrell PT, Sharma A. Pediatric airway management: current practices and future directions. Paediatr Anaesth. 2012;22:1008–15.
5. Arca MJ. The pediatric airway. Handbook of pediatric surgical critical care. Arca M, editor. 1st ed. 2013. https://www.eapsa.org/apsa/media/Documents/APSAHandbookofSurgicalCriticalCare_Jun52014.pdf.
6. Fiadjoe J, Stricker P. Pediatric difficult airway management: current devices and techniques. Anesthesiol Clin. 2009;27:185–95.
7. Lau N, Playfor SD, Rashid A, Dhanarass M. New formulae for predicting tracheal tube length. Paediatr Anaesth. 2006;16:1238–43.
8. Group ALS. Advanced paediatric life support:the practical approach. 5th ed. London: BMJ Books; 2011.
9. Sims C, Ungern-Sternberg v. BS: the normal and the challenging pediatric airway. Paediatr Anaesth. 2012;22:521–6.
10. Arshad A, McCarthy MJ. Management of limb ischaemia in the neonate and infant. Eur J Vasc Endovasc Surg. 2009;38:61–5.
11. Jensen A, Bliss D. Monitoring in the ICU. Handbook of pediatric surgical critical care. Arca MJ, editor. 1st ed. 2013. https://www.eapsa.org/apsa/media/Documents/APSAHandbookofSurgicalCriticalCare_Jun52014.pdf.
12. Kim JH, Lee YS, Kim SH, Lee SK, Lim MK, Kim HS. Does umbilical vein catheterization lead to portal venous thrombosis? Prospective US evaluation in 100 neonates. Radiology. 2001;219:645–50.
13. Coleman MM, Spear ML, Finkelstein M, Leef KH, Pearlman SA, Chien C, Taylor SM, McKenzie SE. Short-term use of umbilical artery catheters may not be associated with increased risk for thrombosis. Pediatrics. 2004;113:770–4.
14. Veldman A, Nold MF, Michel-Behnke I. Thrombosis in the critically ill neonate: incidence, diagnosis, and management. Vasc Health Risk Manag. 2008;4:1337–48.
15. Nowak-Göttl U, von Kries R, Göbel U. Neonatal symptomatic thromboembolism in Germany: two year survey. Arch Dis Child Fetal Neonatal Ed. 1997;76:F163–7.
16. Surgeons ACo. ATLS student course manual: advanced trauma life support. 9th ed. American College of Surgeons; 2012. Chicago, IL
17. Bright futures: guidelines for health supervision of infants, children, and adolescents. 3rd ed. Elk Grove: The American Academy of Pediatrics, 2008.
18. Harris J, Ramelet AS, van Dijk M, Pokorna P, Wielenga J, Tume L, Tibboel D, Ista E. Clinical recommendations for pain, sedation, withdrawal and delirium assessment in critically ill infants and children: an ESPNIC position statement for healthcare professionals. Intensive Care Med. 2016;42:972–86.
19. Franck LS, Harris SK, Soetenga DJ, Amling JK, Curley MA. The withdrawal assessment tool-1 (WAT-1): an assessment instrument for monitoring opioid and benzodiazepine withdrawal symptoms in pediatric patients. Pediatr Crit Care Med. 2008;9:573–80.
20. Merkel SI, Voepel-Lewis T, Shayevitz JR, Malviya S. The FLACC: a behavioral scale for scoring postoperative pain in young children. Pediatr Nurs. 1997;23:293–7.
21. Ista E, van Dijk M, Tibboel D, de Hoog M. Assessment of sedation levels in pediatric intensive care patients can be improved by using the COMFORT "behavior" scale. Pediatr Crit Care Med. 2005;6:58–63.
22. van Dijk M, Peters JW, van Deventer P, Tibboel D. The COMFORT behavior scale: a tool for assessing pain and sedation in infants. Am J Nurs. 2005;105:33–6.
23. Silver G, Traube C, Kearney J, Kelly D, Yoon MJ, Nash Moyal W, Gangopadhyay M, Shao H, Ward MJ. Detecting pediatric delirium: development of a rapid observational assessment tool. Intensive Care Med. 2012;38:1025–31.
24. Smith HA, Fuchs DC, Pandharipande PP, Barr FE, Ely EW. Delirium: an emerging frontier in the management of critically ill children. Anesthesiol Clin. 2011;29:729–50.
25. Alievi PT, Carvalho PR, Trotta EA, Mombelli Filho R. The impact of admission to a pediatric intensive care unit assessed by means of global and cognitive performance scales. J Pediatr. 2007;83:505–11.
26. Fiser DH, Long N, Roberson PK, Hefley G, Zolten K, Brodie-Fowler M. Relationship of pediatric overall performance category and pediatric cerebral performance category scores at pediatric intensive care unit discharge with outcome measures collected at hospital discharge and 1- and 6-month follow-up assessments. Crit Care Med. 2000;28:2616–20.
27. Horswell BB, Jaskolka MS. Pediatric head injuries. Oral Maxillofac Surg Clin North Am. 2012;24:337–50.
28. Tieves K. In: Holcomb III GW, Murphy JP, editors. Pediatric head trauma. Ashcraft's pediatric surgery. 5th ed. Philadelphia: Saunders Elsevier; 2010.
29. Easter JS, Bakes K, Dhaliwal J, Miller M, Caruso E, Haukoos JS. Comparison of PECARN, CATCH, and CHALICE rules for children with minor head injury: a prospective cohort study. Ann Emerg Med. 2014;64:145–52. 52.e1–5.
30. Kuppermann N, Holmes JF, Dayan PS, Hoyle JD, Atabaki SM, Holubkov R, Nadel FM, Monroe D, Stanley RM, Borgialli DA, Badawy MK, Schunk JE, Quayle KS, Mahajan P, Lichenstein R, Lillis KA, Tunik MG, Jacobs ES, Callahan JM, Gorelick MH, Glass TF, Lee LK, Bachman MC, Cooper A, Powell EC, Gerardi MJ, Melville KA, Muizelaar JP, Wisner DH, Zuspan SJ, Dean JM, Wootton-Gorges SL. (PECARN) PECARN: identification of children at very low risk of clinically-important brain injuries after head trauma: a prospective cohort study. Lancet. 2009;374:1160–70.
31. da Silva PS, Reis ME, Aguiar VE. Value of repeat cranial computed tomography in pediatric patients sustaining moderate to severe traumatic brain injury. J Trauma. 2008;65:1293–7.
32. Bata SC, Yung M. Role of routine repeat head imaging in paediatric traumatic brain injury. ANZ J Surg. 2014;84:438–41.
33. Howe J, Fitzpatrick CM, Lakam DR, Gleisner A, Vane DW. Routine repeat brain computed tomography in all children with mild traumatic brain injury may result in unnecessary radiation exposure. J Trauma Acute Care Surg. 2014;76:292–5. discussion 5-6.
34. Farach SM, Danielson PD, Amankwah EK, Chandler NM. Repeat computed tomography scans after pediatric trauma: results of an institutional effort to minimize radiation exposure. Pediatr Surg Int. 2015;31:1027–33.
35. Gasior A, Juang D. Pediatric neurotrauma. Handbook of pediatric surgical critical care. Arca MJ, editor. 1st ed. 2013. https://www.eapsa.org/apsa/media/Documents/APSAHandbookofSurgicalCriticalCare_Jun52014.pdf.
36. Addioui A, Saint-Vil D, Crevier L, Beaudin M. Management of skull fractures in children less than 1 year of age. J Pediatr Surg. 2016;51:1146–50.
37. Powell EC, Atabaki SM, Wootton-Gorges S, Wisner D, Mahajan P, Glass T, Miskin M, Stanley RM, Jacobs E, Dayan PS, Holmes JF, Kuppermann N. Isolated linear skull fractures in children with blunt head trauma. Pediatrics. 2015;135:e851–7.

38. Malhotra A, Wu X, Kalra VB, Goodman TR, Schindler J, Forman HP. Screening for pediatric blunt cerebrovascular injury: review of literature and a cost-effectiveness analysis. J Pediatr Surg. 2015;50:1751–7.
39. Kochanek PM, Carney N, Adelson PD, Ashwal S, Bell MJ, Bratton S, Carson S, Chesnut RM, Ghajar J, Goldstein B, Grant GA, Kissoon N, Peterson K, Selden NR, Tasker RC, Tong KA, Vavilala MS, Wainwright MS, Warden CR, Surgery AAoP-SoN, Surgeons AAoNSCoN, Society CN, Care ESoPaNI, Society NC, Group PNCR, Medicine SoCC, UK PICS, Care SfNiAaC, Societies WFoPIaCC. Guidelines for the acute medical management of severe traumatic brain injury in infants, children, and adolescents--second edition. Pediatr Crit Care Med. 2012;13(Suppl 1):S1–82.
40. Foundation BT. Guidelines for the management of severe traumatic brain injury. 4th ed. 2016. Neurosurg. 2017;80:6–15.
41. Chesnut RM, Temkin N, Carney N, Dikmen S, Rondina C, Videtta W, Petroni G, Lujan S, Pridgeon J, Barber J, Machamer J, Chaddock K, Celix JM, Cherner M, Hendrix T, Group GNR. A trial of intracranial-pressure monitoring in traumatic brain injury. N Engl J Med. 2012;367:2471–81.
42. Tanaka T, Litofsky NS. Anti-epileptic drugs in pediatric traumatic brain injury. Expert Rev Neurother. 2016;16:1229–34.
43. Liesemer K, Bratton SL, Zebrack CM, Brockmeyer D, Statler KD. Early post-traumatic seizures in moderate to severe pediatric traumatic brain injury: rates, risk factors, and clinical features. J Neurotrauma. 2011;28:755–62.
44. Young B, Rapp RP, Norton JA, Haack D, Walsh JW. Failure of prophylactically administered phenytoin to prevent post-traumatic seizures in children. Childs Brain. 1983;10:185–92.
45. Pearl PL, McCarter R, McGavin CL, Yu Y, Sandoval F, Trzcinski S, Atabaki SM, Tsuchida T, van den Anker J, He J, Klein P. Results of phase II levetiracetam trial following acute head injury in children at risk for posttraumatic epilepsy. Epilepsia. 2013;54:e135–7.
46. Lewis RJ, Yee L, Inkelis SH, Gilmore D. Clinical predictors of post-traumatic seizures in children with head trauma. Ann Emerg Med. 1993;22:1114–8.
47. Freeman JM. Febrile seizures: a consensus of their significance, evaluation, and treatment. Pediatrics. 1980;66:1009.
48. Gupta A. Febrile Seizures. Continuum (Minneap Minn). 2016;22:51–9.
49. Epstein LG, Shinnar S, Hesdorffer DC, Nordli DR, Hamidullah A, Benn EK, Pellock JM, Frank LM, Lewis DV, Moshe SL, Shinnar RC, Sun S, team Fs. Human herpesvirus 6 and 7 in febrile status epilepticus: the FEBSTAT study. Epilepsia. 2012;53:1481–8.
50. Steering Committee on Quality Improvement and Management SboFSAAoP. Febrile seizures: clinical practice guideline for the long-term management of the child with simple febrile seizures. Pediatrics. 2008;121:1281–6.
51. Seizures SoF, Pediatrics AAo. Neurodiagnostic evaluation of the child with a simple febrile seizure. Pediatrics. 2011;127:389–94.
52. Oluwabusi T, Sood SK. Update on the management of simple febrile seizures: emphasis on minimal intervention. Curr Opin Pediatr. 2012;24:259–65.
53. Freilich ER, Schreiber JM, Zelleke T, Gaillard WD. Pediatric status epilepticus: identification and evaluation. Curr Opin Pediatr. 2014;26:655–61.
54. Bober J, Rochlin J, Marneni S. Ventriculoperitoneal shunt complications in children: an evidence-based approach to emergency department management. Pediatr Emerg Med Pract. 2016;13:1–22. quiz –3.
55. Fraser JD, Aguayo P, Sharp SW, Holcomb IIIGW, Ostlie DJ, St Peter SD. The safety of laparoscopy in pediatric patients with ventriculoperitoneal shunts. J Laparoendosc Adv Surg Tech A. 2009;19:675–8.
56. Bui CJ, Tubbs RS, Pate G, Morgan T, Barnhart DC, Acakpo-Satchivi L, Wellons JC, Oakes WJ, Blount JP. Infections of pediatric cerebrospinal fluid shunts related to fundoplication and gastrostomy. J Neurosurg. 2007;107:365–7.
57. Gassas A, Kennedy J, Green G, Connolly B, Cohen J, Dag-Ellams U, Kulkarni A, Bouffet E. Risk of ventriculoperitoneal shunt infections due to gastrostomy feeding tube insertion in pediatric patients with brain tumors. Pediatr Neurosurg. 2006;42:95–9.
58. Dellinger RP, Levy MM, Rhodes A, Annane D, Gerlach H, Opal SM, Sevransky JE, Sprung CL, Douglas IS, Jaeschke R, Osborn TM, Nunnally ME, Townsend SR, Reinhart K, Kleinpell RM, Angus DC, Deutschman CS, Machado FR, Rubenfeld GD, Webb S, Beale RJ, Vincent JL, Moreno R, Subgroup SSCGCiTP. Surviving sepsis campaign: international guidelines for management of severe sepsis and septic shock, 2012. Intensive Care Med. 2013;39:165–228.
59. Brierley J, Carcillo JA, Choong K, Cornell T, Decaen A, Deymann A, Doctor A, Davis A, Duff J, Dugas MA, Duncan A, Evans B, Feldman J, Felmet K, Fisher G, Frankel L, Jeffries H, Greenwald B, Gutierrez J, Hall M, Han YY, Hanson J, Hazelzet J, Hernan L, Kiff J, Kissoon N, Kon A, Irazuzta J, Irazusta J, Lin J, Lorts A, Mariscalco M, Mehta R, Nadel S, Nguyen T, Nicholson C, Peters M, Okhuysen-Cawley R, Poulton T, Relves M, Rodriguez A, Rozenfeld R, Schnitzler E, Shanley T, Kache S, Skache S, Skippen P, Torres A, von Dessauer B, Weingarten J, Yeh T, Zaritsky A, Stojadinovic B, Zimmerman J, Zuckerberg A. Clinical practice parameters for hemodynamic support of pediatric and neonatal septic shock: 2007 update from the American College of Critical Care Medicine. Crit Care Med. 2009;37:666–88.
60. Myburgh J, Cooper DJ, Finfer S, Bellomo R, Norton R, Bishop N, Kai Lo S, Vallance S, Investigators SS, Group AaNZICSCT, Service ARCB, Health GIfI. Saline or albumin for fluid resuscitation in patients with traumatic brain injury. N Engl J Med. 2007;357:874–84.
61. Puligandla PS. Shock, low cardiac output, and inotropic support. Handbook of pediatric surgical critical care. Arca MJ, editor. 1st ed. 2013. https://www.eapsa.org/apsa/media/Documents/APSAHandbookofSurgicalCriticalCare_Jun52014.pdf.
62. Cassel-Choudhury GN, Aydin SI, Toedt-Pingel I, Ushay HM, Killinger JS, Cohen HW, Ceresnak SR. Arrhythmias in the paediatric intensive care unit: a prospective study of the rates and predictors of arrhythmias in children without underlying cardiac disease. Cardiol Young. 2015;25:1281–9.
63. Moffett BS, Salvin JW, Kim JJ. Pediatric cardiac intensive care society 2014 consensus statement: pharmacotherapies in cardiac critical care Antiarrhythmics. Pediatr Crit Care Med. 2016;17:S49–58.
64. Hansen JH, Petko C, Bauer G, Voges I, Kramer HH, Scheewe J. Fifteen-year single-center experience with the Norwood operation for complex lesions with single-ventricle physiology compared with hypoplastic left heart syndrome. J Thorac Cardiovasc Surg. 2012;144:166–72.
65. Green DM, Grigoriev YA, Nan B, Takashima JR, Norkool PA, D'Angio GJ, Breslow NE. Congestive heart failure after treatment for Wilms' tumor: a report from the National Wilms' Tumor Study group. J Clin Oncol. 2001;19:1926–34.
66. Huh WW, Jaffe N, Durand JB, Munsell MF, Herzog CE. Comparison of doxorubicin cardiotoxicity in pediatric sarcoma patients when given with dexrazoxane versus as continuous infusion. Pediatr Hematol Oncol. 2010;27:546–57.
67. Agarwala S, Kumar R, Bhatnagar V, Bajpai M, Gupta DK, Mitra DK. High incidence of adriamycin cardiotoxicity in children even at low cumulative doses: role of radionuclide cardiac angiography. J Pediatr Surg. 2000;35:1786–9.
68. Goldberg JM, Scully RE, Sallan SE, Lipshultz SE. Cardiac failure 30 years after treatment containing anthracycline for childhood acute lymphoblastic leukemia. J Pediatr Hematol Oncol. 2012;34:395–7.

69. Kremer LC, van Dalen EC, Offringa M, Voûte PA. Frequency and risk factors of anthracycline-induced clinical heart failure in children: a systematic review. Ann Oncol. 2002;13:503–12.
70. Goorin AM, Chauvenet AR, Perez-Atayde AR, Cruz J, McKone R, Lipshultz SE. Initial congestive heart failure, six to ten years after doxorubicin chemotherapy for childhood cancer. J Pediatr. 1990;116:144–7.
71. Henderson IC, Sloss LJ, Jaffe N, Blum RH, Frei E. Serial studies of cardiac function in patients receiving adriamycin. Cancer Treat Rep. 1978;62:923–9.
72. Medhora M, Gao F, Glisch C, Narayanan J, Sharma A, Harmann LM, Lawlor MW, Snyder LA, Fish BL, Down JD, Moulder JE, Strande JL, Jacobs ER. Whole-thorax irradiation induces hypoxic respiratory failure, pleural effusions and cardiac remodeling. J Radiat Res. 2015;56:248–60.
73. Chen C, Heusch A, Donner B, Janssen G, Göbel U, Schmidt KG. Present risk of anthracycline or radiation-induced cardiac sequelae following therapy of malignancies in children and adolescents. Klin Padiatr. 2009;221:162–6.
74. Burrows FA, Hickey PR, Colan S. Perioperative complications in patients with anthracycline chemotherapeutic agents. Can Anaesth Soc J. 1985;32:149–57.
75. Jonsson T, Mortensen SA, Aabo K. Acute cardiac failure precipitated by anesthesia and surgery in patients treated with adriamycin. Ugeskr Laeger. 1984;146:3837–9.
76. Gadepalli S, Ruzic A, Hirschl RB. Extracorporeal membrane oxygenation/extracorporeal lung support. Handbook of pediatric surgical critical care. Arca MJ, editor. 1st ed. 2013. https://www.eapsa.org/apsa/media/Documents/APSAHandbookofSurgicalCriticalCare_Jun52014.pdf.
77. Thiagarajan RR, Barbaro RP, Rycus PT, Mcmullan DM, Conrad SA, Fortenberry JD, Paden ML, centers Em. Extracorporeal life support organization registry international report 2016. ASAIO J. 2017;63:60–7.
78. Wenger RK, Bavaria JE, Ratcliffe MB, Bogen D, Edmunds LH. Flow dynamics of peripheral venous catheters during extracorporeal membrane oxygenation with a centrifugal pump. J Thorac Cardiovasc Surg. 1988;96:478–84.
79. Hirschl RB, Bartlett RB. In: Coran AG, editor. Extracorporeal life support for cardiopulmonary failure. Pediatric surgery. 7th ed. Philadelphia: Saunders; 2012.
80. Rajagopal H, Karnik R, Sahulee R. Pediatric pulmonary hypertension. Pediatr Rev. 2016;37:129–31.
81. Abman SH, Hansmann G, Archer SL, Ivy DD, Adatia I, Chung WK, Hanna BD, Rosenzweig EB, Raj JU, Cornfield D, Stenmark KR, Steinhorn R, Thébaud B, Fineman JR, Kuehne T, Feinstein JA, Friedberg MK, Earing M, Barst RJ, Keller RL, Kinsella JP, Mullen M, Deterding R, Kulik T, Mallory G, Humpl T, Wessel DL, American Heart Association Council on Cardiopulmonary ACC, Perioperative and Resuscitation, Cardiology CoC, Young CoCDit, Intervention CoCRa, Anesthesia CoCSa, Society atAT. Pediatric pulmonary hypertension: guidelines from the American Heart Association and American Thoracic Society. Circulation. 2015;132:2037–99.
82. Wakeham M, Arca MJ. Mechanical ventilation. Handbook of pediatric surgical critical care. Arca MJ, editor. 1st ed. 2013. https://www.eapsa.org/apsa/media/Documents/APSAHandbookofSurgicalCriticalCare_Jun52014.pdf.
83. Liedel J, Das U. Ventilation in the NICU. Handbook of pediatric surgical critical care. Arca MJ, editor. 1st ed. 2013. https://www.eapsa.org/apsa/media/Documents/APSAHandbookofSurgicalCriticalCare_Jun52014.pdf.
84. Greer SE, McCunn M. High-frequency oscillatory ventilation. Curr Probl Surg. 2013;50:471–8.
85. Ethawi YH, Abou Mehrem A, Minski J, Ruth CA, Davis PG. High frequency jet ventilation versus high frequency oscillatory ventilation for pulmonary dysfunction in preterm infants. Cochrane Database Syst Rev. 2016;CD010548.
86. Rowan CM, Cristea O, Greathouse ST, Coleman JJ, Nitu ME. Preemptive use of high-frequency oscillatory ventilation in pediatric burn patients. J Burn Care Res. 2013;34:237–42.
87. Cortiella J, Mlcak R, Herndon D. High frequency percussive ventilation in pediatric patients with inhalation injury. J Burn Care Rehabil. 1999;20:232–5.
88. Schweiger C, Marostica PJ, Smith MM, Manica D, Carvalho PR, Kuhl G. Incidence of post-intubation subglottic stenosis in children: prospective study. J Laryngol Otol. 2013;127:399–403.
89. Manica D, Schweiger C, Maróstica PJ, Kuhl G, Carvalho PR. Association between length of intubation and subglottic stenosis in children. Laryngoscope. 2013;123:1049–54.
90. Choi SS, Zalzal GH. Changing trends in neonatal subglottic stenosis. Otolaryngol Head Neck Surg. 2000;122:61–3.
91. Overman AE, Liu M, Kurachek SC, Shreve MR, Maynard RC, Mammel MC, Moore BM. Tracheostomy for infants requiring prolonged mechanical ventilation: 10 years' experience. Pediatrics. 2013;131:e1491–6.
92. Ogilvie LN, Kozak JK, Chiu S, Adderley RJ, Kozak FK. Changes in pediatric tracheostomy 1982-2011: a Canadian tertiary children's hospital review. J Pediatr Surg. 2014;49:1549–53.
93. Simma B, Spehler D, Burger R, Uehlinger J, Ghelfi D, Dangel P, Hof E, Fanconi S. Tracheostomy in children. Eur J Pediatr. 1994;153:291–6.
94. Fraga JC, Souza JC, Kruel J. Pediatric tracheostomy. J Pediatr. 2009;85:97–103.
95. Al-Samri M, Mitchell I, Drummond DS, Bjornson C. Tracheostomy in children: a population-based experience over 17 years. Pediatr Pulmonol. 2010;45:487–93.
96. Martinez EE, Mehta NM. The science and art of pediatric critical care nutrition. Curr Opin Crit Care. 2016;22:316–24.
97. Kenney B, Arca MJ. Fluid, electrolytes, and nutrition. Handbook of pediatric surgical critical care. Arca MJ, editor. 1st ed. 2013. https://www.eapsa.org/apsa/media/Documents/APSAHandbookofSurgicalCriticalCare_Jun52014.pdf.
98. Fivez T, Kerklaan D, Mesotten D, Verbruggen S, Wouters PJ, Vanhorebeek I, Debaveye Y, Vlasselaers D, Desmet L, Casaer MP, Garcia Guerra G, Hanot J, Joffe A, Tibboel D, Joosten K, Van den Berghe G. Early versus late parenteral nutrition in critically ill children. N Engl J Med. 2016;374:1111–22.
99. Teitelbaum DH, Btaiche IF, Coran AG. In: Coran A, Adzick NS, Krummel TM, Laberge JM, Caldamone A, Shamberger R, editors. Nutritional support in the pediatric surgical patient. Pediatric surgery. 7th ed. Philadelphia: Saunders; 2012.
100. Araujo TE, Vieira SM, Carvalho PR. Stress ulcer prophylaxis in pediatric intensive care units. J Pediatr. 2010;86:525–30.
101. Reveiz L, Guerrero-Lozano R, Camacho A, Yara L, Mosquera PA. Stress ulcer, gastritis, and gastrointestinal bleeding prophylaxis in critically ill pediatric patients: a systematic review. Pediatr Crit Care Med. 2010;11:124–32.
102. López-Herce J, Dorao P, Elola P, Delgado MA, Ruza F, Madero R. Frequency and prophylaxis of upper gastrointestinal hemorrhage in critically ill children: a prospective study comparing the efficacy of almagate, ranitidine, and sucralfate. The Gastrointestinal Hemorrhage Study Group. Crit Care Med. 1992;20:1082–9.
103. Nithiwathanapong C, Reungrongrat S, Ukarapol N. Prevalence and risk factors of stress-induced gastrointestinal bleeding in critically ill children. World J Gastroenterol. 2005;11:6839–42.
104. Costarino AT, Dai D, Feng R, Feudtner C, Guevara JP. Gastric acid suppressant prophylaxis in pediatric intensive care: current practice as reflected in a large administrative database. Pediatr Crit Care Med. 2015;16:605–12.

105. Sahin S, Ayar G, Yazici MU, Koksal T, Akman AO, Gunduz RC, Kirsacoglu CT, Gulerman F. Stress induced gastrointestinal bleeding in a pediatric intensive care unit: which risk factors should necessitate prophilaxis? Minerva Pediatr. 2016;68:19–26.
106. Terrin G, Passariello A, De Curtis M, Manguso F, Salvia G, Lega L, Messina F, Paludetto R, Canani RB. Ranitidine is associated with infections, necrotizing enterocolitis, and fatal outcome in newborns. Pediatrics. 2012;129:e40–5.
107. Lightdale JR, Gremse DA, Section on Gastroenterology Hp, and Nutrition. Gastroesophageal reflux: management guidance for the pediatrician. Pediatrics. 2013;131:e1684–95.
108. Mohinuddin S, Sakhuja P, Bermundo B, Ratnavel N, Kempley S, Ward HC, Sinha A. Outcomes of full-term infants with bilious vomiting: observational study of a retrieved cohort. Arch Dis Child. 2015;100:14–7.
109. Rönnholm KA, Holmberg C. Peritoneal dialysis in infants. Pediatr Nephrol. 2006;21:751–6.
110. Zaritsky J, Warady BA. Peritoneal dialysis in infants and young children. Semin Nephrol. 2011;31:213–24.
111. Kaiser BA, Polinsky MS, Stover J, Morgenstern BZ, Baluarte HJ. Growth of children following the initiation of dialysis: a comparison of three dialysis modalities. Pediatr Nephrol. 1994;8:733–8.
112. Stewart CL, Acker SN, Pyle LL, Kulungowski A, Cadnapaphornchai M, Bruny JL, Karrer F. Factors associated with peritoneal dialysis catheter complications in children. J Pediatr Surg. 2016;51:159–62.
113. Fraser N, Hussain FK, Connell R, Shenoy MU. Chronic peritoneal dialysis in children. Int J Nephrol Renovasc Dis. 2015;8:125–37.
114. Goldstein SL. Advances in pediatric renal replacement therapy for acute kidney injury. Semin Dial. 2011;24:187–91.
115. Bock KR. Renal replacement therapy in pediatric critical care medicine. Curr Opin Pediatr. 2005;17:368–71.
116. Lacroix J, Hébert PC, Hutchison JS, Hume HA, Tucci M, Ducruet T, Gauvin F, Collet JP, Toledano BJ, Robillard P, Joffe A, Biarent D, Meert K, Peters MJ, Investigators T, Group CCCT, Network PALIaSI. Transfusion strategies for patients in pediatric intensive care units. N Engl J Med. 2007;356:1609–19.
117. Ricca RL, Arca MJ. Transfusion and anticoagulation. Handbook of pediatric surgical critical care. Arca MJ, editor. 1st ed. 2013. p. 214–31. https://www.eapsa.org/apsa/media/Documents/APSAHandbookofSurgicalCriticalCare_Jun52014.pdf.
118. Quinn K, Quinn M, Moreno C, Soundar E, Teruya J, Hui SK. Neonatal transfusion models to determine the impact of using fresh red blood cells on inventory and exposure. Blood Transfus. 2015;13:595–9.
119. Andrew M, David M, Adams M, Ali K, Anderson R, Barnard D, Bernstein M, Brisson L, Cairney B, DeSai D. Venous thromboembolic complications (VTE) in children: first analyses of the Canadian Registry of VTE. Blood. 1994;83:1251–7.
120. Raffini L, Huang YS, Witmer C, Feudtner C. Dramatic increase in venous thromboembolism in children's hospitals in the United States from 2001 to 2007. Pediatrics. 2009;124:1001–8.
121. Monagle P. Diagnosis and management of deep venous thrombosis and pulmonary embolism in neonates and children. Semin Thromb Hemost. 2012;38:683–90.
122. Connelly CR, Laird A, Barton JS, Fischer PE, Krishnaswami S, Schreiber MA, Zonies DH, Watters JM. A clinical tool for the prediction of venous thromboembolism in pediatric trauma patients. JAMA Surg. 2016;151:50–7.
123. Thompson AJ, McSwain SD, Webb SA, Stroud MA, Streck CJ. Venous thromboembolism prophylaxis in the pediatric trauma population. J Pediatr Surg. 2013;48:1413–21.
124. Leeper CM, Vissa M, Cooper JD, Malec LM, Gaines BA. Venous thromboembolism in pediatric trauma patients: ten-year experience and long-term follow-up in a tertiary care center. Pediatr Blood Cancer. 2017. Pediatr. Blood Cancer. 2017;64.
125. Monagle P, Chan AK, Goldenberg NA, Ichord RN, Journeycake JM, Nowak-Göttl U, Vesely SK, Physicians ACoC. Antithrombotic therapy in neonates and children: antithrombotic therapy and prevention of thrombosis, 9th ed: American College of Chest Physicians Evidence-Based Clinical Practice Guidelines. Chest. 2012;141:e737S–801S.
126. Acharya SS. Rare bleeding disorders in children: identification and primary care management. Pediatrics. 2013;132:882–92.
127. Singer M, Deutschman CS, Seymour CW, Shankar-Hari M, Annane D, Bauer M, Bellomo R, Bernard GR, Chiche JD, Coopersmith CM, Hotchkiss RS, Levy MM, Marshall JC, Martin GS, Opal SM, Rubenfeld GD, van der Poll T, Vincent JL, Angus DC. The third international consensus definitions for sepsis and septic shock (Sepsis-3). JAMA. 2016;315:801–10.
128. Ruzic A, Gadepalli S, Hirschl R. Sepsis. Handbook of pediatric surgical critical care. Arca MJ, editor. 1st ed. 2013. https://www.eapsa.org/apsa/media/Documents/APSAHandbookofSurgicalCriticalCare_Jun52014.pdf.
129. Cortese F, Scicchitano P, Gesualdo M, Filaninno A, De Giorgi E, Schettini F, Laforgia N, Ciccone MM. Early and late infections in newborns: where do we stand? A review. Pediatr Neonatol. 2015. Pediatr. Neonatol. 2016;57:265–73.
130. Sur DK, Bukont EL. Evaluating fever of unidentifiable source in young children. Am Fam Physician. 2007;75:1805–11.
131. Sherman JM, Sood SK. Current challenges in the diagnosis and management of fever. Curr Opin Pediatr. 2012;24:400–6.
132. Centers for Disease Control and Prevention NCfIPaC: 10 Leading Causes of Death by Age Group, United States - 2011. http://www.cdc.gov/injury/wisqars/pdf/leading_causes_of_death_by_age_group_2011-a.pdf.
133. Association AH. Pediatric advanced life support (PALS) provider manual. 12th ed. Dallas: American Heart Association; 2016.
134. Leventhal JM, Martin KD, Gaither JR. Using US data to estimate the incidence of serious physical abuse in children. Pediatrics. 2012;129:458–64.
135. Lane WG, Lotwin I, Dubowitz H, Langenberg P, Dischinger P. Outcomes for children hospitalized with abusive versus noninflicted abdominal trauma. Pediatrics. 2011;127:e1400–5.
136. Paul AR, Adamo MA. Non-accidental trauma in pediatric patients: a review of epidemiology, pathophysiology, diagnosis and treatment. Transl Pediatr. 2014;3:195–207.
137. Horowitz L, Kassam-Adams N, Bergstein J. Mental health aspects of emergency medical services for children: summary of a consensus conference. Acad Emerg Med. 2001;8:1187–96.
138. Balluffi A, Kassam-Adams N, Kazak A, Tucker M, Dominguez T, Helfaer M. Traumatic stress in parents of children admitted to the pediatric intensive care unit. Pediatr Crit Care Med. 2004;5:547–53.
139. Muscara F, Burke K, McCarthy MC, Anderson VA, Hearps SJ, Dimovski A, Nicholson JM. Parent distress reactions following a serious illness or injury in their child: a protocol paper for the take a Breath Cohort Study. BMC Psychiatry. 2015;15:153.
140. Davidson JE, Aslakson RA, Long AC, Puntillo KA, Kross EK, Hart J, Cox CE, Wunsch H, Wickline MA, Nunnally ME, Netzer G, Kentish-Barnes N, Sprung CL, Hartog CS, Coombs M, Gerritsen RT, Hopkins RO, Franck LS, Skrobik Y, Kon AA, Scruth EA, Harvey MA, Lewis-Newby M, White DB, Swoboda SM, Cooke CR, Levy MM, Azoulay E, Curtis JR. Guidelines for family-centered care in the neonatal, pediatric, and adult ICU. Crit Care Med. 2017;45:103–28.

Palliative Care in the Surgical Intensive Care Unit

58

Kathleen O'Connell and Zara Cooper

As research evolves and surgical critical care capabilities expand, the line between what we can do to address physiologic derangements and what we should do for patients is increasingly blurred. The shift away from paternalistic surgical care to a patient-centered approach begets heightened expectations for high-quality communication and shared decision-making that have historically been lacking in general surgery training. Current healthcare delivery reform prioritizes care transformation to improve the patient experience, achieve better health outcomes, and control healthcare costs. The incorporation of palliative medicine into surgical care of the critically ill is one approach to successfully target all three of these goals.

Palliative care is a holistic approach to patient care with a focus on the alleviation of pain, psychological suffering, and spiritual unrest to improve quality of life for critically ill patients. As more studies demonstrate that palliative care is associated with improved quality of care, reduced healthcare utilization, and delayed mortality in some cases, the demand for specialized palliative medicine services is increasing [1–3]. In 2005, the American College of Surgeons (ACS) affirmed the need for palliative medicine within the context of chronic illness and injury and rejected palliative care as an approach that should be restricted only to those near the end of life [4]. The American Board of Surgery incorporated palliative care principles within the core competencies of general surgery training, and the ACS has provided educational opportunities for practicing surgeons to learn the basic tenets of palliative care including relief of suffering, prognostication, communication about code status, and identification of patient-centered goals of care. Nonetheless, incorporation of palliative care principles into modern surgical care is lagging compared to other medical specialties [5, 6].

K. O'Connell
Department of Surgery, University of Washington, Seattle, WA, USA

Z. Cooper (✉)
Department of Trauma, Burn, and Surgical Critical Care, Brigham and Women's Hospital, Boston, MA, USA
e-mail: zcooper@partners.org

In this chapter we highlight commonly encountered palliative medicine themes that arise in caring for critically ill patients. Core principles of palliative medicine are outlined in the context of real-life clinical scenarios. Structured communication tools that have been developed for surgical patients and successfully employed by surgeons are described.

Emma was a 79-year-old nursing home patient with dementia, NYHA Class II heart failure, atrial fibrillation, peripheral vascular disease, and mild chronic kidney disease who presented to the emergency department with shortness of breath. She was therapeutically anticoagulated on warfarin, and also on antiplatelet therapy. On arrival she was hypoxic, hypotensive with a systolic blood pressure of 85 mmHg, and a heart rate of 150 beats per minute. The cardiac monitor showed atrial fibrillation with rapid ventricular response. A chest x ray showed bilateral effusions, fluffy bilateral infiltrates and free air under the diaphragm. The surgical team saw her promptly and recommended emergent surgery to her daughter, who was her health care proxy. Although she had a designated health care power of attorney and a living will, identification of goals of care were not established preoperatively despite the high-risk nature of the operation. Emma had an exploratory laparotomy, and a Graham Patch repair for a 0.5 cm perforated post-pyloric duodenal ulcer. Her anticoagulation was held for 24 hours after surgery. The patient's postoperative course was complicated by septic shock, prolonged respiratory failure, congestive heart failure, ventilator associated pneumonia and infectious diarrhea. Because if her hypotension, the team was reluctant to give Emma sedatives and analgesia that could alleviate her pain and agitation. On postoperative day (POD) 10, the surgical team approached Emma's daughter about tracheostomy and she declined. After Emma's daughter conferred with her mother's minister and other relatives, she requested a shift in goals of care to comfort and the patient died on POD 12 after compassionate extubation.

The recent rise in the number of patients 65 years and older with surgical critical care needs is expected to persist over the next 20 years. Hospitalization for acute surgical conditions, including traumatic injury, often marks a downward inflection point in the health trajectory of older adults, marking functional and cognitive decline, increased healthcare utilization, and increased risk of death for years after injury. One third of Medicare beneficiaries have an operation in the last year of life, placing surgeons at the forefront of end-of-life care [7].

A. Salim et al. (eds.), *Surgical Critical Care Therapy*, https://doi.org/10.1007/978-3-319-71712-8_58

Palliative medicine should be routinely provided alongside, or in lieu of, disease-directed treatment in critical illness. Primary palliative care refers to the management of physical symptoms, spiritual and psychosocial distress, and communication with the patients and their families and includes a core set of skills that all clinicians treating seriously ill patients should have. Herein we describe elements of palliative care as they relate to critically ill surgical patients.

Symptom Management

Critically ill patients are at high risk of having undertreated symptoms including pain, thirst, fatigue, constipation, and anxiety. Surgeons are well versed in treatment of acute postoperative pain, but less so in treating total pain which includes physical, spiritual, psychological, and social pain, and can interfere with quality of life and recovery. Pain assessment includes a focused history on the onset, location, quality, and duration of the pain as well as a focused physical exam. Acute physical pain may be somatic (throbbing, aching, localized, sharp), visceral (campy, dull, and poorly localized), or neuropathic (burning, shooting, stabbing, or itching). Somatic pain (e.g., from a fracture) can be treated with acetaminophen or nonsteroidal anti-inflammatories. Opiates are useful for visceral and somatic pain (e.g., a small bowel obstruction), whereas tricyclic antidepressants and anticonvulsant agents are helpful in the treatment of neuropathic pain. During and after surgery, local anesthetics (nerve blocks or epidurals) can help to minimize the use of opiates. Acute care surgeons must understand different pain syndromes; recognize that patients may have somatic, visceral, and neuropathic pain all at once; and be skilled in using multimodal therapy to treat pain. In accordance with the World Health Organization pain ladder [8], oral analgesics are preferable to intravenous medications. Mild pain should be treated with acetaminophen, with or without NSAIDS or COX-2 inhibitors; if pain is moderate, a weak opiate (e.g., tramadol) should be added; and, in the case of severe pain, stronger opiates such as morphine, hydromorphone, or fentanyl can be employed. Patients with continuous pain should receive analgesia around the clock, and as needed, or prn, medications can be used for temporary exacerbations. Prescribers should be mindful of the expected onset and appropriate dosing interval to ensure that pain is adequately controlled. Dosing should be adjusted to minimize side effects. With the heightened focus on opioid abuse in the United States, surgeons must become particularly skilled in understanding and diagnosing different types of pain and the origin of pain, in order to provide the appropriate pharmacologic regimen. Pain that is refractory to multimodal pharmacologic regimens may have a psychosomatic component, in which behavioral interventions or spiritual support may be necessary to alleviate suffering.

Other bothersome symptoms including nausea, vomiting, constipation, dyspnea, and insomnia require aggressive treatment. More insidious symptoms to assess are nonphysical such as anxiety, depression, and spiritual unrest. Formal symptom assessment with the use of a validated tool can help surgeons measure patient's symptoms and support their palliative care needs. The Palliative care Outcome Scale (POS) measures are a set of validated instruments to facilitate prognosis for severely ill patients of with various disease types [9]. The IPOS tool is a streamlined assessment of both physical and nonphysical symptoms and is free to download at https://pos-pal.org/maix/ (Fig. 58.1). Although surgeons may not feel adequately equipped to deal with the emotional, spiritual, and social concerns that frequently accompany critical illness, acknowledging their presence will build trust with the patient and family. The interdisciplinary approach to palliative care is especially valuable when addressing nonphysical symptoms of surgical patients, which can include social work, chaplaincy, and other integrated approaches such as acupuncture and massage.

Prognostication

Prognostic understanding is critical for high-quality decisions for seriously and critically ill patients. Studies show that patients and families want to hear prognostic information and that sharing a poor prognosis does not take away hope or increase the risk of depression. Patients who have accurate prognostic understanding are less likely to choose high-intensity treatments near the end of life. In the acute setting, prognosis is determined by the immediately life-threatening diagnosis as well as the patient's underlying health state. Older patients with chronic medical illnesses or frailty are highly susceptible to complications and functional decline and have increased mortality after trauma and surgery. Chronic diseases tend to have predictable trajectories. For example, the trajectory in cancer is characterized by a rapid decline in function near the end of life, whereas congestive heart failure and COPD frequently include acute exacerbations followed by sudden death. Patients with dementia and frailty typically experience a slow decline over time, colloquially known as the "dwindles." Predictive tools, such as the APACHE score or the Injury Severity Score, are best utilized to estimate prognosis among large populations. In practice, when formulating prognosis surgeons must gather data from the patient, caregivers, and other clinicians to determine the patient's baseline health status, including functional status, expected trajectory, and life expectancy. Web-based prognostic calculators such as e-prognosis and the National Surgical Quality Improvement Program risk calculator can facilitate prognostic estimates. As helpful as numerical estimates can be, uncertainty remains, and clinicians must acknowledge prognostic uncertainty when communicating with patients and their families.

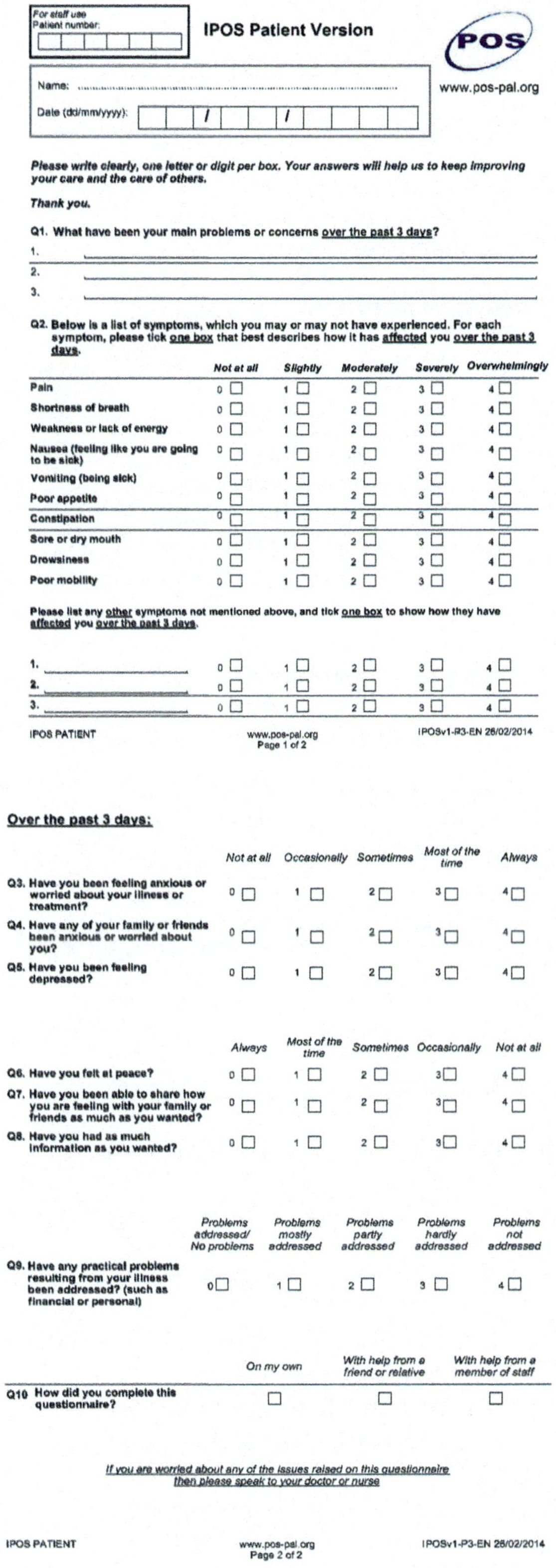

For staff use
Patient number:

IPOS Patient Version

POS

Name: ....

www.pos-pal.org

Date (dd/mm/yyyy): / /

Please write clearly, one letter or digit per box. Your answers will help us to keep improving your care and the care of others.

Thank you.

Q1. What have been your main problems or concerns over the past 3 days?

1.
2.
3.

Q2. Below is a list of symptoms, which you may or may not have experienced. For each symptom, please tick one box that best describes how it has affected you over the past 3 days.

	Not at all	Slightly	Moderately	Severely	Overwhelmingly
Pain	0 ☐	1 ☐	2 ☐	3 ☐	4 ☐
Shortness of breath	0 ☐	1 ☐	2 ☐	3 ☐	4 ☐
Weakness or lack of energy	0 ☐	1 ☐	2 ☐	3 ☐	4 ☐
Nausea (feeling like you are going to be sick)	0 ☐	1 ☐	2 ☐	3 ☐	4 ☐
Vomiting (being sick)	0 ☐	1 ☐	2 ☐	3 ☐	4 ☐
Poor appetite	0 ☐	1 ☐	2 ☐	3 ☐	4 ☐
Constipation	0 ☐	1 ☐	2 ☐	3 ☐	4 ☐
Sore or dry mouth	0 ☐	1 ☐	2 ☐	3 ☐	4 ☐
Drowsiness	0 ☐	1 ☐	2 ☐	3 ☐	4 ☐
Poor mobility	0 ☐	1 ☐	2 ☐	3 ☐	4 ☐

Please list any other symptoms not mentioned above, and tick one box to show how they have affected you over the past 3 days.

1.	0 ☐	1 ☐	2 ☐	3 ☐	4 ☐
2.	0 ☐	1 ☐	2 ☐	3 ☐	4 ☐
3.	0 ☐	1 ☐	2 ☐	3 ☐	4 ☐

IPOS PATIENT www.pos-pal.org Page 1 of 2 IPOSv1-P3-EN 28/02/2014

Over the past 3 days:

	Not at all	Occasionally	Sometimes	Most of the time	Always
Q3. Have you been feeling anxious or worried about your illness or treatment?	0 ☐	1 ☐	2 ☐	3 ☐	4 ☐
Q4. Have any of your family or friends been anxious or worried about you?	0 ☐	1 ☐	2 ☐	3 ☐	4 ☐
Q5. Have you been feeling depressed?	0 ☐	1 ☐	2 ☐	3 ☐	4 ☐

	Always	Most of the time	Sometimes	Occasionally	Not at all
Q6. Have you felt at peace?	0 ☐	1 ☐	2 ☐	3 ☐	4 ☐
Q7. Have you been able to share how you are feeling with your family or friends as much as you wanted?	0 ☐	1 ☐	2 ☐	3 ☐	4 ☐
Q8. Have you had as much information as you wanted?	0 ☐	1 ☐	2 ☐	3 ☐	4 ☐

	Problems addressed/ No problems	Problems mostly addressed	Problems partly addressed	Problems hardly addressed	Problems not addressed
Q9. Have any practical problems resulting from your illness been addressed? (such as financial or personal)	0 ☐	1 ☐	2 ☐	3 ☐	4 ☐

	On my own	With help from a friend or relative	With help from a member of staff
Q10 How did you complete this questionnaire?	☐	☐	☐

If you are worried about any of the issues raised on this questionnaire then please speak to your doctor or nurse

IPOS PATIENT www.pos-pal.org Page 2 of 2 IPOSv1-P3-EN 28/02/2014

Fig. 58.1 Palliative care outcome scale IPOS symptom assessment tool

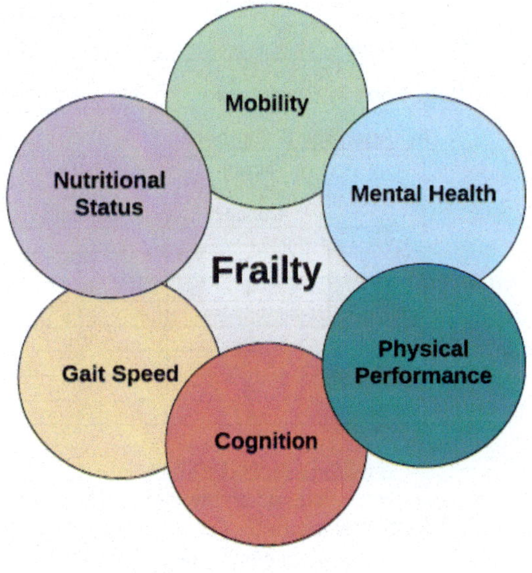

Fig. 58.2 Domains of frailty

In older patients frailty screening is an important component of prognostic assessment. Frailty is a decline in physiologic reserve that predicates an increased risk of dying in 6 months to 5 years [10]. Frailty assessments have been shown to predict postoperative complications, functional decline, need for institutionalized care, and mortality [11–13]. Although there is no gold standard for assessing frailty, experts agree that frailty is a multidimensional construct that consists of the six domains illustrated in Fig. 58.2 [14].

In order to facilitate routine frailty assessments into the preoperative history and physical examinations, a Frailty Screening Tool must be quick and simple to use. With this in mind, Hall et al. developed a novel 14-point frailty index, the Risk Analysis Index (RAI), for use in surgical patients (Fig. 58.3) [18]. The RAI is clinically feasible, taking 1–2 min to complete, and has been prospectively validated to predict postoperative mortality up to 1 year. The RAI provides additional information extending beyond the 30-day window [16].

Ernst et al. implemented a system-wide preoperative frailty screening in a single Veterans Affairs hospital and used frailty as a trigger for palliative medicine referral [1]. Implementation of the frailty screening program significantly increased the number of referrals from surgeons, of which preoperative referrals were associated with a reduction in mortality (OR 0.27; 95% CI, 0.11–0.68) after adjusting for confounding factors. These findings should reassure surgeons that palliative care consultation effectively supplements surgical care and does not hasten mortality by deterring patients from undergoing surgical intervention.

Restructuring the preoperative evaluation of older patients to include a frailty assessment creates a platform for initiating conversations prior to high-risk surgery. The frailty assessment provides the surgeon with a starting point from which to communicate prognostic predictions and engage

Risk Analysis Index (RAI)

Last Name:______________________ Last Four: _________

Date Form is Completed:__________ Date & Type of Anticipated Surgery:_________________

A. Age, Sex & Cancer

Age	Score *without* Cancer	Score *with* Cancer
≤ 69	2	20
70-74	3	19
75-79	4	18
80-84	5	17
85-89	6	16
90-94	7	15
95-99	8	14
100+	9	13

1. Sex Female= 0 Male= 5 ___________
2. Age ___________
3. Does the patient have cancer?
   (Excluding skin cancer,except for melanoma)
   If no, score *without* cancer ___________
   or
   If yes, score *with* cancer ___________

B. Medical Co-Morbidities

4. Have you had unintentional weight loss in the past 3 months (>10 lbs)? No= 0 Yes= 5 ______
5. Renal failure? No= 0 Yes= 6 ______
6. Chronic/congestive heart failure? No= 0 Yes= 4 ______
7. Poor appetite? No= 0 Yes= 4 ______
8. Shortness of breath (at rest)? No= 0 Yes= 8 ______

C. Cognition, Residence & Activity of Daily Living

9. Do you reside in a setting other than independent living?
   If yes, check answer: Skilled nursing facility □ Assisted living □ Nursing home □
   No= 0 Yes= 8 ______
   If yes, were you admitted within the past 3 months? No □ Yes □

D. Activities of Daily Living & Cognitive Decline (*Circle score for each ADL*)

10. Mobility/Locomotion	11. Eating	12. Toilet Use	13. Personal Hygiene
0. Independent	0. Independent	0. Independent	0. Independent
1. Supervised	1. Supervised	1. Supervised	1. Supervised
2. Limited assistance	2. Limited assistance	2. Limited assistance	2. Limited assistance
3. Extensive assistance	3. Extensive assistance	3. Extensive assistance	3. Extensive assistance
4. Total Dependence	4. Total Dependence	4. Total Dependence	4. Total Dependence

14. Have your cognitive skills or status deteriorated over the past 3 months? No □ Yes □ (*see score chart*)

ADL Score *without* Cognitive Decline (*Sum of ADL Scores*)	ADL Score *with* Cognitive Decline
0	ADL Score -2
1,2	ADL Score -1
3,4	ADL Score 0
5-7	ADL Score +1
8,9	ADL Score +2
10,11	ADL Score +3
12,13	ADL Score +4
14-16	ADL Score +5

Score *without* cognitive decline ______________ (0 to 16)
or
Score *with* cognitive decline ______________(-2 to 21)

Total RAI Score: ___________

Scoring Instructions: To calculate the RAI-C score, first look at the Age/Cancer table to determine the single value between 2 and 20 that corresponds to the patient's age and cancer status. Record this single value in the appropriate line for item 3. Next look at the ADL table and sum the scores (0-4) for the four ADLs queried in items 10-13. This sum is the ADL Score and should range between 0 and 16. Next look at the ADL/Cognitive-Decline table to determine the single value between -2 and 21 that corresponds to the patient's ADL Score and cognitive decline. Record the value in the appropriate line for item 14. Finally, sum the values for items 1,3-9, and 14 to yield a final RAI-C score between 0 and 81.

Fig. 58.3 Frailty Screening Tool: Risk Analysis Index [15]

shared decision-making. Although it may be difficult for patients and families to grasp the complexities of an operation or conceptualize the rigors of postoperative care, they do relate to loss of cognitive and functional capabilities that result in loss of independence.

Communication

Surrogates and Advance Directives

Communicating in the acute setting is fraught with challenges. Patients are often unable to communicate and are in extremis with life-threatening emergencies, and patients and their clinicians have no established relationship. In many cases clinicians must engage surrogate decision-makers who are frequently ill-prepared for their role and have inadequate understanding of the patients. The ethical standard for surrogate decision-making is predicated upon using substituted judgment, with a goal to make the same decisions that the patient would. Advance directives (ADs), or living wills, specify treatment limitations in the event the patient can no longer advocate for himself or herself. They are intended to protect patient autonomy and can be invoked when a patient lacks capacity to make their own medical decisions. ADs are associated with less unwanted, non-beneficial treatments for patients who have them and reduce surrogate burden. Unfortunately they are frequently too ambiguous or specific to be useful and often difficult to locate in emergencies. Physician orders for life-sustaining treatments or POLST forms are medical orders that should be honored across institutions in states where they are honored. POLST forms include directives for life-sustaining treatments and hospitalizations.

If the patient's desires for treatment are unknown, surrogates should use the best interest standard, which requires that decisions are what a "reasonable person" would be expected to do in the same situation. Clinicians must keep this ethical standard in mind as the counsel surrogates who may be distressed and inclined to make decisions based on what *they* would want for the patient rather than what the patient would want for themselves.

Decision-Making

Communication with seriously ill patients is a core skill for acute care surgeons that, like other surgical skills, can be taught, learned, refined, and mastered. Critical communication skills include formulating and communicating prognosis, delivering bad news, eliciting goals of care, determining code status, and conducting family meetings. Fear of talking about death, taking away hope, or prognostic uncertainty heightens anxiety around difficult conversations and may lead surgeons to entirely abrogate clinical decisions to patients and surrogates who are ill-prepared to make high-risk existential decisions in the moment.

In seriously ill patients with multiple chronic illnesses or baseline cognitive or functional dependence, provision of primary palliative care should start before surgery with utilization of evidence-based communication techniques. *Shared decision-making* (SDM) is a collaborative process that allows patients/surrogates and clinicians to make healthcare decisions together, taking into account the best scientific evidence available, as well as the patient's values, goals, and preferences [15]. The model for SDM contains three major components including *information exchange*, *treatment option deliberation*, and making a *final treatment decision*. The American College of Critical Care Medicine and the American Thoracic Society established key communication skills to guide physicians in fostering SDM [17] (Table 58.2).

Shared decision-making is particularly relevant in the types of treatment decisions with high risk and high uncertainty that frequently characterize critical illness. The overarching goal is to honor patient autonomy by providing treatments that are aligned with the individual patient's goals and values. It is important that surgeon's recognize that these goals may be dynamic and change with patients' health states. Therefore surgeons should not presume that patients, who agree to surgery at the outset, would automatically agree to additional interventions if complications ensue or if their health status worsens. Instead, goals and values should be revisited at regular intervals and around escalations in care.

Surgical buy-in describes an unspoken, implicit assumption made by surgeons that when patients consent to an operation, they also agree to subsequent life-sustaining interventions (e.g., prolonged mechanical ventilation, repeat operations, feeding tubes, dialysis, etc.) required to ensure survival [18]. One study, a qualitative analysis of preoperative conversations between older patients, or their surrogates, and surgeons before high-risk surgery, found that surgeons did not explicitly discuss patient preferences for treatment limitations [19]. Surprisingly, most patients and their families believed that their surgeon shared their personal values and would act accordingly in the event of a serious complication. Patients reported full confidence that their advance directive would protect their wishes and direct treatment if a serious complication were to occur. However, in most cases advance directives were not addressed. This study also exposed misguided assumptions and misunderstandings in regard to the nature of "life-supporting treatments," the concepts of "brain death" and "vegetative state," and the existence of prognostic uncertainty in cases of unexpected complications. Needless to say, there was a wide range of patient preferences concerning treatment limitations and personally identified goals of care that they had not discussed with their surgeon.

Table 58.1 Best communication practices to facilitate goal-concordant care [20, 21]

Guide	Clinician steps	Clinician prompts
Prognosis	Gather data about illness trajectory and formulate prognosis.	
	Review prior advance directives	
Connect and elicit	Address symptoms, express concern for patient's well-being, elicit patient illness understanding	"How would you describe your overall health? How have you been functioning lately?"
Inform	Disclose information about the acute problem in context of illness trajectory	"It seems that we've hit something today that changes the course of things …"
Summarize	Establish shared understanding of patient's overall condition	"The way I am seeing things is that you have both a serious ongoing medical issue, and a new acute surgical crisis. I think what this means is that …"
Pause	Allow the patient to process the information; respond to patient's emotion	"I can see how upsetting this is …"
Options	Describe the benefits, burdens, and likely outcomes of surgical and nonsurgical options, including palliative treatments, in context of patient's goals	"In your situation, here is what we expect this could look like …"
Goals	Understand patient's goals, priorities, and tradeoffs. Discuss existing advance directives with the patient or designated surrogate	"Have you thought about the kind of medical care you would want if you became very sick?"
		"Are there any treatments or health states that are intolerable to you?"
		"How much are you willing to go through to try to get you over this crisis?"
Recommend	Recommend a course of treatment in the context of the patient's goals. Consider time-limited trials	"Based on your priorities, I would recommend we do *x*. We can meet again in *x* time and see whether things are getting better or worse and reconsider the options then."
Support	Affirm relationship, describe next steps to patient, document the conversation in the medical record, and communicate with clinical team	"We are all committed to taking great care of you, and respecting your goals."

Table 58.2 Key communication skills to involve patients or surrogates in treatment decisions [13]

Communication skill
Establish a trusting partnership
Meet regularly with patients and/or surrogates
Express commitment to patient and family
Involve interdisciplinary team in supporting the family
Provide emotional support
Acknowledge strong emotions
Convey empathy
Explore surrogate's fears and concerns
Assess patient's or surrogates' understanding of the situation
Ask open-ended question about what patient or surrogate has been told
Explain the medical situation
Use simple language to explain patients illness
"Chunk and check" – convey information in small aliquots with frequent pauses to assess understanding
Convey prognosis for both risk of death and risk of functional impairment
Highlight that there is a choice
Explain that there is more than one reasonable treatment choice with different risks/benefits
Explain why surrogates' input is important
When necessary, explain surrogate decision making
Explain surrogate's role to promote patient's values, goals, and preferences
Explain substituted judgment
Assess patient's/surrogate's role preference
Discuss patient's/surrogate's comfort making decisions at that moment
Explain the range of permissible decision-making models
Explain treatment options
Describe the treatment options, as well as their risks and benefits
Elicit patient's values, goals, and preferences
Elicit previously expressed treatment preferences (oral or written)
Elicit patient's values about relevant health states
Ask surrogates what the patient would likely choose if he/she were able to speak for himself/herself
Deliberate with patients and surrogates
Discuss the advantages and disadvantages of various diagnostic and therapeutic options
Explore patients' or surrogates' thoughts and concerns
Correct misperceptions
Provide a recommendation and explain rationale underlying recommendation
Make a decision
Agree on a treatment decision to implement

In recent years, guidelines have been published outlining best communication practices to assist surgeons in facilitating goal-concordant care for older patients. The following structured communication framework was developed for use in emergent surgical situations [20] (Tables 58.1 and 58.2).

Before entering the patient's room or family meeting, the surgeon should gather information on the patient's current condition, underlying diagnosis, and expected illness trajectory to formulate a prognosis of the patient's overall health, with and without surgery.

The discussion is initiated by eliciting the patient/surrogate's understanding of their illness, including anticipated illness trajectory and overall health. This will provide an opportunity to achieve a shared understanding of the patient's overall health and address inaccuracies.

Next, the surgeon should transition into discussing the current acute surgical condition with a "warning shot" phrase signaling to the patient and family that they are about to hear bad news. Examples of such a phrase include "I'm sorry that I don't have better news to discuss with you" or "I'm worried that we have hit something new that changes the course of things." Subsequently, the surgeon informs the patient of the acute surgical condition and how this will impact their overall prognosis and healthcare trajectory.

It is important that after breaking bad news, the surgeon allows a pause. The pause allows the patient or surrogate time to process difficult information, signals the seriousness of the news, and gives the surgeon an opportunity to respond to the patient or surrogate's emotion. A second transition is made into discussing the benefits, burdens, and range of likely outcomes after surgical and nonsurgical treatments. Keeping in mind that the majority of older patients with severe chronic illness report they would decline even a low-risk intervention if the likely outcome were severe functional impairment, a clear description of potential postoperative trajectories (including burdensome treatments, duration of life-sustaining treatments, and the need for institutionalized care) should be thoroughly reviewed [21]. Palliative approaches should be offered along with appropriate procedural or surgical interventions.

Prior to making a treatment recommendation, the surgeon should seek to understand what is an acceptable quality of life for the patient. Are there life or family milestones the patient hopes to achieve? Which activities are necessary for the patient to retain an acceptable quality of life? What is admissible regarding life-extending treatments versus comfort-focused care? The discussion surrounding life priorities will help the surgeon construct a treatment recommendation that is concordant with the patients' goals. In cases of clinical uncertainty, where patients and families do not want to prematurely forgo treatments that might improve the patient's condition but also don't want to risk indefinite commitment to burdensome treatments/care, a **time-limited trial** can be negotiated. A time-limited trial is an agreement between the patient/surrogates and surgeon to use one mode of treatment over a defined period of time to give the patient an opportunity to improve according to mutually defined clinical outcomes [22]. If the patient improves during the time period, next steps are proposed. On the other hand, if the clinical improvements are not achieved, the treatment is discontinued and either a second time-limited trial or transition to a solely palliative approach is pursued. Regardless of the ultimate decision, it is important for the patient/family to feel supported by the surgeon, especially when choosing comfort-focused care.

Scenario planning is a strategy used by corporations for financial planning and to structure thinking about the future. It has also been implemented in medicine to help patients and families envision an array of potential outcomes when the future is uncertain. Using scenario planning as a platform, Schwarze et al. developed the *best case/worst case (BC/WC)* tool to augment SDM in the setting of unpredictable outcomes [23]. This technique supplements the SDM verbal structure with a storytelling narrative and visual outline of potential clinical outcomes.

Using the aforementioned guidelines as a framework, tin BC/WC, the surgeon describes each treatment option including the best and worst possible outcomes as a continuum under each option [24]. Using a pen and paper, the surgeon simply creates a visual scale of the outcomes continuum. The location of the "most likely" indicator along the line (closer to "best case" or "worst case") is determined by the surgeon after considering the patient's values and goals. It is imperative for both the surgeon and family to realize that death is not always the worst possible outcome for some patients, especially elderly patients or those who are neurologically devastated. At the end of the BC/WC discussion, the surgeon is to provide a treatment recommendation that integrates patient preferences with plausible therapeutic options.

Jack was a 22 yo Native American man with a history of morbid obesity, uncontrolled type 2 diabetes, and end-stage renal disease who was non-compliant with dialysis. He presented with several days of pain and foul-smelling drainage from his genital region, and was in septic shock. The patient was diagnosed with Fournier's Gangrene, and underwent emergent surgical debridement and administration of broad-spectrum antibiotic therapy. Post-operatively the patient's clinical status quickly declined with worsening respiratory, hepatic, and circulatory failure. Maximal support was provided for several days with aggressive surgical debridements and supportive care for the multisystem organ failure. Daily family meetings revealed that despite Jack's young age, he had a poor quality of life and would likely not accept living in a nursing home if he were able to survive to hospital discharge. With the full support of the surgical critical care team, the patient's mother elected to transition to comfort-focused care. Do not resuscitate orders were placed and the patient died peacefully with his family performing cultural rituals at the bedside.

Family Meetings

Organized, interdisciplinary family meetings for ICU patients facilitate shared decision-making, improve family satisfaction, and reduce days of life-sustaining treatment for patients who die in the ICU without increasing ICU mortality rates. Evidence also shows that the first family meeting should occur around day 5 of the patients' ICU stay. Patients and families should be reassured that the family meeting is a routine part of ICU care, rather than a hallmark of poor prognosis. Holding a family meeting early helps establish goals of care for the ICU stay and builds rapport with the family that can ease difficult decision-making later in the ICU stay. The VALUE approach is useful to communication with families in the ICU: **v**alue family statements, **a**cknowledge family emotions, **l**isten to the family, **u**nderstand the patient as a person, and **e**licit family questions.

Discussions About Code Status

The timing and urgency of code status discussions are determined by the patient's prognosis but suffice it to say that a sizable portion of patients requiring acute surgical care are at high risk of death and should have their code status clarified. Physicians need to be thoughtful and deliberate in their approach to these discussions. Cardiopulmonary resuscitation is a procedure like any other, with indications, risks, and benefits. When approaching patients about CPR, physicians must set aside their own biases and expectations about what the patient's code status should be and focus their discussion on the patient's goals, values, and desires for treatment. Clinicians should seek to establish shared understating of the patient's prognosis and priorities treatment and then describe the benefits and burdens of resuscitation within that context. Patients with relatively poor understanding of what resuscitation entails should not be asked to choose from a menu of choices (e.g., vasopressors, intubations, shocks, or compressions) nor should they be given choices that include CPR or "doing nothing." The latter signals patient abandonment and causes significant psychological distress for patients and surrogates. Rather the term "allow a natural death" is more acceptable to patients and surrogates, and given this option, they are more likely to forgo CPR. Clinicians should also emphasize that every effort will be made to provide comfort and preserve dignity. Therapies should be offered if they make it possible to achieve the patient's states goals; clinicians are not ethically obligated to offer life-sustaining treatments if they do not think it will improve survival or result in an outcome that is acceptable to the patient. In approaching code status discussions, it can be helpful to use the phrases, "I hope," "I worry," and "I wonder." To start the conversation: "***I hope*** *you get better and can go home, but I do* ***worry*** *that since you've have a history of heart disease and that you've been having irregular heart rhythms after surgery that your heart could stop unexpectedly.* ***I wonder*** *if you became so sick that your heart were to stop what kind of treatments we should provide that would be in keeping with your wishes.*" For patients who are known to be near the end of life, it can be helpful to ask a question such as "*When you think about dying what things are most important to you*?"

Care of the Dying Patient

For seriously ill patients whose death is imminent, palliative care alleviates suffering and provides support for the family. "Comfort-focused care" revolves around immediate relief of symptoms for a patient who is very close to death [25]. Although management of symptoms was discussed previously in relation to primary palliative care in critical illness, it becomes the primary focus near the end of life.

Comfort-focused care constitutes the withdrawal of invasive, life-sustaining therapies with the intent of maximizing the patient's comfort. This includes removal of mechanical ventilation and endotracheal tube, removal of nasogastric/orogastric tubes, and cessation of intravenous fluids, antibiotics, blood pressure support, and artificial nutrition. Intravenous catheters should remain in place to facilitate expeditious delivery of opioids and benzodiazepines as needed. Education of the family regarding the possibility of common symptoms near death will help prepare them for the dying process and reassure them that the surgical team will provide continuity of care to ensure a peaceful death. For a thorough evidence-based review on symptom management in dying patients, please refer to the review by Blinderman and Billings [25].

Equally important to symptom control is granting the family privacy with the patient. Monitors should be removed, medical devices silenced, and interruptions limited. In some cases, the patient may be appropriate to transfer out of the ICU if the dying process is expected to take a few days or even be discharged to home with hospice.

Summary

Surgical ethos is deeply rooted in the fundamental ethical principles of autonomy, beneficence, non-maleficence, and justice. As such, palliative care has an integral and prominent role in surgical care of seriously ill patients and their families. There are currently less than 80 surgeons board certified in hospice and palliative medicine (HPM) in the United States, and the national shortage of non-surgeon HPM providers is estimated at 6000–18,000 and rising [26, 27]. With the workforce shortage of board-certified palliative care providers, provision of primary palliative care to manage physical and nonphysical symptoms defines goals of care within the context of serious illness, and to ensure excellence in end-of-life care is the surgeon's responsibility. By clarifying the limits of what is possible for patients and families and identifying patient treatment preferences in the context of their values, surgeons have an immense impact in decreasing unwanted burdensome treatments at the end of life.

References

1. Ernst KF, Hall DE, Schmid KK, et al. Surgical palliative care consultations over time in relationship to systemwide frailty screening. JAMA Surg. 2014;149:1121–6.
2. Miner TJ, Cohen J, Charpentier K, McPhillips J, Marvell L, Cioffi WG. The palliative triangle: improved patient selection and outcomes associated with palliative operations. Arch Surg. 2011;146:517–22.
3. Lilley EJ, Khan KT, Johnston FM, et al. Palliative care interventions for surgical patients: a systematic review. JAMA Surg. 2016;151:172–83.
4. American College of Surgeons and Task Force on Surgical Palliative Care and Committee on Ethics. Statement of principles of palliative care. Bull Am Coll Surg. 2005;90(8):34–35.
5. Kross EK, Engelberg RA, Downey L, et al. Differences in end-of-life care in the ICU across patients cared for by medicine, surgery, neurology, and neurosurgery physicians. Chest. 2014;145:313–21.
6. Olmsted CL, Johnson AM, Kaboli P, Cullen J, Vaughan-Sarrazin MS. Use of palliative care and hospice among surgical and medical specialties in the Veterans Health Administration. JAMA Surg. 2014;149:1169–75.
7. Kwok AC, Semel ME, Lipsitz SR, et al. The intensity and variation of surgical care at the end of life: a retrospective cohort study. Lancet. 2011;378:1408–13.
8. World Health Organization. Cancer Pin Relief. Geneva: WHO; 1986.
9. Hearn J, Higginson IJ. Development and validation of a core outcome measure for palliative care: the palliative care outcome scale. Palliative Care Core Audit Project Advisory Group. Qual Health Care. 1999;8:219–27.
10. Hall DE, Arya S, Schmid KK, et al. Development and initial validation of the risk analysis index for measuring frailty in surgical populations. JAMA Surg. 2017;152:175–82.
11. Makary MA, Segev DL, Pronovost PJ, et al. Frailty as a predictor of surgical outcomes in older patients. J Am Coll Surg. 2010;210:901–8.
12. Robinson TN, Wu DS, Pointer L, Dunn CL, Cleveland JC Jr, Moss M. Simple frailty score predicts postoperative complications across surgical specialties. Am J Surg. 2013;206:544–50.
13. Hall DE, Arya S, Schmid KK, et al. Association of a frailty screening initiative with postoperative survival at 30, 180, and 365 days. JAMA Surg. 2017;152:233–40.
14. Rodriguez-Manas L, Feart C, Mann G, et al. Searching for an operational definition of frailty: a Delphi method based consensus statement: the frailty operative definition-consensus conference project. J Gerontol A Biol Sci Med Sci. 2013;68:62–7.
15. Kon AA, Davidson JE, Morrison W, Danis M, White DB. Shared Decision-Making in Intensive Care Units. Executive Summary of the American College of Critical Care Medicine and American Thoracic Society Policy Statement. Am J Respir Crit Care Med. 2016;193:1334–6.
16. Bilimoria KY, Liu Y, Paruch JL, et al. Development and evaluation of the universal ACS NSQIP surgical risk calculator: a decision aid and informed consent tool for patients and surgeons. J Am Coll Surg. 2013;217:833–42. e1–3
17. Kon AA, Davidson JE, Morrison W, Danis M, White DB. Shared Decision Making in ICUs: an American College of Critical Care Medicine and American Thoracic Society Policy Statement. Crit Care Med. 2016;44:188–201.
18. Schwarze ML, Bradley CT, Brasel KJ. Surgical "buy-in": the contractual relationship between surgeons and patients that influences decisions regarding life-supporting therapy. Crit Care Med. 2010;38:843–8.
19. Nabozny MJ, Kruser JM, Steffens NM, et al. Patient-reported limitations to surgical buy-in: a qualitative study of patients facing high-risk surgery. Ann Surg. 2017;265:97–102.
20. Cooper Z, Koritsanszky LA, Cauley CE, et al. Recommendations for best communication practices to facilitate goal-concordant care for seriously ill older patients with emergency surgical conditions. Ann Surg. 2016;263:1–6.
21. Fried TR, Bradley EH, Towle VR, Allore H. Understanding the treatment preferences of seriously ill patients. N Engl J Med. 2002;346:1061–6.
22. Quill TE, Holloway R. Time-limited trials near the end of life. JAMA. 2011;306:1483–4.
23. Schwarze ML, Kehler JM, Campbell TC. Navigating high risk procedures with more than just a street map. J Palliat Med. 2013;16:1169–71.
24. Kruser JM, Taylor LJ, Campbell TC, et al. "Best case/worst case": training surgeons to use a novel communication tool for high-risk acute surgical problems. J Pain Symptom Manag. 2017;53:711–9. e5
25. Blinderman CD, Billings JA. Comfort care for patients dying in the hospital. N Engl J Med. 2015;373:2549–61.
26. The American Board of Surgery. Diplomat totals. 2017. http://www.absurgery.org/default.jsp?statsummary. Accessed 13 Apr 2017.
27. Lupu D. Estimate of current hospice and palliative medicine physician workforce shortage. J Pain Symptom Manag. 2010;40:899–911.

Ethics in Critical Care

59

Jessica Ballou and Karen J. Brasel

Introduction

The treatment and subsequent recovery of most ICU patients present few ethical challenges. However, the nature of surgical critical care is such that psychologic and physiologic stress, end-of-life care, caretaker and family dynamics, and limited resources can result in an environment where conflict occurs [1–5]. These difficult times are taxing on patients and providers alike. The purpose of this chapter is to discuss the existing consensus statements and precedents that are associated with the more common ethical dilemmas that may present in an ICU as well as identify the key principles and resources that may be applied to a variety of critical care scenarios to help providers make informed, practical decisions.

The topic of ethics in the critical care setting is immense, and the diversity of experiences and cultural lenses through which ethical dilemmas present make it impossible to cover the appropriate action in each situation. It is therefore beyond the scope of this chapter to delve specifically into the ethical issues associated with vulnerable populations: pediatrics, pregnant women, prisoners, refugees, etc. except where explicitly stated below. However, we describe general principles that can be modified and adapted to specific situations in these vulnerable populations.

J. Ballou
Oregon Health and Science University, Portland, OR, USA

K. J. Brasel (✉)
Department of Surgery, Division of Trauma, Critical Care, and Acute Care Surgery, Oregon Health and Science University, Portland, OR, USA
e-mail: brasel@ohsu.edu

What Is the Purpose of an Intensive Care Unit?

The primary purpose of ICU care is to provide treatment to patients for whom there is a reasonable expectation of survival outside of the acute care setting with sufficient cognitive ability to perceive the benefits of treatment [6]. It is therefore generally understood that the objective of ICU care is to overcome an acute threat and to maintain a certain quality of life. Yet, the changing nature of critical care medicine is such that more than one in five of all deaths occur during or shortly following an ICU admission [7, 8].

ICU utilization by the elderly will continue to increase as the North American population ages [9]. Americans age 65 and older represent the fastest-growing segment of the US population, comprising an estimated 13% of the total population (more than 40 million persons) with an expected doubling of the demographic by 2050 [10]. Similar models also predict a tripling of the over 85 age population during this time [10]. As a result, approximately half of current ICU patients are over age 65 [8, 11].

Admission to an ICU is often a harbinger of generalized health decline. So, while the primary purpose of the ICU is to support life, the reality is that it is often the case that the role of the intensivist is to prepare the patient and their family for death. In one long-term follow-up study, there was only 50% survival among SICU patients after 10 years [12]. Similarly, in a Canadian study of patients over age 80 admitted to the ICU, 35% died in the hospital within just 10 days of an ICU admission [7]. Perhaps not surprisingly, median time to death was longest in family members who were unsure of their treatment preferences [7]. And while nearly 70% of community-dwelling elderly possess advance directives in some areas, the directives that are meant to provide guidance for surrogates do not negate the possibility of conflict [13, 14]. ICU clinicians must therefore be prepared for managing the ethical conflicts that will inevitably arise as the ICU becomes a final destination for an increasing number of elderly patients.

A. Salim et al. (eds.), *Surgical Critical Care Therapy*, https://doi.org/10.1007/978-3-319-71712-8_59

What Is the Role of Ethics and Ethics Committees in an ICU?

Ethics refers to a set of moral principles that govern behavior. A full review of the means and methods by which we have arrived at our current set of principles is a discussion to be had elsewhere, but in brief the healthcare community abides by the agreed upon principles of autonomy, beneficence, non-maleficence, and justice.

Though there are innumerable ways in which ethical conflicts may present in an ICU, there are common themes that tend to make up the majority of ICU ethics consults: withdrawing or withholding life-sustaining treatments, patient and surrogate decision-making concerns, resuscitation issues, informed consent and right to refuse treatment, professional responsibilities, appropriateness of treatment (i.e., futility), interprofessional and family disagreements, advance directives, resource allocation, end-of-life care, and religious/spiritual/cultural issues [15]. Generally, ethics consults in the setting of conflict have been shown to reduce hospital costs and the use of non-beneficial treatments [16]. Proactive ethics consults on long-term ICU patients, however, have not been shown to have the same effect [17].

Providing Palliative Care in the ICU

Although there can be some overlap between ethics committees and palliative care services, generally, ethics committees deal with perceived or actual ethical questions and conflict, while palliative care is focused on provision of clinical care to manage symptoms in concordance with patient goals. According to the World Health Organization, palliative care improves the quality of life of patients and their families dealing with life-threatening illness through the prevention and relief of suffering by means of early identification and treatment of pain and physical, psychosocial, and spiritual problems [18]. Palliative care physicians are in critically short supply, making it the responsibility of all intensivists to attempt to meet the basic palliative needs of their critically ill patients [19].

The first step toward identifying palliative care needs is completing a primary palliative care assessment. This includes identifying physical or psychological symptoms, recognizing social or spiritual concerns affecting daily life, verifying whether the patient comprehends the illness and treatment plan, identifying the goals of care/advanced directives, and transitioning care post-discharge [19]. To the extent that they are available, palliative care consultations are recommended for cases where there are unmet care needs despite best attempts by the primary providers. Patients at high risk of having unmet palliative care needs include those for whom there is a life-limiting or life-threatening condition and one of the following criteria (Table 59.1):

Table 59.1 Identifying patients at high risk for unmet palliative care needs

You would not be surprised if the patient died within 12 months
Difficult to control physical or psychological symptoms
ICU length of stay >7 days
Lack of goals of care clarity and documentation
Disagreements or uncertainty among the patient, staff, and/or family regarding major medical decisions, resuscitation preferences, or use of non-oral feeding or hydration
Patients with long-term critical illness (e.g., transplant, dialysis, LVAD, etc.)

Adapted from Ref. [19]

Ultimately, palliative care is an increasingly integral component of critical care medicine and may be an adjunct, not substitute, for aggressive treatments [20].

Treating Pain: The Principle of Double Effect

Adequate pain management is a central tenet of patient care in an ICU. In 2013 the Society of Critical Care Medicine published its guidelines for the management of pain, agitation, and delirium in ICU patients [21]. Generally, the guidelines recommend that pain be adequately monitored via the behavioral pain scale and the critical-care pain observation tool, not just vital signs, for patients unable to communicate pain. These scales use physical signs, such as facial grimacing, body movements, ventilator compliance, and muscle tension to gauge how comfortable the patient appears. Further, the guidelines recommend intravenous opioids as first line to treat non-neuropathic pain along with non-opioid adjuncts.

However, there may be circumstances where the principle of double effect is employed: where the administration of narcotics and sedatives to ease pain and suffering may hasten death [22, 23]. Euthanasia, which is largely illegal in the USA with few exceptions, refers to the administration of medications with the intention of death. Each state has their own laws regarding the requirements and mechanisms for these practices. Although controversial, the principle of double effect allows for the administration of drugs that cause respiratory depression, even to the point of death, as long as the primary intent is to relieve pain and suffering and as long as the encounter is well-documented [22, 23].

Patient Autonomy and the Role of Surrogates

Multiple legal precedents have established that adult patients have the right to refuse medical treatment [24–26]. With regard to children, the law errs on the side of providing treatment. While not explicitly pertaining to medical care, in *Prince v. Massachusetts* (1944), the Supreme Court ruled that "while parents may feel free to become martyrs themselves they are not free to make martyrs of their children" [27].

When an adult patient lacks decision-making capacity, the responsibility for all decisions falls to the patient's surrogate. Identifying a surrogate is delineated by a hierarchy determined by each state. Generally, there is a consistent pattern of spouse followed by adult children, then parent, and so on. In many states, there is a caveat that any individual identified by the patient as the surrogate takes precedent. It is important to note, however, that not all states designate domestic partners as the same authority as spouses and that there are individual state variations. In addition, a handful of states do not designate an official surrogacy hierarchy but instead state that the surrogate should be the "morally relevant agent." In the case of the individual who has no identifiable surrogate (the "unbefriended" patient), some states have designated the attending physician or other healthcare providers in conjunction with an ethics committee, while others make no such distinction. In these circumstances, it is essential to consult the local legal precedents in conjunction with the hospital ethics committee [28].

The role of the surrogate is to speak for the patient with a goal of adhering to the patient's preferences. When the patient's preferences are known, the surrogate relies on the "substituted judgment standard"—making the decision the patient would have most likely made. If the patient's wishes are unknown, then the "best interests" standard applies—a decision is made in the patient's best interest given the available information [23, 29]. Yet, as well intended as these standards may be, surrogates often have significant difficulty making decisions on behalf of patients. In a prospective study of surrogate decision-makers in an ICU, Boyd et al. [30] found that surrogates report using multiple sources of information, including the patient's strength of character and the patient's history of survival as factors in their interpretation of a physician's prognosis [30]. In only 2% of cases did the surrogates' beliefs about the patient's prognosis entirely reflect the information from the physician. Recognizing that there is likely to be a disconnect between what a surrogate hears from a physician and what they believe to be true about the patient's recovery is therefore an important point of discussion that needs to take place between the physician and the surrogate. Continuing to stress that the surrogate's role is to make the decision that the patient would make, rather than the decision the surrogate wants to make, is an important strategy when the surrogate continues to have difficulty through multiple conversations.

Shared Decision-Making and Family-Centered Care

There is ample support in the critical care literature to incorporate the patient and their family, when present, into medical decision-making in the ICU [6, 23, 27]. However, it is important to note that the emphasis on patient-centered care and respect for patient autonomy does not mean the physician relinquishes decision-making capacity. Placing the burden of decision-making entirely on a patient or a patient's surrogate in a time of acuity has been termed both ethically untenable in some instances and abandonment in others [31, 32]. Rather, a more productive approach to caring for the critically ill is the concept of shared decision-making and family-centered care [6, 32].

Shared decision-making between the patient and provider would seem intuitive, but as a guiding principle, it is complex, nuanced, and challenging. This is particularly true when a patient's ability to comprehend and communicate waxes and wanes with their illness [23]. Shared decision-making does necessarily imply a completely shared *responsibility* for decision-making. This means that following a discussion of treatment options that the physician should not simply ask the patient or surrogate what they would like to do. Once goals have been identified, it is appropriate for the physician to make a recommendation, similar to what would happen in a routine office visit. Some studies have shown that up to 20% of patients or surrogates wish to completely defer important medical decision to physicians [6]. Such transference of decision-making does not imply blanket assent [23]. Rather, it is the clinician's responsibility to ensure continued and ongoing communication with patients and their families to ensure that the care plan reflects the patient's goals and wishes [23].

Additional benefits can be seen with allowing family members increasing access to patients in the ICU and developing protocols for optimizing family support. This includes having family members witness to and participants in family meetings, rounds, and even resuscitations [32]. Having family members present during CPR, for example, has not been shown to have negative effects on resuscitation efforts nor the psychological outcomes of the family members [33–35]. Rather, incorporating patients and their families in their care to the extent that they desire demonstrates respect for the family unit and ensures that the patient's goals and values are upheld [6].

Futility and Potentially Inappropriate or Non-beneficial Interventions

In times of distress, it is not uncommon for physicians to be asked to perform futile/non-beneficial or potentially inappropriate interventions in hope of a recovery. Futile interventions are those that *cannot* accomplish a physiologic goal, which is also known as quantitative futility [6, 36, 37]. Inappropriate treatment, where there is *some* chance of meeting a physiologic goal but not significant or meaningful clinical improvement, is also known as qualitative futility [36]. In one prospective study of ICU clinicians, there was a sense that more than 10% of patients had received some form of futile treatment during their ICU stay [37]. In addition to the impact that potentially harmful or painful interventions may have on the patient, non-beneficial treatment has also been associated with high physician and nursing burnout [38].

In a 2015 official policy statement, multiple critical care societies, including the American Thoracic Society, the Society of Critical Care Medicine, and the American Association of Critical Care Nursing, among others, took a firm stance that *clinicians are not to provide futile interventions* and that they are to clearly communicate the reasons for the refusal [31]. The same holds true for proscribed treatments, which are those that are prohibited by applicable laws, judicial precedent, or widely accepted public policies [6]. An example of a proscribed practice would be altering organ allocation policies or providing lethal medication doses outside of explicitly defined circumstances.

But what should be done when families or surrogates disagree with providers on what is considered futile? With the exception of legally proscribed treatments, the law is variable with regard to the role that courts play in cases of futile interventions. For better or for worse, each state has its own laws regarding how entangled the courts are willing to become in cases of non-beneficial treatment [39]. In the Texas Advance Directives Act of 1999, for example, the only role of the judiciary in these cases is to potentially grant a family more time to find an alternative provider for a disputed treatment if the current provider and ethics committee deem the intervention futile [40]. Ultimately, the Texas law grants unilateral decision-making capacity to the provider and ethics committee in the event of an impasse.

If conflict remains despite initial attempts between providers and patients/surrogates, Bosslet et al. [31] suggests a seven-step process to resolve disagreements about potentially inappropriate treatments (Table 59.2) [31].

Occasionally, the nature of critical illness does not afford the time to complete all seven steps. In these circumstances, it is recommended that physician continue to refuse to provide the requested intervention while simultaneously striving to complete as much of the seven-step process as possible [31].

Table 59.2 Seven steps to conflict resolution

1. Enlist expert consultation to continue negotiation during the dispute resolution process
2. Give notice of the process to surrogates
3. Obtain a second medical opinion
4. Provide review by an interdisciplinary hospital committee
5. Offer surrogates the opportunity to transfer the patient to an alternate institution
6. Inform surrogates of the opportunity to pursue extramural appeal
7. Implement the decision of the resolution process

Adapted from Ref. [31]

Resources for Identifying Potentially Inappropriate Treatments

Estimating survival and outcomes in critically ill patients is a challenge owing to the extreme diversity of age, preexisting conditions, severity of illness, resources, etc. Multiple attempts at critical care prognosis have been made, and each has their own flaws, and even fewer are applicable to the intensive care setting. The largest of these—Acute Physiology and Chronic Health Evaluation (APACHE) I–IV, MPM (mortality probability model), and Simplified Acute Physiology (SAPS 1–3)—are meant to serve as tools for assessing ICU performance, not managing individual patients [41]. More individualized prognostic tools including the Sequential Organ Failure Assessment (SOFA) and the ACS NSQIP Surgical Risk Calculator exist, but they are really only meant to be applied to septic or preoperative patients with a single operative indication [42, 43]. Regardless, Sinuff et al. [44] found that ICU providers more accurately predicted patient mortality in the first 24 h than any scoring system [44].

Because all prognostic systems are flawed, an approach that focuses on goal-concordant care is more appropriate. One approach is the "best case/worst case" framework for organizing and visualizing patient treatment option. To do this, the physician outlines for the patient the "best," "worst," and "most likely" scenarios of various interventions (typically operating or not, although this can be applied to any intervention) based on both experience and best available evidence [45]. The reactions and goals of the patient or surrogate can then be gleaned from the conversations that follow. This allows for a more balanced and grounded discussion of the potential outcomes as they apply to the specific patient.

Improving Physician and Patient/Surrogate Communication

Surveys of families in an ICU cite a physician's communication skills as having equal or higher importance than their clinical skills [46]. Ironically, effective communication amounts to physicians communicating more but talking less. Studies of family conferences show that physicians tend to speak the majority of the time (average 70% of the words spoken), yet the proportion of family speech during these conferences tends to correlate with family members' satisfaction ratings [46]. While these are only associations and likely an oversimplification of a complex and dynamic situations, the importance of frequent, thorough, and honest communication between providers and patients and their families cannot be overstated. Providers tend to view family meetings and conversations as vehicles to transmit information and come to a decision. In this context, the narrative tends to follow a "tell-ask-tell" dynamic in which the provider gives information, asks whether there are questions, and summarizes the decision. A more effective method of communication in these scenarios follows an "ask-tell-ask-ask-ask" dynamic, in which the provider asks what the family understands, communicates additional information and corrects any misconceptions, asks what questions the patient or family has, asks what goals the patient has, and continues to ask questions until a decision emerges.

Allocation of Scarce Resources

Critical care resources, in the form of providers, staff, medications, and equipment, are scarce. The most common example of resource scarcity that critical care physicians will find themselves in is the shortage of ICU beds. In some places, this is an almost daily struggle. Multiple studies have shown that there is an increased mortality rate for patients refused or delayed ICU admission compared to those admitted [47–50]. This finding is likely the result of both delayed essential treatments in some circumstance, while in others admitting providers may have determined that a patient was "too sick to benefit" from intensive care interventions.

There are several strategies for mitigating ICU capacity strain including optimizing bed space, creation of step-down units [51, 52], revised triage policies including the use of rapid response teams [53], and improved discharge planning [51, 54]. Yet, none of these methods have been shown to consistently reduce ICU shortages. Therefore, in 2016, the American College of Critical Care Medicine updated their 1999 guidelines for ICU admission, discharge, and triage [55]. Particular recommendations include limiting ICU admission to those who need hourly or invasive monitoring only (intermediate medical units are for patients who need monitoring every 2–4 h) and that patients who have a higher probability of recovery and would accept intensive care including CPR receive a higher priority for ICU admission than those with a lower probability of recovery who choose not to receive CPR [53]. This is not an age- or diagnosis-specific recommendation; rather, admitting decisions should be based on patient's comorbidities, functional status, and care preferences.

While this is an overarching goal, they note that there are "no conclusive studies showing all-encompassing, definitive criteria for ICU admissions." [53]. ICU admission criteria therefore tend to be variable and based on the personnel, clinical areas of expertise, technologies, and resources available at each specific site. Given the inherent flaws in imperfect patient selection, any ICU admission model will inevitably have a component of over or under triage as patients are either admitted or refused admission to an ICU. In general, clinicians should err toward overtriage (occasionally accepting less critically ill patients who may not have needed the ICU) to reduce life-threatening undertriage when possible. Caution should be particularly applied in mass casualties, however, where the authors note that over triage can siphon care from the truly critically ill [53]. Ultimately, critical care medicine is dynamic, and determining a patient's ongoing need for ICU care and facilitating appropriate transfer out of the ICU is a central to optical resource utilization.

The principles of ICU management also apply to rarer situations of mass casualties or disasters. Planning for mass casualties or disasters, however, requires extensive preparation and collaboration with locoregional resources with critical care physicians providing significant input [56]. Yet, planning for all disasters is not feasible. One method that has been suggested in the 2014 CHEST consensus statement on surge capacity principles is that hospitals recognize the surge needs on a continuum. That is, there is conventional care (an expansion of standard practices), contingency care (utilizing less commonly used spaces, staff, and supplies), and crisis care (not consistent with usual care—i.e., being maximally resourceful). In general, the consensus statement makes the argument that hospitals should have concrete plans in place to be able to expand their critical care resources by at least 20% for a conventional response, 100% for a contingent response, and 200% for a crisis response [56]. An example of conventional response includes utilizing vacant beds, discharging or transferring lower acuity patients, canceling procedures, etc. [56]. Likewise, contingency care would be providing ICU care in an OR or PACU, while crisis care would require access to stockpiles and outside resources. Resources that are likely to be particularly scarce include respiratory and ventilator care, pharmacy, and radiology [57]. In such shortages adaptation, recycling, reallocation, and conservation practices may prolong resources (e.g., titrating oxygen saturations to 89% as opposed to 95%, using feeding tubes by gravity rather than pump, etc.) [57].

But which patients get priority in treatment? In 2008, the Task Force for Mass Critical Care met to establish a set of guidelines and recommendations in the event of a nationwide pandemic [58]. This working group focused on preparing for a flu pandemic, but the principles are the same regardless: emphasize locoregional preparation and maximize triage system at various levels of care and ration care only after expansion and augmentation of available resources have been exceeded [58]. When rationing is absolutely necessary, the Task Force recommends that critical care rationing be uniform, transparent, and abide by "objective medical criteria." The objective criteria to which they refer apply primarily to the methods of assessing lack of potential benefit from critical care intervention: the Sequential Organ Failure Assessment (SOFA) score and severity of chronic illness. A SOFA score is calculated using the patient's P/F ratio, platelet count, need for vasopressors, GCS, and creatinine or urine output. A SOFA score >15 or mean score that is worsening or stably ≥5 for 5 days or has six or more organ failures is associated with at least an 80% risk of mortality and may be considered for exclusion from critical care [58]. It is further recommended that a designated "triage officer," usually an intensivist separate from the primary attending, oversee the critical care inclusion and exclusion criteria.

Rationing of health care is an ethically and emotionally complex scenario for which there is no perfect process. While the focus and attention on what is not available to patients usually take precedence, it is important to note that palliative care is an equally essential and required component of all critical care.

Recommendations for End-of-Life Care in ICU

It is not uncommon that the role of the ICU provider is to guide the patient and their families through the dying process. Early discussions about goals of care, when possible, are associated with better quality of life, reduced use of non-beneficial medical care near death, enhanced goal-consistent care, positive family outcomes, and reduced costs [59]. Yet, eliciting a patient's goals of care can be a challenge, particularly in the acute care setting where providers and patients may meet for the first time in a crisis setting. It is therefore prudent for the ICU provider to make it a regular endeavor to elicit a patient's goals of care so the patient's wishes may be respected if the situation arises. In their 2014 review of best practices, Bernacki and Block provide a conversation guide for eliciting goals of care that centers around having patients answer the following questions [59]:

1. What is your understanding now of where you are with your illness?
2. How much information about what is likely to be ahead with your illness would you like from me? (This then prompts a discussion of prognosis.)
3. If your health situation worsens, what are your most important goals?
4. What are your biggest fears and worries about the future with your health?
5. What abilities are so critical to your life that you can't imagine living without them?
6. If you become sicker, how much are you willing to go through for the possibility of gaining more time?
7. How much does your family know about your priorities and wishes?

Eliciting goals of care is an important first step in discussing end-of-life care with patients and their families. Throughout the dying process, providers ought to be aware of the language that they use in an effort to provide maximal comfort. Providers should refer to decreasing interventions as "withdrawal of life-sustaining interventions" as "withdrawal of care" is inappropriate and may be distressing to patients and families. Further language recommendations include avoiding the term "agonal" as it may be mistaken for "agony" as well as using plain, non-euphemistic language including the words dead, dying, death, or die to communicate a prognosis or pronouncement [23].

Additional actions that may be taken to ease patients through the dying process include discontinuing treatments that do not provide comfort. This includes stopping life-sustaining interventions including blood products, IV fluids, nutritional support, antibiotics, etc. It is important, however, to re-recognize that respiratory support should not be abruptly discontinued as this may worsen dyspnea and make the patient uncomfortable [23]. At this time, palliative care including medications to treat pain, dyspnea, or delirium becomes the primary method of intervention. Family support throughout the dying process by the provider and bereavement experts is the final.

Organ Donation

The Uniform Anatomical Gift Act grant the rights of adults to decide to donate their organs. Surrogates cannot technically override a patient's decision to donate, but all efforts are made to align the patient's decision with the wishes of the family and surrogates. In cases where there is not an explicitly stated decision either through DMV registry, online donor registry, durable power of attorney, or advance directive, then the decision regarding organ donation falls to the surrogate decision-maker. If there is ever a dispute, then the Organ Procurement Organizations (OPO) will most likely honor the surrogate's decision after conversation with the surrogate and family. It is critically important to avoid any real or perceived conflict of interest between providing life-sustaining care and treatment for the patient and preparing for potential organ donation. This is best accomplished by completely separating these two functions and leaving any detailed conversations about organ donation and requests for family consent to the designated OPO personnel rather than a physician involved in the primary managing care team.

Donation After Circulatory Determination of Death (DCDD)

DCDD entails the recovery of organs after cessation of circulation among patients with severe neurological, neuromuscular, or pulmonary disease for whom decisions are made to forego further life-prolonging treatments [60]. DCDD—which is defined as 2 min of mechanical asystole—presents its own ethical challenges as the decision to donate is made *before* the declaration of death, and interventions may still be needed to promote the health of the organs even after the decision has been made to cease life-sustaining measures. These interventions, which are geared toward ensuring organ viability, by definition, occur simultaneously with the provision of end-of-life care for dying patients [60]. Providing therapies to promote organ donation is one of the few times that physicians provide care that is not intended to promote the survival of the patient. Because of this unique circumstance, a multidisciplinary committee comprised of the American Thoracic Society, International Society for Heart and Lung Transplantation, Society of Critical Care Medicine, and UNOS published an official statement on ethical and policy considerations in organ donation after circulatory determination of death in 2013 [60]. Specifically, they state that there are three ethical principles that frame DCDD health policy:

1. Acts that promote the opportunity to donate viable organs respect the patient's potential interest in becoming an organ donor.
2. The legitimacy of surrogate decision-making for critically ill patients whose wishes are unknown extends to decisions regarding organ donation.
3. If real or perceived conflicts arise between the goals of providing optimal end-of-life care and the goals of procuring organs, delivery of quality end-of-life care should take priority.

It should be noted that these policy statements exist for controlled DCDD. Unexpected DCDD raises its own ethical issues and does not carry consistent guidelines. Recommendations at this time regarding unexpected circulatory death are such that each event is to be examined on a case-by-case basis.

There is a general consensus that discussions regarding organ donation should *only* take place following the decision to withdraw life-sustaining measures. This is the policy at the majority of pediatric hospitals and is considered to be standard practice. While direct discussion of donation with the family may be delayed, physicians are encouraged to contact Organ Procurement Organization (OPO) within 1 h of identifying an impending death or decision to withdraw or limit life-sustaining therapies. The early notification provides time for patient evaluation as well as time to relay information about the opportunity to donate to families.

As far as who can obtain consent, the Center for Medicare and Medicaid requires that an OPO representative or a "designated requestor" who has taken an OPO-approved training program obtains consent for donation. Only under rare circumstances should members of the treatment team engage in consent discussions as ICU physicians and staff may have real or perceived conflicts of interest in caring for the patient versus preparing for organ donation.

Antemortem interventions "are ethically appropriate if they contribute to good transplant outcomes and have a low chance of harming the prospective donor" [60]. This may include moving the patient to an operating room to reduce organ recovery time, administering heparin or vasoactive medications, cannulating large vessels (although there is currently no consensus regarding the use of extracorporeal membrane oxygenation, ECMO), and performing bronchoscopy [60]. Certain physiologic parameters and goals (described below) have also been shown to be beneficial for organ preservation (Table 59.3) [61]:

Table 59.3 General physiologic goals for optimizing organ donation

Mean arterial pressure at least 60 mmHg
Maintain urine output at least 1 ml/kg/h
Left ventricle ejection fraction at least 45%
Lower vasopressor dose (e.g., dopamine ≤10 μg/kg/min)
Fluid replacement using hemodynamic parameters, particularly CVP or PAOP, and targeted at maintaining euvolemia of the donor
Recommended isotonic crystalloids are 0.9% saline and lactated Ringer solution

Adapted from Ref. [61]

Conclusion

The ICU is an inherently stressful environment owing to the critical nature of the patients therein. Given this, multiple ethical challenges are bound to arise as patients and providers alike are forced to make emotionally charged decisions often regarding the life or death of a patient. While there is no clear decision pathway for many of the ethical dilemmas that may arise, there are common themes in the literature of giving direct, honest prognoses, including the patient or their surrogate in the medical decision-making to the extent that they wish to be involved, being prepared to have difficult discussions surrounding end-of-life care, and having a low threshold to involve ethics committees if there are complex needs or communication challenges.

References

1. Schuster RA, Hong SY, Arnold RM, White DB. Investigating conflict in ICUs-is the clinicians' perspective enough? Crit Care Med. 2014;42:328–35.
2. Azoulay E, Timsit JF, Sprung CL, et al. Prevalence and factors of intensive care unit conflicts: the conflicus study. Am J Respir Crit Care Med. 2009;180:853–60.
3. Breen CM, Abernethy AP, Abbott KH, Tulsky JA. Conflict associated with decisions to limit life-sustaining treatment in intensive care units. J Gen Intern Med. 2001;16:283–9.
4. Hawryluck L, Sibbald R, Chidwick P. The standard of care and conflicts at the end of life in critical care: lessons from medical-legal crossroads and the role of a quasi-judicial tribunal in decision-making. J Crit Care. 2013;28:1055–61.
5. Studdert DM, Mello MM, Burns JP, et al. Conflict in the care of patients with prolonged stay in the ICU: types, sources, and predictors. Intensive Care Med. 2003;29:1489–97.
6. Kon AA, Davidson JE, Morrison W, et al. Shared decision making in ICUs: an American College of Critical Care Medicine and American Thoracic Society Policy Statement. Crit Care Med. 2016;44:188–201.
7. Heyland D, Cook D, Bagshaw SM, et al. The very elderly admitted to ICU: a quality finish? Crit Care Med. 2015;43:1352–60.
8. Angus DC, Barnato AE, Linde-Zwirble WT, et al. Use of intensive care at the end of life in the United States: an epidemiologic study. Crit Care Med. 2004;32:638–43.
9. Teno JM, Gozalo PL, Bynum JP, et al. Change in end-of-life care for Medicare beneficiaries: site of death, place of care, and health care transitions in 2000, 2005, and 2009. JAMA. 2013;309:470–7.
10. Ortman J, Velkoff V, Hogan H. An aging nation: the older population in the United States. Washington, DC: U.S. Census Bureau; 2014.
11. Marik PE. The cost of inappropriate care at the end of life: implications for an aging population. Am J Hosp Palliat Care. 2015;32:703–8.
12. Timmers TK, Verhofstad MH, Moons KG, Leenen LP. Long-term survival after surgical intensive care unit admission: fifty percent die within 10 years. Ann Surg. 2011;253:151–7.
13. Danis M, Southerland LI, Garrett JM, et al. A prospective study of advance directives for life-sustaining care. N Engl J Med. 1991;324:882–8.
14. Silveira MJ, Kim SY, Langa KM. Advance directives and outcomes of surrogate decision making before death. N Engl J Med. 2010;362:1211–8.
15. Swetz KM, Crowley ME, Hook C, Mueller PS. Report of 255 clinical ethics consultations and review of the literature. Mayo Clin Proc. 2007;82:686–91.
16. Gilmer T, Schneiderman LJ, Teetzel H, et al. The costs of nonbeneficial treatment in the intensive care setting. Health Aff (Millwood). 2005;24:961–71.
17. Andereck WS, McGaughey JW, Schneiderman LJ, Jonsen AR. Seeking to reduce nonbeneficial treatment in the ICU: an exploratory trial of proactive ethics intervention. Crit Care Med. 2014;42:824–30.
18. WHO. Palliative care. 2015. http://www.who.int/mediacentre/factsheets/fs402/en/. Accessed 12 Dec 2016.
19. Weissman DE, Meier DE. Identifying patients in need of a palliative care assessment in the hospital setting: a consensus report from the Center to Advance Palliative Care. J Palliat Med. 2011;14:17–23.
20. Mosenthal AC, Weissman DE, Curtis JR, et al. Integrating palliative care in the surgical and trauma intensive care unit: a report from the Improving Palliative Care in the Intensive Care Unit (IPAL-ICU) Project Advisory Board and the Center to Advance Palliative Care. Crit Care Med. 2012;40:1199–206.
21. Barr J, Fraser GL, Puntillo K, et al. Clinical practice guidelines for the management of pain, agitation, and delirium in adult patients in the intensive care unit. Crit Care Med. 2013;41:263–306.
22. Hawryluck LA, Harvey WR, Lemieux-Charles L, Singer PA. Consensus guidelines on analgesia and sedation in dying intensive care unit patients. BMC Med Ethics. 2002;3:E3.
23. Truog RD, Campbell ML, Curtis JR, et al. Recommendations for end-of-life care in the intensive care unit: a consensus statement by the American College [corrected] of Critical Care Medicine. Crit Care Med. 2008;36:953–63.
24. Schloendorff v. Society of New York Hospital. New York Court of Appeals; 1914.
25. In re Quinlan. New Jersey Supreme Court; 1976.
26. Cruzan v. Director, Missouri Department of Health. United States Supreme Court; 1990.
27. Prince v. Commonwealth of Massachusetts. Supreme Court of the U.S.; 1944. p. 158.
28. American Bar Association Commission on Law and Aging. Default surrogate consent statutes. 2014. http://www.americanbar.org/content/dam/aba/administrative/law_aging/2014_default_surrogate_consent_statutes.authcheckdam.pdf. Accessed 21 Oct 2016.
29. Cooper Z, Courtwright A, Karlage A, Gawande A, Block S. Pitfalls in communication that lead to nonbeneficial emergency surgery in elderly patients with serious illness: description of the problem and elements of a solution. Ann Surg. 2014;260:949–57.
30. Boyd EA, Lo B, Evans LR, et al. "It's not just what the doctor tells me:" factors that influence surrogate decision-makers' perceptions of prognosis. Crit Care Med. 2010;38:1270–5.
31. Bosslet GT, Pope TM, Rubenfeld GD, et al. An official ATS/AACN/ACCP/ESICM/SCCM policy statement: responding to requests for potentially inappropriate treatments in intensive care units. Am J Respir Crit Care Med. 2015;191:1318–30.
32. Davidson JE, Powers K, Hedayat KM, et al. Clinical practice guidelines for support of the family in the patient-centered intensive care unit: American College of Critical Care Medicine Task Force 2004-2005. Crit Care Med. 2007;35:605–22.
33. De Stefano C, Normand D, Jabre P, et al. Family presence during resuscitation: a qualitative analysis from a national multicenter randomized clinical trial. PLoS One. 2016;11:e0156100.
34. Jabre P, Belpomme V, Azoulay E, et al. Family presence during cardiopulmonary resuscitation. N Engl J Med. 2013;368:1008–18.
35. Meyers TA, Eichhorn DJ, Guzzetta CE, et al. Family presence during invasive procedures and resuscitation. Am J Nurs. 2000;100:32–42. quiz 3
36. Schneiderman LJ. Defining medical futility and improving medical care. J Bioeth Inq. 2011;8:123–31.
37. Huynh TN, Kleerup EC, Wiley JF, et al. The frequency and cost of treatment perceived to be futile in critical care. JAMA Intern Med. 2013;173:1887–94.
38. Schwarzkopf D, Rüddel H, Thomas-Rüddel DO, et al. Perceived nonbeneficial treatment of patients, burnout, and intention to leave the job among ICU nurses and junior and senior physicians. Crit Care Med. 2017;45:e265–73.
39. White DB, Pope TM. The courts, futility, and the ends of medicine. JAMA. 2012;307:151–2.
40. Fine RL. Medical futility and the Texas Advance Directives Act of 1999. Proc (Bayl Univ Med Cent). 2000;13:144–7.
41. Breslow MJ, Badawi O. Severity scoring in the critically ill: part 1--interpretation and accuracy of outcome prediction scoring systems. Chest. 2012;141:245–52.
42. Jones AE, Trzeciak S, Kline JA. The Sequential Organ Failure Assessment score for predicting outcome in patients with severe sepsis and evidence of hypoperfusion at the time of emergency department presentation. Crit Care Med. 2009;37:1649–54.
43. American College of Surgery. ACS NSQIP surgical risk calculator. 2017. http://riskcalculator.facs.org/. Accessed 10 Jan 2017.

44. Sinuff T, Adhikari NK, Cook DJ, et al. Mortality predictions in the intensive care unit: comparing physicians with scoring systems. Crit Care Med. 2006;34:878–85.
45. Kruser JM, Nabozny MJ, Steffens NM, et al. "Best case/worst case": qualitative evaluation of a novel communication tool for difficult in-the-moment surgical decisions. J Am Geriatr Soc. 2015;63:1805–11.
46. McDonagh JR, Elliott TB, Engelberg RA, et al. Family satisfaction with family conferences about end-of-life care in the intensive care unit: increased proportion of family speech is associated with increased satisfaction. Crit Care Med. 2004;32:1484–8.
47. Sinuff T, Kahnamoui K, Cook DJ, Luce JM, Levy MM. Force VEaRiCCT. Rationing critical care beds: a systematic review. Crit Care Med. 2004;32:1588–97.
48. Cardoso LT, Grion CM, Matsuo T, et al. Impact of delayed admission to intensive care units on mortality of critically ill patients: a cohort study. Crit Care. 2011;15:R28.
49. Bing-Hua YU. Delayed admission to intensive care unit for critically surgical patients is associated with increased mortality. Am J Surg. 2014;208:268–74.
50. Chalfin DB, Trzeciak S, Likourezos A, Baumann BM, Dellinger RP, DELAY-ED Study Group. Impact of delayed transfer of critically ill patients from the emergency department to the intensive care unit. Crit Care Med. 2007;35:1477–83.
51. Eachempati SR, Hydo LJ, Barie PS. The effect of an intermediate care unit on the demographics and outcomes of a surgical intensive care unit population. Arch Surg. 2004;139:315–9.
52. Prin M, Wunsch H. The role of stepdown beds in hospital care. Am J Respir Crit Care Med. 2014;190:1210–6.
53. Nates JL, Nunnally M, Kleinpell R, et al. ICU admission, discharge, and triage guidelines: a framework to enhance clinical operations, development of institutional policies, and further research. Crit Care Med. 2016;44:1553–602.
54. Mathews KS, Long EF. A conceptual framework for improving critical care patient flow and bed use. Ann Am Thorac Soc. 2015;12:886–94.
55. Blanch L, Abillama FF, Amin P, et al. Triage decisions for ICU admission: report from the Task Force of the World Federation of Societies of Intensive and Critical Care Medicine. J Crit Care. 2016;36:301–5.
56. Hick JL, Einav S, Hanfling D, et al. Surge capacity principles: care of the critically ill and injured during pandemics and disasters: CHEST consensus statement. Chest. 2014;146:e1S–e16S.
57. Einav S, Hick JL, Hanfling D, et al. Surge capacity logistics: care of the critically ill and injured during pandemics and disasters: CHEST consensus statement. Chest. 2014;146:e17S–43S.
58. Devereaux AV, Dichter JR, Christian MD, et al. Definitive care for the critically ill during a disaster: a framework for allocation of scarce resources in mass critical care: from a Task Force for Mass Critical Care summit meeting, January 26–27, 2007, Chicago, IL. Chest. 2008;133:51S–66S.
59. Bernacki RE, Block SD, Force ACoPHVCT. Communication about serious illness care goals: a review and synthesis of best practices. JAMA Intern Med. 2014;174:1994–2003.
60. Gries CJ, White DB, Truog RD, et al. An official American Thoracic Society/International Society for Heart and Lung Transplantation/Society of Critical Care Medicine/Association of Organ and Procurement Organizations/United Network of Organ Sharing Statement: ethical and policy considerations in organ donation after circulatory determination of death. Am J Respir Crit Care Med. 2013;188:103–9.
61. Kotloff RM, Blosser S, Fulda GJ, et al. Management of the Potential Organ Donor in the ICU: Society of Critical Care Medicine/American College of Chest Physicians/Association of Organ Procurement Organizations Consensus Statement. Crit Care Med. 2015;43:1291–325.

Biostatistics and Research Design for Clinicians

60

Tarsicio Uribe-Leitz, Alyssa Fitzpatrick Harlow, and Adil H. Haider

Basic Biostatistics for Clinicians

A broad understanding of the basic concepts of biostatistics is essential for surgeons. This chapter serves as a succinct guide of key biostatistics concepts to help develop sound research questions and evaluate evidence to advance surgical practice.

Basic Concepts

To better understand biostatistics, we first need to define common terminology. Following are some terms that we will frequently use during this chapter.

Population The entire pool of individuals from which our study sample is drawn. If, for example, we are interested in the body mass index (BMI) of patients admitted to the trauma service, the population will consist of all patients admitted to the trauma service, regardless of age or other qualifying variables. A population can be finite or conceptually infinite. If the population measurements are fixed, it is considered finite. Conversely, if there is nonstop succession of measurements, it is considered infinite.

Sample A group of individuals under consideration for a study, drawn from the population. For example, the selected population consists of all patients admitted to the trauma service. If we analyze the BMI of only a fraction of these patients, such as those seen between a specified period of time (e.g., 1 June to 31 July), that is a *sample*.

T. Uribe-Leitz · A. F. Harlow · A. H. Haider (✉)
Center for Surgery and Public Health (CSPH), Brigham and Women's Hospital, Boston, MA, USA
e-mail: ahhaider@partners.org

Inference To reach a conclusion about a population based on the information obtained from the sample drawn from that population.

Types of Data *Continuous (quantitative) variable:* A variable with an unlimited number of possible measurements ranging between a known minimum and maximum. For example, age, height, and blood pressure.

- *Categorical variable:* A variable with a defined number of measurements. Below are the different types and examples of categorical variables.
  - *Binary*: Dichotomous categories. For example, yes/no, disease/no disease, and 0 or 1.
  - *Nominal*: No order to the categories. For example, race, ethnicity, and eye color
  - *Ordinal*: Ordered categories. For example, tumor stage I–IV
- *Dependent variable:* Also known as the outcome variable, or the primary response. For example, survival or complications.
- *Independent variable:* Also known as the predictor, exposure, or risk factor variable when related to the dependent variable. For example, demographics, comorbidities, and physician/hospital characteristics.

Generating and Testing Hypotheses

Defining a Solid Research Question

The first step to any research study is to define your research question: a clear question statement that identifies the specific objectives of the study. The research question serves as a logical construct that will eventually translate a problem area into an operational hypothesis. The steps toward establishing an operational hypothesis are as follows:

A. Salim et al. (eds.), *Surgical Critical Care Therapy*, https://doi.org/10.1007/978-3-319-71712-8_60

1. Begin by defining the general *area* of research you plan to address.
2. The next step is to define the *topic* of interest for your study.
3. Once you have established your topic, define your *research question.*
4. Your research question will lead to a *proposition.*
5. The proposition will ultimately translate into a *hypothesis.*

These steps will help the researcher come up with a very specific question that leads to testing a specific hypothesis. The research question is oftentimes called an objective or aim; however, framing it as a question allows the researcher to begin focusing the hypothesis and thinking about how to find an answer.

We recommend using the **FINER** criteria [8] to support the development of a meaningful research question. According to the FINER criteria, a research question should be:

Feasible: Manageable in time, scope, and cost, with access to the population of interest.
Interesting: To the scientific community and potentially to the public.
Novel: Adds to the surgical and scientific literature.
Ethical: Complies with local, national, and/or international ethical research standards.
Relevant: It must have clinical relevance.

Ineffective or poor research questions are those that are not meaningful to anybody (including yourself), as well as those that are generated from data dredging or "fishing expeditions" (gathering new data with the hopes that it will lead to a research question). Similarly, expecting a research question to emerge from routine clinical records leads to biased and confounded information that lacks the information needed to answer a question reliably, given that the records were originally collected for a purpose other than research.

Once the area and topic of interest are established, how does one focus their research question? The researcher may benefit from a brief literature search for previous evidence, discussing with colleagues or other experts in the field and narrowing the question down to a particular time, place, or group of interest, in order to clearly express what it is that he or she expects to find. The **PICO** [3] format is a useful resource to help in the development of a specific research question. It includes establishing the **P**opulation of interest (e.g., disease or condition, stage/severity, demographic characteristics like age, race, or gender), the **I**ntervention being studied (e.g., type, dose, duration, timing, route), the **C**omparison group (e.g., risk or treatment, placebo or other active treatment), and the **O**utcome of interest (e.g., frequency, risk, benefit, harm, dichotomous or continuous, type mortality, morbidity, quality of life, etc.). **T**iming is oftentimes added to PICO (T) to specify time frame during which the study will take place. Defining the population of interest (and the stringency of inclusion and exclusion criteria) sets the stage for the interpretation, and ultimately the applicability and generalizability, of the research findings. For example, if the study population is restricted, this may limit bias and increase the study's internal validity. However, this is at the expense of external validity, as a restricted population will reduce the generalizability of the findings to the clinical setting. On the other hand, if the study population is broadly defined, the results may be representative of the clinical setting, but there is a chance for increased bias and reduced internal validity [4, 9].

Hypothesis-Generating Vs. Hypothesis-Testing Research

There are two general types of research, hypothesis-generating studies and hypothesis- testing studies. A *hypothesis* can be defined as a prediction statement about expected outcomes. It must include measurable variables and a primary outcome of interest. A good hypothesis should be direct and explicit, have a substantive link to the literature and theory, be testable, and have implications that are understandable and easy to envision. Hypotheses are intended to be tested against actual data relevant to the problem of interest. A *hypothesis-generating study* is intended to spot possible leads worthy of further research; this often takes the form of large-scale studies on a representative population designed to explore cause and effect of a phenomenon. Findings from such studies can generate both specific hypotheses to be tested in future studies or information used to make these studies more cost-effective. A *hypothesis-testing study* aims to confirm or reject a specific hypothesis. For this reason, they are commonly based on a previous hypothesis-generating study, previous observations, or meaningful ramifications of other research. These studies include randomized trials and pre-post studies. Pilot studies are preliminary, hypothesis-testing studies in which research designs intended for hypothesis testing are "tried out." A summary of the steps involved for each type of study is shown in Table 60.1 [2].

Study Design Selection

Choosing the appropriate study design to test the hypothesis is one of the most important steps in a successful research project. Before diving into the different types of study designs, it is important to distinguish between observational and experimental studies ("Study Designs"), as all study designs can be grouped into either one of these categories. As the names imply, an observational study observes,

Table 60.1 Generating and testing a hypothesis in clinical research

Hypothesis generation	Hypothesis testing
Identification of relevant patient population and consent	Gather background information and consent
Generate high-throughput data	Identify subjects
Parse data for patterns	Divide into groups (e.g., cases/controls)
Formulate clinical hypotheses	Apply a biological assay or test to subject
Perform clinical research to refute/support	Interpret data and prove or disprove hypothesis
Interpret data, refine, and extend hypothesis	

Adapted from Biesecker [2]

while an experimental study experiments. Below are more detailed definitions.

Observational studies involve observing natural effects without manipulation on the part of the researcher. This type of study is valuable when the researcher is interested in studying the effects of exposures that are difficult (or unethical) to manipulate. Limitations of observational studies include the potential for sampling bias, a need to control for confounders, and a weaker claim for causality. Case-control, cohort, and some cross-sectional study designs are examples of observational study designs. Scientists who undertake observational studies are sometimes known as *differentialists*.

Experimental studies test the effects of an intervention or treatment. The researcher manipulates the exposure by allocating participants to an intervention (exposure) group and following them under carefully controlled conditions. Sampling must be random and representative. Experimental study designs control for confounders, and therefore the researcher can make strong claims regarding causality. An example of an experimental study design includes a double-blind randomized controlled trial. Scientists who undertake experimental studies are sometimes known as *experimentalists*.

The distinction between observational and experimental studies is important because the study design affects the statistical methods used during analysis. For example, while simpler statistical methods (chi-square or t-test) will suffice for a well-designed experimental study, more complex statistical methods might be required for an observational study. Of note, complex statistical methods contribute to, but do not necessarily guarantee, stronger evidence. A tree of the most basic study designs is shown in Fig. 60.1 ("Study Designs").

Descriptive studies describe what is happening on a population level. These include case reports, case series, qualitative studies, and cross-sectional survey studies. Analytic studies examine the effect of interventions/exposures on outcomes. They compare the frequency of outcomes in a comparison group (known as a control group), with the frequency in the intervention or exposed group, in order to quantify the effect. Analytic studies may be experimental (e.g., parallel group or crossover studies) or observational (e.g., cohort study, cross-sectional and case-control studies).

Figure 60.2 shows the hierarchy of evidence generated from different study designs. At the top of the pyramid are meta-analyses. Meta-analyses are heavily evidence-based and less numerous and thus can only be written once considerable publications on a particular topic exist. The opposite holds true toward the base of the pyramid case reports and cross-sectional studies are the first articles published on new topics, often greater in number, and less evidence-based. The strength of study design drives evidence-based clinical decision-making. Below we provide more detail on each study design.

Case Reports *("Study Design 101")*

Case reports describe and interpret an individual clinical case, including unique or unexplained diseases and syndromes, interesting variations of diseases and conditions, unexpected events in cases that might yield new useful information, and two or more unexpected diseases or disorders in one patient. Case reports represent the first line of evidence and are considered the lowest level of evidence.

Cross-Sectional Study *("Study Design 101")*

Cross-sectional studies examine the relationship between diseases or other health-related characteristics and other variables of interest in a defined population at one particular point or "slice" in time. The exposure and outcomes are measured simultaneously. Cross-sectional designs can quantify prevalence, risk, or diagnostic test accuracy.

Case-Control Study *("Study Design 101")*

Case-control studies compare patients who have a disease or outcome of interest (cases) with patients who do not have the disease or outcome (controls). Past exposures related to the risk factor of interest are then compared between each group: cases and controls. Case-control studies are only able to estimate odds.

Cohort Study *("Study Design 101")*

One or more samples, called cohorts, are established, and data is obtained to determine which members of the cohort have been exposed to the factor of interest (exposure). The cohort is then followed prospectively over time to see which members develop the outcome (disease) of interest. This allows the researcher to determine which initial participant characteristics (risk factors or exposures) are associated with the outcome. No allocation of exposure is made by the researcher. The cohort study is the best study design to establish the effects of risk factors on an outcome.

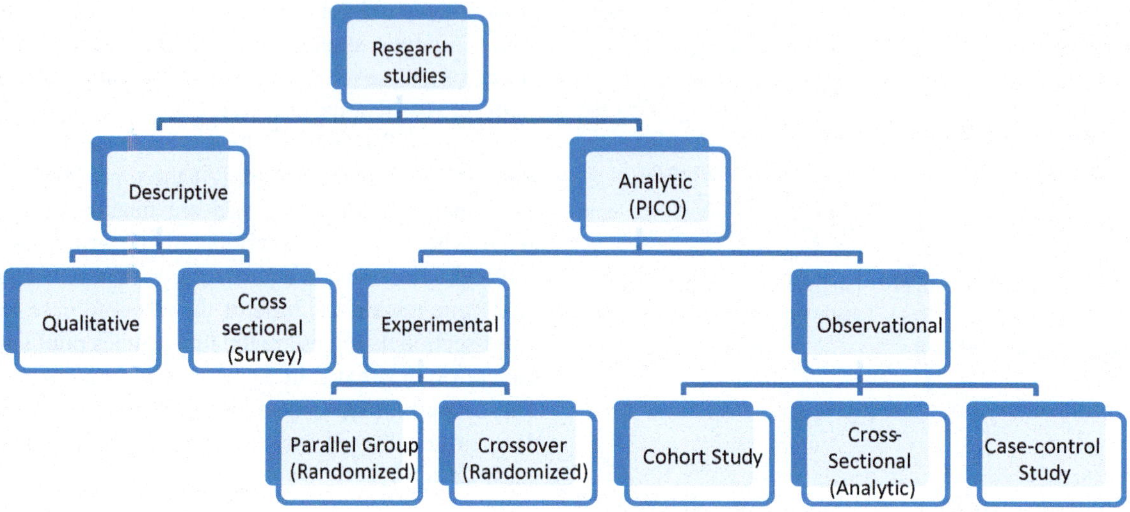

Fig. 60.1 Tree of different study designs (Adapted from Centre for Evidence-Based Medicine (CEBM))

Fig. 60.2 Hierarchy of Evidence. This pyramid shows the strength of different study designs for evidence-based clinical decision-making, with the highest level of evidence at the top

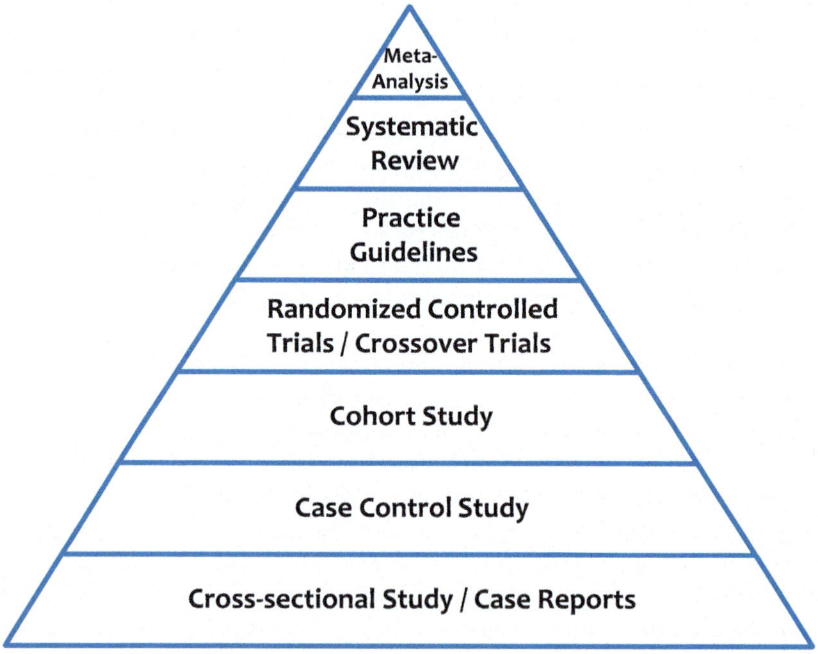

Randomized Controlled Trials (RTC) *("Study Design 101")*

A randomized controlled trial (RCT) is an experimental comparison study in which participants are allocated to either a treatment/intervention group or control/placebo group, using a random mechanism. Randomization serves to balance the treatment and control group in terms of patient characteristics. The only expected difference between groups in a RCT is the exposure/treatment under investigation. The RCT is the best study design for analyzing the effect of an intervention.

Crossover Trials *("Study Design 101")*

Crossover trials are a type of controlled trial in which all participants serve as their own controls. Participants will be in both intervention and placebo groups at some point, after a washout period in between therapies/exposures to ensure there is no residual effect of treatment.

Evidence-Based (Practice) Guidelines *("Study Design 101")*

Evidence-based (practice) guidelines are statements produced by a panel of experts in the relevant field that outline the current gold standards in clinical practice. The statements are produced after an extensive review of the literature and are used to inform health-care professionals and patients during clinical decision-making; they should be reviewed frequently and updated as needed for continued accuracy and relevance.

Systematic Review *("Study Design 101")*

A systematic review is a comprehensive overview of all relevant studies (published or unpublished) on a particular clinical or health-related topic or question.

Meta-Analysis *("Study Design 101")*

Meta-analyses are systematic combinations of pertinent qualitative and quantitative study data from numerous selected studies; the goal is to develop a single conclusion that has greater statistical power than a single study. Meta-analyses are statistically stronger than the analysis of any single study due to bigger sample sizes, more diversity, and accumulated effects and results. Combining several selected RCTs would be the highest level of evidence on the evidence hierarchy.

The study design used impacts how the researcher will deal with confounders (variables associated with both the exposure and outcome that distort the true association, biasing the results). For instance, RCTs minimize differences between groups in known and unknown confounders. Therefore, simpler statistical univariate analyses such as chi-square or student's t-test can be performed. On the other hand, observational cohort studies adjust for confounders during analysis and therefore require more complex statistical methods such as multiple logistic or linear regression analyses. Finally, case-control studies match based on important confounders, requiring regression analyses for matched pairs, such as conditional logistic regression. The key pros and cons of each study design are highlighted in Table 60.2.

Several systems have been created to rank evidence by quality in order to inform evidence-based clinical decision-making. Table 60.3 shows one system proposed by the US Preventive Service Task Force (USPSTF) for ranking evidence about the effectiveness of treatments or screening [6]. Level I is the highest level of evidence, and level III the lowest. Furthermore, recommendations to guide clinical decision-making have been developed by classifying and balancing the risks and benefits of different levels of evidence. Table 60.4 shows the system used by the USPSTF. Of note, recommendations are intended for specific populations and are followed by rational statements.

Analysis Plan: The Twofold Approach

Approaching the analysis plan using a "twofold approach" helps to formulate a clear and comprehensive analysis plan. The twofold approach includes using descriptive statistics followed by inferential statistics.

Descriptive Statistics

Once the raw data from the sample is available for analyses, the researcher seeks to arrange, organize, and summarize in order to make sense of it all. The summarization of the data to a single measure is defined as a *descriptive measure* [5]. Descriptive statistics are important when generalizing to the population and usually constitute Table 60.1 of most studies. Descriptive statistics provide researchers with an understanding of the basic features of their data. This includes information on measures of central tendency, distribution of the data, and measures of dispersion.

Measures of Central Tendency

Measures of central tendency tell the researcher where the middle of their data lies. In other words, measures of central tendency transmit information in relation to the average of a set of values. The three most commonly used measures of central tendency are the *mean*, the *median*, and the *mode*.

- *Mean*: The sum of a set of values in a population or a sample divided by the total number of values added.
  - Population mean: $\mu = (\Sigma X_i)/N$, where N = number of values in the population
  - Sample mean: $\bar{x} = (\Sigma X_i)/n$, where n = number of values in the sample
- *Median*: The value that separates a set of values into two even parts (top 50% from the bottom 50%). If the number is odd, the median will be the middle value after arranging the values by order of magnitude. If the number is even, the median is the average of the two middle values. Median is preferred for nonsymmetric data because it is less sensitive to outliers than the mean.
- *Mode*: The most frequently occurring value in a set of observations. It is possible to have more than one mode, or no mode, in the case where all values are different.

Distribution of the Data

The distribution of the data shows the researcher the overall shape, spread, and center of their data. A normal distribution is the probability that a continuous outcome will follow a bell-shaped curve (a.k.a. Gaussian distribution). In a normal distribution, the mean = median = mode and the distribution are symmetric about the mean. The empirical rule suggests that approximately 68% of the values fall between the mean and one standard deviation; approximately 95% of the values fall between the mean and two standard deviations; and 99.9% of the values fall between the mean and three standard deviations, as shown in Fig. 60.3.

Measures of Dispersion

Measures of dispersion convey information regarding the amount of variability present in a set of data. Below are some commonly used measures of dispersion.

Table 60.2 Study design pros and cons

Study design	Pros	Cons
Case reports	Useful to identify new trends or diseases Helpful to discover rare manifestations of disease	Challenging generalizability Lowest level of evidence
Cross-sectional study	Cost-effective and simple Relatively free form ethical restrictions	Establishes association but not causality Potential sources of bias: recall bias, social desirability bias, researcher's bias Unequal group sizes are possible Unequal distribution on confounders likely
Case-control study	Beneficial when dealing with rare conditions or diseases Requires less time to conduct the study, the condition or disease has already occurred Allows the study of multiple risk factors at simultaneously Oftentimes initial study to establish an association	Relies on recall or records to determine exposure status Potential for confounders Selection of suitable control groups can be challenging Potential bias: recall bias and selection bias
Cohort study	Ethically safe Participants can be matched (helping to limit confounding variables) Can establish temporality and directionality of events Eligibility criteria and outcome assessments can be standardized Less costly and complicated to conduct RTC's	Confounding variables can make identifying cohorts difficult Imbalances in patient characteristics between groups could exist due to lack of randomization Complicated blinding or masking Outcome of interest could take a long time to occur
Randomized controlled trials	Population bias taken care of with a successful Easier to blind or mask Statistical analysis of results can be performed with common statistical tools Clearly identified participating populations	Time and resource expensive Volunteer biases: population participating may not be representative of the whole Causation cannot be ascertained Attrition of participating individuals related to treatment
Crossover trials	Since all participants serve as their own controls, error variance is reduced requiring smaller sample sizes All participants receive treatment	Randomization can be implied for statistical purposes Blinding/masking can be maintained All participants receive placebo or alternative treatment Washout period can take a long time Not adequate for treatments with permanent effects Potential for carryover effects to confound results
Evidence-based (practice) guidelines	Developed by experts in the field Founded on scientific published literature Provides useful guidance for clinicians Evidence-based resource	Guidelines may be slow to change or be updated Limited data on controversial topics Costly and time-intensive to produce Recommendations can vary depending on the type of organization creating the guidelines
Systematic review	Exhaustive review of the up-to-date available evidence, including current literature, unpublished studies, and ongoing research More efficient, reliable, accurate, and generalizable than creating new study Evidence-based resource	Requires a lot of time Can be challenging to combine studies
Meta-analysis	Superior statistical power Confirmatory data analysis Increased capacity to transfer to general population Evidence-based resource	Complex and prolonged identification of right studies Studies may not provide sufficient data for inclusion and analysis Entails complex statistical techniques Often heterogeneity of study populations

Adapted from Himmelfarb Health Sciences Library [7]

Range Difference between the minimum and maximum values in a set of observations.

Variance Average squared deviation from the mean. Not an appropriate measure of dispersion when looking to express original units, since it represents square units and not the original units of the data.

$$s^2 = \frac{\Sigma\left(X - \bar{X}\right)^2}{N-1}$$

Standard Deviation (SD) Square root of the variance. Most commonly used measure of dispersion provides a measure of dispersion in the original units used in the data.

$$\sigma = \sqrt{\frac{1}{N}\sum_{i=1}^{N}\left(x_i - \mu\right)^2}$$

Percentiles and Quartiles Percentiles are values in the distribution that hold a specified percentage of the popula-

Table 60.3 US Preventive Service Task Force (USPTF) ranking of evidence quality

Level	Strength of study design for evidence-based clinical decision-making
I	Evidence obtained from at least one properly designed randomized controlled trial
II-1	Evidence obtained from well-designed controlled trials without randomization
II-2	Evidence obtained from well-designed cohort or case-control analytic studies, preferably from more than one center or research group
II-3	Evidence obtained from multiple time series with or without the intervention. Dramatic results in uncontrolled trials might also be regarded as this type of evidence
III	Opinions of respected authorities, based on clinical experience, descriptive studies, or reports of expert committees

Adapted from Harris et al. [6]

Table 60.4 Preventive Service Task Force (USPTF) recommendations for clinical service

Recommendation	Language
Level A	Good scientific evidence suggests that the benefits of the clinical service substantially outweigh the potential risks. Clinicians should discuss the service with eligible patients
Level B	At least fair scientific evidence suggests that the benefits of the clinical service outweigh the potential risks. Clinicians should discuss the service with eligible patients
Level C	At least fair scientific evidence suggests that there are benefits provided by the clinical service, but the balance between benefits and risks is too close for making general recommendations
Level D	At least fair scientific evidence suggests that the risks of the clinical service outweigh potential benefits. Clinicians should not routinely offer the service to asymptomatic patients
Level I	Scientific evidence is lacking, of poor quality, or conflicting, such that the risk versus benefit balance cannot be assessed. Clinicians should help patients understand the uncertainty surrounding the clinical service

Adapted from Harris et al. [6]

tion below it. Quartiles are values that divide a distribution into four equally sized groups.

Interquartile Range (IQR) Difference between the third and first quartiles, as shown in Fig. 60.4.

$$\text{IQR} = Q_3 - Q_1$$

Inferential Statistics

Inferential statistics are used to reach a conclusion about a population based on the information contained in a sample drawn from that population. The goal of inferential analyses is to describe the effects or patterns of correlations between variables. It contains both univariate and multivariate analyses.

Univariate Analyses Univariate analyses are used when the researcher is interested in analyzing one dependent outcome variable and one independent predictor variable. An example of a univariate analysis would be to determine the association between functional deficit (dependent variable) and age (independent variable) in patients after trauma surgery.

Determining which type of univariate statistical test to use will vary depending on factors such as the type of variables (categorical vs. continuous), the number of groups being compared, if the data are paired or dependent, and if the data are normally distributed (when dealing with continuous data). The following are examples of univariate statistical test: chi-square (Fisher's exact test), McNemar test (non-independent data), student's t-test, and analysis of variance (ANOVA). Table 60.5 can help determine which type of analysis to use depending on the nature of the data.

Multivariate Analyses Multivariate analyses are used when the researcher must assess one dependent outcome variable and multiple independent predictor variables. For example, if the researcher is interested in determining the association between functional deficit and age in patients after trauma surgery, but would like to adjust for other factors such as duration of surgery, nutrition status, BMI, or existing comorbidities, then a multivariate analysis would be appropriate.

Multiple regression analysis is the most common type of multivariate statistical test. Multiple regression is used when one needs to evaluate the effect of an intervention (or exposure) while adjusting for multiple confounders, such as with an observational cohort study. It is also used to assess for an interaction (effect modification) of one variable on another. A confounder is a variable that is associated with the exposure or the predictor and the outcome, but is not in the causal pathway. Multiple regression includes both logistic and linear regression models. If the outcome variable is continuous, a linear regression is the appropriate analysis to run. If the outcome variable is categorical, a logistic regression should be used to analyze the data. When the dependent variable is dichotomous (outcome is 1 or 0), the prediction probabilities of an outcome result can range from $-\infty$ to $+\infty$. The solution in this case is to perform a logistic transformation.

There are multiple methods one can use to select which variables should be included in a regression model. Two of the most common approaches are forward selection and backward elimination to evaluate fit and performance. Forward selection, as its name implies, begins with one variable and adds extra variables one at a time. The backward elimination method begins with all potential variables, and followed by eliminating variables one

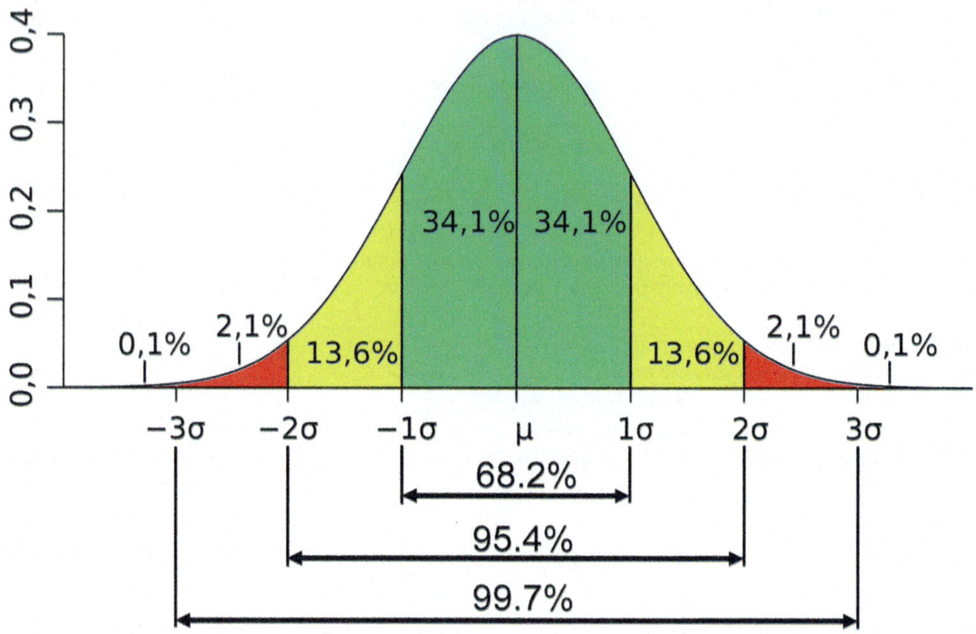

Fig. 60.3 Normal (Gaussian) distribution or bell curve where μ is the mean (median and/or mode), and σ is the standard deviation. The figure illustrates the percentage of the study population that would fall within one, two, or three standard deviations from the mean

at a time. The ultimate goal is to obtain a parsimonious model that includes all key variables. The abovementioned analyses are usually performed using statistical packages (i.e., SAS, STATA, R) which have built-in procedures for these purposes.

Beyond the Basics: Working with Missing Data

Below we present additional analysis approaches that are valuable when working with datasets that may contain substantial missing data or analyses that require advanced methods for controlling known and unknown confounders.

Propensity Score Analysis Propensity score analysis is an alternative method of risk adjustment. Propensity scores compare outcomes across groups that have a similar probability (or propensity) of receiving the treatment or therapy of interest. Outcomes of interest can be compared thorough matching, stratified analyses, or regression (adjusting for propensity) [10]. Propensity scores are useful if the number of confounders is high compared to the number of events (<10 events per covariate) which would otherwise result in an underpowered regression analysis. Propensity scores can also be used if there is no interest in the association between adjustment factors and outcome and when the association between exposure and propensity for treatment can be estimated with higher precision than the association between the exposure and outcome [1].

Instrumental Variable Analysis Instrumental variable analysis consists of controlling for all potential confounding variables (known and unknown) associated with the outcome and exposure of interest by selecting and including a variable exogenous to the study subject, which the study subject has no control over. This exogenous variable should be strongly associated with the exposure but not the outcome [10].

Missing Data Missing data can compromise the power of a study, or likely bias the results, if subjects with missing data are excluded from the analysis. Missing data can be categorized as missing at random (MAAR), missing not at random (MNAR), and missing completely at random (MCAR). Depending on the nature of the missing data, there are several methods to address missing data, such as multiple imputation. However, special considerations need to be taken into account when dealing with MCAR data [10].

Essentials for Sound Evidence

The Grading of Recommendations, Assessment, Development, and Evaluations (GRADE) Working Group ("What is GRADE?" [12]) developed a systematic point-based approach to judge the quality of data and strength of recommendations produced by research studies. The final GRADE score falls under one of the following four categories: high (at least 4 points overall), moderate (3 points), low (2 points), and very low (one or less).

It is composed of five criteria to be scored:

1. *Type of evidence*: Higher score for RCTs (4 points) and lower for observational studies (2 points)

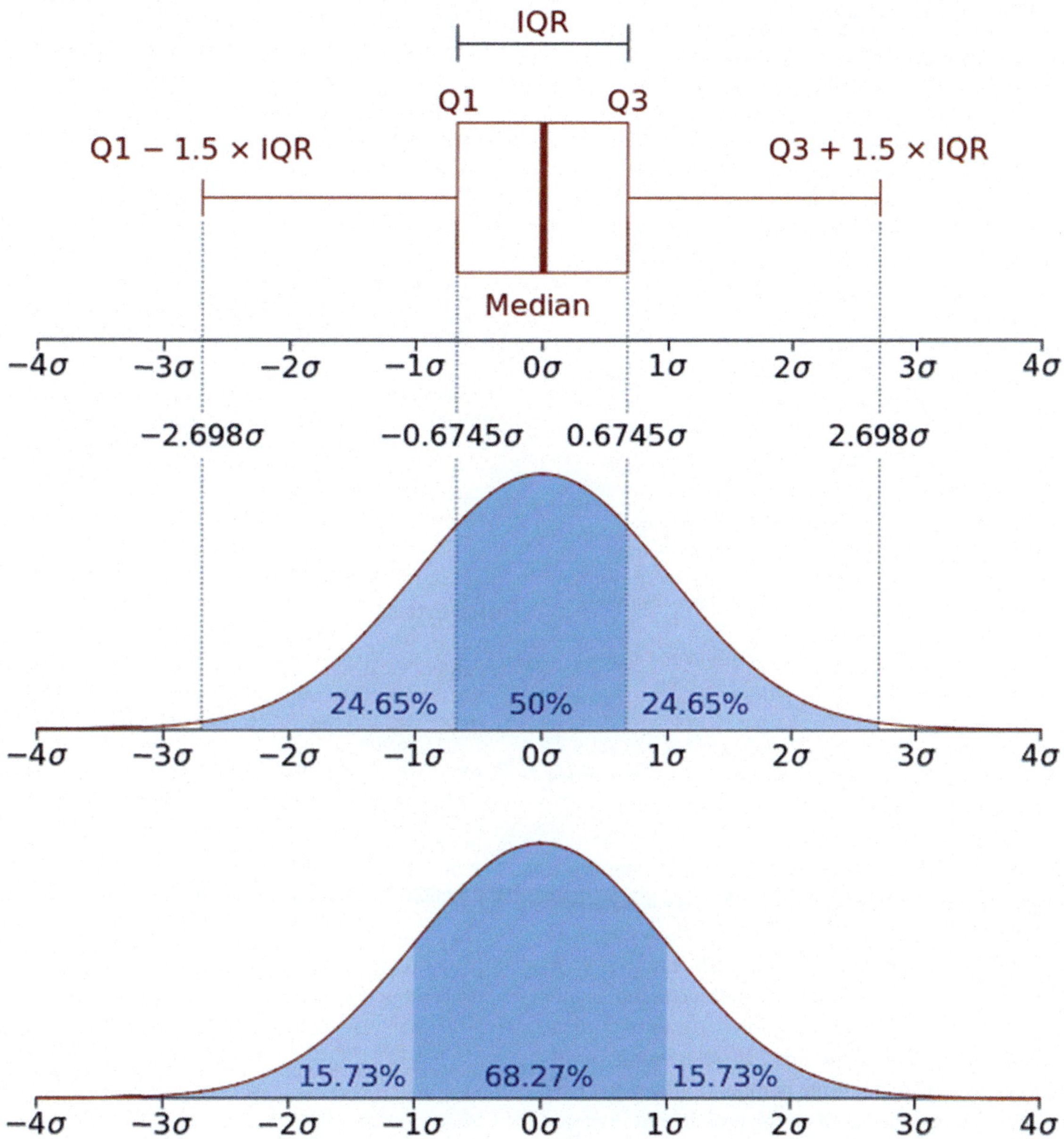

Fig. 60.4 Interquartile range (IQR). This figure illustrates median, IQR, and the percentage of the population that would fall under it and how this compares to standard deviations

2. *Quality*: Refers to blinding, allocation concealment, sparseness of data, follow-up, withdrawals, incomplete reporting of results, and other quality issues
3. *Consistency*: Determines the degree of uniformity of effect between or within studies
4. *Directness*: Refers to the generalizability of population and outcomes from each study to the population of interest
5. *Effect size*: The reported odds ratio (OD), risk ratio (RR), and hazard ratio (HR)

For an observed effect to be considered evidence, it must be accurate and reliable and hold statistical and/or clinical significance. We define each term below.

Accuracy Refers to the veracity of test measurements (validity). Systematic error reduces accuracy.

Reliability Refers to the consistency and reproducibility and the absence of random variation. In other words, that repeated measures are as closely clustered as possible.

***P*-value** The probability of obtaining the observed effect (or more extreme), assuming the null hypothesis is true. The *p*-value is used to determine the statistical significance of the data [5, 11]. A result is generally deemed statistically significant if the *p*-value is less than 0.05. When statistically significant, it means that there is a less than 5%

Table 60.5 Univariate statistical tests

Data type	Characteristics and tests			
Continuous	How many groups are being compared?	(≥2)	Analysis of variance (ANOVA)	
		(2)	*Student's t-test* or appropriate variant	
Categorical	*Chi-square* or appropriate variant			
Independent data?	(Yes)	Is the expected frequency of any cell less than 5	(Yes)	*Fisher's exact test*
			(No)	*Chi-square test*
	(No)	*McNemar test*		
Two groups of continuous data	Normally distributed data and independent data	(Yes, Yes)	*Student's t-test*	
		(Yes, No)	*Paired t-test*	
		(No, Yes)	*Wilcoxon rank sum test or Mann-Whitney U test*	
		(No, No)	*Wilcoxon signed rank test*	

possibility that an observed result (or more extreme) occurred by chance.

Confidence Interval (CI) A range of possible values for a population parameter, to determine that there is a specified probability that the value of the parameter falls within this range. This range is defined as the "confidence level." A 95% CI, for example, means that with infinite measures, the resulting intervals would include the unknown parameter (true population parameter) 95% of the time. In other words, if the study were to be repeated an infinite number of times, the true parameter would be included 95% of the time in that interval. The CI is dependent partially on the sample size and reflects the precision of the results. Larger sample sizes will result in narrower (more precise) CIs and smaller sample sizes will result in larger (not as precise) estimates. A CI is considered not statistically significant if it crosses 1 (the null value) when expressing a risk ratio (RR) or an odds ratio (OR).

Statistical significance Provides information regarding the veracity of the observed differences: whether the observed differences are real. For example, a 5-point systolic blood pressure (SBP) difference with Drug X. A result can be statistically significant, but not be clinically significant.

Clinical significance Reflects how meaningful the translation of observed differences will be toward desired patient effects. For example, is a 5-point SBP difference (from 135 to 140) clinically meaningful to a patient's health?

Summary

In conclusion, a basic understanding of statistics is essential to achieving meaningful research results. A well-defined study design early on will set a strong foundation for a robust analysis that will ultimately translate into sound evidence. When in doubt, talk to a biostatistician or epidemiologist!

Acknowledgment Dr. Haider would like to thank the Career Development Course of the Association for Academic Surgery where he has lectured on this topic over the past several years. Most of the concepts presented here have been discussed during the course of these presentations.

References

1. Austin PC. An introduction to propensity score methods for reducing the effects of confounding in observational studies. Multivar Behav Res. 2011;46(3):399–424. https://doi.org/10.1080/00273171.2011.568786.
2. Biesecker LG. Hypothesis-generating research and predictive medicine. Genome Res. 2013;23(7):1051–3. https://doi.org/10.1101/gr.157826.113.
3. Brian Haynes R. Forming research questions. J Clin Epidemiol. 2006;59(9):881–6. https://doi.org/10.1016/j.jclinepi.2006.06.006
4. Counsell C. Formulating questions and locating primary studies for inclusion in systematic reviews. Ann Intern Med. 1997;127(5):380–7.
5. Daniel WW, Cross CL. Biostatistics: a foundation for analysis in the health sciences. 10th ed. Hoboken: Wiley; 2013.
6. Harris RP, Helfand M, Woolf SH, Lohr KN, Mulrow CD, Teutsch SM, Atkins D. Current methods of the U.S. Preventive Services Task Force: a review of the process. Am J Prev Med. 2001;20(3 Supplement):21–35. https://doi.org/10.1016/S0749-3797(01)00261-6
7. Himmelfarb Health Sciences Library. Study Design 101. Washington, DC: George Washington University. 2011. https://himmelfarb.gwu.edu/tutorials/studydesign101/. Retrieved 24 Mar 2017.
8. Hulley SB, Cummings SR, Browner WS, Grady DG, Newman TB. Designing clinical research. 3rd ed. Philadelphia: Lippincott Williams and Wilkins; 2007.
9. Richardson WS, Wilson MC, Nishikawa J, Hayward RS. The well-built clinical question: a key to evidence-based decisions. ACP J Club. 1995;123(3):A12–3.
10. Simianu VV, Farjah F, Flum DR. Evidence-based surgery: critically assessing surgical literature. In: Sabiston textbook of surgery: the biological basis of modern surgical practice. 20th ed. Philadelphia: Elsevier; 2013.
11. Sullivan LM. Essentials of biostatistics in public health. 2nd ed. Sudbury: Jones & Bartlett Learning; 2012.
12. What is GRADE? BMJ Clinical Evidence. London. 2012. http://clinicalevidence.bmj.com/x/set/static/ebm/learn/665072.html. Retrieved 29 Mar 2017.

Organizational Innovation in Surgical Critical Care

61

Brian C. Beldowicz and Gregory J. Jurkovich

Highly specialized medical attention is a finite resource. Relative to its demand, it can be the scarcest resource in American healthcare, outstripping the available supply of critical care units and specialty trained physicians. The concentration of specialized attention is precisely what differentiates patient care provided in a critical care environment from that on a general hospital ward, so the goal of any critical care organization should be to concentrate this precious resource on those patients most likely to benefit from increased scrutiny of every aspect of their illness and every facet of its care.

Properly directed, critical care serves two essential needs within a patient care organization. First, it is the ultimate arbiter of patient safety. All medical care incurs a variable level of risk. It is estimated that 11% of admission to medical ICUs is related directly to complications of medical care [1]. Unsurprisingly, this rate doubles to nearly 20% in units that also admit surgical patients [2]. Critical care helps mitigate the risks inherent to the practice of medicine, providing a crucial means of preserving favorable outcomes even in patients that suffer substantial complications. In this regard, critical care functions as the safety net that enables all other medical interventions to be performed responsibly.

Second, critical care expands the possibility of meaningful survival to disease processes, injury patterns, and patient populations where such would otherwise be unsalvageable. It achieves this through the laborious pursuit of more subtle therapeutic benefits that collectively influence outcomes. Distributing the resources required for this level of attention can be a moral and ethical challenge. A critical care system reflects a hospital's ability to rescue from death patients with failing organ systems, and increasingly this capacity to salvage good outcomes in the most challenging patients is recognized as the principle means of distinguishing the best hospitals from their peers.

With specialized medical attention its most distinguishing resource, modern critical care has become more of an organizational innovation than a technological development [3], allocating capabilities to meet its missions of mitigating medical risk and conferring improved outcomes to the most acutely ill patients. Within any institution, the organization and administration of critical care should therefore be guided by the primary intention of assembling, coordinating, and distributing specialized attention effectively, reliably, and efficiently. The organization must also ensure that its ability to meet its missions evolves alongside its population of patients and wider standards of care.

The Competing Priorities of Efficiency and Responsiveness

One popular model adapted from industrial management describes an organization as a collection of structures, processes, and outcomes [4]. Structure includes some of the least pliable aspects of an organization such as its physical space and layout, and it also houses aspects most influenced by extrinsic factors such as labor contracts, human resource functions, and budgetary constraints. Too often, however, less obvious elements of organizational structure are ignored, sacrificing efficiency, responsiveness, or both. To optimize performance, the critical care organization must define standards of accessibility, responsibility, and accountability as part of their organizational structure. Structural decisions often must prioritize either efficiency or responsiveness, as most interventions that enhance one will do so at the expense of the other. Identifying the proper balance of efficiency and responsiveness to fit the patient volume, acuity and demographics of a particular institution will be invaluable in guiding decisions regarding the structure of critical care.

B. C. Beldowicz · G. J. Jurkovich (✉)
Department of Surgery, Division of Trauma, UC Davis Health, Acute Care Surgery and Surgical Critical Care, Sacramento, CA, USA
e-mail: gjjurkovich@ucdavis.edu

A. Salim et al. (eds.), *Surgical Critical Care Therapy*, https://doi.org/10.1007/978-3-319-71712-8_61

Standards of Accessibility: Open and Closed ICUs

Standards of accessibility identify those with authority to admit patients to the ICU and discharge them from it, balancing the resources available in the ICU with the needs of individual patients. In "open" ICUs, patients are admitted under the authority of a primary attending that retains considerable care obligations outside of the unit. By contrast, "closed" ICUs specify independent providers who evaluate and approve patients for admission. These providers are generally protected from outside obligations during the periods for which they are responsible for critical care triage. Admission decisions require consideration of critical care demand, capacity, and capability and must be commensurate with the capabilities of an institution's general wards. There is often a gap between the needs that require critical care and those which medical-surgical wards can meet. For example, patients that require close observation due to delirium, titratable infusions, elaborate wound car, or intravenous medications for blood pressure management will sometimes require a level of nursing attention not consistently available on medical-surgical wards. Such patients may be transferred to the more closely monitored setting of a critical care unit without requiring the breadth of attention provided by the balance of the critical care team. Oftentimes the relative demand for one level of care or the other will dictate such a patient's disposition, but the organization should recognize such inconsistency as a source of risk and inefficiency.

Standards of Responsibility: Low-Intensity and High-Intensity Staffing Models

Standards of responsibility establish a reliable hierarchy of decision-making and order-writing authority that is essential to the seamless flow of pertinent clinical information and the reliable communication and timely execution of the ever-evolving clinical plan. Low-intensity staffing models privilege individual providers to independently administer patient care within critical care units. Such staffing emphasizes efficiency by minimizing the number of healthcare providers involved in a patient's care throughout their hospital course and preserves the autonomy of the provider most familiar with the patient and his or her disease process. In contrast, high-intensity staffing models require participation of certified critical care intensivists, either as the principle medical provider or as a mandatory consultant for the comprehensive, multisystem management of complex patients.

A landmark 2002 study published in JAMA demonstrated marked improvements in patient outcomes associated with high-intensity physician staffing models. Specifically, the study reported a 29% reduction in in-hospital mortality, a 39% reduction in ICU mortality, and reduced hospital and ICU lengths of stay [5].

The reason for this observed benefit is multifactorial. Intensivists (board certified and fellowship trained in critical care medicine) bring a unique set of skills and characteristics that not only compliment the care of challenging patients but also should enhance the function of a clinical care team and optimize the performance of a critical care system. In addition, intensivists afford two components of medical attention that other physicians find challenging to replicate in modern practice: responsiveness and objectivity.

Availability is an essential component of responsiveness. To fulfill the demands of productivity, physicians at all levels and types of hospitals must maintain busy elective practices and considerable commitments outside of the critical care unit. These obligations make physicians less available to respond to unanticipated developments in the course of their patients' care and illness. Designated intensivists enable other physicians to maintain efficiency in their independent practices by shouldering the demand for responsiveness required for the care of complicated patients.

The second component, objectivity, is particularly valuable in the care of surgical patients. Surgeons are often biased by their own experience of a patient's clinical course. While this perspective and continuity can be beneficial to comprehensive patient care, it leaves providers prone to misappropriating the relative importance of clinical data. Surgeons may be particularly susceptible to subjective assessments of clinical developments. Some are more inclined to a posture of denial, reluctant to accept any clinical change as indicating a complication of their procedure. Others, meanwhile, are prejudiced to a posture of guilt, where every untoward development is a complication of their intervention until proven otherwise. The subjectivity of the former predisposes patients to delays in diagnosis and treatment. The bias of the latter subjects patients to unwarranted testing, consultations, and interventions. Designated intensivists are best when they are positioned to approach clinical changes without a tendency toward denial or guilt, objectively evaluating patients with no such predisposition.

The Leapfrog Group, a consortium of high-volume purchasers of health insurance wielding ever-expanding influence in patterns of referral and healthcare reimbursement, has advocated for high-intensity staffing practices in an effort to improve the value and safety of the healthcare they are purchasing [6]. By requiring intensivists to be physically present during daytime hours with clinical responsibilities limited exclusively to the ICU, Leapfrog optimizes both the objectivity and responsiveness of care provided to the most ill. Their guidelines ensure that objectivity informs the interdisciplinary development of the patient care plan each day and that the care team will be responsive to acute developments without distractions or competing clinical obligations outside of the unit. This is of increasing importance as interventions for high-mortality conditions such as shock, trauma, stroke, myocardial infarction, and sepsis have all proven time-sensitive.

To overcome budgetary constraints and the well-documented shortfall of certified intensivists, many ICUs following a high-intensity staffing model utilize personnel that augment intensivist presence and influence. These augmenters, including residents, nurse practitioners, or physician's assistants, can be remotely supervised by intensivists during overnight hours with no apparent decrement in patient outcomes so long as clinical plans of care were devised and executed by intensivists during the day [7]. Studies have demonstrated no significant detriment in patient outcome or care efficiency when comparing one class of augmenter to another [8], and the presence of one or more of these classes of healthcare providers enhances the care team's flexibility. Projecting and distributing the appropriate level of specialized attention enables the team to address multiple acute issues simultaneously while also maintaining the detail-oriented discipline that differentiates critical care from non-intensive inpatient care.

Some institutions maximize the efficiency of low-intensity staffing and the responsiveness of high-intensity models by implementing intermediate care or "step-down" units. Such units allow primary physicians to take advantage of enhanced nursing attention without syphoning the finite resource of specialized, interdisciplinary critical care teams from needier patients. Developing intermediate care units, formulating ward care policies, allocating critical care unit bed space, and implementing ICU staffing models are elements of institutional structure that should not be considered individually. All must be considered collectively to balance the competing demands for efficiency and responsiveness that pervade healthcare today.

Standards of Accountability: Multidisciplinary and Interdisciplinary Care Teams

Leadership sets the tone of an organization's culture, and as the leader of a sophisticated team, an intensivist must interact synergistically with team members. Interactions with consultants and primary operating surgeons are a key component of the life of a surgical intensivist, and the structure of the ICU organization can help with those interactions. Professional inter-provider relationships limit personal bias and challenge assumptions that unduly influence patient care. Such an attitude elevates each consultant's accountability to the rest of the team. Consultants accountable to peer-level oversight must be prepared to substantiate their recommendations and are more likely to adhere to published guidelines and evidence-based best practices.

A dangerous tendency when surrounded by consultants in the ICU is for the intensivist to defer critical management decisions to these highly focused and specialized professionals. This erodes the intensivist's practical expertise and disrupts the development of a functioning critical care team. Isolating patient care into a collection of independent silos impairs the team's ability to anticipate and identify problems or adapt to unexpected developments.

The intensivist should be capable of anticipating the implications of management decisions on all organ systems and as such should assimilate data from multiple sources into a comprehensive understanding of each patient's clinical state. But coordinating consultations from multiple disciplines also requires expertly managing relationships. Incorporating expectations for relationships and communication into the defined structure of an ICU enables members of the team to overcome numerous obstacles that are inherent to complex tasks in large organizations. This begins with understanding the nature of the relationship between the intensivist and associated consultants, physician augmenters, and bedside staff. Recognizing the difference between a multidisciplinary relationship and an interdisciplinary relationship helps to define expectations and to delineate roles, responsibilities, and authorities, lessening the chance for miscommunication or misunderstanding.

In a multidisciplinary team, each consultant approaches the clinical situation from his or her own independent perspective. These consultants then either document recommendations for the primary provider or are given independent order-writing authority to independently pursue their plan of care for the particular medical problem for which they were consulted.

The benefit of this type of organization is its logistical feasibility. A multidisciplinary relationship does not require coordination of provider schedules, and communication can be exchanged indirectly through more available intermediaries such as nurses or physician assistants or through clinical documentation in the medical record. This arrangement enables consultants to commit only the time necessary to evaluate the patient and initiate a plan and then refocus their attention on competing demands. Though multidisciplinary care can often be sufficient, its convenience does come at the expense of more thorough collaboration.

An interdisciplinary team, by contrast, integrates the impressions of all team members into a shared mutual understanding of each patient. In such a system, each consultant is required to consider the concerns of all other stakeholders and to incorporate those perspectives into their own recommendations. The role of the SCC intensivist is to facilitate identification and reconciliation of interdisciplinary conflicts in order to arrive at a treatment plan that prospectively incorporates all points of view. While substantially more time-consuming and resource demanding, this method has the advantage of better integrating all perspectives to develop suitable compromises and risk mitigation strategies required by complex clinical problems.

Due to logistical constraints and competing demands, interactions with physician-centric teams of various medical specialties in open ICUs often adopt a multidisciplinary approach whereas an ICU-based clinical care teams in closed ICUs with high-intensity staffing embrace an interdisciplinary relationship. The care of critically ill and injured patients in many institutions incorporates a hybrid of these relationships. The primary provider must differentiate and manage multiple relationships of each type to ensure the maximum benefit is realized in terms of both patient care and organizational culture.

Playing the Orchestra[1]: Interdisciplinary Rounds

To characterize an organization as a mere collection of structures, processes, and outcomes ignores the importance of organizational culture to performance. While structure can be quite inflexible owing to its dependence on outside concerns, culture is often the organizational element most inherently resistant to change. A critical care team is a convergence of individual perspectives, each with its own professional concerns, departmental hierarchies, and role in institutional bureaucracies competing for prioritization. Such subgroups of large organizations are often prone to status quo bias, interpreting any change to existing practices as a challenge to previous performance. Additionally, practice changes often incur learning and implementation curves that may transiently increase risks of mistakes, misunderstandings and miscommunication, and, occasionally, patient outcome.

A critical care organization can overcome this tendency toward stagnation by promoting a culture of perpetual collaboration and learning, but this requires establishing structured lines of communication. Allowing communication to proceed in an unstructured, ad hoc fashion is not consistent with the demands of critical care medicine. Sufficient time and resources for inter-provider communication should be incorporated in the daily routine, and both responsibilities and expectations for this interaction should be clearly defined. It is unreasonable to assume that the care team will develop and maintain effective communication if such practices are not standardized, prioritized, and exercised routinely.

Table 61.1 Content and process of interdisciplinary critical care rounds

Patient plan of care
Main problem
Diagnostic plan
Provisional goals
Intermediate (beyond today) and long-term (beyond ICU) therapies
Highest perceived risks (both in likelihood and severity)
Interdisciplinary process
Clarify consultant expectations of critical care team
Assessment and questions from house staff
Assessment and questions from bedside staff
Plan of care summary
Closed-loop clarification of task priority and responsibility

(Adapted from *The Scientific World Journal* 2015, Article ID 951924)

Interdisciplinary rounds are a process, but because of the level of coordination required among providers and consultants, rounds are also an essential component of the communication structure in most ICUs. The productivity of ICU rounds will invariably be proportional to the quality of its input and the expectations of its output. High-intensity staffing models benefit from the consistency and reliability of rounds under the leadership of a single SCC intensivist. Low-intensity models suffer from variance of practices and communication styles inherent in having a diverse cadre of physicians providing primary care decisions. In either instance, the critical care organization should establish explicit expectations regarding responsibility for the collection of data, the conveyance of information, and the process by which knowledge is shared and decisions communicated among all members of the team.

An interdisciplinary rounding team facilitates a shared understanding of the patient including short, intermediate, and long-term goals of care. The team should be designed after considering which care providers and consultants can consistently contribute to this understanding and which can better execute their role by participating in the interdisciplinary process. The leader of such rounds has some important structural roles. They must minimize nonessential interruptions and distractions, ensure that all stakeholders have the opportunity to voice their concerns for each patient, and clearly assign responsibilities for the agreed upon plan. Undisciplined and disorganized discussions are too often left open-ended with no clear plan of care and no specified delegation of tasks. The process of rounds must assure that such doubts are not left lingering. Table 61.1 illustrates one checklist for both the structure and process of conducting bedside rounds in critically ill patients.

There is no more sensitive indicator of subtle alterations in a patient's clinical course than prolonged patient

[1] "Musicians play their instruments; I play the orchestra." *Steve Jobs*. Screenplay by Aaron Sorkin. Dir. Danny Boyle. Perf. Michael Fassbender. Universal Pictures, 2015. Film.

observation at the bedside. This makes the critical care nurse an essential component of every patient assessment. Physicians and other specialized consultants are restricted to a limited collection of clinical snapshots when focusing only on their own bedside observations; nurses can offer a far more panoramic, time-lapsed perspective. Their perspective should be incorporated in discussions of both pertinent events and the evolution of pertinent findings on the clinical examination. Additionally, nurses are often privy to psychosocial details that influence patient care.

Presence of a clinical pharmacist on the critical care team reduces prescribing errors by two-thirds [9]. In addition to simply catching prescribing errors, clinical pharmacists safeguard against drug-drug interactions, recommend regimens for acute pain management, guide renal and hepatic dose adjustments, enforce antibiotic stewardship programs, and advise physicians regarding cost discrepancies between similar therapies.

Malnourishment is a problem that continues to plague critically ill patients despite mounting evidence that early feeding improves outcomes. Reasons for the discrepancy between evidence and practice include inaccurate nutritional assessments, lack of education pertaining to tube feed interruption, and uncertainty regarding tube feed tolerance. This can be ameliorated by the regular participation of a nutritionist. Discussions with the nutritionist will enhance team understanding of when to initiate, titrate, hold, and discontinue nutritional supplementation, improving consistency with evidence-based best practice [10].

At any point in time, approximately 40% of ICU inhabitants are dependent on mechanical ventilation [11], and while standard ventilator management is sufficient for most critically ill patients with respiratory failure, respiratory therapists can help facilitate continuity and consistency in ventilator weaning for patients requiring prolonged intubation. Their focused perspective developed over a greater amount of time spent with each patient can help clue intensivists into which patients may require deeper investigation into the etiology of their pulmonary failure.

Early mobility remains a key element in management of many critically ill patients. This has proven to be an invaluable tool for improving respiratory mechanics, decreasing delirium, and decreasing rehabilitation time after patients recover from their acute illness. Ensuring that the perspective of physical and occupational therapists is incorporated into daily rounds, either directly or through nursing, will help maximize their utilization and ensure that activity restrictions such as spinal precautions or weight-bearing limitations are dispensed with as soon as appropriate.

To maximize a system's throughput and optimize its efficiency, discharge planning should begin immediately upon admission. This must include early decisions regarding end of life care and a priori decision in this regard. Social workers and case managers provide a valuable perspective of the relationship between a patient, his family and social support structures, and the care team. Incorporation of the social and economic realities of a patient's situation into the care plan will help alleviate sources of friction and identify barriers to eventual disposition.

In developing both a structure and a process for interdisciplinary rounds, it is essential to balance the attention to detail required of critical care with demands for team efficiency and responsiveness. Not every perspective will demand input on every patient every day, but it is important that a structure and process is in place to ensure each perspective is consistently considered and has a forum to reliably voice its concerns.

Total Quality Management

In complex systems such as surgical critical care, measures of performance and outcomes are an essential component of organizational culture, incorporating elements of both systems-based performance improvement with events-based quality assurance. As in industrial systems engineering, performance management seeks to improve the efficacy, efficiency and reliability of healthcare delivery through reductions in process variance and error commission. While this approach is not always widely accepted ("my patients are different…; *or "the most cost effective care is no care"*), [12] there is strong evidence that cost effective care is both quality care and less expensive care, and that avoiding unnecessary variability is a key component of this process [13].

Start from the M&M Podium… and Work Your Way Backward

Event-Based Quality Assurance

Event-based quality assurance is a reactive systems management tool intended to identify lapses in performance. The actions that this identification invokes range from singling out the individuals involved for punishment to ignoring the event as "an outlier." However, in order to reduce the incidence and severity of errors, an approach somewhere in between those extremes is likely to be more effective. Quality improvement programs are present at all hospitals, taking the form of hospital risk management committees, departmental morbidity and mortality conferences, and leadership-directed root cause analyses. With in-depth assessment of errors, a system should be able to identify the location, source, and cause of errors. One report of unanticipated trauma deaths demonstrated that the

Table 61.2 Triggers for morbidity and mortality conference consideration

Iatrogenic injuries related directly to ICU procedures
Major medication errors
Mortality
Occurrence of a *National Quality Forum* "never event"
Unplanned re-admission after transfer from ICU
Unplanned re-intubation
Unplanned return to OR

ICU setting is the major source of errors responsible for such outcomes [14].

Morbidity and mortality (M&M) conferences are the most pervasive form of event-based quality assurance on a departmental level, but the structure, process, and outcome of the conference affect its ability to positively influence organizational culture and performance. M&M conference should be reliably scheduled at a frequency commiserate with patient volume and complexity. An organized list of cases to be presented should be maintained and made available throughout the department in a non-identifying, protected format. For the process to be objective, referral for M&M presentation must go beyond simply self-reporting. A department should establish a system for identifying patients for presentation, whether by reviewing admission rosters, hospital censuses, or provider case logs. The key to a useful process is the identification and tracking of *all* errors, whether or not they are "presented" in a formal process. Selecting out only a limited number of events as "good discussions" will fail to identify subtle and pervasive problems in care delivery. Table 61.2 lists a set of institutional triggers that should automatically warrant consideration for presentation at an M&M conference.

Time allotted for case discussion should be protected from distractions and outside interference. A minimum attendance rate for staff members should be required and tracked. Cases should only be presented only when all stakeholders are present and prepared.

Presentations should be structured, so there should be a prescribed format for case write-ups and discussion. Facts presented as facts, whether in terms of the patient's specific clinical course or medical literature that guided decision-making, should be verified from either the medical record or peer-reviewed publications, respectively. All presenters suffer from recall bias and are therefore more likely to misremember data or events in a way that could compromise the validity of the case review process. Requiring substantive write-ups ensures sufficient preparation and facilitates meaningful discussion of unambiguous conditions surrounding the patient's clinical course. These write-ups are also a valuable reference when communicating recommendations to other institutional boards or medical services.

The attitude of the conference should not be confrontational but rather professional and respectful though still direct and objective. All observers are subject to both hindsight bias and outcome bias, and these biases can be a source of conflict between presenter and audience. Hindsight bias overestimates the predictability of an outcome by subconsciously incorporating information not available prospectively. Outcome bias is an inappropriate judgment of the quality of decision-making after the outcome of the decisions has been determined. In addition to undermining the constructiveness of the forum, these biases can spark interpersonal conflicts that could damage team culture and cohesiveness. Biases are virtually inevitable in conferences with broad participation; however, those individuals conducting the conference must constantly indicate the presence of recall, hindsight, and outcomes biases in order to minimize their influence on individual presentations and collective attitudes. Consistently unproductive conferences are often an indicator of a culture of blame or lack of accountability. These issues demand disciplined leadership to ensure the conference is focused on serving departmental goals rather than individual disputes and agendas.

Humility is a key component in any quality assurance discussions, and the first priority of all M&M cases should focus on the role of attendees in preventing a similar complication in the future. As a matter of course, only after one or more opportunities for internal improvements have been identified should the discussion then turn to the responsibilities of extrinsic services and personnel. Even when the complication is the direct result of improper execution of an extrinsic care provider, there will often be an opportunity for improved education, communication, or oversight. All recommendations should become part of the case's formal write-up for local filing or forwarding to other appropriate institutional bodies such as other involved care services, an ethics committee, hospital leadership, or risk management. If open peer review is difficult or impossible because of competition between providers, a blinded voting system regarding the impact and severity of the error may be required.

Event-based quality assurance has expanded beyond identifying unanticipated outcomes to include incidents described as "near misses." This adjustment in attitude acknowledges the role of chance in translating errors into outcomes. Examining only the lapses in performance that result in bad outcomes ignores numerous missed opportunities for improvement. Hence, an event-based process of quality assurance is insufficient for the high-stakes complexity of modern critical care organizations. A parallel curriculum that strives for evidence-based systems performance improvement is essential. While medical quality of care indicators as championed by the Agency for Healthcare Research and Quality, the National Surgical Quality Improvement Program, and the Leapfrog Group, among others, are good starting points, the best of critical care units have in addition their own proactive, anticipatory goals of improving care based on their individual problem areas.

You Can't Change What You Don't Measure: Systems-Based Performance Improvement

The first step required for systems-based performance improvement is benchmarking. This involves the collection and regular analysis of organizational data, comparing it to both historical institutional performance and contemporary peer performance. In benchmarking, it is necessary to first identify data points that serve as meaningful surrogates for process quality or reliability. Benchmarks not only indicate what within the system needs to be changed but also what the system is capable of changing. Table 61.3 lists a selection of metrics that can accurately represent pertinent critical care processes when measured consistently and objectively. Identifying relationships between different metrics is valuable as identifying trends in any individual metric.

A list of benchmarks should remain consistent but not stagnant. Change in the healthcare environment, emergence of scientific evidence, observation of new threats, and alterations in team member behavior can render old metrics obsolete or new measurements more representative. Benchmarks better identify worrisome trends only when performance is compared in two dimensions, both over time and across peers. Comparisons over time control for institutional variables. Comparisons across peers control for changes in practice standards.

Inconsistency undermines the validity of metrics for representing processes. Total Quality Management is a systems management strategy that seeks to reduce unnecessary variability as a means of improving the reliability of both a process and the metrics that represent it.

Dealing with Cats[2]: The Role of Protocols and Guidelines

High-quality processes are those in which unnecessary variance has been eliminated. Variance is a product of individual provider autonomy (physicians and others), yet it introduces additional variables to the care process resulting in outcomes that are inconsistent and incomparable. This makes for identification of areas the need improvement difficult to identify. Processes for which there has been clearly demonstrated benefit in terms of efficiency or efficacy should be translated into a carefully considered and meticulously maintained set of institutional protocols. Protocols are effective tools for communication, continuity, and consistency. They strengthen team-building and organizational resilience by standardizing expectations and processes. Treatment errors, particularly

[2]"Anyone who considers protocol unimportant has never dealt with a cat." – Robert A. Heinlein. *The Cat Who Walks Through Walls*. G. P. Putnam & Sons, New York, 1985.

Table 61.3 Risk-stratified benchmarks of ICU performance

Unit census/throughput
Number of admissions each day
Number of transfers each day
Number of direct from ICU discharges
Length of stay: ICU and total hospital
Catheter-associated urinary tract infections
Number of patients admitted with catheter in place
Number of catheters discontinued
Number of catheters replaced for urinary retention
Total number of catheter days for each patient
Number of patients initiated on antibiotics for suspected UTI based on urinalysis
Number of urine culture confirmed CAUTI
Ratio of catheterized patients to total patients
Central line-associated bloodstream infections
Number of patients admitted with central line in place
Number of new initial central lines placed within ICU
Number of central lines changes performed in ICU (new site and re-wire)
Number of culture confirmed bloodstream infections
Number confirmed in patients with central lines
Number objectively confirmed to be directly related to central line
Decubitus ulcers
Absolute number, by stage (not present on admission)
Emergency response
Total number of activated codes
Noninvasive ventilation
Intubation/positive pressure ventilation
ACLS procedures
Number of activated codes that resulted in death
Falls
Absolute number
GI prophylaxis
Number of days
Glycemic control
Absolute number of severe hypoglycemic events (blood glucose <70)
Number of blood glucose measurements >180 mg/dL per patient per day
Mechanical ventilation
Number of patients admitted on ventilator
Number of ventilator days per patient
Number of unplanned re-intubations
Mortality
ICU mortality
In-hospital mortality
30-day all-cause mortality
90-day all-cause mortality
Narcosis reversal (naloxone, flumazenil)
Absolute number of incidents
Nutrition
Time from admission to initiation
Time from admission to goal caloric intake
Caloric intake relative to calories required for patients on supplemental nutrition

(continued)

Table 61.3 (continued)

Pneumonia	
	Number of patients initiated on antibiotics for suspected VAP/HAP
	Number of culture confirmed VAP/HAP
Restraints	
	Number of patients admitted with restraint order
	Number of patients in whom restraint days relative to total ICU days
VTE prophylaxis	
	Time from admission to initiation
	Number of doses held or delayed per patient

what are called treatment intent actions, are prevalent contributors to unanticipated deaths. Protocols have been shown to reduce such errors [14] and improve patient care and outcomes [15].

One of the greatest challenges in unifying the care team is developing a shared understanding of priorities and responsibilities, particularly when there are multiple areas requiring simultaneous attention. By allowing for reflexive, regimented management of common critical care issues such as glycemic control, electrolyte replenishment, or initiation of enteral feeding, protocols can ensure that the benefit to be gained from less urgent issues is not surrendered in the face of more acute concerns.

In healthcare, greater responsibility often results in more enthusiasm and increased job satisfaction. Teams practicing such reductionism tend to be more collaborative than authoritative, fostering both cooperation and communication. Protocols help decentralize management responsibilities so that the demand for attention can be more evenly distributed to qualified personnel across the entirety of the team, and patients can continue to receive the comprehensive, detail-oriented care their condition requires despite episodic distractions throughout their clinical course.

The single greatest obstacle to protocol adoption is the perception of some providers that protocols are a restriction of their autonomy, and, to be fair, this is true. Academically, with more than 800,000 articles published in the medical literature each year, the expanse of medical knowledge has far surpassed any reasonable threshold of command for a single healthcare provider. A 2000 study examined the malfunction of "passive diffusion" for incorporation of medical evidence into practice, estimating it takes an average of 17 years for clinical evidence to be incorporated into the practice of half of active physicians [16].

Part of the specialization of the intensivist is to be able to identify where those knowledge gaps are most likely to exist, which of the gaps are most likely to influence patient outcomes, and whether a protocol is an appropriate means of bridging such gaps at the expense of provider autonomy. Performance issues suitable for protocol-based solutions may present as practice patterns that conflict with prevailing published observations, substantial inter-provider variability, or as a deviation of institutional data from anticipated outcomes. Part of the benefit of mandatory intensivist involvement is his or her ability to detect such troubling trends across a larger patient population than independent providers are capable of perceiving.

The key to effective protocol implementation lies in an appreciation for their limitations. No protocol can account for all pertinent clinical variables, so it remains the responsibility of individual providers to not only ensure that protocols are valid, current, and properly understood and executed but to also understand when each should be initiated, aborted, or ignored [15]. Protocols differ from guidelines in that guidelines remain more respectful of provider autonomy and serve merely as prompts supporting a preferred management strategy. Compliance with guidelines is considered voluntary; compliance with protocols is considered more compulsory, and providers are held more to account for deviation from protocols when it results in a poor outcome. An appreciation for when objective data is insufficient to justify restriction of physician autonomy will help determine when a guideline is a more appropriate strategy to reduce inter-provider variance than a protocol, and these limitations underscore the importance of the manner in which protocols are developed.

A Protocol for Protocols

To begin, the intensivist must first identify a clinical management problem and determine the suitability of a protocol as an effective solution. To facilitate adoption and utilization, an effective protocol should be developed by those who will employ it. The intensivist must identify relevant stakeholders, specifically those members of the healthcare team qualified to contribute to the development process and those directly invested in its outcome. Balance at this stage is important. Soliciting too much input invites conflict between perspectives, inviting too little compromises objectivity and transparency.

A representative collection of stakeholders should then be charged with assembling pertinent data from both published literature and institutional experience. Administrative personnel can assist this effort, and the utility of medical librarians should not be overlooked. During data collection, it is important to restrict input to objective facts so as not to mischaracterize personal preferences or anecdotal experience as scientific evidence. Published systematic reviews and guidelines of professional organizations serve as a good foundation as they often have already assembled and objectively graded available published experience. It is imperative that a protocol's designers ensure that any available guideline has remained consistent with data that has emerged since its publication.

The unbiased data should then be presented to a larger collection of stakeholders and feedback solicited. It is at this point that subjective preferences and experience can be incorporated into the process, but should be limited to considerations that help navigate unique institutional challenges. Segregating this input from scientific evidence ensures it will not be given equal emphasis. A detailed proposal is then drafted and subject to review before ultimately a final product is disseminated.

A good protocol should be brief and easy to follow and should use common terminology, avoiding unnecessary acronyms or abbreviations, when possible, it should be depicted graphically or should fit on a single side of a sheet of paper, and it should be widely disseminated and easy to access for point-of-care referencing. Structures and processes should be designed to ensure that adherence to an adopted protocol is the easiest means of managing common care issues, so translating the protocol into a standardized order set removes one significant obstacle to adoption and can help ensure consistent compliance with accreditation requirements. For the sake of space and ease of reading, references should not be included in the protocol; however, a repository for a more comprehensive description including a relevant bibliography should be made available to facilitate process transparency and support ongoing education.

The benefit of adequately addressing less acute concerns does not evaporate in the face of more pressing issues; in fact, the value of incremental progress only becomes more valuable when other things are going wrong. Physicians caring for the critically ill cannot afford to surrender these benefits simply because they are unable to independently provide them sufficient attention. Effective protocols can decrease the demand for attention or distribute that demand over a greater portion of the healthcare team.

Admittedly there is not an evidence-based best practice for the management of all disease processes or clinical variables encountered in the critically ill. But standardizing practices across providers also reduces the risk of miscommunication between ordering providers and team members responsible for order execution. Standardization also enables consistent orientation and education of team members, further reducing the likelihood of misunderstanding or improper implementation. Provider variability also complicates the care of already complicated patients, and unstandardized processes can make it exceptionally difficult to monitor trends in care quality and outcomes making it difficult to conduct performance comparisons over time and across peers.

A Case for Surgical Intensivists

While all intensive care involves a balancing of conflicting interventions, critical care of the surgical patients adds an additional layer of complexity in the timing and performing operative procedures in a manner that optimizes benefit while mitigating risks. This additional complexity can benefit from an intensivist with surgical training, integrating uniquely surgical considerations into the organized system of care [17].

Critical care surgeons are recognized by the American Board of Surgery for having completed ACGME-approved training in surgery (5 clinical years) and surgical critical care (1–2 years). This cadre comprises only one-fifth of the intensivist workforce [18], but they are uniquely qualified to both organize and deliver the care required by the most acutely ill and injured surgical patients. First, given their (near universal) background in trauma, surgical intensivists are accustomed to the design and function of a trauma system, namely, developing, maintaining, and functioning within regionalized multi-institutional systems that demand coordinated distribution of patients to specifically qualified locations that enable concentration of extremely limited and highly specialized capabilities. Second, surgeons are uniquely accustomed to operating within multi-discipline, multi-profession teams, in which levels of training, experience, and expertise may vary considerably. This experience in high-acuity situations demands that they be adept at appropriately distributing responsibility across a diverse collection of team members in time-sensitive situations while still maintaining overall accountability for team performance, patient outcome, and the overall perception of care. Third, surgeons benefit from a broad understanding of both medical and surgical disciplines, enabling effective communication and collaboration in an environment where competing priorities can have substantial consequences. The intensivist is the ultimate arbiter in balancing the beneficial effects of one therapy and its potential influence on another discipline's morbidity. Additionally, surgeons are best suited to detect subtle changes in the postoperative patient's status that may signify an underlying complication related to the operation. Lastly, surgeons regularly function within systems designed to measure and monitor care quality and efficiency. The National Surgery Quality Improvement Project and the Trauma Quality Improvement Project enable individual providers, departments, and institutions to trend their performance over time and compare that performance to local, regional, and national peers, enhancing their ability to identify and implement best practices. This experience will prove invaluable as our evolving healthcare system demands the adoption of similar requirements for critical care.

Organization and Culture in Surgical Critical Care

At a time when more medical care is being performed outside of the hospital, the demand and expectations for critical care are increasing [19]. Critical care is increasingly viewed as a measure of overall institutional quality, as it is often the ultimate arbiter of patient salvage. Critical care capacity or performance cannot be improved through technology alone. Aligning organizational structures, processes, and outcomes within a performance-based culture will ensure that critical care resources are assembled, coordinated, and distributed in a manner that is effective, efficient, and reliable.

References

1. Darchy B, Le Miere E, Figueredo B, Bavoux E, Domart Y. Iatrogenic diseases as a reason for admission to the intensive care unit: incidence, causes, and consequences. Arch Intern Med. 1999;159(1):71–8.
2. Mercier E, Giraudeau B, Ginies G, Perrotin D, Dequin PF. Iatrogenic events contributing to ICU admission: a prospective study. Intensive Care Med. 2010;36(6):1033–7. https://doi.org/10.1007/s00134-010-1793-9.
3. Rubenfeld GD, Scales DC. Organizational change in critical care: the next magic bullet? In: Scales DC, Rubenfeld GD, editors. The organization of critical care: an evidence-based approach to improving quality. Respiratory medicine. New York: Humana Press; 2014. p. 3–8.
4. Donabedian A. Continuity and change in the quest for quality. Clin Perform Qual Health Care. 1993;1(1):9–16.
5. Pronovost PJ, Angus DC, Dorman T, Robinson KA, Dremsizov TT, Young TL. Physician staffing patterns and clinical outcomes in critically ill patients: a systematic review. JAMA. 2002;288(17):2151–62.
6. The Leapfrog Group (2016) Factsheet: ICU Physician Staffing. http://www.leapfroggroup.org/sites/default/files/Files/IPS Fact Sheet.pdf. Accessed 3/2/2017.
7. Kerlin MP, Small DS, Cooney E, Fuchs BD, Bellini LM, Mikkelsen ME, Schweickert WD, Bakhru RN, Gabler NB, Harhay MO, Hansen-Flaschen J, Halpern SD. A randomized trial of nighttime physician staffing in an intensive care unit. N Engl J Med. 2013;368(23):2201–9. https://doi.org/10.1056/NEJMoa1302854.
8. Costa DK, Wallace DJ, Barnato AE, Kahn JM. Nurse practitioner/physician assistant staffing and critical care mortality. Chest. 2014;146(6):1566–73. https://doi.org/10.1378/chest.14-0566.
9. Leape LL, Cullen DJ, Clapp MD, Burdick E, Demonaco HJ, Erickson JI, Bates DW. Pharmacist participation on physician rounds and adverse drug events in the intensive care unit. JAMA. 1999;282(3):267–70.
10. Behara AS, Peterson SJ, Chen Y, Butsch J, Lateef O, Komanduri S. Nutrition support in the critically ill: a physician survey. JPEN J Parenter Enteral Nutr. 2008;32(2):113–9. https://doi.org/10.1177/0148607108314763.
11. Wunsch H, Wagner J, Herlim M, Chong DH, Kramer AA, Halpern SD. ICU occupancy and mechanical ventilator use in the United States. Crit Care Med. 2013;41(12):2712–9. https://doi.org/10.1097/CCM.0b013e318298a139.
12. Barzel US. Cost-effective medical care--real or oxymoron? N Engl J Med. 1990;322(23):1676. https://doi.org/10.1056/NEJM199006073222319.
13. Drexler M, Weinstein M. Can cost-effective health care = better health care? Harvard School of Public Health. 2010. https://www.hsph.harvard.edu/news/magazine/winter10assessment/. Accessed Winter 2010 2017.
14. Gruen RL, Jurkovich GJ, McIntyre LK, Foy HM, Maier RV. Patterns of errors contributing to trauma mortality: lessons learned from 2,594 deaths. Ann Surg. 2006;244(3):371–80. https://doi.org/10.1097/01.sla.0000234655.83517.56.
15. Chang SY, Sevransky J, Martin GS. Protocols in the management of critical illness. Crit Care. 2012;16(2):306. https://doi.org/10.1186/cc10578.
16. Balas EA, Boren SA. Managing clinical knowledge for health care improvement. Yearb Med Inform 2000: Patient-Cent Syst. 2000;2000(2000):65–70.
17. Nathens AB, Rivara FP, MacKenzie EJ, Maier RV, Wang J, Egleston B, Scharfstein DO, Jurkovich GJ. The impact of an intensivist-model ICU on trauma-related mortality. Ann Surg. 2006;244(4):545–54. https://doi.org/10.1097/01.sla.0000239005.26353.49.
18. Frankel HL, Butler KL, Cuschieri J, Friese RS, Huynh T, Mohr AM, Schinco MA, Napolitano LM, Britt LD, Coimbra R, Croce MA, Davis JW, Jurkovich GJ, Moore EE, Morris JA Jr, Peitzman AB, Pruitt BA, Rozycki GS, Scalea TM, Meredith JW. The role and value of surgical critical care, an essential component of acute care surgery, in the Affordable Care Act: a report from the Critical Care Committee and Board of Managers of the American Association for the Surgery of Trauma. J Trauma Acute Care Surg. 2012;73(1):20–6. https://doi.org/10.1097/TA.0b013e31825a78d5.
19. Halpern NA, Pastores SM. Critical care medicine in the United States 2000–2005: an analysis of bed numbers, occupancy rates, payer mix, and costs. Crit Care Med. 2010;38(1):65–71. https://doi.org/10.1097/CCM.0b013e3181b090d0.

Billing

62

R. Lawrence Reed II

Background

Physicians and other professional care providers are paid for their services through professional billing. In contrast to earlier times when professionals billed independently and charged their patients whatever the market would bear, current billing practices are governed by rules set by so-called "third-party" carriers, which are health insurance providers, including the Centers for Medicare and Medicaid Services (CMS), an arm of the federal government. In this system, physicians are paid based upon the number of relative value units (RVUs) they generate from the provision of their professional services. Those services are catalogued in the American Medical Association's Current Procedural Terminology (CPT) manual, which is updated annually. The CPT manual provides a listing of codes that correspond to various professional services, which are grouped into two basic types: (1) procedures and (2) evaluation and management (E&M) services. Procedures involve technical services such as operations, bedside procedures, endoscopies, radiographic interpretation, and others. E&M services include history and physical examinations, daily inpatient management, clinic visits, and others, including critical care. Professional services for critical care are both E&M services and procedures, often performed on the same patient during the same day. To effectively and appropriately bill for critical care services, therefore, it is necessary to understand the rules governing billing during the surgical global periods for procedures.

R. L. Reed II (✉)
Revenue Cycle Services, IU Heatlh, Department of Surgery, IU Health Methodist Hospital, Indianapolis, IN, USA
e-mail: rreed8@iuhealth.org

Evaluation and Management Services

Evaluation and management services are provided by physicians when they obtain the patient's medical history, perform a physical examination, identify one or more current diagnoses needing medical attention, and construct a plan of treatment for those conditions. There are several different categories of E&M services, including outpatient clinic visits, emergency department visits, initial hospital admission history and physical examinations, daily hospital visits, and so forth.

Any E&M service can be provided by an intensivist, but, most commonly, intensivists bill for critical care E&M services using CPT codes 99291 with or without additional 99292 codes. These E&M services are unique as they do not depend upon the extent of the patient's history, physical examination, or medical decision-making as do the majority of E&M CPT codes. Rather, they are used when the physician's note is able to provide documentation of two criteria: (1) the patient is critically ill and (2) the cumulative amount of time spent by the physician in providing critical care services (exclusive of any time spent performing procedures on the patient during a 24-h day).

Establishing that the patient is critically ill is a key component of the documentation. The patient's location in a critical unit does not necessarily mean that the patient is critically ill. If a patient is critically ill, their care (i.e., critical care) can be provided wherever the patient is located, whether it be in the emergency department, a hospital floor, a waiting room, the operating room, or an intensive care unit. The Centers for Medicare and Medicaid Services (CMS) states that "Critical care is defined as the direct delivery by a physician(s) medical care for a critically ill or critically injured patient. A critical illness or injury acutely impairs one or more vital organ systems such that there is a high probability of imminent or life threatening deterioration in the patient's condition. Critical care involves high complexity decision making to assess, manipulate, and support vital system functions(s) to treat single or multiple vital organ system failure and/or to

A. Salim et al. (eds.), *Surgical Critical Care Therapy*, https://doi.org/10.1007/978-3-319-71712-8_62

prevent further life threatening deterioration of the patient's condition." [1].

Documentation of Critical Illness

The first requirement for coding a critical care encounter, therefore, is to identify the specific organ system(s) that is impaired and which provides the potential for imminent or life-threatening deterioration. The physician's documentation should identify the nature of the organ dysfunction and the potential adverse consequences of inadequate monitoring and treatment. Physicians have been denied payment for their critical care management because their documentation fails to stress the severity of the patient's condition. In a real sense, a physician's experience and comfort with managing the critically ill patient can set them at a disadvantage for reimbursement because they fail to emphasize the severity of the patient's condition adequately.

As an example, an experienced intensivist may provide the following documentation for a patient trying to recover from severe adult respiratory distress syndrome (ARDS):

> Patient remains stable on PRVC at 60% O_2 with 8 cm of PEEP. Po_2 65, Pco_2 33. Will try some permissive hypercapnia.

While accurate, this documentation fails to convey the severity of the patient's pulmonary condition to a coder or reviewer responsible for determining the accuracy of the physician's charges. The same condition could also be represented by the following statement:

> The patient remains in critical condition requiring constant attention. Oxygenation is severely impaired by the lung's impaired physiology, requiring an increased F_IO_2 of 60% and 8 cm H_2O of positive end-expiratory pressure (PEEP), and even then only generating a marginally adequate P_aO_2 of 65 mm Hg (P:F ratio = 108). In addition, the patient is currently being hyperventilated with a P_aCO_2 of 33 mm Hg. As this could be unnecessarily damaging to the pulmonary parenchyma, we will start a trial of permissive hypercapnia to reduce that potential. No efforts at weaning mechanical ventilation are possible given the current status of the patient's pulmonary function, as such efforts will lead to further pulmonary compromise with potential additional organ failure and death.

The additional information makes the critical condition of the patient clear to the coding personnel and reviewers who not only may be inexperienced in critical care but are usually not clinically trained individuals. While the increased verbiage can take the clinician extra time to document, there are two important perspectives to understand: (1) documentation can now be facilitated by automation, and (2) the total time spent in critical care is reimbursed, including the time spent in writing the note.

In electronic medical record systems, documentation can be significantly facilitated by automating repetitive functions. Unfortunately, many clinicians make the terrible mistake of copying a previous note and pasting it as the current note without updating the information in the new note. Such behavior is routinely condemned, primarily because of the great potential for (and experience with) inaccurate documentation if conditions have changed but the documentation has not. However, copying, pasting, and editing are the appropriate actions employed in the effective use of electronic documentation.

More effectively, electronic templates can be produced that provide the structure of the necessary documentation, with manual editing of the individual components. Many of the phrases (if not entire paragraphs) in such notes can be automated as macros in electronic medical record systems. Moreover, EMR systems provide the ability to insert special characters (i.e., an underscore, "_", in Cerner, or 3 asterisks, "***", in EPIC) into macros, thereby enabling the user to quickly insert the specific data (such as the blood gas values for that patient encounter example above). Pressing the F2 key in EPIC or the F3 key in Cerner will take the author to the wildcard placeholder so the author can enter the specific data for that patient.

The effective use of EMR templates can facilitate and speed up the time quality documentation takes. However, the wise intensivist realizes that the quality of the note, not the speed with which it is produced, is the important aspect. The overwhelming majority of professional clinical documentation rules were developed (and often enforced) by CMS. Moreover, reimbursement for professional services is primarily based upon the documentation provided. In a very real sense, the clinician's note in the patient record serves as the invoice for payment. Therefore, it is very important that the severity of the patient's critical illness be accurately and thoroughly documented in order to establish the fact that the patient is critically ill.

Documentation of Time

As previously mentioned, the other key component in billing 99291/99292 codes is the total time spent in delivering the service. The time consists of the cumulative time spent by a single physician (and his colleagues in the same group and the same specialty) in providing critical care to the patient. That time is exclusive of any time spent in the performance of procedures on that patient, which are charged separately. The intensivist must document that number of minutes in providing critical care services in his or her clinical note for each day of service. Again, the time spent in documentation is also included in the total time spent in evaluation and management of the patient.

The 99291 code purportedly covers the first hour of critical care time spent during the day and thus can only be used once daily by each specialty, whereas the 99292 code covers each additional half hour. Specifically, however, the 99291 code cannot be charged unless at least 30 min have been spent in the critical care of the patient, and the 99292 code cannot be charged until at least 15 min of its time has been spent providing critical care. So if an intensivist provides up to 74 min of critical care time on a patient, only one 99291 can be charged. If the intensivist provides 75–104 min of critical care, then both a 99291 and a 99292 can be charged. For 105–134 min of critical care, a 99291 and two 99292s are billed. In short, 99291 covers up to the first 30–74 min of critical care for the day and each 99292 covers additional 15–30 min blocks.

Noncritical Care E&M Code Billing

For situations where the patient's condition does not meet the definition of critical illness or the physician's total time with the patient is less than 30 min for the entire day, standard hospital daily visit codes (99231, 99232, or 99233) should be used. With these codes, in contrast to the billing requirements for critical care documentation, there is no requirement for the patient to be critically ill and there is no requirement for a minimal amount of time spent. However, the documentation requirements for daily visit codes are more rigorous than the documentation requirements for critical care services (where only establishment of the patient's critical illness and documentation of time spent is required).

In contrast to the critical care documentation, documentation for daily visit E&M services must provide an interval history, a physical examination, and medical decision-making. The level of service determined from this documentation ranges from low (99231) to intermediate (99232) to high (99233) levels, and the documentation rules are very specific regarding the requirements to meet each level.

For example, to meet a high-level daily visit code (99233), the clinician must document at least two of the following three components: a detailed interval history, a detailed examination, and/or medical decision-making of high complexity. Each of these components is further specified. A detailed interval history is defined as one that contains a chief complaint, and extended history of present illness, a problem pertinent system review extended to include a review of a limited number of additional systems, and pertinent past, family, and/or social history directly related to the patient's problems. A detailed examination requires documentation of an extended examination of the affected body area(s) and other symptomatic or related organ system(s). And, finally, medical decision-making of high complexity requires documentation of an extensive number of diagnoses or management options, an extensive amount of or complexity of data to review, and a high risk of complications and/or morbidity or mortality.

To employ these rules effectively, it is important to understand that only two of the three sectional components of the note need to be documented. Thus, for a patient with multiple medical conditions that are being addressed (which is often the case in patients who require management in an ICU), the physical examination and medical decision-making components are likely the most effectively used, especially if there are several body areas that are examined and multiple lab and imaging results along with multiple diagnoses or conditions to manage. On the other hand, if a patient only has only one significant clinical problem, such as may be seen with an emergency general surgery patient (as opposed to a multiply injured trauma patient), then it may be more productive and appropriate to provide a detail interval history along with a thorough physical examination.

Complying with those documentation requirements generates 2.00 work RVUs (2.95 total RVUs) for a high-level (99233) daily visit charge but only 1.39 wRVUs (2.04 total RVUs) for a 99232 and 0.76 wRVUs (1.11 total RVUs) for a 99231. Compare that to the 4.5 work RVUs (7.75 total RVUs) that are generated with a 99291 critical care charge, which only requires documentation that establishes the nature of the patient's critical illness and that the total time spent on the patient was at least 30 min of the day. Thus, if a patient meets the standard of being critically ill and the physician has spent at least 30 min in the critical care of the procedure, billing a critical care code should always be the preferred option. However, if those criteria are not met, then the daily visit documentation and coding rules apply.

Procedures

Many critically ill patients require procedures during their critical care stay. Common critical care procedures include the placement of central venous catheters, arterial catheters, chest tubes, feeding catheters, endotracheal tubes, tracheostomies, and others. Many procedures performed on a critically ill patient are billable, but there are issues that must be understood to bill appropriately and optimally.

First, there are several procedures that would otherwise be separately billable, but if 99291/99292 codes are billed, the procedures listed in Table 62.1 cannot be billed [2]. Payment for those procedures are considered to be included in the payment for the 99291/99292 critical care E&M services, and therefore billing for them in addition to billing for 99291 would constitute "double-dipping." It is interesting to note, however, that 99291 generates 4.5 wRVUs (7.75 total RVUs), whereas the cumulative valuation of the procedures listed in Table 62.1 provides 9.31 wRVUs (and 17.24 total

Table 62.1 Procedures included in 99291 and 99292 payments and cannot be separately billed [2]

Description	CPT Code(s)
Interpretation of blood gases	82800, 82810, 82803, 82805
Interpretation of chest films	71010, 71015, 71020
Measurement of cardiac output	93561-93562
Interpretation of other computer stored information	99090
Pulse oximetry	94760-94762
Gastric intubation	43752-43753
Transcutaneous pacing, temporary	92953
Venous access, arterial puncture	36000, 36410, 36415, 36591, 36600
Ventilation assistance and management includes CPAP, continuous negative pressure (CNP) ventilation	94002-94004, 94660, 94662

RVUs), ranging from 0 wRVUs (and 0 total RVUs) to 1.99 wRVUs (2.63 total RVUs) each.

As previously mentioned, the time spent performing critical care E&M services (i.e., 99291 or 99292) is independent of any time spent performing procedures (other than those procedures listed in Table 62.1).

Global Package Issues

Aside from those procedures listed in Table 62.1, all other procedures can be billed as long as they are legitimately performed and documented by a credentialed provider. However, intensivists from any primary specialty (surgery, internal medicine, pulmonology, nephrology, anesthesiology) other than pediatrics must be aware of the concept of the surgical global package [3]. When the Health Care Financing Agency (now CMS) developed the current system for physician reimbursement, they defined a surgical global package (SGP) for all procedures. Conceptually, the SGP provides a bundled payment to the physician; this bundled payment can also be paid to an advanced practice provider when he or she performs the procedure instead of a physician. The package payment includes payment for the procedure as well as the preoperative, intraoperative, and postoperative E&M services provided to the patient in the perioperative period. However, despite CMS' claims that payment for routine E&M services is included in global package payments, critical analysis has revealed that there are deep discounts in the actual amount paid for those E&M services such that in many cases – especially those patients who have a long length of stay – surgeons would fare better financially if they didn't bill for the surgical procedure but instead only billed for the daily inpatient visits [4].

Surgical global package periods are in effect for a variable number of days, depending on the procedure. Global package periods currently are assigned as 90-day, 10-day, or 0-day global periods, meaning that the global package rules apply for 90 days from the date of the procedure, 10 days from the procedure, or only on the date of the procedure, respectively. Some procedures, such as insertion of a central venous catheter in an adult (CPT 36556), carry a 0-day global package, which means that any other procedure or service performed on the same day is considered to be included in the procedure unless a modifier is provided to indicate otherwise. Thus, if an intensivist performs a central venous catheter insertion, he or she should bill the 36556 code because it is not included in the list in Table 62.1. However, if the intensivist also writes a clinical note that day – either a critical care service note (99291/99292) or a daily inpatient visit note (99233/99232/99231) – no payment for that E&M service will be provided because of the global surgical package being active on that day, *unless a modifier is provided* (see below).

There are currently 1223 CPT codes that are assigned a zero (0)-day global package period as in the example above. Listing of all of these codes and procedures is beyond the scope of this publication, but the information can be downloaded at any time and at no charge from the CMS website at https://www.cms.gov/Medicare/Medicare-Fee-for-Service-Payment/PhysicianFeeSched/PFS-Relative-Value-Files.html. There are several 0-day global package procedures that are frequently performed in the practice of critical care, listed in Table 62.2.

There are 472 CPT codes that carry a 10-day global package period and 3785 CPT codes that carry a 90-day global package period. Most of these are not typical or standard ICU procedures and are rarely performed in the ICU setting. However, a surgical intensivist and his or her surgical intensivist colleagues usually perform operative procedures on whom they or their surgical partners also provide critical care services. It is therefore necessary to know that a procedure with a global package was performed on that patient so that appropriate modifiers can be applied to the E&M as well as other procedure codes throughout the effective global period, although, again, it is important to check on any procedures done during a patient's hospitalization to determine their global package durations. For example, most simple laceration repairs carry a 10-day global period. Repairing a patient's laceration in the ED or ICU and knowing to provide a 25 modifier to the admission note are commonly understood. However, that laceration repair will invalidate billing for the subsequent 9 days of critical care for unrelated conditions such as respiratory failure or coagulopathy unless a 24 modifier is applied to the billing for each of those daily visit or critical care codes during that period.

Table 62.2 Examples of 0-day global package period procedures commonly performed in critical care

CPT code	Description	Comment	Work RVUs
10030	Image-guided fluid collection drainage by catheter (e.g., abscess, hematoma, seroma, lymphocele, cyst), soft tissue (e.g., extremity, abdominal wall, neck), percutaneous	Note that percutaneous drainage of pleural, peritoneal, transrectal, or transvaginal drainage collections are not billed using this code. It definitely covers percutaneous image-guided (i.e., via fluoroscopy, ultrasound, plain films, etc.) drainage of other soft tissue fluid collections	2.75
31500	Intubation, endotracheal, emergency procedure	Emergency endotracheal intubation	3.00
31502	Tracheotomy tube change prior to establishment of fistula tract	This would be reasonable for any tracheostomy tube changes during the first week following the performance of tracheostomy. Subsequent use of this code should be supported by documentation that the patient has not yet established a stable tracheocutaneous fistula tract	0.65
31600	Tracheostomy, planned (separate procedure)	Elective tracheostomy (can be done at bedside)	7.17
31603	Tracheostomy, emergency procedure; transtracheal	Emergency tracheostomy	4.14
31605	Tracheostomy, emergency procedure; cricothyroid membrane	Emergency cricothyrotomy	3.57
31612	Tracheal puncture, percutaneous with transtracheal aspiration and/or injection	Also known as a "minitracheostomy," [5–8] this is the placement of a transtracheal catheter (often using the Seldinger technique) for intermittent stimulation of cough reflex	0.91
31623	Bronchoscopy, rigid or flexible, including fluoroscopic guidance, when performed; with brushing or protected brushings	Diagnostic bronchoscopy	2.63
31624	Bronchoscopy, rigid or flexible, including fluoroscopic guidance, when performed; with bronchial alveolar lavage	Bronchoscopy with bronchoalveolar lavage (BAL)	2.63
31720	Catheter aspiration (separate procedure); nasotracheal	Nasotracheal suctioning	1.06
32551	Tube thoracostomy includes connection to drainage system (e.g., water seal), when performed, open (separate procedure)	Standard chest (thoracostomy) tube insertion	3.04
32554	Thoracentesis, needle or catheter, aspiration of the pleural space; without imaging guidance	Bedside needle/catheter thoracentesis	1.82
36556	Insertion of non-tunneled centrally inserted central venous catheter; age 5 years or older	Standard percutaneous central venous catheter insertion	2.50
36620	Arterial catheterization or cannulation for sampling, monitoring or transfusion (separate procedure); percutaneous	Insertion of indwelling percutaneous arterial catheter	1.15
36625	Arterial catheterization or cannulation for sampling, monitoring or transfusion (separate procedure); cutdown	Cutdown insertion of indwelling arterial catheter	2.11
43241	Esophagogastroduodenoscopy, flexible, transoral; with insertion of intraluminal tube or catheter	EGD with tube insertion	2.49
43246	Esophagogastroduodenoscopy, flexible, transoral; with directed placement of percutaneous gastrostomy tube	EGD with PEG insertion	3.56
43761	Repositioning of a naso- or orogastric feeding tube, through the duodenum for enteric nutrition	Repositioning of nasogastric or orogastric tube into duodenum for enteral nutrition	2.01
93503	Insertion and placement of flow-directed catheter (e.g., Swan-Ganz) for monitoring purposes	Pulmonary artery (Swan-Ganz) catheter insertion	2.91

Modifiers

Modifiers are critical to appropriate payment for complicated patients requiring multiple procedures and the management of multiple conditions. Without a modifier, the global package concept provides the default attitude for payment, which is that payment for a procedure covers all services and procedures performed on the patient during the global period. Thus, there will be no payments to the same physician who performed the original procedure (including his or her partners in the same group and specialty) for any other procedures or services they perform during that global period. It's as though the only reason the patient saw a physician on that day or – in the case of a 90-day global package – for those 3 months was for the performance of that procedure. In essence, without modifiers, a large volume of appropriate care is unpaid.

However, in the case of complicated acute care surgery, there are often multiple services and procedures that are necessary during the patient's intensive care stay, which is often during the global package postoperative period following one or more procedures. In order to receive payment for those services and procedures, modifiers must be applied to the additional procedure(s) and/or service(s) the patient is receiving during the global period.

In order to qualify for payment, in addition to providing the modifier, there should also be sufficient documentation to indicate that the service or procedure is unrelated to the global package's procedure. For example, the management of a preexisting condition (i.e., diabetes, hypertension, chronic renal failure) is separately payable during the postoperative period even if it is performed by the same physician (or the physician's partner in the same group and specialty) who performed the operation. However, management of conditions "typically" associated with the operation (i.e., wound care, incisional pain management, suture removal) is not separately payable.

Unfortunately, there is some confusion related to the concept of what constitutes a "typical" condition during the postoperative period, because CMS' guidance, published in Chap. 12 of the Medicare Claims Processing Manual [3], is actually unclear. In one section, it states that the global package payment covers treatment for postoperative complications that do not require a return trip to the operating room. Thus, opening an infected wound postoperatively at the bedside would likely not be separately paid. However, elsewhere in the same document, treatment for a condition that is "above and beyond the usual preoperative and postoperative care associated with the procedure or service that was performed" is payable as long as the appropriate modifier is applied for the additional E&M service. Of course, in most cases, opening a postoperative wound infection at the bedside is not "usual" postoperative care for most procedures but distinctly unusual (although not extremely rare). Nevertheless, billing for opening an infected wound at bedside is often a futile effort, as payments for such procedures are usually denied.

Because of the confused guidance, therefore, if a physician provides a service or procedure during the postoperative period and the physician wishes to be paid for that service, it is important to document clearly how it is that the condition being treated is unrelated to the procedure for which a global package period is in effect. For example, if a patient develops pneumonia following an operation for major liver trauma, it is important to document that the pneumonia is related to the patient's rib fractures, pulmonary contusion, or heavy sedation requirements and not specifically to the operative procedure performed to control the liver hemorrhage. (Note that it is also important to do so from the hospital's standpoint, as the hospital gets penalized if the pneumonia is attributed to the patient's mechanical ventilation.)

The modifiers applied by the intensivist should be applied to the E&M service billing and to any procedural billing performed during the global package procedures. There may, in fact, be overlapping global package periods in some patients. These don't affect the need for modifiers, but documentation must provide evidence that the postoperative procedures and services are unrelated to the procedures with active global periods.

While there are currently 379 modifiers that have been established for CPT codes, only a few are commonly used in critical care:

1. Modifier 24 ("Unrelated Evaluation and Management Service by the Same Physician or Other Qualified Health Care Professional During a Postoperative Period"). This indicates that the E&M service is being performed during a global package period of a procedure that was performed by the same physician (or his or her partner from the same specialty), but the E&M service (e.g., clinical note such as 99291/99292) is unrelated to the procedure. In order to meet the latter criterion, it is most effective if the physician's note focuses on the management of diagnoses that are different from the diagnoses related to the operation.
2. Modifier 25 ("Significant, Separately Identifiable Evaluation and Management Service by the Same Physician or Other Qualified Health Care Professional on the Same Day of the Procedure or Other Service"). This modifier is applied to an E&M service that is provided on the same day as a procedure but is unrelated to the procedure. Typically, this is used in cases where the procedure has a 0-day or 10-day global package period. Again, the note for which the E&M code is being applied should refer to conditions or diagnoses unrelated to the condition for which the procedure is being performed. For example, a central venous catheter (CPT 36556) is introduced for hypovolemia (ICD-10-CM E86.1), while the daily critical care note covering 38 min of time (CPT 99291) refers to the patient's other conditions of respiratory failure, hyponatremia, oliguria, and hypotension (ICD-10-CM codes J96.20, E87.1, R34, and I95.89, respectively).
3. Modifier 57 ("Decision for Surgery"). This is applied for any E&M service where the patient is evaluated, and it is determined that the patient should undergo operative surgery. The code is usually applied in cases of major (i.e., 90-day global surgery package periods) operations and is needed for E&M services applied the day before or the day of the operation. In contrast to the other E&M service modifiers listed here, the diagnosis for the E&M service can (and probably should) be the same as the diagnosis for the operation. In other words, this is a "related" E&M service as opposed to an unrelated E&M service. This modifier is rarely, if ever, appropriate for admission

history and physical examinations performed on the day of admission for a patient undergoing a scheduled elective operation; the decision an elective operation was made previously, for example, in the clinic, and that E&M service should have already been billed.

4. Modifier 59 ("Distinct Procedural Service"). In contrast to the modifiers described above, this is a modifier applied to procedural CPT codes instead of E&M service CPT codes. It specifies that the procedure for which it is being applied was done on the same patient during the same day by the same physician (or that physician's partner of the same specialty and the same group), but it was performed at a different time, or on a different site, through a different incision, or on a different body area. For example, if a tracheostomy (CPT 31600) is performed by the same physician who also subsequently performs a percutaneous endoscopic gastrostomy (PEG) insertion (CPT 43246), a 59 modifier should be applied to the PEG procedure, as it is the lesser valued procedure (3.56 vs. 7.17 work RVUs).

References

1. Medicare Claims Processing Manual, Chapter 12 – Physicians/ Nonphysician Practitioners, Section 30.6.12 – Critical Care Visits and Neonatal Intensive Care (Codes 99291–99292), Subsection A: Use of Critical Care Codes.63–64. https://www.cms.gov/Regulations-and-Guidance/Guidance/Manuals/Downloads/clm104c12.pdf. Accessed 8 June 2017.
2. Medicare Claims Processing Manual, Chapter 12 – Physicians/ Nonphysician Practitioners, Section 30.6.12 – Critical Care Visits and Neonatal Intensive Care (Codes 99291–99292), Subsection J: Critical Care Services and Other Procedures Provided on the Same Day by the Same Physician as Critical Care Codes 99291–99292.74. https://www.cms.gov/Regulations-and-Guidance/Guidance/Manuals/Downloads/clm104c12.pdf. Accessed 13 June 2017.
3. Medicare Claims Processing Manual, Chapter 12 – Physicians/ Nonphysician Practitioners, Section 40.1: Definition of a Global Surgical Package.90–94. https://www.cms.gov/Regulations-and-Guidance/Guidance/Manuals/Downloads/clm104c12.pdf. Accessed 6/8/2017.
4. Reed RL 2nd, Luchette FA, Esposito TJ, Pyrz K, Gamelli RL. Medicare's "global" terrorism: where is the pay for performance? J Trauma. 2008;64(2):374–83; discussion 383–374.
5. Beach L, Denehy L, Lee A. The efficacy of minitracheostomy for the management of sputum retention: a systematic review. Physiotherapy. 2013;99(4):271–7.
6. Bonde P, Papachristos I, McCraith A, et al. Sputum retention after lung operation: prospective, randomized trial shows superiority of prophylactic minitracheostomy in high-risk patients. Ann Thorac Surg. 2002;74(1):196–202; discussion 202–193.
7. Corke C, Cranswick PA. Seldinger technique for minitracheostomy insertion. Anaesth Intensive Care. 1988;16(2):206–7.
8. Randell TT, Tierala EK, Lepantalo MJ, Lindgren L. Prophylactic minitracheostomy after thoracotomy: a prospective, random control, clinical trial. Eur J Surg. 1991;157(9):501–4.

Tracheostomy in the ICU

63

Maher M. Matar, Stephen A. Fann, and Bruce A. Crookes

Introduction

A tracheostomy is a surgical procedure that establishes a stoma between the trachea and the overlying skin of the anterior neck. Technical proficiency in this procedure is required by all trauma and acute care surgeons involved in the management of critically ill patients. Knowledge of the indications, contraindications, potential complications, and the optimal timing of the procedure is crucial and will be discussed herein. A discussion of the pertinent landmarks and surface anatomy will be addressed in the procedure portion of the chapter (Fig. 63.1).

The modern day, open tracheostomy was first described in detail by Chevalier Jackson in 1909, but the procedure dates to Egypt, 3600 BC. Percutaneous tracheostomy was popularized by Pasquale Ciaglia in 1980s and, since then, has evolved into the most popular method of performing the procedure, with the introduction of prepackaged "tracheostomy kits" such as the Ciaglia Blue Rhino® and the Portex® GRIGGS®, to mention a few.

Indications

The indications for performing a tracheostomy are threefold: ventilator "dependence," upper airway obstruction, and facilitation of pulmonary toilet. The clinical settings in which these indications might manifest include an inability to protect the airway due to vocal cord trauma or paralysis, severe traumatic brain injury leading to a low Glasgow Coma Scale score, complex tracheal surgeries, and high cervical spine injury, to mention a few. In addition, there exists a group of patients that require prolonged mechanical ventilator support due to an inability to wean from the ventilator. Most trauma and acute care surgeons agree that this group would benefit from tracheostomy as well, although there is little consensus on this indication as to its benefit and its timing. Tracheostomy also enhances two-way communication with the patient, facilitating oral hygiene and pulmonary toilet.

M. M. Matar
Department of Surgery, Division of General Surgery, The Ottawa Hospital, Ottawa, Ontario, Canada

S. A. Fann · B. A. Crookes (✉)
Department of Surgery, General Surgery Division, Medical University of South Carolina, Charleston, SC, USA
e-mail: crookes@musc.edu

Complications

Complications can be divided into early and late. In general, open surgical tracheostomy exhibits an overall complication rate of 10% during the procedure and 3% post-procedure. Percutaneous tracheostomy exhibits an overall complication rate of 10% and 7%, during and post-procedure, respectively [1].

Early Complications

Early delineates a period of up to 7- days post tracheostomy. The most common complications in this period are post-procedure hemorrhage and pneumothorax. Major bleeding is estimated at 0–7% in open tracheostomy, whereas minor bleeding occurred in up to 2% of patients receiving either open or percutaneous tracheostomy. Other complications include pneumomediastinum (0–4%), subcutaneous emphysema (0–4%), tracheal fracture during dilation of the tract, airway fires due to cautery use, unplanned decannulation, and loss of airway and mucus or hematoma plug leading to airway obstruction. One unique complication of percutaneous tracheostomy is false passage of the tracheostomy tube into the subcutaneous space anterior to the trachea which occurs in up to 4% of cases. In rare instances, early opportunistic skin infections may occur as well [1–3].

A. Salim et al. (eds.), *Surgical Critical Care Therapy*, https://doi.org/10.1007/978-3-319-71712-8_63

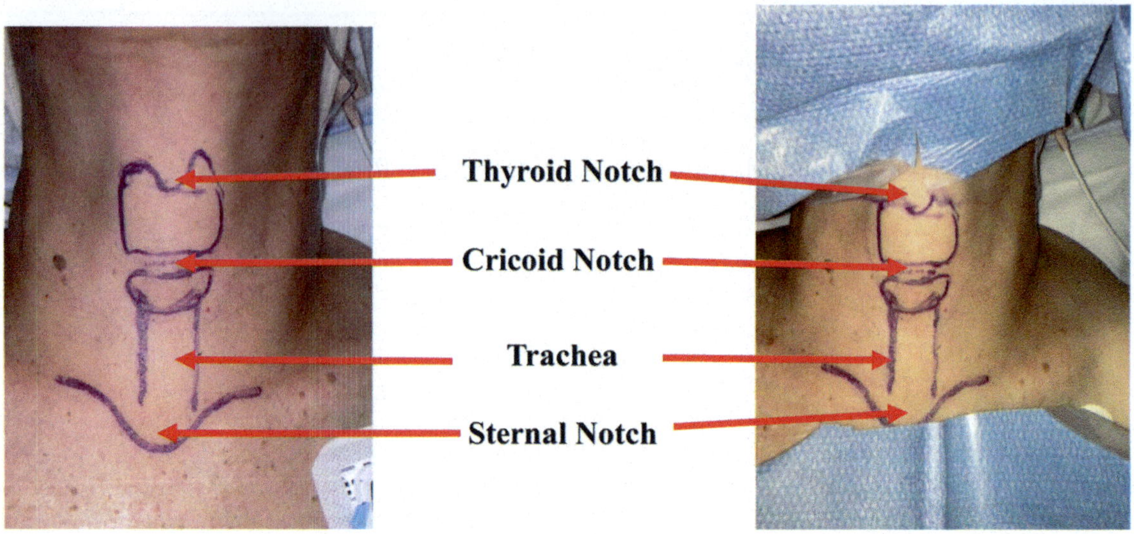

Fig. 63.1 Relevant anatomy for tracheostomy placement drawn on the skin before (left panel) and after (right panel) sterile draping of the area

Delayed Complications

Delayed complications can include any of the above complications occurring 7 days after the procedure, along with some unique issues that may arise beyond this time point. Delayed complications include wound infection, which can lead to inflammatory changes in the trachea resulting in stenosis in the long term, fistula formation between the trachea and surrounding structures (such as the esophagus and arterial structures), and failure of wound closure.

Granulation tissue accumulation as a result of infection and inflammation leads to laryngotracheal stenosis. This may be avoided by limiting the size of the initial incision and maintaining cuff pressures below 25 mmHg. Furthermore, ensuring proper tracheostomy care and minimizing infection are also crucial to avoid the formation of excessive granulation tissue.

Probably the most dreaded complication with tracheostomies, and one that thankfully occurs in less than 1% of patients, is the tracheoinnominate artery fistula (TIAF) formation. In this complication, whose peak incidence is at 7–14 days post-procedure, a fistulous tract forms between the innominate artery, which resides below the sternum, and the trachea as a result of pressure necrosis. This complication usually results in immediate life-threatening hemorrhage. To avoid this complication, the tracheostomy should remain above the fourth tracheal ring. Fifty percent of these cases will present with a self-limiting sentinel bleed; as a result, any bleeding that occurs 3–6 days after insertion of a tracheostomy should be assumed to be a tracheoinnominate fistula until proven otherwise.

If a fistula is suspected after a sentinel bleed, the tracheal tube cuff should be maximally inflated, to allow for compression of the fistula and artery against the sternum, bronchoscopy should be performed to assess for the bleeding source, and the amount of blood in the trachea and bronchi should be noted. This also allows for pulmonary toilet and clearing the blood from the bronchi, to optimize ventilation. Of note, the bronchoscope can be passed through the nasopharynx to examine the tracheal tissue surrounding the tube as well. If the concern for TIAF persists, a computed-tomography angiography of the neck and chest should be performed.

In the actively bleeding patient, orotracheal intubation should be established, and the tracheostomy tube removed, allowing for a finger to pass through the tracheostomy site and press the artery against the sternum, known as the Utley maneuver, at which point emergency surgical intervention is required [4]. Mortality is extremely high due to an inability to ventilate and properly oxygenate the patient [5]. There have been multiple reports of successful repair of TIAF via endovascular and/or interventional radiologic approaches published in the literature.

Timing of Tracheostomy

One of the controversial questions that a clinician tending to the care of critically ill patients is challenged with is the timing of tracheostomy. In 2005, Rumbak and colleagues randomly assigned 128 patients prospectively into an early tracheostomy group (48 h) versus late tracheostomy (14–16 days) in patients that were predicted to require >16 days of mechanical ventilation. The early tracheostomy group showed significantly lower mortality rates at 30 days, lower rates of pneumonia, decreased sedation requirements, less time on ventilator, and a shorter length of stay in the ICU [6]. A well-executed systematic review and meta-analysis by Siempos and colleagues, published in the Lancet in 2015, sought to address this issue once again. Their analysis showed statistically significantly less cases of ventilator-associated pneumonia, shorter time on ventilator, earlier patient mobilization, and a decrease length of stay in the ICU. They failed to show an improvement in mortality outcomes between early tracheostomy (<48 h) and late (>15 days) [7]. In many intensive care units, *time to tracheostomy* is being used as a quality indicator by administrators, despite the controversy surrounding the subject.

Open Surgical Tracheostomy Versus Percutaneous Tracheostomy

The choice of performing an open or a percutaneous tracheostomy depends strictly on individual patient characteristics and the surgeon's comfort with the technique. Patients with a previous history of mantle radiation, neck trauma, neck surgery, tracheal surgery, or any condition that would lead to an anatomic deviation from normal should be taken to the operating room for an open tracheostomy. However, one common misconception is to automatically assume that any adverse anatomic factor will make the decision weigh more heavily in favor of an open tracheostomy. The most common of these is obesity, and particularly in severely obese patients with very short and thick necks. While this does increase the difficulty of performing a percutaneous tracheostomy, it arguably has a more significant adverse impact on the performance of an open tracheostomy than the percutaneous approach. We do not consider obesity to be a contraindication to percutaneous tracheostomy, and in fact have found the percutaneous approach to be significantly faster and less technically difficult than performing an open tracheostomy in this patient population.

A recent Cochrane Review conducted by Brass and colleagues in 2015 looking at the literature surrounding open and percutaneous tracheostomies showed that there exists no difference in the mortality rates or hemorrhage rates between the two procedures. Furthermore, the review showed no difference in the rate of tracheostomy tube occlusion, accidental decannulation, or difficulty in tube change between the two groups. The review did, on the other hand, show that rates of wound infection and stomatitis, and rates of unfavorable scarring, were decreased in the patients receiving percutaneous tracheostomy by 76% and 75%, respectively [8].

The authors would strongly recommend that any surgeon performing tracheostomy be comfortable with both techniques. Knowledge of the skills required for both types of procedures allows the surgeon the ability to use the alternative technique as a *rescue procedure*, in the event of a complication during the procedure. If the surgeon and surgical assistant are not comfortable with manipulation of the endotracheal tube and performing emergent rapid reintubation if the tube is prematurely dislodged, then an additional airway expert should be present for assistance during the critical parts of the procedure.

Prophylactic Antibiotics

Surgical and percutaneous tracheostomy is considered to be *clean-contaminated* cases, due to the necessary violation of the airway, but there is a scant body of literature surrounding the topic of prophylactic antibiotics. Surgical site infections in percutaneous tracheostomy are cited at up to 7%. One recent study by Hagiya and colleagues retrospectively examined patients in their ICU that had received prophylactic antibiotics prior to percutaneous tracheostomy and compared them to those that did not receive antibiotics. The authors found that the overall surgical site infection (SSI) rate was 7.25%, and patients who received prophylactic antibiotics had statistically significantly less cases of SSI, as compared to those who did not receive antibiotics (0.88% and 7.25%, respectively) [9]. Our practice is to not administer pre-procedural antibiotics.

Cricothyroidotomy Conversion to Tracheostomy

The classical surgical teaching has been to convert an emergent cricothyroidotomy into a tracheostomy to avoid subglottic stenosis, as described by Chevalier and Jackson in 1921. A recent review published by Talving and colleagues reported that the actual incidence of tracheal stenosis post cricothyroidotomy was 2.2% overall and 1.1% in trauma patients specifically [10]. This finding challenges the need to expose critically the critically ill patient to further manipulation of the airway once cricothyroidotomy has been established.

Procedure

To-do Checklist Prior to Procedure

- Review the patient's history for contraindications of percutaneous tracheostomy and for history of neck trauma that may impede neck mobility.
- Review existing imaging for high-riding innominate artery.
- Review patient chart for list of medications and identify coagulation status (heparin, low molecular weight heparin, aspirin, novel anticoagulants, etc.).
- Patient consent.

Equipment Checklist

- Medications:
  - Pain management including local analgesia
  - Sedative agent
  - Paralytic agent
- Bronchoscope with suction

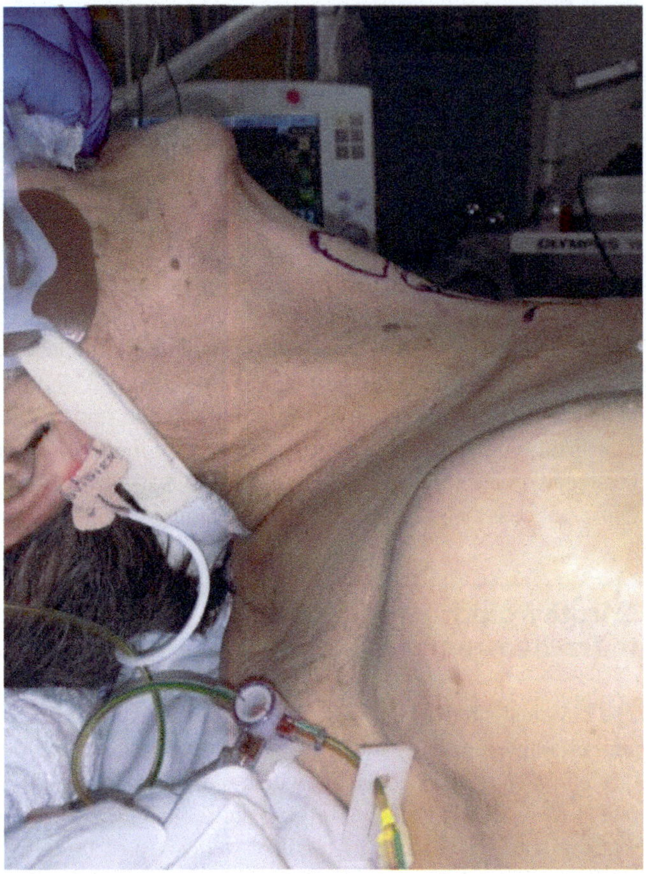

Fig. 63.2 Neck position in extension with pillow below shoulders, brings trachea anterior

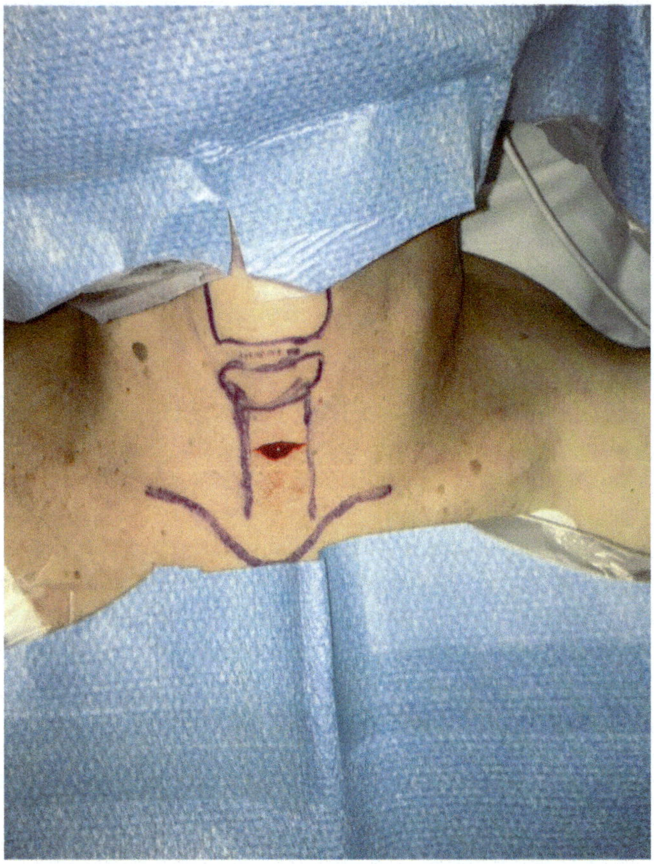

Fig. 63.3 Incision two fingerbreadths from the sternal notch

- Sterile gloves, gowns, hair net, face mask, and drape
- Percutaneous tracheostomy set
- Cuffed tracheostomy tube (multiple sizes, balloon tested)
- Tracheostomy kit with Army-Navy retractors, hemostats, tracheal hook, and tracheal dilator (on standby)
- Backup endotracheal airway kit

Step-by-Step Technique

Positioning

- If the patient is not on C-spine precautions, place a 5-inch rolled towel behind the upper back to allow for a mild extension of the neck, displacing the trachea anteriorly (Fig. 63.2). This is particularly critical in patients with obesity and/or shorter neck lengths.
- The patient should be up high in the bed to allow for bronchoscopy and reintubation if needed.
- Patients in C-spine precautions should have the collar removed and C-spine precautions maintained by a dedicated individual. The use of roles on either side of the head can be helpful.

Administer medications

- Vitals should be continuously monitored throughout the procedure.

Perform bronchoscopy

- Ensure that the endotracheal tube does not move with the bronchoscope, as the patient may become inadvertently extubated.
- Clear out the airway by suctioning the trachea and tube clear from mucus, and collect samples for culture if needed.
- Identify the second tracheal space from within the tube with the bronchoscope.

Using sterile technique

- Identify the anatomy of the trachea using external landmarks and transillumination from the bronchoscope aiming for the second or third inter-tracheal space (Fig. 63.3).
- Inject local anesthetic.
- Make a vertical or horizontal incision approximately 2 fingerbreadths above the sternal notch (Fig. 63.3).

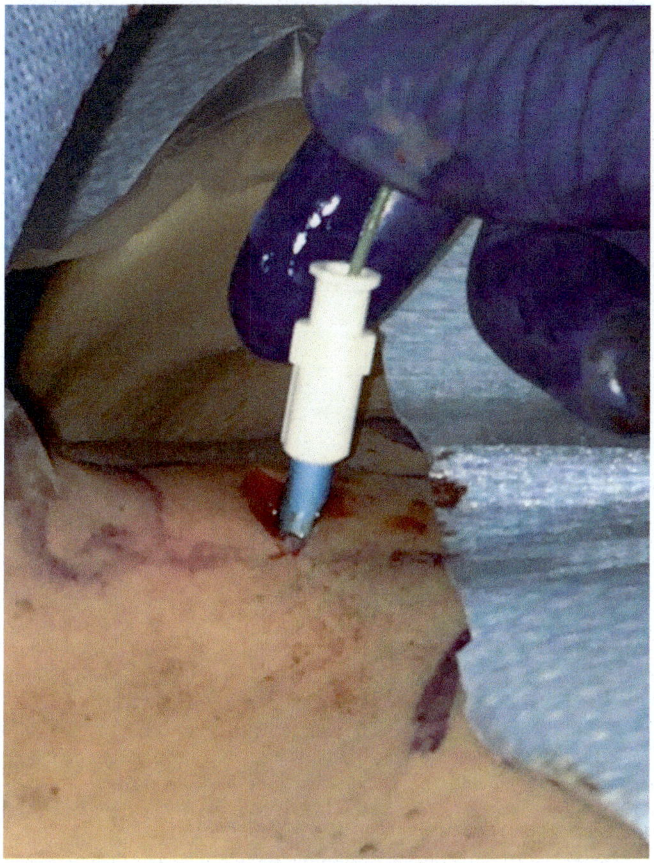

Fig. 63.4 Initial dilator with guidewire in place

- – Ensure that the incision is big enough to accommodate the dilators and the cuffed tracheostomy tube.
- – Note: horizontal incisions deliver best aesthetic results with risk of injuring the anterior jugular veins that travel on either side of the trachea, while vertical incisions allow for the needle to be repositioned if need be.
- With the incision made through the skin, identify the tracheal anatomy using your finger.
- Have the endotracheal tube pulled back until you can feel its tip at the second tracheal ring.
- Insert the finder needle under bronchoscopic guidance to ensure that the needle is in the midline.
- Pass the guidewire through the needle and then remove the needle (Fig. 63.4).
- Pass the series of dilators provided in the kit under direct visualization, and keep the trachea stable in the midline with the non-dominant hand as you do this. You may need to pass the dilator a few times to facilitate the insertion of the tracheostomy tube (Fig. 63.5).
- Place the tracheostomy tube with the introducer (obturator) into the tracheostomy under direct visualization. This may require some gentle pressure (Fig. 63.6).
- Remove the introducer (obturator) and the guidewire and insert the inner cannula.

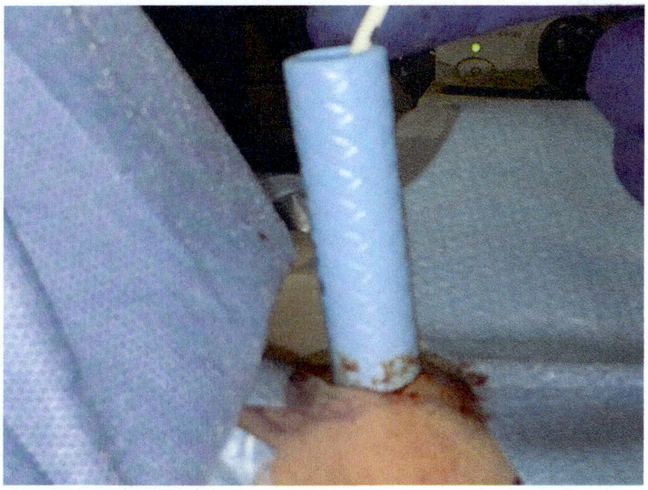

Fig. 63.5 Subsequent Blue Rhino® dilator with guidewire in place

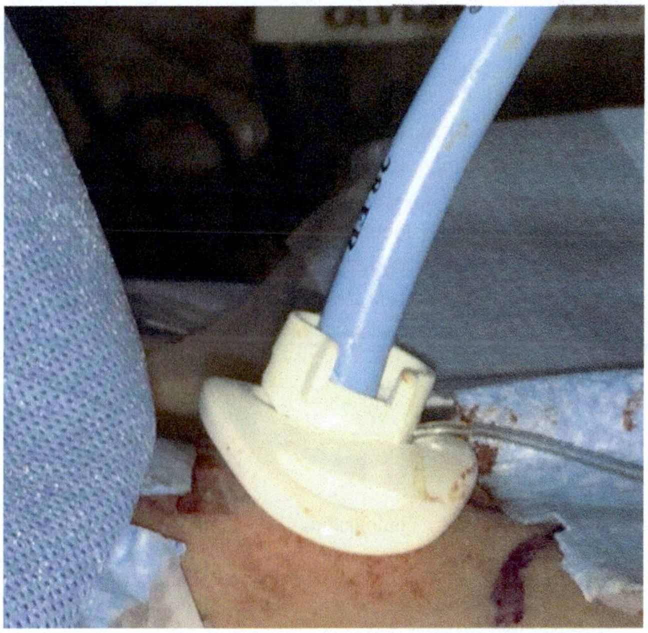

Fig. 63.6 Tracheostomy tube introduced with 28 Fr dilator

- Pass the bronchoscope into the tracheostomy tube to confirm placement and position by identifying the carina and suction out blood that may be in the trachea (Fig. 63.7).
- Inflate the balloon and connect the patient to the ventilator – look for return of end-tidal CO_2 on the ventilator.
- Secure the tracheostomy tube with the neck strap provided, along with sutures to the skin (sutures are optional).
- Gauze may be placed around the tracheostomy tube to control bleeding, ensuring that it does not elevate the tracheostomy tube significantly off the skin.

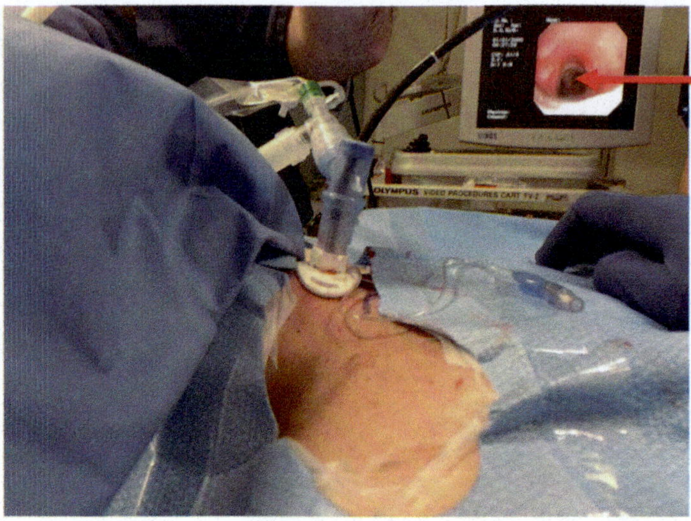

Fig. 63.7 Final bronchoscopy to confirm position and clear secretions

Post-placement items

- Obtain a portable chest x-ray to confirm position and depth of the tracheostomy tube, and rule out any complications such as pneumothorax or lobar collapse.
- Assess for any signs of a cuff-leak, usually manifest as audible gurgling with respirations. If present this usually indicates the cuff was damaged during insertion, and the tube should be replaced.
- Document the procedure, the postoperative x-ray findings, and any guidance for tracheostomy care in a detailed procedure or operative note on the chart.

References

1. Dubrin CGJ. Early complications of tracheostomy. Respir Care. 2005;50(4):511–5.
2. Tobler WD, Agarwal S. Tracheostomy. In: Cameron JL, Cameron AM, editors. Current surgical therapy. 11th ed. Philadelphia: Elsevier Inc.; 2014. p. 1238–41.
3. Sifir Z, Mohr A. Surgical procedures in the surgical intensive care unit. In: Asensio JA, Trunkey DD, editors. Current therapy of trauma and surgical critical care. 2nd ed. Philadelphia: Elsevier; 2016. p. 755.
4. Utley J, Singer M, Roe B, Fraser D, Dedo H. Definitive management of innominate artery hemorrhage complicating tracheostomy. JAMA. 1972;220(4):577–9.
5. Grant CA, Dempsey G, Harrison J, Jones T. Tracheo-innominate artery fistula after percutaneous tracheostomy: three case reports and a clinical review. Br J Anaesth. 2006;96(1):127–31.
6. Rumbak MJ, Newton M, Truncale T, Schwartz SW, Adams JW, Hazard PB. A prospective, randomized, study comparing early percutaneous dilational tracheotomy to prolonged translaryngeal intubation (delayed tracheotomy) in critically ill medical patients. Crit Care Med. 2004;32(8):1689–94.
7. Siempos II, Ntaidou TK, Filippidis FT, Choi AMK. Effect of early versus late or no tracheostomy on mortality and pneumonia of critically ill patients receiving mechanical ventilation: a systematic review and meta-analysis. Lancet Respir Med [Internet] Elsevier Ltd. 2015;3(2):150–8. Available from: https://doi.org/10.1016/S2213-2600(15)00007-7
8. Brass P, Hellmich M, Kullmer B, Ladra A, Ladra J. Percutaneous technique versus surgical techniques for tracheostomy. Cochrane Database Syst Rev [Internet]. 2009;(4). Available from: http://www.mrw.interscience.wiley.com/cochrane/clsysrev/articles/CD008045/frame.html LK - Link%7Chttp://www.mrw.interscience.wiley.com/cochrane/clsysrev/articles/CD008045/frame.html%7C FG - 0
9. Hagiya H, Naito H, Hagioka S, Okahara S, Morimoto N, Kusano N, et al. Effects of antibiotics administration on the incidence of wound infection in percutaneous dilatational tracheostomy. Acta Med Okayama. 2014;68(2):57–62.
10. Talving P, DuBose J, Inaba K, Demetriades D. Conversion of emergent cricothyrotomy to tracheotomy in trauma patients. Arch Surg. 2010;145(1):87–91.

64 Feeding Gastrostomy Tubes

Brittany K. Bankhead-Kendall and Jayson Aydelotte

Oftentimes enteral feedings need to be transitioned from the nasogastric tube or orogastric tube to a gastrostomy tube. This form of nutrition is often most suitable for patients who are physiologically or anatomically unable to swallow safely. This chapter addresses the indications for feeding gastrostomy tubes, techniques of placement, and potential complications.

Indications

Feeding gastrostomy tubes are most often indicated when patients have a functional swallowing problem or have a structural anomaly that prevents safe, effective swallowing, most commonly head and neck tumors or cerebral dysfunction. Neurologic deficits caused by stroke, subarachnoid hemorrhage, severe traumatic brain injury, or anoxic injury can lead to dysphagia and need for an alternative, more long-term route of enteral nutrition. The most common indication for gastrostomy is dysphagia secondary to stroke [1]. Norton et al. randomized patients who suffered debilitating strokes to receive tube feedings via percutaneous endoscopic gastrostomy (PEG) or prolonged nasogastric tube (NGT) feedings. Patients who required enteral tube feeds 14 days poststroke were randomized. Patients who underwent early gastrostomy placement had a lower 6-month mortality (12% vs 57%), received a higher proportion of their goal tube feed volume (94% vs 78%), and had a significantly better improvement in their serum albumin concentration at 6 weeks [2].

A more recent study, the "Feed or Ordinary Diet" ("FOOD") trial was a family of three separate multicenter prospective trials. Trial 1 incorporated patients who could swallow within 30 days of admission and were randomized to normal diet or normal diet plus oral nutritional supplements. Trial 2 evaluated patients with dysphagia who were assigned an early enteral tube feeding vs waiting at least 1 week for enteral feeding. The third arm of the trial evaluated patients with dysphagia who were randomized to nasogastric tube feedings or PEG tube feedings. This third trial included 321 patients in 47 hospitals across 11 countries. Outcomes included overall mortality, survival with a poor functional outcome, and survival with a good overall functional outcome. There was no statistically significant difference between the NGT feeding group and PEG tube feeding group for any of the outcome measures [3].

Head and neck cancers, as well as proximal esophageal tumors, may also necessitate more distal feeding access. As tumors enlarge and either cause mass effect or invasion of the esophageal lumen, food is unable to successfully pass these areas. Gastrostomy tubes are a reasonable alternative method of nutrition, provided an appropriate operative approach is taken while taking into consideration the primary tumor. A systematic review in 2014 evaluated several randomized controlled trials, as well as non-experimental studies comparing PEG tube feeding to NG tube feeding. Overall, the review showed that PEG tubes and NG tubes had equivalent outcomes when comparing weight maintenance in patients with head and neck cancers, as well as no difference in disease-free or overall survival [4].

Technique

Four general forms of gastrostomy tube placement exist: open gastrostomy placement, percutaneous endoscopic gastrostomy ("PEG"), laparoscopic gastrostomy, and radiologic placement. Open gastrostomy tubes are created using an upper midline incision; the stomach is directly visualized and a gastrostomy is made. A feeding tube is placed through the abdominal wall and into the lumen of the stomach through a separate incision. The laparoscopic approach is very similar.

B. K. Bankhead-Kendall
Dell Medical School, University of Texas at Austin, Austin, TX, USA

J. Aydelotte (✉)
Department of Surgery and Perioperative Care, Dell Medical School at the University of Texas-Austin, Austin, TX, USA
e-mail: JDAydelotte@seton.org

A. Salim et al. (eds.), *Surgical Critical Care Therapy*, https://doi.org/10.1007/978-3-319-71712-8_64

Laparoscopic access is obtained and the stomach directly visualized. The gastrostomy tube is generally placed through a separate stab incision in the abdominal wall or through a 5 mm working port into the abdomen and then again into the stomach. In both the laparoscopic and open procedures, the gastrostomy is typically fixed with a purse-string-type suture, and then the stomach is fixed to the abdominal wall with suture around the opening for the tube.

A meta-analysis of 22 studies comprising 5752 patients compared open gastrostomy, laparoscopic gastrostomy, and percutaneous gastrostomy tubes in children. There were no differences in major complications (death or reoperations) between open gastrostomy and PEG or between open gastrostomy and laparoscopic gastrostomy. However, there was a statistically significantly lower likelihood of major complications between laparoscopic gastrostomy tube placement and PEG [5].

Oliveira et al. performed a retrospective evaluation of all feeding gastrostomies performed in a single institution over a 13-year period. In general there was a preponderance increasing frequency of PEGs versus other surgical approaches over that time period. There were no significant differences between laparoscopic and PEG major complications. However, there was an increased mortality and major complication rate in open gastrostomy placement over PEG. But these open gastrostomies were almost all done as a part of other major surgeries as an adjunct and not a primary feeding procedure, as were nearly all the PEGs and laparoscopic gastrostomy tubes in this study [6].

Another study comparing PEG vs open gastrostomy in lung transplant recipients evaluated the National Inpatient Sample as a large retrospective analysis over a 5-year period. A total of 215 patients were included. There was no difference in venothromboembolic complications, urinary tract infection, surgical site infection, or myocardial infarction between the two groups. However, there was a statistically significant increase in mortality acute renal failure in the PEG group [7].

Mizrahi et al. retrospectively evaluated all the open and laparoscopic gastrostomy tubes in a single institution over an 8-year period. 71 patients were included in the study, 46 open gastrostomy tube patients and 25 laparoscopic gastrostomy tube placement patients. While laparoscopic placement took significantly longer 77 min vs 56 min, there were no differences in major complications including mortality [8].

PEG tubes are placed using the "push" or "pull" method. In both techniques, an endoscope is placed into the stomach and the stomach insufflated with air. An assistant then palpates the upper abdomen with one finger, and the indentation is seen with the gastroscope. The abdominal wall is transilluminated, and the light is seen by the assistant looking at the abdominal wall skin. The "pull" method requires a needle to be placed through the abdominal wall and into the stomach. A wire is then placed through the needle, grasped by the endoscope, and pulled out of the mouth. The actual gastrostomy tube is then placed over the wire or connected to the wire, and the wire/tube is then "pulled" through the needle gastrotomy and the abdominal wall. In this technique the tube is fixed to a seamless dilator system that dilates the needle gastrotomy as it's being pulled through. The lumen end of the tube is flanged, and the flange is held against the stomach wall and the stomach against the abdominal wall by friction when a soft bumper is placed around the tube on the skin side of the abdominal wall. The "push" technique is done under direct visualization with the endoscope as well. A needle is inserted into the stomach, and oftentimes the stomach is fixed against the peritoneal surface of the abdominal wall with fasteners under direct visualization. A wire is placed through the needle and a system of dilators is used from the skin side of the abdominal wall going into the stomach lumen. The tube is then placed into the gastrostomy from the skin side and held in place with a similar bumper system.

Kohler et al. performed a single-institution retrospective review of both types of PEG placement, 131 "pull" PEGs and 100 "push" PEGs. A total of 231 patients received a PEG. The overall complication rate (33% vs 21.4%), tube dislocation (12% vs 3.8%), and PEG occlusion (10% vs 0.8%) were significantly higher in the "push" method vs the "pull" method [9]. This is in contrast to an earlier study retrospectively comparing the two techniques. In a much smaller sample size, the push technique had significantly fewer (0%) overall complications than the pull technique (30%) [10]. Pull-PEGs were more likely to have tube dislocation, and push-PEGs were associated with more occlusions over a 10-day follow-up period. Notably, only 2.2% of patients required a reoperation due to a complication of either method [1]. Overall, it does not appear as though there is a definitive answer to which type of method should be employed on a regular basis. Taking into account the patient's pathology and current anatomy, as well as surgeon and endoscopist's comfort level with either technique, would be appropriate factors to take into consideration when deciding on type.

Radiologic gastrostomy tubes are placed by an interventional radiologist. Different methods have been described using fluoroscopic, CT, or ultrasound guidance. A nasogastric tube is often placed for administration of air for better visualization of the gastric bubble during the procedure, and occasionally contrast is given as well in order to potentially aid in identification of the colon during placement. The technique is generally to percutaneously access the stomach and then use a modified "push" technique with or without gastropexy with fasteners [1]. A recent single-institution retrospective review comparing radiologic versus endoscopically placed gastrostomy tubes failed to show a difference in overall or major complications [11].

Complications

Complications of gastrostomy tubes can be both early and late and usually range from 3% to 8%. Technical complications of the procedure fall into the early category and vary by how the gastrostomy tube was placed. All procedure types can be complicated by bleeding or infection; additionally, leaking around the tube is common, especially immediately after placement. Poor nutritional status among all patients can lead to delayed wound healing.

Tube site wound infection is one of the more common complications: the literature reports a very wide range of these, between 5% and 65%. These mild infections (not merely erythema, but with evidence of purulent drainage) are usually treated with topical antibiotics and daily dressing changes. However, intravenous cephalosporin is the gold standard for treatment of these wound infections [12]. Peristomal leakage is another complication of gastrostomy tubes; this can be hastened by the reason for the tube placement, most commonly malnutrition. Trying to place a larger tube usually leads to more problems, so recommendations are generally to remove the tube and allow complete healing and/or place a feeding tube in a separate site.

Tube dislodgement is a common reason for emergency room visit among patients with PEG tubes. If the tube slides in, it could cause a gastric outlet obstruction; if it slides out, the tract could theoretically close or, worse, could be lodged in the abdominal wall or peritoneal cavity and cause sepsis, even death. If the tube is inadvertently pulled and the tract is mature (over 1 week old), a new one can be safely replaced and a fluoroscopic tube study done to confirm placement.

Aspiration pneumonia is one of the common complications following PEG tube placement, especially in elderly patients with dementia. Rates can be as high as 18% (higher than that of site infection in the same study). Mortality following PEG tubes is exceedingly rare and most often attributed to the underlying illness for which the PEG tube was placed [12].

Another potential complication in patients undergoing PEG placement for enteral feeding access with head and neck cancers is seeding of the abdominal wall with metastatic cancer cells, ostensibly drug through the wound during the actual procedure. Fung et al. retrospectively reviewed 777 cases of PEG tube placement in patients with head and neck cancer over a 5-year period in two separate academic institutions. Five patients (<1%) had identified abdominal wall metastases with an average follow-up of 27.55 months; all were via the pull technique. All of the patients with stomal metastases also presented at the time with widespread distant metastases and had initial presentations of stage IV cancer [13].

Open gastrostomy tubes have an adjacent larger incision which necessitates keeping the wounds separate and ensuring no leaking of stomach contents into the nearby wound. Additionally, laparoscopic and open procedure necessitate general anesthesia which often carries a higher perioperative cardiopulmonary risk. PEG tubes and radiologic tubes are not placed under direct visualization and as such could inadvertently traverse adjacent structures, including the colon. This is best avoided by confirmation of transillumination using the endoscope before the initial needle placement. PEG tubes may be complicated by iatrogenic esophageal perforation secondary to the endoscopic portion of the procedure. Late complications can include leaking of tube feeds or enteral contents, eroding bumper, and displacement of feeding tube.

Overall, gastrostomy tube placement is a relatively safe procedure that can be very helpful in maintaining good nutrition in those patients who cannot safely swallow. The various techniques for placement are all relatively safe, and there is no concrete data suggesting one particular method of placement is more or less safe.

References

1. Lyon S, et al. Percutaneous gastrostomy and gastrojejunostomy. Semin Interv Radiol. 2004;21(3):181–9.
2. Norton B, et al. A randomised prospective comparison of percutaneous endoscopic gastrostomy and nasogastric tube feeding after acute dysphagic stroke. Br Med J. 1996;312(7022):13–6.
3. Dennis M. FOOD: a multicentre randomised trial evaluation feeding policies in patients admitted to hospital with a recent stroke. Health Technol Assess. 2006;10(2):iii–v, ix–x, 1–120
4. Jinfeng W, et al. Percutaneous endoscopic gastrostomy versus nasogastric tube feeding for patients with head and neck cancer: a systematic review. J Radiat Res. 2014;55(3):559–67.
5. Baker L, et al. A systematic review and meta-analysis of gastrostomy insertion techniques in children. J Pediatr Surg. 2015;50(5):718–25.
6. Oliveira GP, et al. The role of surgical gastrostomy in the age of endoscopic gastrostomy: a 13 years and 543 patients retrospective study. Revista espanola de enfermedades digestivas: organo oficial de la Sociedad Espanola de Patologia Digestiva. 2016;108(12):776–9.
7. Taghavi S, et al. Comparison of open gastrostomy tube to percutaneous endoscopic gastrostomy tube in lung transplant patients. Ann Med Surg. 2015;5:76–80.
8. Mizrahi I, et al. Comparison of laparoscopic versus open approach to gastrostomy tubes. J Soc Laparoendosc Surg. 2014;18(1):28–33.
9. Kohler G, et al. Comparison of 231 patients receiving either "pull-through" or "push" percutaneous endoscopic gastrostomy. Surg Endosc. 2015;29(1):170–5.
10. Tucker AT, et al. 'Push' versus 'pull' percutaneous endoscopic gastrostomy tube placement in patients with advanced head and neck cancer. Laryngoscope. 2003;113(11):1898–902.
11. Galaski A, et al. Gastrostomy tube placement by radiological versus endoscopic methods in an acute care setting: a retrospective review of frequency, indications, complications, and outcomes. Can J Gastroenterol. 2009;23(2):109–14.
12. Rahnemai-Azar A, et al. Percutaneous endoscopic gastrostomy: indications, technique, complications, management. World J Gastroenterol. 2014;20(24):7739–51.
13. Fung E, et al. Incidence of abdominal wall metastases following percutaneous endoscopic gastrostomy placement in patients with head and neck cancer. Surg Endosc. 2016;30:1–5.

Central Line Placement

65

Marc D. Trust and Pedro G. R. Teixeira

Introduction

Establishing intravenous access is an essential and early step in most acute care situations. Cannulation of peripheral veins with short- and large-bore catheters is the initial choice as it provides quick access for initial resuscitation allowing rapid infusion of fluids and medications. Patients admitted to the intensive care unit, however, frequently require central venous access. Central venous catheters (CVCs) not only provide a route to administer a wide variety of medications necessary for the critically ill patient but can also be used to obtain hemodynamic and physiologic information at the bedside that aids in treatment decision making. Table 65.1 lists many of the common indications for CVC placement; however, a comprehensive discussion of all these indications is beyond the scope of this chapter.

It is estimated that 5–7 million CVCs are placed in the United States each year, leading to an estimated 15 million days of CVC exposure [1–3]. While CVCs are an essential tool in the intensive care setting, they do not come without risks, both mechanical and infectious, that not only lead to increased length of hospital stay and costs but also have the potential for severe morbidity and mortality [4–6]. The technical aspects of CVC insertion are of paramount importance, considering that a sixfold increase in mechanical complications has been described when more than two attempts are necessary for line insertion [4]. For that reason, excellent knowledge of the anatomy and operative technique are essential. In this chapter, we will discuss appropriate catheter site selection, review the pertinent anatomy and technique for insertion of CVCs, and discuss the potential complications and their management.

M. D. Trust · P. G. R. Teixeira (✉)
Department of Surgery and Perioperative Care, University of Texas at Austin, Dell Medical School, Austin, TX, USA
e-mail: pgteixeira@austin.utexas.edu

Catheter Type and Insertion Site Selection

Numerous types of catheters for central insertion are available. Multi-lumen catheters are convenient for patients requiring infusion of multiple types of fluids and drugs and have not been found to increase the risk of septic complications compared to single-lumen catheters [7]. Because these catheters are relatively long and each individual lumen has a small diameter, they are not suitable for rapid fluid infusion. If the main purpose for the CVC is rapid fluid administration, an introducer sheath should be selected instead. These sheaths are usually 8.5 Fr in diameter and significantly shorter than the multi-lumen catheters. They were originally designed to allow introduction of additional intravascular devices such as pulmonary artery catheters, but the side arm of the sheath can be connected to an IV line and used for rapid fluid infusion.

For those patients in whom central access is intended for hemodialysis, large-bore dual-lumen catheters specifically designed to provide the high flow rates required for dialysis should be used. Because these patients may need long-term hemodialysis and eventually require a definitive dialysis access such as an arteriovenous fistula or graft created in the upper extremities, the subclavian vein should be avoided to reduce the risk of central venous stenosis compromising the upper extremities as potential sites for dialysis access creation. In most instances, tunneling of CVC is not necessary during the acute phase in intensive care setting.

The sites available for direct percutaneous CVC insertion include the internal jugular, subclavian, and femoral veins. When selecting which of these sites to access, one must consider multiple factors such as infectious risk, existing wounds and injuries such as those found in burn and trauma patients, the presence of appliances such as cervical collars, suspicion of underlying venous thrombosis, accessibility, and patient comfort. Because of the important implications of central line-associated blood stream infections (CLABSI), site-specific infection risks have become the main determinant of CVC site choice for patients in the intensive care unit. The

A. Salim et al. (eds.), *Surgical Critical Care Therapy*, https://doi.org/10.1007/978-3-319-71712-8_65

Table 65.1 Indications for central venous catheter placement

Vasopressor infusion
Infusion of hypertonic solutions
Central total parenteral nutrition
Central venous oxygenation monitoring
Invasive cardiovascular monitoring
Inability to obtain peripheral venous access
Rapid resuscitation

Centers for Disease Control and Prevention (CDC) currently recommends that the subclavian site be the primary option for central venous access due to this lower infectious risk [2]. The femoral site is associated with the highest rates of infection [8] and is usually not routinely recommended as a CVC insertion site unless central access is required emergently and the subclavian and jugular veins are not available for access. The CDC strongly recommends against the use of femoral vein for central venous access [2].

Anatomy

As with most major venous structures in the body, the three possible sites for central venous catheterization have paired arteries that run in close proximity to the veins. The internal jugular vein is located bilaterally in the neck just lateral to the common carotid within the carotid sheath, with the vagus nerve running between these two structures. The junction of the sternal and clavicular heads of the sternocleidomastoid muscle just cephalad to the clavicular head marks the external landmark for access.

The axillary vein becomes the subclavian vein as it enters the thoracic outlet crossing over the lateral edge of the first rib. The subclavian vein then runs from lateral to medial between the first rib and the clavicle, anteriorly to the anterior scalene muscle, and then joins the ipsilateral internal jugular vein to form the brachiocephalic vein. The subclavian artery lies just posterior and slightly cephalad to the vein. Typically, the appropriate puncture site is the junction of the medial and lateral thirds of the clavicle, which lies just lateral to the clavicle curvature found in many people. This area can also be quickly identified at the deltopectoral groove.

The boundaries of the femoral triangle are the inguinal ligament superiorly, the adductor longus medially, and the sartorius muscle laterally. It is within this triangle that the femoral structures can be found, with the lateral to medial orientation of the nerve, artery, and vein. During CVC insertion in this location, care must be taken to ensure that the puncture is positioned caudal to the inguinal ligament, as injury to a vessel above this ligament could result in retroperitoneal hemorrhage that is not easily controlled with direct pressure.

Technique

Continuous monitoring with electrocardiography and pulse oximetry during the procedure is recommended. All equipment needed for the procedure should be available at the bedside. Most commercially available CVCs come in a set including sterile garment for prepping and draping, local anesthetics, needles, syringes, the catheter with wire and dilator, saline flushes, sutures and surgical instruments for securing the catheter to the skin, and supplies for sterile dressing application at the end of the procedure. Because of the variety of CVC kits available, the operator's familiarity with the kit being used should be confirmed. If ultrasound-guided access is planned, the ultrasound machine should be tested to confirm proper function, and a sterile sleeve for probe coverage should be available.

Aseptic measures and technique are essential to preventing CLABSI. The CDC recommends that hands must be cleansed with either conventional soap or alcohol-based hand rubs before and after placement of a CVC. The skin overlying the area of insertion should be widely prepped with a chlorhexidine solution and allowed to dry prior to proceeding with placement. Full sterile barrier precautions including cap, mask, sterile gown, gloves, and full-body drapes should be used throughout the entire procedure (Fig. 65.1). A sterile cover should also be used over the ultrasound probe if one is used to assist with placement. Prophylactic antibiotics are not indicated to prevent infections.

Modified Seldinger technique is used for CVC placement, irrespective of site chosen. For subclavian access site, the patient should be placed in the Trendelenburg position, which results in venodilation facilitating access with the needle, as well as theoretically reducing the chances of air embolism during the procedure. Placement of a towel roll positioned longitudinally under the patient's thoracic spine results in lowering of the shoulders and can facilitate subclavian vein catheterization. As mentioned previously in the anatomy section, the insertion site is typically at the junction of the lateral and middle thirds of the clavicle, approximately 2 cm inferior and 2 cm lateral to this point. The operator should stand by the patient at the side of the subclavian vein being accessed. The skin and subcutaneous tissue of the insertion track should be anesthetized with a lidocaine solution. Using a sharp 18-gauge needle on a syringe, the needle is inserted through the skin with an angle almost parallel to the frontal plane (practically, parallel to the floor), with the tip of the needle directed toward the sternal notch (Fig. 65.2). The vein is typically just posterior to the clavicle, and a flat angle of the needle to the skin is necessary. A steeper angle increases the chances of complications such as arterial puncture or pneumothorax. Maintaining constant negative pressure applied on the syringe, the needle should be advanced underneath the

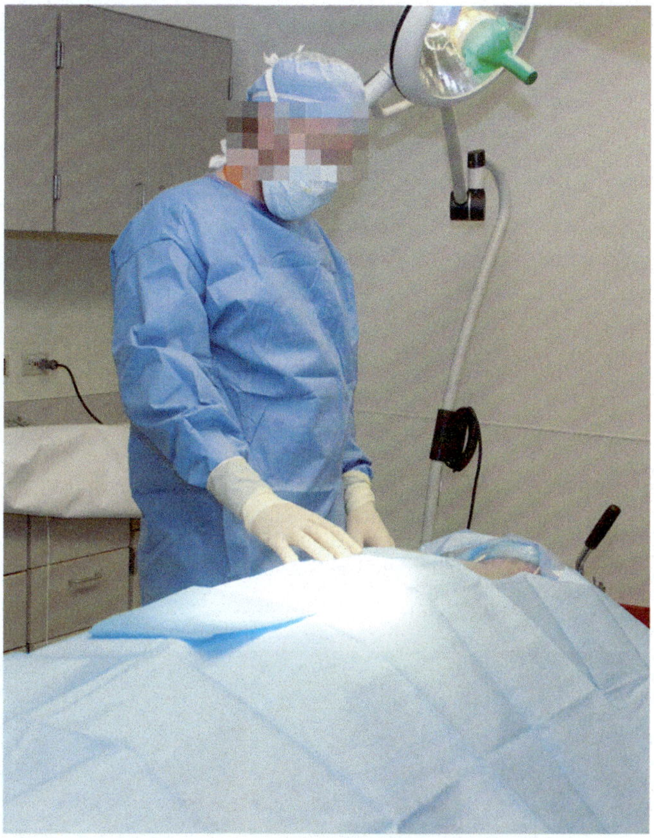

Fig. 65.1 Maximal sterile barrier precautions including cap, mask, gown, sterile gloves, and full-body drape for placement of CVC

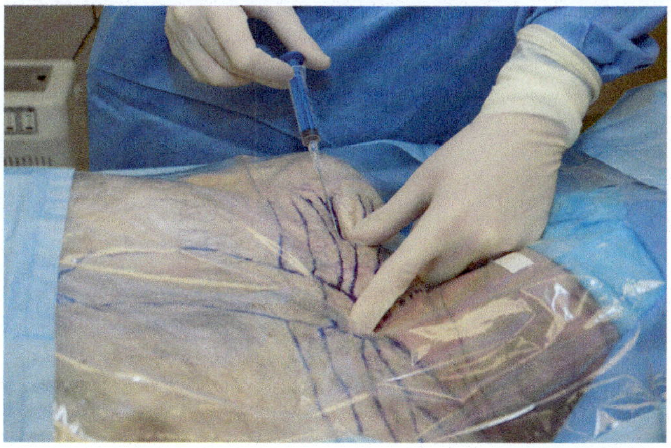

Fig. 65.2 Technique for subclavian vein access: the needle is inserted below the clavicle and advanced between the clavicle and the first rib maintaining an angle almost parallel to the frontal plane and pointing toward the sternal notch

clavicle until a flash of dark blood is aspirated (Fig. 65.3). While steadying the needle with the non-dominant hand, the syringe is then removed from the needle, which is digitally capped to prevent air embolism. The J-tip end of the wire is then introduced through the needle (Fig. 65.4), and the wire is carefully advanced paying attention to the electrocardiographic monitor. Ectopies suggest intracardiac position of the wire tip. Wire advancement should not meet resistance. If resistance is encountered, both wire and needle may need to be withdrawn as a unit and the procedure restarted. Withdrawal of the wire through the needle may result in wire fragmentation and embolization. With the wire successfully positioned into the vein, the needle is removed maintaining the wire in place (Fig. 65.5), and a small skin incision with an 11 blade is made at the puncture site. A dilator is advanced over the wire through the subcutaneous tract and removed. The catheter is then inserted over the wire carefully maintaining wire position (Fig. 65.6) to avoid the risk of wire embolization. The wire is then removed and its removal noted for the records. All ports on the catheter should be tested to ensure they easily aspirate and flush with sterile saline solution (Fig. 65.7). The

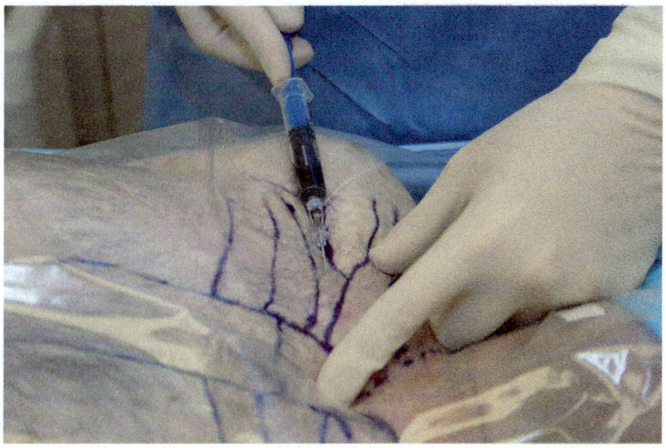

Fig. 65.3 Technique for subclavian vein access: negative pressure is constantly applied to the syringe as the needle advanced until a flush of dark blood is identified

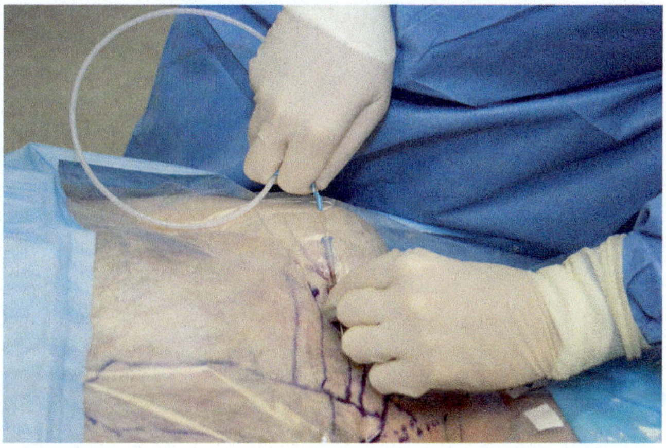

Fig. 65.4 Technique for subclavian vein access: the syringe is disconnected from the needle, and a J-tip wire is inserted through the needle. Because of the risk of air embolism during this step, attention should be paid not to leave the needle open and have the wire close to the operative field to minimize the amplitude of movement required for this step. Trendelenburg position also should help reduce the risk of air embolism

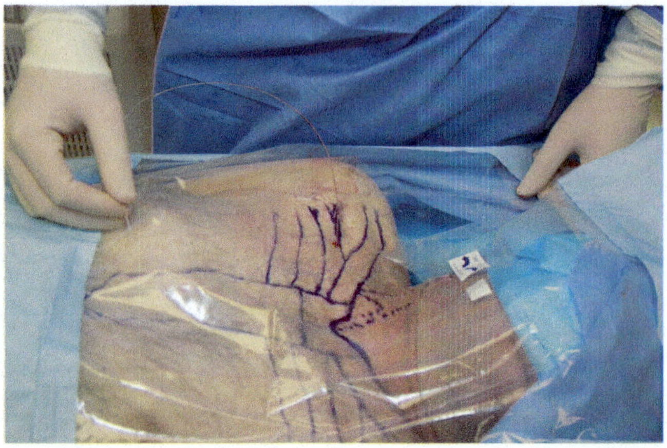

Fig. 65.5 Technique for subclavian vein access: the needle is withdrawn over the wire and removed, leaving the wire in position

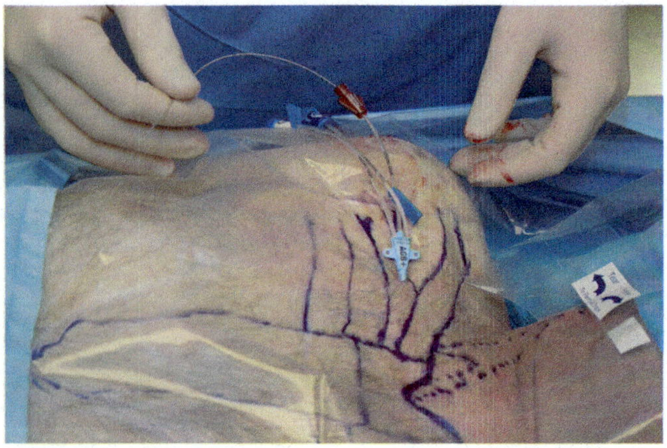

Fig. 65.6 Technique for subclavian vein access: after the skin and subcutaneous tract have been dilated, the CVC is inserted over the wire carefully maintaining wire control throughout the insertion step. The wire is then removed and the catheter remains in place

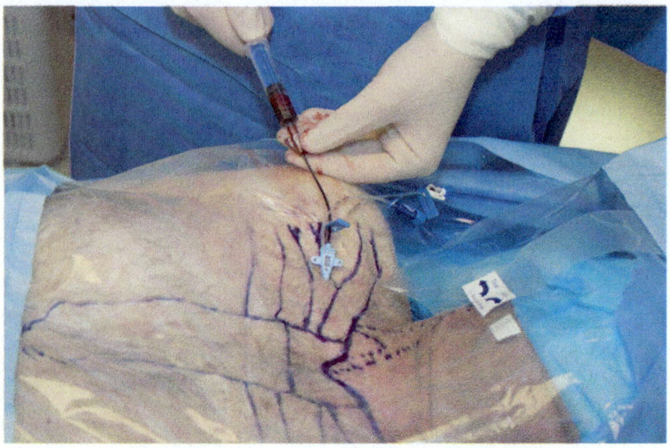

Fig. 65.7 Technique for subclavian vein access: all ports of the CVC should be aspirated and flushed to confirm proper functioning of the catheter. After flushed, each port should be capped. The catheter is then secured to the skin with sutures, and a sterile dressing is applied prior to drape removal

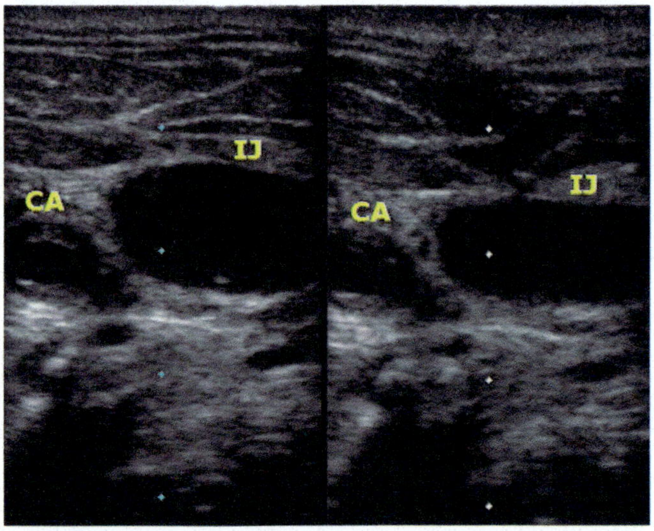

Fig. 65.8 Ultrasound images of the neck vessels demonstrating a transversal view of the carotid artery and the internal jugular vein. Gentle pressure with the probe over the vessels is used for confirmation of the anatomy as it results in compression of the vein but not the artery (Image on the left: no compression. Image on the left: with compression). CA carotid artery, IJ internal jugular vein

catheter is then secured in place with sutures and a sterile dressing placed over the puncture site.

For placement of the catheter in the internal jugular sites, the patient's head should be turned away from the access site, and the patient should be placed in a 15-degree Trendelenburg position. The operator should stand at the head of the bed. If ultrasound guidance is to be used, the probe is placed over the insertion site and the ultrasonographic anatomy identified. The internal jugular vein and carotid artery can be differentiated by application of gentle pressure, which results in compression of the vein but not the artery (Fig. 65.8). The angle of ultrasound visualization and insertion should follow a route that does not place the artery immediately posterior to the vein, as this can result in inadvertent arterial puncture. The distance from the skin to the jugular vein should be noted on ultrasound and guide the depth of needle introduction during puncture. After local anesthetic injection, an 18-gauge needle connected to a syringe is introduced at an approximately 30–45 degree angle to the skin, while the ultrasound probe is held in place (Fig. 65.9). The needle should be identified on the ultrasound screen and advanced under visualization until intraluminal position is achieved (Fig. 65.10) and a flash of dark blood is aspirated into the syringe. The hand holding the ultrasound probe is then used to stabilize the needle, and the syringe is removed and a J-tip wire is advanced as described above for the subclavian access. Confirmation of intraluminal position of the wire with the ultrasound is recommended prior to dilation of the puncture site (Fig. 65.11). After confirmation of wire position with the ultrasound, the

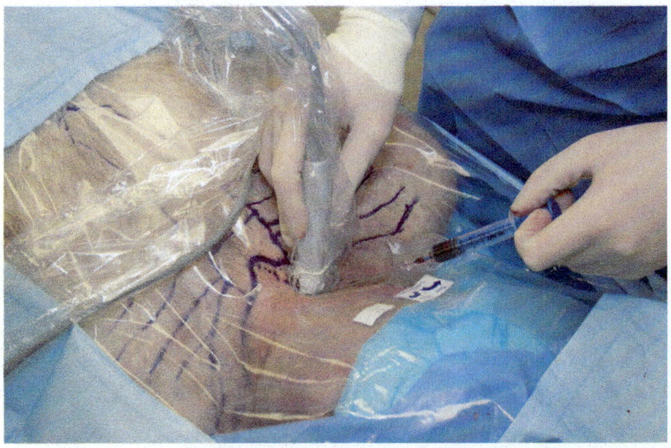

Fig. 65.9 Technique for internal jugular vein access: with the ultrasound probe being held in position, the needle is advanced at a 45-degree angle under ultrasound guidance while maintaining continuous negative pressure on the syringe

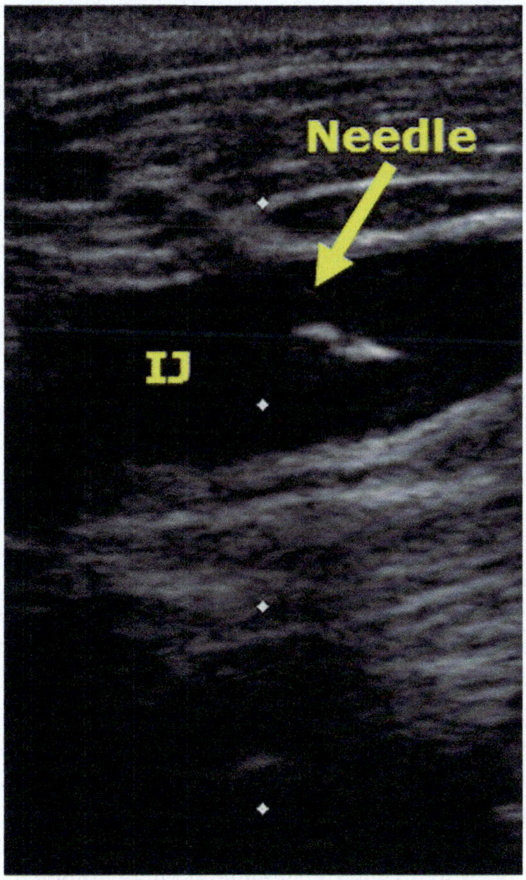

Fig. 65.10 Technique for internal jugular vein access: the needle is visualized with the ultrasound while being advanced. This longitudinal ultrasound view demonstrates the tip of the needle in the lumen of the internal jugular vein. IJ internal jugular vein

subcutaneous tract is dilated, the catheter is inserted over the wire, the wire is removed, and the catheter is flushed and secured in place as described above.

Differently from the positioning for subclavian and jugular access, femoral vein access is facilitated by a reverse Trendelenburg position. The inguinal ligament position is estimated by tracing a line from the anterior superior iliac spine to the pubic tubercle. The femoral pulse is then identified just caudal to the inguinal ligament. The needle insertion site for femoral vein access should be approximately 1–2 cm caudal to the inguinal ligament and 1 cm medial to the femoral pulse. Ultrasound guidance can facilitate femoral access and decrease the risk of inadvertent arterial puncture, particularly in hemodynamically unstable patients, in whom palpation of the femoral pulse may be difficult. For emergent placement in a patient without a palpable pulse, we recommend starting 3 cm medial to the midpoint of the inguinal ligament, and then do serial needle passes moving laterally until the vein is accessed. The needle should be inserted at a 45-degree angle to the skin and directed cephalad and with a slightly medial angle. After successful puncture of the femoral vein, the Seldinger technique principles are followed as described above.

Use of Ultrasound

Although historically performed using anatomical landmarks for guidance, the use of ultrasound guidance decreasing complication rates during CVC placement has been well documented. [9] Two recently published Cochrane Reviews including randomized and quasi-randomized trials comparing ultrasound guidance versus an anatomic landmark technique for CVC placement demonstrated that the highest benefit was seen at the internal jugular site, where the use of ultrasound guidance resulted in an overall 71% reduction in complications and an increase in success rates by 12% [10, 11]. On the other hand, no evidence was found for a difference in overall complication rates for the subclavian and femoral vein sites.

Complications and Management

Complications of central venous catheters can be placed into mechanical, infectious, and thrombotic categories (Table 65.2).

Mechanical Complications

Mechanical complications associated with CVC insertion include pneumothorax, hemothorax, arterial puncture, venous laceration, central vein stenosis, air embolism, and catheter misplacement.

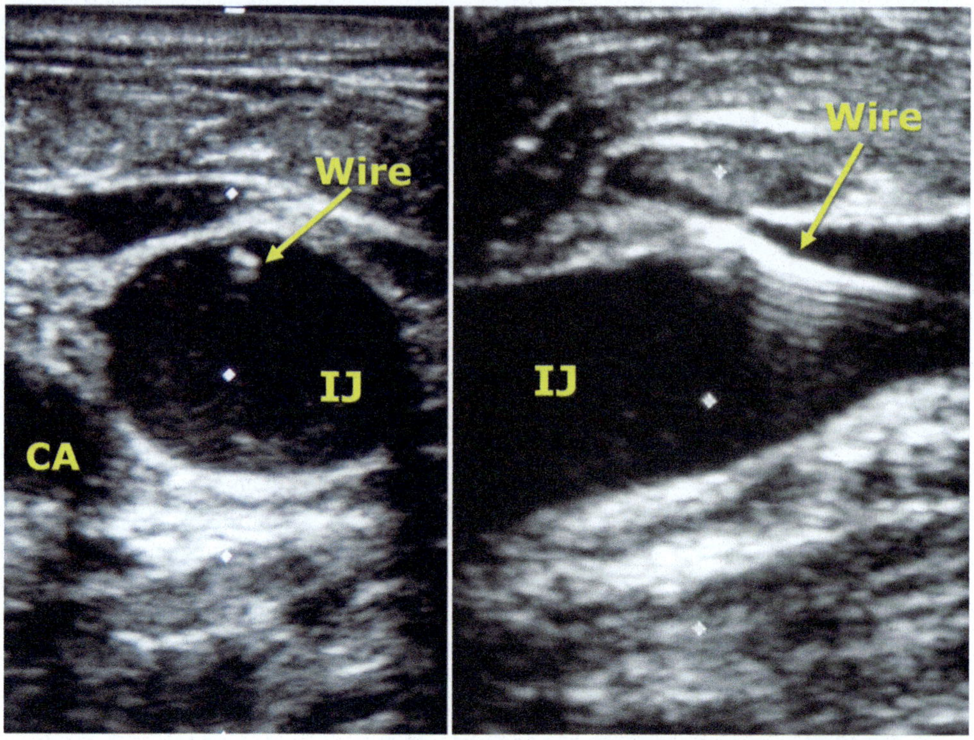

Fig. 65.11 Technique for internal jugular vein access: ultrasound confirmation of intraluminal wire position is recommended prior to dilation of the access site. These ultrasound images demonstrate the intraluminal position of the wire (Image on the left: transversal view; image on the right: longitudinal view). CA carotid artery, IJ internal jugular vein

Table 65.2 Complications of central venous catheter placement

Mechanical
Pneumothorax
Hematoma
Vascular injury (venous laceration, arterial pseudoaneurysm)
Chylothorax
Air embolism
Arrhythmia
Central venous stenosis
Thrombotic
Deep/central vein thrombosis
Embolism
Catheter fracture
Superior vena cava syndrome
Infectious
Central line-associated blood stream infection

Pneumothorax is a commonly reported complications of CVC placement and is highest after CVC insertions at the subclavian site at 1.5–3.1% incidence [12]. Risk factors for pneumothorax include multiple insertion attempts, operator inexperience, larger catheter size, and emergency situations [13]. These are typically diagnosed on post-insertion plain film chest X-ray, but bedside ultrasonography can also be used. A small pneumothorax does not necessarily require intervention if the patient is asymptomatic, but a surveillance plan should be established, and one should have a low threshold for intervention if enlargement of the pneumothorax or symptoms such as hypoxia or difficulty ventilating occur.

Arterial complications can be a significant source of morbidity and mortality and are more common for femoral vein access and least common for subclavian vein access [12]. Inadvertent arterial puncture, even if quickly identified and managed with removal of the needle and compression, may still result in secondary complications such as hematoma, pseudoaneurysm, AV fistula, and thromboembolic sequelae such as stroke. Although less common, arterial laceration or cannulation especially poses a major risk. [1] It is critical to assess for arterial quality blood from a needle prior to dilation and catheter placement. Unless significant hypoxemia is present, arterial blood can be readily identified by its bright red color. If unclear if an arterial puncture has been made, an 18 G angiocatheter can be introduced over the wire and connected to a transducer for evaluation of the waveform, which should allow clear identification of arterial pressure and wave pattern. It is also important to note that if an attempt at entering the vein is not successful, the needle is withdrawn back to the superficial subcutaneous tissue to reposition the needle angle prior to a subsequent attempt, as realignment in the perivascular space can result in laceration. If arterial cannulation does occur, treatment options include immediate removal and compression, endovascular therapy (Figs. 65.12 and 65.13), and surgical repair. Decision of therapy must weigh the ease of compression based on access site, availability of a vascular surgeon, resources at ones institution including endovascular suite and device availability, and patient stability.

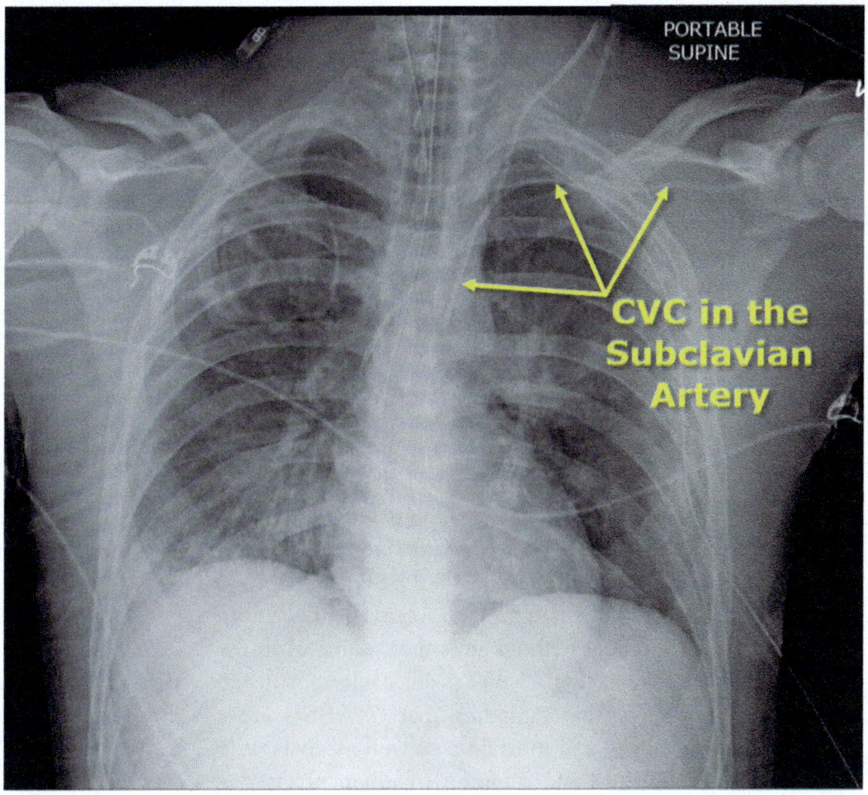

Fig. 65.12 Plain chest X-ray demonstrating a catheter inadvertently inserted into the left subclavian artery

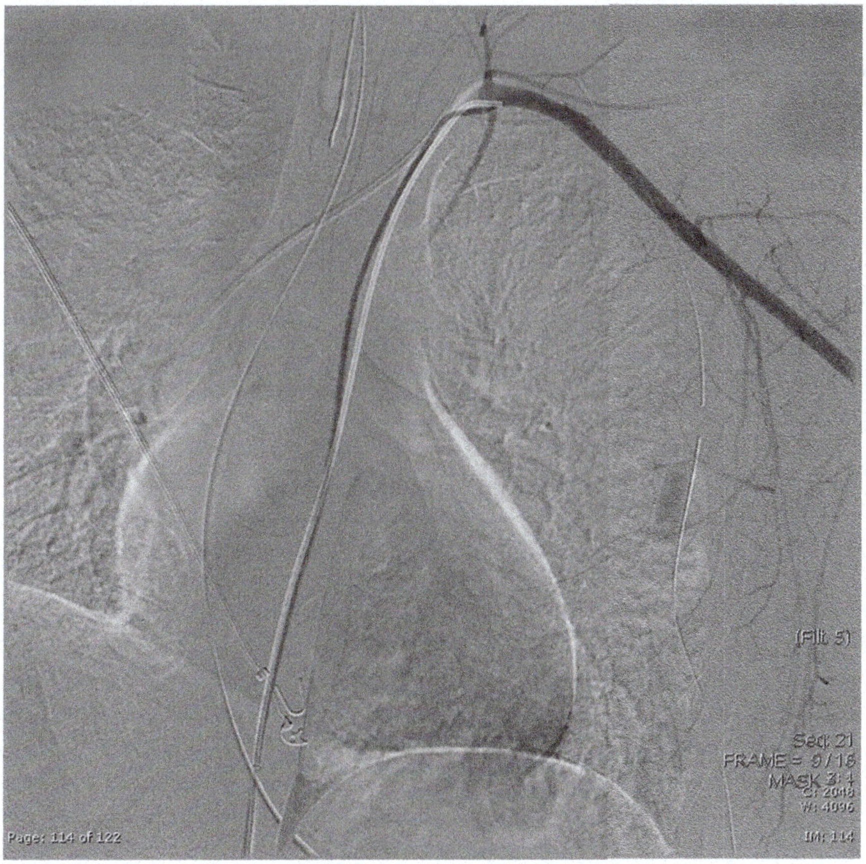

Fig. 65.13 Completion angiogram after the arterial catheter showed in Fig. 65.12 was removed over a wire in the angiography site and hemostasis at the puncture site achieved with a percutaneous closure device. The images demonstrate patency of the subclavian artery, without evidence of residual stenosis or contrast extravasation

Major vascular and mechanical complications can be related to the wire and dilator, as the wire can become lodged against a lumen wall and manipulation can cause a laceration or puncture with the related passing of the dilator [1]. While inserting the dilator or catheter, the wire must be able to easily slide back and forth without any resistance to ensure this lodging has not occurred to prevent further injury. Another major mechanical complication worth mentioning, although rare, is perforation from an indwelling catheter. Predictors of perforation include a curled catheter or tip of the catheter abutting the wall of vein and should be repositioned [13].

Infectious Complications

Infectious complications have garnered a great deal of attention over the last two decades. The CDC defines central line-associated blood stream infections (CLABSIs) as a blood stream infection in a patient who had a central line within 48 h prior to development without any other source of infection, and it is estimated that 41,000 occur each year in the United States. [8] The understanding that CLABSIs are a significant of morbidity and mortality, as well as costs with increased length of stay and required treatment, caused a shift of focus to prevention. Table 65.3 outlines the CDC recommendations for prevention of CLABSI. The subclavian site is associated with the lowest infectious rate and is currently the recommended site by the CDC, when available, while the femoral site is associated with the highest rate of infection. [2]

Table 65.3 Prevention of CLABSI

Use subclavian site
Use ultrasound to reduce cannulation attempts and minimize mechanical complications
Early removal of catheter when no longer needed
Replace catheter within 48 h when aseptic technique not used for placement
Hand hygiene with either washing or alcohol-based rub prior to inserting or manipulating catheter
Maintain aseptic technique for insertion
Maximal barrier precautions including cap, mask sterile gloves, gown, and full-body drape when inserting catheter
Prepare skin with chlorhexidine preparation before placement
Use sterile dressing to cover the catheter site
Replace dressing if it becomes damp, loosened, or soiled
Replace transparent dressings every 7 days
Use chlorhexidine-impregnated sponge dressing
Do not replace catheters to prevent infections
Do not remove catheters based on fever alone

Patients in whom a CVC is inserted without strict adherence to sterile technique should ideally have the catheter replaced within 48 h. However, planned routine replacement of CVCs that have been inserted in compliance with aseptic techniques is not recommended [2]. If a patient with a CVC develops signs of an infection and no other obvious source is identified, a high index of suspicion for CLABSI is needed. Paired blood samples drawn from a peripheral vein and from the CVC should be obtained prior to broad-spectrum antimicrobial therapy initiation. Definitive confirmation of CLABSI requires two blood cultures positive for the same microorganism (one from a peripheral venipuncture and one from the CVC) or a positive blood culture and positive culture of the CVC tip, both also growing the same microorganism [14].

In patients with suspected CLABSI, immediate CVC removal is not universally necessary, and catheter salvage may be attempted unless one of the following conditions is present: severe sepsis, suppurative thrombophlebitis, endocarditis, or infections due to *Staphylococcus aureus*, *Pseudomonas aeruginosa*, fungi, or mycobacteria. Catheter salvage failure is determined if blood cultures remain positive after 72 h of appropriate antimicrobial therapy [14]. The decision to remove the CVC should also take into account other factors such as vascular accessibility and the risk of mechanical complications associated with another access. [15]

Thrombotic Complications

At 10%, the rate of catheter-related thrombosis for subclavian CVCs is significantly lower compared to the rates observed for the femoral and jugular sites, which have an incidence of up to 21–33% [5, 16]. Thrombosis may manifest clinically as a CVC not functioning properly, an edematous and painful extremity, evidence of central venous obstruction, or central embolism. Systemic anticoagulation is often needed for CVC-associated thrombosis, and the need to remove the CVC should be evaluated according to the clinical scenario and balanced against the risks of new central access [17].

Conclusion

Central venous catheters are an essential tool for the care of critically ill patients. The technical aspects of CVC insertion are of paramount importance, and excellent knowledge of the anatomy and operative technique are essential requirements to prevent morbidity from this necessary procedure. Understanding of both immediate and delayed complications of CVC and their management is fundamental to patient safety.

References

1. Kornbau C, Lee KC, Hughes GD, Firstenberg MS. Central line complications. Int J Crit Illn Inj Sci. 2015;5(3):170–8.
2. O'Grady NP, Alexander M, Burns LA, Dellinger EP, Garland J, Heard SO, et al. Guidelines for the prevention of intravascular catheter-related infections. Am J Infect Control. 2011;39(4):S1–S34.
3. Raad I. Intravascular-catheter-related infections. Lancet. 1998;351:893–8.
4. Mansfield PF, Hohn DC, Fornage BD, Gregurich MA, Ota DM. Complications and failures of subclavian-vein catheterization. N Engl J Med. 1994;331(26):1735–8.
5. Merrer J, De Jonghe B, Golliot F, Lefrant JY, Raffy B, Barre E, et al. Complications of femoral and subclavian venous catheterization in critically ill patients: a randomized controlled trial. JAMA. 2001;286(6):700–7.
6. Sznajder JI, Zveibil FR, Bitterman H, Weiner P, Bursztein S. Central vein catheterization. Failure and complication rates by three percutaneous approaches. Arch Intern Med. 1986;146(2):259–61.
7. Farkas JC, Liu N, Bleriot JP, Chevret S, Goldstein FW, Carlet J. Single- versus triple-lumen central catheter-related sepsis: a prospective randomized study in a critically ill population. Am J Med. 1992;93(3):277–82.
8. Baldea AJ Jr, Cocanour CS. Central line-associated blood stream infections. In: Cameron JL, Cameron AM, editors. Current surgical therapy. 11th ed. Philadelphia: Elsevier; 2014. p. 1259–62.
9. Randolph AG, Cook DJ, Gonzales CA, Pribble CG. Ultrasound guidance for placement of central venous catheters: a meta-analysis of the literature. Crit Care Med. 1996;24(12):2053–8.
10. Brass P, Hellmich M, Kolodziej L, Schick G, Smith AF. Ultrasound guidance versus anatomical landmarks for internal jugular vein catheterization. Brass P, editor. Cochrane Database Syst Rev. 1996;13(4):213.
11. Brass P, Hellmich M, Kolodziej L, Schick G, Smith AF. Ultrasound guidance versus anatomical landmarks for subclavian or femoral vein catheterization. Brass P, editor. Cochrane Database Syst Rev. 1996;111(3):S80.
12. Graham AS, Ozment C, Tegtmeyer K, Lai S, Braner DAV. Central venous catheterization. N Engl J Med. 2007;356(21):e21.
13. Kusminsky RE. Complications of central venous catheterization. J Am Coll Surg. 2007;204(4):681–96.
14. Mermel LA, Allon M, Bouza E, Craven DE, Flynn P, O'Grady NP, et al. Clinical practice guidelines for the diagnosis and management of intravascular catheter-related infection: 2009 update by the Infectious Diseases Society of America. Clin Infect Dis. 2009;49(1):1–45.
15. Lorente L, Martín MM, Vidal P, Rebollo S, Ostabal MI, Solé-Violán J, et al. Should central venous catheter be systematically removed in patients with suspected catheter related infection? Crit Care. 2014;18(5):564.
16. Timsit JF, Farkas JC, Boyer JM, Martin JB, Misset B. Central vein catheter-related thrombosis in intensive care patients: incidence, risks factors, and relationship with catheter-related sepsis. Chest. 1998;114(1):207–13.
17. Bodenham A, Babu S, Bennett J, Binks R, Fee P, Fox B, et al. Association of anaesthetists of Great Britain and Ireland: safe vascular access 2016. Anaesthesia. 2016;71(1):573–85.

Pulmonary Artery Catheter

66

Matthew J. Eckert and Matthew J. Martin

Background

The pulmonary artery catheter (PAC) or Swan-Ganz catheter as it is commonly referred to today was first described in the right heart catheterization of a patient in 1970 [1]. The flow-directed balloon-tipped catheter that until recently was ubiquitous in most intensive care units (ICU), and particularly in surgical/trauma ICUs, evolved during the early twentieth century as clinicians studied normal and abnormal cardiac physiology. Doctors Swan and Ganz and colleagues developed this device and technique to provide safer and more efficient means to access the heart and pulmonary artery for hemodynamic monitoring and blood sampling in patients suffering myocardial infarction, without the requirement for image guidance during placement. Subsequent modifications of the catheter allowed for intermittent or continuous measurement of cardiac output and mixed venous oxygen saturation, as well as electrocardiac pacing.

Pulmonary Artery Catheters

Numerous types of PACs are available for use today in both adult and pediatric patients. The typical catheter is a multi-lumen device with a small-volume distal balloon located just before the catheter tip (Fig. 66.1). A proximal port opens roughly in the right atrium and allows measurement of right atrial and/or central venous pressures, sampling of blood, and delivery of medications or fluid for cardiac output measurement. An additional proximal infusion port is often located nearby to allow administration of medications, fluids, or injectate for cardiac output calculation. Finally, the distal pulmonary artery (PA) port opens at the catheter tip to allow PA pressure measurement (also called "wedge pressure") and sampling of blood for mixed venous oxygen saturation. A micro thermistor located near the catheter tip rapidly calculates blood temperature changes after injection of a "cold" fluid bolus in a proximal infusion port. The temperature change over time is used to calculate the cardiac output and cardiac index (cardiac output indexed to body surface area).

Advanced catheters may be equipped with mechanisms of continuous cardiac output, core body temperature, and mixed venous oxygen saturation measurement. Additional variations of the PAC allow for electrocardiac pacing of single or dual chambers for short-term pacing requirements or when transcutaneous pacing fails to capture. Further modifications of the PAC allow for measurement of right ventricular end-diastolic volume and ejection fraction. Lastly, a variety of catheter lengths and tip shapes are available to allow placement from internal jugular/subclavian vein access sites or transfemoral access in both adults and children.

PAC Function and Hemodynamic Measurements

The flow-directed balloon-tipped PAC used today is placed through a large single-lumen central venous access device (typically a "cordis" line) and subsequently guided through the right atrium and ventricle and into a branch of the pulmonary artery where the balloon becomes "wedged" and obstructs further flow in that vessel. This "wedge" pressure is known as the pulmonary artery occlusion pressure (PAOP). In theory, a continuous column of blood extends from the distal tip of the catheter to the pulmonary arterial and venous tree and to the left atrium, thus allowing measurement of the left atrial (LA) pressure. At the end of diastole and prior to the mitral valve closing, the pressure in the LA and LV should be equivalent. Thus, this measurement should also reflect left ventricular end-diastolic pressure (LVEDP),

M. J. Eckert (✉)
Department of Surgery, Madigan Army Medical Center, Joint Base Lewis-McChord, Tacoma, WA, USA

M. J. Martin
Trauma and Emergency Surgery Service, Legacy Emanuel Medical Center, Portland, OR, USA

A. Salim et al. (eds.), *Surgical Critical Care Therapy*, https://doi.org/10.1007/978-3-319-71712-8_66

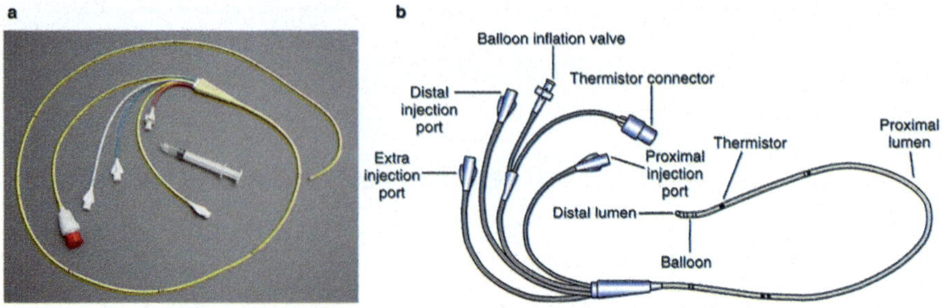

Fig. 66.1 Pulmonary artery catheter (**a**) and basic catheter components (**b**) (Panel A from https://lifeinthefastlane.com/wp-content/uploads/2012/07/PAC-1.jpg and panel B from Wilkins et al. [15])

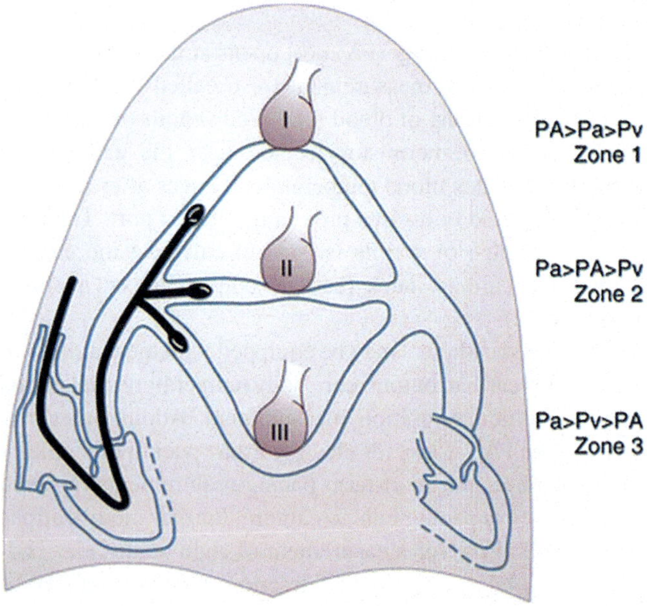

Fig. 66.2 West lung zones figure: lung zones and relation to pulmonary artery pressure (Pa), alveolar pressure (PA). and pulmonary vein pressure (Pv) (From Marini [16], with permission)

Table 66.1 Measured and calculated cardiovascular and oxygenation data with normal reference range values

Cardiovascular functions
Cardiac output (L/min) = 4–8 L/min
CVP (mmHg) = 2–6 mmHg
PCWP (mmHg) = 8–12 mmHg
PAP (mmHg) = 15–30/8–15 mmHg
Cardiac index (L/min/m^2) = 2.5–4 L/min/m^2
Stroke volume (L/beat) = 0.06–0.1 L/beat
Stroke volume index (L/beat/m^2) = 0.033–0.047 L/beat/m^2
SVR (dyne-sec-cm^{-5}) = 800–1200 dyne-sec-cm^{-5}
SVRI ([dyne-sec-cm^{-5}]/m^2) = 1970–2390 [dyne-sec-cm^{-5}]/m^2
PVR (dyne-sec-cm^{-5}) = <250 dyne-sec-cm^{-5}
PVRI ([dyne/sec/cm^{-5}]/m^2) = 255–285 [dyne-sec-cm^{-5}]/m^2
LVSWI (g-m/m^2/beat) = 50–62 g-m/m^2/beat
RVSWI (g-m/m^2/beat) = 5–10 g-m/m^2/beat
Oxygenation
SvO2 = 65–70%
DO_2 (mL/min/m^2) = 500–600 mL/min
VO_2 (mL/min) = 200–250 mL/min
O_2ER = 25–30%

BSA body surface area, *CaO_2* arterial O_2 content, *CI* cardiac index, *CO* cardiac output, *CVP* central venous pressure, *DO_2* oxygen delivery, *Hb* hemoglobin, *HR* heart rate, *LVSWI* left ventricular stroke work index, *MAP* mean arterial pressure, *O_2 ER* oxygen extraction ratio, *PAP* pulmonary artery pressure, *PCWP* pulmonary capillary wedge pressure, *PVR* pulmonary vascular resistance, *PVRI* pulmonary vascular resistance index, *RAP* right atrial pressure, *RVSWI* right ventricular stroke work index, *SV* stroke volume, *SVI* stroke volume index, *SvO_2* mixed venous saturation, *SVR* systemic vascular resistance, *SVRI* systemic vascular resistance index, *VO_2* oxygen consumption (Adapted with permission from Gidwani [14])

which is used clinically as a surrogate for left ventricular end-diastolic volume. The identical principles hold true on the right side of the heart, with the measured CVP being used as a surrogate for right ventricular end-diastolic pressure, or the "filling pressure" of the heart. Both the CVP and the PAOP are commonly interpreted as reflecting the intravascular volume status of the patient and the adequacy of preload in the right and left sides of the heart.

It is important to note, and frequently overlooked, that the catheter tip must be placed into West's Zone III of the lung for optimal measurement of left atrial pressure (Fig. 66.2). This position ensures that the pulmonary arterial and venous pressures exceed alveolar pressure and prevent compression of the continuous column of blood between the catheter tip and left atrium, thus avoiding erroneous pressure measurements. With the catheter tip wedged in the appropriate position, the measured pressure reflects that of a point of transition between flowing and non-flowing blood in the downstream pulmonary venous circuit. Under ideal conditions, the measured PAOP correlates with the mean left atrial pressure, which reflects the left ventricular end-diastolic pressure. These pressure relationships allow for the calculation and study of left heart pressures and function, and theoretically not influenced by pulmonary or alveolar pressures if the catheter is positioned appropriately. A complete listing of the cardiopulmonary functions and oxygen dynamic variables both measured and derived from the PAC is shown in Table 66.1.

Table 66.2 Common alterations of PAC-derived variables in different categories of shock

Cause	CVP/RA	PCWP	CO/CI	SVR/SVRI	Intervention
Hypovolemic, hemorrhagic	⇓⇓	⇓	⇓	⇑	IV fluids, blood products, bleeding control
Cardiogenic, tamponade	⇑	⇑	⇓⇓	⇑	Treat reversible causes, relief of tamponade, inotropes
Septic (early)	⇓	⇓	⇑⇑	⇓⇓	IV fluids, vasopressors
Septic (late)	⇓	⇓	⇓	⇓	IV fluids, vasopressor + inotropes
Neurogenic	⇓	⇓	⇑	⇓⇓	IV fluids, vasopressor

CVP/RA central venous pressure/right atrial, *PCWP* pulmonary capillary wedge pressure, *CO/CI* cardiac output/cardiac index, *SVR/SVI* systemic vascular resistance/systemic vascular resistance index, *IV* intravenous

The PAC allows calculation of the pulmonary and systemic vascular resistances that may be indexed to body surface area. These resistance measures are commonly used to guide vasoactive medication use and the assessment and management of pulmonary hypertension, right heart function, and distributive shock states. Calculations of stroke volume and stroke work may also be derived from the cardiac output and measured pressures. These data provide a surrogate for the examination of cardiac contractility. Right and left ventricular function can be assessed using the calculated ejection fractions and ventricular stroke work, which can also be indexed to the body surface area to allow for a more accurate individual assessment and comparisons between patients of different sizes.

Direct intermittent or continuous measurement of mixed venous oxygen saturation (SmvO2) from the pulmonary artery provides important information about the balance of oxygen delivery and consumption in the body and is required to calculate both the oxygen consumption and the oxygen extraction ratio (the percent of delivered oxygen that is extracted by the tissues). When oxygen demand increases, an increased tissue extraction leads to lower venous oxygen content in the pulmonary artery and central veins. A decrease in SmvO2 may reflect the increase in tissue demand or possibly increased oxygen extraction due to limitations in delivery. This may be reflective of inadequate arterial oxygen content, decreased cardiac output, shunt, or downstream impediments of arterial flow. An abnormally elevated SmvO2 indicates either a significant decrease in peripheral oxygen extraction/consumption, the presence of a shunt bypassing major peripheral tissue beds, or a left-to-right cardiac shunt as seen with a patent foramen ovale.

Lastly, a sampling of central venous blood from the most proximal port allows determination of the central venous oxygen saturations (ScvO2). Venous sampling from this location has been shown to approximate trends in the SmvO2 in numerous studies but not necessarily individual measurement correlation, assuming the absence of a significant cardiac shunt and normal myocardial function [2, 3]. Abnormal gradients between the ScvO2 and SmvO2 may suggest impaired myocardial function or the presence of an intracardiac shunt. Over the past decade as the standard indications and utilization of the PAC has sharply declined, the ScvO2 has become more widely used as a standard marker of adequacy of resuscitation, particularly among patients with sepsis or septic shock.

The correct analysis and interpretation of the measured values, calculated values, and extrapolated data obtained from a PAC is an area of significant controversy and debate. The failure of the PAC to show evidence of a patient benefit in multiple randomized controlled trials has frequently been attributed to misinterpretation of the data and erroneous decision-making based on those interpretations. A complete description of the interpretation and recommended actions for every PAC value or patterns of values is beyond the scope of this chapter. Table 66.2 shows the common interpretations and recommended actions for the most frequently encountered scenarios in a trauma or surgical ICU population. As noted, the filling pressures (CVP and PAOP/wedge) are typically low in shock states that are associated with loss of intravascular volume (bleeding, dehydration) or systemic vasodilation (early sepsis). The SVR will then be the next important variable which will distinguish between these two conditions, with a high SVR associated with intravascular volume loss and a low SVR with sepsis. For any source of cardiogenic shock (infarction, CHF exacerbation, cardiac contusion, tamponade, tension pneumothorax), the key primary finding is a significantly decreased cardiac output/cardiac index, typically with elevated filling pressures. Another key specific to tamponade or tension pneumothorax is "equalization of filling pressures," with the CVP and wedge values becoming equal or near equal. Finally, it is important to note that although sepsis is typically thought of as a hyperdynamic pattern of elevated heart rate and cardiac output with low SVR, it can also present like cardiogenic shock. This is typically seen with late sepsis or with overwhelming early sepsis (and often with gram positive organisms) and can be attributed to multi-organ failure and the production of myocardial depressant factors resulting in significant cardiac dysfunction. Additional conditions that can be diagnosed by relatively straightforward interpretation of PAC values or patterns include pulmonary hypertension (elevated PA pressures), severe mitral stenosis or regurgitation (typically PAOP/wedge will be higher than PA diastolic pressure), and left-to-right cardiac shunts (elevated mixed venous oxygen saturation, often above 90%).

Confounding Variables and PAC Data Validity

Ideal conditions must be present for accurate PAOP measurement and calculation of left heart pressures and function. The model assumes a low-resistance pulmonary vascular distribution. Under pathologic conditions such as systemic acidosis, hypoxemia, pulmonary hypertension, pulmonary artery embolism, vasoconstrictive medication use, and elevated downstream pressures in the setting of left heart failure or mitral valvular disease, the measured pressure may not accurately reflect the left atrial pressure and the LVEDP. For the most accurate measure of PA pressures, the distal port lumen must be in the middle of the PA vessel where balloon occlusion occurs. Potential malposition such as contacting the vessel wall, location near a confluence of vessels, or partial occlusion by the balloon can all affect the accuracy of PA and PAOP measurement. Before any measurements are performed, the PAC must be appropriately calibrated and pressure zeroed at the level of the right atrium, or phlebostatic axis. One of the most common sources of erroneous and inconsistent PAC measurements and calculations is not properly leveling and calibrating the device. This is particularly important any time the patient is moved in and out of bed, repositioned, or transported.

High intrathoracic pressures can also affect the accuracy of the PAOP. In the setting of positive pressure ventilation with elevated levels of positive end-expiratory pressure (PEEP) or decreased pulmonary and chest wall compliance, the pulmonary vascular hydrostatic pressure may be significantly impacted by the transmural pleural pressures. Optimal measurement of the PAOP is timed to occur at end expiration, thus mitigating the effects of pleural pressure. It is important to note that the point of measurement of the PAOP from the PA waveform should always be at end expiration, but this will be different in spontaneously ventilating patients versus those on positive pressure ventilation. With positive pressure ventilation, expiration results in a depression in the waveform, and thus PAOP is measured from the low point, or "valley." But with spontaneous breaths, end expiration will be at the peak of the PAOP waveform. In situations where high PEEP is used for lung recruitment and facilitation of gas exchange, such as acute respiratory distress syndrome, the circuit pressure may need to be transiently released to allow for accurate PAOP measurement. Estimated adjustments for high levels of PEEP have also been performed to avoid lung de-recruitment by releasing the circuit pressure for PAOP measurement.

Factors potentially influencing the accuracy of cardiac output measurement using thermodilution include the presence of a cardiac shunt, severe right heart failure, significant tricuspid or mitral valve regurgitation, and systemic therapeutic hypothermia [4]. PAC data calculations require complex algorithms with unique coefficients that must be correctly entered into the computer used for accurate data analysis and display. The patient's height and weight must also be entered correctly to obtain an accurate cardiac index or other measures that are indexed to body surface area. Additional factors that may impact the accuracy of data include catheter tip or port contact with the vessel wall, adherent clot, and adjacent high-flow or temperature discordant fluid infusions. Finally, it is important to remember which PAC measures are being directly measured, which are extrapolations, and which are calculated values based off of PAC or patient measures. The usual directly measured results are the CVP, the pulmonary artery systolic and diastolic pressures, and the PAOP or wedge pressure. The cardiac output is a calculated value, but it is from a directly measured change in the temperature of a cold infusate bolus. The major extrapolations from PAC data are the use of the CVP and PAOP or the right and left "filling pressures" as a reflection of end-diastolic volume and therefore volume status. And finally, the primary calculated values include the systemic vascular resistance, the pulmonary vascular resistance, the right and left heart stroke volume indices, and the measures that are indexed to body surface area (cardiac index, SVR index, etc.).

One of the most important confounders or misassumptions to understand involves the above stated extrapolation of the PAC-obtained right and left heart filling pressures (CVP and PAOP) as representing end-diastolic volume and overall intravascular volume status. The assumption relies on multiple prerequisites, including the correct calibration and leveling of the device, the correct measurement on the waveform, the lack of significant valvular pathology that is affecting the atrioventricular pressure relationships, the lack of confounding by pulmonary airway pressures, and the presence of a regular heart rhythm with consistent stroke volumes and cardiac output. Even if all the above are normal and the filling pressures are actually reflective of end-diastolic pressure, there is now ample evidence that this may not have a reliable relationship or standard dynamic response to ventricular volumes. This is primarily due to the fact that the resultant pressure for any given ventricular volume will be highly dependent on the ventricular compliance, which can vary widely between patients or even between measurements in the same patient. A low compliance ventricle may falsely elevate filling pressures even in the absence of any increased intravascular volume, and the opposite effect can be seen with highly compliant ventricles. In addition, ventricular compliance may change rapidly over time, particularly among the critically ill patient population, and thus wide variations in the measured filling pressures may be seen even where there is no corresponding significant change in intravascular volume status. Thus, these filling pressures should be interpreted with caution, should be assessed and evaluated in accordance with the global picture of the patient's evolving cardiopulmonary status, and should not be taken as the definitive measure of intravascular volume status or end-diastolic volume.

Indications and Contraindications

While initial enthusiasm for the PAC resulted in widespread multispecialty critical care adoption, multiple subsequent clinical studies, including randomized trials, have questioned its utility. Numerous trials investigating PAC-guided therapy have demonstrated no improvement or worse outcomes across a variety of clinical conditions: acute coronary syndrome [5–8], ARDS [9], hypovolemic and septic shock [10–12], and heart failure [13]. There is still an ongoing debate on the reasons for the lack of a proven benefit and the remaining indications (if any) for use of a PAC. One common argument against the current level 1 evidence is that the PAC-guided protocols were faulty or that the PAC data was misinterpreted and misused by the managing intensivists. We find these arguments to lack merit, as evidenced by the number and diversity of studies assessing PAC use and PAC interpretation and management by ICU physicians, all of which showed no benefit.

With this lack of robust evidence supporting the routine use of a PAC for most indications in the intensive care unit, are there any acceptable current indications? We believe there is still a defined but significantly decreased role for the PAC in the modern ICU. This would include any patient with complex or rapidly changing/evolving cardiac performance measures and the lack of other readily available methods (such as ultrasound) to assess and frequently reassess cardiac performance. Additional indications would include patients requiring active titration of cardiotropic medications based on cardiac output/index, those with an unclear intravascular volume status despite standard evaluations and measures, and those with an anatomic or physiologic abnormality that requires direct measurement of a true mixed venous oxygen saturation. Admittedly, the majority of surgical ICU patients are unlikely to benefit from placement of a PAC and PAC-guided management, but the information can be useful in highly select patient populations or in unique situations where other measures are not available or feasible.

One of the most important concepts regarding the use and utility of the PAC in the modern ICU is an appreciation of both the value and the limitations of the data that is provided with this device. It is a mathematical certainty that as you increase the number of variables or amount of data that must be integrated into complex decision-making, there will correspondingly be an increased chance for errors due to either bad data or bad interpretation of the data. The ICU physician and care team must be meticulous in using the PAC, including the initial positioning and confirmation of an adequate PAOP waveform, leveling and calibration of the device with frequent recalibration, and obtaining the key measures in a standard and uniform fashion every time. With the rise of the electronic medical record and automated data capture, it is tempting to evaluate and interpret the PAC parameters purely through a review of the recorded numbers, rather than through actual bedside assessment. We strongly recommend that the managing physician visually assess the waveform and the measurement of the key pressures, as well as the injection procedure for determining cardiac output and index. This is particularly important if there is wide variation of the PAC data and results recorded in the electronic record. And finally, the PAC should be thought of and utilized as a means for continuous assessments and guided titration of therapy and for situations where that information is not easily obtained via other less invasive means. One of the most common misapplications of the PAC we have observed is when it is used as a "wedge-ometer." This refers to placing the device because of a question about volume status, obtaining a wedge pressure as the only piece of actionable data, and then not using it for any continuous titration or assessment of therapy. In this example, the data could have been more easily obtained, and likely with more reliable results, via a standard bedside echocardiogram.

Placement of the Pulmonary Artery Catheter

A central venous access introducer sheath (typically a "cordis" catheter) must be placed prior to pulmonary artery catheterization. While all central veins are in theory candidate sites for access, the right internal jugular vein and the left subclavian vein are the preferred points of access for subsequent passage of the PAC due to their favorable positioning and angulation to the superior vena cava and right atrium. The pressure transducing system is connected to a visual waveform display allowing continuous observation of the distal port waveform and pressure. Prior to catheter placement, all channels are flushed with sterile fluid, and the catheter pressure is zeroed at the phlebostatic access point to ensure accurate measurements. A gentle shaking motion of the catheter tip should be represented by a 1:1 responsive waveform motion on the screen readout that has been designated for the pulmonary arterial pressures. Of note, the correct calculation coefficient must be entered into the monitoring system or the measured data and calculations will not be valid.

Under sterile conditions, the PAC is passed into the introducer sheath using a sterile protective sleeve that allows for subsequent catheter manipulation without catheter or central line contamination. A traditional method of catheter advancement called for estimating the position of the catheter tip by 10 cm increments (10 cm to clear the sheath, 20 cm to the

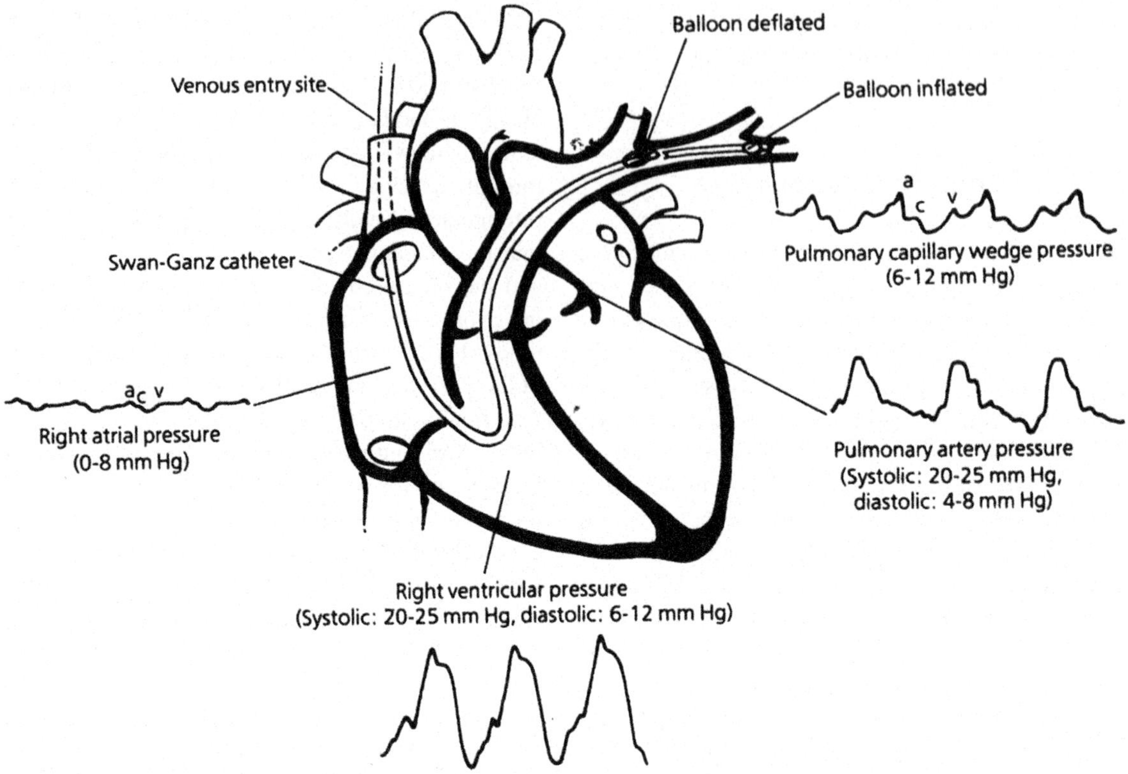

Fig. 66.3 Typical waveforms and pressures encountered during passage of the pulmonary artery catheter and corresponding anatomic locations (With permission from Disease-a-month [17])

right atrium, 30 cm to the right ventricle, etc.). However, safe catheter passage and accurate data interpretation require the proceduralist to be familiar with the expected pressure ranges and waveforms encountered along the catheter en route to the pulmonary artery (Fig. 66.3). Characteristic waveforms representing the right atrium, right ventricle, pulmonary artery, and finally pulmonary artery wedge position must be identified to ensure appropriate placement in this non-radiologic image-guided approach. All forward movement of the catheter should be performed with the balloon fully inflated to 1.5 mL once it has cleared the introducer sheath. Furthermore, the balloon must be completely deflated prior to any withdrawal of the catheter to avoid injury to valvular structures.

There are several key points to successful and accurate placement of a PAC. First is ensuring that the pressure transducers are connected correctly and the corresponding waveforms are correctly labeled and identified on the monitor. It is relatively common to have the distal port waveform showing as the CVP/RA waveform on the monitor and vice versa. This means either the transducers are connected to the wrong port on the PAC or the monitor labels are reversed. Next, the PAC is inserted into the central line lumen with the balloon completely deflated and advanced to at least the 10–15 cm marking. This should produce a low amplitude CVP tracing, which will remain unchanged as the catheter is advanced through the right atrium. The PAC balloon is then slowly inflated and then advanced in 5–10 cm increments while continuously watching the monitor for a change in the waveform signifying entry into the right ventricle. This is characterized by a high-amplitude arterial waveform with a peak typically of 20–30 mmHg and then a complete return to baseline (see Fig. 66.3, bottom). The catheter is then advanced until the RV waveform is replaced by a pulmonary arterial waveform, most easily identified by a peak that is approximately equivalent to the RV but an elevated trough that does not return to the baseline seen with the RV tracing. The catheter should now be slowly advanced until a pulmonary capillary wedge tracing is obtained, typically characterized by small and fine deflections, which may even appear close to a flatline on the monitor. The final step to assure proper positioning is to now deflate the balloon, and the tracing should return to a pulmonary artery waveform. If it does not, then the catheter likely needs to be slightly withdrawn. With the catheter now located in the pulmonary artery, a chest radiograph is performed to confirm location and evaluate the West lung zone position as well as any mechanical complications such as pneumothorax, pulmonary artery rupture, or catheter malposition. The depth of insertion should be noted and recorded in case of inadvertent manipulation of the catheter during patient movement, and the PAC should be locked in position by rotating the fastener knob on the PAC sterile sheath.

There are relatively common problems encountered during the "floating" of a PAC, which are almost always related to getting the catheter into the PA or getting from the PA tracing to a wedge pressure tracing. If a normal CVP/RA tracing is obtained but advancing does not result in transition to an RV tracing, then the catheter is likely going into the subclavian vein (from the IJ) or across to the contralateral subclavian vein. If an RV tracing is obtained but then changes back to a CVP tracing with advancement of the catheter, then the catheter has gone through the RV and into the inferior vena cava. This is commonly seen with forgetting to inflate the balloon prior to advancing. Finally, if there is a persistent RV tracing despite advancing to an appropriate distance (40–50 cm), then the catheter is curling up in the RV. The solution to most of these issues is withdrawal of the catheter to the starting point and repeat attempts. Varying the speed of advancement and distance with each advance will often help. Having the patient reposition from supine to lateral decubitus position can also help in difficult cases. Finally, advancing the catheter under direct fluoroscopic visualization is a final alternative for particularly difficult cases. It is critical to remember that the balloon should only remain inflated during measurement of the PAOP and forward movement of the catheter and that once the catheter is "wedged," the balloon should be inflated slowly and only to the point where a clear pulmonary capillary wedge pressure tracing is obtained.

Several common mechanical and system difficulties may prevent achieving the wedge position or cause errors in the pressure and waveform interpretation (Table 66.3). Inability to access the RA from the central vein can usually be

Table 66.3 Sources of error in pulmonary artery catheter data

Problem	Potential causes	Troubleshooting
Dampened waveform	Incorrect scale on monitor Incorrect referencing Air in the system Spontaneous wedging of catheter	Ensure the correct scale is in use Check referencing and pressure bag Check for loose connections Remove air bubbles in system Flush system (see below-spontaneous wedge)
Overdamping (diminished systolic peak, loss of dicrotic notch, rounder waveforms)	Compliant tubing Large air bubbles Clots/blood in system Loose connections Kinked catheter or tip against vessel wall	Check tubing Check for loose connections Flush tubing Perform square wave test Reposition/remove catheter as indicated
Underdamping (falsely high systolic peak, falsely low diastolic value, artifact)	Pressure tubing is too long Too many components (i.e., stopcocks) Small air bubbles Defective transducer	Ensure correct tubing is in use Eliminate tubing extensions Remove extra components Remove air bubbles Change transducer
Erratic waveform with highly variable pressures	Catheter whip	Reposition catheter to a less turbulent area of vessel
Spontaneous wedge	Catheter is advanced too far or is too flexible	Do not flush catheter Assess for other causes of dampened waveform (see above) Reposition catheter
Unable to obtain wedge	Air returns to syringe—Catheter is probably not advanced far enough into the PA Air does not return to syringe – balloon is probably ruptured	Reposition catheter Replace catheter
Overwedging	Excessive air in balloon catheter is advanced too far	Observe waveform on monitor while injecting air—Stop injecting as soon as the waveform dampens reposition catheter
Absent waveform	Disconnect of monitoring system Incorrect scale in use Faulty transducer dome or air in dome Defective transducer Inadequate pressure in pressure bag Check for kinks in the system Catheter tip or lumen totally occluded	Check connections Set correct scale on monitor Change transducer Adjust pressure to 300 mmHg Change transducer Add appropriate pressure to bag Remove kinks Slowly aspirate to check for blood—If no blood return, may need to remove catheter

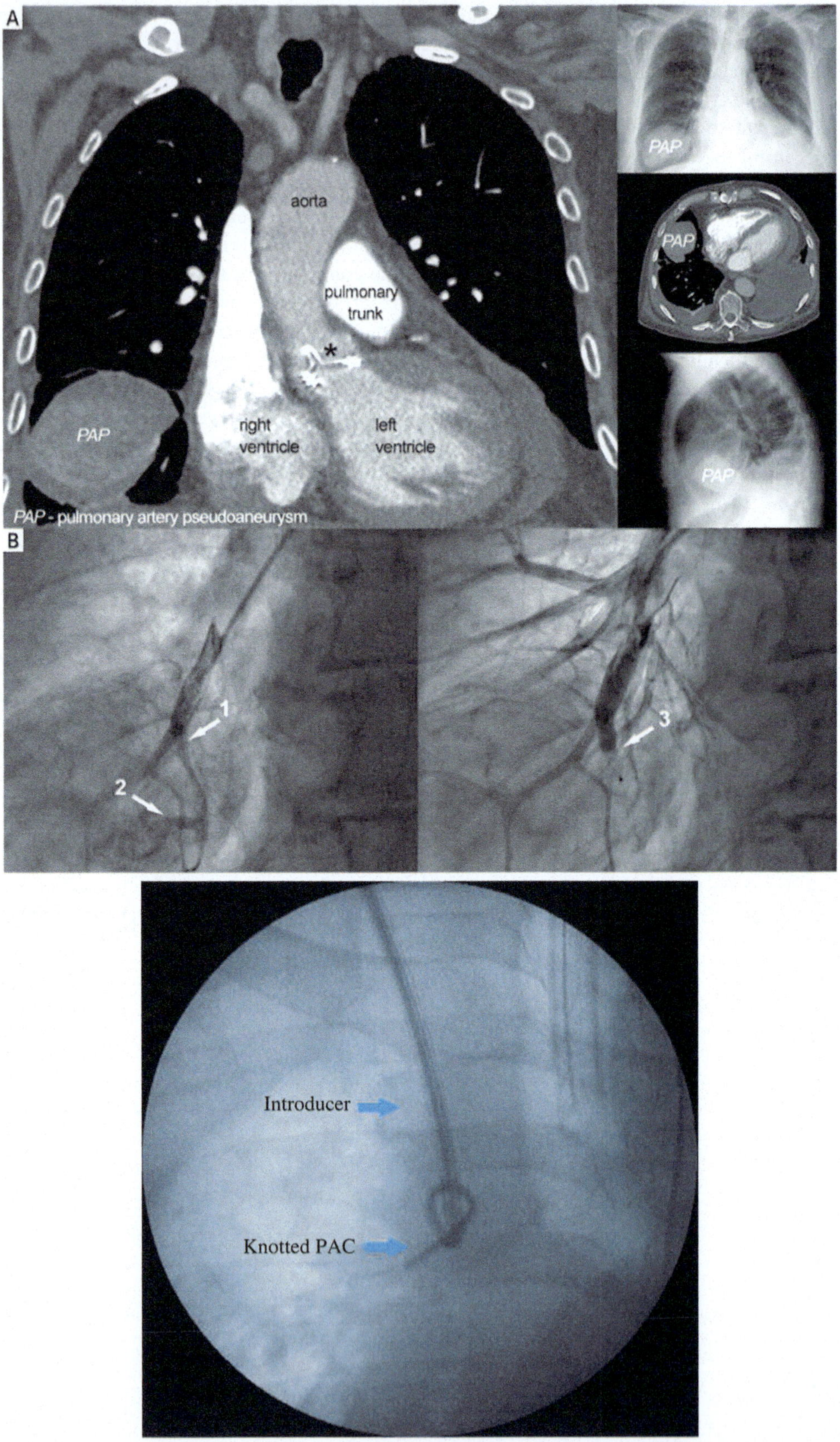

Fig. 66.4 Major PAC-related complications: pulmonary artery rupture due to PAC balloon inflation (**a**) and knotted pulmonary artery catheter (**b**) (Panel A from Rudziński et al. [18] and panel B from Smith et al. [19])

prevented by utilizing one of the preferred central venous access sites and carefully placing the gently curving catheter tip such that it will favorably curve into the RA with the balloon inflated. Over extended periods of catheter position in the bloodstream, the body temperature will cause the catheter tip to lose the gentle curve that facilitates RA access. Placing the patient in Trendelenburg position may also increase the right heart venous inflow and facilitate access to the RA (keeping in mind potential postural effects upon the zeroed catheter position). Failure to advance to the next chamber may be due to turbulent flow or hyperdynamic conditions, incorrect interpretation of the waveform, catheter coiling, catheter tip lodging in cardiac structures, inadvertent balloon deflation, and excessively rapid catheter advancement.

When the PAC passes through the RV, it is not uncommon to see transient arrhythmia. In this event, the balloon should be deflated and the catheter withdrawn until return to previous or sinus rhythm. Theses arrhythmias are almost always transient and related to brief mechanical irritation from catheter passage or due to coiling of the catheter in the RV. Failure of arrhythmia resolution should prompt appropriate cardiac assessment and intervention as indicated. A chest radiograph should be performed to help rule out other mechanical complications.

Complications of the Pulmonary Artery Catheter

While it may be argued that the most common complication of the PAC is incorrect data interpretation or accuracy, most reported complications are either mechanical in nature or related to prolonged use. Common mechanical complications include associated central access problems such as pneumothorax, hematoma, vascular injuries, and arrhythmias. Complications related to prolonged use may include bloodstream infection, thrombosis, pulmonary infarction, and pulmonary artery injury. Rare complications include refractory arrhythmias, catheter fragmentation and embolization, catheter knotting, valvular injuries, and damage to the coronary sinus or myocardial wall.

Pulmonary artery rupture is a rare but potentially catastrophic complication likely due to balloon inflation or progressive vessel wall injury in high-risk patients such as the elderly or those with pulmonary hypertension. Classic signs of this complication include sudden hypotension and hypoxia, hemoptysis, and signs of rupture on chest radiograph (Fig. 66.3a). If recognized promptly, the balloon should be deflated, slightly withdrawn, and carefully reinflated to tamponade the hemorrhage. The "damaged" lung should be positioned downward after selective intubation of the opposite main stem bronchus or use of a dual lumen endotracheal tube with bronchial blocker. Interventional arterial embolization or emergent surgery may be required for control of complete ruptures.

Coiling of the PAC within the RV may result in knotting of the catheter during difficult or novice placement (Fig. 66.3b and 66.4). Any unexpected resistance encountered during catheter advancement should prompt balloon deflation and gentle withdrawal. If any further resistance is encountered, a chest radiograph should be performed prior to any further PAC manipulation. Catheter knotting can frequently be resolved using interventional vascular radiology techniques but may require cardiac surgery for removal.

Summary

The pulmonary artery catheter has played a key role in the advancement of contemporary critical care medicine and should continue to have a defined role within a subset of critically ill medical and surgical patients. While catheter utilization and expertise with this device have declined in recent decades for numerous reasons, there remain several indications for continued selective use today. Successful catheter placement, data capture and interpretation, and application of the diverse information available from the PAC remain a necessary skill for many professional critical care practitioners.

References

1. Swan H, Ganz W, Forrester J, Marcus H, Diamond G, Chonette D. Catheterization of the heart in man with use of a flow-directed balloon-tipped catheter. N Engl J Med. 1970;283:447–51.
2. Gasparovic H, Gabelica R, Ostojic Z, Petricevic M, Ivancan V, Biocina B. Diagnostic accuracy of central venous saturation in estimating mixed venous saturation is proportional to cardiac performance among cardiac surgery patient. J Crit Care. 2014;29(5):828–34.
3. Dueck MH, Klimek M, Appenrodt S, Weigand C, Boerner U. Trends but not individual values of central venous oxygen saturation agree with mixed venous oxygen saturation during varying hemodynamic conditions. J Am Soc Anesthesiol. 2005;103(2):249–57.
4. Marini JJ, Wheeler AP, editors. Critical care medicine: the essentials. 3rd ed. Philadelphia: Lippincott Williams and Wilkins; 2006. p. 33–4.
5. Weiner RA, Welch HG. Trends in the use of the pulmonary artery catheter in the United States, 1993–2004. JAMA. 2007;298:423–9.
6. Gore JM, Goldberg RJ, Spodick DH, Alpert JS, Dalen JE. A community-wide assessment of the use of pulmonary artery catheters in patients with acute myocardial infarction. Chest. 1987;92:721–7.

7. Cohen MG, Kelly RV, Kong DF, Menon V, Shah M, Ferreira J, Pieper KS, Criger D, Poggio R, Ohman EM, et al. Pulmonary artery catheterization in acute coronary syndromes: insights from the GUSTO IIb and GUSTO trials. Am J Med. 2005;118:482–8.
8. Ruisi CP, Goldberg RJ, Kennelly BM, Goodman SG, Lopez-Sendon J, Granger CB, Avezum A, Eagle KA, Fitzgerald G, Gore JM, et al. Pulmonary artery catheterization in patients with acute coronary syndromes. Am Heart J. 2009;158:170–6.
9. Wheeler AP, Bernard GR, Thompson BT, Schoenfeld D, Wiedemann HP, de Boisblanc B, Connors AF Jr, Hite RD, Harabin AL. National Heart, Lung, and Blood Institute Acute Respiratory Distress Syndrome (ARDS) Clinical Trials Network: Pulmonary-artery versus central venous catheter to guide treatment of acute lung injury. N Engl J Med. 2006;354:2213–24.
10. Sandham JD, Hull RD, Brant RF, Knox L, Pineo GF, Doig CJ, Laporta DP, Viner S, Passerini L, Devitt H, et al. A randomized, controlled trial of the use of pulmonary artery catheters in high-risk surgical patients. N Engl J Med. 2003;348:5–14.
11. McKinley BA, Sucher JF, Todd SR, Gonzalez EA, Kozar RA, Sailors RM, Moore FA. Central venous pressure versus pulmonary artery catheter-directed shock resuscitation. Shock. 2009;32:463–70.
12. Barmparas G, Inaba K, Georgiou C, Hadjizacharia P, Chan LS, Demetriades D, Friese R, Rhee P. Swan-Ganz catheter use in trauma patients can be reduced without negatively affecting outcomes. World J Surg. 2011;35:1809–17.
13. Binanay C, Califf RM, Hasselblad V, O'Connor CM, Shah MR, Sopko G, Stevenson LW, Francis GS, Leier CV, Miller LW. Evaluation study of congestive heart failure and pulmonary artery catheterization effectiveness: the ESCAPE trial. JAMA. 2005;294:1625–33.
14. Gidwani UK, Goel S. The pulmonary artery catheter in 2015: the swan and the phoenix. Cardiol Rev. 2016;24(1):1–13.
15. Wilkins RL, Stoller JK, Kacmarek RM. Egan's fundamentals of respiratory care. 9th ed. St Louis: Mosby; 2009.
16. Marini JJ. Respiratory medicine and intensive care for the house officer. Baltimore: Williams & Wilkins; 1991.
17. Disease-a-month. The Swan-Ganz Catheter. Dis Mon. 1991;37(8):509–43.
18. Rudziński PN, et al. Pulmonary artery rupture as a complication of Swan-Ganz catheter application. Postępy W Kardiologii Interwencyjnej = Adv Interv Cardiol. 2016;12(2):135–9. https://doi.org/10.5114/aic.2016.59364.
19. Smith M, et al. Nonsurgical removal of knotted pulmonary artery catheter. J Med Cases [Online]. 2013;4(3):163–5.

Extracorporeal Membrane Oxygenation: How Do We Do It?

67

Pablo G. Sanchez and Aaron M. Cheng

Indications for ECMO

ECMO support should be considered whenever a critically ill patient has severe respiratory or cardiorespiratory failure and conventional circulatory or respiratory therapy has failed or is anticipated to be inadequate to support vital organ function. Intuitively, like most acute life-supportive interventions, the earlier ECMO support is initiated when required, the more likely a desired clinical outcome can be achieved. Patients considered appropriate for ECMO support should have reversible clinical conditions that are expected to have realistic chances of recovery or have available options for more durable, long-term support when the primary indication is for circulatory failure.

The variety of different clinical scenarios in which ECMO support has been utilized has markedly expanded over the last two decades, particularly as management of critically ill patients has improved and ECMO technology continues to evolve and is applied by a wider clinical audience. Acute refractory hypoxemic respiratory failure and cardiogenic shock remain the most common diagnoses for which ECMO support is instituted, but as shown by the illustration below (Fig. 67.1), the role of ECMO continues to expand.

Patients who decompensate due to progressive deterioration of chronic diseases which have failed treatment, those who have suffered acute devastating neurocognitive injury, and patients who have terminal illnesses with poor life expectancy are generally not considered appropriate for ECMO support. Also, the initiation of ECMO would be inappropriate for individual patients whose known goals of care would be clearly incompatible with ECMO support. As such, there currently remains no clearly defined standard in which ECMO support should or should not be utilized in critically ill patients. The Extracorporeal Life Support Organization (ELSO), a nonprofit international consortium for ECMO education and implementation, has presented its organizational guidelines for general indications and contraindications for ECMO support as outlined in Table 67.1 and available on their website: www.elso.org.

ECMO Circuit and Configurations

All current ECMO circuits consist of the following basic components: (1) large-diameter cannula(s) for drainage of deoxygenated venous blood from the patient, (2) cannula(s) for returning oxygenated blood back to the patients' circulatory system, (3) an extracorporeal regulated pump to "circulate" blood between the patient and (4) gas-exchange device (aka, oxygenator), and a (5) heat exchanger to help regulate body temperature; these components are connected with circuit blood tubing. Additional devices can increase the complexity of the basic ECMO circuit and include various monitoring and measuring devices and different connectors to allow access for additional therapeutic modalities such as hemofiltration and renal replacement therapy.

Establishing good vascular access for cannula insertion and positioning is critical to achieving adequate ECMO support. The selection of vascular access is determined by various factors which should take into account the patient's age and size, the type and amount of support required, and the individual clinical scenario. The sites of vascular access for

P. G. Sanchez
University of Pittsburgh, Department of Cardiothoracic Surgery, Division of Lung Transplant and Lung Failure, University of Pittsburgh Medical Center, Associate Director of Lung Transplant and ECLS, Pittsburgh, PA, USA
e-mail: Sanchezpg@upmc.edu

A. M. Cheng (✉)
University of Washington, Department of Surgery, Division of Cardiothoracic Surgery Co-Director, Cardiothoracic ICU, University of Washington Medical Center Director, Thoracic Surgery, Harborview Medical Center, Seattle, WA, USA
e-mail: chengam@uw.edu

A. Salim et al. (eds.), *Surgical Critical Care Therapy*, https://doi.org/10.1007/978-3-319-71712-8_67

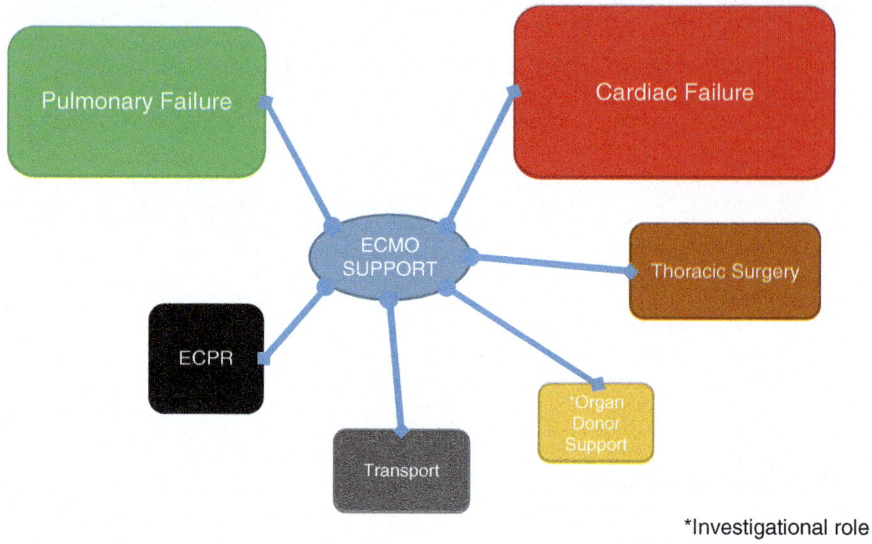

Fig. 67.1 Contemporary ECMO utilization

Table 67.1 Indications and contraindications for ECMO in hypoxic respiratory failure

Indications
Any cause
Consider when the risk of mortality ≥50%
P/F ratio less than 150 on >90% FiO2 and/or Murray score 2–3
Indicated when the risk of mortality is ≥80%
P/F ratio less than 100 on >90% FiO2 and/or Murray score 3–4
CO2 retention despite high plateau pressures (>30)
Severe air leak syndromes
Need for intubation in a patient on lung transplant list
Immediate cardiac/respiratory collapse (PE, blocked airway, unresponsive to optimal care)
Contraindications
No absolute contraindication but several relative contraindications
Requiring high ventilator settings >7 days (FiO2 > 90%, Pplat > 30)
Major pharmacologic immunosuppression (ANC < 400/mm^3)
CNS bleeding that is recent or expanding
Nonreversible major comorbidity such as severe brain injury and terminal cancer
No absolute age cutoff, but consider the increasing risk with increasing age

ECMO support determine the ECMO configuration: whether it is for respiratory support only via venovenous ECMO (VV-ECMO) or for both cardiorespiratory support via veno-arterial ECMO (VA-ECMO). In VV-ECMO, vascular access for cannulation of the drainage cannula for deoxygenated blood and of the return cannula for oxygenated blood to the patient are both in the venous system (Fig. 67.2). In VA-ECMO, vascular access for the drainage cannula is in the patient's venous system, but the return cannula is inserted in the arterial system, typically the femoral artery.

Typically, the large peripheral vessels are cannulated for VV-ECMO or VA-ECMO in the adult patient, and most commonly the common femoral vein (CFV) or the internal jugular vein (IJ) and the common femoral artery (CFA) are chosen. In some circumstances where VA-ECMO support is required, transthoracic ECMO cannulation may be preferred. Typically, this occurs when patients are unable to be weaned from cardiopulmonary bypass after cardiac surgery or after post-sternotomy resuscitation. Under these circumstances, access to the right atrium for inserting a drainage cannula and the ascending aorta for the return cannula is readily available. Frequently the same vascular access used for cannulation during cardiopulmonary bypass can be used. However, since these cannulation techniques are not routinely performed by non-cardiothoracic surgeons or surgical intensivists, the procedure of transthoracic or central cannulation for VA-ECMO will not be further discussed. Procedural and technical details will focus on peripheral cannulation, which is most commonly utilized in general/trauma surgical critical care patients requiring ECMO support.

Procedure and Technique

Cannula Selection

Ideally the largest diameter and shortest drainage cannula that can be inserted in the vein is chosen. The drainage cannula usually has both end and side holes to allow blood flow to the ECMO pump and oxygenator even if the end hole becomes blocked. Various cannula manufacturers report tested flow rates with associated pressure gradients according to their cannula diameters. However, for most adult patients, our size selection ranges from 23 Fr to 29 Fr for the drainage cannula: usually for patients with smaller body habitus and BMI or those patients whom high ECMO flows are not required for cardiorespiratory support, we choose a

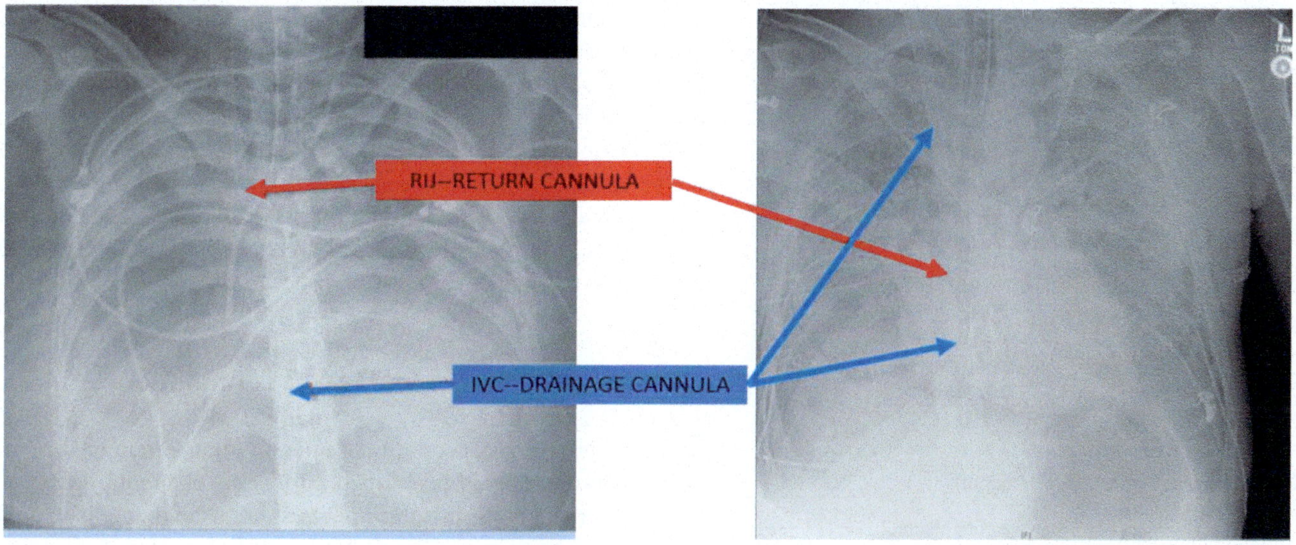

Fig. 67.2 Chest X-ray after venovenous ECMO. (**a**) Separate cannulas for VV-ECMO: RIJ cannula and IVC cannula. (**b**) Dual-lumen single cannula for VV-ECMO

size 23 Fr or 25 Fr cannula. We prefer a size 27 Fr or 29 Fr drainage cannula for male patients, and those we anticipate will need higher ECMO flows. The venous drainage cannula is commercially available in different lengths, and the length should be selected based on the distance of from the planned insertion site to the right atrium, which will vary depending on the patient's torso length.

The arterial or return cannulas are smaller in diameter, and we keep available sizes from 17 Fr to 23 Fr. We customarily prefer to use a 17Fr or 19Fr size cannula for the artery for VA-ECMO and a 21 Fr or 23 Fr size return cannula for VV-ECMO, depending on the body size of the patient and the flow requirements anticipated to be required for respiratory support.

A dual-lumen single cannula (Avalon Elite®, Maquet, Wayne, NJ, USA) is also commercially available for VV-ECMO support. This single catheter cannula inserted in the right internal jugular vein has two lumens: one to allow venous drainage of deoxygenated blood from the SVC and IVC and a second lumen to allow simultaneous reinfusion of oxygenated return blood directed toward the tricuspid valve of the right atrium (Fig. 67.2b). For adult patients, the cannula sizes used typically range from 19 Fr to 31 Fr. Generally, we reserve insertion of this particular cannula in patients who we anticipate will require a long duration of VV-ECMO support, are able to be ambulatory, and can have this cannulation procedure performed in a nonurgent/emergent fashion with the availability of transesophageal echocardiography and fluoroscopy (e.g., pre-lung transplant candidate patients who acutely decompensate and are already on the waiting list). In most cases of VV-ECMO, we prefer to use separate single-lumen cannulas given the simpler technical considerations for percutaneous insertion at the patient's bedside (Fig. 67.2a).

Cannula Insertion Site

The most common sites for peripheral cannulation for VV-ECMO and VA-ECMO in adults are the common femoral vein for drainage of deoxygenated blood and either the internal jugular vein or the common femoral artery for VV-ECMO and VA-ECMO, respectively. The direct route of the right internal jugular vein to the superior vena cava makes this vein preferred over the left internal jugular vein. Likewise, for VA-ECMO, we prefer to insert the drainage cannula via the right common femoral vein whenever possible and use the opposite left groin for the return arterial cannula. Other sites for peripheral ECMO cannulation can also be used but are less common. For VA-ECMO, axillary artery has been described for the arterial access, and for VV-ECMO, the use of both left and right common femoral veins have also been used, particularly whenever access to the left or right internal jugular vein is not available for insertion of the return cannula. The subclavian vein is uncommonly used for vascular access in VV-ECMO given the challenges with applying direct pressure to the vein during cannula removal once ECMO support is no longer required.

Vascular access of these vessels can be achieved by the percutaneous Seldinger technique or by the open cut-down approach. For obvious reasons, the percutaneous approach is preferred, but preparation and equipment to convert to an

Table 67.2 Vascular access tray for ECMO cannulation

Instrument description	Quantity per tray
Weitlaner retractor (regular size 5.5–6.5″ sharp teeth)	1
Army-navy retractor	1
Vessel loops	4
Metzenbaum scissors	1
Debakey forceps (9.5″)	2
Adson forceps w/teeth	2
Mosquito clamps curved 5″	2
Kelly clamps curved 6.25″	2
Needle drivers – 6″ Mayo-Hegar	2
Scalpel handles #3, 5″	2
Scalpel blades #15	
Scalpel blades #10	
Richardson retractor (small, 1″ depth)	1
Skin stapler	1
Straight blunt/sharp suture scissors	1

open incision approach should always be readily available at the patient's bedside. Difficulties encountered during percutaneous insertion may warrant expedited conversion to direct open cannulation techniques. A list of basic equipment we keep in our vascular access tray is listed in Table 67.2.

Pre-ECMO Cannulation Preparation

Once a patient has been decided to be placed on ECMO support and the decision for either VV-ECMO or VA-ECMO support has been made, it is important to optimize conditions for cannulation. Frequently, decisions will have to be made about whether first obtaining additional vascular access for administration of necessary medications and fluid therapy and hemodynamic and laboratory monitoring is necessary. Whenever feasible, it is often easier to have inserted the additional central venous catheters and invasive arterial monitoring lines needed before rather than after the ECMO cannulation procedure. This opportunity often depends on the urgency of requiring ECMO support, however. It is also important to ensure that the ECMO circuit is primed and ready to use and the ECMO personnel who will manage the ECMO device and circuit are also present and available. The provider team that will provide analgesia and sedation during the cannulation procedure should also have vasoactive medications and fluids readily available to administer as it is not uncommon that patients manifest labile hemodynamics during ECMO initiation.

The patient should be positioned supine and flat, and comfortable access to the planned vascular access sites should be prepared. Vascular access and ECMO cannulation should be performed as sterilely as possible, and therefore the skin sites should be widely prepped with chlorohexidine or other antibacterial, antiseptic topical agent. One should consider antiseptic skin prep for alternative vascular access sites should one be unsuccessful in percutaneously accessing the intended vessel for cannulation. Like any other central venous line access procedure, the patient should be fully covered with a sterile surgical drape to reduce the incidence of cannula site infection. Full personal protective equipment should be worn by those individuals who will be actually performing the cannulation procedure.

Vascular Access and ECMO Cannulation

Percutaneous access of the internal jugular vein or common femoral vein is performed similar to obtaining access for central venous line placement using the Seldinger technique. We administer of an intravenous bolus of unfractionated heparin before we start the cannulation procedure, usually 3000–5000 units, if not contraindicated by bleeding concerns. Although not required, safe practice for central venous line placement would recommend that vessel puncture should be carried out under ultrasound guidance whenever circumstances allow. Ultrasound imaging provides visual assessment of the relationship of the vein to the adjacent artery and idea of the relative depth the catheter needle trocar needs to traverse from the skin to puncture the vessel. Importantly, ultrasound allows an assessment of the vessel diameter relative to the cannula chosen. Ultrasound visualization of the needle in the desired vessel and subsequently also the guidewire is obtained. We specifically try to avoid the "through-and-through" technique with vessel puncture; purposefully "backwalling" the artery, in particular, and then slowly withdrawing the needle into the lumen has been associated with troublesome hematoma formation and subsequent difficulty passing the guidewire smoothly. We use the 6 Fr micropuncture set (Micropuncture introducer kit, Cook Medical) to obtain initial percutaneous access of the vessel initially. The 6 Fr needle trocar can accommodate a 0.035 in. guidewire which is then inserted in the vessel to be cannulated. For venous cannulation, we use a 150 cm guidewire; for cannulation of the common femoral artery, a 100 cm length guidewire is usually sufficient. It is particularly important to ensure that guidewire inserts easily through the needle catheter and passes proximally easily within the vessel.

Once sufficient guidewire length has been passed into the vessel; we use hydrophilic dilators to sequentially enlarge the vessel over the guidewire (Sorin Vascular Dilator Kit, LivaNova, USA). In our experience, it is important to dilate the vessel in a stepwise fashion and avoid skipping dilator sizes; the vessel should be dilated to the size of the intended diameter of the cannula to inserted. Care should be taken to avoid kinking the guidewire anywhere along its length when passing the dilators over the guidewire, and it is crucial to check that the guidewires move back and forth easily as the dilator is progressively inserted over the wire. Important areas where the guidewire frequently kinks is at the level of the skin, at the enveloping vascular sheath, and with the internal jugular vein, at the level of the sternocleidomastoid muscle and at the level of the sternal notch where the vessel passes through the thoracic inlet. We find it occasionally useful to enlarge the skin incision where the guidewire passes across the skin to facilitate smooth insertion of the dilators. This is especially true in obese individuals with groin cannulation. If the guidewire becomes kinked, it can be difficult to pass subsequent dilators and the cannula itself without excessive force and unsafe to do so; when this does occur, it is often easier to proceed by first exchanging the kinked guidewire for new guidewire.

The selected cannula should be able to pass along the guidewire without undue pressure. It is customary to insert the venous drainage cannula first, followed by insertion of the return/arterial cannula. If the same groin side is being cannulated for VA-ECMO, it is often easier to first obtain vascular access of both the vein and artery before proceeding with dilation and insertion of the venous cannula.

The length of venous cannula insertion can be estimated by the patient's surface anatomy. For venous cannulation from the groin, the length to be inserted can be estimated by summing the measured distance from the groin skin puncture site to the umbilicus and then to a point just superior to the level of xiphoid. For cannula insertion of the internal jugular vein, the distance to be inserted can be estimated by the distance to the level of the sternomanubrial junction. With cannulation of the femoral artery and the cannula has side holes, it is critical that the most proximal hole is well within the vessel. We always prefer to insert the cannula deeper and have to pull the cannula back rather than have to push the cannula that has been inserted too short, particularly once the introducer and guidewire have been removed.

Once the cannula is inserted to its desired length, we remove the tapered cannula introducer and guidewire, verify that there is appropriate blood backflow into the cannula, and then occlude the proximal end of the cannula with a large atraumatic straight clamp. After both the drainage and return cannulas have been inserted, we connect and secure the proximal end of the drainage cannula to the ECMO circuit tubing, followed by next connecting the return cannula to the ECMO circuit. This is all done sterilely and taking necessary precautions to avoid introducing air bubbles inside the circuit.

Next, we confirm that there are no air bubbles detected along the circuit and cannulas, the clamp on the drainage cannula is removed first, followed by removing the clamp on the return cannula, and the ECMO flow is initiated. For VA-ECMO, we like to ensure that the ACT measurement before starting the ECMO flow is ≥220; if there is concern that the ACT level may be too low, we will empirically administer another heparin bolus (usually 2000 units) just before ECMO initiation. We are less particular with the anticoagulation with VV-ECMO flow initiation given the decreased risk of arterial system embolization. The ECMO cannulas then are sutured securely to the skin.

Cannulation with the dual-lumen, single cannula for VV-ECMO is technically more challenging. This cannula is inserted in the right internal jugular vein and is typically placed percutaneously. To achieve the necessary ECMO flow rates, the cannula needs to be larger in diameter than the single-lumen cannula sizes that are typically inserted in the RIJ vein for VV-ECMO. We typically select a 27 Fr cannula with the general size used ranging from 23 Fr to 31 Fr in adult patients. Vascular access is obtained by Seldinger technique under ultrasound guidance as is typically performed for central venous catheter insertion. Ultrasound evaluation is useful in gauging whether inserting this larger diameter cannula in the patient's jugular vein is feasible. Once the guidewire is inserted in the jugular vein, we visualize the trajectory of the guidewire down to the infradiaphragmatic IVC. We rely on fluoroscopy to ensure that the guidewire does not unintentionally loop in the heart or traverse the tricuspid valve. If fluoroscopy is not readily available, plain X-ray films can be obtained serially as required, but it is critical that the guidewire course be direct from the R internal jugular vein across the right atrium and into the inferior vena cava without redundancy or loops. In our opinion, relying solely on echocardiography to determine guidewire location can be misleading; we have experienced circumstances where the guidewire appears by transesophageal echo to pass directly from the SVC across the right atrium and into the IVC, but when fluoroscopy is used, there is actually a loop in the guidewire.

Once guidewire access is obtained and confirmed by fluoroscopy, serial dilation of the insertion tract is performed. It useful to use a hemostat to spread and stretch the skin and subcutaneous tissue at the insertion site alongside the guidewire with each serial dilation. After the last dilator has been used, the cannula is then inserted over the guidewire with its introducer and followed directly with fluoroscopy as the cannula is guided into correct position. Again, fluoroscopy is used to ensure that the cannula and its introducer do not kink the guidewire as they pass over the wire and inadvertently cause right atrial or ventricular wall injury. The tip of the cannula should reside just caudal to the IVC-RA junction within the IVC, and the outflow opening should be rotated toward the tricuspid valve with use of echo. When the dual-lumen cannula is oriented correctly, the outflow arm of the return cannula should be directed medially and lie toward the right ear of the patient.

Cannulation Complications

Cannula placement complications are primarily related to the proficiency with the Seldinger technique and the imaging method utilized to guide percutaneous access to the vessel. In addition, some patient circumstances, such as the placement of an arterial cannula during active CPR, can lead to higher complication rates.

As part of our bedside cannulation strategy, venous access to the internal jugular and common femoral veins is consistently preformed under direct ultrasound guidance. A J-wire is then advanced and stopped when premature ventricular contractions are triggered. We then preform sequential dilations to the diameter of the selected cannula. The most frequent technical complication that we observe during this process is bending the J-wire. In our experience this occurs due to differences between the puncture access angle and the angle in which the dilators are being progressed. As a result, a false path is created. Under these circumstances the wire will need to be exchanged which may require accessing the vein at a different level or choosing a different vessel. This can be particularly challenging if the wire is compromised when trying to access the right internal jugular vein. Under these circumstances, bifemoral VV-ECMO may be the only exit strategy. We normally avoid the use of stiffer guidewires, i.e., Amplatz; in our experience, they are associated with increased vascular injury. Pneumothoraxes, right ventricle rupture, pericardial tamponade, and perforation of the IVC are some of the other complications associated with VV-ECMO cannulation.

Once ECMO is initiated, migration of the cannula can result in lower oxygenation and flow, particularly with the use of bi-caval dual-lumen cannulas. Migration of the distal lumen into the right atrium can increase recirculation and decrease flow. Reduced drainage can be observed when the cannula advances into the suprahepatic veins.

Gaining access to the common femoral artery (CFA) for VA-ECMO initiation can result in hematomas, artery dissection, limb ischemia, and, in severe cases, amputation. To reduce arterial complications, we have a consistent approach to cannulation of the CFA and the superficial femoral artery (SFA). Using ultrasound, we identify the common, the superficial, and the profunda femoral arteries. Then we place a micropuncture into the SFA and a micropunture into the CFA. By wire exchange, a 6F wire reinforced cannula is placed in the SFA. Now, we advance a J-wire 30–40 cm into the abdominal aorta via the micropunture in the CFA. After sequential dilation, again ensuring that the wire is not bending or a false path is created, we insert our arterial cannula and connect the 6 F cannula to its side port (Fig. 67.3).

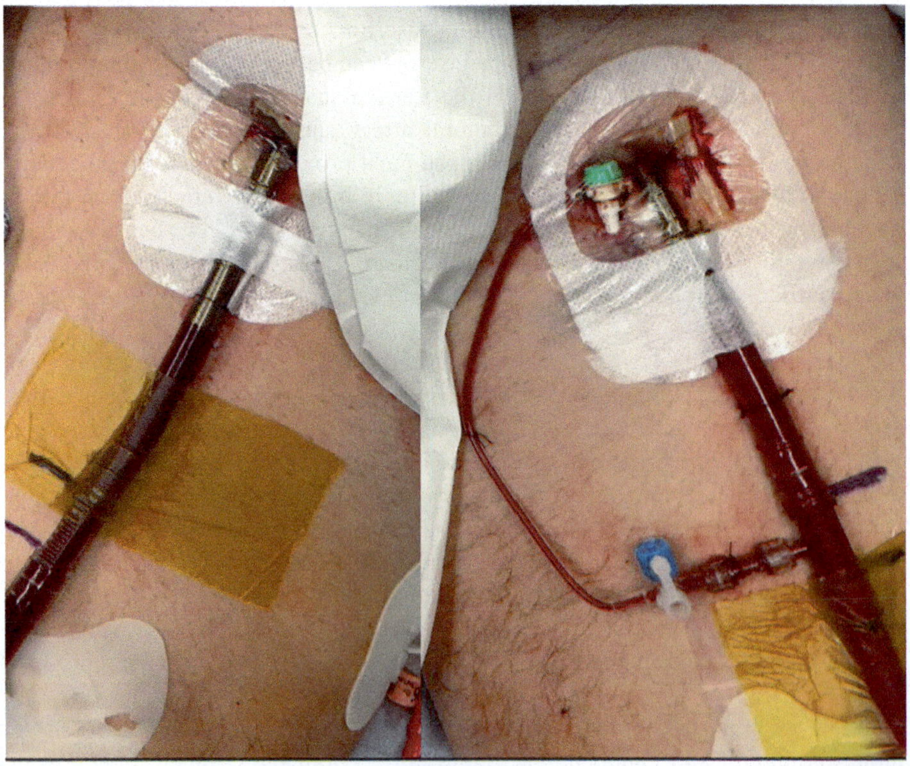

Fig. 67.3 Femoral vessel cannulation sites for venoarterial ECMO (VA-ECMO)

By following this technique and in cases in which urgent arterial cannulation is not necessary, CPR, our rate of arterial complications is lower than 5%.

ECMO Initiation

Once the cannulas are connected and secured to the ECMO circuit and air bubbles have been purged, we increase ECMO flows gradually to achieve the highest flow rates possible. Flow is defined by a negative pressure not > −100 mmHg in the drainage cannula to avoid endothelial injury and hemolysis. We set the oxygen delivery at 100%, and the sweep is set to match the flow rates 1:1. We carefully monitor the decrease of pCO2 to normal values over the next 24 h. Acute shifts in pCO_2 after ECMO initiation have been associated with brain injury. ECMO flows are adjusted to maintain a cardiac index greater than 2 L/m^2 and a mixed venous oxygen saturation >60%. When a patient is placed on VA-ECMO, we perform a transthoracic ECHO to define flows. ECMO flows are determined by evaluating right heart drainage and degree of left ventricular distention. In addition, inotropic support can be initiated to promote contractility. In cases where left ventricular distention and low contractility persist, the need for left ventricular venting is discussed.

As ECMO flows are optimized and if the patient is intubated, we initiate a lung-protective strategy using bi-level settings with a PEEP of 10, a peak airway pressure lower than 25 cmH_2O, and FiO_2 of 40% .

ECMO Weaning

We base our decision to wean from VV-ECMO on improving lung compliance, in the setting of an improving arterial pO_2 and decreasing sweep gas for CO_2 clearance. In most cases, decannulation from VV-ECMO can be accomplished at bedside with a purse string around the cannula insertion site and moderate compression of the area for 15 min.

Weaning from VA-ECMO in cases which ECMO was used as a bridge to recovery requires resolution or improvement of the pathology that triggered cannulation. For example, in cases of massive pulmonary embolism, emboli resolution is necessary before the patient can be weaned from ECMO. This is also the case in myocarditis, post-cardiectomy, ischemic myocardiopathy, or graft failure after transplant. In these cases contractility needs to be reestablished to the point that the patient's perfusion can be achieved without or with minimal ECMO and inotropic support. Improvement in pulsatility and right brachial artery waveform and improving ejection fraction evaluated by transthoracic ECHO (TTE) or transesophageal ECHO (TEE) are good indicators to define VA-ECMO weaning. Our ECHO studies include a stepwise approach of reducing VA-ECMO flows and simultaneously evaluating contractility.

The most simple method to remember how to approach weaning from ECMO is to remember that the goal to VV-ECMO is to wean sweep and in VA-ECMO is to wean flow. Weaning sweep in VA-ECMO can result in decreased oxygenation and end-organ dysfunction.

Ultrasound Imaging for the Surgical Intensivist

68

Charity H. Evans and Samuel Cemaj

Background

The use of ultrasound (US) in medicine dates back to 1942, the year Austrian psychiatrist and neurologist Dr. Karl Theodore Dussik published his work on US investigation of the brain [1]. US as a diagnostic tool was further developed in the 1940s and 1950s, with expanded use in radiology, gynecology, obstetrics, and echocardiography. With advancements in technology, US experienced further dissemination during the 1960s, 1970s, and 1980s into surgery and emergency medicine. By the 1990s, point-of-care US became a part of nearly every specialty's practice [2].

Point-of-care US (POCUS) differs from comprehensive US in its intent and use. POCUS is performed bedside by a clinician, employed to detect acute and often life-threatening conditions to facilitate treatment or to guide performance of an invasive procedure. It is quick and usually only focuses on a single or limited set of organs. Its clinical applications can be viewed as procedural guidance, diagnostics, monitoring, or resuscitation (see Fig. 68.1). Guidelines for the appropriate use of bedside ultrasound in the ICU have been set forth by the Society of Critical Care Medicine [3, 4]. By following evidence-based recommendations regarding the appropriate use of ultrasound in the ICU, clinicians can provide selected patients with effective and efficient care. POCUS has gained significant popularity in the intensive care unit (ICU) for a number of reasons. One, it is portable, allowing for bedside use. Two, results are quick, allowing for expedited decision making and patient care. Three, it is noninvasive with minimal risk, providing important information without radiation or contrast. Four, it is dynamic, allowing for monitoring of conditions over time.

Despite its clear benefits in the ICU, POCUS has its challenges and limitations related to clinician training, patient factors, and US equipment. Teaching a highly educated and specialized surgical critical care specialist to use a novel technique can be challenging. Published guidelines from the American Society of Echocardiography, the Society of Critical Care Medicine, and the American College of Chest Physicians suggest that training should include didactics, hands-on image acquisition, and interpretation with repetition. The number of practice exams and images obtained and interpreted required to achieve an acceptable skill level varies by exam [5, 6] and is outlined in Table 68.1. Furthermore, a competency-based approach to accreditation and maintenance of certification will ensure accuracy and safety. From a medicolegal standpoint, clinicians practicing POCUS in the ICU need to provide the expected standard of care. A structured certification program based on the guidelines mentioned will equip clinicians with the cognitive and procedural skills to perform US. However, a program should also document competence, which is the required endpoint for standard of practice [7].

Patient factors, including body habitus, positioning, and consequences of acute illness (i.e., pleural effusions, subcutaneous emphysema, anasarca, ascites) can limit bedside US studies. For example, US waves are attenuated by adipose tissue in the morbidly obese. Switching to a lower frequency probe will allow for deeper penetration but results in a lower-resolution image. Positioning in the left lateral decubitus allows for a better apical cardiac view; however, this may not be possible in a patient requiring flat bedrest. While US assists in identifying consequences of acute illness, these same conditions can limit the evaluation of other conditions.

Technical factors, including the US machine, probes, and settings, can be barriers to US application in the ICU. Some US machines are designed for point of care with preset applications. Others require setting manipulation. Regardless, the clinician must be familiar with basic operations, including entering the patient's information, selecting a probe and imaging mode, and adjusting the image depth and gain.

C. H. Evans (✉) · S. Cemaj
Department of Surgery, University of Nebraska Medical Center, Omaha, NE, USA
e-mail: charity.evans@unmc.edu

A. Salim et al. (eds.), *Surgical Critical Care Therapy*, https://doi.org/10.1007/978-3-319-71712-8_68

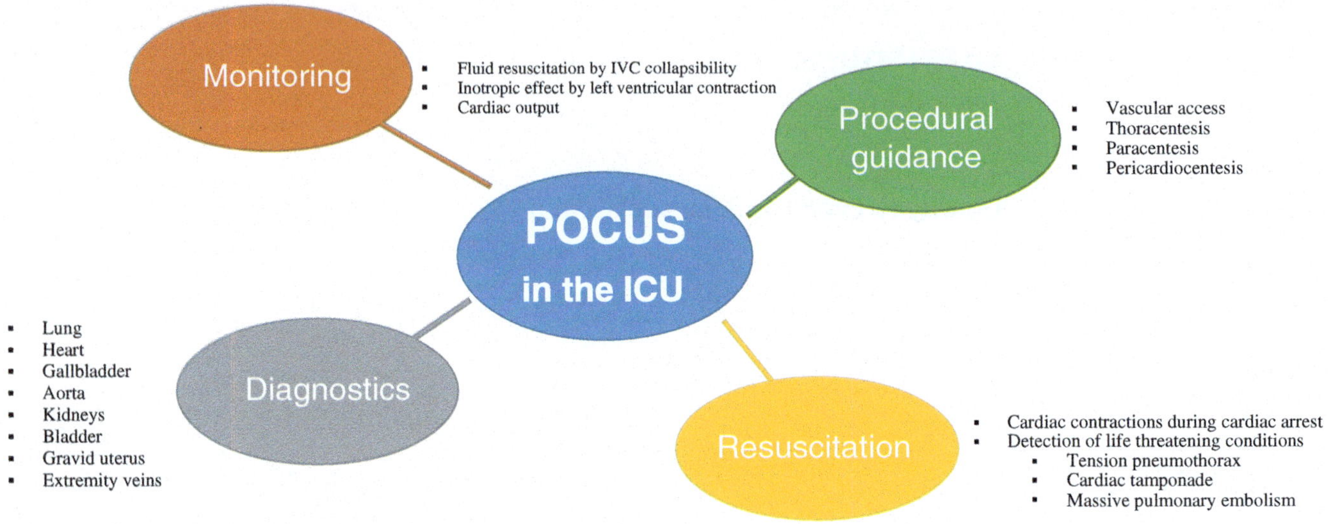

Fig. 68.1 Clinical applications of POCUS in the ICU

Getting Started

US uses sound waves, which are described by their frequency (number of repetitions per second, in hertz), wavelength (distance between waves, in decibels), and period (time it takes for one cycle to occur, in seconds). Sound waves are emitted by piezoelectric material in the US transducer. Mechanical properties of the piezoelectric material determine the range of sound waves frequencies produced, which is why different probes exist. The speed with which a sound wave moves through a medium is dependent upon the density and resistance of the medium. Furthermore, the path of the soundwave is altered as it passes through a medium with two or more interfaces, described as reflection, scattering, refraction, and attenuation. US images are created by sound waves reflected and scattered back to the transducer.

Choosing a probe is centered around maximizing resolution while maintaining adequate penetration. US waves with shorter wavelengths have higher frequency and produce higher-resolution images, with shallower penetration. US waves with longer wavelengths have lower frequency and produce lower-resolution images, with deeper penetration. US has three main probes: linear, phased array, and curvilinear (see Table 68.2).

Image acquisition is determined by the selected ultrasound mode. US has three main modes to choose from and that the operator should be familiar with: B-mode, M-mode, and Doppler mode. B-mode, or brightness, is the default of most machines and displays varying echogenicity of returning echoes as varying degrees of brightness. Anechoic structures appear black, as sound waves return without reflection (i.e., a fluid-filled cyst). Hypoechoic structures appear gray, as the structure reflects some soundwaves but less than the surrounding structures (i.e., soft tissue structures). Hyperechoic structures appear white, as all sound waves are reflected (i.e., calcified vessel wall). Images in B-mode are static. M-mode, or motion, analyzes movement of structures over time. M-mode utilizes a single axis beam emitted along a select line then gathers data on movement of all tissues along that line. This is useful when evaluating inferior vena cava (IVC) diameter during respiration for fluid status or lung-pleura interface for pneumothorax. Doppler mode evaluates the change in frequency of sound waves due to movement in the medium. For example, blood flowing toward the transducer shifts echoes to a higher frequency, whereas blood flowing away shifts echoes to a lower frequency. With spectral Doppler, the movement in the medium is plotted as velocity over time for a quantitative assessment of velocities as pulsed or continuous waves.

There are several common basic steps to starting any US study. These steps ensure a proper setup, which is key to a successful study. Spending a few extra minutes on setting up the ultrasound machine, correct probe selection, and proper patient positioning can produce significant overall time savings as well as enhancing the image quality and the diagnostic or therapeutic yield of the study. Several of the most important basic steps include:

1. Clean the US machine, keyboard, and transducers with a hospital-approved antiseptic wipe.
2. Inspect transducers to ensure no damage to probe or cables.
3. Position yourself on the patient's right side with the US machine directly in front of you. For cardiac US, some feel positioning yourself on the patient's left side allows for higher-quality images.
4. Select the most appropriate probe for your study.
5. Plug in the US machine to a wall electrical outlet, and turn it on.
6. Enter the patient's name, weight, height, and medical record number, and select exam type.

Table 68.1 Number of practice exams and images obtained and interpreted required to achieve an acceptable skill level by exam [5, 6]

Modality	#	Expected standard of care
Core applications: Basic echocardiography, pleural study, lung study, guidance of vascular access, and identification of free abdominal fluid		
Basic echocardiography	30	Global LV size and systolic function
		LV contraction pattern
		Global RV size and systolic function
		Assessment for pericardial fluid/tamponade
		IVC size and respiratory variation
		Basic color Doppler assessment for severe valvular regurgitation
Pleural study	20	Identify hypoechoic or echo-free space surrounded by anatomic boundaries: Diaphragm, chest wall, ribs, visceral pleura, normal/consolidated/atelectatic lung
		Identify liver and ascites, spleen, kidney, heart, pericardium and pericardial effusion, spinal column, aorta, IVC
		Identify characteristic dynamic findings of pleural fluid (i.e., diaphragmatic motion, floating lung, dynamic fluid motion, changes with respiration)
		Characterize fluid: Anechoic, echogenicity, homogeneous or heterogeneous, presence of strands/debris/ septations
		Identify other findings (i.e., pleural masses or thickening)
		Perform assessment of fluid volume
		Recognize specific limitations of US to identify pleural fluid
Lung study	20	Knowledge of the basic semiology of lung US: A-lines, B-lines, sliding lung, lung point
		Identify and characterize consolidated lung
		Identify and characterize air artifacts suggestive of the normal aeration pattern: A- lines with sliding lung
		Identify and characterize air artifacts suggestive of alveolar interstitial pattern: Number and location of B-lines
		Knowledge of the limitations of not visualizing lung sliding/B lines
		Identify and characterize air artifacts to rule out pneumothorax: Presence of sliding lung, presence of B-lines
		Identify and characterize findings that rule in pneumothorax: Presence of lung point (both by 2D imaging and M-mode)
Guidance of vascular access	10	Identify relevant veins and arteries: Internal jugular, carotid, subclavian, axillary, brachial, radial, femoral, and peripheral veins such as basilic, cephalic, external jugular
		Differentiate vein from artery based on anatomic position, compressibility, changes with respiration
		Identify normal anatomic variability (i.e., vascular hypoplasia, variability of carotid artery position relative to internal jugular)
		Identify vascular thrombosis by direct visualization or by compression study
		Identify adjacent nonvenous structures (i.e., sternocleidomastoid muscle, mass, lymph node)
		Knowledge of the effects of patient positioning on anatomic topography: Head/lower extremity rotation effects on overlap of the artery by the vein, effects of Trendelenburg position on vascular distention
Identification of free abdominal fluid	10	Assess for intraperitoneal fluid
		Identify echo-free space surrounded by typical anatomic boundaries: Abdominal wall, diaphragm, liver, gallbladder, spleen, kidney, bladder, bowel, uterus, spinal column, aorta, IVC
		Identify abdominal wall, diaphragm, liver, gallbladder, spleen, kidney, bladder, bowel, uterus, spinal column, aorta, IVC
		Identify characteristic dynamic findings of intraperitoneal fluid, such as diaphragmatic motion, floating bowel, bowel peristalsis, dynamic fluid motion, and respirophasic shape change, compressibility
		Characterize fluid: Anechoic, echogenicity, homogeneous or heterogeneous, presence of strands/debris/ septations
		Qualitative assessment of intraperitoneal fluid volume
		Recognize specific limitations of US to identify intraperitoneal fluid such as inadequate image quality due to technical limitations, hemoperitoneum, echo-dense purulent fluid

Table 68.2 Characteristics of US probes

Probe		Frequency	Wavelength	Depth	Resolution	Application
Linear	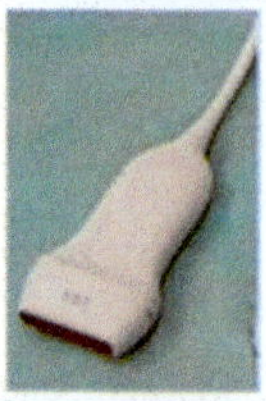	5–10 MHz	Shorter	Superficial, less than 9 cm	Best in axial and lateral dimensions	Muscles, nerves, joints Arteries/veins, US-guided procedures
Phased-array	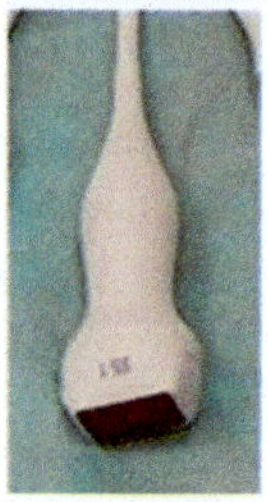	4–7 MHz	Long	Deep, up to 35 cm	Ideal for moving structures with phasing, allowing for velocity measurements	Cardiac Thoracic including pleura Inferior vena cava
Curvilinear	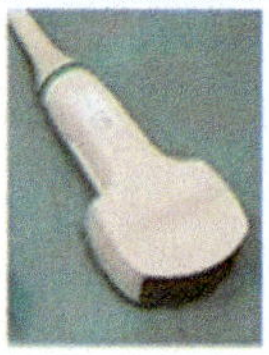	2–5 MHz	Longer	Deeper, 5 cm up to 30 cm	Broader beam images larger volume of structure	Gallbladder, liver, kidney bladder, aorta Abdominal free fluid

7. Position the patient. With most studies, the patient will be supine. However, many cardiac views are best obtained with the patient in left lateral decubitus. Posterior thoracic views may be best obtained with the patient in the seated position.
8. If doing an echocardiogram, place EKG electrodes so that cardiac velocities are timed with the cardiac cycle.
9. Ensure patient privacy. Dim the overhead lights.
10. Orient transducer to screen. Transducer should be held like a pencil, with the thumb, index, and middle finger, with the fourth and fifth fingers resting on the patient for stabilization. The transducer has a long notch on one side, which corresponds to the left side of the screen.
11. Apply gel to transducer. Use a sterile transducer cover, if doing an US-guided procedure.
12. Adjust depth to ensure structure of interest is in the center of the screen. Start a greatest depth to see surrounding structures, then reduce depth to center the area of interest.
13. Adjust gain so that fluid appears black and solid tissues appear gray to white. Increased gain results in a brighter image, whereas decreased gain results in a darker image. As depth is increased, gain must also be adjusted.
14. Review the measurement and calculation capabilities of your US machine before obtaining the needed images. Some calculations are programmed in the software (i.e., bladder volume, cardiac output), whereas others requires some manipulation (i.e., measurement of peak velocities using Doppler mode).
15. Save images in the machine's internal memory, and then download to include in the patient's chart for both documentation and billing.

Basic Echocardiography

The ACCP/SRLF Statement of Competence[5] defines basic echocardiography in the ICU with transthoracic echocardiography (TTE) as acquisition of five views: the parasternal long- and short-axis views, the apical four-chamber view, the subcostal long-axis four-chamber view, and the inferior vena cava (IVC) longitudinal view. The ACCP/SRLF Statement of Competence also provides key cognitive skills in image interpretation of basic echocardiography in the ICU (see Table 68.2). Basic echocardiography is a standard tool in the assessment of a patient with hemodynamic instability. Echo allows for identification of life-threatening conditions, categorization of shock state, and selection of initial therapies, responses to therapies, and identification of coexisting diagnosis (see Table 68.1 – Basic Echocardiography and Table 68.3)

Parasternal Long-Axis View (PLAX) (Fig. 68.2)

1. Patient should be positioned supine, in the left tilt or left lateral decubitus position, if possible.
2. Place the phased-array transducer to the left of the sternum in the third or fourth (images can be attained anywhere from second to fifth, slide transducer up or down as needed for best image) intercostal space.
3. With the transducer notch pointed to the patient's right shoulder, images are sectioned through the long axis of the heart, with the aortic valve (AV) and mitral valve (MV) clearly visualized and positioned just to right of

Table 68.3 Competence in basic echocardiography: required cognitive skills in recognition of clinical conditions

Severe hypovolemia	Small, hyperdynamic ventricles, small IVC with wide respiratory variations
LV failure	Global LV systolic dysfunction, heterogeneous contractility pattern suggestive of myocardial ischemia LV cavity dilatation suggestive of chronic cardiac disease
RV failure	Acute cor pulmonale; RV dilatation and paradoxical septal motion, isolated RV dilatation suggestive of RV infarct, associated findings; dilated, noncollapsible IVC
Tamponade	Pericardial effusion (regardless of size), right atrial/RV diastolic collapse, associated findings: Dilated, noncollapsible IVC
Acute massive left-sided valvular regurgitation	Normal LV cavity size (acute valvulopathy), normal/hyperdynamic LV systolic function (LV volume overload), massive color Doppler regurgitant flow
Circulatory arrest	
During resuscitation	Tamponade or acute cor pulmonale LV systolic function global LV systolic dysfunction
After successful	Heterogeneous contractility pattern suggestive of myocardial ischemia

center of the screen. The apical portion of the heart will be to the left and base to the right of screen and right ventricle (RV) seen anteriorly.
4. Tilt transducer until base comes into view, then slightly rotate transducer to see LV to fullest extent.
5. Tilt the tail of the transducer toward the left shoulder to view the right atrium (RA), tricuspid valve (TV), and RV. The right ventricular outflow tract (RVOT) and chest wall will appear at the top of the screen.

Structures imaged	Echocardiographic findings
RV, AV, MV, LA, RVOT, LVOT, root of aorta, portions of ascending and descending aorta, anterior and posterior pericardium The anteroseptal and inferolateral walls of the left ventricle (LV) Color Doppler can be used to view the interventricular septum, AV, and MV	Qualitative assessment of ejection fraction (EF) RVOT/LV wall thickness, size, and function LV segmental wall functions Septal kinetics LA chamber size Evaluation of AV/MV anatomy with color Doppler, descending aorta, and pericardial space

Parasternal Short-Axis View (PSAX) (Fig. 68.3)

1. From the parasternal long-axis view, the probe is turned clockwise 90 degrees toward the right shoulder until the short axis is obtained with the transducer index mark pointing toward the left shoulder.
2. The image seen is at the midventricular tomographic plane at the level of the papillary muscle.

Structures imaged	Echocardiographic findings
RVOT, AV, LV, TV, PV The anteroseptal and inferolateral walls of the left ventricle (LV) Pulse-wave Doppler can be used to measure Doppler velocity at the RVOT Continuous wave Doppler can be used to assess TV and PV regurgitation	Qualitative assessment of ejection fraction EF RV/LV wall thickness, chamber size, and function LV segmental wall function Septal kinetics Pericardial space

Apical Four-Chamber View (A4C) (Fig. 68.4)

1. Ideally, patient is in the left lateral decubitus position.
2. Place probe inferolaterally to the nipple at the point of maximal heart impulse with transducer index mark pointing 3–4 o'clock position.
3. The septum will be oriented vertically in center of screen, with the LV in orthogonal view, showing the inferoseptal and anterolateral walls, MV, and TV.
4. View allows for qualitative assessment of LV systolic function (endocardial excursion, myocardial thickening, and septal motion of anterior leaflet of MV) as normal, reduced, or severely reduced.

Structures imaged	Echocardiographic findings
LV, RV, LA, RA, TV Pericardial space Continuous wave Doppler can be used to assess TV and MV anatomy	Qualitative assessment of ejection fraction EF RV/LV wall thickness, chamber size, and function LV segmental wall function Septal kinetics RA and LA chamber size

Apical Five-Chamber View (A5C)

1. From the A4C view, tilt the tail of the probe down toward the patient's left hip.
2. View shows LV outflow tract (LVOT), allowing for measurement of velocity time interval (VTI) and stroke volume using pulse-wave Doppler.

Subcostal Long-Axis Four-Chamber View (S4C)

1. Ideally, patient is in the supine position.
2. Place probe just inferior to the xiphoid process with transducer index mark pointing 3 o'clock position.
3. With the liver in the background, all four chambers are seen in the tomographic plane sectioning the heart from right to left. The right-sided structures will be closest to the liver.
4. View allows for assessment of pericardial effusion, specifically adjacent to RV and RA, and ideal to assess diastolic chamber collapse in cardiac tamponade.

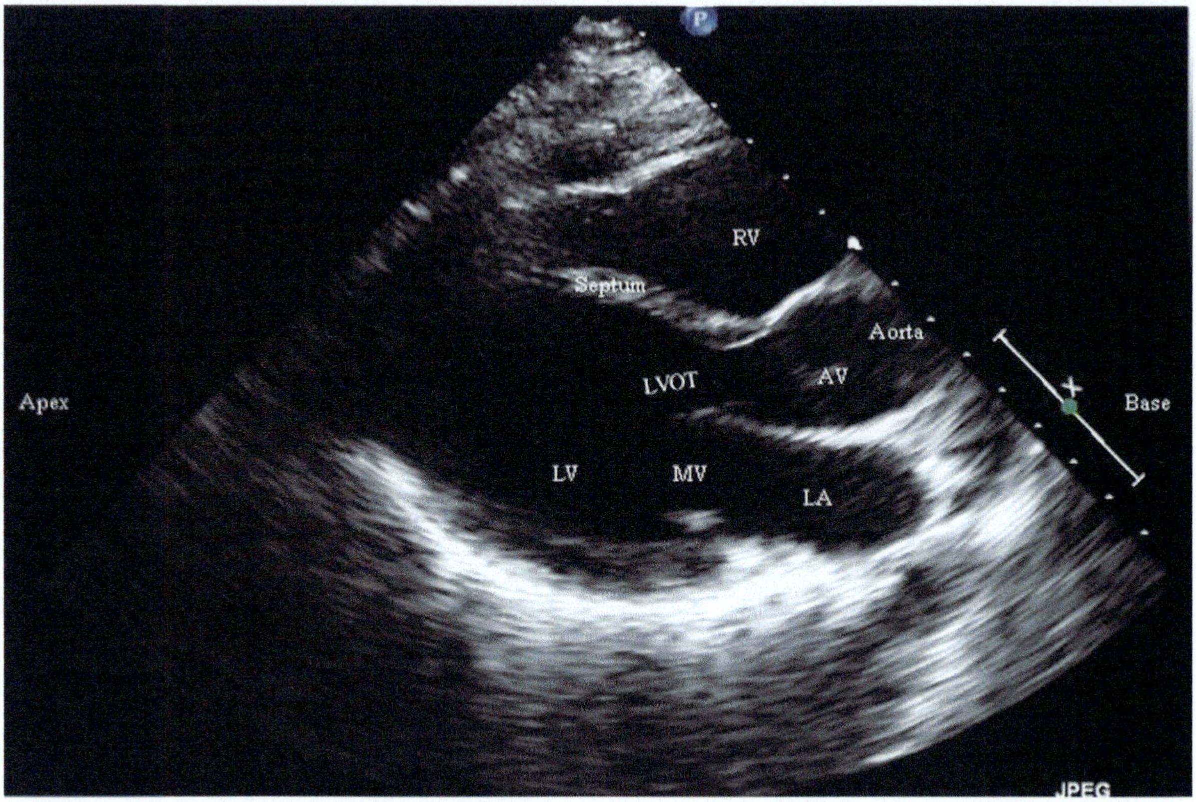

Fig. 68.2 Parasternal long-axis view shown at the end of diastole

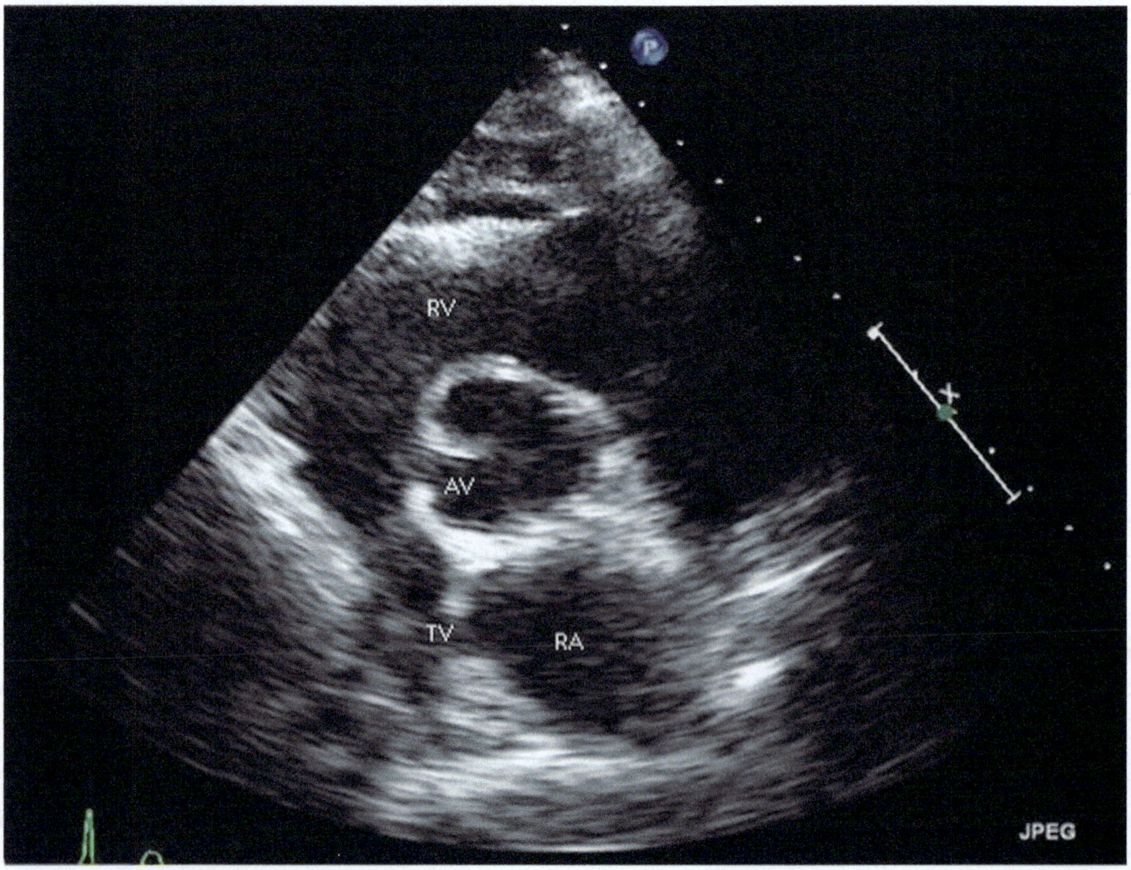

Fig. 68.3 Parasternal short-axis view at the mitral valve level at the end of diastole

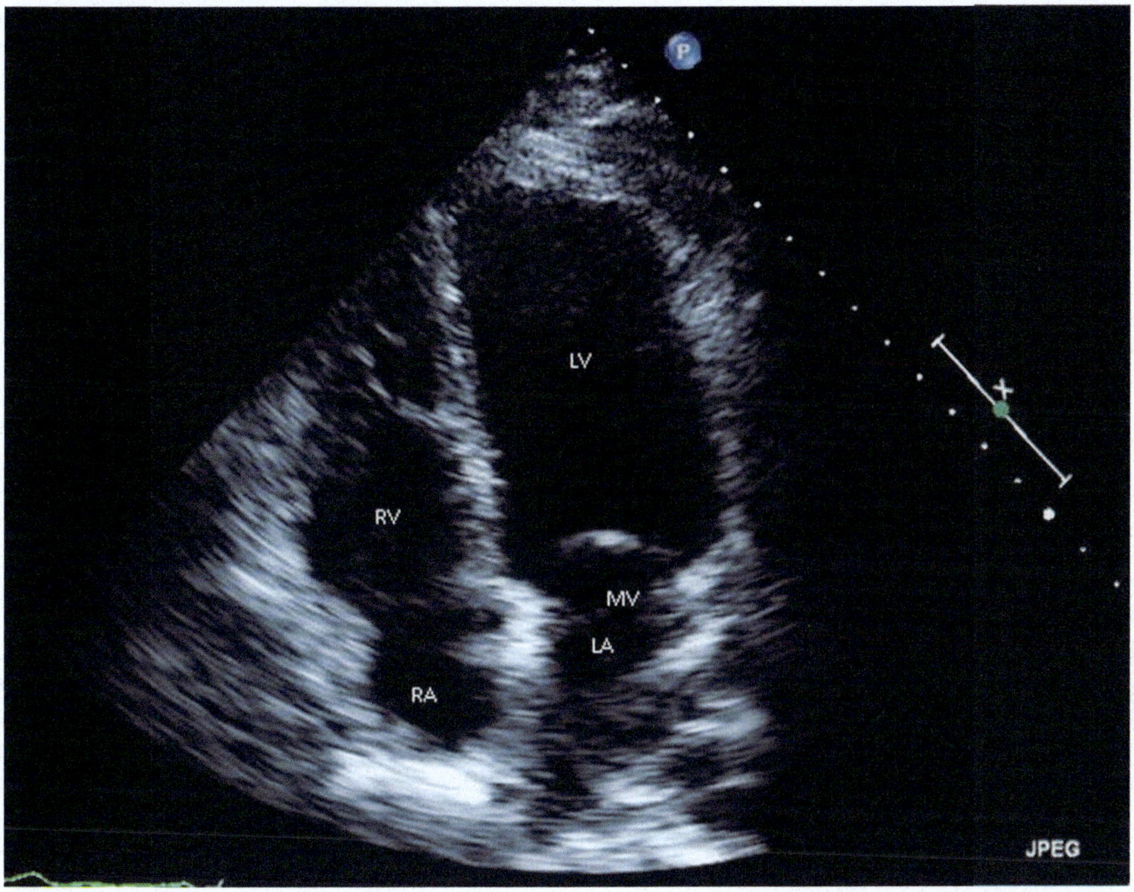

Fig. 68.4 Apical four-chamber view

Structures imaged	Echocardiographic findings
LV, RV, LA, RA, pericardium, interatrial septum Continuous wave Doppler can be used to assess TV and MV anatomy and regurgitation	Qualitative assessment of ejection fraction EF RV/LV wall thickness, chamber size, and function LV segmental wall function Septal kinetics Pericardial space

Structures imaged	Echocardiographic findings
Liver, IVC, hepatic veins, RA, diaphragm Pulse-wave Doppler can be used to confirm IVC versus aorta M-mode can be used to check for IVC collapsibility	Assessment of IVC diameter Assessment of volume responsiveness Assessment of IVC diameter and collapsibility and central venous pressure

Subcostal IVC Longitudinal View

1. Ideally, patient is in the supine position.
2. Place probe just inferior to the xiphoid process with transducer index mark pointing at the 3 o'clock position.
3. Rotate transducer 90 degrees counterclockwise to point transducer index mark cephalad, and then tilt transducer to aim US beam posteriorly.
4. Slight adjustments may be required to center the RA-IVC junction on screen. Ideally, one will see the hepatic vein emptying into the IVC and IVC draining into the RA to avoid mistaking the aorta for the IVC.
5. Cross section of IVC's maximal diameter is measured just distal to the hepatic vein-IVC junction or 2 cm from the IVC-RA junction.

Assessment of RV Strain Secondary to Pulmonary Embolism Using US

RV strain, as seen in large pulmonary emboli, can be difficult to view on basic echocardiography. Yet US can be a fast, noninvasive, diagnostic study in an unstable patient suspected of having a pulmonary embolism. Obtaining adequate views of the RV, PV, and parts of the pulmonary artery allows one to assess for RV strain related to a large pulmonary embolism.

1. Obtain parasternal long-axis view, as above.
2. In PLAX, achieve a view of the RV, PV, and part of the pulmonary artery.
3. Signs consistent with right heart strain related to a pulmonary embolism:

(a) Pulmonary artery dilatation
(b) RV strain
(c) RV dilatation with free wall hypokinesis
(d) Clot in transit on PA (rarely seen)
(e) McConnell's sign: hyperdynamic motion of RV apex with akinesis of RV wall
(f) Paradoxic septal movement (appears "D" shaped), better seen in parasternal short-axis view [8, 9]

Assessment of Cardiac Output Using US

1. Obtain apical five-chamber view, as above.
2. In PLAX, freeze image in systole.
3. Measure diameter of LVOT.
4. Switch to A5C in M-mode.
5. Trace LVOT VTI (cone-shaped cylinder representing stroke volume (SV), where the base is formed by the LVOT).
6. US machine is set to calculate VTI.
7. Calculate SV = 3.14 × (LVOT diameter/2)2 × LVOT VTI (mL).
8. Calculate CO = heart rate × SV (L/min).
9. Note: LVOT VTI may not be accurate when cardiac rhythm is irregular.

Assessment of Systolic Function Using US

US in the ICU provides clinically useful information that may alter the plan of care. US is noninvasive and can be repeated as often as necessary to reevaluate a critically ill patient. This is especially useful after a fluid challenge or initiation of an inotropic agent. Two alternatives for a quick assessment and calculation of the systolic function are the fractional shortening of the LV and the E-point septal separation.

Fractional Shortening of the Left Ventricle

1. Obtain parasternal short-axis view, as above. Switch to M-mode.
2. Measure the LV just beyond the tips of the mitral leaflets at the end of systole and diastole, where FS = EDD-ESD/EDD × 00 (EDD = end diastolic diameter of LV, and ESD = end diastolic diameter).
3. FS is a basic estimate of LV global function, where normal is 25–45%0.2

E-Point Septal Separation

1. Obtain parasternal long-axis view, as above. Switch to M-mode.
2. During diastole, observe the tip of the anterior mitral leaflet.
3. As diastolic dysfunction progresses and the LV contracts less, the distance between the tip of the anterior leaflet of the MV increases toward the LV septum.
4. Normal <7 mm, abnormal >10 mm [10].

The measurement of IVC diameter and its collapsibility and distensibility gives the clinician additional information about a patient's volume status. When measured during the respiratory cycle, this information can be used to infer fluid responsiveness and central venous pressure (CVP).

Assessment of Inferior Vena Cava (IVC) Diameter

1. Obtain subcostal IVC longitudinal view, as above.
2. Freeze image of IVC at largest diameter.
3. Use calipers to measure diameter perpendicular to the long axis of the vein approximately 2 cm from the RA-IVC junction.
4. IVC is normally 1.5–2.5 cm in diameter, such that:

IVC diameter	Clinical inference
<1 cm in trauma	Hemorrhagic shock, requiring transfusion
<1.5 cm	Volume depletion
>2.5 cm	Volume overload

Assessment of Volume Responsiveness

1. Switch to M-mode.
2. Measure IVC diameter at largest diameter (end expiration) and at smallest diameter (end inspiration).
3. Freeze image of IVC at largest diameter (end expiration) and at smallest diameter (end inspiration).
4. Use calipers to measure diameter perpendicular to the long axis of the venin approximately 2 cm from the RA-IVC junction.
5. Measurements should be taken in an identical manner.
6. Calculate IVC distensibility index = IVCmax − IVCmin /IVCmin.
7. IVC distention of at least 18% is predictive of fluid responsiveness, and patient is likely to benefit from a fluid bolus.

Assessment of IVC Diameter and Collapsibility and Central Venous Pressure

1. Switch to M-mode.
2. Measure IVC diameter at end inspiration and end expiration or before and after a "sniff."

3. Calculate IVC collapsibility = IVCmax − IVCmin/IVCmax * 100.
4. Change with respiration or "sniff" estimates RA pressure, such that:

IVC diameter and % collapse	Estimated CVP (mmHg)
Normal: ≤1.5 cm and >50%	0–5
Intermediate: 1.5–2.5 cm and >50%	5–10
High: >2.5 cm and <50%	10–20

Relation between IVC/RA junction and central venous pressure (CVP) (*Adapted from Jones Handbook of Ultrasound in Trauma and Critical Care Illness, 2003*)

Pericardiocentesis

Pericardial tamponade is an emergency requiring rapid diagnosis and treatment. Clinical signs such as hypotension, jugular venous distention, muted heart sounds, chest pain, tachypnea, and dyspnea suggest a hemodynamically significant cardiac effusion and should prompt a sonographic investigation. The subcostal long-axis four-chamber view is most commonly used for diagnosis of pericardial tamponade. US findings seen in pericardial tamponade include a circumferential pericardial effusion, RA systolic and diastolic collapse, increase in RV volume with inspiration, and decrease in RV volume with expiration. Pericardial drainage is indicated for effusions >20 mm by US. The use of US in pericardiocentesis increases procedural success rate and decreases complications.

1. Obtain the subcostal long-axis four-chamber view, as above.
2. Identify location of largest fluid collection.
3. Insert a long 16- or 18-gauge needle between the xiphoid process and left costal margin at a shallow angle with the needle aimed toward the left shoulder while aspirating, under direct US guidance.
4. Once pericardium is entered, proceed with one-time drainage.
5. Before placement of a pigtail catheter over a guidewire, ensure that the needle is in the pericardial space by injecting agitated saline and visualizing turbulent flow within the pericardial space on US.

Thoracentesis

The use of US during thoracentesis improves overall success and decreases the risk for complications. Thoracentesis is indicated in new pleural effusions not related to heart failure or other determined diagnosis. In heart failure, a thoracentesis should be considered when bilateral effusions are of different sizes, pleurisy, fever or signs of infection, absence of other signs of heart failure (i.e., cardiomegaly, echo findings, low B-type brain natriuretic peptide), or effusion that does not resolve with effective heart failure therapy.

1. Patient in sitting position, with arms resting on a surface (i.e., bedside table). Thoracentesis can be done with the patient in the lying position if US identifies a safe needle insertion site.
2. Place the phased-array transducer along the back (at least 6 cm from the spinous processes) at the level of the diaphragm with the index mark pointing cephalad and corresponding screen indicator on the upper left side of the image.
3. Identify the diaphragm, liver or spleen, and lung. Pleural fluid should be visible (will appear black and without stippling) adjacent to the parietal pleura with sufficient distance from the diaphragm and lung throughout the respiratory cycle.
4. Mark the access site on the skin.
5. Measure distance between skin surface and parietal and visceral pleura to estimate depth of needle penetration required (a minimum pleural effusion depth of 1.5 cm is recommended to safely perform this procedure).
6. Advance needle on a syringe over top of the rib while aspirating until return of pleural fluid.
7. Withdraw fluid into syringe for sample.
8. If placing a pigtail catheter:
   (a) Remove syringe and pass wire through needle just enough to clear end of needle.
   (b) Remove needle.
   (c) Use scalpel to make a small incision in the skin where wire enters.
   (d) Pass dilator over wire and into pleural space, and then remove dilator.
   (e) Insert trocar into pigtail catheter, and pass pigtail catheter on trocar over wire, ensuring that last side hole is within the pleural space.
   (f) Remove trocar and guide wire, leaving pigtail catheter in place.
   (g) Suture pigtail catheter to chest wall.
   (h) Attach to Heimlich flutter valve or chest drainage system container.
9. Document lung sliding before and after procedure to exclude post-procedure pneumothorax.

Paracentesis

The use of US during paracentesis also improves overall success and decreases the risk for complications. Indications for paracentesis include new ascites or evaluation of new symptoms in patients with known ascites and therapeutic relief of abdominal distention related to ascites.

1. The bladder should be emptied by voiding or insertion of catheter to prevent bladder injury.
2. Patient in supine position with head of bed elevated to 30–45 degrees so ascites pools in the bilateral lower quadrants.
3. Place the phased-array transducer along the lower abdomen in a longitudinal plane with the transducer index mark pointing cephalad.
4. Scan lateral to the rectus abdominis muscles to localize largest collection of fluid (if only small amount of fluid is viewed, paracentesis cannot be safely completed).
5. Use color-flow Doppler mode to ensure insertion site is not over the inferior epigastric, subcostal, circumflex iliac arteries and veins, and thoracoepigastric veins.
6. Mark site and anesthesize skin and subcutaneous tract to peritoneum under direct visualization.
7. Advance large bore needle on a syringe under real ultrasound guidance through the abdominal wall into peritoneal cavity while aspirating.
8. Complete diagnostic aspiration or therapeutic drainage.

POCUS is performed bedside by a clinician, employed to detect acute and often life-threatening conditions to facilitate treatment or to guide performance of an invasive procedure. It is portable, results are quick, noninvasive with minimal risk, and it is dynamic. There are basic steps to starting any US study, ensuring a proper setup and successful study. Basic echocardiography in the ICU with transthoracic echocardiography (TTE) as acquisition of five views: the parasternal long- and short-axis views, apical four-chamber view, subcostal long-axis four-chamber view, and inferior vena cava (IVC) longitudinal view. An apical five-chamber view is necessary to calculate VTI, SV, and CO and should be considered in the evaluation of a hemodynamically unstable patient. RV strain, as seen in large pulmonary emboli, can be evaluated using POCUS. CO and systolic function can be calculated using select images obtained during POCUS. The measurement of IVC diameter and its collapsibility and distensibility gives the clinician additional information about a patient's volume status. When measured during the respiratory cycle, this information can be used to infer fluid responsiveness and CVP. The addition of US-guided imaging to procedures, such as pericardiocentesis, thoracentesis, and paracentesis, increases procedural success rate and decreases complications. POCUS has its challenges and limitations related to clinician training, patient factors, and US equipment. Yet, its benefits outweigh these challenges, advocating POCUS as a near gold standard in the ICU.

Conclusions

The past decade has seen an explosion in the utilization of ultrasound imaging and the migration of this technology to a multitude of medical and surgical specialties. The portability, size, image quality, and assistive ultrasound software have improved to the point where POCUS can literally be used in applications from the head to toes of any patient. In the intensive care setting, having a rapid and reliable imaging technology that can provide real-time patient assessment, diagnosis, and procedural guidance is an incredible force multiplier for the ICU care team. In addition, the excellent safety profile and noninvasive nature of ultrasound imaging provides additional benefits over many standard radiologic imaging modalities and more invasive monitoring devices. Ultrasound is becoming increasingly integrated into many residency training programs and critical care fellowships, and we anticipate that ultrasound proficiency will soon be an absolute requirement for any board-certified intensivist. Fortunately, the ability to perform most of the bedside assessments and procedural guidance studies outlined in this chapter can be obtained by any interested provider who is willing to invest time and effort into initial training. Once the basic ultrasound skillsets are acquired, continued frequent use and evaluation through a thorough quality assurance program are key components of maintaining this skillset and improving over time. Future generations of ultrasound hardware and software will undoubtedly continue to foster the expansion of this technology to new applications and to enhance the ease and reliability of current applications in the ICU setting.

References

1. Dussik KT. Uber die moglichkeit hochfrequente mechanische schwingungen als diagnostisches hilfsmittel zu verwerten. Zeitschrift für die gesamte Neurologie und Psychiatrie. 1942;174(1):153–68.
2. Levitov A, Mayo P, Slonim A. Critical care ultrasound. 2nd ed. New York: McGraw Hill; 2014.
3. Frankel H, Kirkpatrick A, Elbarbary M, et al. Guidelines for the appropriate use of bedside general and cardiac ultrasonography in the evaluation of critically ill patients part I: general ultrasonography. Crit Care Med. 2015;43(11):2479–502.
4. Levitov A, Frankel H, Blaivas M, et al. Guidelines for the appropriate use of bedside general and cardiac ultrasonography in the evaluation of critically ill patients part II: cardiac ultrasonography. Crit Care Med. 2016;44(6):1206–27.
5. Mayo P, Beaulieu Y, Doelken P, et al. American College of Chest Physicians/La Société de Réanimation de Langue Française Statement on Competence in Critical Care Ultrasonography*. Chest. 2009;135:1050–60.
6. Mayo P, Vieillard-Baron A. International consensus statement on training standards for advanced critical care echocardiography. Intensive Care Med. 2014;40(5):654–66.
7. Huang SJ, McLean AS. Do we need a critical care ultrasound certification program? Implications from an Australian medical-legal perspective. Crit Care. 2010;14:313.
8. McConnell MV, Solomon SD, Rayan ME, Come PC, Goldhaber SZ, Lee RT. Regional right ventricular dysfunction detected by echocardiography in acute pulmonary embolism. Am J Cardiol. 1996;78:469–73.
9. Goldhaber S. Echocardiography in the management of pulmonary embolism. Ann Intern Med. 2002;136:691–700.
10. Perera PH, et al. Cardiac echocardiography. Crit Care Clin. 2014;30:47–92.

Intra-aortic Balloon Pump

69

Daniel Dante Yeh

Introduction

In the twenty-first century, there are several mechanical options for the support of a failing heart. One of the oldest methods is intra-aortic balloon pump (IABP), also known as "counterpulsation." The term "counterpulsation" refers to volume displacement of aortic blood proximally into the coronary arteries and distally into the aorta, occurring out of phase from the normal cardiac cycle [1–4]. Despite the proliferation of other options, IABP remains the most common assist device for several reasons: it is minimally invasive, does not require extracorporeal handling of blood, causes minimal hemolysis, and can be inserted in multiple settings (catheterization lab, operating room, intensive care unit, etc.) by both surgeons and interventional cardiologists [3, 5]. Each year, there are approximately 200,000 IABP insertions worldwide [6].

Although animal studies date back to the 1950s [2, 7], the first description of use of an intra-aortic balloon pump in human patients appeared in 1968 when Kantrowitz et al. reported their clinical experience with IABP in two patients with cardiogenic shock [8]. The IABP, inserted via surgical cutdown on the femoral artery, favorably improved the systemic arterial pressure and urine output. The technique of percutaneous insertion was not described until 1980 [9], though it is now, by far, the most common insertion method [2, 10]. This chapter will review the indications for IABP counterpulsation, describe the physiologic mechanisms supporting its use, describe the technique of insertion as well as potential complications, and finally describe the outcomes reported by clinical trials.

D. D. Yeh (✉)
Department of Surgery, Ryder Trauma Center, Miami, FL, USA
e-mail: dxy154@miami.edu

Indications and Contraindications

Indications

IABP has been described for use in a variety of scenarios, some with stronger supporting evidence than others (Table 69.1). Common FDA-approved indications include cardiogenic shock or mechanical complications of acute myocardial infarction (AMI) and weaning from cardiopulmonary bypass (CPB), while less common indications include prophylaxis for "high-risk" patients, refractory unstable angina, acute right ventricular support, acute mitral valve regurgitation, congestive heart failure secondary to cardiomyopathy, myocardial depression secondary to septic shock, intractable ventricular arrhythmias, mechanical bridge to other alternative assist devices or transplantation, posttransplantation support, and heart transplant rejection [3, 10–12].

Acute Myocardial Infarction (AMI) Without Cardiogenic Shock

Although animal studies have reported decreased infarct size and more salvaged myocardium when IABP has been used prior to reperfusion [13–15], human studies have not been able to translate this into improved clinical outcomes. While earlier studies (predating the era of routine percutaneous coronary intervention [PCI]) did suggest better outcomes [16, 17], more contemporary studies did not report benefits of IABP combined with PCI compared to PCI alone in patients without cardiogenic shock [18, 19]. The Counterpulsation to Reduce Infarct Size Pre-PCI Acute Myocardial Infarction (CRISP AMI) enrolled 337 patients (30 sites, 9 countries) with acute anterior STEMI without cardiogenic shock. Infarct size, as measured by cardiac magnetic resonance imaging 3–5 days after revascularization, was not significantly different between groups, nor were there any differences in secondary endpoints such as all-cause mortality at 6 months [18]. Furthermore, a *post hoc* analysis demonstrated a nonsignificant trend toward larger

A. Salim et al. (eds.), *Surgical Critical Care Therapy*, https://doi.org/10.1007/978-3-319-71712-8_69

Table 69.1 Indications and contraindications for intra-aortic balloon pump

Indications	Contraindications
AMI with cardiogenic shock	Aortic valve regurgitation
Mechanical complication of AMI	Aortic dissection
Weaning from CPB	Aortic aneurysm
Prophylactic for "high-risk" PCI	Poor neurologic outcome expected
Prophylactic for "high-risk" CABG	Severe PVD
Refractory unstable angina	Active bleeding
Intractable ventricular arrhythmia	Uncontrolled coagulopathy
Mechanical bridge to heart transplantation	
Posttransplantation support	
Heart transplant rejection	
Acute RV support	
Acute mitral regurgitation	
Congestive heart failure	
Myocardial depression secondary to septic shock	

AMI acute myocardial infarction, *CABG* coronary artery bypass graft, *CPB* cardiopulmonary bypass, *PCI* percutaneous coronary intervention, *PVD* peripheral vascular disease, *RV* right ventricle

infarct size in patients randomized to IABP (p = 0.06). At this time, routine IABP is **not recommended** in acute myocardial infarction without cardiogenic shock [20].

AMI with Cardiogenic Shock

Hemodynamic support during or after PCI is one of the most common indications for IABP insertion in contemporary practice [12]. The evidence supporting this indication is mixed, though likely due to methodological concerns. The TACTICS study (n = 57) did not demonstrate any benefit in all-cause mortality, though subgroup analysis suggested that patients in the most severe shock may potentially benefit [21]. Another small randomized trial (n = 40), the IABP SHOCK trial, did not show any improvement in APACHE II score or hemodynamic parameters compared to medical therapy alone [22]. Importantly, the IABP was inserted after thrombolysis in both the TACTICS and SHOCK studies. The IABP-SHOCK II trial was the largest randomized controlled trial, enrolling 600 subjects with cardiogenic shock complicating acute MI [23]. At 30 days, there was no significant difference in 30-day all-cause mortality between those randomized to IABP and those for whom IABP was not initially offered. Similarly, there was no improvement in 12-month survival [24].

Several criticisms of this study deserve mention. First, the study population was relatively low risk (mild degrees of shock), and about one-third of the enrolled subjects had non-STEMI. Patients with mechanical complications of MI were excluded [1]. Second, there was a relatively high rate of crossover (10%) from the control arm and increased use of ventricular assist devices in the control group. This may have diluted any signal of treatment benefit. Third, when considering the average recruitment across the sites, there was only a mean annual IABP insertion rate of 1.7 per center. This may have influenced the outcomes, as lower insertion rate is associated with worse outcomes [25]. Fourth, timing of IABP insertion was left to clinician discretion, and nearly 90% of the IABP insertions occurred *after* revascularization. There is controversy regarding whether the IABP should be inserted before or after PCI. Proponents of pre-procedural counterpulsation argue that the IABP can provide invaluable assistance during the procedure, decreasing the amount of inotropic support required. For example, one retrospective study reported significantly decreased in-hospital mortality and overall incidence of major adverse cardiac and cerebrovascular events (MACCE) associated with IABP inserted before PCI as compared to after PCI [26]. Contrarily, supporters of post-procedural counterpulsation argue that placing an IABP may lead to worse outcomes by delaying reperfusion [20]. In a nonrandomized study, Cheng et al. reported higher levels of peak creatine kinase concentrations in patients receiving IABP before PCI in patients with cardiogenic shock, possibly indicating larger infarct size [27]. Finally, nearly 40% of patients underwent induced hypothermia after revascularization, which portends a poor outcome regardless of the use of IABP.

The IABP-SHOCK II trial did not report any harm associated with IABP, and the benefit of counterpulsation *prior* to revascularization in moderate-to-severe cardiogenic shock remains unknown. Therefore, the 2013 American College of Cardiology (ACC)/American Heart Association (AHA) guidelines give a IIa/B recommendation for this indication (downgraded from class I in previous versions). The European Society of Cardiology (ESC) similarly gave this indication a class IIb recommendation [28, 29]. ESC recommends IABP insertion *before* primary PCI [30].

Mechanical Complications of AMI

The use of IABP to support an unstable patient suffering from mechanical complications of AMI is relatively uncontroversial and is strongly supported by current guidelines [28, 31]. Currently, this indication accounts for >10% of all IABP insertions [12].

Cardiogenic Shock

Independent of acute MI, cardiogenic shock remains the most common indication for which IABP is used in contemporary practice, accounting for approximately 25% of all IABP insertions [11, 12].

Prophylaxis for "High-Risk" PCI

In animal models, pre-procedural elective IABP has been demonstrated to significantly reduce total infarct size as a percentage of threatened myocardium [32]. IABP counterpulsation may be used to support a "high-risk" patient undergoing PCI, though there are only a few supporting human trials [10, 33]. The balloon pump-assisted coronary intervention study (BCIS-1) was the first randomized trial to evaluate this indication, enrolling 301 patients with an ejection fraction <30% and severe coronary disease, randomized to undergo PCI with or without elective IABP support [34]. While the study did not show a significantly improved rate of MACCE at 28 days or 6-month mortality with elective IABP, long-term follow-up reported a 34% relative reduction in mortality at a median of 51 months [35]. It is important to note that procedural complications were more common in the control group (10.7% vs. 1.3%, $p < 0.001$) and that >10% required rescue crossover to IABP. Other human trials in high-risk patients have not shown clinical benefit associated with routine IABP use, though some only inserted IABP *after* PCI [36, 37]. Meta-analyses suggest that, similar to normal-risk PCI patients, high-risk PCI patients seem to have a mortality benefit only if they present in cardiogenic shock, though at the cost of increased stroke and major bleeding [38–40]. While it seems likely that routine *post*-procedural IABP is not indicated, it is still unclear whether *pre*-procedure IABP in this population is beneficial.

While there are no universal definitions for this patient cohort, most would consider prophylactic IABP for patients meeting one or more of the following criteria: age > 70, left main coronary artery disease, multivessel angioplasty, prior history of CABG, pharmacologically refractory angina, and severe left ventricular dysfunction [6]. The AHA/ACC considers it reasonable to place an elective IABP as an adjunct to PCI in high-risk patients (class IIb recommendation, level of evidence C) [41].

Coronary Artery Bypass Grafting (CABG): Weaning from Cardiopulmonary Bypass

IABP counterpulsation to assist with weaning from cardiopulmonary bypass (CBP) after cardiac surgery was among the first applications [8, 42] and remains a well-established and uncontroversial indication [10]. Postoperative support accounts for nearly 15% of all IABP insertions [11].

CABG: Prophylactic IABP for "High-Risk" Patients

Prophylactic IABP prior to "high-risk" surgery in stable patients represents approximately 11% of all IABPs inserted in contemporary practice [12]. However, data from randomized trials are conflicting. While a 2011 Cochrane systematic review (6 trials, 255 patients) reported fewer in-hospital deaths associated with IABP use for high-risk "on-pump" bypass surgery, 5 of the 6 trials originated from a single center and investigator [43–47], thus raising the concern about broad generalizability [48]. If IABP is planned, the existing evidence supports preoperative insertion rather than intraoperative or postoperative IABP insertion [49–55].

Bridge to Heart Transplantation and Posttransplantation Support

Long-term IABP has been demonstrated to be feasible, especially when inserted through a site other than the femoral artery [5, 56–58]. The reported rate of complications is as low as 0.13 per patient-week of support [59]. Gjesdal et al. reported the outcomes of 32 patients bridged via IABP to heart transplantation (mean IABP duration 21 days) [60]. Renal and liver function improved, and 30-day and 1-year posttransplantation mortality were similar when compared to elective transplanted patients who did not receive IABP. IABP-related complications were minor and rare.

After transplantation, IABP may be used to support early postoperative low cardiac output syndrome caused by right ventricular failure. Arafa et al. first reported that all 5 patients treated by IABP for this indication were successfully weaned off support, with 4 surviving long-term [61].

Acute Right Ventricular (RV) Infarction with Shock

In patients suffering cardiogenic shock secondary to RV infarction, IABP insertion results in immediate improvement in hemodynamic parameters. Although no trials have been performed, available evidence suggests that the degree of augmentation is predictive of survival [62].

Intractable Ventricular Arrhythmias

IABP counterpulsation has been long described for the treatment of intractable ventricular arrhythmias; however, this remains a very uncommon indication in clinical practice [5, 63, 64].

Contraindications

Absolute

Aortic Valve Regurgitation

It is widely acknowledged that intra-aortic counterpulsation in the setting of moderate-to-severe aortic regurgitation will worsen the condition and thus most consider this an absolute contraindication.

Severe Aortic Pathology (Dissection and Aneurysm)

In cases of known or suspected aortic dissection, IABP insertion and counterpulsation use may cause dissection extension or aortic rupture. Similarly, thoracic aortic aneurysm may be exacerbated or ruptured through the mechanical action of the IABP. Abdominal aortic aneurysm is not necessarily an absolute contraindication, though tortuosity of the vessel may preclude the femoral approach.

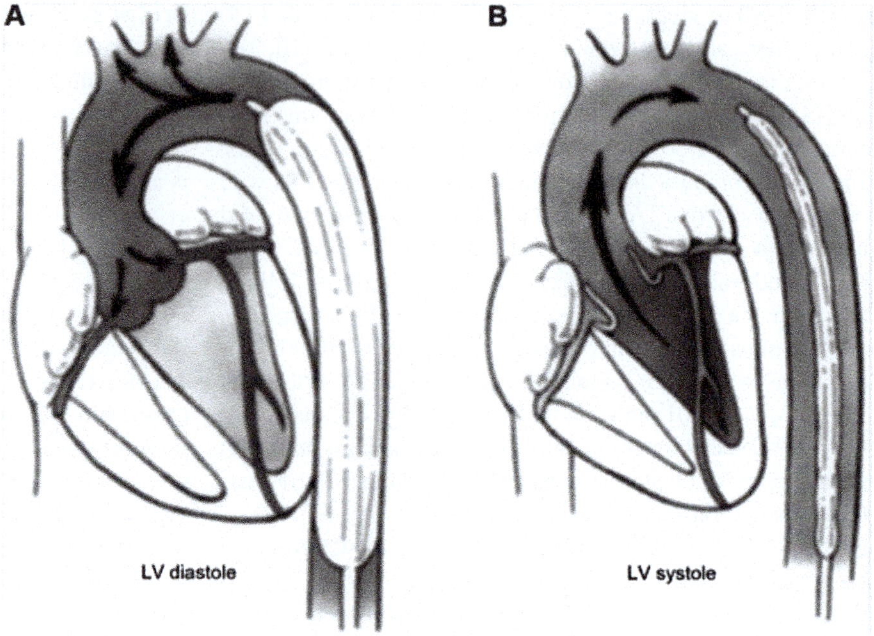

Fig. 69.1 Positioning and functioning of the IABP [86]. The IABP is positioned distal to the left subclavian origin and inflates in diastole (**a**), increasing aortic root and coronary perfusion, then deflates in systole (**b**), reducing LV afterload

Poor Prognosis

As with any invasive procedure and medical treatment, IABP is not recommended for patients who are not expected to have a meaningful recovery (e.g., severe anoxic brain injury) regardless of treatment.

Relative

Severe Peripheral Vascular Disease (PVD)

The main concerns regarding severe PVD mainly relate to access-related difficulties and complications. In these cases, alternate insertion methods may be considered.

Other

Additional relative contraindications to IABP counterpulsation include sepsis and uncontrolled coagulopathy or active bleeding. However, these cases should be evaluated on a case-by-case basis, as support of temporary sepsis-induced myocardial depression may be considered, and counterpulsation without active anticoagulation has been described as safe and effective.

Physiologic Effects

Numerous animal studies and some human studies have been performed to provide a relatively solid mechanistic foundation supporting the use of IABP to improve various physiologic functions. Through IABP inflation during diastole and deflating during systole, at the most fundamental level, it is believed that counterpulsation improves myocardial oxygen supply (via coronary blood flow augmentation) and decreases myocardial demand (via afterload reduction) [1, 33, 65, 66] (Fig. 69.1). Systemic perfusion may also be slightly improved through transformation of the elastic potential energy (stored in the aortic root) into kinetic energy (i.e., the "Windkessel effect") [65]. These effects are evident within a few heartbeats after the initiation of counterpulsation.

Myocardial Oxygen Supply

Inflation of the IABP dramatically increases the diastolic blood pressure, anywhere between 30% and 80% [67, 68]. Additionally, the *diastolic pressure time index (DPTI)*, or the pressure differential between the LV and the aorta, is also augmented. This leads to increased blood flow into the coronary arteries [33, 65]. However, studies have shown that the extent of coronary blood flow (CBF) improvement is dependent upon the degree of luminal narrowing and coronary vascular resistance. CBF proximal to a critical stenosis is significantly increased to nearly double, and this effect is most dramatic in hypotensive patients [67, 69]. Importantly, coronary blood flow distal to a critical stenosis is *not* augmented by IABP. Collateral circulation is also minimally affected. In these patients, it is hypothesized that the benefit is due to afterload reduction rather than CBF improvement [6, 70]. Furthermore, some have argued that diastolic augmentation is less effective when the coronary circulation autoregulation is intact (i.e., reflexive vasoconstriction in response to increased blood flow) [71].

Thus, van Nunen et al. propose that improvements in coronary blood flow are only expected in the following scenarios: (1) critical stenosis, (2) ischemic myocardium (including myocardial "stunning" after infarction and weaning from extracorporeal support), and (3) hypotension below the autoregulatory range [71].

Myocardial Oxygen Demand

IABP deflation during systole reduces the afterload of the left ventricle (LV) by up to 25% [33, 65, 69]. LV end-systolic pressure, LV end-diastolic pressure, and LV end-diastolic volume are all decreased, while stroke volume and ejection fraction are increased [3, 6, 33, 68]. Heart rate, systolic blood pressure, and pulmonary capillary wedge pressure are all decreased [3, 67, 69, 72]. Mean arterial blood pressure (MAP) is unchanged or slightly increased. These changes occur within 20 min of IABP initiation and ultimately lead to reductions in peak LV wall stress and decreased myocardial oxygen consumption, as estimated by the *tension time index (TTI)* [3, 5, 6, 68]. The greatest benefit is seen in hypotensive patients with low cardiac output, with the benefits decreasing as cardiac function improves [3]. In a canine regional infarct model, decreasing LV afterload during ischemia/reperfusion resulted in significant salvage of myocardium compared to reperfusion only [73].

Right Ventricle

In addition to the aforementioned LV mechanisms, IABP may also favorably affect RV function and perfusion via complex interactions between the LV, pulmonary circulation, and RV [65]. For example, through septal-mediated systolic interactions, RV cardiac output may be significantly augmented as the LV function improves [6]. Additionally, the right coronary artery perfusion improves with IABP diastolic augmentation similarly as the left coronary artery.

Factors Affecting Augmentation

The sum total of all these physiologic changes results in a modest increase in cardiac output (up to 1 L/min), cardiac index, and corresponding improvements in organ perfusion [6, 67, 68]. However, the degree of physiologic alteration is also dependent upon several other factors [2, 65]:

1. *Balloon volume* – greater balloon volume will result in greater blood displacement.
2. *Heart rate* – a faster HR results in less filling time and less effective balloon augmentation.
3. *Aortic compliance* – as compliance increases, the magnitude of augmentation decreases, as blood volume is displaced radially into the aorta rather than proximally and distally into the coronary and systemic circulation, respectively.

Technique

The basic components of the IABP have changed very little since their original description over half a century ago: a dual-chamber balloon and a pump console. The balloon's outer lumen is used for gas delivery, and the inner lumen may be used for hemodynamic monitoring. Helium gas is used to inflate the balloon for two reasons: its low density allows for rapid inflation/deflation; it is inert and easily absorbed into the blood (in case of balloon rupture) [2, 4, 6]. Technical modifications include progressive decrease in catheter profile and timing devices to improve synchronization of balloon inflation/deflation, especially in cases of irregular heart rhythms [3, 74].

Insertion

The catheter is usually inserted percutaneously through an introducer sheath via modified Seldinger technique. While the femoral site is most commonly employed, other sites such as iliac, brachial, axillary, or subclavian may be considered. Generally speaking, the limb with the largest artery should be chosen. Alternatively, the catheter may be surgically inserted via a transthoracic or translumbar approach.

The position of the catheter must be confirmed prior to use. This is usually achieved using fluoroscopic guidance or transesophageal echocardiogram. Ideally, the proximal tip of the balloon should reside 2–3 cm distal to the left subclavian artery [2]. The distal extent of the balloon must not occlude the mesenteric or renal arteries.

Initiation

Once the balloon has been successfully inserted and proper positioning confirmed, the IABP is initially set to inflate every other beat (1:2) to allow the clinician to compare assisted to unassisted heart beats [2]. Full support consists of IABP augmentation of every beat (1:1).

The fully expanded balloon diameter should not be greater than 80–90% of the diameter of the descending thoracic aorta. One may also consider adjusting the inflation volume to approximately 50% of ideal stroke volume [6]. It is recommended to ensure continued proper positioning and functioning with daily chest X-ray and continuous hemodynamic monitoring.

While there are no formal recommendations for routine systemic anticoagulation, in the absence of contraindications, most clinicians usually do provide systemic anticoagulation in the form of unfractionated heparin infusion, targeting an activated partial thromboplastin time (aPTT) between 50 and 70 [2]. However, some authors have reported that therapeutic anticoagulation may not be required during active counterpulsation [75, 76].

Next, the console is programmed for balloon inflation during diastole and deflation during systole. The two most common triggers are ECG waveform and systemic arterial pressure waveform.

ECG waveform trigger Balloon inflation begins in the middle of the T wave and deflation occurs at the peak of the R wave. Irregular rhythms with obscured T and R waves (as in atrial fibrillation) may result in only intermittent balloon inflation, and use of this trigger may not be possible in case of electrical interference or poor ECG quality [2, 65].

Systemic arterial pressure waveform trigger Balloon inflation begins after the dicrotic notch (i.e., aortic valve closure), and deflation occurs just prior to the systolic arterial upstroke [2, 6].

Internal trigger Balloon inflation is manually set without regard to synchronization with the heart. This mode is utilized only in cases where there is no cardiac output or electrical activity, for example, during cardiopulmonary bypass or resuscitation.

Pacer trigger Balloon kinetics are synchronized to the ventricular spike in patients who have a 100% paced rhythm.

If timed correctly, the arterial waveform should appear as in Fig. 69.2. Immediately following the dicrotic notch, a second peak (known as *diastolic augmentation*) should be evident. This augmented peak should be higher than the native systolic pressure [65].

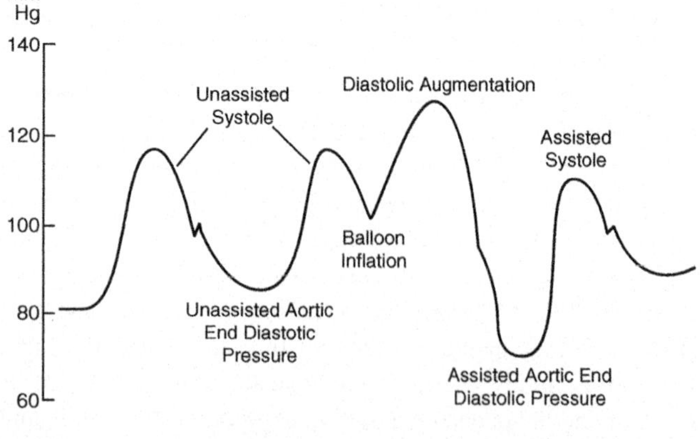

Fig. 69.2 Arterial waveform [2]. The appearance of the arterial waver form on assisted and unassisted heart beats

Weaning from IABP Support

As the patient's cardiac function recovers, weaning from the IABP may be initiated. This is usually achieved by gradually decreasing the ratio of assisted beats from 1:1 to 1:2 and to 1:3 over a period of up to 12 h. Lower ratios (down to 1:8) may be considered, though the IABP may be considered for removal if the patient can tolerate a 1:3 ratio [33]. Additionally, the balloon volume may be gradually decreased to gradually withdraw the level of augmentation [65]. After at least 30 min at the lower setting, cardiac function and perfusion data (e.g., mixed venous saturation, cardiac output, cardiac index, serum lactate, etc.) may be compared to pre-weaning values to determine readiness for liberation. Additionally, SBP will usually increase as the degree of afterload reduction is withdrawn.

Heparin infusion should be discontinued at least 2 h prior to removal so as to minimize bleeding complications at the time of IABP removal. However, without systemic anticoagulation, a defunctionalized balloon begins to form clot within 20 min. Therefore, in order to prevent thrombosis, the balloon should continue to be inflated at least once every eight beats (preferably more frequently) leading up to removal [2, 6, 65]. After sheath removal, manual pressure should be applied for at least 30 min.

Troubleshooting and Complications

There are a myriad of potential complications (Table 69.2), though in modern practice, major IABP-related complications (severe bleeding, limb ischemia, balloon malfunction) are rare, occurring in <3% of cases [11].

Timing

Because balloon inflation/deflation is a highly choreographed event, there are multiple potential errors in timing that may occur, some with more severe consequences than others [2, 6]. It is useful to set the ratio to 1:2 so that assisted and unassisted waveforms may be compared. If the balloon kinetics are optimally timed, both assisted diastolic and systolic pressure should be *lower* than their unassisted counterparts, and the peak diastolic augmentation should be higher than the unassisted systolic pressure [77].

Early Inflation IABP inflation before the aortic valve is fully closed may have severe counterproductive effects. The

Table 69.2 Complications associated with IABP

Timing
Inflation – too early or too late
Deflation – too early or too late
Limb ischemia
Limb loss
Transient loss of pulse
Access site related
Pseudoaneurysm
Bleeding or hematoma
Hematologic
Thromboembolic
Thrombocytopenia
Hemolysis
Infection
Mechanical
Balloon entrapment
Balloon rupture
Anatomic
Cardiac tamponade
Malpositioning leading to cerebral, mesenteric, or renal ischemia
Aortic dissection
Compartment syndrome

valve may be forced closed prematurely or aortic regurgitation may be induced. LV afterload and myocardial oxygen demand are both *increased*, while stroke volume and cardiac output are *decreased* [4, 78]. This error is recognized on the waveform by the absence of a dicrotic notch and encroachment of the diastolic augmentation into systole (Fig. 69.3a).

Late Inflation Delayed IABP inflation will result in less-than-ideal coronary artery perfusion and afterload reduction, but will not have the same counterproductive consequences as early inflation [4]. This error is recognized on the waveform by prolonged dip after the dicrotic notch combined with a blunted diastolic augmentation (Fig. 69.3b).

Early Deflation IABP deflation before the end of diastole will result in less-than-ideal diastolic augmentation and potentially increased myocardial demand. Additionally, the decrease in aortic pressure may actually cause retrograde flow from the carotid or coronary arteries [4]. This error is recognized on waveform by prolonged dip of assisted end-diastolic pressure with no change in assisted (vs. unassisted) systolic pressure. The drop-off after diastolic augmentation will appear nearly vertical, and the assisted systolic pressure will approach the unassisted systolic pressure (Fig. 69.3c).

Late Deflation If the IABP balloon does not deflate until after the start of systole, the same disastrous effects may occur as in early inflation: myocardial oxygen demand will be increased, and cardiac output will be decreased as the LV is forced to contract against an increased afterload [4]. This error is recognized on waveform by the assisted end-diastolic pressure being *higher* than the unassisted end-diastolic pressure. Additionally, the span of diastolic augmentation will be widened, and the slope or rise of the assisted systole beat will be noticeably less steep (Fig. 69.3d).

Other

Vascular complications account for the vast majority (>90%), and about half of all vascular complications occur around insertion or removal [53]. However, limb loss occurs in only about 0.5% and IABP-related mortality occurs in <0.1% [10, 79]. Not surprisingly, the presence of peripheral vascular disease has been demonstrated to be the most reliable predictor of complications. Other predictors include female sex, diabetes mellitus, and tobacco use [80–82].

Real-World Utilization and Outcomes

Several large trials and registries provide insight into the actual usage of IABP in clinical practice. The GUSTO-I study enrolled patients presenting within 6 h of chest pain onset and randomized subjects to one of four thrombolytic treatment protocols [83]. Only 22% of patients presenting with shock received IABP, a significant underutilization of a treatment modality that previously had a class I indication for cardiogenic shock after AMI. In this study, early IABP insertion (within 1 day of enrollment) was associated with a trend toward improved 30-day and 1-year survival. The British Columbia Cardiac Registry reported that only 36% of patients with cardiogenic shock complicating AMI received IABP [84]. Similarly, in the largest registry of AMI (the National Registry of Myocardial Infarction, NRMI-2), only about one-third of patients with cardiogenic shock were treated with IABP [25]. The combination of IABP and thrombolytic therapy decreased the odds of death by 18% [85]. Although most of the patients developed cardiogenic shock after initial presentation to the hospital, less than half of the 750 participating hospitals actually performed IABP. As with other complex procedures and operations, IABP outcomes are improved when performed at high-volume hospitals by experienced providers. A *post hoc* analysis of the NRMI-2 study divided the hospitals performing IABP into three tertiles by annual volume: low-, intermediate-, and high-volume groups performed a median of 3.4, 12.7, and 37.4 IABPs per year. The mortality rate for patients receiving IABP was significantly lower at the high vs. low-volume hospital (51% vs. 65%), and this remained significant when controlling for baseline patient characteristics, hospital characteristics, and other hospital procedures [25].

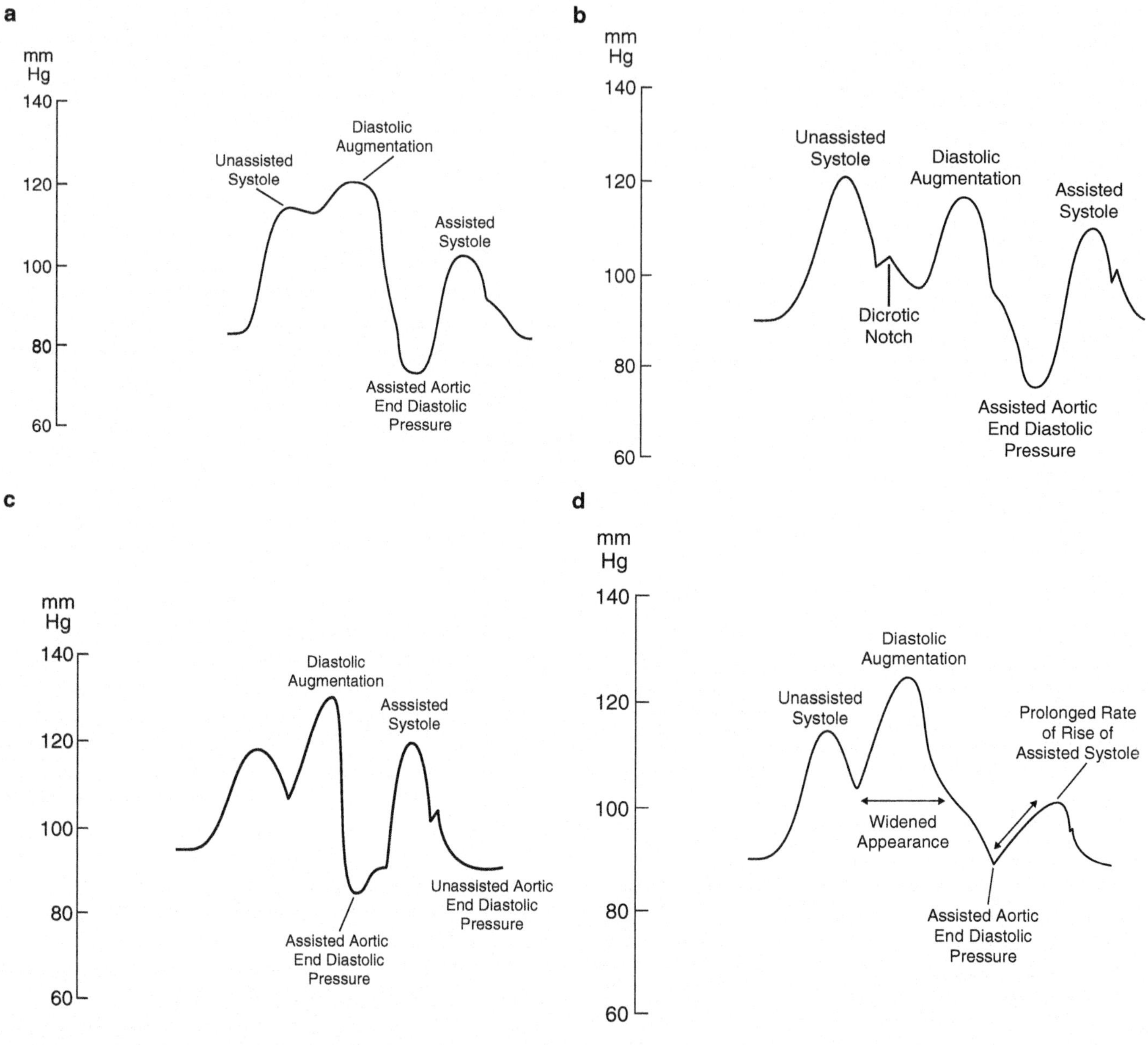

Fig. 69.3 (**a**) Early inflation: absence of a dicrotic notch and encroachment of the diastolic augmentation into systole. (**b**) Late inflation: prolonged dip after the dicrotic notch combined with a blunted diastolic augmentation. (**c**) Early deflation: prolonged dip of assisted end-diastolic pressure with no change in assisted (vs. unassisted) systolic pressure. (**d**) Late deflation: (1) assisted end-diastolic pressure is higher than unassisted end-diastolic pressure; (2) diastolic augmentation is widened; (3) slope of assisted systole beat is less steep (Ref. [2])

Benchmark Registry

The largest repository of IABP experience is the Benchmark registry, which collected 16,909 patient case records from over 200 hospitals worldwide from 1996 to 2000. Review of this database provides insight into IABP practice. Balloon insertion success rates were very high (98%), and the most common indications for IABP were to provide support during or after PCI (21%), cardiogenic shock (19%), weaning from cardiopulmonary bypass (16%), preoperative support for high-risk patients (13%), and refractory unstable angina (12%) [11].

In the Benchmark registry, the majority of IABP insertions occurred in the cardiac catheterization lab (64%) or operating room (24%), with only 4% of insertions occurring in the ICU [11]. Over 95% of insertions were performed percutaneously, with the right femoral artery (65%) preferred over the left femoral artery (36%). Only 1% of percutaneous insertions were via other alternative sites. The median duration of IABP support was 41 h [11].

Overall in-hospital mortality was 21%, with the highest rates seen in cardiogenic shock (28%) and weaning from cardiopulmonary bypass (28%) [79]. Additionally, IABP insertion after more than five inpatient hospital days was strongly predictive of mortality. In comparison, mortality rates for cardiogenic shock without IABP range between 50% and 80%.

Conclusion

IABP is the oldest and most widely used mechanical assist device for the failing heart. The most common indications for appropriate use include hemodynamic support during or after PCI in unstable patients, cardiogenic shock, weaning from cardiopulmonary bypass, and prophylaxis for "high-risk" patients before PCI or cardiac surgery. However, despite relatively strong recommendations from the ACC/AHA and ESC, actual utilization for cardiogenic shock complicating AMI is low, averaging between 25% and 35%. Vigilance must be maintained to guard against balloon inflation/deflation timing errors. When utilized by experienced clinicians, procedural success is very high, and complication rates are low.

References

1. White JM, Ruygrok PN. Intra-aortic balloon counterpulsation in contemporary practice - where are we? Heart Lung Circ. 2015;24(4):335–41.
2. Trost JC, Hillis LD. Intra-aortic balloon counterpulsation. Am J Cardiol. 2006;97(9):1391–8.
3. Moulopoulos SD. Intra-aortic balloon counterpulsation 50 years later: initial conception and consequent ideas. Artif Organs. 2011;35(9):843–8.
4. Hanlon-Pena PM, Quaal SJ. Intra-aortic balloon pump timing: review of evidence supporting current practice. Am J Crit Care. 2011;20(4):323–33; quiz 334.
5. Kapelios CJ, et al. Counterpulsation: a concept with a remarkable past, an established present and a challenging future. Int J Cardiol. 2014;172(2):318–25.
6. Webb CA, Weyker PD, Flynn BC. Management of intra-aortic balloon pumps. Semin Cardiothorac Vasc Anesth. 2015;19(2):106–21.
7. Kantrowitz A. Experimental augmentation of coronary flow by retardation of the arterial pressure pulse. Surgery. 1953;34(4):678–87.
8. Kantrowitz A, et al. Initial clinical experience with intraaortic balloon pumping in cardiogenic shock. JAMA. 1968;203(2):113–8.
9. Bregman D, et al. Percutaneous intraaortic balloon insertion. Am J Cardiol. 1980;46(2):261–4.
10. Abnousi F, et al. The evolution of temporary percutaneous mechanical circulatory support devices: a review of the options and evidence in cardiogenic shock. Curr Cardiol Rep. 2015;17(6):40.
11. Ferguson JJ 3rd, et al. The current practice of intra-aortic balloon counterpulsation: results from the benchmark registry. J Am Coll Cardiol. 2001;38(5):1456–62.
12. Stone GW, et al. Contemporary utilization and outcomes of intra-aortic balloon counterpulsation in acute myocardial infarction: the benchmark registry. J Am Coll Cardiol. 2003;41(11):1940–5.
13. Achour H, et al. Mechanical left ventricular unloading prior to reperfusion reduces infarct size in a canine infarction model. Catheter Cardiovasc Interv. 2005;64(2):182–92.
14. Azevedo CF, et al. The effect of intra-aortic balloon counterpulsation on left ventricular functional recovery early after acute myocardial infarction: a randomized experimental magnetic resonance imaging study. Eur Heart J. 2005;26(12):1235–41.
15. LeDoux JF, et al. Left ventricular unloading with intra-aortic counter pulsation prior to reperfusion reduces myocardial release of endothelin-1 and decreases infarction size in a porcine ischemia-reperfusion model. Catheter Cardiovasc Interv. 2008;72(4):513–21.
16. Ohman EM, et al. Use of aortic counterpulsation to improve sustained coronary artery patency during acute myocardial infarction. Results of a randomized trial. The Randomized IABP Study Group. Circulation. 1994;90(2):792–9.
17. Kono T, et al. Aortic counterpulsation may improve late patency of the occluded coronary artery in patients with early failure of thrombolytic therapy. J Am Coll Cardiol. 1996;28(4):876–81.
18. Patel MR, et al. Intra-aortic balloon counterpulsation and infarct size in patients with acute anterior myocardial infarction without shock: the CRISP AMI randomized trial. JAMA. 2011;306(12):1329–37.
19. Vijayalakshmi K, et al. Intra-aortic counterpulsation does not improve coronary flow early after PCI in a high-risk group of patients: observations from a randomized trial to explore its mode of action. J Invasive Cardiol. 2007;19(8):339–46.
20. Ihdayhid AR, Chopra S, Rankin J. Intra-aortic balloon pump: indications, efficacy, guidelines and future directions. Curr Opin Cardiol. 2014;29(4):285–92.
21. Ohman EM, et al. Thrombolysis and counterpulsation to improve survival in myocardial infarction complicated by hypotension and suspected cardiogenic shock or heart failure: results of the TACTICS Trial. J Thromb Thrombolysis. 2005;19(1):33–9.
22. Prondzinsky R, et al. Hemodynamic effects of intra-aortic balloon counterpulsation in patients with acute myocardial infarction complicated by cardiogenic shock: the prospective, randomized IABP shock trial. Shock. 2012;37(4):378–84.
23. Thiele H, et al. Intraaortic balloon support for myocardial infarction with cardiogenic shock. N Engl J Med. 2012;367(14):1287–96.
24. Thiele H, et al. Intra-aortic balloon counterpulsation in acute myocardial infarction complicated by cardiogenic shock (IABP-SHOCK II): final 12 month results of a randomised, open-label trial. Lancet. 2013;382(9905):1638–45.
25. Chen EW, et al. Relation between hospital intra-aortic balloon counterpulsation volume and mortality in acute myocardial infarction complicated by cardiogenic shock. Circulation. 2003;108(8):951–7.
26. Abdel-Wahab M, et al. Comparison of hospital mortality with intra-aortic balloon counterpulsation insertion before versus after primary percutaneous coronary intervention for cardiogenic shock complicating acute myocardial infarction. Am J Cardiol. 2010;105(7):967–71.
27. Cheng JM, et al. Impact of intra-aortic balloon pump support initiated before versus after primary percutaneous coronary intervention in patients with cardiogenic shock from acute myocardial infarction. Int J Cardiol. 2013;168(4):3758–63.
28. O'Gara PT, et al. 2013 ACCF/AHA guideline for the management of ST-elevation myocardial infarction: executive summary: a report of the American College of Cardiology Foundation/American Heart Association task force on practice guidelines: developed in collaboration with the American College of Emergency Physicians and Society for Cardiovascular Angiography and Interventions. Catheter Cardiovasc Interv. 2013;82(1):E1–27.
29. Task Force on the management of, S.T.s.e.a.m.i.o.t.E.S.o.C, et al. ESC Guidelines for the management of acute myocardial infarction in patients presenting with ST-segment elevation. Eur Heart J. 2012;**33**(20):2569–619.

30. Task Force on Myocardial Revascularization of the European Society of, C, et al. Guidelines on myocardial revascularization. Eur Heart J. 2010;**31**(20):2501–55.
31. Nieminen MS, et al. Executive summary of the guidelines on the diagnosis and treatment of acute heart failure: the task force on acute heart failure of the European Society of Cardiology. Eur Heart J. 2005;26(4):384–416.
32. Nanas JN, et al. Myocardial salvage by the use of reperfusion and intraaortic balloon pump: experimental study. Ann Thorac Surg. 1996;61(2):629–34.
33. Santa-Cruz RA, Cohen MG, Ohman EM. Aortic counterpulsation: a review of the hemodynamic effects and indications for use. Catheter Cardiovasc Interv. 2006;67(1):68–77.
34. Perera D, et al. Elective intra-aortic balloon counterpulsation during high-risk percutaneous coronary intervention: a randomized controlled trial. JAMA. 2010;304(8):867–74.
35. Perera D, et al. Long-term mortality data from the balloon pump-assisted coronary intervention study (BCIS-1): a randomized, controlled trial of elective balloon counterpulsation during high-risk percutaneous coronary intervention. Circulation. 2013;127(2):207–12.
36. Stone GW, et al. A prospective, randomized evaluation of prophylactic intraaortic balloon counterpulsation in high risk patients with acute myocardial infarction treated with primary angioplasty. Second primary angioplasty in myocardial infarction (PAMI-II) trial investigators. J Am Coll Cardiol. 1997;29(7):1459–67.
37. van 't Hof AW, et al. A randomized comparison of intra-aortic balloon pumping after primary coronary angioplasty in high risk patients with acute myocardial infarction. Eur Heart J. 1999;20(9):659–65.
38. Bahekar A, et al. Cardiovascular outcomes using intra-aortic balloon pump in high-risk acute myocardial infarction with or without cardiogenic shock: a meta-analysis. J Cardiovasc Pharmacol Ther. 2012;17(1):44–56.
39. Cassese S, et al. Intra-aortic balloon counterpulsation in patients with acute myocardial infarction without cardiogenic shock. A meta-analysis of randomized trials. Am Heart J. 2012;164(1):58–65 e1.
40. Sjauw KD, et al. A systematic review and meta-analysis of intra-aortic balloon pump therapy in ST-elevation myocardial infarction: should we change the guidelines? Eur Heart J. 2009;30(4):459–68.
41. Levine GN, et al. ACCF/AHA/SCAI guideline for percutaneous coronary intervention. A report of the American College of Cardiology Foundation/American Heart Association task force on practice guidelines and the Society for Cardiovascular Angiography and Interventions. J Am Coll Cardiol. 2011;58(24):e44–122.
42. Buckley MJ, et al. Intra-aortic balloon pump assist for cardiogenic shock after cardiopulmonary bypass. Circulation. 1973;48(1 Suppl):III90–4.
43. Christenson JT, et al. Preoperative intraaortic balloon pump enhances cardiac performance and improves the outcome of redo CABG. Ann Thorac Surg. 1997;64(5):1237–44.
44. Christenson JT, Licker M, Kalangos A. The role of intra-aortic counterpulsation in high-risk OPCAB surgery: a prospective randomized study. J Card Surg. 2003;18(4):286–94.
45. Christenson JT, et al. Evaluation of preoperative intra-aortic balloon pump support in high risk coronary patients. Eur J Cardiothorac Surg. 1997;11(6):1097–103; discussion 1104.
46. Christenson JT, et al. The effect of preoperative intra-aortic balloon pump support in patients with coronary artery disease, poor left-ventricular function (LVEF < 40%), and hypertensive LV hypertrophy. Thorac Cardiovasc Surg. 1997;45(2):60–4.
47. Christenson JT, et al. Optimal timing of preoperative intraaortic balloon pump support in high-risk coronary patients. Ann Thorac Surg. 1999;68(3):934–9.
48. Theologou T, et al. Preoperative intra aortic balloon pumps in patients undergoing coronary artery bypass grafting. Cochrane Database Syst Rev. 2011;(1):CD004472. http://onlinelibrary.wiley.com/doi/10.1002/14651858.CD004472.pub3/full
49. Dyub AM, et al. Preoperative intra-aortic balloon pump in patients undergoing coronary bypass surgery: a systematic review and meta-analysis. J Card Surg. 2008;23(1):79–86.
50. Kang N, Edwards M, Larbalestier R. Preoperative intraaortic balloon pumps in high-risk patients undergoing open heart surgery. Ann Thorac Surg. 2001;72(1):54–7.
51. Zangrillo A, et al. Preoperative intra-aortic balloon pump to reduce mortality in coronary artery bypass graft: a meta-analysis of randomized controlled trials. Crit Care. 2015;19:10.
52. Torchiana DF, et al. Intraaortic balloon pumping for cardiac support: trends in practice and outcome, 1968 to 1995. J Thorac Cardiovasc Surg. 1997;113(4):758–64; discussion 764–9.
53. Christenson JT, et al. Trends in intraaortic balloon counterpulsation complications and outcomes in cardiac surgery. Ann Thorac Surg. 2002;74(4):1086–90; discussion 1090–1.
54. Arafa OE, et al. Intraaortic balloon pump in open heart operations: 10-year follow-up with risk analysis. Ann Thorac Surg. 1998;65(3):741–7.
55. Marra C, et al. Coronary artery bypass grafting in patients with severe left ventricular dysfunction: a prospective randomized study on the timing of perioperative intraaortic balloon pump support. Int J Artif Organs. 2002;25(2):141–6.
56. Cochran RP, et al. Ambulatory intraaortic balloon pump use as bridge to heart transplant. Ann Thorac Surg. 2002;74(3):746–51; discussion 751–2.
57. Russo MJ, et al. Intra-aortic balloon pump inserted through the subclavian artery: a minimally invasive approach to mechanical support in the ambulatory end-stage heart failure patient. J Thorac Cardiovasc Surg. 2012;144(4):951–5.
58. Estep JD, et al. Percutaneous placement of an intra-aortic balloon pump in the left axillary/subclavian position provides safe, ambulatory long-term support as bridge to heart transplantation. JACC Heart Fail. 2013;1(5):382–8.
59. Manord JD, et al. Implications for the vascular surgeon with prolonged (3 to 89 days) intraaortic balloon pump counterpulsation. J Vasc Surg. 1997;26(3):511–5; discussion 515–6.
60. Gjesdal O, et al. Intra-aortic balloon counterpulsation as a bridge to heart transplantation does not impair long-term survival. Eur J Heart Fail. 2009;11(7):709–14.
61. Arafa OE, et al. Intraaortic balloon pumping for predominantly right ventricular failure after heart transplantation. Ann Thorac Surg. 2000;70(5):1587–93.
62. McNamara MW, Dixon SR, Goldstein JA. Impact of intra-aortic balloon pumping on hypotension and outcomes in acute right ventricular infarction. Coron Artery Dis. 2014;25(7):602–7.
63. Culliford AT, et al. Intra-aortic balloon counterpulsation. Refractory ventricular tachycardia. JAMA. 1978;239(5):431–2.
64. Willerson JT, et al. Intraaortic balloon counterpulsation in patients in cardiogenic shock, medically refractory left ventricular failure and/or recurrent ventricular tachycardia. Am J Med. 1975;58(2):183–91.
65. Krishna M, Zacharowski K. Principles of intra-aortic balloon pump counterpulsation. Contin Educ Anaesth Crit Care Pain. 2009;9(1):24–8.
66. de Waha S, et al. Intra-aortic balloon counterpulsation – basic principles and clinical evidence. Vasc Pharmacol. 2014;60(2):52–6.
67. Kern MJ, et al. Enhanced coronary blood flow velocity during intraaortic balloon counterpulsation in critically ill patients. J Am Coll Cardiol. 1993;21(2):359–68.
68. Capoccia M, et al. Evidence of clinical efficacy of counterpulsation therapy methods. Heart Fail Rev. 2015;20(3):323–35.

69. Mueller H, et al. The effects of intra-aortic counterpulsation on cardiac performance and metabolism in shock associated with acute myocardial infarction. J Clin Invest. 1971;50(9):1885–900.
70. Williams DO, et al. The effect of intraaortic balloon counterpulsation on regional myocardial blood flow and oxygen consumption in the presence of coronary artery stenosis in patients with unstable angina. Circulation. 1982;66(3):593–7.
71. van Nunen LX, et al. Usefulness of intra-aortic balloon pump counterpulsation. Am J Cardiol. 2016;117(3):469–76.
72. Scheidt S, et al. Intra-aortic balloon counterpulsation in cardiogenic shock. Report of a co-operative clinical trial. N Engl J Med. 1973;288(19):979–84.
73. Smalling RW, et al. Improved regional myocardial blood flow, left ventricular unloading, and infarct salvage using an axial-flow, transvalvular left ventricular assist device. A comparison with intra-aortic balloon counterpulsation and reperfusion alone in a canine infarction model. Circulation. 1992;85(3):1152–9.
74. Schreuder JJ, et al. Automatic intraaortic balloon pump timing using an intrabeat dicrotic notch prediction algorithm. Ann Thorac Surg. 2005;79(3):1017–22; discussion 1022.
75. Pucher PH, et al. Is heparin needed for patients with an intra-aortic balloon pump? Interact Cardiovasc Thorac Surg. 2012;15(1):136–9.
76. Jiang CY, et al. Anticoagulation therapy in intra-aortic balloon counterpulsation: does IABP really need anti-coagulation? J Zhejiang Univ Sci. 2003;4(5):607–11.
77. Boehmer JP, Popjes E. Cardiac failure: mechanical support strategies. Crit Care Med. 2006;34(9 Suppl):S268–77.
78. Schreuder JJ, et al. Beat-to-beat effects of intraaortic balloon pump timing on left ventricular performance in patients with low ejection fraction. Ann Thorac Surg. 2005;79(3):872–80.
79. Urban PM, et al. In-hospital mortality associated with the use of intra-aortic balloon counterpulsation. Am J Cardiol. 2004;94(2):181–5.
80. Parissis H, Soo A, Al-Alao B. Intra aortic balloon pump: literature review of risk factors related to complications of the intraaortic balloon pump. J Cardiothorac Surg. 2011;6:147.
81. Funk M, Gleason J, Foell D. Lower limb ischemia related to use of the intraaortic balloon pump. Heart Lung. 1989;18(6):542–52.
82. Cohen M, et al. Sex and other predictors of intra-aortic balloon counterpulsation-related complications: prospective study of 1119 consecutive patients. Am Heart J. 2000;139(2 Pt 1):282–7.
83. Anderson RD, et al. Use of intraaortic balloon counterpulsation in patients presenting with cardiogenic shock: observations from the GUSTO-I study. Global utilization of streptokinase and TPA for occluded coronary arteries. J Am Coll Cardiol. 1997;30(3):708–15.
84. Iqbal MB, et al. Intra-aortic balloon pump counterpulsation during primary percutaneous coronary intervention for ST-elevation myocardial infarction and cardiogenic shock: insights from the British Columbia Cardiac Registry. PLoS One. 2016;11(2):e0148931.
85. Barron HV, et al. The use of intra-aortic balloon counterpulsation in patients with cardiogenic shock complicating acute myocardial infarction: data from the National Registry of myocardial infarction 2. Am Heart J. 2001;141(6):933–9.
86. Jones HA, et al. Left ventricular assist for high-risk percutaneous coronary intervention. J Invasive Cardiol. 2012;24(10):544–50.

Index

A. Salim et al. (eds.), *Surgical Critical Care Therapy*, https://doi.org/10.1007/978-3-319-71712-8

C

T

The manufacturer's authorised representative in the EU is Springer Nature Customer Service Centre GmbH, Europaplatz 3, 69115 Heidelberg, Germany. If you have any concerns regarding our products, please contact ProductSafety@springernature.com

Printed and bound by CPI Group (UK) Ltd, Croydon, CR0 4YY
30/09/2026
02225479-0003